The Macrophage
Second edition

OXFORD MEDICAL PUBLICATIONS

The Macrophage
Second edition

Edited by

BERNARD BURKE

University of Leicester, Leicester, UK

and

CLAIRE E. LEWIS

University of Sheffield Medical School, Sheffield, UK

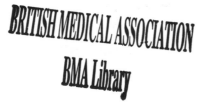
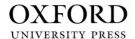

OXFORD
UNIVERSITY PRESS

OXFORD

UNIVERSITY PRESS

Great Clarendon Street, Oxford OX2 6DP

Oxford University Press is a department of the University of Oxford.
It furthers the University's objective of excellence in research, scholarship,
and education by publishing worldwide in

Oxford New York

Auckland Bangkok Buenos Aires Cape Town Chennai
Dar es Salaam Delhi Hong Kong Istanbul Karachi Kolkata
Kuala Lumpur Madrid Melbourne Mexico City Mumbai Nairobi
Sao Paulo Shanghai Taipei Tokyo Toronto

Oxford is a registered trade mark of Oxford University Press
in the UK and in certain other countries

Published in the United States
by Oxford University Press Inc., New York

A catalogue record for this title is available from the British Library

Library of Congress Cataloging in Publication Data
(Data available)

ISBN 0 19 263197 7 (Hbk)

10 9 8 7 6 5 4 3 2 1

Typeset by EXPO Holdings, Malaysia
Printed in Great Britain
on acid-free paper by
Biddles Ltd, Guildford and King's Lynn

Foreword

The macrophage is a highly adaptive and responsive cell, able to recognize alterations in its micro-environment and maintain tissue homeostasis. If this proves beyond its immediate capacity, it will mobilize and orchestrate other cellular systems, in attempts to restore normal function. Therefore, macrophages play a central role in a remarkable range of biological and pathological processes.

Since the first edition of this book, there has been a great deal of progress in our understanding of the molecular and cellular basis for diverse macrophage functions, yet a need remains for overall perspective, and to remind us of some relatively neglected, though important areas of investigation. This volume updates our knowledge admirably and systematically; starting from basic descriptions of the life history and properties of macrophages, and then reviewing a range of interactions with foreign invaders (bacteria, viruses, and parasites), as well as endogenous derangements in which macrophages respond to excessive or abnormal host constituents (Alzheimer's disease, atherosclerosis, and autoimmune antigens). The as-yet mysterious contribution of macrophages to tumorigenesis is explored, as is their essential role in wound repair. Not surprising, but often not appreciated, is the unusual impact of the central nervous system on macrophage behaviour, and the contribution of resident and activated microglia to neuronal dysfunction. Above all, looms the ability of the macrophage to modulate its gene expression in appropriate response to diverse stimuli and to induce acquired immunity or tolerance. We are reminded of macrophage contributions to reproduction (although alas not to the male aspect of this complex physiologic process). Finally, we look ahead to opportunities for future gene therapy, using macrophages as biosynthetically active somatic cell vehicles, of suitably limited life span.

We know more about this one specialized cell than many others, so macrophages lend themselves to general analysis. One such example is explored, the application of mathematical modelling to cellular phenomena.

This book will instruct the beginner and delight the expert, secure in the knowledge that a feast is on offer. Enjoy!

Siamon Gordon
Oxford, May 2002

Preface

In the decade since the first edition of this book was published, the number of scientific papers devoted wholly or partly to this intriguing cell type has increased markedly. We believe that the detailed information available now on macrophage structure and function, the molecular regulation of macrophages (including the range of genes expressed under certain conditions) and their role in various healthy and diseased states warrant a new edition of this book. All the chapters are written by internationally acknowledged leaders in their field, with each being asked to review the topic in a comprehensive, balanced and critical way. We have extended the scope of the book to include chapters on important new facets of macrophage biology, including their possible use in gene therapies, and the use of mathematical models to increase our understanding of their role in disease etiology and progression. We hope this new edition will provide a comprehensive and thought-provoking text for a wide range of readers—from undergraduates in biology or medicine to scientists and clinicians working on macrophage-related topics.

Dr Bernard Burke
Research Fellow and Honorary Lecturer, Department of Microbiology and Immunology, School of Biological Sciences, Faculty of Medicine and Biological Sciences, University of Leicester, Leicester, UK

Professor Claire Lewis
Head, Tumour Targetting Group, Academic Unit of Pathology, Division of Genomic Medicine, University of Sheffield Medical School, Sheffield, UK

Contents

Contributors

R. Andreesen Department of Hematology and Oncology, University of Regensburg, D-93042 Regensburg, Germany.

M.J. Auger Department of Haematology, Kingsmill Centre for Healthcare Services, Mansefield Road, Sutton-in-Ashfield, Nottingham NG17 4JL, UK.

A. Baoutina Centre for Thrombosis and Vascular Research, University of New South Wales, Sydney, NSW 2062, Australia.

C.E. Branecki Center for Neurovirology and Neurodegenerative Disorders, University of Nebraska Medical Center, Omaha, Nebraska 68198-5215, USA.

B. Bresnihan Consultant Rheumatologist, St. Vincent's University Hospital and Professor of Rheumatology, St. Vincent's University Hospital, Elm Park, Dublin 4, Ireland.

B. Burke Department of Microbiology and Immunology, University of Leicester, Leicester LE1 9HN, UK.

H.M. Byrne School of Mathematical Sciences, University of Nottingham, Nottingham, UK.

K.A. Carlson Center for Neurovirology and Neurodegenerative Disorders, University of Nebraska Medical Center, Omaha, Nebraska 68198-5215, USA.

M.P. Colombo Immunotherapy and Gene Therapy Unit, Department of Experimental Oncology, Istituto Nazionale Tumori, Via Venezian 1, 20133 Milano, Italy.

R.L. Cotter Center for Neurovirology and Neurodegenerative Disorders, University of Nebraska Medical Center, Omaha, Nebraska 68198-5215, USA.

L.A. DiPietro Burn and Shock Trauma Institute, Department of Surgery, Loyola University Medical Center, Maywood, Illinois, USA.

J. Fritsche Department of Hematology and Oncology, University of Regensburg, D-93042 Regensburg, Germany.

H.E. Gendelman Department of Medicine, University of Nebraska Medical Center, Omaha, Nebraska 68198-5215, USA.

T.A. Hamilton Department of Immunology, Lerner Research Institute, Cleveland Clinic Foundation, Cleveland, Ohio, USA.

J.-P. Heale The Research Centre, 950 West 28th Avenue, Vancouver, British Columbia, V5Z 4H4 Canada.

W. Jessup Centre for Thrombosis and Vascular Research, University of New South Wales, Sydney, NSW 2062, Australia.

H.-S. Jun Deptartment of Microbiology and Infectious Disease and Laboratory of Viral and Immunopathogenesis of Diabetes, Julia McFarlane Diabetes Research Centre, Faculty of Medicine, The University of Calgary, 3330 Hospital Drive N.W., Calgary, Alberta T2N 4N1, Canada.

H. Kanzaki Department of Obstetrics and Gynecology, Kansai Medical University, Moriguchi 570-8507, Japan.

H. Katabuchi Department of Obstetrics and Gynecology, Kumamoto University School of Medicine, Kumamoto 860-8556, Japan.

M. Kreutz Department of Hematology and Oncology, University of Regensburg, D-93042 Regensburg, Germany.

L. Kritharides Centre for Thrombosis and Vascular Research, University of New South Wales, Sydney, NSW 2062, Australia.

C.E. Lewis Tumour Targeting Group, Academic Unit of Pathology, Division of Genomic Medicine, University of Sheffield Medical School, Beech Hill Road, Sheffield S10 2RX, UK.

P.C. Mahon Institute of Genetic Medicine, The Johns Hopkins University School of Medicine, CMSC-1004, 600 N. Wolfe Street, Baltimore, Maryland 21287-3914, USA.

M.K. Matyszak Department of Medicine, Level 5, Addenbrooks Hospital, Cambridge CB2 2QQ, UK.

H. Okamura Department of Obstetrics and Gynecology, Kumamoto University School of Medicine, Kumamoto 860-8556, Japan.

M.R. Owen Nonlinear and Complex Systems Group, Mathematics Department, Loughborough University, Loughborough LE11 3TU, UK.

P. Paglia Euroclone Ltd., Via Figino, 20/22-20016, Pero (MI), Italy.

V.H. Perry CNS Inflammation group, School of Biological Sciences, University of Southampton, Southampton S016 7PX, UK.

J.A. Ross Molecular Immunology Group, Lister Research Laboratories, University of Edinburgh, Department of Clinical and Surgical Sciences, Royal Infirmary, Edinburgh EH3 9YW, UK.

L. Ryan Departments of Pathology and Microbiology, University of Nebraska Medical Center, Omaha, Nebraska 68198-5215, USA.

D.P. Speert Department of Pediatrics, University of British Columbia, Vancouver, British Columbia, Canada.

R.M. Strieter Division of Pulmonary and Critical Care Medicine, Department of Medicine, UCLA School of Medicine, Los Angeles, California, USA.

S. Sumner Nuffield Department of Clinical Laboratory Sciences, John Radcliffe Hospital, University of Oxford, Oxford OX3 9DU, UK.

B. Vray Laboratoire d'Immunologie Expérimentale (CP 615), Faculté de Médecine, Université Libre de Bruxelles, 808 route de Lennik, B-1070 Brussels, Belgium.

C.E. Williams Center for Neurovirology and Neurodegenerative Disorders, University of Nebraska Medical Center, Omaha, Nebraska 68198-5215, USA.

J.-W. Yoon Department of Microbiology and Infectious Disease and Laboratory of Viral and Immunopathogenesis of Diabetes, Julia McFarlane Diabetes Research Centre, Faculty of Medicine, The University of Calgary, 3330 Hospital Drive N.W., Calgary, Alberta T2N 4N1, Canada and The Department of Internal Medicine, Yonsei University College of Medicine, 134 Shin-Chon Dong, Seo-Dae-Moon Ku, Seoul, Korea.

P. Youssef The Department of Rheumatology, Royal Prince Alfred Hospital, Sydney; The School of Pathology, The University of New South Wales, Sydney, Australia.

J. Zheng Center for Neurovirology and Neurodegenerative Disorders, University of Nebraska Medical Center, Omaha, Nebraska 68198-5215, USA.

W. Zink Center for Neurovirology and Neurodegenerative Disorders, University of Nebraska Medical Center, Omaha, Nebraska 68198-5215, USA.

Abbreviations

Aβ	amyloid beta
AD	Alzheimer's disease
ADCC	antibody-dependent cellular cytotoxicity
ADE	antibody-dependent enhancement
AGE	advance glycation endproduct
APC	antigen-presenting cell
Apo	apolipoprotein
APP	amyloid precursor protein
BCG	bacille Calmette–Guérin
CD40L	CD40 ligand
CMV	cytomegalovirus
CNS	central nervous system
CNTF	ciliary neurotrophic factor
CR	complement receptor
CTL	cytotoxic T lymphocyte
DAF	decay-accelerating factor
DC	dendritic cell
EAE	experimental autoimmune encephalitis
EBV	Epstein–Barr virus
ECM	extracellular matrix
EGF	epidermal growth factor
ELAM	endothelial–leukocyte adhesion molecule
ER	endoplasmic reticulum
FGF	fibroblast growth factor
G-CSF	granulocyte colony-stimulating factor
GM-CSF	granulocyte–macrophage colony stimulating factor
GPCR	G-protein-coupled receptor
HCMV	human cytomegalovirus
HGF	hepatocyte growth factor
HHV	human herpesvirus
HIV	human immunodeficiency virus
HSP	heat shock protein
HSV	herpes simplex virus
ICAM	intercellular cell adhesion molecule
IDDM	insulin-dependent diabetes mellitus
IFN	interferon

IL	interleukin
iNOS	inducible nitric oxide synthase
IRE	interferon regulatory factor
ISRE	IFN-α/β-stimulated regulatory element
JAK	Janus family kinase
KS	Kaposi's sarcoma
LBP	lipopolysaccharide-binding protein
LC	Langerhan cell
LDL	low-density lipoprotein
LFA-1	liver function-associated antigen 1
LIF	leukemia inhibitory factor
LPS	lipopolysaccharide
LT	leukotriene
MAF	macrophage-activating factor
MAP	mitogen-activated protein
MCMV	murine cytomegalovirus
MCP	monocyte chemotactic protein
M-CSF	macrophage colony-stimulating factor
MDP	muramyl dipeptide
MFR	mannosyl–fucosyl receptor
MHC	major histocompatibility complex
MHV	mouse hepatitis virus
MIF	migration inhibitory factor
MIIC	MHC-II-enriched compartment
MIP	macrophage inflammatory protein
MMP	matrix metalloproteinase
MP	mononuclear phagocyte
MPS	mononuclear phagocyte system
MS	multiple sclerosis
MTC	macrophage-mediated tumor cytotoxicity
NFT	neurofibrillary tangle
NF-kB	nuclear factor-kB
NK	natural killer
NMDA	N-methyl-D-aspartate
NO	nitric oxide
NP	neuritic plaque
Nramp	natural resistance-associated macrophage protein
OA	osteoarthritis
ORF	open reading frame
PAF	platelet-activating factor
PBMC	peripheral blood mononuclear cell
PDGF	platelet-derived growth factor
PGE	prostaglandin E
PHF	paired helical filament
PI3K	phosphatidylinositol 3-kinase
PPAR	peroxisome proliferator-activated receptor

PV	parasitophorous vacuole
RA	rheumatoid arthritis
RANTES	regulated on activation, normal T cell-expressed and secreted protein
ROI	reactive oxygen intermediate
ROS	reactive oxygen species
SCF	stem cell factor
SCR	short consensus repeat
SR	scavenger receptor
STAT	signal transducer and activator of transcription
TAM	tumor-associated macrophage
TCR	T-cell receptor
TGF	transforming growth factor
TIMP	tissue inhibitor of metallo-proteinase
TLR	Toll-like receptor
TMEV	Theiler's murine encephalomyelitis virus
TNF	tumor necrosis factor
TSP	thrombus poudin
UTR	untranslated region
VCAM	vascular cell adhesion molecule
VEGF	vascular endothelial growth factor
VLDP	very low-density lipoprotein

1 *The biology of the macrophage*

J.A. Ross and M.J. Auger

1 Introduction

The macrophage is the major differentiated cell of the mononuclear phagocyte system. This system comprises bone marrow monoblasts and promonocytes, peripheral blood monocytes and tissue macrophages. Macrophages are widely distributed throughout the body, displaying great structural and functional heterogeneity. They are to be found in lymphoid organs, the liver, lungs, gastrointestinal tract, central nervous system (CNS), serous cavities, bone, synovium and skin, and participate in a wide range of physiological and pathological processes.

The term 'macrophage' was first used more than 100 years ago by Elie Metchnikoff in Messina to describe the large mononuclear phagocytic cells he observed in tissues (Karnovsky, 1981). In 1924, Aschoff assigned these cells to the reticuloendothelial system (RES), a broad system of cells which included reticular cells, endothelial cells, fibroblasts, histiocytes and monocytes (Aschoff, 1924). However, because the RES included cells of non-macrophage lineage, it did not constitute a true system; in 1969, it was agreed to replace this term with the current title mononuclear phagocyte system (MPS), on the basis that macrophages shared important functional characteristics *in vivo* and were derived from monocytes (van Furth *et al.*, 1972), whereas endothelial cells and fibroblasts were not. Phylogenetically, the mononuclear phagocyte is a very primitive cell type, with related cells being found in early life forms, and some single-cell protozoa exhibiting features similar to the mammalian macrophage. Ontogenetically, the macrophage originates in the yolk sac (Moore and Metcalf, 1970), but in adult man arises from the bone marrow (van Furth, 1989).

2 Macrophage origin and kinetics

Macrophages originate in the bone marrow (Figure 1.1). In man, the bone marrow contains resident macrophages, as well as their precursors; monocytes, promonocytes and monoblasts.There is considerable evidence to suggest that monocytes and neutrophils share a common progenitor cell in the bone marrow (Metcalf, 1971). This common progenitor is called the colony-forming unit, granulocyte–macrophage (CFU-GM) because of its ability to give rise to colonies of monocytes and neutrophils in semi-solid marrow cultures. It is likely that at a level of maturity preceding the promonocyte and promyelocyte stage, a progenitor cell becomes committed to either monocytic or granulocytic differentiation. However, the human promyelocytic leukemia cell line HL-60 differentiates to monocytes and macrophages in the presence of certain phorbol esters but to neutrophils in the presence of dimethylsulfoxide, suggesting that cells may switch at a later point (Koeffler and Golde, 1980).

The monoblast is the least mature cell of the mononuclear phagocyte system. This immaturity is reflected in the morphology and ultrastructure (see Section 5). The monoblast is positive for lysozyme and non-specific esterase, although these enzymes are only present in relatively small amounts. All monoblasts have receptors for IgG and are able to phagocytose IgG-coated red blood cells, but not C3b-coated red blood cells and only rarely ingest opsonized bacteria (van Furth *et al.*, 1980). Division of a monoblast gives rise to two promonocytes, the latter cell type being the direct precursor of the monocyte. Promonocytes stain for lysozyme and non-specific esterase, and in addition

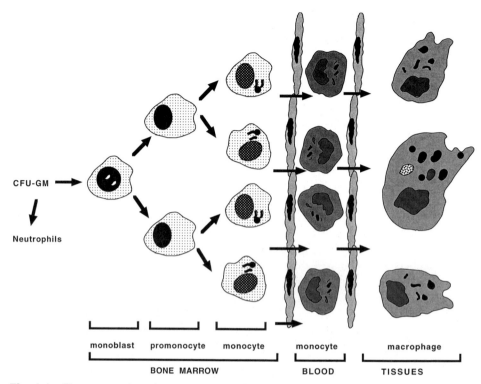

CFU-GM

Neutrophils

| monoblast | promonocyte | monocyte | monocyte | macrophage |

| BONE MARROW | BLOOD | TISSUES |

Fig. 1.1   The mononuclear phagocyte system, showing the origin of macrophages in the bone marrow.

have peroxidase-positive granules. The majority of promonocytes have IgG Fc receptors and C3b receptors, and ingest IgG-coated red blood cells and opsonized bacteria, but relatively few C3b-coated red cells (van Furth and Diesselhoff-den Dulk, 1970; van Furth *et al.*, 1980) (Figure 1.2). Unlike monoblasts, they appear to pinocytose greatly. It is believed that each dividing promonocyte gives rise to two monocytes. The cycle of monoblastic division in mice has been calculated to be 11.9 h and for promonocytes 16.2 h.

Newly formed monocytes probably remain in the bone marrow for less than 24 h before entering the peripheral blood, where they are distributed between circulating and marginating pools (Meuret and Hoffmann, 1973; van Furth and Sluiter, 1986). Studies in mice have shown that monocytes have a half-time in the circulation of 17.4 h under normal circumstances (van Furth and Cohn, 1968), giving an average transit time in the circulation of 25 h. A longer monocyte half-time has been reported in man and may be up to 70 h (Whitelaw, 1966). In the normal adult, the relative peripheral blood monocyte count is generally between 1 and 6 per cent of the total white blood cell count and rarely exceeds 10 per cent. The absolute monocyte count in the adult therefore ranges between 300 and 700 cells per microliter of blood. The migration of peripheral blood monocytes into extravascular tissues to become macrophages involves adherence to the endothelium, diapedesis between endothelial cells and subsequent migration through subendothelial structures. Adherence of monocytes (see Section 8) to endothelium involves high molecu-

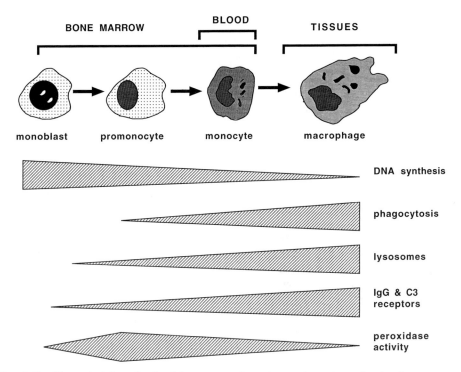

Fig. 1.2   Characteristics of cells of the mononuclear phagocyte system, showing the development of phagocytic activity, lysosomes, IgG and C3 receptors, and peroxidase activity.

lar weight glycoproteins such as LFA-1 (lymphocyte function-associated antigen 1; CD11a/CD18) which interacts with ICAM-1 (intercellular adhesion molecule-1; CD54) present on vascular endothelial cells (Dustin *et al.*, 1986; Rothlein *et al.*, 1986). Cytokines such as interleukin-1 (IL-1) and interferon-γ (IFN-γ) increase the expression of CD54 by endothelial cells and can therefore facilitate monocyte margination and migration to sites of inflammation (Dustin *et al.*, 1986). CD31 is also involved in the transendothelial migration of monocytes (Muller and Randolph, 1999). The proportion of monocytes migrating to various organs is apparently random and corresponds roughly to the size of the organ. Having arrived at their target organ, the monocytes differentiate into macrophages (van Furth and Cohn., 1968). Once monocytes leave the circulation, they do not return, remaining in the tissues as macrophages for several months.

Mononuclear phagocytes are to be found in a variety of locations throughout the body, in addition to the bone marrow (Table 1.1). Though more than 95 per cent of tissue macrophages derive from monocytes, evidence exists which suggests that the remaining 5 per cent of macrophages derive from the local division of mononuclear phagocytes in the tissues. The latter are not resident macrophages, but have arrived in the tissues and body cavities from the bone marrow within the previous 24 h, before completion of cell division (van Furth, 1989). Macrophages in tissues and body cavities are not a constant population of cells, but are being renewed regularly by the influx of monocytes.

The ultimate fate of tissue macrophages is uncertain. The number of macrophages that die must be considerable, because the total monocyte production in the mouse is approxi-

Table 1.1   Distribution of mononuclear phagocytes

Site	Cell
Bone marrow	Monoblasts
	Promonocytes
	Monocytes
	Macrophages
Peripheral blood	Monocytes
Tissues	Liver (Kupffer cells)
	Lung (alveolar macrophages)
	Connective tissue (histiocytes)
	Spleen (red pulp macrophages)
	Lymph node
	Thymus
	Bone (osteoclasts)
	Synovium (type A cells)
	Mucosa-associated lymphoid tissue
	Gastrointestinal tract
	Genitourinary tract
	Endocrine organs
	Central nervous system (microglia)
	Skin (histiocytes/Langerhans cells)
Serous cavities	Pleural macrophages
	Peritoneal macrophages
Inflammatory tissues	Epithelioid cells
	Exudate macrophages
	Multinucleate giant cells

mately 1.5×10^6 cells per 24 h, and all of these cells will eventually leave the bone marrow and become tissue macrophages (van Furth, 1989). Macrophages from liver, lung and gut are known to migrate to nearby draining lymph nodes, but the lymph efferent from these nodes does not contain macrophages or monocytes, making it probable that macrophges die in lymph nodes. It is also conceivable that cell death occurs in tissues and body cavities. Mononuclear phagocytes have different kinetics during inflammatory episodes. During an acute inflammatory reaction, the number of circulating monocytes increases due to an enhanced bone marrow production (van Furth *et al.*, 1973). However, the time spent in the circulation is shorter than under normal conditions, due to an efflux of monocytes from the circulation into inflammatory exudates. Except for the relatively small share taken by local production during acute inflammation, most of the increase in the number of macrophages in the inflammatory exudate is brought about by this influx of monocytes (van Furth, 1988).

3 Humoral control of monocytopoiesis

Despite a great deal of information from *in vitro* studies, relatively little was known about the humoral control of monocytopoiesis *in vivo* until recently. Macrophages themselves appear to synthesize and secrete at least two hematopoietic growth factors, macrophage colony-stimulating factor (M-CSF) (Flanagan and Lader, 1998) and granulocyte– macrophage colony-stimulating factor (GM-CSF) (Quesniaux and Jones, 1998), which stimulate the production and function of mononuclear phagocytes (Jones and Millar,

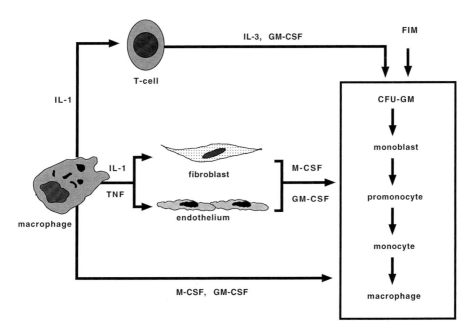

Fig. 1.3   The humoral regulation of monocytopoiesis. (FIM = factor inducing monocytopoiesis).

1989). M-CSF and GM-CSF production by macrophages is stimulated by exposure to external stimuli such as phagocytosable particles and endotoxin. Macrophages also produce and release cytokines that induce non-hematopoietic cells to elaborate M-CSF and GM-CSF. Thus, the release of IL-1 and tumor necrosis factor (TNF) from macrophages can induce fibroblasts and endothelial cells to produce M-CSF and GM-CSF, which in turn stimulate the production of mononuclear phagocytes (Figure 1.3). Similarly, GM-CSF can stimulate TNF synthesis by mononuclear phagocytes (Cannistra *et al.*, 1987). Receptors for granulocyte colony-stimulating factor (G-CSF) and GM-CSF are known to be present on mononuclear phagocytes.

M-CSF (or CSF-1) is a glycoprotein with a molecular weight of 85 kDa which stimulates macrophage colony formation of bone marrow cells in a semi-solid agar culture system. The CSF-1 receptor is the homodimeric, tyrosine kinase product of the c-*fms* proto-oncogene, which contains a kinase insert domain (Hamilton, 1997). M-CSF stimulates differentiation of progenitor cells to mature monocytes, and prolongs the survival of monocytes (Motoyoshi, 1998). It enhances expression of differentiation antigens and stimulates the chemotactic, phagocytic and killing activities of monocytes. M-CSF also stimulates production of several cytokines such as GM-CSF, G-CSF and IL-6 by priming monocytes, and directly stimulates production and secretion of IL-8 and reactive nitrogen intermediates. In addition to the stimulation of hematopoiesis, M-CSF also stimulates differentiation and proliferation of osteoclast progenitor cells.

Mononuclear phagocyte production and activity can also be influenced by certain products of T lymphocytes such as GM-CSF and IL-3, and these factors are probably important in the delayed hypersensitivity reaction (Cannistra *et al.*, 1987). Serum collected during an inflammatory reaction contains a factor that stimulates monocytopoiesis in the bone marrow of mice and rabbits, yet has no M-CSF or IL-1 activity. This has been called 'factor increasing monocytopoiesis' (FIM) and is probably a cocktail of cytokines and growth factors (Golde and Groopman, 1990). GM-CSF and IL-3 are probably important in regulating monocytopoiesis during inflammatory responses, but M-CSF is felt to be a more likely candidate for regulation of monocytopoiesis in the steady state. IL-3 (Mangi and Newland, 1999) was cloned in 1986 and is a multipotent hematopoietic growth factor produced by activated T cells, monocytes/macrophages and stroma cells. The human IL-3 gene is located on chromosome 5 and the high-affinity receptor for human IL-3 is composed of α- and β-subunits, sharing a common β-subunit with GM-CSF and IL-5 (CDw131). The CDw131 subunit has been mapped to chromosome 22q13.1. IL-3 induces proliferation, maturation and probably self-renewal of pluripotent hematopoietic stem cells and cells of myeloid, erythroid and megakaryocytic lineages. Less is understood about the humoral inhibitors of monocytopoiesis. The best studied candidates are prostaglandins of the E series, which are produced by mononuclear phagocytes (Kurland *et al.*, 1978; Pelus *et al.*, 1979), and α-, β- and γ-interferons (Trinchieri and Perussia, 1983).

Recent research has begun to identify key transcription factors involved in monocytopoiesis (Valledor *et al.*, 1998) including AP-1 (fos/jun dimer) (also see Section 8.2) which may play multiple roles in functional development of hematopoietic precursor cells into mature blood cells along the hematopoietic cell lineages. This includes the monocyte/macrophage, granulocyte, megakaryocyte and erythroid lineages. The transcription factors Pu.1 and C/EBPα (Behre *et al.*, 1999) are responsible for normal myeloid differentiation from stem cells to monocytes or granulocytes. The *PU.1* gene (Oikawa *et al.*, 1999) encodes an Ets family transcription factor which controls expression of many B-cell- and macrophage-specific genes. Expression of the gene is critical for development of lymphoid and myeloid cell lineages, since Pu.1-deficient mice exhibit defects in the development of these cell lineages. In particular, Pu.1 induces expression of the M-CSF receptor and the development of monocytes, whereas C/EBPα increases the expression of the G-CSF receptor and leads to mature granulocytes. Studies (Hume *et al.*, 1997) of the *cis*-acting elements of the c-*fms* promoter have indicated a key role for collaboration between the macrophage-specific transcription factor, Pu.1 and other members of the Ets transcription factor family. This appears to be a common pattern in macrophage-specific promoters.

4 Terminology

- Mononuclear phagocytes: includes monoblasts, promonocytes, monocytes and macrophages.
- Resident macrophages: macrophages occurring in specific sites in normal, non-inflamed tissues. However, they may also be observed in small numbers in an inflammatory exudate. They are sometimes called 'normal macrophages'.
- Exudate macrophages: macrophages occurring in an exudate and identifiable on the basis of peroxidase activity, immunophenotype and cell kinetics. They derive from monocytes and have many of the characteristics of the latter. Exudate macrophages are felt to be the precursors of resident macrophages.

- Elicited macrophages: macrophages attracted to a given site because of a particular stimulus. An elicited population of macrophages is heterogeneous both developmentally and functionally.
- Activated macrophages: macrophages exhibiting an increase in one or more functional activities, or the appearance of a new functional activity. Both resident and exudate macrophages can be activated (van Furth, 1989).

5 Morphology of mononuclear phagocytes

5.1 Light microscopy

5.1.1 Macrophages

Macrophages are generally large, irregularly shaped cells measuring 25–50 µm in diameter (Figure 1.4). They often have an eccentrically placed, round or kidney-shaped nucleus with one or two prominent nucleoli and finely dispersed nuclear chromatin. There is often a clearly defined juxtanuclear Golgi complex in an abundant cytoplasm. The cytoplasm contains fine granules and multiple large, azurophilic granules. Cytoplasmic vacuoles are seen frequently near the cell periphery, reflecting the active pinocytosis of macrophages. Characteristically, the surface of these cells appears ruffled. Phase contrast microscopy reveals large cells with a propensity to adhere to and spread on glass sufaces, leaving cell organelles concentrated within the central region of the cell and with an intense ruffling of the membrane borders (Douglas and Hassan, 1990).

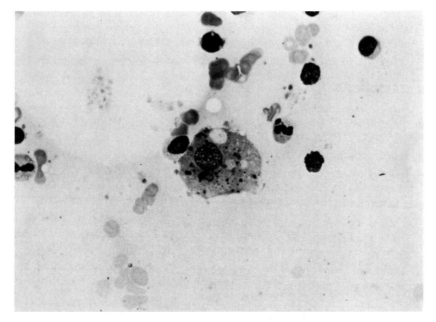

Fig. 1.4   Light micrograph of a human bone marrow macrophage (×1000).

5.1.2 Monocytes and their precursors

Monocytes appear on stained blood films as smaller cells (12–15 μm diameter) with an eccentrically placed nucleus occupying at least 50 per cent of the cell's area (Figure 1.5). The nucleus may be kidney-shaped, round or irregular with a fine chromatin pattern. The cytoplasm contains both fine granules and large azurophilic granules, as well as clear cytoplasmic vacuoles (Goldman, 1989). Phase contrast microscopy reveals gentle undulating movements of the cytoplasm and a prominent ruffled plasma membrane (Douglas and Hassan, 1990).

The bone marrow precursors of peripheral blood monocytes are the promonocytes and monoblasts. Promonocytes are intermediate between monoblasts and monocytes, measure 12–18 μm in diameter and are characterized by the appearance of several immature and mature azurophilic granules and deeply indented and irregularly shaped nuclei. The monoblast is indistinguishable from the myeloblast by light microscopy and is present in very small numbers in normal stained bone marrow specimens (Goldman, 1989).

5.2 Ultrastructure

5.2.1 Macrophages

Macrophage ultrastructure varies with their location, degree of activation and the procedures employed during their isolation and preparation for microscopy. However, certain general features of macrophage ultrastructure may be outlined.

Electron microscopy demonstrates an eccentric nucleus of variable shape, with chromatin disposed in fine clumps. Clear spaces between membrane-fixed chromatin clumps mark the site of nuclear pores. The cytoplasm contains scattered strands of rough endoplasmic reticulum, a well-developed Golgi complex in a juxtanuclear position, variable numbers of vesicles, vacuoles and pinocytic vesicles, large mitochondria and electron-dense membrane-bound lysosomes which can be seen fusing with phagosomes to form secondary lysosomes. Within the secondary lysosomes, ingested cellular, bacterial and non-cellular material can be seen in various stages of degradation and digestion (Figure 1.6). The surfaces of macrophages and monocytes are covered in ruffles and micrivilli, and small surface blebs. Microtubules and microfilaments are prominent in macrophages and form a well-organized, three-dimensional cytoskeleton which surrounds the nucleus and extends throughout the cytoplasm to the cell periphery. Actin microfilaments immediately beneath the cell membrane are responsible for the prominent ruffling, locomotion and pseudopod formation, as well as influencing endocytotic events (Stossel, 1981, 1988; Hartwig and Shelvin, 1986) and establishing the polarity of migration in response to chemotactic stimuli.

5.2.2 Monocytes and their precursors

The monocyte nucleus generally contains one or two small nucleoli surrounded by nucleolar associated chromatin. The cytoplasm is relatively abundant and contains scattered rough endoplasmic reticulum and a prominent Golgi apparatus which is frequently located in the area of nuclear indentation. Small vesicles are scattered throughout the cytoplasm, but are often particularly numerous in the Golgi region and near the cell surface, where they represent pinocytotic vacuoles. Small mitochondria are abundant in the cytoplasm, and inconspicuous bundles of fibrils are often seen in a perinuclear position. Cytoplasmic granules measuring 0.05–0.2 μm are seen, which are dense, homoge-

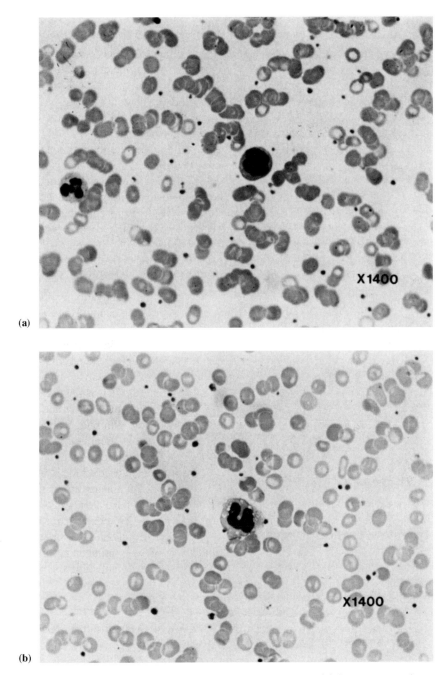

Fig. 1.5   Light micrographs of human peripheral blood monocytes. (a) A monocyte and neutrophil are present; (b) a monocyte with a typically kidney-shaped nucleus.

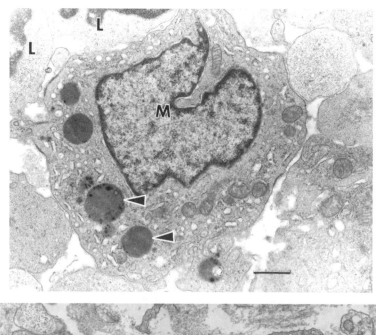

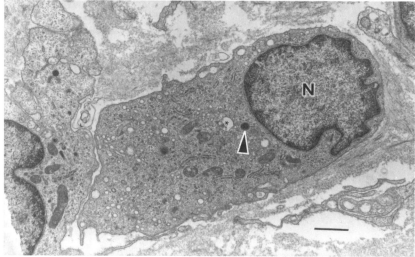

Fig. 1.6 (a) Electron micrograph of a dermal macrophage (M) in contact with two lymphocytes (L) during a delayed type hypersensitivity reaction in skin. Membrane-bound secondary lysosomes (phagosomes) (arrowheads) containing material of various electron densities are present in the cytoplasm. Bar = 1 μm. (b) A recent monocyte recruit into the dermis showing rounded nucleus (N), development of vesicles, a multivesicular vesicle (*) and a dense granule (arrowhead). Bar = 1 μm.

neous and surrounded by a limiting membrane (Figure 1.7). It is not possible on ultra-structural examination alone to recognize distinct subpopulations of monocyte granules, but ultrastructural cytochemical studies suggest that such subpopulations may exist (Hayhoe and Quaglino, 1988).

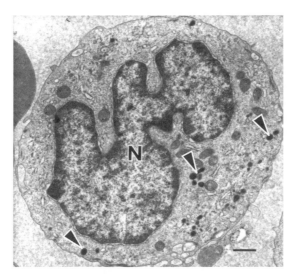

Fig. 1.7 Electron micrograph of a human peripheral blood monocyte. The cell has a lobulated nucleus (N) and the cytoplasm contains populations of dense granules (arrowheads). Bar = 1 μm.

Marrow promonocytes are the first clearly identifiable members of the mononuclear phagocyte system. They are characterized by the presence of distinctive cytoplasmic granules which are quite different from granulocyte granules. Promonocytes contain a moderate sized nucleus with one or more nucleoli and sometimes slight peripheral chromatin condensation. A well-developed Golgi apparatus, plentiful ribosomes and moderate numbers of mitochondria are seen. The maturation sequence from promonocytes through to later monocyte forms consists of increasing nuclear chromatin condensation, reduced numbers of ribosomes and a reduction in the amount of rough endoplasmic reticulum. In more mature cells, the nucleus assumes a kidney—or horseshoe—shape and nucleoli are less frequent.

6 Histochemistry of mononuclear phagocytes

Various hydrolytic enzymes have been isolated from macrophages and monocytes, including acid phosphatase, α-glucuronidase, N-acetylglucosaminidase, lysozyme, ±-naphthyl butyrate esterase and peroxidase. Monocytes also stain weakly for polysaccharides in the periodic acid–Schiff (PAS) reaction and for lipids in the Sudan black B reaction. Macrophages are generally PAS negative, but following phagocytosis they may show globular PAS-positive intracytoplasmic deposits. They may also contain Sudan black-positive material, hemosiderin and other substances (Schmalzl and Braunsteiner, 1970). Non-specific esterase is an enzyme on the external surface of the plasma membrane of macrophages and monocytes (Yam *et al.*, 1971). It is the most commonly used cytochemical marker for monocytes. The reaction with non-specific esterase is fluoride sensitive. Acid phosphatase is contained in the primary lysosomes of monocytes and macrophages. Several isoenzymes of acid phosphatase exist in macrophages. A granular cytoplasmic staining for 5′-nucleotidase is evident in most macrophages (Ginsel *et al.*, 1983).

Human bone marrow promonocytes and blood monocytes contain granules that comprise two functionally distinct populations (Nichols and Bainton, 1973; Hayhoe and Quaglino, 1988). One population contains acid phosphatase, aryl sulfatase and peroxidase; these granules are modified primary lysosomes and are analogous to the azurophilic granules of the neutrophil. The content of the other population of monocyte granules is unknown, but they lack alkaline phosphatase and hence are not strictly analogous to the specific granules of neutrophils. The lysosome granules have a digestive function, whereas the function of the second population is unknown.

7 Composition and metabolism

The composition and metabolism of mononuclear phagocytes alter during differentiation. Concurrent with the transition from monocyte to macrophage, there is an increase in the number of mitochondria, activity of mitochondrial enzymes and rate of cellular respiration (Cohn, 1968). Both glucose oxidation and lactate production increase with cellular maturation. There is also an increase in the number of lysosomes, with increases in lysosomal enzymes. Even in an apparent resting state, however, macrophages are extremely active metabolically. For example, they are estimated to turn over the equivalent of their entire plasma membrane every 30 min (Steinman *et al.*, 1983). Aerobic glycolysis provides the energy required by mammalian monocytes (Oren *et al.*, 1963). The mature macrophage employs both glycolysis and oxidative phosphorylation in the generation of energy, though the predominant source of energy depends on the origin of the macrophage. The ATP generated by glycolysis is stored in a large pool of creatine phosphate, which provides the immediate source of energy for mobility-dependent function (Loike *et al.*, 1979). Even under anaerobic conditions, however, most macrophages are effective phagocytes. This anaerobic phagocytic capability is obviously advantageous to cells that are required to function in granulomas or abscess cavities remote from oxygenated blood. However, the pulmonary alveolar macrophage of man is incapable of phagocytosis under severely anaerobic conditions and requires a partial pressure of oxygen greater than 25 mmHg for phagocytosis and energy production (Cohen and Cline, 1971; Hocking and Golde, 1979).

The basal metabolism of macrophages can be significantly affected by receptor–ligand interactions (Adams and Hamilton, 1984) (see Section 8), which often result in a 'respiratory burst' with the metabolism of large quantities of glucose by way of the hexose monophosphate shunt and an increased oxygen consumption. This respiratory burst results in altered activity of the membrane-bound oxidase complex and the reduction of molecular oxygen to superoxide (Babior, 1984). The superoxide thus generated is rapidly converted to hydrogen peroxide and hydroxyl radicals, which provide most of the microbicidal oxidative activity both within the phagosome and in the extracellular environment. The molecular oxygen is reduced ultimately to water, but the superoxide anion, hydrogen peroxide and hydroxyl radicals are referred to as the reactive oxygen intermediates (ROIs).

$O_2 \rightarrow$	$O_2^{2-} \rightarrow$	$H_2O_2 \rightarrow$	$OH^- \rightarrow$	H_2O
Oxygen	Superoxide anion	Hydrogen peroxide	Hydroxyl radical	Water

The magnitude of the respiratory burst decreases markedly when monocytes mature into macrophages (Klebanoff, 1988). Resident macrophages, for example, have only a weak respiratory burst, though this may be increased severalfold when they are activated *in vivo*. *In vitro*, an increased respiratory burst can be induced by recombinant IFN-γ (Nathan *et al.*, 1984) and migration inhibitory factor (MIF) (Nishihira, 1998).

A second consequence of receptor–ligand interaction is the release of arachidonic acid by phospholipase A2, from cellular stores of phospholipids, and its subsequent conversion via either lipooxygenases or cyclooxygenases to a series of leukotrienes or prostaglandins, respectively (Pawlowski *et al.*, 1983).

Lysosomal enzymes involved in degradation of phagocytosed material are synthesized in the endoplasmic reticulum and packaged by the Golgi apparatus into structures called primary lysosomes (Schmalzl and Braunsteiner, 1970). These primary lysosomes may fuse with phagocytic or pinocytic vacuoles (phagosomes) containing ingested materials. These structures are termed secondary lysosomes (phagolysosomes).

Activation of macrophages (see also Chapter 2) refers to a state of enhanced cellular metabolism, mobility, lysosomal enzyme activity and cytocidal capacity (Adams and Hamilton, 1984). Macrophage activation is usually accompanied by increased elaboration of important products of mononuclear phagocytes, including lysosomal neutral proteases, acid hydrolases, complement components, enzyme inhibitors, binding proteins, IL-1, TNF and factors promoting hematopoiesis. Most forms of activation, however, include down-regulation of certain physiological characteristics as well as up-regulation of others. It is clear that CpG DNA and lipopolysaccharide (LPS) induce distinct patterns of activation in human monocytes (Hartmann and Krieg, 1999) which may have important implications for gene therapy approaches.

Transmembrane signal transduction has been studied in mononuclear phagocytes. For example, it has been suggested that chemoattractant oligopeptides binding to the appropriate receptor on the mononuclear phagocyte surface activate a phospholipase—possibly phospholipase C. This then degrades phosphatidylinositol and releases arachidonic acid. Phosphatidylinositol, phosphatidylinositol-4-phosphate and phosphatidylinositol-4,5-bisphosphate are converted into diacylglycerol and the corresponding phosphoinosides—all of which can mobilize intracellular calcium stores. Calcium, together with arachidonate and diacylglycerol, can activate protein kinase C. In addition, conditions that lead to the activation of the respiratory burst may translocate this kinase from the cytosol to the cell membrane (Myers *et al.*, 1984); this will influence the substrates it phosphorylates and, therefore, determine which biological response will be triggered by the chemoattractants (e.g. chemotactic as distinct from secretory).

Transcriptional regulation has been examined in relation to a number of signaling pathways (see also Section 3) including nuclear factor-κB (NF-κB), NF-IL-6, signal transducer and activator of transcription (STAT) 3 and peroxisome proliferator-activated receptors (PPARs). NF-κB is one of the key transcription factors regulating genes involved in the immune and inflammatory response and in the regulation of growth (Ghosh *et al.*, 1998). LPS and TNF can both trigger activation of NF-kB with subsequent transcription of pro-inflammatory cytokines such as IL-6 and IL-8. NF-IL-6 is phosphorylated by a Ras-dependent mitogen-activated protein (MAP) kinase cascade, while STAT3/APRF is tyrosine phosphorylated directly by JAK kinases which are associated with the cytoplasmic portion of the receptor. STAT3 dimerizes and translocates to the nucleus where it binds to the consensus sequences of responsive genes and activates transcription (i.e. the JAK–STAT pathway). STAT3 is also tyrosine phosphorylated in response to epidermal growth factor (EGF), G-CSF, leptin and other IL-6-type cytokines including ciliary neurotrophic factor (CNTF), oncostatin M and leukemia inhibitory factor (LIF). Mice deficient in NF-IL-6 are highly susceptible to facultative intracellular bacteria due to ineffective killing of the pathogens by macrophages (Akira, 1997). In addition, the tumor cytotoxicity of macrophages from NF-IL-6 knockout mice is severely impaired, indicating a crucial role for NF-IL-6 in macrophage bactericidal and tumoricidal activities. PPARs are ligand-dependent transcription factors of the nuclear hormone receptor superfamily, which includes the steroid, retinoid and thyroid hormone receptors. The PPARs can be activated by various fatty acids and eicosanoid metabolites (Ross *et al.*, 1999), and have been considered primarily as regulating genes involved in lipid and glucose homeostasis. Recent research has also implicated PPAR-γ in macrophage biology, regulation of inflammatory responses and atherosclerosis (Ricote *et al.*, 1999).

8 Macrophage surface receptors

Receptors on the surface of the macrophage determine the control of activities such as growth, differentiation, activation, recognition, endocytosis, migration and secretion. Numerous ligands have been reported as binding to the surface of the macrophage (Table 1.2), and a selection are discussed below. Subsequent chapters will cover this topic in greater depth.

8.1 Fc and complement receptors

The first macrophage receptors to be identified were those for the Fc region of the IgG molecule (Berken and Benacerref, 1966) and for the cleavage product of the third component of complement (C3) (Lay and Nussenzweig, 1968).The attachment of the Fc portions of immunoglobulin molecules to the surface of the macrophage via Fc receptors may trigger various functions such as endocytosis, the generation of transmembrane signals, resulting in the reorganization of cytoskeletal microfilaments at the site of attachment facilitating phagocytosis, and the secretion of potent mediators. Among these Fc receptors are those for IgG: FcγRI (CD64) with high affinity for monomeric IgG, and other receptors, FcγRII (CDw32) and FcγRIII (CD16) which have only low affinity for monomeric IgG but that can effectively bind immune complexes by multiple receptor–ligand interactions (Unkeless *et al.*, 1988). Macrophages also possess the low-affinity receptor for IgE, FcεRIIb (CD23), following IL-4 induction, and a role for CD23 in host defense mechanisms against IgE-inducing parasites has been suggested. Unlike other Fc receptors which have been sequenced, CD23 is not a member of the Ig superfamily (Table 1.3) but belongs to a primitive superfamily of invertebrate and vertebrate lectins (Kinet, 1989). The gene for CD23 has been assigned to chromosome 19.

In recent years, it has become clear that other members of the lectin family are important in complement activation mediated by the mannose-binding lectin (MBL) (Vasta *et al.*, 1999). This has been described as a key mechanism for the mammalian acute phase response to infection, and the complement activation pathway is initiated by binding of MBL (a humoral C-type lectin) to microbial surfaces bearing distinct carbohydrate deter-

Table 1.2   Surface receptors of monocytes and macrophages

Fc receptors
        IgG_{2a}, IgG_{2b}/IgG_1, IgG_3, IgA, IgE
Complement receptors
C3b, C3d, C3bi, C5a, C1q
Cytokine receptors
        MIF, MAF, LIF, CF, MFF, IL-1, IL-2, IL-3, IL-4, IL-6, IL-7, IL-10, IL-13, IL-16, IL-17, leptin, HGF
        Interferon-α, -β, -γ
        Colony-stimulating factors (GM-CSF, M-CSF/CSF-1)
Chemokine receptors
        CCR1, CCR2, CCR5, CCR8, CCR9, CXCR1, CXCR2, CXCR4, CX3CR1
Receptors for peptides and small molecules
        H_1, H_2, 5-HT
        1,2,5-Dihydroxy vitamin D3
        N-Formylated peptides
        Enkephalins/endorphins
        Substance P
        Arg-vasopressin
Hormone receptors
        Insulin
        Glucocorticosteroids
        Angiotensin
Transferrin and lactoferrin receptors
Lipoprotein lipid receptors
        Anionic low-density lipoproteins
        PGE_2, LTB4, LTC4, LTD4, PAG
        Apolipoproteins B and E (chylomicron remnants, VLDL)
Receptor for coagulants and anticoagulants
        Fibrinogen/fibrin
        Coagulation factor VII
        α1-Antithrombin
        Heparin
Fibronectin receptors
Laminin receptors
Mannosyl, fucosyl, galactosyl residues,
AGE receptors
α_2-Macroglobulin–proteinase complex receptors
Others
        Cholinergic agonists
        α-Adrenergic agonists
        β-Adrenergic agonists

Abbreviations: AGE = advanced glycation endproduct; C = complement; CSF = colony-stimulating factor; GM = granulocyte—macrophage; H = histamine; 5-HT = 5-hydroxytryptamine; Ig = immunoglobulin; IL = interleukin; LIF = leukocyte migration inhibition factor; LT = leukotriene; MAF = macrophage-activating factor; MFF = macrophage fusion factor; MIF = macrophage inhibitory factor; PG = prostaglandin; VLDL = very low-density lipoprotein.
It is important to remember that there may be overlap among cytokines and 'factors' which may comprise several active molecular species, for example MAF activity is partly due to IFN-γ.

minants. MBL is associated with a serine protease which, following binding, activates the complement component C3, leading to either humoral cell killing, via assembly of the membrane attack complex, or phagocytosis of the opsonized target via the complement receptor. Galectins (formerly S-type lectins) modulate the activity of CR3 and can mediate macrophage adhesion to lymphocytes which are activated by signaling through another C-type lectin, L-selectin. The functional interactions of the galectins, MBL and

Table 1.3 Selected macrophage surface molecules related to known superfamilies

Superfamily	Molecule	Mol. wt (kDa)
Integrin		
LFA-1	CD11a/CD18	180/95
CR3	CD11b/CD18	170/95
CR4–2	CD11c/CD18	150/95
VLA-4	CD49d/CD29	150/130
VNR	CD51/CD61	140/110
SCRs		
CR1	CD35	160–250
DAF	CD55	70
MCF	CD46	45–70
Immunoglobulin		
FcγRI	CD64	75
FcγRII	CDw32	40
FcγRIII	CD16	50–65
MHC class I		45
MHC class II		27–33
β_2-Microglobulin		12
CSF-1R	CD115	150
ICAM-1	CD54	92
CD4	59	
Cytokine receptor		
IL-2R	CD25	55
IL-3R	CD123, CD131	70, 140
IL-4R	CD124, CD132	140, 64–70
IL-6R	CD126, CD130	80, gp130
GM-CSFR	CD116	80
IL-7R		49.5
Leptin-R		
IL-13R	CD213a,b	145
Lectin-like		65
B-Glucan		
FcεRIIb (CD23)		45
MFR		175
AGE-R		90
Thrombomodulin	CD141	75
Chemokine receptors		
CCR1		
CCR2		
CCR5	CD195	
CCR8		
CCR9		
CXCR1	CDw128	67–70
CXCR2	CDw128	67–70
CXCR4	CD184	
CX3CR1		

Abbreviations: AGE = advanced glycation endproduct; CD = cluster of differentiation; CR = complement receptor; CSF = colony-stimulating factor; DAF = decay-accelerating factor; FN = fibronectin; GM = granulocyte–macrophage; ICAM = intercellular cell adhesion molecule; IL = interleukin; LFA = leukocyte function antigen; MCF = membrane cofactor protein; MHC = major histocompatibility complex; MFR = mannosyl–fucosyl receptor; SCR = short consensus repeat; VLA = very late antigen; VN = vitronectin. For a comprehensive analysis of cell surface molecule families see Barclay and Brown (1997) and PROW (protein reviews on the web) at http://www.ncbi.nlm.nih.gov.prow/.

L-selectin in the acute phase response therefore assist in combating any microbial challenge.

Complement receptors on the macrophage are involved in the binding and ingestion of opsonized particles. CR1 (CD35) recognizes C3b and CR3, the Mac-1 molecule (CD11b/CD18) recognizes C3bi; the ligand for CR4 is still unclear but may also be C3bi. CR3 is an α/β-heterodimeric glycoprotein, non-covalently linked and a member of the integrin supergene family of adhesion molecules, as is CR4 (CD11c/CD18). CR1 is a member of a group of proteins, including the complement proteins, C1r, C1s, C2, factor H, C4-binding protein, factor B, monocyte chemotactic protein (MCP; CD46) and decay-accelerating factor (DAF; CD55), having structural elements called short consensus repeats (SCRs). Complement regulatory proteins accelerate the decay of C3 convertases or act as cofactors for proteolytic cleavage, thereby limiting the activity of C3 convertases. In this way, they inhibit complement activation on autologous tissues (Hourcade *et al.*, 1989). CR1 (CD35), MCP (CD46) and DAF (CD55) are membrane bound while C4-binding protein and factor H operate in the extracellular fluid.

8.2 Cytokine receptors

Macrophages, in addition to elaborating a large variety of cytokines, possess receptors for many cytokines (see Tables 1.2 and 1.3). There is a structural relationship between cytokine receptors, with most showing homology with either the cytokine receptor family (IL-2R, IL-3R, IL-4R and GM-CSFR) or the Ig superfamily. Second messenger systems are gradually being implicated in the intracellular signaling induced by cytokine binding to receptors. Phosphorylation of proteins has been one of the earliest changes detected in cells stimulated by IL-2, IL-3, TNF and CSF-1, implying regulation through alterations in protein kinase activity. Some cytokine receptors may be coupled to G-proteins since interaction with ligand induces increased binding and hydrolysis of GTP in the cell membrane. A few of the transcriptional pathways involved in signaling have been mentioned, but detailed consideration of these is not possible in this chapter.

A wide variety of biological effects are generated by the interaction of ligands with their receptors. Individual cytokines or combinations of cytokines interacting with specific receptors modulate the function of macrophages (Table 1.4). A number of cytokines, including IFN-γ (Gonwa *et al.*, 1986), IFN-α (Dinarello and Mier, 1987), TNF (Talmadge *et al.*, 1988), IL-2 (Malkovsky, 1987), IL-4 (Paul and Ohara, 1987), M-CSF (Flanagan and Lader, 1998) and GM-CSF (Quesniaux and Jones, 1998), all having pleiotropic effects, are involved in the activation of macrophages (see Chapter 2). Many of the functions carried out by macrophages, including the destruction of intracelllular parasites and, *in vitro*, the destruction of some malignant cells, are enhanced by this activation (Table 1.5). IFN-γ, for example, has been found to be a major constituent of macrophage-activating factor (MAF) and also up-regulates class II expression. It has also been reported that binding of TNF, IL-4, GM-CSF or IL-2 to receptors on the macrophage promotes MAF activity.

GM-CSF stimulates proliferation of monocyte precursors, and platelet-activating factor (PAF) stimulates chemotaxis and bactericidal activity. M-CSF induces proliferation of monocyte/macrophage progenitor cells and can also activate some functions of mature cells. The c-*fms* proto-oncogene encodes the CSF-1 (M-CSF) receptor (Flanagan and Lader, 1998). IL-3 has been reported as having macrophage-activating properties, in a

Table 1.4   Effects of cytokines on monocytes/macrophages

Cytokine	Source	Action on monocytes/macrophages
IL-1	Macrophages, others	Release of IL-1, TNF, CSFs
IL-2 and	Activated T cells	Proliferation and differentiation of precursors, enhances cytolytic tumoricidal activity
IL-3	T cells	Growth and differentiation
IL-4	CD4+ T cells	Fusion, increased MHC II expression, dendritic morphology, antigen presentation, induction of mannose receptor (CD206), Fcε receptor (CD23), CD13 and CD11a/CD18, down-regulates CD14, blocks ADCC
IL-6	Macrophages, others	Maturation
IL-7	Stromal cells, others	Increases immune effector functions
IL-8	Macrophages, NK cells, others	Increase in $[Ca^{2+}]i$, weak respiratory burst, enhances integrin expression
IL-10	Macrophages, activated T and B cells	Inhibits production of IL-1, IL-6, IL-8, Il-10, IL-12, GM-CSF, G-CSF, M-CSF, NF, MIP1-α, MIP1-β, MIP2, RANTES, LIF; enhances production of IL-1RA, TNFRp55 and p75; inhibits expression of MHC II, CD54, CD80, CD86 and CD23; enhances expression of FcR (CD16 and CD64)
IL-11	EC, others	Promotes GM colony formation
IL-13	T cells, others	Similar effects to IL-4; up-regulates adhesion molecules including CD116, CD11c, CD18, CD29, CD49e and MHC II, CD80, CD86, mannose receptor; promote fusion and formation of giant cells; inhibits synthesis of IL-1, IL-6, IL-12, TNF, IL-8, MIP1-α, MIP1-β, MCP-3, PGE_2, NO; enhances production of IL-1RA, decoy IL-1RII; induces expression of 15S-HETE, lipoxin A4
IL-16	T cells	Increased chemotaxis, enhanced MHC II expression
IL-17	Activated T cells, stromal cells	Up-regulates IL-6, IL-1, MCP-1
TNF-α	Macrophages, others	Release of IL-1, PAF, PGE_2, chemotaxis
M-CSF	Fibroblasts, macrophages	Growth and differentiation, urokinase induction
GM-CSF	T cells, macrophages	Growth, differentiation and ?activation of endothelium
IFN-α	Leukocytes	Antiviral and activation
IFN-β	Fibroblasts	Antiviral and activation
IFN-γ	T cells	Antiviral and activation (e.g. enhanced MHC II expression, respiratory burst, down-regulation of MFR)
TGF-β	Platelets, macrophages	Chemotaxis, growth factor release, macrophage deactivation

Abbreviations: EC = endothelial cells; GM-CSF = granulocyte—macrophage colony-stimulating factor; IFN = interferon; IL = interleukin; M-CSF = macrophage colony-stimulating factor; MFR = mannosyl–fucosyl receptor; NO = nitric oxide; PAF = platelet-activating factor; PGE = prostaglandin E; TGF = transforming growth factor; TNF = tumor necrosis factor.

murine system, which are distinct from those of IFN-γ and IL-4. IL-3 (Gonwa *et al.*, 1986; Mangi and Newland, 1999) has MAF activity and can regulate the expression of class II major histocompatibility complex (MHC) molecules and the cellular interaction molecule LFA-1, and induces IL-1 mRNA expression, although IL-1 bioactivity was only demonstrated after the addition of suboptimal amounts of LPS.

Table 1.5   Major alterations of activated macrophages

Increased
    Size
    Phagocytosis for C3b- and IgG-coated particles
    Secretion of collagenase, elastase, plasminogen activator
    Prostaglandin release
    Rate of spreading
    Adherence to glass
    Rate of fluid phase pinocytosis
    Cellular ATP
    Plasmalemmal alkaline phosphodiesterase
    Glucose consumption
    O_2 consumption
    O_2 radical release
    H_2O_2 release
    NO release
    Microbicidal activity
    Tumoricidal and tumoristatic ability
    Expression of class II molecules
Decreased
    Mannose–fucose receptor sites
    Leukotriene production
    Plasmalemmal 5′ nucleotidase
    Secretion of apolipoprotein E

Abbreviations: ATP = adenosine triphosphate; C = complement;.Ig = immunoglobulin.

Hepatocyte growth factor (HGF) (Beilmann *et al.*, 2000) is a pluripotent cytokine with mitogenic, migration and morphogenic activity for epithelial and endothelial target cells. The HGF receptor, Met, is induced in stimulated peripheral blood monocytes. Stimulation of monocytes with recombinant HGF results in modulation of genes involved in cell movement. HGF-stimulated monocytes demonstrate significantly increased matrigel invasion, suggesting a pro-inflammatory role for HGF and an important role for the HGF/Met signaling system in the activation of the non-specific cellular inflammatory response. Recent work also suggests that leptin (Lee *et al.*, 1999) may influence macrophage biology. Cells with leptin receptors have been identified outside of the appetite regulatory centers in the brain. Macrophages express leptin receptors which are signaling competent (long form); these cells may be altered during chronic leptin deficiency. Several phenotypic abnormalities are apparent in macrophages from ob/ob mice, including decreased steady-state levels of uncoupling protein-2 mRNA, increased mitochondrial production of superoxide and hydrogen peroxide, constitutive activation of CCAAT enhancer-binding protein (C/EBP)—an oxidant-sensitive transcription factor—increased expression of IL-6 and cyclooxygenase (COX)-2, two C/EBP target genes, and increased COX-2-dependent production of prostaglandinn E_2 (PGE_2). Another molecule which appears to tread a fine line between hormone and cytokine is macrophage MIF (Swope and Lolis, 1999) which possesses pleiotropic pro-inflammatory properties and has been demonstrated to be glucocorticoid inducible. This observation has the potential to explain key aspects of the biphasic regulation of the inflammatory response by endogenous glucocorticoids.

Macrophages express IL-4, IL-10 and IL-13 receptors and their function can be modulated by these cytokines. Among those effects described (Essner *et al.*, 1989) is the influence of IL-4 and IL-10 on macrophage production of other cytokines such as IL-1,

TNF and IL-6, with possible implications for control of, for example, the acute phase protein response (see Section 11.1). Th2 cells secrete IL-4, IL-10 and IL-13 which are important in the control of macrophage function (Table 1.4). Recent studies demonstrate that IL-11 has potent anti-inflammatory activity (Trepicchio and Dorner, 1998) and reduces production of pro-inflammatory mediators such as TNF-α and IL-12 from activated macrophages. This effect on pro-inflammatory cytokine production is mediated at the transcriptional level by inhibition of the transcription factor, NF-kB.

8.3 Chemokine receptors

In addition to the increasing number of cytokine receptors described, there are now many chemokine receptors (Bacon *et al.*, 1998, Chantry *et al.*, 1998; Wuyts *et al.*, 1998) which have been identified on the surface of the moncyte/macrophage lineage. The rapidly increasing amount of information on chemokine biology makes it difficult to introduce even a small part of this subject in the present chapter. The superfamily of chemokines now exceeds 60 members and includes representatives of the C, CC, CXC and CX3C subclasses. A number of CC receptors (CCRs) and CXC receptors (CXCRs) have been identified on the macrophage, including CCR1 which binds MIP-1α, RANTES and monocyte chemotactic protein (MCP)-3; CCR2 which binds MCP-1, -2, -3 and -4; CCR5 (now CD195) which can bind RANTES, MIP-1α and MIP-1β; CXCR-1 and CXCR-2 which both bind IL-8; CXCR4 (now CD184) which binds SDF-1; and CX3CR1 which binds fractalkine. Some of the ability of human immunodeficiency virus type 1 (HIV-1) isolates to infect macrophages (Berger *et al.*, 1999) has also been attributed to the expression of CXCR4 or CCR5 (see Chapters 4 and 8).

8.4 Macrophage lipoprotein receptors

The macrophage has specific receptors which allow them to take up and digest cholesterol-containing lipoproteins, low-density lipoproteins (LDLs) (Herijgers *et al.*, 2000), and has various mechanisms for the oxidation of lipoproteins (Guy *et al.*, 1999; Egan and Carding, 2000). These receptor-mediated mechanisms differ from those in other cell types such as fibroblasts and smooth muscle cells. There are several types of lipoprotein receptors on macrophages: the LDL receptor recognizes apolipoprotein E and apolipoprotein B-100 and is regulated by intracellular cholesterol levels; the β- VLDL (very low-density lipoprotein) receptor which is not very responsive to cellular cholesterol levels; and 'scavenger' receptors. Modified (acetylated) LDLs are recognized by scavenger receptors. The macrophage scavenger receptors (Shirai *et al.*, 1999) have an unusually broad binding specificity. Ligands include modified LDL and some polyanions. The scavenger receptor type I has three principal extracellular domains that could participate in ligand binding: two fibrous coiled-coil domains (α-helical coiled-coil domain IV and collagen-like domain V) and the 110-amino acid, cysteine-rich, C-terminal domain VI. The type II scavenger receptor has also been cloned. This receptor is identical to the type I receptor, except that the cysteine-rich domain is replaced by a six-residue C-terminus. Despite this truncation, the type II receptor mediates endocytosis of chemically modified LDL with high affinity and specificity, similar to that of the type I receptor. Therefore, one or both of the extracellular fibrous domains are responsible for the unusual ligand-binding specificity of the receptor. Type I and II macrophage scavenger receptors are implicated in the pathological deposition of cholesterol during atherogenesis (see Section 11.7). The charged collagen structure of type I and II receptors can recognize a wide range of negatively charged macromolecules including oxidized LDL as well as damaged or apoptotic cells and pathogenic microorganisms. Under physiological conditions, scavenger receptors are believed to scavenge or clean up cellular debris and other related materials, as well as playing a role in host defense.

8.5 AGE receptors

Proteins of the extracellular matrix undergo over time multiple reactions with glucose to form advanced glycation endproducts (AGEs) which are highly active in protein cross-linking (Sano *et al.*, 1999). A macrophage/monocyte receptor for AGE moieties, which have been implicated in tissue damage associated with aging and diabetes, mediates the uptake of AGE-modified proteins by a process that also induces IL-1 and TNF secretion. TNF can induce a severalfold enhancement of binding, endocytosis and degradation of AGE-modified bovine serum albumin by both murine peritoneal macrophages and human blood monocytes *in vitro*, and also enhances the rate of disappearance of AGE-modified red blood cells *in vivo*. These data suggest that TNF, in addition to influencing tissue regeneration and remodeling, may also normally regulate the disposal of tissue-damaging AGE proteins through an autocrine mechanism.

8.6 Lectin-like receptors

Macrophages express a variety of lectin-like (see Tables 1.2 and 1.3 and Section 8.1) proteins which are specific for oligosaccharides terminating in fucose, mannose, galactose and sialic acid (Weis *et al.*, 1998; Vasta *et al.*, 1999). Protein–carbohydrate interactions serve multiple functions in the immune system. Many lectins mediate both cell–cell interactions and pathogen recognition using structurally related calcium-dependent carbohydrate recognition domains. Pathogen recognition by the macrophage cell surface mannose receptor is effected by binding of terminal monosaccharide residues which are characteristic of bacterial and fungal cell surfaces. The broad selectivity of the monosaccharide-binding sites and the geometrical arrangement of multiple recognition domains in the intact lectin explain the ability of the proteins to mediate discrimination between self and non-self. Sugar-specific recognition is therefore an important determinant of cell–cell interaction. The mannose receptor (Stahl and Ezekowitz, 1998) has a role in macrophage receptor-mediated endocytosis and can mediate phagocytosis independently of Fc and C3 receptors. CD141 (thrombomodulin) is a member of the C-type lectin family which can be up-regulated by heat shock and is critical for the thrombin-mediated activation of protein C. The lectin-like domain in CD141 may possibly also be involved in adhesion.

8.7 Adhesion receptors and migration

There is considerable overlap in the categorization of adhesion receptors on the cell surface, and published information on monocyte migration lags behind studies of the neutrophil. New light has been shed on macrophage migration by the elucidation of the chemokines and their receptors (see Section 8.3). Monocytes are more difficult to isolate in sufficient numbers to study their adhesive interactions. Monocytes share a number of adhesion molecules (see Tables 1.3 and 1.6) with both neutrophils, for example

CD11b/CD18 (Mac1), the PADGEM/GMP140 (CD62) ligand, and lymphocytes, for example CD11a/CD18 (LFA-1) and CD49d/CD29 (VLA-4), probably indicating that similar mechanisms of migration are utilized. Inflammatory mediators, including LPS, IFN-γ, IL-1 and TNF, cause strong induction of ICAM-1 (CD54) in a wide variety of tissues and greatly increase the binding of monocytes and lymphocytes through their cell surface LFA-1. This contributes to the infiltration of mononuclear cells into sites of inflammation, for example in delayed-type hypersensitivity reactions in skin (Vejlsgaard *et al.*, 1989). CD54 is also used as a receptor by the major group of human rhinoviruses. LFA-1 (CD11a/CD18) is a member of the integrin family of cell adhesion molecules which comprise α- and β-subunits. Three subfamilies are distinguished by their α-subunits which are the α1 (CD29), α2 (CD18) and α3 (CD61) integrins. LFA-1 belongs to the α2 family and is most closely related to two other integrins Mac-1 (CD11b/CD18) and p150,95 (CD11c/CD18). These two are particularly important in adhesion of myeloid cells to ligands which become insolubilized during activation of the complement and clotting cascades (Kishimoto *et al.*, 1989) and in binding to other cells. The importance of the α2 family of leukocyte integrins is illustrated by individuals who lack the common α2 subunit and whose phagocytes are unable to traverse the endothelium at sites of infection. This is a congenital leukocyte adhesion deficiency (LAD) in which the patients are prone to recurring infections and is often fatal in childhood unless corrected by bone marrow transplantation.

VLA-4 (CD49d/CD29) is an unusual α1 integrin expressed on monocytes, resting lymphocytes and neural crest-derived cells, funtioning as both a cell and a matrix receptor (Hemler, 1990). It binds to a region of fibronectin distinct from the binding site of VLA-5 (Guan and Hynes, 1990) and also binds to the cell receptor vascular cell adhesion molecule 1 (VCAM-1) (Elices *et al.*, 1990). The complexities of the integrin family are described in recent reviews of adhesion molecules (Gonzalez-Amaro and Sanchez-Madrid, 1999; Jones and Walker, 1999).

As well as the integrins, macrophages also possess adhesion molecules belonging to the lectin-like and Ig superfamilies and are capable of binding to molecules of the selectin family. The selectins described thus far [Mel-14/LAM-1 (CD62L), ELAM-1 (CD62E) and PADGEM (CD62P)] help regulate leukocyte binding to endothelium at inflammatory sites. One of the selectins mentioned above, called PADGEM, GMP-140 or CD62P, is contained within the Weibel–Palade bodies of endothelial cells and α-granules of platelets, and quickly appears on the surface of these cells after stimulation by products of the clotting cascade where it mediates adhesion of monocytes and neutrophils (Johnston *et al.*, 1989).

Of the Ig superfamily (Marchalonis *et al.*, 1998), a number of molecular species are present on the macrophage membrane and include LFA-3 (CD58), ICAM-1 (CD54), CD86, CD100, CD147, CD166 and MHC class I and class II. MHC class I and class II molecules are the ligands for CD8 and CD4, respectively. CD54 is the ligand for LFA-1 and CD58 is the ligand for CD2, another member of the Ig superfamily, which is present on T cells. Thus the molecules in the Ig superfamily are important in macrophage–T cell interactions. Members of the Ig superfamily share the Ig domain which comprises 90–100 amino acids arranged in a sandwich of two sheets of antiparallel α-strands usually joined by a disulfide bond. ICAM-1, in contrast to the MHC and Ig molecules, has unpaired domains.

Neurothelin/basigin (CD147) (Tachikui *et al.*, 1999) is a developmentally regulated Ig-like surface glycoprotein which has been detected previously on blood–brain barrier endothelium, epithelial tissue barriers and neurons. CD166 (CD6 ligand) interactions have been implicated in the regulation of T-cell adhesion and activation. CD6 is a member of the scavenger receptor family, whereas its human ligand [ALCAM (CD166)] (Bowen and Aruffo, 1999) belongs to the Ig superfamily. A number of homologs of CD166 have been identified including BEN in the chicken, and neurolin in the zebrafish. The presence of the CD6 ligand molecule on macrophages may be of interest with regard to T-cell stimulation in inflammatory conditions. CD165 (AD2) is another molecule present on the macrophage which has been implicated in interactions with T cells.

8.8 Surface antigens

A large number of cell surface molecules are present on the surface of monocytes and macrophages by which the macrophage interacts with its environment. Some of these are growth factor receptors, others recognition or adhesion molecules important in cellular interactions, and others are enzymes or receptors for specific ligands important in the role of the macrophage. During differentiation and activation, this mosaic of antigens is constantly changing in a way which is orchestrated by genetic programming in response to signals from the extracellular environment. Many of these antigens are not lineage specific but are also common to other cell types, for example CD44 (Borland *et al.*, 1998) and the MHC class I and II molecules. MHC class II molecules, products of the HLA-DR, -DP and -DQ loci, are expressed discoordinately by monocytes (Guy *et al.*, 1984), with DR molecules expressed at a high surface density. All peripheral monocytes can be induced to express HLA-DQ and -DP molecules in the presence of IFN-γ (Gonwa *et al.*, 1986).

A large number of other molecules are present which are more restricted in their cell-specific expression and are obviously important in the cellular interactions in which the macrophage engages (Gordon, 1999). Through the production of monoclonal antibodies and the vehicle of international workshops on human leukocyte differentiation antigens, a plethora of information on cell surface regulatory molecules has been generated. Some surface antigens (Table 1.6) have relatively well-defined functions, while little is known of the functions of others. Although most receptors described above are also cell surface structures, this section concentrates on antigens primarily identified by the availability of monoclonal antibodies rather than by function. The following selection is by no means exhaustive, and many more remain to be described or ascribed a function.

The CD14 molecule (Schutt, 1999) is one of the most characteristic surface antigens of the monocyte lineage and comprises 356 amino acids anchored to the plasma membrane by a phosphoinositol linkage. It is expressed at high density and is an excellent marker of monocytes and tissue macrophages, but is also present at lower density on a proportion of granulocytes (heterogeneous expression), Langerhans cells (LCs), follicular dendritic cells (DCs), histiocytes and high endothelial venules. Antibodies against the CD14 molecule induce oxidative burst formation. A soluble form of this molecule, of molecular weight 53 kDa, identical to the surface-linked form, is also present in urine. The CD14 gene is located on the long arm of chromosome 5 (5q32) in a region containing a cluster of genes encoding growth factors and receptors (GM-CSF, IL-3, IL-5, ECGF, CSF-1, CSF-1R and PDGFR) (Goyart *et al.*, 1988). This chromosomal region is deleted in a

Table 1.6 Cluster of differentiation antigens present on the monocyte/macrophage series

Cluster	Main cellular reactivity	Recognized membrane component
CD4	T subset (M)	Class II/HIV receptor, gp59
CD9	Pre-B, M, platelets	p24
CD11a	Leukocytes	LFA-1, gp180/95
CD11b	M,G,NK	C3bi receptor, gp155/95
CD11c	M, G, NK, B subset	gp150, 95
CDw12	M, G, Plt	(p90–120)
CD13	M,G	Aminopeptidase N, gp150
CD14	M, (G), LHC	gp55
CD15	G, (M)	3-FAL, X-hapten
CD16	NK, G, M	FcRIII, gp50–65
CD17	G, M, Plt	Latosylceramide
CD18	Leukocytes broad	β-Chain to CD11a, b, c
CD19	B (some M leukemias)	gp95
CD23	B subset, activated M, Eo	FcεRII, gp45–50
CD25	Activated B, T, M	IL-2R β-chain, gp55
CD29	Broad	VLA-b, integrin β-chain, Plt.GPIIa
CD31	Plt, M, G, B, (T)	gp140, Plt.GPIIIa
CDw32	M, G, B	FcRII, gp40
CD33	M, Prog., AML	gp67
CD34	Prog.	gp105–120
CD35	G, M, B	CR1
CD36	M, Plt, (B)	gp90, Plt.GPIV
CD37	B, (T, M)	gp40–52
CD43	T, G, M, brain	Leukosialin, gp95
CD44	Leukocytes, brain, RBC	Pgp-1, gp80–95, Hermes-1
CD45	Leukocytes	LCA, T200
CD45RA	T subset, B, G, M	Restricted LCA, gp220, exon A
CD45RB	T subset, B, G, M	Restricted LCA, gp200, exon B
CD45RO	T subset, B, G, M	Restricted LCA, gp180, exons spliced out
CD46	Leukocytes	MCF, gp66/56
CD47	Broad	gp47–52, N-linked glycan
CD48	Leukocytes	gp41, PI-linked
CDw49d	M, T, B, (LC), Thy	VLA-a 4 chain, gp150
CDw50	Leukocytes	gp148/108
CDw52	Leukocytes	Campath-1, gp21–28
CD53	Leukocytes	gp32–40
CD54	Broad, activation	ICAM-1
CD55	Broad	DAF
CD58	Leukocytes, epithelium	LFA-3, gp40–65
CD59	Broad	gp18–20
CD62L	B, T, M, G	74–95
CD63	Plt activ., M, (G, T, B)	gp53
CD64	M	FcRI, gp75
CDw65	G, M	Ceramide-dodecasaccharide 4c
CD68	M	gp110
CD71	Proliferating cells, Mac.	Transferrin receptor
CD74	B, M	Class II-associated invariant chain, gp41/35/33
CD81	Hemopoietic cells	Target for anti-proliferative antigen-1
CD82	Hemopoietic cells	– (tetraspan molecule)
CD85	Hemopoietic cells (M)	–
CD86	DC, LC, (B) (M)	B7.2
CD87	M, T, NK, G, EC, others	Urokinase plasminogen activator receptor
CD88	G, M, DC	C5a receptor
CD89	G, M	IgA Fc receptor

Table 1.6   Continued

Cluster	Main cellular reactivity	Recognized membrane component
CD91	M, others	α_2-Macroglobulin receptor
CD92	G, M, others (weak)	–
CD93	M, G, EC	–
CD95	Activated T, activated B, M (weak)	Fas antigen
CD97	Activated T, activated B, M, G	– (EGF-TM7 family)
CD98	Broad	4F2
CD100	Hemopoietic	– (semaphorin family)
CD101	M, G, DC, activated T	–
CD116	M, G, DC	GM-CSF receptor
CDw119	Broad	Interferon-γ receptor
CD120a, b	Broad	TNF receptor type I/II (p55/p75)
CD121a	Broad	IL-1 receptor type I
CD121b	B, T (M)	IL-1 receptor type II
CD122	T, B, NK, M	IL-2 receptor β-chain
CDw123	G, M (EC)	IL-3 receptor α-subunit
CD124	Broad	IL-4 receptor
CD126	T, M, activated B, hepatocytes, others	IL-6 receptor
CDw128	G, M, NK, others	IL-8 receptor type A: CXCR1, type B: CXCR2
CD130	Broad	gp130 signaling molecule
CDw131	Most myeloid, early B	Common β-subunit of IL-3R, IL-5R and GM-CSFR
CD132	T, B, NK, M, G	Common γ-subunit
CD139	B, M, G	–
CD140b	G, M	Platelet-derived growth factor-β receptor
CD141	G, M, EC, others	Thrombomodulin
CD142	Epithelial, (M) (EC)	Tissue factor
CD147	Leukocytes, EC, RBC, platelets	Basigin, neurothelin
CD148	G, M, T, DC, others	PTPase 1
CDw149	Lymphocytes, G, M	MEM-133
CD153	Activated T, activated M, G, B	CD30 ligand
CD155	M, possibly others	Poliovirus receptor
CD156	G, M	ADAM (a disintegrin and metalloprotease)
CD157	G, M, (T), (B), stromal	BST-1 (cyclic ADP-ribose hydrolase)
CD161	NK, (T), (M)	NKR-P1A (a C-type lectin–group V)
CD162	T, M, G	P-selectin ligand, sialomucin
CD163	(M)	M130 (member of scavenger receptor family)
CD164	M	MGC-24 ?adhesion molecule
CD165	(Lymphocytes), [M]	AD2 adhesion molecule
CD166	Activated T, activated M, others	ALCAM, BEN (chicken), neurolin (zebrafish)
CD169	M (others)	Sialoadhesin
CD204	M	Macrophage scavenger receptor
CD206	M	Macrophage mannose receptor

Abbreviations: (brackets denote reactivity with a subset of cells); B = B cell; DAF = decay-accelerating factor; DC = dendritic cell; EC = endothelial cell; Eo = eosinophil; G = granulocyte; LC = Langerhans cell; LCA = leukocyte common antigen; M = monocyte/macrophage; MCF = membrane cofactor protein; NK = natural killer cells; Plt =platelet; Prog. = progenitor cells; T = T cell; Thy = thymocyte.
Adapted from Kishimoto *et al.* (1997) with permission. Some new information has also been incorporated from the 7th Workshop on human leukocyte differentiation antigens (HLDA7) held in Harrogate, 2000.

number of acute myeloid leukemias and pre-leukemic conditions. CD14 is the receptor for endotoxin, with the serum protein LPS-binding protein (LBP) facilitating the binding of LPS to CD14. Toll-like receptor 2 (TLR2) has been suggested to be involved in LPS-mediated signaling, with evidence that human TLR2 could interact with CD14 to form the LPS receptor complex. TLR2 binds LPS in the presence of LBP and CD14 and induces NF-κB activation. Recently, mutations of the mouse *Lps* locus (Beutler, 2000) have been shown to abolish responses to LPS. Positional cloning work has revealed that *Lps* encodes the Toll-like receptor 4 (TLR4), which functions as the transmembrane component of the LPS receptor complex and appears to be an unduplicated pathway for the detection of endotoxin. The structurally related protein Tlr2 appears to make no contribution to LPS signal transduction in the murine system. It has also been suggested (Gregory, 2000) that macrophage CD14 serves as a receptor involved in the recognition and phagocytosis of cells undergoing apoptosis, mediating clearance of apoptotic cells without inciting inflammation.

The CD68 antigen is a specific marker of monocytes and macrophages. Antibodies against this antigen label macrophages and other members of the mononuclear phagocyte lineage in routinely processed tissue sections and have been used to stain a range of lymphoid, histiocytic and myelomonocytic proliferations (Warnke *et al.*, 1989). The antigen recognized is present in intracellular granules but can exist in the extracellular environment. This may provide some clue as to its function.

The CD33 molecule is restricted to myeloid cells and is at least expressed on some multipotent progenitor cells (CFU-GEMM) and early erythroid progenitors (BFU-E). Virtually all granulocyte–macrophage progenitor cells (CFU-GM) are identified by CD33 antibodies. It is presumed that the function of this molecule relates specifically to the function of cells of the myelomonocytic lineage (Peiper and Guo, 1997), but the function has remained enigmatic. Binding of antibodies against this molecule has been detected in sections of the spleen, testis, placenta, liver (Kupffer cells), lung (alveolar macrophages) and in the dermis of skin. LCs in the epidermis also possess surface CD33 at low density. The molecule is a member of the sialoadhesin family which are sialic acid-dependent adhesion molecules, and CD33 has lectin activity for sugar chains containing sialic acid.

CD91 is the α_2-macroglobulin receptor which is restricted, within hemopoietic cells, to the cells of the monocytic lineage and to erythroblasts/reticulocytes. It is a member of the LDL receptor family and is synthesized as a single-chain molecule but is processed into a two-chain molecule by cleavage in the Golgi. The cellular function of CD91 is thought to involve mediating endocytosis in coated pits in the cell membrane. High expression of CD91 is observed in atherosclerotic lesions and in plaques of Alzheimer's disease. Targeted disruption of the gene in mice is lethal.

CD163 (van den Heuvel *et al.*, 1999) is a member of the group B scavenger receptor cysteine-rich (SRCR) superfamily and has almost exclusive expression on resident macrophages such as red pulp macrophages and alveolar macrophages. CD163 expression is inducible on monocyte-derived macrophages by glucocorticoids but not by IFN-γ, GM-CSF or IL-4. Cross-linking of CD163 induces a protein tyrosine kinase-dependent signal resulting in inositol triphosphate production, calcium mobilization and the secretion of IL-6 and GM-CSF.

9 Macrophage heterogeneity

The seeding of monocytes to different tissues (Werb and Goldstein, 1987; Gordon *et al.*, 1988; Law, 1988; Papadimitriou and Ashman, 1989; Wintergerst *et al.*, 1998) where they remain as macrophages is apparently random since there is no evidence that the tissue destination is pre-programmed. Resident macrophages are distributed constitutively throughout the normal body in the absence of any inflammatory signal and display regional heterogeneity. Functional, morphological and phenotypic heterogeneity may reflect these cells' environments and involvement in many disease processes.

9.1 Alveolar macrophages

Macrophages are a major cellular component of the lung, with a life span suggested by bone marrow transplant studies of approximately 3 months (Thomas *et al.*, 1976) . Several functionally and biochemically distinct subpopulations of alveolar macrophage have been demonstrated in normal human and pathological (sarcoid) lung (Sandron *et al.*, 1986). The most characteristic ultrastructural feature of alveolar macrophages is the abundance of membrane-bound cytoplasmic inclusions (Nakstad *et al.*, 1989) containing proteolytic enzymes. Analysis of tissue distribution of a novel monocyte subpopulation, forming about 13 per cent of circulating monocytes (Passlick *et al.*, 1989), revealed large numbers of these CD14$^+$,CD16$^+$ cells in the alveolar space. Alveolar macrophages may represent a self-replicating population as they proliferate readily to colony-stimulating factors *in vitro* and maintain their numbers after bone marrow ablation. Macrophages are the predominant defense cell in the normal lung and conditions associated with chronic inflammation such as chronic obstructive pulmonary disease (Shapiro, 1999). Macrophages in the lung are involved in local defense against a variety of pathogenic and particulate entrants via the airway and play an early role in inflammation and the control of infection. Alveolar and recruited macrophages have a central role in chronic granulomatous conditions such as sarcoidosis (Section 11.8), silicosis and asbestosis, and in infections such as tuberculosis and *Legionella* .

9.2 Kupffer cells

The resident macrophages of the liver are involved in the clearance of particulate and soluble substances and express Fc and other receptors such as the mannosyl–fucosyl receptor (MFR), CD14 and CD33. It is believed that Kupffer cells' responses to LPS and other gut-derived stimuli may be important in their interactions with hepatocytes. Indeed these cells may be at least partially responsible for regulating the acute phase response in injury and malignancy, possibly producing IL-6 which appears to deliver the final signal to hepatocytes in initiating the altered metabolism associated with the acute phase response (see Section 11.1). Large numbers of monocytes are recruited to the liver following uptake of microorganisms by Kupffer cells and contribute to the immune response against the invaders.

Kupffer cells are also believed to be involved in reperfusion injury after liver preservation for transplantation (Lemasters and Thurman, 1997). Activated Kupffer cells release a number of inflammatory mediators including TNF-α, IL-1, IL-6, prostaglandins and nitric oxide (NO), and subsequent changes in endothelial cell, leukocyte and platelet behavior may contribute to the ischemic process. With regard to the role of liver macrophages in malignancy, Daemen *et al.* (1989) have demonstrated that although the macrophage population of the liver is heterogeneous with respect to endocytic and lysosomal enzyme activity, all liver macrophages in the rat can be activated to a tumoricidal state by the i.v. injection of liposomal muramyl dipeptide (MDP).

9.3 Spleen

The spleen contains a heterogeneous population of macrophages and related cells. Differences reported in phenotype and appearance (Buckley *et al.*, 1987) probably reflect the different functions they undertake: trapping and processing of foreign antigens in the marginal zone, specialized interactions with T and B cells in the lymphoid areas, and phagocytosis and degradation of red blood cells in the red pulp.

9.4 Bone marrow

Macrophages play an integral role in the support of hemopoiesis. Bone marrow and fetal liver contain a network of mature macrophages which ramify through the stroma. These stromal macrophages make intimate contact with a 'nest' of surrounding developing hemopoietic cells (Crocker and Gordon, 1985) which can be isolated intact. The stromal macrophages appear to be essential for maintaining the growth and differentiation of hemopoietic precursors *in vitro* and possess adhesion molecules for maintaining contact with developing hemopoietic cells (Hanspal, 1997).

9.5 Intestine

The gut lamina propria in both the large and small intestine contains a large population of macrophages (Mikkelsen and Thuneberg, 1999). They are also present in the specialized gut-associated lymphoid tissue with a well-defined structure, such as the tonsils and Peyers patches (Hume *et al.*, 1987).

9.6 Other sites

Macrophages are present in many other areas of the body such as the subendothelium of the greater arteries. Morphological, histochemical and ultrastructural results have shown that these are mainly metabolically quiescent, resident macrophages, their number being regulated by influences depending on endothelium and intimal factors. The major signal for subendothelial macrophage accumulation in man appears to be intimal deposition of lipids. Many macrophages also penetrate the blood–brain barrier under normal circumstances, first entering the nervous system during embryonic development, and comprise the microglia whose function is unknown. Macrophages, other than the microglia, are common inhabitants of the choroid plexus and leptomeninges. An interesting aspect of macrophage and microglia phenotype is the presence of CD4 molecules on their surface which make them susceptible to invasion by HIV with a possible bearing on the transport of virus across the blood–brain barrier and the development of encephalopathy reported in AIDS; see also Chapters 4 and 8. The control of expression of CD4 on monocytes, macrophages and microglia in rats has been investigated (Perry and Gordon, 1987).

9.7 Relationship to Langerhans cells and other 'professional' antigen-presenting cells

It is now clear that there is a close relationship between macrophages and certain professional antigen-presenting cells (APCs) such as DCs in lymph nodes and LCs (Figure 1.8) in the epithelium of skin. Some studies, based on the reactivity of monoclonal antibodies (Murphy *et al.*, 1986), would indicate that precursors of human LCs express myeloid antigens upon entry into the epidermis, losing many of these surface molecules in residence. However, these myeloid antigens are expressed on LCs in disease states (Groh *et al.*, 1988). It is now clear that monocytes can generate immunostimulatory DCs after treatment with GM-CSF and IL-4 (Caux *et al.*, 1999), displaying the phenotype of an immature DC (low levels of CD80, CD86, CD58 and MHC II within cytoplasmic compartments, and monocyte markers CD11b, CD36, CD68 and CD115). Such DCs can take up antigen efficiently and have a weak capacity to prime naive T cells. Maturation can be induced by LPS, TNF-α, IL-1 or CD40 ligand. DCs are a thousandfold more potent APCs than macrophages but are poorly phagocytic in comparison (see Chapter 3). Classical tissue macrophages are present in the dermis of skin, often invading the epidermis during inflammatory responses (Figure 1.9). Recently, Langerin (CD207) (Valladeau *et al.*, 2000), a novel C-type lectin specific to LCs, which is an endocytic receptor that induces the formation of Birbeck granules, has been described.

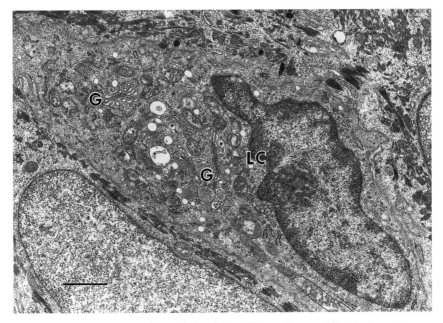

Fig. 1.8   Electron micrograph of part of an epidermal Langerhans cell (LC) between keratinocytes in the skin. The Langerhans cell has a well-developed Golgi (G) and distinctive tennis-raquet-shaped Birbeck granules (*) in the cytoplasm. Bar = 1 μm.

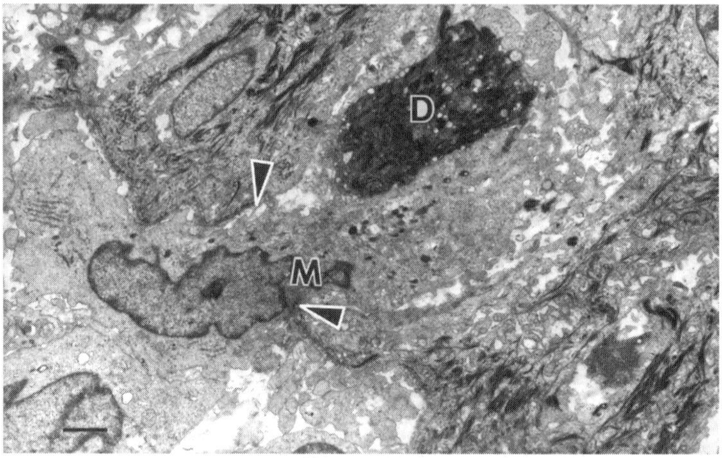

Fig. 1.9   A macrophage (M) breaching the basal lamina (arrowheads) of the skin to engulf a dead keratinocyte (D) during a secondary contact allergic response to dinitrochlorobenzene. Bar = 2 μm.

9.8 Giant cells

Epithelioid cells (EpCs) and their fusion products, the multinucleated giant cells (MnGC) are members of the mononuclear phagocyte system. They are considered to be a terminal stage of development of the macrophage system and, in contrast to other macrophages, are poorly phagocytic but exhibit increased lysosomal and respiratory enzyme activity (Anderson, 2000). EpCs and MnGCs have reduced numbers of cell surface Ig and complement receptors (Papadimitrou and van Bruggen, 1986) and are common in granulomatous lesions. The histogenesis of the multinucleated cells that characterize myeloma cast nephropathy ('myeloma kidney') has long been a subject of debate. Recent studies have implicated monocyte/macrophage-derived cells rather than tubular EpCs as the progenitors of these multinucleated cells. Some studies (Alpers *et al.*, 1989) claim to have confirmed the macrophage origin of the multinucleated cells in this form of renal injury. Giant cells containing lipid vacuoles (Figure 1.10) are common in xanthoma and lipid storage diseases.

10 Macrophage functions

10.1 Phagocytosis and destruction of microorganisms

10.1.1 Recognition and phagocytosis

Mononuclear phagocytes and neutrophils provide a defense against microbial invasion. The neutrophil, in general, is a more efficient phagocyte, except when the particle is large in relation to the cell or when the particle load is great (Cohn, 1968). Under these circumstances, mononuclear phagocytes (Aderem and Underhill, 1999) are more effective than neutrophils. Macrophages thus represent a major defense against invasion of the host by a wide variety of microorganisms, including bacteria, viruses, fungi and protozoa. Macrophages move toward the microbial particles guided by a gradient of chemotactic molecules emanating from them (see Section 10.2) (Metchnikoff, 1905). Engulfment then

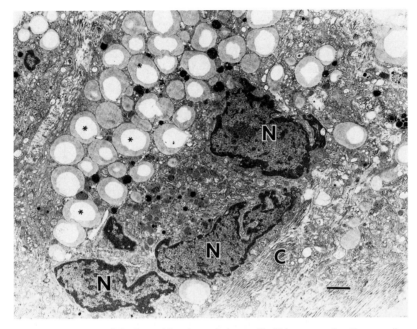

Fig. 1.10 Multiple nuclei (N) of a multinucleated giant cell within connective tissue collagen (C) from a patient with xanthoma. Large lipid-containing vacuoles (*) occupy much of the cytoplasm. Bar = 2 μm.

occurs, beginning with the macrophage advancing pseudopodia over regions of the microorganism that are linked to recognition molecules, opsonins, which bind to specific sites on both invading microorganisms and macrophages. Opsonins are of various types, but those most studied are IgG and fragments of the third component of complement. Receptors that bind specifically to the Fc domain of various subclasses of IgG and to several isotypes of C3 are present on the macrophage surface (see Section 8.1) (Adams and Hamilton, 1988). Many microorganisms are capable of activating the complement cascade and generating complement fragments that coat the organism and opsonize it. Furthermore, the macrophage itself is an important source of complement components, and macrophage-derived complement factors can opsonize microorganisms for subsequent destruction in the absence of other sources. After binding with the appropriate ligand, initiation of the process of internalization and microbial destruction occur (Nathan *et al.*, 1980). Adsorption can also occur without opsonization if the microorganisms possess surface determinants that can be recognized directly by the macrophage; an example is the interaction of the macrophage MFR with carbohydrate residues (Sung *et al.*, 1983).

The protrusive pseudopodial movement underlying phagocytosis represents events within only a localized region of membrane and peripheral cytoplasm (Griffin *et al.*, 1975, 1976). Granule movements then become prominent at the base of the forming phagocytic vacuole, and exocytosis of granule contents into the phagosomal vacuole is thought to occur (Hirsch, 1962). The pseudopodial actin cytoskeleton plays a major role in phagocytosis (Stossel, 1988).

Fc receptor-mediated phagocytosis results in the release of large amounts of oxygen and arachidonic acid metabolites by macrophages (Rouzer *et al.*, 1980; Klebanoff, 1988). In contrast, ligation of C3 receptors fails to release either arachidonic or oxygen metabolites from mononuclear phagocytes (Platt *et al.*, 1998; Aderem and Underhill, 1999). Macrophages also have receptors for C5a. Occupancy of this receptor induces secretion of IL-1 and initiates chemotactic phenomena (Goodman *et al.*, 1982). Particle ingestion by mononuclear phagocytes may occur over a broad pH range and is accompanied by enhanced glucose oxidation similar to that which occurs with phagocytosis by neutrophils (Cline *et al.*, 1978).

Although many microorganisms are phagocytosed and destroyed with comparable ease by macrophages, there are certain pathogens that parasitize macrophages and replicate within them (see Chapter 6). When the macrophage is activated, these intracellular pathogens may be inhibited or destroyed. *Listeria, Salmonella, Brucella, Mycobacteria, Chlamydia, Rickettsia, Leishmania, Toxoplasma, Trypanosoma* and *Legionella pneumophilia* have been found capable of invading and inhabiting non-activated macrophages (Nathan *et al.*, 1980). *Mycobacterium tuberculosis* may release certain substances such as sulfolipids that interfere with fusion of primary lysosomes with phagosomes and thereby avoid exposure to the macrophages' lysosomal enzymes (Shurin and Stossel, 1978). *Leishmania* and *Mycobacterium lepraemurium* survive within secondary lysosomes despite exposure to lysosomal enzymes; this may be due to the resistance of the microbial cell wall to the macrophages' degradative enzymes (Nathan *et al.*, 1980). HIV has also been demonstrated to infect and replicate within monocytes and macrophages. Infection with HIV occurs by binding of the virus to the CD4 molecule and other molecules (see Section 8.3, and Chapters 4 and 8) present at a low density on monocytes and macrophages (Cohen *et al.*, 1997).

10.1.2 Microbicidal mechanisms

The production and intracellular release of ROIs are a major microbicidal mechanism employed by monocytes and macrophages (see Section 7). As monocytes mature into macrophages, there is evidence of decreased microbicidal activity. This may be due to a reduction in the respiratory burst or to the decreased content of granule peroxidase as monocytes mature into macrophages (Nakagawara *et al.*, 1981). In addition to oxygen-dependent cytotoxic systems, phagocytes are equipped with oxygen-independent means of killing microorganisms. A variety of granule-associated proteins of macrophages have been shown to possess antimicrobial activity. These include elastase, collagenases, lipases, deoxyribonucleases, polysaccharidases, sulfatases, phosphatases and the defensins (Elsbach and Weiss, 1988). The latter are a group of small cationic proteins that have distinct antimicrobial properties and have been isolated from rabbit alveolar macrophages and human peripheral blood neutrophils (Elsbach and Weiss, 1988). The primary lysosomes fuse with phagocytic vacuoles (phagosomes) containing ingested materials to form secondary lysosomes or phagolysosomes (Myers *et al.*, 1984). The mechanism of fusion of the primary lysosome and the phagosome is not known, but it is clear that formation of the secondary lysosome is necessary for degradation of the ingested material (Henson *et al.*, 1988). Mononuclear phagocytes are also capable of interferon production, which may aid in protection against viral infection (Smith and Wagner, 1967), as does NO production (MacMicking *et al.*, 1997). Monocyte cationic proteins other than peroxidase have been shown to have fungicidal activity (Vazquez-Torres and Balish, 1997). Macrophages activated by cytokines such as IFN-γ, TNF or IL-1 have greater microbicidal capacities than non-activated cells (Nathan, 1987).

There are differences in the mechanisms by which blood monocytes and tissue macrophages kill some microbes. For example, human monocytes kill *Candida albicans* readily, whereas macrophages do not; macrophages do, however, kill *Candida pseudotropicalis* since this organism does not require peroxidase activity in order to be destroyed (Vazquez-Torres and Balish, 1997). Sustained production of NO also endows macrophages with cytostatic or cytotoxic activity against viruses, bacteria, fungi, protozoa, helminths and tumor cells (MacMicking *et al.*, 1997).

The relatively long life span of the macrophage and its sustained biosynthetic capacity permit the continued production of antimicrobial proteins and continued microbicidal activity. See also Chapters, 4, 5 and 6 for further detail on the mechanisms used by macrophages to destroy microorganisms.

10.2 Chemotaxis

Chemotaxis refers to the directed movement of cells along a concentration gradient of a 'chemotactic factor' (Jones *et al.*, 1998). Leukocyte responses to chemotactic stimuli are vital for host defense and, in the past 10 years, a great deal of insight has been gained into the mechanisms of chemotaxis in mononuclear phagocytes (Luster and Rothenberg, 1997). Chemotactic factors, or chemoattractants, initiate a leukocyte response after binding to specific receptors on the cell surface. Specific receptors have been characterized for a number of chemoattractants including *N*-formylated peptides, C5a and leukotriene B4 (LTB4) (Brown and Gallin, 1988) and the macrophage chemotactic proteins (Berger *et al.*, 1999) (see Section 8.3). *N*-formylated peptide receptors are internalized following chemoattractant binding. The mononuclear phagocytes involved must bear receptors for chemoattractants which can be up- or down-regulated, and the binding of chemoattractants must activate certain transduction pathways for cell activation, resulting in such abilities as attachment to the endothelial cell surface, proper orientation of the cell, shape change due to cytoskeletal rearrangement and movement across the endothelial cell layer towards the inflammatory focus (diapedesis) (Brown and Gallin, 1988).

In 1975, Schiffmann discovered the synthetic chemotactic peptide *N*-formyl methionylleucylphenylalanine (FMLP) (Schiffmann *et al.*, 1975) and described its receptor on leukocytes one year later. This is the most extensively studied chemoattractant receptor (Snyderman and Fudman, 1980; Panaro and Mitolo, 1999). Phagocytes have been shown to express surface receptors for FMLP and, in addition to initiating locomotion, the FMLP receptor has been linked to respiratory burst activation and lysosomal enzyme degranulation (Snyderman and Pike, 1984). A high density of receptors is located along the leading edge of the cell, presumably to optimize detection of low concentrations of chemoattractants. The FMLP receptor appears to exist in two different affinity states on macrophages, high and low affinity, which are regulated by a guanine-binding protein (Snyderman *et al.*, 1984). In addition to FMLP, intracellular receptor pools exist for the complement chemotactic factor CR3 (or iC3b), which co-purifies with specific granules in neutrophils (Fearon and Collins, 1983). Other mediators of phagocyte chemotaxis include C5a (Snyderman *et al.*, 1971) and LTB$_4$ (Brown and Gallin, 1988), and it has also been shown that IFN-γ stimulates monocyte chemotaxis (Sechler and Gallin,

1987). This chemotactic effect is turned off with prolonged exposure to IFN-γ. An increasing number of factors chemotactic for macrophages and their receptors (Bacon *et al.*, 1998, Chantry *et al.*, 1998; Wuyts *et al.*, 1998; Berger *et al.*, 1999) are being described, including the MCP family (see Section 8.3). Recently, the peptide Trp-Lys-Tyr-Met-Val-D-Met has been shown to be a chemoattractant for human phagocytic cells (Bae *et al.*, 1999).

Once receptors are occupied and the cell responds to a stimulus, there is some adaptation, and chemotactic activity is decreased in the face of the same concentration of chemoattractant. Multiple controls exist for termination of chemoattractant signaling. The agonist can be hydrolyzed externally or internalized and degraded within the cell. Elevation of intracellular cAMP levels also attenuates the chemoattractant-induced activation of leukocytes, perhaps through inhibitors of calcium influx or subsequent responses (Chantry *et al.*, 1998; Snyderman and Uhing, 1988).

Although specific receptors are present for the various chemoattractants, they appear to utilize common mechanisms for stimulating phosphoinositide hydrolysis. Binding of the chemoattractant to the receptor activates the protein kinase C pathway of the mononuclear phagocyte. Results demonstrate that phosphatidylinsoitol 3-kinase (PI3K)-γ is a crucial signaling molecule required for macrophage accumulation in inflammation (Hirsch *et al.*, 2000). Temporal studies show rapid (<5 s) increases in phosphoinositide metabolism and cytosolic calcium levels, followed by changes in physiological functions, e.g. shape change, degranulation and superoxide production (Chantry *et al.*, 1998; Snyderman and Uhing, 1988). However, the ability of macrophages to participate in the inflammatory response is also regulated by another second messenger system involving cAMP. PGE_1, PGE_2 and histamine elevate cAMP concentrations in leukocytes through receptor-mediated activation of adenylate cyclase (Takenawa *et al.*, 1986). The increased cAMP levels attenuate chemoattractant-induced macrophage activation. Chemoattractants also increase cellular cAMP levels, by a calcium-mediated inhibition of cAMP degradation. This may serve as an autoregulatory action in chemoattractant-induced leukocyte activation (Chantry *et al.*, 1998; Snyderman and Uhing, 1988).

Mononuclear phagocytes must attach to a surface before moving in response to the sensing of the FMLP and other factors, and in recent years much interest has focused on the leukocyte–endothelial cell interaction. Endothelial cell adhesiveness for neutrophils can be markedly enhanced by pre-treatment with endotoxin, phorbol esters and IL-1 (Schleimer and Rutledge, 1986). The increased adhesion appears to involve the LFA-1–MAC-1–p150,95 (CD 11/18) complex on phagocytes, as well as one or more inducible factors on the endothelial cell surface important for emigration, e.g. ICAM-1 (Dustin *et al.*, 1986; Rothlein *et al.*, 1986; Gonzalez-Amaro and Sanchez-Madrid, 1999).

After attachment to endothelium, mononuclear phagocytes move across the endothelial cell layer towards the inflammatory focus. Chemotactic disorders of phagocytes can lead to dramatic and often life-threatening host defense problems (Brown and Gallin, 1988). Chemokines or chemotactic cytokines represent an expanding family of structurally related proteins and may be important in various disease states. MCP-1, for example, is highly expressed in human atherosclerotic lesions (Reape and Groot, 1999) and is postulated to be central in monocyte recruitment into the arterial wall and developing lesions.

10.3 Antigen processing and presentation

Antigen presentation by macrophages is covered in greater detail in Chapter 3 but, for completeness, a brief summery is also presented here. Several different types of cells may take up antigen when it enters the body. The APC for regulatory T cells may be an MHC class II-expressing DC, B cell or a professional phagocyte, the macrophage, which can phagocytose antigen with or without the help of Fc receptors. Indeed one of the major functions of the macrophage is to assist in initiating and facilitating cell-mediated immune responses against pathogens. After uptake, antigen is processed inside the cell and, in the case of protein antigens, peptides are generated and recycled to the cell surface in association with glycoproteins encoded by the class II (HLA-DR, -DP, -DQ) (Guy *et al.*, 1984) genes of the MHC.

However, intracellular processing of antigen may allow the appearance of peptides on the cell surface in association with not only class II, but also class I molecules for recognition by the appropriate MHC class II- (CD4-expressing T cell) or class I- (CD8-expressing T cell) restricted antigen-specific T cells.

There appear to be fundamental differences not only in the processing of endogenous and exogenous antigens but also in the processing for class I-restricted presentation and class II-restricted presentation. Most endogenous proteins are degraded by non-lysosomal proteolytic mechanisms. The cytosolic ubiquitin-dependent system is the best characterized and depends on proteins being conjugated initially to ubiquitin before degradation by specific proteases. For exogenous protein, there is evidence that the proteins are enclosed in endosomal vesicles containing proteases which later fuse with Golgi-derived endosomes containing acidic proteases. Transport of the phagocytosed and degraded antigens, and processed peptides derived from these molecules, into the endoplasmic reticulum appears to be essential for proper processing and the presentation of peptides on the surface of cells.

10.3.1 Processing for class I-restricted antigen presentation

The primary requirement for presentation in the context of class I molecules is cytoplasmic localization of the antigen as described above. Synthesis of new class I molecules does not appear to be necessary. Reports have suggested (Nuchtern *et al.*, 1989; Yewdell and Bennik, 1989) that processed cytoplasmic antigens associate with class I molecules before their release from the endoplasmic reticulum. The macrophage in this instance, in expressing the antigen in the context of class I molecules on its surface, may be targeted by class I-restricted cytotoxic T cells and be destroyed.

10.3.2 Processing for class II-restricted antigen presentation

It seems that antigens endocytosed and degraded in endosomes intersect the biosynthetic pathway of class II molecules (Cresswell, 1985) and this is necessary for presentation in the context of class II molecules. In contrast, endocytosed antigen cannot be presented in the context of class I molecules (Morrison *et al.*, 1986; Moore *et al.*, 1988). The epitope recognized by responding T cells appears to be created when a peptide fragment associates with the MHC molecule. It has also been suggested that for some exogenous antigens, the invariant chain (CD74), associated with class II molecules, is necessary for processing and presentation to occur.

In summary, for the macrophage to be capable of presenting antigen to T cells for the initiation of an immune response, it must fulfill certain criteria:

(1) it must be able to internalize antigen, for example by phagocytosis, to allow processing to occur;

(2) it must be capable of processing antigen by proteolysis, the primary mode of antigen degradation;

(3) it must be capable of transcribing the products of MHC class II (and/or class I) genes and expressing these at the cell surface in sufficient quantity;

(4) it must be capable of associating the processed peptide fragments, several amino acids long, with the MHC molecules and expressing these on the cell surface; and

(5) it must be capable of providing the necessary regulatory signals in the form of cytokines to responding cells.

10.3.3 T-cell activation

T cell interaction with the class II/peptide conformation is required but not sufficient for T-cell activation to occur. T-cell activation requires a second signal—the presence of IL-1 which stimulates T-cell growth and differentiation by inducing receptors for IL-2 and by stimulating IL-2 production—and, as is becoming apparent, may also require other macrophage–T cell interactions through cell surface adhesion molecules. Various experimental approaches have suggested or demonstrated that the type of response generated by presenting cell and T cell interaction can be radically altered by blocking of other cell surface receptors besides class II (Qin *et al.*, 1989).

10.4 Secretion

It has become apparent that mononuclear phagocytes, in addition to their phagocytic and immune-modulating properties, have an extensive secretory capability that includes secretion not only of enzymes but of many other biologically active substances (Table 1.7). Over 100 substances have been reported to be secreted by mononuclear phagocytes, with molecular mass ranging from 32 Da (superoxide anions) to 440 000 Da (fibronectin), and biological activity ranging from induction of cell growth to cell death (Nathan, 1987). Secretion includes both release of constituents of these cells into the external milieu and also discharge of these materials into the phagocytic vacuole. These two processes are thought to be related.

Three points concerning macrophage secretory products are worth making.

1. A single macrophage product can have diverse activities.

2. A single activity can reflect the action of many macrophage products.

3. Few, if any, macrophage secretory products arise solely from macrophages.

Macrophage secretion involves synthesis on the rough endoplasmic reticulum, co-translational glycosylation and translocation into the lumen of the endoplasmic reticulum, transport to the Golgi and vesicle transport to the plasma membrane. After an intracellular triggering event causes the translocation of secretory vesicles to the inner surface of the plasma membrane, repulsive forces are overcome, enabling contact of the two opposing membranes. Fusion of the secretory vesicle membrane and the plasma membrane then occurs, with re-establishment of the membrane bilayer structure, thereby maintaining the

Table 1.7   Macrophage secretory products

Enzymes	Nitric oxide
Lysozyme	Peroxynitrite
Lysosomal acid hydrolases:	
Lipases	*Arachidonic acid intermediates*
proteases	Cyclooxygenase products:
(deoxy)ribonuclease	PGE$_2$, prostacyclin, thromboxane
phosphatases	Lipooxygenase products:
glycosidases	hydroxyeicosotetranoic acids
sulfatases	leukotrienes
Neutral proteases:	Platelet-activating factors
collagenase	
elastase	*Coagulation factors*
myelinase	Tissue factor
angiotensin convertase	Prothrombin activator
plasminogen activator	Coagulation factors II, VII, IX, X, XIII
cytolytic proteinase	Plasminogen activator
Lipases	Plasminogen activator inhibitors
lipoprotein lipase	
phospholipase A2	*Cytokines*
Arginase	IL-1, IL-6, IL-10, IL-12, IL-15, IL-18
	TNF-α
Enzyme and cytokine inhibitors	Interferons-α and -γ
Protease inhibitors:	Platelet-derived growth factors
α_2-Macroglobulin	Fibroblast growth factor
α1-Antitrypsin inhibitor	Transforming growth factor-β
plasminogen activator inhibitor	GM-CSF
collagenase inhibitor	M-CSF
Phospholipase inhibitor	Erythropoietin
IL-1 inhibitors	Factor inducing monocytopoiesis
	Angiogenesis factor
Complement components	CXC chemokines (IL-8, GRO, ENA-78, IP-10)
Classical pathway:	
C1, C4, C2, C3, C5	*Others*
Alternative pathway:	Thrombospondin
factor B, factor D, properdin	Fibronectin
Active fragments:	Lipocortin
C3a, C3b, C5a, Bb	Transcobalamin II
Inhibitors:	Transferrin
C3b inactivator, β-1H	Ferritin
	Haptoglobin
Reactive oxygen intermediates	Glutathione
Superoxide	Uric acid
Hydrogen peroxide	Apolipoprotein E
Hydroxyl radical	Neopterin

integrity of the cell while expelling vesicle contents to the external milieu (Henson *et al.*, 1988).

Some secretory products such as lysozyme (Gordon *et al.*, 1974), complement components and apolipoprotein E are synthesized and secreted continuously (constitutive secretion) whereas others are only released upon appropriate stimulation (regulated or induced secretion) (Gordon, 1978; Henson *et al.*, 1988; Bresnihan, 1999). Stimulation of synthesis could occur at the level of transcription/translation or at the level of packaging, processing, transport or membrane fusion. Probably different proteins are controlled by one or both of these broad mechanisms (Bresnihan, 1999).

10.4.1 Enzymes

Lysozyme mediates digestion of the cell walls of some bacteria and is a well-documented secretory product of macrophages (Gordon *et al.*, 1974; Osserman, 1975). However, its biological usefulness is uncertain as relatively few bacteria are susceptible to hydrolysis by lysozyme. Furthermore, naturally occurring substrates for lysozyme, other than bacterial cell wall polysaccharides, have not been recognized. Lysozyme is secreted constitutively, and essentially all populations of macrophages produce and secrete large amounts. Lysozyme secretion is more marked in macrophages and monocytes than in monoblasts and promonocytes (Cohn and Benson, 1965).

Lysosomal acid hydrolases are released by macrophages in response to numerous appropriate exogenous stimuli (Page *et al.*, 1978). These enzymes were once regarded solely as intracellular digestive enzymes, but are now known to be secreted actively into the extracellular fluid in response to engagement of macrophage Fc receptors or complement receptors, activation of macrophages by cytokines or exposure to bacterial products (Pantalone and Page, 1975; Gabig and Babior, 1981). Acid hydrolases can degrade collagen, basement membrane and other components of connective tissue. They can also hydrolyze complement, immunoglobulins and kinins (Lasser, 1983). The enzymes include proteases, lipases, (deoxy)ribonucleases, phosphatases, glycosidases and sulfatases (Nathan, 1987). They are active when the pH is low.

Neutral proteases include collagenase, elastase, angiotensin convertase, plasminogen activator and a cysteine protease (Werb and Gordon, 1975a,b; Siverstein *et al.*, 1979; Nathan, 1987). They are active at a neutral pH and their secretion is closely and differentially regulated during activation (Gordon, 1978). Elastase and collagenase have no clear-cut independent antibacterial activity, though they may react synergistically with other enzymes (Elsbach and Weiss, 1988). While resident macrophages are poor secretors of most proteases, inflammatory macrophages secrete substantial amounts. In the case of collagenase and plasminogen activator, low secretory cells have very low levels of intracellular enzyme, suggesting that appropriate signals induce both synthesis and secretion of these products. Release of neutral proteases is regulated in two steps—an initial priming signal and a subsequent signal which triggers actual release/secretion of the product in question (Gordon, 1978). Priming for neutral protease secretion can be induced by cytokines, endotoxin and proteases themselves. Secretion by primed macrophages can be triggered by acetylated proteins, endotoxin or a phagocytic challenge (Gordon, 1978; Johnson *et al.*, 1982). Secretion of this same set of neutral proteases can be shut off by binding of α_2-macroglobulin–protease complexes to their specific receptor (Johnson *et al.*, 1982). This effect is observed most readily in fully activated macrophages where protease secretion is highest.

Lipases such as lipoprotein lipase and phospholipase A2 are also secreted by macrophages (Nathan, 1987).

10.4.2 Enzyme inhibitors

Secretion of proteases can be reduced dramatically by binding of α2-macroglobulin–protease complexes to their surface receptor (Johnson *et al.*, 1982) with subsequent internalization and degradation of the enzymes. As well as the large molecule α_2-macroglobulin which inhibits not only plasmin but also plasminogen activator, collagenase, elastase and kallikrein, macrophages secrete inhibitors of plasmin of low and intermediate molecular weight (Nathan *et al.*, 1980). α1-Antitrypsin inhibitor, plasminogen activator inhibitors, collagenase inhibitor as well as a phospholipase inhibitor and inhibitors of IL-1 have been found within macrophages (Nathan, 1987).

10.4.3 Complement components

Macrophages secrete numerous components of the complement system, including members of both classical and alternative pathways. These include C1, C4, C2, C3, C5, factor B, factor D, properdin, C3b inactivator and α-IH (Whaley, 1980; Strunk *et al.*, 1985). Furthermore, active fragments generated by macrophage proteases such as C3a, C3b, C5a and Bb are secreted (Brade and Bentley, 1980). Elevated complement secretion can be induced in various populations of macrophages by host infection with *Listeria monocytogenes* or bacille Calmette–Guérin (BCG). Cholinergic and adrenergic receptor agonists stimulate synthesis and secretion following *in vitro* exposure (Whaley *et al.*, 1981). In addition to synthesizing and secreting numerous complement components, macrophages can bind activated complement through at least two types of complement receptor and degrade complement. After interaction with receptors on the macrophage surface, complement may affect the migratory, endocytic and secretory behavior of the cells. For example, C3a and C5a stimulate macrophage migration, but a product of the alternative pathway (Bb) suppresses migration and promotes cell spreading (Nathan *et al.*, 1980).

10.4.4 Reactive oxygen intermediates

When exposed to certain stimuli, phagocytes undergo marked changes in the way they handle oxygen. Their rates of oxygen uptake increase greatly and they begin to produce ROIs, such as superoxide, hydrogen peroxide and hydroxyl groups (Babior, 1984) (see Section 7). Because of the sharp increase in oxygen uptake, this series of changes has come to be known as the 'respiratory burst', though its purpose is to generate cytotoxic agents rather than to produce energy (Babior, 1984; Vazquez-Torres and Balish, 1997). Secretion of ROIs is incompletely understood at the molecular level. Engagement of Fc receptors, complement receptors, receptors for mannose terminal glycoproteins and phorbol 12-myristate 13-acetate (PMA) can stimulate an oxidative burst (Nathan and Root, 1977; Johnston, 1981). Induction of the secretion of ROIs does not correlate precisely with induction of tumoricidal function (Adams and Hamilton, 1984), neither is phagocytosis necessarily accompanied by a respiratory burst. Generation of ROIs by external stimuli requires the activation of an NADPH oxidase, and the rapidity of enzyme activation (within seconds in some instances) essentially rules out its *de novo* synthesis (McPhail and Snyderman, 1983). It has therefore been suggested that macrophage activation may lead to modification of existing oxidase molecules rather than to generation of new ones. Reactive nitrogen intermediates should also be added to the well-established ROIs of macrophages (Vazquez-Torres and Balish, 1997). Furthermore, what were thought to be two independent pathways, nitric oxide and superoxide anion, have now been shown to combine to form a potent macrophage molecule, peroxynitrite, important in killing microorganisns such as *Candida* (Vazquez-Torres and Balish, 1997).

10.4.5 Arachidonic acid intermediates

Macrophages are a major source of these products, and their release constitutes an important aspect of their function (Bonney and Davies, 1984). For example, prostaglandins of the E series can play an autoregulatory role by limiting certain aspects of tumor cytolysis by macrophages. The biochemical pathways involved in the synthesis of the various arachidonic acid products are well known (Sammuelson *et al.*, 1978) although there is evidence of alternative pathways (Balsinde *et al.*, 2000). Arachidonic acid metabolites include prostacyclin, thromboxane, PGE2 and LTB4 (Pawlowski *et al.*, 1983). The enzymes responsible for metabolism of arachidonic acid are targets for regulation of arachidonic acid metabolism. For example, availability of arachidonic acid for metabolism depends on phospholipase A2, which cleaves arachidonic acid from its stored form in the cells' pool of neutral phospholipid. Levels of cyclooooxygenase and lipooxygenase control the pattern of metabolism for the released arachidonic acid. Lipoxins are lipoxygenase-derived eicosanoids generated during inflammation which inhibit polymorphonuclear neutrophil (PMN) chemotaxis and adhesion and are putative braking signals for PMN-mediated tissue injury. Lipoxin A4 (Godson *et al.*, 2000) promotes phagocytosis of apoptotic PMN by monocyte-derived macrophages, an important step in the resolution phase of inflammation (see Section 11.11). This bioactivity was reproduced by stable synthetic lipoxin A4 analogs but not by other eicosanoids.

10.4.6 Coagulation factors

Mononuclear phagocytes have been known for some time to synthesize coagulation factors. Different 'procoagulant' factors have been described in cells from different species, different anatomical sites, stimulated by different agonists under different conditions either *in vitro* or *in vivo*. Peripheral blood monocytes have been studied much more extensively than tissue macrophages due to the relative ease of access. The procoagulant which has been found most consistently in human mononuclear phagocyte populations is tissue factor, which is expressed on the cell surface (Prydz and Allison, 1978). Active tissue factor, in the presence of adequate phospholipid, greatly enhances the ability of factor VII to activate the extrinsic coagulation cascade (Nemerson, 1966). Stimulation of monocytes by a variety of agents, including endotoxin, immune complexes, complement component C5a and inflammation-inducing particles, strongly increases tissue factor synthesis by the cell in a dose- and time-dependent manner (Edwards and Rickles, 1984). Unstimulated monocytes express little if any tissue factor, but after stimulation tissue factor is expressed within 2 h (Prydz and Allison, 1978). Little is known concerning the biosynthesis and intracellular transport of tissue factor, although it seems likely that changes in intracellular concentrations of calcium, cyclic nucleotides and arachidonic acid metabolites as well as transmethylation reactions are of importance and modulate the integrated response which leads to altered gene expression, *de novo* synthesis of apoprotein III (the protein component of tissue factor) and the intracellular transport of this by a vesicular route to the cell membrane, where it is inserted (Edwards and Rickles, 1984). Other procoagulants synthesized by monocytes are described, including a prothrombin activator (Hogg, 1983) and coagulation factors II, VII, IX, X and XIII (van Dam-Mieras *et al.*, 1985).

Human moncytes have been found to synthesize a plasminogen activator (Stephens and Golder, 1984). One study suggested that the nature of the plasminogen activator produced by human monocytes depends on the differentiation of the cell: mature, differentiated macrophages producing urokinase and granulocyte/macrophage progenitors producing tissue-type plasminogen activator (Wilson and Francis, 1987). Urokinase receptors have been found on the surface of monocytes and a monocytoid cell line and linked to cell motility and growth (Stoppelli *et al.*, 1985). It has been suggested that urokinase binding to monocyte membranes may represent a mechanism whereby monocytes develop migratory properties. A rapid plasminogen activator inhibitor, called minactivin, is also produced by monocytes (Stephens *et al.*, 1985).

10.4.7 Cytokine secretion

Following recognition of antigen, both T and B cells become susceptible to activation by cytokines, which can be defined as soluble peptide factors influencing function, growth and differentiation. Cells of the macrophage lineage are responsible for the secretion of many cytokines and assist in the control and fine tuning of the immune response. The identification of different cytokines generally began with the description of a biological action and the isolation of a peptide(s) that mediated this action. It soon emerged that one cytokine might be responsible for many different actions, depending on such criteria as target cell, local concentration and the combination of other cytokines present, and also that many cytokines had overlapping activities. For largely historical reasons, several groupings of cytokines have emerged, including the TNF, transforming growth factor (TGF), CSF, IFN, IL and chemokine families. The criteria for designation as an interleukin (production by leukocytes, known primary structure and action during immune responses) are so broad that many of the cytokines described above would now be termed interleukins.

TNF was first identified in serum from mice primed with BCG and challenged with endotoxin. On transfer to tumor-bearing animals, there was evidence of tumor necrosis. TNF-α, produced by the macrophage, was later shown to be identical to cachectin, responsible for wasting in neoplastic and parasitic diseases. The genes encoding both TNF-α (Shirai *et al.*, 1985) and TNF-β (produced by lymphocytes) have been cloned, sequenced and assigned to chromosome 6 near the MHC loci. The stimuli for production are LPS and other microbial agents, IL-2, GM-CSF and IL-1. TNFs *in vivo* are involved in the necrosis of tumors, endotoxic shock-like syndrome, cachexia, fever, the acute phase protein response and may have some antiparasitic effects. TNF-α has been shown to have cytostatic and cytotoxic effects *in vitro* against a variety of human tumors and to be involved in the induction of IL-1, GM-CSF, IL-6 and ICAM-1 (CD54) production (Cerami and Beutler, 1988).

Macrophages are known to produce IFN-α in response to viruses, bacteria and tumor or foreign cells (Pestka *et al.*, 1987). The biological actions of IFN-α include antiviral and antimitotic effects, up-regulation of MHC class II expression and an increase in natural killer (NK) cell activity.

Following stimulation by LPS or IL-1, cells of the monocyte/macrophage series produce M-CSF, GM-CSF and G-CSF (Metcalf, 1987) (see Section 3). M-CSF induces the formation of monocyte precursor colonies and also induces production of PGE_2, plasminogen activator, IL-1, IFN-γ and TNF-α. GM-CSF induces the formation of granulocyte, eosinophil and monocyte colonies, is involved in radioprotection of marrow, fighting bacterial and parasitic infections by enhancing eosinophil and neutrophil function, and influences IL-1 and TNF production. G-CSF promotes the formation of granulocyte colonies, the terminal differentiation of myeloid cells and enhances mature neutrophil function.

Monocytes, together with many other cells, produce IL-1, which is involved in immunoregulation, influencing IL-2, IL-4, IL-6 and TNF production. IL-1 represents a family of polypeptides with a wide range of biological activities including augmentation of cellular immune responses (T, B and NK cells), proliferation of fibroblasts, chemotaxis of monocytes, neutrophils and lymphocytes; stimulation of PGE$_2$, increased numbers of peripheral blood neutrophils and neutrophil activation (Dinarello, 1985). IL-1 plays a role in fever, the acute phase protein response, hypotension and slow wave sleep, the production of collagenase from mesenchymal cells and also influences bone and cartilage resorption. IL-1 is known to synergize with IFN and IL-2 in enhancing tumor killing by NK cells and stimulates myeloid progenitor cells to proliferate in long-term bone marrow cultures (Fibbe *et al.*, 1987).

Cells of the monocyte/macrophage series are the main source of IL-6, although this cytokine is also produced by activated T cells and fibroblasts. Cardiac myxoma cells and cervical adenocarcinoma cell lines and also (Hutchins *et al.*, 1990) some human B-cell lines have also been shown to produce IL-6. There is evidence that IL-1 and TNF induce the up-regulation of IL-6 production (Zhang *et al.*, 1989); platelet-derived growth factor (PDGF) is also a stimulus, and autocrine production has been reported in some cell lines. IL-6 (Heinrich, 1990) is the cytokine primarily involved in delivering the final signal for an alteration in the regulation of protein synthesis to hepatocytes (see Section 11.1) during the acute phase protein response. The effect of IL-6 on hepatocytes can be profoundly altered by insulin, dexamethasone and the counter-regulatory hormones (O'Riordain *et al.*, 1995). Macrophages express IL-4 receptors, and IL-4 has been shown to down-regulate IL-6 production (Lee *et al.*, 1990). IL-6 induces the proliferation of immature and mature T cells (Matsuda *et al.*, 1989) and the expression of the IL-2 receptor on these cells. Proliferation of hemopoietic cells due to the IL-3- and GM-CSF-like action of IL-6 has also been reported, and IL-6 will support the growth of plasmacytoma and hybridoma cells *in vitro* . IL-6 acts on B lymphocytes as a differentiation factor, inducing Ig secretion, and as both a positive and negative regulator of growth acting through IL-6 receptors on these cells.

Human monocytes, together with lymphocytes, hepatocytes, endothelial cells, dermal fibroblasts and other cell types, produce IL-8 (Tables 1.7 and 1.8). This cytokine is a member of the rapidly expanding chemokine family (Bacon *et al.*, 1998; Chantry *et al.*, 1998; Wuyts *et al.*, 1998). IL-8 stimulates the chemotaxis of both neutrophils and T cells, and inhibits IFN-γ release by human NK cells *in vitro* (Lewis *et al.*, 1991). The expression of the IL-8 gene in monocytes is regulated by known inflammatory agents such as LPS, PGE$_2$, IL-1, TNF-α and IFN-γ. IL-8 is also capable of inducing an acute phase response from isolated human hepatocytes (Wigmore *et al.*, 1997) presumably via an alternative pathway to the gp130 signaling pathway.

TGF-β (types 1, 2 and 3) is also produced by macrophages (Assoian *et al.*, 1987) and has a myriad of properties (Chieftez *et al.*, 1987) including immunosuppressive consequences such as inhibition of all known IL-2 effects including IL-2 receptor expression. TGF-β is chemotactic for monocytes and plays a role in fibrosis and wound healing, with increased gene expression of collagen I, III and IV and induction of osteoblast prolifera-

Table 1.8 Cytokines secreted by macrophages

Cytokine	Other names	Stimuli for production	Biological action
IFN-α	Viral IFN, Type I IFN	Viruses, bacteria	Antiviral; antimitotic; MHC class II (+); NK activity (+); decreased c-*myc* expression
M-CSF	MGF, CSF-1, MGI-1M	LPS, IL-1	Macrophage colonies; antiviral; induces PGE_2, plasminogen activator, IL-1, IFN-γ, TNF-α
GM-CSF	MGI-1GM, CSF-2, NIF-T, pluripoietin-α	LPS, IL-1, TNF, retroviral infection	Granulocyte, eosinophil, macrophage colonies; radioprotection; protection from bacterial and parasitic infections; enhances neutrophil and eosinophil functions; PGE_2, IL-1, TNF and O_2 induction.
G-CSF	MGI-2, DF, CSF-β	LPS, IL-1	Granulocyte colonies; terminal differentiation of myeloid cells; enhancement of neutrophil function.
TNF-α	Cachectin, TNF	LPS and other microbial agents, IL-2, GM-CSF, IL-1	Necrosis of tumors; endotoxic shock-like syndrome; cachexia; fever; IL-1; acute phase protein response; antiparasitic; *in vitro* induction of CD54, IL-1, GM-CSF, IL-6; up-regulation of MHCI and II expression.
IL-1	BAF, ETAF, LAF	Microbial products, TNF, GM-CSF, IL-2, antigen presentation	Immunoregulation (induction of IL-2, IL-4, IL-6, TNF); fever; acute phase protein response; hypotension; slow wave sleep; induction of collagenase and PGE_2 bone cartilage resorption in culture.
IL-6	BSF-2, IFNβ2, HSF	IL-1, TNF, PDGF	Proliferation of myeloma cell lines and hemopoietic cells (GM-CSF and IL-3-like action); induces IL-2R in T cells; induces Ig production in B cells; induces acute phase production by hepatocytes (influenced by hormones); fever.
IL-8	NAF, MONAP, MDCNF	IL-1, IL-2, IL-3, IL-7, IL-13, TNF-α, GM-CSF, LPS	Neutrophil chemotaxis, shape change, degranulation (release of elastase, myeloperoxidase, gelatinase); enhances phagocytosis of opsonized particles; increases microbicidal activity; induces acute phase proteins in hepatocytes.
IL-10	CSIF	T and B-cell activation; LPS, immune complexes, CD23 cross-linking	Inhibits granulocyte cytokine and chemokine production; co-factor for IL-3- or IL-4-induced proliferation of mast cells; enhances MHC II on B cells; inhibits T-cell cytokine production and proliferation; profound effects on macrophage function (see Table 1.4)
IL-12	NKSF, CLMF	LPS, IFN-γ, poly(I:C), CD40 ligation, HIV gp120, bacteria and bacterial products	Promotes expansion of activated T cells, TIL and NK-LAK cells; synergizes with IL-2 or IL-15 to promote proliferation of activated memory T cells; promotes anti-tumor activity; induces IL-10 production by T cells; profound role in antigen presentation/processing—influences Th1 or Th2 bias of immune response.
IL-15	IL-T	LPS, BCG, *M.tuberculosis*, *Toxoplasma gondii*, herpes virus 6	Can substitute for IL-2 in induction of cytotoxic T cells and LAK cell activity; induction of facets of perforin and Fas-dependent cytolysis pathways; potent growth factor for activated T cells; effects on B cells, neutrophils, mast cells and others.

Table 1.8 Continued

Cytokine	Other names	Stimuli for production	Biological action
IL-16	LCF	N	Chemotactic for CD4 T cells; up-regulates IL-2R, MHC II; inhibits CD3-dependent activation.
IL-18	IGIF activity	LPS, microbial products	Increases IFN-γ and GM-CSF production and stimulates Th1 cells; decreases IL-10 production; multiple regulatory functions increasing antitumor activity.
TGF-βb	(multiple types: TGF-β1, TGF-β2, TGF-β3)	–	Inhibition of IL-2 effects; role in fibrosis and wound healing *in vivo*; anti-proliferative effects on hepatocytes, epithelial cells, T cells and B cells; influences integrin expression and differentiation; inhibits proliferative actions of EGF, PDGF, IL-2 and FGF.
Basic FGF	HBGF, MDGF	–	Endothelial cell chemotaxis and growth; IFN-γ induction; angiogenesis *in vivo*, myoblast and cortical neuron growth.
PDGF	PDGF I, PDGF II	Activated by thrombin, coagulation, LPS, lectins, zymosan	Induction of IL-1, IL-1R, IFN-γ, IFN-β, PGE$_2$, LDL receptor, c-myc, c-fos, amino acid transport; neutrophil activation; intracellular actin reorganization; augments synthesis of collagen; chemotaxis and proliferation of mesenchymal cells.
EGF	β-Urogastrone	–	Proliferation and differentiation of basal layer in epithelia; angiogenic; wound healing.
MIP-1α	Macrophage inflammatory protein 1	LPS	Regulation of hemopoiesis; neutrophil recruitment.
MDC	Macrophage-derived chemokine	–	Chemoattractant for dendritic cells, T cells, and natural killer cells.

The above are only a selection of the activities associated with individual cytokines. A few chemokines are noted above but this is a rapidly expanding area and is not covered in detail: see, for example, Bacon *et al.* (1998); Chantry *et al.* (1998); Wuyts *et al.* (1998).

BAF = B cell-activating factor; BSF-2 = B cell stimulatory factor; CLMF = cytotoxic lymphocyte maturation factor; CSF = colony-stimulating factor; EGF = epidermal growth factor; ETAF = epidermal cell-derived T cell-activating factor; FGF = fibroblast growth factor; G = granulocyte; HBGF = heparin-binding growth factor; HSF = hepatocyte-stimulating factor; ICAM = intercellular cell adhesion molecule; IFN = interferon; IGIF = interferon-g-inducing factor; IL-T = interleukin supporting proliferation of IL-2-dependent T cells; LAF = lymphocyte-activating factor; M = macrophage; MDCNF = monocyte-derived neutrophil chemotactic factor; MGI = macrophage/granulocyte factor; MGI = macrophage/granulocyte inducer; MONAP = monocyte-derived neutrophil-activating peptide; NAF = neutrophil-activating factor; NIF-T = neutrophil-inhibiting factor; NKSF = natural killer stimulatory factor; PDGF = platelet-derived growth factor; T = T cell-derived; TGF = transforming growth factor.

tion, fibroblast chemotaxis and production of collagenase. There are also general cellular effects (Massague, 1987), and TGF-β appears to deliver an anti-proliferative message for hepatocytes, epithelial cells, keratinocytes, and T and B cells. TGF-β also influences the expression of integrins and cell adhesion–cytoskeleton interactions and inhibits some actions of other cytokines such as EGF, PDGF, IL-2 and fibroblast growth factor (FGF).

Heparin-binding growth factors (HBGFs) of the basic type (FGF) are produced by macrophages and play a role in angiogenesis and in neuron, myoblast and endothelial cell growth (Ignotz and Massague, 1987). PDGF and EGF, also produced by monocytes, both have numerous effects. PDGF is involved in vasoconstriction, wound healing and vascular permeability (Ross, 1987). EGF is involved in the proliferation and differentiation of basal cell layers in epithelia and in wound healing (Carpenter, 1987). Macrophage inflammatory protein-2 (MIP-2) is also a heparin-binding protein and is a member of a large family of proteins having the ability to modulate the inflammatory response. The murine MIP-2 and its human homologs have been cloned (Tekamp-Olson *et al.*, 1990).

Macrophages are also capable of secreting a number of the more recently described cytokines including IL-12 (Sinigaglia *et al.*, 1999), IL-15 (Carson and Caligiuri, 1998) and IL-18 (Akira, 2000). IL-12 is required for the development of Th1 cells (Sinigaglia *et al.*, 1999), which are important for the cell-mediated immune responses against a variety of intracellular pathogens. Expression of the IL-12R β2 receptor subunit in humans is critically influenced by IL-12 and type I interferons. IL-12 signaling results in STAT4 activation and interferon IFN-γ production and modulation of a number of genes involved in leukocyte trafficking. Thus, IL-12 is an important pro-inflammatory cytokine, inducing production of IFN-γ and subsequent activation of phagocytic cells. IL-12 may also play a major role in regulating the migration and positioning of effector cells. IL-15 (Carson and Caligiuri, 1998) is a recently described cytokine which is produced by activated monocytes usually early in the course of the innate immune response. IL-15 is able to bind to components of the IL-2R, despite the fact that it has no sequence homology with IL-2, and can substitute for IL-2 in some circumstances. IL-15 can stimulate human NK cell cytokine production proliferation and cytotoxicity. IL-18 (Akira, 2000), formerly called IFN-γ-inducing factor, has potent IFN-γ-inducing activities and plays an important role in the Th1-mediated immune response in collaboration with IL-12. IL-18 is a member of the IL-1 family, and the receptor and signal transduction pathway are analogous to those of the IL-1 receptor. Mice lacking IL-18 have suppressed IFN-γ production, despite the presence of IL-12, and are deficient in their *in vivo* Th1 response and in NK cell activity.

10.5 Tumor cell control

Macrophages infiltrate tumors, and lysis of tumor cells by monocytes and macrophages is believed to be a mechanism of host defense against tumors (Wood and Gollahon, 1977). Cultured human monocytes have been reported to kill tumor cells when activated with cytokines and endotoxin. Several modes of tumor cell control by macrophages have been reported (Figure 1.11). See also Chapter 11 for more information on the role of macrophages in tumor biology.

10.5.1 Inhibition of tumor cell division

Inhibition of tumor cell division may occur by mediators secreted by macrophages which act on all proliferating cells present. These mediators are largely uncharacterized, but

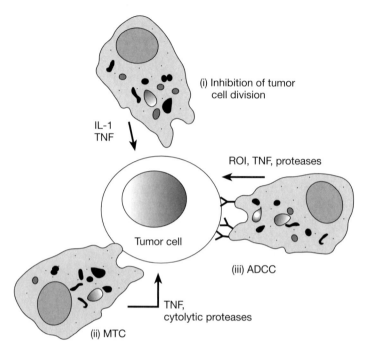

Fig. 1.11   Mechanisms of tumor cell control by macrophages. MTC = macrophage-mediated tumor cytotoxicity; ADCC = antibody-dependent cellular cytotoxicity.

include prostaglandins, IL-1 and TNF. This inhibition is not thought to require cell contact and occurs rapidly (Steplewski *et al.*, 1983).

10.5.2 Macrophage-mediated tumor cytotoxicity

Macrophage-mediated tumor cytotoxicity (MTC) is a contact-dependent, non-phagocytic process which occurs very slowly over 1–3 days. It is selective for neoplastic cells and is independent of antibody production. After recognition of the neoplastic cells, binding to macrophages occurs followed by the secretion of toxic substances, which result in the eventual lysis of the bound tumor cells. TNF and a novel serine protease are the major candidates for the toxic mediators. ROIs can probably potentiate MTC (Adams and Hamilton, 1988).

10.5.3 Antibody-dependent cellular cytotoxicity

Antibody-dependent cellular cytotoxicity (ADCC) is a process whereby macrophages are able to lyse antibody-coated tumor cells (Adams and Hamilton, 1984, 1988). The classical form of ADCC by macrophages is rapid and mediated by polyclonal antisera. However, in experimental systems in both mice and humans, monoclonal antibodies against tumor cells direct and enhance macrophage cytotoxicity (Steplewski *et al.*, 1983; Adams *et al.*, 1984; Johnson *et al.*, 1986). The Fab portion of the Ig binds to antigens on the surface of tumor cells and the Fc portion binds to surface receptors on the macrophage. After binding, lysis occurs. Secretion of lytic mediators by macrophages occurs upon occupancy and cross-linking of the Fc receptor. ROIs, especially hydrogen peroxide, play a major role in cytolysis, but other mediators may also be important, such as complement components, neutral protease and TNF. ADCC may occur rapidly over 5–6 h, or slowly over 1–2 days. Cytokines, such as recombinant human M-CSF (Munn *et al.*, 1990), may enhance monocyte differentiation into macrophages that have increased antitumor ADCC.

Though TNF appears to be an important mediator of the cytotoxicity of human mononuclear phagocytes *in vitro*, and IFN-γ can increase this cytotoxicity by sensitizing tumor cells to its lytic action (Feinman *et al.*, 1987), Phase 1 trials in patients with various types of cancer given recombinant TNF systemically have shown response rates of less than 5 per cent (Blick *et al.*, 1987). However, direct injection into the tumor has given more encouraging results (Taguchi, 1987).

As well as macrophages exerting some control over tumor cells, some tumor cells can interfere with mononuclear phagocyte function. Reduced monocyte chemotaxis and phagocytosis are well recognized in subjects with malignant disease (Sokol and Hudson, 1983). The mechanisms whereby the tumor suppresses the antitumor activity of the macrophage are of great interest and probably involve both regulatory T cells and substances derived from tumor cells themselves.

11 Introduction to the role of mononuclear phagocytes in health and disease

11.1 Role in the acute phase protein response

The acute phase protein response results from disturbances to homeostasis due to neoplastic growth, tissue injury, infection or immunological disorders. It comprises fever, tachychardia, shock and changes in concentration of circulating proteins such as C-reactive protein, serum amyloid-A and fibrinogen. In 1951, it was shown that the liver is the major organ for the synthesis of the acute phase proteins (Miller *et al.*, 1951). As this altered protein turnover in the liver is related to trauma in other parts of the body, the existence of mediators, probably released by leukocytes, which control the acute phase protein response was proposed. The monocyte/macrophage was later shown to be central to this response (Sipe *et al.*, 1979), and at least three monocyte products are important in the control of the acute phase protein response: IL-1, TNF and IL-6 (Heinrich, 1990). IL-1 may induce fever through triggering the release of PGE acting on the hypothalamus to reset the hypothalamic thermoregulatory receptor. IL-1 and TNF also mediate the accelerated catabolism of muscle protein and negative nitrogen balance, which result in the myalgia and impaired physical performance seen in acute infection and malignancy.

Increased circulating levels of TNF and IL-6 have been observed in tumor-bearing rodents (Jablons *et al.*, 1989; Stovroff *et al.*, 1989), and repeated injection of TNF (Tracey *et al.*, 1988) or the transplantion of transfected cells secreting TNF (Oliff *et al.*, 1987) has been shown to induce a syndrome similar to that of cancer cachexia. TNF previously was proposed as a key mediator of catabolism in cancer patients, but the results of many studies suggest that IL-6 rather than TNF may be important in delivering the signal to hepatocytes for altered protein metabolism. It has been shown (Fearon *et al.*, 1998) that IL-6 is elevated in the serum of weight-losing patients with advanced colon cancer and pancreatic cancer, and that this relates to profound changes in hepatic protein metabolism (fixed hepatic protein synthesis was suppressed and acute phase protein production increased). IL-6-induced (Tamm, 1989; Heinrich, 1990) transcriptional activation of a set of human acute phase proteins (Morrone *et al.*, 1988) and nuclear transcription factors which interact with the C-reactive protein promoter (Majello *et al.*, 1990) have been described.

The mechanisms which lead to enhanced cytokine release in cancer patients are poorly understood, as too are the factors which control cytokine release in normal individuals. There appears to be some correlation between increased monocyte cytokine release and depressed T-cell function in patients with advanced cancer. Cancer cachexia is associated with an elevated hepatic acute phase protein response, poor outcome and elevated cytokine production from peripheral blood mononuclear cells (Falconer *et al.*, 1994ab). The *n*-3 fatty acids show some promise as both anti-catabolic agents and regulators of monocyte/macrophage function (Ross *et al.*, 1999).

11.2 Role in hematopoiesis

The growth of committed hematopoietic progenitor cells *in vitro* requires factors that may be derived from macrophages (Sadahira and Mori, 1999), mesenchymal cells and T lymphocytes. These factors may only act locally within the bone marrow and not be detected in plasma (Flanagan and Lader, 1998). GM-CSF is secreted by normal human macrophages and monocytes, and highly purified natural or recombinant human GM-CSF stimulates granulocyte/macrophage and eosinophil colony formation *in vitro*. In addition to its effect on progenitor differentiation, GM-CSF also induces a variety of functional changes in mature macrophages and neutrophils. For example, it has been shown that GM-CSF stimulates the oxidative metabolism and Fc-dependent phagocytic activity of peritoneal macrophages (Coleman *et al.*, 1988).

Macrophage synthesis of G-CSF appears to depend on induction with endotoxin, and this may be an important factor in inducing increased hematopoiesis during stress (Sieff, 1987). Furthermore, macrophages produce both IL-1 and TNF in response to endotoxin. These monokines may induce circulating T lymphocytes to produce both GM-CSF and IL-3 which stimulate hematopoiesis. Monocyte-derived IL-1 and/or TNF may also induce fixed bone marrow stromal cell populations (endothelial and fibroblasts) to produce GM-CSF and G-CSF as well (see Section 3). Basal hematopoiesis, on the other hand, is probably maintained by local production of growth factors by fixed stromal cells (endothelial cells, fibroblasts and perhaps macrophages).

Mononuclear phagocytes also appear to participate in the regulation of early erythroid development (Sadahira and Mori, 1999). GM-CSF, in the presence of erythropoietin, induces the formation of colonies derived from early erythroid burst-forming units (BFU-E) and from mixed colony-forming units that comprise granulocytes, erythroid cells, macrophages and megakaryocytes (CFU-GEMM). Cultured macrophages have been found to express the erythropoietin gene and it has been postulated that a subpopulation of resident bone marrow macrophages may be responsible for producing erythropoietin under adult steady-state conditions. The kidney may only function as an erythropoietin-producing organ under conditions of erythropoietic stress (Rich, 1988).

11.3 Role in hemostasis

A host response to infection, tumors or injury may be to activate the coagulation system within the circulation, resulting in disseminated intravascular coagulation. One of the most severe examples of this occurs in meningococcal septicemia (Dennis *et al.*, 1968), though it occurs less severely but more commonly with solid tumors (Auger and Mackie, 1987). Monocytes and macrophages synthesize and express tissue factor and possibly other coagulation factors (see Section 10.4.6). Mononuclear cells taken from the peripheral blood of patients with tumors of the breast (Auger and Mackie, 1988) and lung (Edwards *et al.*, 1981), inflammatory bowel disease (Edwards *et al.*, 1987) and meningococcal septicemia (Osterud and Flaegstad, 1983) synthesize increased amounts of tissue factor *in vitro* and a strong positive correlation has been found between the generation of monocyte tissue factor *in vitro* and *in vivo* blood coagulation in patients with certain solid tumors (Edwards *et al.*, 1981; Auger and Mackie, 1988) and inflammatory bowel disease (Edwards *et al.*, 1987).

The monokines IL-1 and TNF can induce tissue factor synthesis and expression by endothelial cells lining blood vessels, thereby having a potentially important role in thrombogenesis. Furthermore, they have been shown to down-regulate the activity of the protein C pathway on endothelial cells, thereby reducing natural anti-coagulant mechanisms and further supporting thrombogenesis (Bevilacqua *et al.*, 1984; Nawroth and Stern, 1986).

11.4 Role in destruction of microorganisms

Mononuclear phagocytes play a prominent role in the defense against a variety of infectious agents, including viruses (see Chapter 4), bacteria (Chapter 5), protozoa and parasites (Chapter 6). Having been attracted in increased numbers to an infected focus by a variety of substances (see Section 10.2) including bacterial components and endotoxins, complement components, immune complexes and collagen fragments (Lasser, 1983), they remain there under the influence of a migration inhibition factor released by T lymphocytes (Rocklin *et al.*, 1980). After arriving at the infected focus, the mononuclear cells phagocytose the infectious agent (see Section 10.1). Once ingested, the organism may be killed by both oxygen-dependent and oxygen-independent mechanisms. It is clear that not all organisms are killed by the same mechanism. Oxygen-dependent mechanisms include the production and intracellular release of reactive oxygen species, such as superoxide, hydrogen peroxide and hydroxyl ions derived from the respiratory burst. Indeed, the ability of murine macrophages to kill or inhibit the intracellular replication of the protozoa *Toxoplasma gondii* and *Trypanosoma cruzi* correlates closely with their oxidative capacity, as judged by release of hydrogen peroxide (Klebanoff, 1988). Oxidized halogens have been shown to destroy many bacterial components including nucleotides and redox enzymes at a very rapid rate, but they kill bacteria even more quickly (Babior, 1984). Superoxide and hydrogen peroxide are only weakly microbicidal and the peroxidase–H_2O_2–halide system, which results in the production of oxidized halogens, appears to be important. Generation of NO may also be an important mechanism (MacMicking *et al.*, 1997).

Some organisms are killed by oxygen-independent mechanisms, when there is acidification of the phagocytic vacuole itself to a pH of about 4.5 after lysosomal fusion

(Gabig and Babior, 1981). This acidification occurs within 15 min. However, killing of organisms is probably not solely due to acidification of the phagocytic vacuole, but is also likely to be related to the pH optima of lysosomal acid hydrolases which themselves kill some species.

Certain microorganisms are able to escape the potent microbicidal activity of mononuclear phagocytes (Sangari *et al.*, 1999). *Mycobacterium tuberculosis* may release substances that interfere with the fusion of primary lysosomes with phagosomes. *Leishmania* and *M.lepraemurium* survive within secondary lysosomes due to the resistance of the microbial cell wall to the macrophages' degradative enzymes (see Section 10.1). *Mycobacterium avium* is an environmental microorganism that is adapted to live both in the environment and in fish, bird and mammal hosts. In humans, *M.avium* infection (Sangari *et al.*, 1999) is seen in patients with some sort of immunosuppression, such chronic lung disease or AIDS. *Mycobacterium avium* can enter and survive within macrophages and monocytes. Entry seems to be dependent on binding to the complement receptor *in vitro*, but *in vivo* the bacterium appears to enter macrophages by alternative mechanisms.

11.5 Role in disposal of damaged or senescent red cells

Macrophages phagocytose aged erythrocytes during their circulation through the spleen. The mechanism whereby macrophages recognize senescent cells is unknown. Senescent red cells are sequestered in the spleen and their destruction presumably occurs because of a subtle abnormality detected by splenic macrophages. However, the relevant abnormalities are uncertain. Furthermore, splenectomy does not enhance red cell survival in otherwise normal people. Hypotheses have ranged from aging cells progressively losing sialic acid, cation and water loss, loss of red cell membrane surface, altered membrane lipid and proteins, through to the concept that as the normal erythrocyte ages its membrane nonspecifically binds increasing quantities of Ig until it may be sufficiently coated to be recognized by the macrophage Fc receptors and phagocytosed (Kay, 1975). It is possible that effete leukocytes (see Section 11.10) and platelets are removed by similar mechanisms (Lasser, 1983). Once ingested by macrophages, the erythrocyte is degraded to liberate iron from heme, which is then stored in protein complexes and transferred to developing erythroblasts (Hershko, 1977).

11.6 Role in wound healing, tissue repair and remodeling

Macrophages are rapidly present in wounds after injury, where they can synthesize and secrete collagenase and elastase, helping to debride the wound (Werb and Gordon, 1975a,b). Macrophages also participate in wound healing and tissue remodeling by releasing substances that induce fibroblast proliferation and neovascularization and in remodeling bone through resorption by osteoclasts (Nathan, 1987; Knighton and Fiegel, 1989). The role of macrophages in wound healing is dealt with in greater detail in Chapter 10.

11.7 Role in atherogenesis

The nature of the role of the macrophage in atherogenesis is still uncertain. Some evidence points to an important role for the macrophage in plaque development, whilst equally convincing evidence suggests they act as a defense against plaque progression (Wissler *et al.*, 1987). Attention is now being given to the involvement of chemokines in the inflammatory recruitment of monocytes/macrophages (Reape and Groot, 1999) and also to their role in the related local immune responses and vascular remodeling which occur during the formation of unstable atherosclerotic plaques. Macrophages are usually present in small numbers in human atheromatous plaques, but in certain experimental models it is the predominant cell type. This leads to difficulties in extrapolating between the two situations. Macrophages may become loaded with lipid and cholesterol, and when they die this may become deposited in the blood vessel wall (Stary, 1983). In addition, it has been suggested that monocyte-derived foam cells may leave the artery wall and whilst re-entering the circulation may cause endothelial injury. The latter could then result in platelet adhesion and aggregation, as well as allowing lipid influx (Gerrity, 1981). Conversely, macrophages may be equally important as scavenger cells in removing excess cholesterol and other fatty substances from intimal lesions. The lipases, collagenase and elastase they synthesize and secrete may accelerate plaque regression (Wissler *et al.*, 1987). Whether the macrophages in atherosclerotic plaques are important primarily in plaque progression or regression is the subject of current investigations. The role of the macrophage in atherogenesis and cardiovascular disease is discussed in greater detail in Chapter 12.

11.8 Role in autoimmunity

The macrophage plays a role in many autoimmune diseases in humans. The role of the macrophage in autoimmunity is described in detail in Chapter 8. However, it is also appropriate to mention several examples here. In rheumatoid arthritis (Cutolo, 1990; Bresnihan, 1999) (see Chapter 9), macrophages and other 'professional' APCs are the first cells to be involved: processessing and presenting antigen to antigen-specific T cells. The initial stimulus for the disease remains unknown but may be due to a single virus or several viruses, possibly possessing epitopes cross-reactive with self-antigens, which are the object of the immune response. A majority of patients with rheumatoid arthritis have HLA-DR4- and/or HLA-DR1-expressing cells but these two haplotypes are not the only genetic components of the disease. The immune response gradually becomes organized in the perivascular areas of the synovial membrane, with the accumulation of T cells leading to the proliferation of B cells within a network of new blood vessels and synovial cell proliferation. Macrophages appear to be responsible for the angiogenesis and thus the development of the extensive network of new blood vessels in the synovial membrane essential to the evolution of rheumatoid synovitis. Cytokines originating from macrophages within the rheumatoid synovial membrane have been demonstrated. Thus macrophages, by their production of cytokines, may orchestrate the disease process with the alteration in endothelial cell adhesion and the subsequent influx of neutrophils. Eventually severe inflammation and synovial hyperplasia result in an invasive advance that affects cartilage, tendons and subchondral bone. Macrophages and synoviocytes at the cartilage–pannus junction (Bresnihan, 1999) express matrix metalloproteinase and cathepsin mRNA from the earliest stage of rheumatoid arthritis. The role of the macrophage in rheumatoid arthritis is covered in greater detail in Chapter 9.

In Hashimoto's, spontaneous and experimental autoimmune thyroiditis, the thyroid gland is infiltrated diffusely by lymphocytes (which may aggregate to form secondary lymphoid follicles), plasma cells and macrophages (Charriere, 1989). The role of macrophages is not clear, but they may have a role in the initial processing and presentation of the self-antigen involved. The serum of patients with Hashimoto's disease usually contains antibodies to thyroglobulin.

Macrophages play a central role in sarcoidosis, which is a multisystem disorder of unknown etiology manifesting initially as inflammation of the alveolar structures followed by the development of granulomas. Autoantibodies reactive with T cells are often present. The active sarcoid granuloma consists of a tightly packed central follicle of macrophages, epithelioid cells and multinucleated giant cells surrounded by a perimeter of lymphocytes, monocytes and fibroblasts (Kataria and Holter, 1997). It has been suggested that the central follicle of the granulomata contains activated macrophages whose primary function is the secretion of cytokines rather than phagocytosis. Although the lungs are the primary organ affected, granulomas are often present in other sites.

11.9 Role in central nervous system diseases

A role for the macrophage in both the induction and effector phases of multiple sclerosis (MS) (see Chapter 8) has been suggested. Inappropriate induction of antigen-specific helper T cells resulting in altered regulation of the immune response is postulated to be one of the factors in the mechanism of autoimmune disease. In MS (Bar-Or *et al.*, 1999), once autoreactive T cells have been presented with the relevant antigen and received the appropriate cytokine stimuli, they become activated and cross into the CNS across the blood–brain barrier. Subsequent proliferation of these autoreactive T cells may occur following presentation by indigenous macrophages, microglia or possibly astrocytes. CNS damage and edema following the release of cytokines and macrophages, which are known to strip myelin from nerve sheaths, play a role in the subsequent demyelination. See also Chapter 13 for a more detailed examination of the role of macrophages in the CNS.

11.10 Role in inflammatory bowel disease

A large population of macrophages reside in the normal intestinal mucosa where they represent a major APC population. Various studies suggest that intestinal macrophages cannot easily be induced to mediate acute inflammatory responses. In inflammatory bowel disease, however, there is an increase in the mucosal macrophage population where the recruited macrophages are phenotypically disparate from the resident macrophages (Mahida, 2000). These recruited macrophages appear to perform a major role in mediating the chronic mucosal inflammation seen in patients with ulcerative colitis and Crohn's disease. There is evidence that the recruited macrophages release reactive metabolites of oxygen and nitrogen and proteases which degrade the extracellular matrix. There is also evidence that the recruited macrophages may be primarily responsible for the secretion of cytokines which are important in the pro-inflammatory process, including TNF-α, IL-1, IL-6, IL-8, IL-12 and IL-18.

11.11 Role in resolution of inflammation

The resolution of inflammation involves the death of excess or effete inflammatory cells by a process of physiological programmed cell death (apoptosis) and the subsequent recognition and removal of apoptotic cells by phagocytes (Ward *et al.*, 1999). Engulfment by a phagocyte is probably the final common event in the life of most apoptotic cells. Phagocytosis of apoptotic bodies prior to their lysis prevents the release of potentially toxic or immunogenic intracellular contents and activates an anti-inflammatory response in macrophages (Fadok, 1999). The neutrophil, for example, is a vital component in the defense against infectious agents. However, during the resolution phase of an inflammatory reaction, an uncontrolled release of toxic substances from the neutrophil may damage surrounding tissue and further promote the inflammatory response (Haslett, 1999), leading to scarring and tissue destruction. See also Chapter 10 for more details on the role of macrophages in wound healing. Neutrophil granulocytes and their granule contents have been implicated in the pathogenesis of a variety of inflammatory diseases including the adult respiratory distress syndrome, idiopathic pulmonary fibrosis, ulcerative colitis and rheumatoid arthritis. The mechanisms by which macrophages and other phagocytes recognize apoptotic cells *in vitro* have been the subject of intense study in recent years (Platt *et al.*, 1998) as have the changes which occur on the surface of the granulocyte during apoptosis (Hart *et al.*, 2000). A number of mechanisms or receptors have been implicated in the recognition and ingestion of dying cells including class A scavenger receptors (Platt *et al.*, 1999), the CD36/thrombospondin hypothesis (Ren and Savill, 1998) and CD14 (Gregory, 2000). There is still a considerable gap in knowledge concerning the process of clearance of apoptotic cells *in vivo*. Recently, lipoxin A4 (see Section 10.4.5) has been shown to trigger rapid, concentration-dependent uptake of apoptotic PMN (Godson *et al.*, 2000). Lipoxin A4-triggered phagocytosis did not provoke IL-8 or MCP-1 release. Lipoxin A4-induced phagocytosis was attenuated by anti-CD36, $\alpha vb3$ and CD18 antibodies. Compounds such as lipoxin A4 may provide the basis for a new class of anti-inflammatory compounds which promote macrophage clearance of neutrophils from inflammatory sites.

11.12 Role in the response to environmental particles

Chronic inhalation of various dusts can cause a variety of lung disorders. The inhalation of coal dust (Schins and Borm, 1999), for example, can cause chronic bronchitis, lung function loss, simple coal workers pneumoconiosis (CWP), progressive massive fibrosis (PMF) and emphysema. Macrophages and neutrophils are the key inflammatory cells in such disorders with the release of cytokines, ROIs and growth factors. In vitro and *in vivo* studies with coal dusts have shown the up-regulation of important leukocyte-recruiting factors such as MCP-1, LTB4, PDGF and TNF-α, as well as CD54 (ICAM-1). Coal dust particles are also known to stimulate macrophage production of various factors, with the potential capacity to modulate lung cells and/or extracellular matrix, including ROIs, fibroblast chemoattractants (PDGF, TGF-β and fibronectin) and a number of factors that have been shown to influence fibroblast growth and collagen production such as PDGF, insulin-like growth factor, TNF-α, TGF-β and PGE2. Asbestosis is a diffuse pulmonary fibrotic process caused by the inhalation of asbestos fibers (Kamp and Weitzman, 1997) but the precise mechanisms regulating asbestos-induced lung damage are not fully understood. Once again, the physical properties of the fibers, iron-catalyzed ROIs, and macrophage-derived cytokines and growth factors appear to be important.

11.13 Role in gene therapy

There is considerable interest in the use of gene therapy to modify macrophages for the treatment of tumors (and other diseases) as the use of activated macrophages in the treatment of cancer has been largely ineffectual. By providing these cells with the ability to express a therapeutic gene, there may be significant benefits in the efficacy of this approach (see Chapter 15 for information on the potential uses of macrophages in gene therapy). A hypoxia-regulated adenoviral vector (Griffiths *et al.*, 2000) has been employed to transduce human macrophages with either a reporter or a therapeutic gene encoding human cytochrome P450 2B6 (CYP2B6). Infiltration of transduced macrophages into a tumor spheroid results in induction of gene expression and significant tumor cell killing in the presence of cyclophosphamide. This offers the hope of targeting tumors via hypoxia-regulated gene expression. Other workers (Kluth *et al.*, 2000) have demonstrated gene transfer into inflamed glomeruli using macrophages transfected with adenovirus with encouraging results. Retrovirally mediated IFN-β transduction (Cremer *et al.*, 2000) of macrophages induces resistance to HIV, and this correlates with up-regulation of RANTES production and down-regulation of C-C chemokine receptor-5 expression.

Gene insertion has also been employed to study pluripotent hematopoietic stem cells (Faust *et al.*, 2000) and the events that occur during their differentiation. In a novel approach, myelomonocytic cells were labeled with green fluorescent protein (GFP) *in vivo*. This was achieved by knocking the enhanced GFP (EGFP) gene into the murine lysozyme M (lys) locus and using a targeting vector which contained a neomycin resistance gene flanked by LoxP sites. This allowed analysis of the blood and bone marrow and differentiation of multipotent progenitors, and may provide models for the accurate analysis of macrophage differentiation and function.

12 Summary

The macrophage is the major differentiated cell of a phylogenetically primitive system of cells termed the mononuclear phagocyte system. In adult man, macrophages originate in the bone marrow but become widely distributed throughout the body, being particularly prominent in the lymph nodes and spleen, liver, lungs, gastrointestinal tract, serous cavities, bone, synovium, skin and CNS. Once thought of as solely phagocytic, it is now known that they have many important and diverse functions. They have a prominent role in defense against many infectious agents and, following attraction to an infected focus by chemoattractants, they remain there under the influence of migration inhibition factors. After arrival at the infected focus, the macrophage may phagocytose the infectious agent and kill it by a variety of mechanisms. Macrophages also play an important role in inducing and regulating the immune response, by taking up protein antigens and generating immunogenic fragments from them which may be used to activate T cells (see Chapter 3). Macrophages frequently are found to infiltrate tumors and they may form an important mechanism of host defense against the tumor cell, either inhibiting tumor cell division or killing the cells following secretion of soluble mediators (see Chapter 11). Macrophages are known to secrete a large number of other substances *in vitro* though the physiological significance is sometimes uncertain. However, some appear to have a role in the induction of the acute phase response, regulation of hematopoiesis, cleansing and healing of injured tissue, clearance of apoptotic cells, regulation of hemostasis as well as a role in the pathogenesis of atherosclerosis (see Chapter 12), autoimmune (Chapter 8) and CNS diseases (Chapter 13). The more that is learned of macrophage biology, the more remarkable and fundamental this group of cells appear to be.

Acknowledgments

The authors would like to thank A. Ross, MRC Human Genetics Unit and J. Spencer, Department of Dermatology, Royal Infirmary, Edinburgh for help with the electron micrographs. Work in the author's (J.A.R.) laboratory is supported by the BBSRC, Wellcome Trust and by the CSO.

References

Adams D.O. and Hamilton, T.A. (1984). The cell biology of macrophage activation. *Annual Review of Immunology*, **2**, 283–318.

Adams, D.O. and Hamilton, T.A. (1988). Phagocytic cells. Cytotoxic activities of macrophages. In Galin, J.I., Goldstein, I.M. and Snyderman, R. (ed.), *Inflammation Basic Principles and Clinical Correlates*. Raven Press, New York, pp. 471–92.

Adams, D.O., Hall, T., Steplewski, Z. and Koprowski, H. (1984). Tumours undergoing rejection induced by monoclonal antibodies of the IgG_{2a} isotype contain increased numbers of macrophages activated for a distinctive form of antibody-dependent cytolysis. *Proceedings of the National Academy of Science USA*, **81**, 3506–10.

Aderem, A. and Underhill, D.M. (1999). Mechanisms of phagocytosis in macrophages. *Annual Review of Immunology*, **17**, 593–623.

Akira, S. (1997). IL-6-regulated transcription factors. *International Journal of Biochemistry and Cell Biology*, **29**, 1401–8.

Akira, S. (2000). The role of IL-18 in innate immunity. *Current Opinion in Immunology*, **12**, 59–63.

Alpers, C.E., Magil, A.B. and Gown, A.M. (1989). Macrophage origin of the multinucleated cells of myeloma cast nephropathy. *American Journal of Clinical Pathology*, **92**, 662–5.

Anderson, J.M. (2000). Multinucleated giant cells. *Current Opinion in Hematology*, **7**, 40–47.

Aschoff, L. (1924). Das reticulo-endotheliale system. *Ergeb. Inn. Med. Kinderheilkd.*, **26**, 1–118.

Assoian, R.K., Fleurdelys, B.E., Stevenson, H.C., Miller, P.J., Madtes, D.K., Raines, E.W. *et al.* (1987). Expression and secretion of type β transforming growth factor by activated human macrophages. *Proceedings of the National Academy of Sciences USA*, **84**, 6020–4.

Auger, M.J. and Mackie, M.J. (1987). Monocyte procoagulant activity in breast cancer. *Thrombosis Research*, **47**, 77–84.

Auger, M.J. and Mackie, M.J. (1988). Haemostasis in malignant disease. *Journal of the Royal College of Physicians London*, **22**, 74–9.

Babior, B.M. (1984). The respiratory burst of phagocytes. *Journal of Clinical Investigation*, **73**, 599–601.

Bacon, K.B., Greaves, D.R., Dairaghi, D.J. and Schall, T.J. (1998). The expanding universe of C, CX3C and CC chemokines. In Thomson, A. (ed.), *The Cytokine Handbook*, 3rd edn. Academic Press, San Diego, pp. 753–75.

Bae, Y.S., Kim, Y., Kim, Y., Kim, J.H., Suh, P.G. and Ryu, S.H. (1999). Trp-Lys-Tyr-Met-Val-D-Met is a chemoattractant for human phagocytic cells. *Journal of Leukocyte Biology*, **66**, 915–22.

Balsinde, J., Balboa, M.A. and Dennis, E.A. (2000). Identification of a third pathway for arachidonic acid mobilization and prostaglandin production in activated P388D1 macrophage-like cells. *Journal of Biological Chemistry*, **275**, 22544–9.

Barclay, A.N and Brown, M.H. (1997). *The Leucocyte Antigens FactsBook*, 2nd edn. Academic Press, San Diego.

Bar-Or, A., Oliveira, E.M., Anderson, D.E. and Hafler, D.A. (1999). Molecular pathogenesis of multiple sclerosis. *Journal of Neuroimmunology*, **100**, 252–9.

Behre, G., Zhang, P., Zhang, D.E. and Tenen, D.G. (1999). Analysis of the modulation of transcriptional activity in myelopoiesis and leukemogenesis. *Methods*, **17**, 231–7.

Beilmann, M., Vande Woude, G.F., Dienes, H.-P. and Schirmacher, P. (2000). Hepatocyte growth factor-stimulated invasiveness of monocytes. *Blood*, **95**, 3964–9.

Berger, E.A., Murphy, P.M. and Farber, J.M. (1999). Chemokine receptors as HIV-1 coreceptors: roles in viral entry, tropism, and disease. *Annual Review of Immunology*, **17**, 657–700.

Berken, A. and Benacerref, B. (1966). Properties of antibodies cytophilic for macrophages. *Journal of Experimental Medicine*, **123**, 119–44.

Beutler, B. (2000). Tlr4: central component of the sole mammalian LPS sensor. *Current Opinion in Immunology*, **12**, 20–6.

Bevilacqua, M.P., Pober, J.S., Majeau, G.R., Cotran, R.S. and Gimrone, M.A. (1984). Interleukin 1 induces biosynthesis and cell surface expression of procoagulant activity in human vascular endothelial cells. *Journal of Experimental Medicine*, **160**, 618–21.

Blick, M., Sherwin, S.A., Rosenblum, M. and Gutterman, J. (1987). Phase I study of recombinant tumour necrosis factor in cancer patients. *Cancer Research*, **47**, 2986–9.

Bonney, R.J. and Davies, P. (1984). Possible autoregulatory functions of the secretory products of mononuclear phagocytes. *Contempary Topics in Immunobiology*, **14**, 199–223.

Borland, G., Ross, J.A. and Guy, K. (1998). Forms and functions of CD44. *Immunology*, **93**, 139–48.

Bowen, M.A. and Aruffo, A. (1999). Adhesion molecules, their receptors, and their regulation: analysis of CD6-activated leukocyte cell adhesion molecule (ALCAM/CD166) interactions. *Transplantation Proceedings*, **31**, 795–6.

Brade, V. and Bentley, C. (1980). Synthesis and release of complement components by macrophages. In van Furth, R. (ed.), *Mononuclear Phagocytes: Functional Aspects*. Martinus Nijhoff, Boston.

Bresnihan, B. (1999). Pathogenesis of joint damage in rheumatoid arthritis. *Journal of Rheumatology*, **26**, 717–9.

Brown, C.C. and Gallin, J.I. (1988). Chemotactic disorders. In Curnutte, J.T. (ed.), *Hematology/Oncology Clinics of North America. Phagocytic Defects. I. Abnormalities Outside of the Respiratory Burst*. W.B. Saunders Co., Philadelphia.

Buckley, P.J., Smith, M.R., Braverman, M.F. and Dickson, S.A. (1987). Human spleen contains phenotypic subsets of macrophages and dendritic cells that occupy discrete microanatomic locations. *American Journal of Pathology*, **128**, 505–20.

Cannistra, S.A., Rambaldi, A., Spriggs, D.R., Herrmann, F., Kufe, D. and Griffin, J.D. (1987). Human granulocyte–macrophage colony stimulating factor induces expression of the tumour necrosis factor gene by the U937 cell line and by normal human monocytes. *Journal of Clinical Investigation*, **79**, 1720–8.

Carpenter, G. (1987). Receptors for epidermal growth factor and other polypeptide mitogens. *Annual Reviews of Biochemistry*, **56**, 881–914.

Carson, W. and Caligiuri, M.A. (1998). Interleukin-15 as a potential regulator of the innate immune response. *Brazilian Journal of Medical and Biological Research*, **31**, 1–9.

Caux, C., Lebeque, S., Liu, Y.-J. and Banchereau, J. (1999). Developmental pathways of human myeloid dendritic cells. In Lotze, M. and Thomson, A.W. (ed.), *Dendritic Cells*. Academic Press, San Diego, pp. 63–92.

Cerami, A. and Beutler, B. (1988). The role of cachectin/TNF in endotoxic shock and cachexia. *Imunology Today*, **9**, 28–31.

Chantry, D., DeMaggio, A.J., Brammer, H., Raport, C.J., Wood, C.L., Schweickart, V.L. *et al.* (1998). Profile of human macrophage transcripts: insights into macrophage biology and identification of novel chemokines. *Journal of Leukocyte Biology*, **64**, 49–54.

Charriere, J. (1989). Immune mechanisms in autoimmune thyroiditis. *Advances in Immunology*, **46**, 263–334.

Chieftez, S., Weatherbee, J.A., Tsang, M.L.S., Anderson, J.K., Mole, J.E., Lucas, R. *et al.* (1987). The transforming growth factor-β system, a complex pattern of cross-reactive ligands and receptors. *Cell*, **48**, 409–15.

Cline, M.J., Lehrer, R.I., Territo, M.C. and Golde, D.W. (1978). Monocytes and macrophages: functions and diseases. *Annals of Internal Medicine*, **88**, 78–88.

Cohen, A.B. and Cline, M.J. (1971). The human alveolar macrophage: isolation, cultivation *in vitro*, and studies of morphologic and functional characteristics. *Journal of Clinical Investigation*, **50**, 1390–8.

Cohen, O.J., Kinter, A. and Fauci, A.S. (1997). Host factors in the pathogenesis of HIV disease. *Immunological Reviews*, **159**, 31–48.

Cohn, Z.A. (1968). The structure and function of monocytes and macrophages. *Adances in Immunology*, **9**, 163–214.

Cohn, Z.A. and Benson, B.A. (1965). The differentiation of mononuclear phagocytes: morphology, cytochemistry and biochemistry. *Journal of Experimental Medicine*, **121**, 153–70.

Coleman, D.L., Chodakewitz, J.A., Bartiss, A.H. and Mellors, J.W. (1988). Granulocyte–macrophage colony-stimulating factor enhances selective effector functions of tissue-derived macrophages. *Blood*, **72**, 573–8.

Cremer, I., Vieillard ,V. and De Maeyer, E. (2000). Retrovirally mediated IFN-β transduction of macrophages induces resistance to HIV, correlated with up-regulation of RANTES production and down-regulation of C-C chemokine receptor-5 expression. *Journal of Immunology*, **164**, 1582–7.

Cresswell, P. (1985). Intracellular class II HLA antigens are accessible to transferrin–neuraminadase conjugates internalised by receptor-mediated endocytosis. *Proceedings of the National Academy of Sciences USA*, **82**, 8188–92.

Crocker, P.R. and Gordon, S. (1985). Isolation and characterisation of resident stromal macrophages and haemopoietic cell clusters from mouse bone marrow. *Journal of Experimental Medicine*, **162**, 993–1014.

Cutolo, M. (1999). Macrophages as effectors of the immunoendocrinologic interactions in autoimmune rheumatic diseases. *Annals of the New York Academy of Sciences*, **22**, 32–41.

Daemen, T., Veninga, A., Roerdink, F.H. and Scherphof, G.L. (1989). Endocytic and tumoricidal heterogeneity of rat liver macrophage populations. *Sel. Cancer Ther.*, **5**, 157–67.

Dennis, L.H., Cohen, R.J. and Schachner, S.H. (1968). Consumptive coagulopathy in fulminant meningococcaemia. *Journal of the American Medical Association*, **205**, 183–5.

Dinarello, C.A. (1985). An update on human interleukin-1: from molecular biology to clinical relevance. *Journal of Clinical Immunology*, **5**, 287–97.

Dinarello, C.A. and Mier, J.W. (1987). Lymphokines. *New England Journal of Medicine*, **317**, 940–5.

Douglas, S.D. and Hassan, N.F. (1990). Morphology of monocytes and macrophages. In Williams, W.J., Beutler, E., Erslev, A.J. and Lichtman, M.A. (ed.), *Haematology*, 4th edn., pp. 858–68 McGraw-Hill.

Dustin, M.L., Rothlein, R., Bhan, A.K., Dinarello, C.A. and Springer, T.A. (1986). Induction by IL-1 and interferon-γ: tissue distribution, biochemistry and function of a natural adherence molecule (ICAM-1). *Journal of Immunology*, **137**, 245–54.

Edwards, R.L. and Rickles, F.R. (1984). Macrophage procoagulants. In Spaet T.H. (ed.), *Progress in Haemostasis and Thrombosis*, Vol. 7, pp. 183–209. Grune and Stratton, New York.

Edwards, R.L., Rickles, F.R. and Cronlund, M. (1981). Abnormalities of blood coagulation in patients with cancer. Mononuclear cell tissue factor generation. *Journal of Laboratory and Clinical Medicine*, **98**, 917–28.

Edwards, R.L., Levine, J.B., Green, R., Duffy, M., Mathews, E., Brande, W. *et al.* (1987). Activation of blood coagulation in Crohn's disease. Increased plasma fibrinopeptide A levels and enhanced generation of monocyte tissue factor activity. *Gastroenterology*, **92**, 329–37.

Egan, P.J. and Carding, S.R. (2000). Multiple, distinct pathways exist through which monocytes–macrophages can promote LDL oxidation. *Journal of Experimental Medicine*, **191**, 2145–58.

Elices, M.J., Osborn, L., Takada, Y., Crouse, C., Luhowskyj, S., Hemler, M.E. *et al.* (1990). VCAM-1 on activated endothelium interacts with the leucocyte integrin VLA-4 at a site distinct from the VLA-4/fibronectin binding site. *Cell*, **60**, 577–84.

Elsbach, P. and Weiss, J. (1988). Phagocytic cells: oxygen-independent antimicrobial systems. In Gallin, J.I., Goldstein, I.M. and Snyderman, R. (ed.), *Inflammation: Basic Principles and Clinical Correlates*, pp. 445–70. Raven Press, New York.

Essner, R., Rhoades, K., McBride, W.H., Morton, D.L. and Economou, J.S. (1989). IL-4 down regulates IL-1 and TNF gene expression in human monocytes. *Journal of Immunology*, **142**, 3857–61.

Fadok, V.A. (1999). Clearance: the last and often forgotten stage of apoptosis. *Journal of Mammary Gland Biology and Neoplasia*, **4**, 203–11.

Falconer, J.S., Fearon, K.C.H., Plester, C.E., Ross, J.A. and Carter, D.C. (1994a). Cytokines, the acute phase response, and resting energy expenditure in cachectic patients with pancreatic cancer. *Annals of Surgery*, **219**, 325–31.

Falconer, J.S., Ross, J.A. and Fearon, K.C.H. (1994b). A phase II study of γ-linolenic acid in pancreatic cancer and its effect on immune function and cytokine production. In Horrobin, D. (ed.), *New Approaches to Cancer Treatment*. Churchill-Livingstone, pp. 68–78.

Faust, N., Varas, F., Kelly, L.M., Heck, S. and Graf T. (2000). Insertion of enhanced green fluorescent protein into the lysozyme gene creates mice with green fluorescent granulocytes and macrophages. *Blood*, **96**, 719–26.

Fearon, D.T. and Collins, L.A. (1983). Increased expression of C3b receptors on polymorphonuclear leucocytes induced by chemotactic factors and by purification procedures. *Journal of Immunology*, **130**, 370–5.

Fearon, K.C.H., Barber, M.D., Falconer, J.S., McMillan, D.C., Ross, J.A. and Preston, T. (1998). Pancreatic cancer as a model: inflammatory mediators, the acute phase response and cancer cachexia. *World Journal of Surgery*, **23**, 584–8.

Feinman, R., Henriksen-De Stephano, D., Tsujimoto, M. and Vilcek, J. (1987). Tumour necrosis factor is an important mediator of tumour cell killing by human monocytes. *Journal of Immunology*, **138**, 635–40.

Fibbe, W.E., van Damme, J., Billiau, A., Goselink, H.M., van Eden, G., Voogt, P.J. *et al.* (1987). Interleukin-1 (IL-1) stimulates myeloid progenitor cells to proliferate in long term bone marrow cultures. *Blood*, **70** (Supplement 1), 172a.

Flanagan, A.M. and Lader, C.S. (1998). Update on the biologic effects of macrophage colony-stimulating factor. *Current Opinion in Hematology*, **5**, 181–5.

Gabig, T.G. and Babior, B.M. (1981). The killing of pathogens by phagocytes. *Annual Review of Medicine*, **32**, 313–26.

Gerrity, R.G. (1981). The role of the monocyte in atherogenesis. I. Transition of blood borne monocytes into foam cells in fatty lesions. *American Journal of Pathology*, **103**, 181–90.

Ghosh, S., May, M.J. and Kopp, E.B. (1998). NFkB and Rel proteins: evolutionarily conserved mediators of immune responses. *Annual Review of Immunology*, **16**, 225–60.

Ginsel, L.A., Onderwater, J.J.M., De Water, R., Block, J. and Daems, W.T. (1983). 5′ Nucleotidase activity in mouse peritoneal macrophages. *Histochemistry*, **79**, 295–309.

Godson, C., Mitchell, S., Harvey, K., Petasis, N.A., Hogg, N. and Brady, H.R. (2000). Cutting edge: lipoxins rapidly stimulate nonphlogistic phagocytosis of apoptotic neutrophils by monocyte-derived macrophages. *Journal of Immunology*, **164**, 1663–7.

Golde, D.W. and Groopman, J.E. (1990). Production, distribution and fate of monocytes and macrophages. In Williams, W.J., Beutler, E., Erslev, A.J. and Lichtman, M.A. (eds.), *Haematology*, 4th edn., pp. 869–73. McGraw-Hill.

Goldman, J.M. (1989). Granulocytes, monocytes and their benign disorders. In Hoffbrand, A.V. and Lewis, S.M. (ed.), *Postgraduate Haematology,* pp. 294–324. Heinemann Professional Publishing, Oxford.

Gonwa, T.A., Frost, J.P. and Karr, R.W. (1986). All human monocytes have the capability of expressing HLA-DQ and HLA-DP molecules on stimulation with interferon-γ. *Journal of Immunology*, **137**, 519–24.

Gonzalez-Amaro, R. and Sanchez-Madrid, F. (1999). Cell adhesion molecules: selectins and integrins. *Critical Reviews in Immunology*, **19**, 389–429.

Goodman, M.G., Chenoweth, D.E. and Weigle, W.O. (1982). Induction of interleukin 1 secretion and enhancement of humoral immunity by binding of human C5a to macrophage surface C5a receptors. *Journal of Experimental Medicine*, **156**, 912–7.

Gordon, S. (1978). Regulation of enzyme secretion by mononuclear phagocytes: studies with macrophage plasminogen activator and lysozyme. *Federation Proceedings*, **37**, 2754–8.

Gordon, S. (1999). Macrophage-restricted molecules: role in differentiation and activation. *Immunology Letters*, **65**, 5–8.

Gordon, S., Todd, J. and Cohn, Z.A. (1974). *In vitro* synthesis and secretion of lysozyme by mononuclear phagocytes. *Journal of Experimental Medicine*, **139**, 1228–48.

Gordon,S., Keshav,S. and Chung,L.P. (1988). Mononuclear phagocytes: tissue distribution and functional heterogeneity. *Current Opinion in Immunology*, **1**, 26–35.

Goyart, S.M., Ferrero, E., Rettig, W.J., Yenamandra, A.K., Obata, F. and Le Beau, M.M. (1988). The CD14 monocyte differentiation antigen maps to a region encoding growth factor receptors and receptors. *Science*, **239**, 497–500.

Gregory, C.D. (2000). CD14-dependent clearance of apoptotic cells: relevance to the immune system. *Current Opinion in Immunology*, **12**, 27–34.

Griffin, F.M., Jr, Griffin, J.A., Leider, J.E. and Silverstein, S.C. (1975). Studies on the mechanism of phagocytosis. I Requirements for circumferential attachment of particle-bound ligands to specific receptors on the macrophage plasma membrane. *Journal of Experimental Medicine*, **142**, 1263–82.

Griffin, F.M., Griffin, J.A. and Silverstein, S.C. (1976). Studies on the mechanism of phagocytosis. II The interaction of macrophages with anti-immunoglobulin IgG-coated bone marrow derived lymphocytes. *Journal of Experimental Medicine*, **144**, 788–809.

Griffiths, L., Binley, K., Iqball, S., Kan, O., Maxwell, P., Ratcliffe, P. *et al.* (2000). The macrophage—a novel system to deliver gene therapy to pathological hypoxia. *Gene Therapy*, **7**, 255–62.

Groh, V., Gadner, H., Radaszkiewicz, T., Rappersberger, K., Konrad, K., Wolff, K. *et al.* (1988). The phenotypic spectrum of histiocytosis X cells. *Journal of Investigative Dermatology*, **90**, 441–7.

Guan, J.-L. and Hynes, R.O. (1990). Lymphoid cells recognise an alternatively spliced segment of fibronectin via the integrin receptor $\alpha_4\beta_1$. *Cell*, **60**, 53–61.

Guy, K., Ritchie, A.S. and van Heyningen, V. (1984). Anomalous expression of MHC class II antigens on human monocytes. *Disease Markers*, **2**, 283–5.

Guy, M. Chisolm, G.M., Hazen, S.L., Fox, P.L. and Cathcart, M.K. (1999). The oxidation of lipoproteins by monocytes–macrophages. Biochemical and biological mechanisms. *Journal of Biological Chemistry*, **274**, 25959–62.

Hamilton, J.A. (1997). CSF-1 signal transduction. *Journal of Leukocyte Biology*, **62**, 145–155.

Hanspal, M. (1997). Importance of cell–cell interactions in regulation of erythropoiesis. *Current Opinion in Hematology*, **4**,142–27.

Hart, S.P., Ross, J.A., Ross, K., Haslett, C. and Dransfield, I. (2000). Molecular characterisation of the surface of apoptotic neutrophils: implications for functional down-regulation and recognition by phagocytes. *Cell Death and Differentiation*, **7**, 493–503.

Hartmann, G. and Krieg, A.M. (1999). CpG DNA and LPS induce distinct patterns of activation in human monocytes. *Gene Therapy*, **6**, 893–903.

Hartwig, J.H. and Shelvin, P.A. (1986). The architecture of actin filaments and the ultrastructural location of actin binding protein in the periphery of lung macrophages. *Journal of Cell Biology*, **103**, 1007–20.

Haslett, C. (1999). Granulocyte apoptosis and its role in the resolution and control of lung inflammation. *American Journal of Respiratory and Critical Care Medicine*, **160**, S5–11.

Hayhoe, F.G.J. and Quaglino, D. (1988). *Haematological Cytochemistry*, 2nd edn. Churchill Livingstone, Edinburgh.

Heinrich, P.C. (1990). Interleukin-6 and the acute phase protein response. *Biochemical Journal*, **265**, 621–36.

Hemler, M.E. (1990). VLA proteins in the integrin family: structures, functions and their role on leucocytes. *Annual Review of Immunology*, **8**, 365–400.

Henson, P.M., Henson, J.E., Fittschen, C., Kimani, G., Bratton, D.L. and Riches, D.W.H. (1988). Phagocytic cells: degranulation and secretion. In Gallin, J.I., Goldstein, I.M. and Snyderman, R. (ed.), *Inflammation: Basic Principles and Clinical Correlates*, pp. 363–90. Raven Press, New York.

Herijgers, N., Van Eck, M., Korporaal, S.J.A., Hoogerbrugge, P.M. and Van Berkel, T.J.C. (2000). Relative importance of the LDL receptor and scavenger receptor class B in the β-VLDL-induced uptake and accumulation of cholesteryl esters by peritoneal macrophages. *Journal of Lipid Research*, **41**, 1163–71.

Hershko, C. (1977). Storage iron regulation. In Brown, E.B. (ed.), *Progress in Haematology*, Vol. X, pp. 105–48. Grune and Stratton, New York.

Hirsch, E., Katanaev, V.L., Garlanda, C., Azzolino, O., Pirola, L., Silengo, L. *et al.* (2000). Central role for G protein-coupled phosphoinositide 3-kinase g in inflammation. *Science*, **287**, 1049–53.

Hirsch, J.G. (1962). Cinemicrophotographic observations on granule lysis in polymorphonuclear leucocytes during phagocytosis. *Journal of Experimental Medicine*, **116**, 827–33.

Hocking, W.G. and Golde, D.W. (1979). The pulmonary alveolar macrophage. *New England Journal of Medicine*, **301**, 580 and 639.

Hogg, N. (1983). Human monocytes have prothrombin cleaving activity. *Clinical and Experimental Immunology*, **53**, 725–30.

Hourcade, D., Holers, V.M. and Atkinson, J.P. (1989). The regulators of complement activation (RCA) gene cluster. *Advances in Immunology*. **45**, 381–

Hume, D.A., Allan, W., Hogan, P.G. and Doe, W.F. (1987). Immunohistochemical characterisation of macrophages in the liver and gastrointestinal tract: expression of CD4, HLA-Dr, OKM1 and the mature macrophage marker 25F9 in normal and diseased tissue. *Journal of Leucokyte Biology*, **42**, 474–84.

Hume, D.A., Yue, X., Ross, I.L., Favot, P., Lichanska, A. and Ostrowski, M.C. (1997). Regulation of CSF-1 receptor expression. *Molecular Reproduction and Development*, **46**, 46–52.

Hutchins, D., Cohen, B.B. and Steel, C.M. (1990). Production and regulation of interleukin 6 in human B lymphoid cells. *European Journal of Immunology*, **20**, 961–8.

Ignotz, R.A. and Massague,J. (1987). Cell adhesion protein receptors as targets for transforming growth factor-β action. *Cell*, **51**, 189–97.

Jablons, D.M., McIntosh, J.K., Mule, J.J., Nordan, R.P., Rudikoff, S. and Lotze, M. (1989). Induction of interferon-β$_2$/interleukin-6 by cytokine administration and detection of circulating IL-6 in the tumour bearing state. *Annals of the New York Academy of Science*, **557**, 157–61.

Johnson, W.J., Pizzo, S.V., Imber, M.J. and Adams, D.O. (1982). Receptors for maleylated proteins regulate secretion of neutral proteases by murine macrophages. *Science*, **218**, 574–6.

Johnson, W.J., Steplewski, Z., Matthews, T.J., Hamilton, T.A., Koprowski, H. and Adams, D.O. (1986). Cytolytic interactions between murine macrophages, tumour cells, and monoclonal antibodies: characterization of lytic conditions and requirements for effector activation. *Journal of Immunology*, **136**, 4704–13.

Johnston, R.B. (1981). Enhancement of phagocytosis-associated oxidase metabolism as a manifestation of macrophage activation. *Lymphokines*, **3**, 33–56.

Johnston, G.I., Cook, R.G. and McEver, R.P. (1989). Cloning of GMP140, a granule membrane protein of platelets and endothelium: sequence similarity to proteins involved in cell adhesion and inflammation. *Cell*, **56**, 1033–44.

Jones, A.L. and Millar, J.L. (1989). Growth factors in haemopoiesis. In Gordon-Smith, E.C. (ed.), *Clinical Haematology: Aplastic Anaemia*. Vol.2, pp. 83–111. Bailliere Tindall, London.

Jones, G.E., Allen, W.E. and Ridley, A.J. (1998). The Rho GTPases in macrophage motility and chemotaxis. *Cell Adhesion and Communication*, **6**, 237–45.

Jones, J.L. and Walker, R.A. (1999). Integrins: a role as cell signalling molecules. *Molecular Pathology*, **52**, 208–13.

Kamp, D.W. and Weitzman, S.A. (1997). Asbestosis: clinical spectrum and pathogenic mechanisms. *Proceedings of the Society for Experimental Biology and Medicine*, **214**, 12–26.

Karnovsky, M.L. (1981). Metchnikoff in Messina: a century of studies on phagocytosis. *New
England Journal of Medicine*, **304**, 1178–80.

Kataria, Y.P. and Holter, J.F. (1997). Immunology of sarcoidosis. *Clinics in Chest Medicine*, **18**,
719–39.

Kay, M.M.B. (1975). Mechanism of removal of senescent cells by human macrophages *in situ*.
Proceedings of the National Academy of Sciences USA, **72**, 3521.

Kinet, J.-P. (1989). Antibody–cell interactions: Fc receptors. *Cell*, **57**, 351–4.

Kishimoto, T.K., Larson, R.S., Corbi, A.L., Dustin, M.L., Staunton, D.E. and Springer, T.A. (1989).
The leucocyte integrins. *Advances in Immunology*, **46**, 149–82.

Kishimoto, T., Kikutani, H., von der Borne, A.E.G., Kr., Goyert, S.M., Mason, D.Y., Miyasaka, M.
et al. (ed.) (1997). *Leucocyte Typing VI*. Garland Publishing Inc., New York.

Klebanoff, S.J. (1988). Phagocytic cells: products of oxygen metabolism. In Gallin, J.I., Goldstein,
I.M. and Snyderman, R. (ed.), *Inflammation: Basic Principles and Clinical Correlates*,
pp. 391–444. Raven Press, New York.

Kluth, D.C., Erwig, L.P., Pearce, W.P. and Rees, A.J. (2000). Gene transfer into inflamed glomeruli
using macrophages transfected with adenovirus. *Gene Therapy*, **7**, 263–70.

Knighton, D.R. and Fiegel, V.D. (1989). The macrophages: effector cell wound repair. *Progress in
Clinical and Biological Research*, **299**, 217–26.

Koeffler, H.P. and Golde, D.W. (1980). Human myeloid leukaemia cell lines: a review. *Blood*, **56**,
344–50.

Kurland, J.I., Bockman, R.S., Broxmeyer, H.E. and Moore, M.A.S. (1978). Limitation of excessive
myelopoiesis by the intrinsic modulation of macrophage-derived prostaglandin E. *Science*, **199**,
552–5.

Lasser, A. (1983). The mononuclear phagocyte system: a review. *Human Pathology*, **14**, 108–26.

Law, S.K.A. (1988). C3 receptors on macrophages. *Journal of Cell Science*, **9** (Suppl.), 67–97.

Lay, W.H. and Nussenzweig, V. (1968). Receptors for complement on leukocytes. *Journal of
Experimental Medicine*, **128**, 991–1009.

Lee, F.-Y.J., Li, Y., Yang, E.K., Yang, S.Q., Lin, H.Z., Trush, M.A. *et al*. (1999). Phenotypic abnormalities in macrophages from leptin-deficient, obese mice. *American Journal of Physiology*,
276, C386–94.

Lee, J.D., Swisher, S.G., Minehart, E.H., McBride, W.H. and Economou, J.S. (1990). Interleukin-4
downregulates interleukin-6 production in human peripheral blood mononuclear cells. *Journal
of Leukocyte Biology*, **47**, 475–9.

Lemasters, J.J. and Thurman, R.G. (1997). Reperfusion injury after liver preservation for transplantation. *Annual Reviews of Pharmacology and Toxicology*, **37**, 327–38.

Lewis, C.E., McCracken, D., Ling, R., Richards, P.S., McCarthy, S.P. and McGee, J.O'D. (1991).
Analysis of cytokine release at the single cell level: use of the reverse haemolytic plaque assay.
Immunological Reviews, **119**, 23–39.

Loike, J.P., Kozler, V.F. and Silverstein, S.C. (1979). Increased ATP and creatine phosphate turnover
in phagocytosing mouse peritoneal macrophages. *Journal of Biological Chemistry*, **254**,
9558–64.

Luster, A.D. and Rothenberg, M.E. (1997). Role of the monocyte chemoattractant protein and
eotaxin subfamily of chemokines in allergic inflammation. *Journal of Leukocyte Biology*, **62**,
620–33.

MacMicking, J., Xie, Q.-W. and Nathan, C. (1997). Nitric oxide and macrophage function. *Annual Review of Immunology*, **15**, 323–50.

Mahida,Y.R. (2000). The key role of macrophages in the immunopathogenesis of inflammatory bowel disease. *Inflammatory Bowel Diseases*, **6**, 21–33.

Majello, B., Arcone, R., Toniatto, C. and Ciliberto, G. (1990). Constitutive and IL-6-induced nuclear factors that interact with the human C-reactive protein promoter. *EMBO Journal*, **9**, 457–65.

Malkovsky, M. (1987). Recombinant IL-2 directly augments the cytotoxicity of human monocytes. *Nature*, **325**, 262–5.

Mangi, M.H. and Newland, A.C. (1999). Interleukin-3 in hematology and oncology: current state of knowledge and future directions. *Cytokines, Cellular and Molecular Therapy*, **5**, 87–95.

Marchalonis, J.J., Schluter, S.F., Bernstein, R.M., Shen, S. and Edmundson, A.B. (1998). Phylogenetic emergence and molecular evolution of the immunoglobulin family. *Advances in Immunology*, **70**, 417–506.

Massague, J. (1987). The TGF-β family of growth and differentiation factors. *Cell*, **49**, 437–8.

Matsuda, T., Suematsu, S., Kawano, M., Yoshizaki, K., Tang, B., Tanabe, O. *et al.* (1989). IL-6/BSF2 in normal and abnormal regulation of immune responses. *Annals of the New York Academy of Science*, **557**, 466–76.

McPhail, L.C. and Snyderman, R. (1983). Activation of the respiratory burst enzyme in human polymorphonuclear leucocytes by chemoattractants and other soluble stimuli: evidence that the same oxidase is activated by different transductional mechanisms. *Journal of Clinical Investigation*, **72**, 192–200.

Metcalf, D. (1971). Transformation of granulocytes to macrophages in bone marrow colonies *in vitro*. *Journal of Cell Physiology*, **77**, 277–80.

Metcalf, D. (1987). The molecular control of normal and leukaemic granulocytes and macrophages. *Proceedings of the Royal Society (Biology)*, **230**, 389–423.

Metchnikoff, E. (1905). *Immunity in Infective Disease*. Cambridge University Press.

Meuret, G. and Hoffmann, G. (1973). Monocyte kinetic studies in normal and disease states. *British Journal of Haematology*, **24**, 275–85.

Mikkelsen, H.B. and Thuneberg, L. (1999). Op/op mice defective in production of functional colony-stimulating factor-1 lack macrophages in muscularis externa of the small intestine. *Cell and Tissue Research*, **295**, 485–93.

Miller, L.L., Bly, C.G., Watson, M.L. and Bale, W.F. (1951). The dominant role of the liver in plasma protein synthesis. *Journal of Experimental Medicine*, **94**, 431–53.

Moore, M.A.S. and Metcalf, D. (1970). Ontogeny of the haemopoietic system: yolk sac origin of *in vivo* and *in vitro* colony forming cells in the developing mouse embryo. *British Journal of Haematology*, **18**, 279–96.

Moore, M.W., Carbone, F.R. and Bevan, M.J. (1988). Introduction of soluble protein into the class I pathway of antigen processing and presentation. *Cell*, **54**, 777–85.

Morrison, L.A., Lukacher, A.E., Braciale, V.L., Fan, D.P. and Braciale, T.J. (1986). Differences in antigen presentation to MHC class I- and class II-restricted influenza virus-specific cytolytic T lymphocyte clones. *Journal of Experimental Medicine*, **163**, 903–21.

Morrone, G., Ciliberto, G., Oliviero, S., Arcone, R., Dente, L., Content, J. and Cortese, R. (1988). Recombinant interleukin-6 regulates the transcriptional activation of a set of human acute phase genes. *Journal of Biological Chemistry*, **263**, 12554–8.

Motoyoshi, K. (1998). Biological activities and clinical application of M-CSF. *International Journal of Hematology*, **67**, 109–22.

Muller, W.A. and Randolph, G.J. (1999). Migration of leukocytes across endothelium and beyond: molecules involved in the transmigration and fate of monocytes. *Journal of Leukocyte Biology*, **66**, 698–704.

Munn, D.H., Garnick, M.B. and Cheung, N.-K.V. (1990). Effects of parenteral recombinant human macrophage colony-stimulating factor on monocyte number, phenotype, and antitumour cytotoxicity in nonhuman primates. *Blood*, **75**, 2042–8.

Murphy, G.F., Messadi, D., Fonferko, E. and Hancock, W.W. (1986). Phenotypic transformation of macrophages to Langerhans cells in the skin. *American Journal of Pathology*, **123**, 401–6.

Myers, M.A., McPhail, L.C. and Snyderman, R. (1984). Protein kinase C activity in human lymphocytes and monocytes: phorbol myristate acetate stimulation shifts activity from cytosol to membrane components. *Clinical Research*, **32**, 353A.

Nakagawara, A., Nathan, C.F. and Cohn, Z.A. (1981). Hydrogen peroxide metabolism in human monocytes during differentiation *in vitro*. *Journal of Clinical Investigation*, **68**, 1243–1252.

Nakstad, B., Lyberg, T., Skjorten, F. and Boye, N.P. (1989). Subpopulations of human alveolar macrophages: an ultrastructural study. *Ultrastructural Pathology*. **13**, 1–13.

Nathan, C.F. (1987). Secretory products of macrophages. *Journal of Clinical Investigation*, **79**, 319–26.

Nathan, C.F. and Root, R.K. (1977). Hydrogen peroxide release from mouse peritoneal macrophages. Dependence on sequential activation and triggering. *Journal of Experimental Medicine*, **146**, 1648–62.

Nathan, C.F., Murray, H.W. and Cohn, Z.A. (1980). The macrophage as an effector cell. *New England Journal of Medicine*, **303**, 622–6.

Nathan, C.F., Prendergast, T.J., Wiebe, M.E., Stanley, E.R., Platzer, E., Remold, H.G. *et al.* (1984). Activation of human macrophages: comparison of other cytokines with interferon-γ. *Journal of Experimental Medicine*, **160**, 600–5.

Nawroth, P.P. and Stern, D.M. (1986). Modulation of endothelial cell haemostatic properties by tumour necrosis factor. *Journal of Experimental Medicine*, **163**, 740–5.

Nemerson, Y. (1966). The reaction between bovine brain tissue factor and factor VII and X. *Biochemistry*, **5**, 601–8.

Nichols, B.A. and Bainton, D.F. (1973). Differentiation of human monocytes in bone marrow and blood: Sequential formation of two granule populations. *Laboratory Investigation*, **29**, 27–40.

Nishihira, J. (1998). Novel pathophysiological aspects of macrophage migration inhibitory factor. *International Journal of Molecular Medicine*, **2**, 17–28.

Nuchtern, J.G., Bonifacino, J.S., Biddison, W.E. and Klausner, R.D. (1989). Brefeldin A implicates egress from the endoplasmic reticulum in class I-restricted antigen presentation. *Nature*, **339**, 223–6.

Oikawa, T., Yamada ,T., Kihara-Negishi, F., Yamamoto, H., Kondoh, N., Hitomi, Y. *et al.* (1999). The role of Ets family transcription factor PU.1 in hematopoietic cell differentiation, proliferation and apoptosis. *Cell Death and Differentiation*, **6**, 599–608.

Oliff, A., Defoe-Jones, D., Boyer, M., Martinez, D., Kiefer, D., Vuocolo, G. *et al.* (1987). Tumours secreting human TNF/cachectin induce cachexia in mice. *Cell*, **50**, 555–63.

Oren, R., Franham, A.E., Saito, K., Milofsky, E. and Karnovsky, M.L. (1963). Metabolic patterns in three types of phagocytosing cells. *Journal of Cell Biology*, **17**, 487–501.

O'Riordain, M.G., Ross, J.A., Fearon, K.C.H., Maingay, J.P., Farouk, M., Garden, O.J. *et al.* (1995). Insulin and the counter-regulatory hormones influence acute phase protein production in the human hepatocyte. *American Journal of Physiology*, **269**, E323–30.

Osserman, E.F. (1975). Lysozyme. *New England Journal of Medicine*, **292**, 424–5.

Osterud, B. and Flaegstad, T. (1983). Increased tissue thromboplastin activity in monocytes of patients with meningococcal infection: related to an unfavourable prognosis. *Thrombosis and Haemostasis*, **49**, 5–7.

Page, R.C., Davies, P. and Allison, A.C. (1978). The macrophage as a secretory cell. *International Review of Cytology*, **52**, 119–57.

Panaro, M.A. and Mitolo, V. (1999). Cellular responses to FMLP challenging: a mini-review. *Immunopharmacology and Immunotoxicology*, **21**, 397–419.

Pantalone, R.M. and Page, R.C. (1975). Lymphokine-induced production and release of lysosomal enzymes by macrophages. *Proceedings of the National Academy of Sciences USA*, **72**, 2091–4.

Papadimitriou, J.M. and Ashman, R.B. (1989). Macrophages: current views on their differentiation, structure and function. *Ultrastructural Pathology*, **13**, 343–72.

Papadimitriou, J.M. and van Bruggen, I. (1986). Evidence that multinucleate giant cells are examples of mononuclear phagocyte differentiation. *Journal of Pathology*, **148**, 149–57.

Passlick,B., Flieger,D. and Loms Ziegler-Heitbrock, H.W. (1989). Identification and characteristics of a novel monocyte population in human peripheral blood. *Blood*, **74**, 2527–34.

Paul, W.E. and Ohara, J. (1987). B-cell stimulatory factor-1/interleukin 4. *Annual Review of Immunology*, **5**, 429–59

Pawlowski, N.A., Kaplan, G., Hamill, A.L., Cohn, Z.A. and Scott, W.A. (1983). Arachidonic acid metabolism by human monocytes. Studies with platelet-depleted cultures. *Journal of Experimental Medicine*, **158**, 393–412.

Peiper, S.C. and Guo, H.-H. (1997). CD33 workshop panel report: biochemical and genetic characterisation of gp67. In Kishimoto, T., Kikutani, H., von der Borne, A.E.G., Kr, Goyert, S.M., Mason, D.Y., Miyasaka, M. *et al.* (ed.), *Leucocyte Typing VI.*, pp. 972–4. Garland Publishing Inc., New York.

Pelus, L.M., Broxmeyer, H.E., Kurland, J.I. and Moore, M.A.S. (1979). Regulation of macrophage and granulocyte proliferation: specificities of prostaglandin E and lactoferrin. *Journal of Experimental Medicine*, **150**, 277–92.

Perry,V.H. and Gordon ,S. (1987). Modulation of CD4 antigens on macrophages and microglia in rat brain. *Journal of Experimental Medicine*, **166**, 1138–43.

Pestka, S., Langer, J.A., Zoon, K.C. and Samuel, C.E. (1987). Interferons and their actions. *Annual Review of Biochemistry*, **56**, 727–77.

Platt, N., da Silva, R.P. and Gordon, S. (1998). Recognizing death: the phagocytosis of apoptotic cells. *Trends in Cell Biology*, **8**, 365–72.

Platt, N., da Silva, R.P. and Gordon, S. (1999). Class A scavenger receptors and the phagocytosis of apoptotic cells. *Immunology Letters*, **65**, 15–9.

PROW (Protein Reviews on the Web). http://www.ncbi.nlm.nih.gov/prow/.

Prydz, H. and Allison, A. (1978). Tissue thromboplastin activity of isolated human monocytes. *Thrombosis and Haemostasis*, **39**, 582–91.

Qin, S., Cobbold, S., Benjamin, R. and Waldmann, H. (1989). Induction of classical tolerance in the adult. *Journal of Experimental Medicine*, **169**, 779–94.

Quesniaux, V.F.J. and Jones, T.C. (1998). Granulocyte–macrophage colony stimulating factor. In Thomson, A. (ed.), *The Cytokine Handbook*, 3rd edn. Academic Press, San Diego, pp. 635–70.

Reape, T.J. and Groot, P.H. (1999). Chemokines and atherosclerosis. *Atherosclerosis*, **147**, 213–25.

Ren, Y. and Savill, J. (1998). Apoptosis: the importance of being eaten. *Cell Death and Differentiation*, **5**, 563–8.

Rich, I.N. (1988). The macrophage as a production site for haematopoietic regulator molecules: sensing and responding to normal and pathophysiological signals. *Anticancer Research*, **8**, 1015–40.

Ricote, M., Huang, J.T., Welch, J.S. and Glass, C.K. (1999). The peroxisome proliferator-activated receptor (PPARg) as a regulator of monocyte/macrophage function. *Journal of Leukocyte Biology*, **66**, 733–9.

Rocklin, R.E., Benzden, K. and Greineder, D. (1980). Mediators of immunity: lymphokines and monokines. *Advances in Immunology*, **29**, 55–136.

Ross, J.A., Moses, A.G.W. and Fearon, K.C.H. (1999). Anti-catabolic effects of *n*-3 fatty acids. *Current Opinion in Clinical Nutrition and Metabolic Care*, **2**, 219–26.

Ross,R. (1987). Platelet-derived growth factor. *Annual Review of Medicine*, **38**, 71–79.

Rothlein, R., Dustin, M.L., Marlin, S.D. and Springer, T.A. (1986). A human intercellular adhesion molecule (ICAM-1) distinct from LFA-1. *Journal of Immunology*, **137**, 1270–4.

Rouzer, C.A., Scott, W.A., Kempe, J. and Cohn, Z.A. (1980). Prostaglandin synthesis by macrophages requires a specific receptor–ligand interaction. *Proceedings of the National Academy of Sciences USA*, **77**, 4279–82.

Sadahira, Y. and Mori, M. (1999). Role of the macrophage in erythropoiesis. *Pathology International*, **49**, 841–18.

Sammuelsson, B., Goldyne, M., Granstrom, E., Hamberg, M., Hammarstrom, S. and Malmsten, C. (1978). Prostaglandins and thromboxanes. *Annual Reviews of Biochemistry*, **47**, 997–1029.

Sandron, D., Reynolds, H.Y., Laval, A.M., Venet, A., Israel-Biet, D. and Chretein, J. (1986). Human alveolar macrophage subpopulations isolated on discontinuous albumin gradients: cytological data in normals and sarcoid patients. *European Journal of Respiratory Diseases*, **68**, 177–85.

Sangari, F.J., Parker, A. and Bermudez, L.E. (1999). *Mycobacterium avium* interaction with macrophages and intestinal epithelial cells. *Frontiers in Bioscience*, **15**, D582–8.

Sano, H., Nagai, R., Matsumoto, K. and Horiuchi, S. (1999). Receptors for proteins modified by advanced glycation endproducts (AGE)—their functional role in atherosclerosis. *Mechanisms of Ageing and Development*, **107**, 333–46.

Schiffmann, E., Corcoran, B and Wahl, S. (1975). *N*-Formylmethionyl peptides as chemoattractants for leucocytes. *Proceedings of the National Academy of Sciences USA*, **72**, 1059–62.

Schins, R.P. and Borm, P.J. (1999). Mechanisms and mediators in coal dust induced toxicity: a review. *Annals of Occupational Hygiene*, **43**, 7–33.

Schleimer, R. and Rutledge, B. (1986). Cultured human vasular endothelial cells acquire adhesiveness for neutrophils after stimulation with interleukin 1, endotoxin and tumour-promoting phorbol esters. *Journal of Immunology*, **136**, 649–54.

Schmalzl, F. and Braunsteiner, H. (1970). The cytochemistry of monocytes and macrophages. *Ser. Haematology*, **3**, 93–131.

Schutt, C. (1999). CD14. *International Journal of Biochemistry and Cell Biology*, **31**, 545–9.

Sechler, J. and Gallin, J.I. (1987). Recombinant g interferon is a chemoattractant for human monocytes. *Federation Proceedings*, **46** (abstract 5523).

Shapiro, S.D. (1999). The macrophage in chronic obstructive pulmonary disease. *American Journal of Respiratory and Critical Care Medicine*, **160**, S29–32.

Shirai, H., Murakami, T., Yamada, Y., Doi, T., Hamakubo, T. and Kodama T. (1999). Structure and function of type I and II macrophage scavenger receptors. *Mechanisms of Ageing and Development*, **111**, 107–21.

Shirai,T., Yamaguchi,H., Ito,H., Todd, C.W. and Wallace, R.B. (1985). Cloning and expression in *Escherichia coli* of the gene for tumour necrosis factor. *Nature*, **313**, 803–6.

Shurin, S.B. and Stossel, T.P. (1978). Complement (C3)-activated phagocytosis by lung macrophages. *Journal of Immunology*, **120**, 1305–12.

Sieff, C.A. (1987). Haematopoietic growth factors. *Journal of Clinical Investigation*, **79**, 1549–57.

Sinigaglia, F., D'Ambrosio, D., Panina-Bordignon, P. and Rogge, L. (1999). Regulation of the IL-12/IL-12R axis: a critical step in T-helper cell differentiation and effector function. *Immunological Reviews*, **170**, 65–72.

Sipe, J.D., Vogel, S.N., Ryan, J.L., McAdam, K.P.W.J. and Rosenstreich, D.L. (1979). Detection of a mediator derived from endotoxin stimulated macrophages that induces the acute phase serum amyloid A response in mice. *Journal of Experimental Medicine*, **150**, 597–606.

Siverstein, E., Friedland, J. and Setton, C. (1979). Angiotensin converting enzyme: induction in rabbit alveolar macrophages and human monocytes in culture. *Advances in Experimental and Medical Biology*, **121**, 149–56.

Smith, T.J. and Wagner, R.R. (1967). Rabbit macrophage interferons. I. Conditions for biosynthesis by virus-infected and uninfected cells. *Journal of Experimental Medicine*, **125**, 559–77.

Snyderman, R. and Fudman, E.J. (1980). Demonstration of a chemotactic factor receptor on macrophages. *Journal of Immunology*, **124**, 2754–7.

Snyderman, R. and Pike, M.C. (1984). Chemoattractant receptors on phagocytic cells. *Annual Review of Immunology*, **2**, 257–81.

Snyderman, R and Uhing, R.J. (1988). Phagocytic cells: stimulus–response coupling mechanisms. In Gallin, J.I., Goldstein, I.M. and Snyderman, R. (ed.), *Inflammation: Basic Principles and Clinical Correlates*, pp. 309–24. Raven Press, New York.

Snyderman, R., Phillips, J.K. and Mergenhagen, S.E. (1971). Biological activity of complement *in vivo*. Role of C5 in accumulation of polymorphonuclear leucocytes in inflammatory exudates. *Journal of Experimental Medicine*, **134**, 1131–43.

Snyderman, R., Pike, M.C., Edge, S. and Lane, B. (1984). A chemotactic receptor on macrophages exists in two affinity states regulated by guanine nucleotides. *Journal of Cell Biology*, **98**, 444–8.

Sokol, R.J. and Hudson, G. (1983). Disordered function of mononuclear phagocytes in malignant disease. *Journal of Cliical. Pathology*, **36**, 316–23.

Stahl, P.D. and Ezekowitz, R.A. (1998). The mannose receptor is a pattern recognition receptor involved in host defense. *Current Opinion in Immunology*, **10**, 50–5.

Stary, H.C. (1983). Macrophages in coronary artery and aortic intima and in atheroclerotic lesions of children and young adults up to age 29. In Schettler, G., Gotto, A.M., Middelhoff, G., Habenicht, A.S. and Jurutka, K.R. (ed.), *Atherosclerosis VI*, pp. 237–9. Springer-Verlag, Berlin.

Steinman, R.M., Mellman, J.S., Muller, W.A. and Cohn, Z.A. (1983). Endocytosis and the recycling of plasma membrane. *Journal of Cell Biology*, **96**, 1–27.

Stephens, R.W. and Golder, J.P. (1984). Novel properties of human monocyte plasminogen activator. *European Journal of Biochemistry*, **139**, 253–8.

Stephens, R.W., Golder, J.P., Fayle, D.R.H., Hume, D.A., Hapel, A.J., Allan, W. *et al.* (1985). Minactivin expression in human monocyte and macrophage populations. *Blood*, **66**, 333–7.

Steplewski, Z., Lubeck, M.D. and Koprowski, H. (1983). Human macrophages armed with murine immunoglobulin G2a antibodies to tumours destroy human cancer cells. *Science*, **221**, 865–7.

Stoppelli, M.P., Corti, A., Soffientini, A., Cassani, G., Blasi, F. and Assoian, R.K. (1985). Differentiation-enhanced binding of the amino-terminal fragment of human urokinase plasminogen activator to a specific receptor on U937 monocytes. *Proceedings of the National Academy of Sciences USA,* **82**, 4939–43.

Stossel, T.P. (1981). Actin filaments and secretion. The macrophage model. *Methods in Cell Biology,* **23**, 215–30.

Stossel, T.P. (1988). The mechanical responses of white blood cells. In Gallin, J.I., Goldstein, I.M. and Snyderman, R. (ed.), *Inflammation: Basic Principles and Clinical Correlates,* pp. 325–42. Raven Press, New York.

Stovroff, M.C., Fraker, D.L. and Norton, J.A. (1989). Cachectin activity in the serum of cachectic tumour-bearing rats. *Archives of Surgery,* **124**, 94–9.

Strunk, R.C., Whitehead, A.S. and Cole, F.S. (1985). Pretranslational regulation of the synthesis of the third component of complement in human mononuclear phagocytes by the lipid A portion of lipopolysaccharide. *Journal of Clinical Investigation,* **76**, 985–90.

Sung, S.S., Nelson, R.S. and Silverstein, S.C. (1983). Yeast mannans inhibit binding and phagocytosis of zymosan by mouse peritoneal macrophages. *Journal of Cell Biology,* **96**, 160–6.

Swope, M.D. and Lolis, E. (1999). Macrophage migration inhibitory factor: cytokine, hormone, or enzyme?. *Reviews of Physiology, Biochemistry and Pharmacology,* **139**, 1–32.

Tachikui, H., Kurosawa, N., Kadomatsu, K. and Muramatsu, T. (1999). Genomic organization and promoter activity of embigin, a member of the immunoglobulin superfamily. *Gene,* **240**, 325–32.

Taguchi, T. (1987). Clinical studies on recombinant human tumour necrosis factor. *Immunobiology,* **175**, 37.

Takenawa, T., Ishitoya, J. and Nagai, Y. (1986). Inhibitory effect of prostaglandin E2, forskolin and dibutyryl cAMP on arachidonic acid release and inositol phospholipid metabolism in guinea pig neutrophils. *Journal of Biological Chemistry,* **261**, 1092–8.

Talmadge, J.E., Phillips, H., Schneider, M., Rowe, T., Pennington, T., Bowersox, O. *et al.* (1988). Immunomodulatory properties of recombinant murine and human tumour necrosis factor. *Cancer Research,* **48**, 544–50.

Tamm, I. (1989). IL-6: current research and new questions. *Annals of the New York Academy of Sciences.* **557**, 478–89.

Tekamp-Olson, P., Gallegos, C., Bauer, D., McLain, J., Sherry, B., Fabre, M. *et al.* (1990). Cloning and characterisation of cDNAs for murine macrophage inflammatory protein 2 and its human homologues. *Journal of Experimental Medicine,* **172**, 911–9.

Thomas, E.D., Ramberg, R.E., Sale, G.E., Sparkes, R.S. and Golde, D.W. (1976). Direct evidence for a bone marrow origin of the alveolar macrophage in man. *Science,* **192**, 1016–8.

Tracey, K.J., Wei, H.E. and Manogue, K.R. (1988). Cachectin/tumour necrosis factor induces cachexia, anaemia and inflammation. *Journal of Experimental Medicine,* **167**, 1211–27.

Trepicchio, W.L. and Dorner, A.J. (1998). Interleukin-11. A gp130 cytokine. *Annals of the New York Academy of Sciences,* **856**, 12–21.

Trinchieri, G. and Perussia, B. (1983). Immune interferon: a pleitropic lymphokine with multiple effects. *Immunology Today,* **6**, 131–6.

Unkeless, J.C., Scigliono, E. and Freedman, V.H. (1988). Structure and function of human and murine receptors for IgG. *Annual Review of Immunology,* **6**, 251–81.

Valladeau, J., Ravel, O., Dezutter-Dambuyant, C., Moore, K., Kleijmeer, M., Liu, Y. *et al.* (2000). Langerin, a novel C-type lectin specific to Langerhans cells, is an endocytic receptor that induces the formation of Birbeck granules. *Immunity,* **12**, 71–81.

Valledor, A.F., Borras, F.E., Cullell-Young, M. and Celada, A.(1998). Transcription factors that regulate monocyte/macrophage differentiation. *Journal of Leukocyte Biology,* **63**, 405–17.

Van Dam-Mieras, M.C.E., Muller, A.D., van Deijk, W.A. and Hemker, H.C. (1985). Clotting factors secreted by monocytes and macrophages: analytical considerations. *Thrombosis Research*, **37**, 9–19.

van den Heuvel, M.M., Tensen, C.P., van As, J.H., Van den Berg, T.K., Fluitsma, D.M., Dijkstra, C.D. *et al.* (1999). Regulation of CD163 on human macrophages: cross-linking of CD163 induces signaling and activation. *Journal of Leukocyte Biology*, **66**, 858–66.

van Furth, R. (1988). Phagocytic cells: development and distribution of mononuclear phagocytes in normal steady state and inflammation. In Gallin, J.I., Goldstein, I.M. and Snyderman, R. (ed.), *Inflammation: Basic Principles and Clinical Correlates,* pp. 281–96 Raven Press, New York.

van Furth, R. (1989). Origin and turnover of monocytes and macrophages. *Current Topics in Pathology,* **79**, 125–50.

van Furth, R. and Cohn, Z.A. (1968). The origin and kinetics of mononuclear phagocytes. *Journal of Experimental Medicine*, **128**, 415–35.

van Furth, R. and Diesselhoff-den Dulk, M.M.C. (1970). The kinetics of promoncytes and monocytes in the bone marrow. *Journal of Experimental Medicine,* **132**, 813–28.

van Furth, R. and Sluiter, W. (1986). Distribution of blood monocytes between a marginating and a circulating pool. *Journal of Experimental Medicine*, **163**, 474–9.

van Furth, R., Cohn, Z.A., Hirsch, J.G., Humphry, J.H., Spector, W.G. and Langevoort, H.L. (1972). The mononuclear phagocyte system: a new classification of macrophages, monocytes and their precursor cells. *Bulletin of the World Health Organisation*, **46**, 845–52.

van Furth, R., Diesselhoff-den Dulk, M.M.C. and Mattie, H. (1973). Quantitative study on the production and kinetics of mononuclear phagocytes during an acute inflammatory reaction. *Journal of Experimental Medicine*, **138**, 1314–30.

van Furth, R., Diesselhoff-den Dulk, M.M.C., Raeburn, J.A., van Zwet, Th.L., Crofton, R. and Bluss van Oud Alblas, A. (1980). Characteristics, origin and kinetics of human and murine mononuclear phagocytes. In van Furth, R. (ed.), *Mononuclear Phagocytes. Functional Aspects,* pp. 279–98 Martinus Nijhoff Publishers, The Hague.

Vasta, G.R. Quesenberry, M., Ahmed, H. and O'Leary, N. (1999). C-type lectins and galectins mediate innate and adaptive immune functions: their roles in the complement activation pathway. *Developmental and Comparative Immunology*, **23**, 401–20.

Vazquez-Torres, A. and Balish, E. (1997). Macrophages in resistance to candidiasis. *Microbiology and Molecular Biology Review*, **61**, 170–92.

Vejlsgaard, G.L., Ralfkaier, E., Avnstrop, C., Czajkowski, M., Marlin, S.D. and Rothlein, R. (1989). Kinetics and characterisation of intercellular adhesion molecule-1 (ICAM-1) expression on keratinocytes in various inflammatory skin lesions and malignant cutaneous lymphoma. *Journal of the American Academy of Dermaology*, **20**, 782–90.

Ward, I., Dransfield , I., Chilvers, E.R., Haslett, C. and Rossi, A.G. (1999). Pharmacological manipulation of granulocyte apoptosis: potential therapeutic targets. *Trends in Pharmacological Sciences*, **20**, 503–9.

Warnke, R.A., Pulford, K.A., Pallesen, G., Ralfkiaer, E., Brown, D.C., Gatter, K.C. *et al.* (1989). Diagnosis of myelomonocytic and macrophage neoplasms in routinely processed tissue biopsies with monoclonal antibody KP1. *American Journal of Pathology*, **135**, 1089–95.

Weis, W.I., Taylor, M.E. and Drickamer, K. (1998). The C-type lectin superfamily in the immune system. *Immunological Reviews* **163**, 19–34.

Werb, Z. and Goldstein, I.M. (1987). Phagocytic cells: chemotactic and effector functionsof macrophages and granulocytes. In Stites, D.P., Stoba, J.D. and Wells, J.V. (ed.), *Basic and Clinical Immunology*, 6th edn. Appleton and Lange, Norwalk, pp. 96–113.

Werb, Z. and Gordon, S. (1975a). Secretion of a specific collagenase by stimulated macrophages. *Journal of Experimental Medicine*, **142**, 346–60.

Werb, Z. and Gordon, S. (1975b). Elastase secretion by stimulated macrophages: characterization and regulation. *Journal of Experimental Medicine*, **142**, 361–77.

Whaley, K. (1980). Biosynthesis of the complement components and the regulatory proteins of the alternative complement pathway by human peripheral blood monocytes. *Journal of Experimental Medicine*, **151**, 501–16.

Whaley, K., Lappin, D. and Barkas, T. (1981). C2 synthesis by human monocytes is modulated by a nicotinic cholinergic receptor. *Nature*, **293**, 580–3.

Whitelaw, D.M. (1966). The intravascular lifespan of monocytes. *Blood*, **28**, 445–64.

Wigmore, S.J., Fearon, K.C.H., Maingay, J.P., Lai, P.B.S. and Ross, J.A. (1997). Interleukin-8 can mediate acute phase protein production by isolated human hepatocytes. *American Journal of Physiology*, **273**, E720–6.

Wilson, E.L. and Francis, G.E. (1987). Differentiation-linked secretion of urokinase and tissue plasminogen activator by normal human haemopoietic cells. *Journal of Experimental Medicine*, **165**, 1609–23.

Wintergerst, E.S., Jelk, J. and Asmis R. (1998). Differential expression of CD14, CD36 and the LDL receptor on human monocyte-derived macrophages. A novel cell culture system to study macrophage differentiation and heterogeneity. *Histochemistry and Cell Biology*, **110**, 231–41.

Wissler, R.W., Vesselinovitch, D. and Davis, H.R. (1987). Cellular components of the progressive atherosclerotic process. In Olsson, A.G. (ed.), *Atherosclerosis. Biology and Clinical Science,* pp. 57–74. Churchill Livingstone.

Wood, G.W. and Gollahon, K.A. (1977). Detection and quantitation of macrophage infiltration into primary tumours with the use of cell surface markers. *Journal of the National Cancer Institute*, **59**, 1081–7.

Wuyts, A., Proost, P. and Van Damme, J. (1998). Interleukin-8 and other CXC chemokines. In Thomson, A. (ed.), *The Cytokine Handbook,* 3rd edn. Academic Press, San Diego, pp. 271–311.

Yam, L.T., Li, C.Y. and Crosby, W.H. (1971). Cytochemical identification of monocytes and granulocytes. *American Journal of Clinical Pathology*, **55**, 283–90.

Yewdell, J.W. and Bennik, J.R. (1989). Brefeldin A specifically inhibits presentation of protein antigens to cytotoxic T lymphocytes. *Science*, **244**, 1072–5.

Zhang, Y., Lin, J.-X., Yip, Y.K. and Vilcek, J. (1989). Stimulation of interleukin-6 mRNA levels by tumour necrosis factor and Interleukin-1. *Annals of the New York Academy of Sciences*, **557**, 548–9.

2 *Molecular basis of macrophage activation: from gene expression to phenotypic diversity*

T.A. Hamilton

1 Introduction

1.1 Concepts of macrophage activation

Mononuclear phagocytes represent a host-wide system of cells which provide a broad range of physiologically important services (Adams and Hamilton, 1984, 1992a; Nathan and Cohn, 1995; Van Rooijen *et al.*, 1996; Bosque *et al.*, 1997; Gordon, 1998). Not surprisingly, members of this cell system can exhibit a diverse array of characteristics. The mononuclear phagocyte lineage develops in the bone marrow and, following entry into the circulation, seeds essentially all tissues. Thus, under resting conditions, the differences between macrophages in different organ locations are likely to result from developmental signals encountered within individual tissue sites. Such differences are not the consequence of 'activation' as they reflect the specific physiology of each tissue and are stable over time. Examples of such developmentally distinct mononuclear phagocyte populations include microglia, Kupffer cells, splenic macrophages and the spectrum of myeloid dendritic cells.

In addition to these differentiated phenotypes, each macrophage can also change characteristics quite dramatically in response to stimuli encountered transiently in the tissue microenvironment (Adams and Hamilton, 1984, 1992a; Nathan and Cohn, 1995; Van Rooijen *et al.*, 1996; Bosque *et al.*, 1997; Gordon, 1998). This stimulus-induced acquisition of new functional capacities can be broadly defined as activation and generally serves the organism to restore pre-stimulus homeostatic balance. Some well-recognized examples of enhanced or altered functions which represent the consequences of macrophage activation include increased phagocytic capacity, enhanced cytokine and chemokine expression, acquisition of antimicrobial or antitumor functions, response to chemoattractant signals and both qualitative and quantitative modulation of the capacity to process or present specific antigens.

The activation of macrophages for enhanced function occurs within two broadly defined categories (Adams and Hamilton, 1984, 1992a; Hamilton, 1988). *Acute* changes utilize existing cellular structures, the activity of which can be triggered within seconds to minutes by rapidly engaged signaling pathways. Acute forms of macrophage activation include the generation of reactive oxygen species, the release of arachidonic acid and its metabolism, enhanced phagocytic activity and directed cell mobility. In contrast to acute changes, *adaptive* change requires modulation of gene expression and generally occurs over a period of hours to days. Though acute and adaptive changes may involve very different molecular events, both forms of activation may be initiated by the same stimulus and may share at least some components in the signal transduction pathways.

The adaptive forms of macrophage activation are determined largely by the modulation of gene expression (Adams and Hamilton, 1984; Ohmori and Hamilton, 1994b). These changes are initiated in response to a complex array of stimuli and involve multiple pathways of intracellular signal transduction. Though there are many extracellular stimuli, there are a limited number of intracellular signaling pathways which are commonly used by all cells to interpret changes in the environment. Furthermore, the relatively limited complexity of the signaling machinery must translate the extracellular stimulus complexity into even more diverse patterns of altered gene expression. This requirement for signal transduction using a limited alphabet defines a major problem in cell biology in general and in macrophage activation specifically; how does the cell integrate complex signals into well-orchestrated functional outcomes?

1.2 Scope of the chapter

In this chapter, I will first discuss the need for diversity in macrophage activity, the magnitude or extent of such diversity, its physiological relevance and the general mechanisms through which such diversity may be achieved. In the next sections, the major mechanistic determinants of macrophage activation will be considered. First, the spectrum of stimuli to which macrophages can respond will be presented in the context of three stages of response to injury and/or microbial challenge. Secondly, intracellular signaling pathways through which prototypic macrophage activating agents modulate cell behavior will be discussed. In the final section, the molecular mechanisms through which signaling molecules regulate gene expression will be described. This will include consideration of transcriptional initiation, stabilization of mRNA transcripts and translation of specific mRNA products.

2 Diversity in macrophage activation

2.1 Magnitude and physiology

A central function for the mononuclear phagocyte system is the provision of host defense against environmental challenge (Adams and Hamilton, 1992b; Nathan and Cohn, 1995). The scope of environmental threats is tremendously diverse and therefore requires cell-mediated protective functions which are not only diverse but subject to precise modulation based upon the specific circumstance. Thus the establishment of mechanisms for generating a diverse activation profile for mononuclear phagocytes was no doubt a high priority during the evolution of multicellular organisms, and the evolutionary age of the mononuclear phagocyte system serves as testimony to its central importance.

As the understanding of macrophage participation in response to microbial challenge and in immunoregulation has expanded, it has become clear that the diversity of functional states is extensive (Adams and Hamilton, 1992b; Hamilton *et al.*, 1992). Early models of macrophage activation were based upon the sequential acquisition of a particular functional competence (e.g. the ability to destroy microbes or tumor cells) (Adams and Hamilton, 1984, 1992b; Hamilton *et al.*, 1992). In concert with the discovery and classification of extracellular stimuli which can modulate the state of macrophage activity, a number of laboratories defined a two-stage model of activation (see Figure 2.1A) (Ruco and Meltzer, 1978; Russell *et al.*, 1978; Adams and Hamilton, 1984). The first stage was a priming signal [prototypically interferon-γ (IFN-γ)] which, though capable of inducing a number of changes, was insufficient to endow the responding cell with full functional competence. Exposure to a second triggering signal [lipopolysaccharide (LPS)] was sufficient to complete the functional activation process. These individual stages could be defined experimentally and linked with specific molecular correlates (Adams and Hamilton, 1984, 1992a,b). Roles for interleukin (IL)-4 and IL-10 in regulating pro-inflammatory responses to IFN-γ and LPS respectively were also incorporated into this concept. Though this model is still a useful predictive paradigm for macrophage activation, the dramatic increase in knowledge of extracellular stimulus complexity

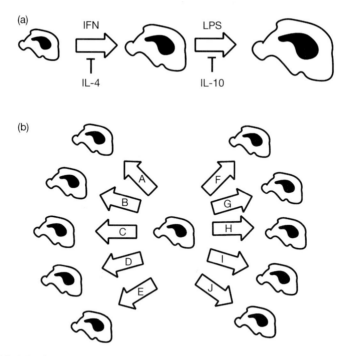

Fig. 2.1 Models of macrophage activation. (A) A classical model depicting the sequential linear response of macrophages to pro-inflammatory stimuli, prototypically IFN-γ and LPS. These agents are known to act cooperatively, and the sequence of stimulus exposure can alter qualitatively the subsequent response to a second stimulus. These prototypic pro-inflammatory responses can be blocked or diminished by the action of prototypic anti-inflammatory agents such as IL-4 and IL-10. This model is a useful predictor for patterns of response in general terms but cannot account for the diversity of macrophage phenotypic status when analyzed in molecular detail. (B) A model of macrophage activation depicting the potential diversity of phenotypic states which can be developed following exposure to a large number of agents. The number of individual phenotypic states will be a product of the number of genes which contribute and the freedom with which each can be expressed. The response will be influenced by the complexity of the stimulus pool found in the tissue microenvironment, the sequence of exposure and the state of macrophage differentiation at the time of exposure. Since many genes are regulated by similar (though distinguishable) mechanisms, patterns of response emerge which suggest coordinate control.

(including the range of cellular receptors through which they act) and in understanding the molecular pathways which regulate expression of individual genes compels consideration of the true potential for diversity in cellular activation responses.

Indeed, substantial diversity is observed routinely among different macrophage populations; both mononuclear phagocytes resident in tissues and those which enter tissues upon initiation of an inflammatory reaction exhibit many different levels of function (Van Rooijen *et al.*, 1996; Bosque *et al.*, 1997; Goerdt and Orfanos, 1999). The most obvious examples include pro-inflammatory versus anti-inflammatory phenotypes and, indeed, the concept of type I and type II immune response patterns has clear parallels in macrophage activation. Further diversity may be evident in the temporal sequence of an inflammatory reaction (e.g. recruitment of inflammatory cells, antimicrobial action, resolution of injury and repair of tissue) and each may involve the participation of mononuclear phagocytes

(Van Rooijen *et al.*, 1996; Bosque *et al.*, 1997; Goerdt and Orfanos, 1999). Thus the state of macrophage activation must be varied so as to provide an appropriate range of functions. A model more consistent with the observed diversity of activation-induced phenotypes is presented in Figure 2.1B where a macrophage may be induced by a multiple stimuli to develop a broad spectrum of functional capacities through selective control of the pattern of gene expression.

2.2 Generation of diversity

There undoubtedly are many different sources of diversity in macrophage functional activation (Adams and Hamilton, 1992a; Hamilton *et al.*, 1992). The following discussion will consider two features of the inflammatory response that contribute to such diversity and the general mechanisms through which they function. First, the stimulus composition of the extracellular microenvironment is highly complex and variable. Nevertheless, most studies of macrophage activation have considered the effects of an individual stimulus in isolation; this is, of course, not a natural circumstance and, indeed, the response to any particular agent may be modulated both qualitatively and quantitatively when it occurs in the context of other stimuli. The complexity of such response patterns will be increased markedly if both time and sequence of exposure are also considered. For example, it has been demonstrated in several laboratories that IL-4 can either inhibit or potentiate LPS-induced tumor necrosis factor (TNF) production depending upon the time of exposure to IL-4 and the IL-4/LPS exposure sequence (D'Andrea *et al.*, 1995).

A second contributing variable is the developmental state of the macrophage at the time of stimulation. Thus the different populations of macrophages found in different tissue and organ sites can exhibit very different patterns of response to identical stimulatory conditions (McCormack *et al.*, 1992; Walker *et al.*, 1995; Askew *et al.*, 1996). The variable response is likely to result from alterations in the composition of signaling components in the cell; a given cell will be predisposed for response to a particular stimulus/receptor pair with a subset of possible downstream endpoints.

Both of these determinants of diverse response (stimulus complexity and the state of macrophage differentiation) function through the ability of the cell to transduce the extracellular signal into modulated gene expression. The number and variety of stimulus/receptor combinations which impinge on mononuclear phagocytes in the course of host defense function is large. The complexity and repertoire of biological responses which occur as a consequence of ligand receptor engagement is, however, substantially larger (perhaps by as much 10- to 100-fold) (Adams and Hamilton, 1992a). The mechanisms involved in transducing extracellular signals and regulating gene expression provide several mechanistic opportunities to achieve this expansion. First, it is clear that a single stimulus/receptor pair can initiate signals through more than one pathway and these pathways may operate at least partially independently. Secondly, there are multiple opportunities for cross-talk between pathways, thus providing some restriction on independence but greatly increasing the potential for one stimulus to modify the response to a second stimulus. Thirdly, most signaling pathways involve cascades which are composed of multiple sequential stages and, at each stage, there may be multiple options. Finally, the expression of genes is controlled at multiple levels (e.g. transcription, post-transcription and translation), and at each stage multiple regulatory sequences may provide the opportunity for linkage with a variety of upstream signaling pathways. When these variables are assembled in combinatorial fashion, the potential number of distinct endpoints becomes remarkably large.

3 Initiating stimuli in macrophage activation

3.1 Categories of stimuli

The modulation of macrophage function serves many different physiological goals and the number of different physiological/pathophysiological conditions in which macrophages may respond to transient signals is correspondingly large. Thus a detailed presentation of macrophage-activating stimuli covering this topic is clearly beyond the scope of this chapter. Rather, the following discussion will arbitrarily separate signals which initiate macrophage activation into three distinct categories based upon the temporal sequence of a prototypic response to injury: these include (1) early injury and chemotaxis; (2) response to microbial invasion; and (3) the interface between macrophages and lymphocytes in the development of acquired immunity. The discussion will focus on well-studied examples of macrophage stimulation; there are many additional forms of stimulation which will not be discussed but which are, nevertheless, important determinants of macrophage function.

3.2 Early injury and chemotaxis

From the perspective of mononuclear phagocytes, the immediate response to tissue injury will result in several important forms of stimulation. Chemotactic agents are likely to be the initial form of stimulus encountered by macrophages entering sites of tissue injury, and these materials will promote the directed migration of macrophages through the endothelium and into the tissue. The spectrum of biological products which are capable of stimulating chemotaxis in inflammatory leukocytes is remarkably diverse. Perhaps the first chemoattractants generated during injury are proteolytic fragments of the coagulation and complement fixation cascades (Goldstein, 1992). For example, the C5a complement fragment exhibits potent chemoattractant activities for both neutrophils and macrophages. Multiple members of the chemokine gene family will also be induced. This family includes more than 50 individual members, many of which target monocytes and macrophages (Rollins, 1997; Baggiolini, 1998; Luster, 1998). Following extravasation from the circulation, macrophages may encounter one or both of the pro-inflammatory cytokines TNF and/or IL-1 which are often produced and released rapidly upon tissue injury (Luster, 1998). For example, in the skin, IL-1α is stored in inactive form in epidermal keratinocytes and, upon injury, may flood the surrounding tissue (Camp *et al.*, 1990; Wood *et al.*, 1996). Both IL-1α and IL-1β are also produced *de novo* in resident tissue cells during this phase. These broad-acting agents will in turn stimulate other cells, including macrophages, to produce additional cytokines and chemokines. TNF, IL-1 and chemoattractants can all induce the release and metabolism of arachidonic acid (Davies and MacIntyre, 1992; Lam and Austen, 1992). Stimulated phospholipase A2 activity releases arachidonic acid from membrane phospholipids providing the primary substrate for cyclooxygenases and lipooxygenases. The spectrum of archidonate metabolites is quite large, and both chemoattractant as well as suppressive functions are commonly ascribed to these substances.

The receptors involved in mediating the response to most chemoattractants are members of the G-protein-coupled receptor (GPCR) family (Snyderman and Uhing, 1992; Rollins, 1997; Baggiolini, 1998; Luster, 1998). This gene family contains more than 1000 members which serve a remarkably broad range of physiological roles (Baldwin, 1994; Strader *et al.*, 1995). In macrophages and other inflammatory leukocytes, these receptors frequently not only are coupled to chemotaxis but also signal the production of reactive oxygen intermediates and degranulation (Snyderman and Uhing, 1992). While the intracellular signaling events linked with GPCRs can impact on gene expression, most GPCR-initiated responses can be categorized as acute or immediate and do not depend upon alterations in gene expression. There are two receptors for TNF (TNFR1 and TNFR2) which are members of a larger gene family; these ligands are coupled with both pro-inflammatory and apoptotic responses (Tartaglia *et al.*, 1991; Smith *et al.*, 1994). While there are two defined IL-1 receptors (IL-1R1 and IL-1R2), only the type 1 receptor is able to signal; the type 2 receptor appears to serve as a decoy (Auron, 1998; Dinarello, 1998; O'Neill and Greene, 1998). The IL-1R1 is a member of the Toll-like receptor (TLR) family, the founding member of which (TOLL) was identified in *Drosophila* and functions in embryogenesis as well as host defense in the adult (Gay and Kubota, 1996; O'Neill and Greene, 1998; Rock *et al.*, 1998).

3.3 Microbial stimuli

The most intensely studied macrophage-activating stimulus is LPS, a structurally heterogeneous material which marks the cell wall of Gram-negative bacteria (Morrison and Ryan, 1979; Ulevitch and Tobias, 1999). LPS is recognized by multicellular organisms as a molecular correlate of Gram-negative bacterial invasion and is capable of promoting a very vigorous inflammatory response in which mononuclear phagocytes play a central role (Adams and Hamilton, 1992b; Hamilton *et al.*, 1993). LPS and other bacterial products induce a complex array of responses including the expression of many new genes encoding chemokines and cytokines which collectively amplify the response by recruitment of additional inflammatory cells. These secondary products also provide complex immunoregulatory function and promote a broad array of antimicrobial activities. Though there are many variants of LPS in the bacterial world, the primary structure recognized is a membrane-active lipid in which the diacylglycerol backbone has been substituted with a diacylglucosamine (Morrison and Ryan, 1979; Ulevitch and Tobias, 1999). This structure, termed lipid A, can reproduce virtually the full spectrum of biological responses seen with intact LPS. The mononuclear phagocyte system also recognizes a wide variety of additional structures which are found associated with various potentially pathogenic microbes. These include peptidoglycans, lipotechoic acid, lipoarabinomannan and others (Weidemann *et al.*, 1997; Underhill *et al.*, 1999; Yoshimura *et al.*, 1999). Though most of these agents produce similar dramatic changes in macrophage gene expression, each individual agent can have distinct characteristics.

Despite intense study, knowledge of responses to microbial stimuli in molecular terms remains limited. Collectively, many of the proteins which participate in host recognition of microbial invasion are termed pattern recognition receptors (Krieger, 1997; Fraser *et al.*, 1998; Medzhitov and Janeway, 1998). There appear to be at least three functional stages which, in combination, provide high sensitivity and precise selectivity in the recognition of and response to bacterial products. The first stage involves high-affinity recognition and binding of bacterial products such as LPS by secreted recognition proteins whose elevated expression following injury or infection constitute a portion of the acute phase response (Fenton and Golenbock, 1998; Tapping *et al.*, 1998; Tobias *et al.*, 1999). These include such products as LPS-binding protein (LBP) and C-reactive protein. Soluble complexes composed of host protein and bacterial product can bind with one or more cell surface pattern recognition protein which serves to concentrate the microbial stimulus on the cell surface. Prototypic of this second stage is CD14, a glycolipid-anchored surface protein with specificity for lipid A but which does not itself trigger a response (Kielian and Blecha, 1995; Ulevitch and Tobias, 1995, 1999; Tobias *et al.*, 1999). Other pattern recognition receptors which may also participate in this stage of recognition include the integrin CD18/CD11b, the mannose receptor and various members of the scavenger receptor families (Krieger, 1997; Fraser *et al.*, 1998; Medzhitov and Janeway, 1998). The third stage involves delivery of bacterial product to one or more signaling proteins. This last group includes at least two members of the TLR gene family (Medzhitov and Janeway, 1998; O'Neill and Greene, 1998; Poltorak *et al.*, 1998; Underhill *et al.*, 1999; Yoshimura *et al.*, 1999). TLRs are now known to confer selective sensitivity to LPS and other bacterial cell wall products, and detailed knowledge of the signaling pathways is now emerging (O'Neill and Greene, 1998). While all three stages of microbial recognition by macrophages are important, all three may not be essential for response. Indeed, mice in which genes for either LBP or CD14 have been deleted retain some, albeit reduced, sensitivity to LPS (Wurfel *et al.*, 1997; Fenton and Golenbock, 1998; Haziot *et al.*, 1998; Vogel *et al.*, 1998). In contrast, deletion of the *TLR4* gene produces complete loss of LPS sensitivity, indicating that the last of the three recognition stages is absolutely required (Poltorak *et al.*, 1998). Nevertheless, this multiple-stage combinatorial process provides the host with high sensitivity and selectivity such that a limited number of receptors can produce broad but highly precise recognition and response.

3.4 Macrophages and acquired immunity

The acquired immune response requires days to develop as compared with the minutes or hours associated with early injury and microbe-driven responses (Medzhitov and Janeway, 1998). The participation of lymphocytes in host defense often occurs under circumstances where other mechanisms have already failed. The proper development and resolution of the antigen-specific immune response is a highly complex process involving multiple cell types and a nearly bewildering array of secreted regulatory molecules. Members of the mononuclear phagocyte lineage are important participants in this process: macrophage products induced by injury and in response to microbial stimuli help to promote the development of an acquired immune response, and macrophages are the frequent target of natural killer (NK)-, T and B cell-derived lymphokines. The latter serve to modulate macrophage responses in either pro- or anti-inflammatory directions.

The pro-inflammatory and anti-inflammatory aspects of macrophage activation reflect macrophage participation in immune-mediated injury through the well accepted paradigm of type I and type II T cell-mediated immune responses (O'Garra and Murphy, 1996; Mosmann and Sad, 1996; Romagnani, 1997). Type I and type II responses have clear parallels in macrophage activation; pro-inflammatory macrophage-activating agents promote a macrophage phenotype which supports Th1 cell development while anti-inflammatory agents are comparably linked to the type II response (O'Garra and Murphy, 1996; Goerdt and Orfanos, 1999). While these categories of response have often been referred to as either stimulatory or suppressive, the responses are indeed multifactorial and more recently have been termed classical (stimulatory) and alternative (suppressive) macrophage activation (Gordon *et al.*, 1995; Gordon, 1998; Goerdt and Orfanos, 1999). Thus, in a *classical* activation pattern, macrophages produce products which drive type I responses such as IL-12, while type I T and NK cell products such as IFN-γ, IL-2, TNF-α, leukotriene (LT)-α and LT-β, CD40 and IL-18 can act on macrophages to enhance this pattern of response further. In contrast, IL-4, released by subsets of NK cells, mast cells and type II T cells, not only diminishes the ability of LPS-stimulated macrophages to further the type I response but also promotes a pattern of activation that helps to drive a type II T-cell response. *Alternative* activation responses can be induced by type II lymphokines in addition to IL-4 including IL-13, IL-5 and IL-10. Interestingly, in the same way that IL-4 can diminish macrophage responses to IFN-γ and other type I lymphokines, IFN-γ has comparable suppressive activity targeting the alternative response patterns induced by IL-4 (Fenton *et al.*, 1992; Dickensheets and Donnelly, 1997, 1999). While early responses in host defense function may be appropriately pro-inflammatory, later events must promote the resolution of inflammation and restoration of normal tissue integrity and thus might be predicted to exhibit anti-inflammatory character.

Most cytokine responses are mediated by cytokine family receptors (CFRs) (Goodwin *et al.*, 1994; Ihle *et al.*, 1995, 1998; Onishi *et al.*, 1998). Cytokine receptors occur as monomers, homodimers, heterodimers and as oligomeric structures containing three distinct subunits. Some subunits are found as components of multiple distinct receptors. For example, the GP130 chain is involved in receptors for IL-6, incostatin M, leukemia inhibitory factor (LIF) and others, while the common γ-chain participates in receptors mediating response to IL-2, IL-4, IL-7 and IL-15. Members of the TNF receptor family, discussed above, are also important participants in immune-driven macrophage responses.

4 Intracellular signaling pathways in macrophage activation

The current state of our descriptive knowledge of receptor-coupled signaling pathways is extensive, and a full discussion is clearly beyond the scope of this chapter. It is important, however, to appreciate mechanisms through which different stimuli and their cognate receptor/signaling pathways interact to provide the complexity which leads to biological diversity. In the following section, signaling events associated with four sets of prototypic ligand–receptor pairs involved in macrophage activation will be considered. These will include chemoattractant/GPCR signaling, TNF receptor signaling, LPS/TLR signaling and signaling initiated by CFRs. A summary of basic signaling components which have been associated with each of these ligand–receptor systems are outlined in Figure 2.2. Two important concepts are apparent in this comparison. First, each stimulus can initiate multiple signaling pathways at the same time, thereby creating the opportunity for linking stimuli with more than one functional endpoint. Secondly, though each receptor system contains some unique features, there are also often shared components. This is particu-

G Protein Coupled Receptors	Toll-Like Receptors	TNF Receptors	Cytokine Family Receptors

Trimeric G proteins (αβγ)
  Phospholipases (A,C,D)
  adenylyl cyclase
  phosphodiesterase
  PI3K
Small GTPases
  Rho, Rac, cdc42
MAPKKK, PKc
MAPKK
MAPK (ERK,JNK,p38)
	MYD88, IL-1RacP,RAS
	IRAK
	TRAF6
	NIK, RAF,MAPKKK
	IKK, MAPKK
	IκB, MAPK (ERK, JNK, p38)
		TRADD, RIP,FADD,(TNFR1)
		TRAF1,2 (TNFRII)
		TRAF6
		NIK, MAPKKK
		IKK, MAPKK
		IκB, MAPK (JNK, p38)
			JAK, IRS1,2
			STAT,PI3K
			RAF,MAPKKK
			MAPKK
			MAPK (ERK,JNK, p38)

Fig. 2.2   Signaling pathways in macrophage activation. The signaling events which are likely to participate in macrophage responses to four prototypic extracellular stimuli are presented. These include G-protein-coupled chemoattractant receptors, TNF receptors, Toll-like receptors and cytokine family receptors. While each class of receptor can signal through pathways which are at least partially unique, there is substantial use of common signaling components. This overlap provides the opportunity for diverse groups of extracellular stimuli to initiate intracellular signaling sequences which communicate with each other and create potential for remarkable diversity in the biological response.

larly notable with respect to the mitogen-activated protein (MAP) kinase pathways which participate in all of the receptor systems under consideration. This feature provides a direct opportunity for cross-talk between receptor systems and may also provide the means to introduce specificity into individual responses.

4.1 Chemoattractant signaling

GPCRs are linked to the broadest spectrum of signaling pathways and functional outcomes (Baldwin, 1994; Murphy, 1994; Gilman, 1995; Strader *et al.*, 1995; Post and Brown, 1996). GPCRs couple through interaction with a trimeric G-protein complex which is regulated by ligand-dependent GTP binding and hydrolysis. These receptors have been clearly linked with activation of phospholipases which catalyze phospholipid hydrolysis. Products of phospholipase action can directly mediate intracellular Ca^{2+} mobilization and secondary activation of several multimember protein kinase families including protein kinase B and protein kinase C (Nishizuka, 1995; Nakamura, 1996). In addition, GPCRs are able, by modulating adenylate cyclase or cyclic nucleotide phosphodiestersase activities, to enhance or diminish the activities of the cyclic nucleotide-dependent protein kinase A (Gilman, 1995). GPCRs are also now well recognized to activate MAP kinases, including the extracellular signal-regulated kinases (ERKs), ERK1 and ERK2 (p44 and p42, respectively); stress-activated protein kinases (SAPKs, also termed Jun N-terminal kinase or JNK); and members of the p38 kinase family. These enzyme systems, collectively termed the MAP kinases, are all regulated through at least a three-stage cascade. The terminology for the first stage is the MAP kinase kinase kinase (MAPKKK) which phosphorylates the second stage (MAPKK) which in turn targets the third stage (MAPK). At each stage, there are multiple members which exhibit relatively restricted specificity for their immediate downstream substrate. Recent data indicate that the stimulation of the ERK kinases is mediated by both α- and β/γ-subunits of the primary coupling G-protein and involves activation of phosphatidylinositol 3-kinase (PI3K), and functional association among adaptor proteins including Shc, Grb2 and Sos. SAPKs/JNKs and p38 are activated through G-protein β/γ-subunits and involve intermediate small GTP-binding proteins including RhoA, Rac1 and Cdc42 (Lopez-Ilasaca, 1998; Dikic and Blaukat, 1999).

4.2 TNF receptor signaling

Though there are multiple receptors in the TNF receptor family, the prototypes are TNFR1 and TNFR2 (Tartaglia *et al.*, 1991; Smith *et al.*, 1994). These receptors are known to both produce pro-inflammatory responses and initiate apoptosis; TNFR1 can signal both endpoints while TNFR2 is most frequently linked with the pro-inflammatory response (Grell *et al.*, 1994; Baker and Reddy, 1998; Natoli *et al.*, 1998; Warzocha and Salles, 1998). The two receptors use distinct signaling pathways though both involve a cascade of protein–protein interactions which ultimately link to several different protein kinase systems (Darnay and Aggarwal, 1997; Malek *et al.*, 1998; Natoli *et al.*, 1998; Warzocha and Salles, 1998; Wajant *et al.*, 1999). The intracellular domain of the TNFR1 contains a protein–protein interaction sequence region termed the death domain which initiates signal transduction through interaction with a series of adaptor proteins which also contain the death domain (Schulze-Osthoff *et al.*, 1998). The most thoroughly studied include TRADD, FADD/Mort1 and RIP; TRADD can signal both inflammation (NF-kB activation) and apoptosis, FADD signals exclusively apoptosis and RIP is most potent in activation of NF-kB. The determination of outcome will be influenced by the abundance of each component in a particular cell type. TNFR2 utilizes a different protein–protein interaction domain which signals through a separate family of adaptor proteins known as the TNF receptor-associated factors (TRAFs) which includes at least six members (Darnay and Aggarwal, 1997; Wajant *et al.*, 1999). TRAFs 1 and 2 are responsible for TNFR2 signaling and can also participate with TNFR1 (by interaction with TRADD or RIP). TRAFs can couple to MAPKKKs including NF-kB-inducing kinase (NIK). Either directly or indirectly, these enzyme systems can stimulate the IkB kinase complex (IKK), resulting in sequential phosphorylation, ubiquitination and proteosome-mediated degradation of IkBs and release of active NF-kB (Finco and Baldwin, 1995; Pahl and Baeuerle, 1996; Baichwal and Baeuerle, 1997; Ghosh *et al.*, 1998; May and Ghosh, 1998). TNF-α is well known to provide both life (pro-inflammatory) and death (apoptosis) signals; when both responses are intact, the apoptosis pathway is blocked, at least in part, by the NF-kB-dependent expression of anti-apoptotic gene products (Baichwal and Baeuerle, 1997). If the cell phenotype exhibits reduced NF-kB activation, the apoptosis pathways predominate. It is noteworthy that in mouse macrophages, stimuli which promote TNF expression also up-regulate the expression of TNFR2 which might serve to protect such cells from the autocrine/paracrine apoptotic effect (Tannenbaum *et al.*, 1993; Bethea *et al.*, 1997).

4.3 LPS/TLR signaling

Within the last 2 years, our understanding of intracellular signaling pathways coupled with LPS stimulation has progressed tremendously. This is a result of two important contributions. First was the identification of the Toll-like receptor (TLR) family based upon homology with the *Drosophila* TOLL protein (Gay and Kubota, 1996; O'Neill and Greene, 1998; Rock *et al.*, 1998). The second important finding was the demonstration that LPS sensitivity in mice was encoded in the *TLR4* gene (Poltorak *et al.*, 1998; Qureshi *et al.*, 1999). TLR2 has also been implicated in signaling from LPS and from a subset of other microbial products known to stimulate robust pro-inflammatory macrophage activation responses (Kirschning *et al.*, 1998; Lien *et al.*, 1999; Schwandner *et al.*, 1999; Takeuchi *et al.*, 1999). The first member of this family identified in vertebrates was IL-1 receptor type I (O'Neill and Greene, 1998). The predominant feature of the IL-1R1 and other TLR family members is a protein–protein interaction domain (Toll domain) which is essential for initiation of the signaling cascade following receptor aggregation (O'Neill and Greene, 1998). The TLR domain mediates binding of a second TLR domain-containing factor termed MYD88. Downstream sequential components include one or more members of the IL-1 receptor-associated kinase (IRAK) and TRAF6. The latter can couple with several protein kinase cascades including NIK and similar MAP kinase modules, RAS, RAF and downstream targets (Hambleton *et al.*, 1995, 1996; O'Neill and Greene, 1998). This divergence provides at least one opportunity for generating multiple, partially independent response pathways. NIK and potentially MAPK module components are able to activate the IkB kinase complex, leading to release of active NF-kB (May and Ghosh, 1998; O'Neill and Greene, 1998; Wajant *et al.*, 1999). These protein kinase cascades no doubt lead to the activation of multiple additional factors which regulate the process of gene expression by both transcriptional and post-transcriptional mechanisms. Many components of the IL-1 signaling pathway are shared, with TNF-initiated events accounting for the substantial overlap in functional responses to these two agents.

4.4 Cytokine family receptor signaling

The central signaling pathways utilized by CFRs have been well characterized over the last 6–8 years (Ihle, 1996; Darnell, 1997; Horvath and Darnell, 1997; Stark *et al.*, 1998; Ihle *et al.*, 1998). These receptors depend upon protein tyrosine phosphorylation but possess no inherent kinase activity. Instead they initiate signaling through utilization of a distinct family of non-receptor protein tyrosine kinases (the Janus or JAK kinases) which phosphorylate one or more members of the signal transducing and activator of transcription (STAT) family. Phosphorylated STATs can dimerize (predominantly as homodimers) and, via mechanisms not fully understood, translocate to the nucleus where they can bind to cognate nucleotide sequence motifs in target genes and modulate transcription. There are four members of the JAK family and seven members of the STAT family which collectively serve to mediate responses through more than 20 distinct cytokine ligand–receptor pairs. Utilization of both JAK kinases and STATs is generally promiscuous and thus our understanding of the determinants of specificity in response to cytokine stimuli remains incomplete. IFN-γ is linked closely to STAT1, while STAT6 is the sole mediator of response to IL-4. In contrast, many other receptors have been shown to stimulate two or more STATs. In this regard, CFRs have also been shown to couple through additional pathways and these may provide the opportunity for cytokines to initate multiple independent signaling routes and/or for specific modulation of responses involving common JAKS and STATs. For example, CFRs are known to link with the insulin receptor substrates (IRS), RAS, RAF and PI3 kinase and to signal selectively to subsets of the MAP kinase modules, one or more isoforms of protein kinase C, and to protein kinase B (White, 1996; Stancato *et al.*, 1997; Uddin *et al.*, 1997; Goh *et al.*, 1999; Kovarik *et al.*, 1999). The molecular details of such coupling and the physiological significance of each remain to be fully appreciated.

5 Regulation of gene expression

Many stimuli induce changes in cell function which do not require new gene expression, and such responses utilize pre-existing cell components and systems. In contrast, altering the pattern of macrophage gene expression provides a means to tailor precisely the cell's function to new environmental circumstances and is the mechanistic foundation for induced activation (Adams and Hamilton, 1984, 1992a; Hamilton, 1988). The control of gene expression is a product of the interaction between two molecular structures: (1) regulatory nucleotide sequences encoded within the non-expressed and expressed portions of the genome; and (2) proteins which recognize such regulatory sequences. The regulatory sequences in the genome serve as the final interpreter of the signaling cascades initiated by extracellular stimulation. Proteins which recognize regulatory sequence are often the final substrates of signaling pathways involving protein phosphorylation, and such modification endows them with new functional potential. These proteins fall into a variety of functional categories including transcription factors as well as factors regulating mRNA stability and/or translation. These multiple stages in the process of gene expression can each be an important determinant of the final macrophage phenotype. The following sections will discuss mechanisms through which prototypic macrophage-activating agents modulate gene expression by altering the frequency of transcriptional initiation, the stability of mature cytoplasmic mRNAs and their translation.

5.1 Transcription

5.1.1 Basic mechanisms

The transcriptional activity of a gene is controlled by assembly of the RNA polymerase complex at sites immediately upstream of the transcription start site (Isner and Dietz, 1988; Ogbourne and Antalis, 1998; Tsuruta *et al.*, 1998; Huang *et al.*, 1999). This appears to be a process which is regulated by the activity of transcription factors which can recognize and bind to precise nucleotide sequences in the promoters of target genes. The mechanisms by which transcription factors function are only now being elucidated in biochemical terms but are likely to involve opening the chromatin structure through the action of histone acetyltransferases and/or deacetylases thereby altering chromatin structure and access to transcription start sites (Grunstein, 1997; Ogbourne and Antalis, 1998; Struhl, 1998; Davie and Spencer, 1999). Sequences which provide such regulatory function are often 10–15 nucleotides in length and generally serve to provide high-affinity specific binding sites for cognate transcription factors. Individual transcription factor families often contain multiple members, and the individual isoforms may exhibit variable recognition of and function through corresponding sites. Furthermore, there often is functional diversity within the collection of sequences recognized by individual members of a particular transcription factor family. Inducible genes are often regulated by multiple sequence motifs arranged within their promoter regions. Though the binding of an individual transcription factor may produce some change in transcription initiation, the combination of multiple factors simultaneously binding to a collection of sites is often necessary for optimal transcriptional activity. The assembly of several regulatory sequence motifs within a promoter can provide further opportunity for differential control of gene expression. Indeed inflammatory gene expression in macrophages may be regulated by a small number of regulatory sequence/transcription factors pairs that can,

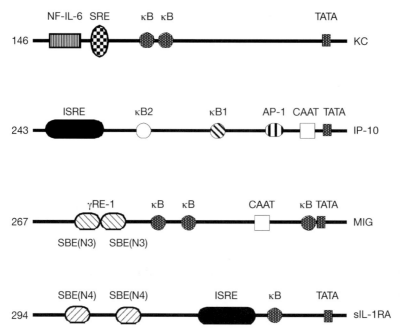

Fig. 2.3 Gene promoters exhibit stimulus-specific sensitivity through multiple regulatory sequence motifs. The regulatory sequence motifs found in four prototypic gene promoters are depicted. These include the promoters for the IP-10, MIG, IRF-1 and soluble IL-1 receptor antagonist genes. Each promoter contains a selection of functional sequence elements which serve as the binding sites for stimulus-sensitive transcription factors. Combinatorial use provides for differential gene sensitivity where each stimulus may initiate the activation of a distinct collection of transcription factors. Thus fine specificity control of inflammatory gene expression is achieved.

through variable combinatorial action, differentially control many individual genes (Ernst and Smale, 1995). Transcriptional initiation of one gene may also depend upon the sequential activation of other genes which themselves encode transcription factors. This provides for the important feature of temporal control. The following paragraphs will describe transcriptional mechanisms operating in macrophages stimulated with LPS, IFN-γ and IL-4. In addition, the routes through which these agents may act in synergistic or antagonistic fashion will be presented. In Figure 2.3, the promoters for four inflammation-associated genes (KC, IP-10, MIG and sIL-1Ra) are shown. The array of regulatory sites within each promoter and their use to control transcription serve to illustrate the concepts described above and in the following sections.

5.1.2 LPS-stimulated transcription

LPS and other comparable bacterial products, acting through one or more TLRs, can stimulate multiple transcription factors via distinct signaling pathways (Hamilton *et al.*, 1993; Hamilton and Ohmori, 1996; Sweet and Hume, 1996). The prototypic transcription factor associated with inflammatory responses is NF-kB (Ghosh *et al.*, 1998). The kB sequence motif originally was identified as a regulator of k immunoglobulin light chain gene transcription in B lymphocytes and is now recognized as a critical determinant of inflammatory responses in many cell types (Ghosh *et al.*, 1998; May and Ghosh, 1998).

kB sites are important determinants of transcriptional control in many genes but their function can be variable. For example, activation of NF-kB by TNF, IL-1 or LPS is sufficient to stimulate strong expression of the *KC* gene but only low level transcription of the *IP-10* gene. Though the *MIG* promoter has NF-kB sites which are important in cooperative function, NF-kB activation alone has no effect on *MIG* gene transcription (T.A. Hamilton, unpublished) (see Figure 2.3).

NF-kBs are homo- or heterodimers composed of one or more members of the Rel homology family, which, following release from a cytoplasmic inhibitor, IkB, freely translocate to the nucleus (Finco and Baldwin, 1995; Pahl and Baeuerle, 1996; May and Ghosh, 1998). The activity of NF-kB is controlled not only through interaction with IkBs but also by serine phosphorylation sites probably located within the transactivation domain (Ghosh *et al.*, 1998). LPS is also known to modulate transcription through the action of other factors including members of the AP-1 (fos/jun heterodimers) and c/EBP families (Hamilton *et al.*, 1993; Hamilton and Ohmori, 1996; Sweet and Hume, 1996). Both of these events are probably controlled through the action of the JNK and p38 kinase pathways. Recently, several laboratories have also demonstrated a role for Sp1, best known as a regulator of constitutive gene transcription, in LPS-dependent transcriptional regulation (Bethea *et al.*, 1997; Brightbill *et al.*, 2000).

LPS is known to induce expression of multiple cytokine genes in macrophages, and the autocrine role of these products has been recognized for some time. Indeed, a substantial subset of genes described as LPS-inducible (including *IP-10*) are, in fact, secondary products of LPS-induced type I IFN production (Pace *et al.*, 1985; Hattori *et al.*, 1996; Tebo *et al.*, 1998). In addition to pro-inflammatory cytokines, LPS also induces the expression of the anti-inflammatory cytokine IL-10 which may serve as a negative feedback circuit to limit macrophage inflammatory function (Barsig *et al.*, 1995; Brightbill *et al.*, 2000).

5.1.3 IFN-γ-stimulated transcription

IFN-γ was identified as the principle form of macrophage-activating factor (MAF) in 1984 and is now known to control transcription of a variety of genes associated with a type I or pro-inflammatory response in macrophages (Farrar and Schreiber, 1993; Schreiber *et al.*, 1983; Adams and Hamilton, 1984; Ohmori and Hamilton, 1994b). Indeed, though virtually all cells are responsive to IFN-γ, its activity on macrophages may represent one of its more important effector functions in immunoregulation (Vilcek *et al.*, 1985; Young and Hardy, 1995; Boehm *et al.*, 1997; Stark *et al.*, 1998). IFNg-regulated genes involve at least three kinds of sites (Decker *et al.*, 1997; Stark *et al.*, 1998). The first group are those recognized by STAT1 α, the primary direct signaling mediator and transcription factor activated by IFN-γ (Decker *et al.*, 1997). The *MIG* gene promoter contains two tandemly arrayed STAT1 α-binding elements (SBEs) which together are termed the γRE, and this site is necessary though perhaps not sufficient for optimal MIG transcription (Wong *et al.*, 1994; Ohmori and Hamilton, 1998). The second group of sites are those recognized by members of the IRF family of transcription factors (ISREs, IREs). Included within this group is the type I IFN-stimulated gene factor 3 (ISGF3) which is composed of STAT1, STAT2 and p48 (an IRF-1 family member) (Stark *et al.*, 1998). The IFN-responsive site in the IP-10 promoter is an ISRE and provides opportunity for both IFN-γ and IFN-α/β to drive transcription; this feature distinguishes the IFN sensitivity of the *IP-10* and *MIG* genes (Ohmori and Hamilton, 1993, 1995, 1998).

Another IRF family member, ICSBP, is expressed exclusively in macrophages and mediates both positive and negative responses to IFN-γ (Driggers *et al.*, 1990; Scharton-Kersten *et al.*, 1997). Finally, class II major histocompatibility complex (MHC) expression is regulated uniquely through the concerted action of a set of constitutive DNA-binding factors which recognize the promoter sites and which are in turn bound by an inducible protein (class II transactivator, CIITA) (Ting and Baldwin, 1993; Wright *et al.*, 1998). The expression of CIITA, IRF-1 and ICSBP is regulated by IFN-γ through the action of STAT1 (Sims *et al.*, 1993; Politis *et al.*, 1994; Piskurich *et al.*, 1999).

5.1.4 IL-4-stimulated transcription

IL-4 has emerged as one of the prototypic lymphokines responsible for alternative macrophage activation (Stein *et al.*, 1992; Gordon, 1998; Goerdt and Orfanos, 1999). IL-4 results in highly selective phosphorylation, dimerization and nuclear translocation of STAT6 (Kotanides and Reich, 1993; Hou *et al.*, 1994; Mikita *et al.*, 1996). Interestingly, STAT6 exhibits the broadest specificity among the STATs in nucleotide sequence recognition (Schindler *et al.*, 1995; Seidel *et al.*, 1995). While most STATs bind only nine nucleotide sites (TTCNNNGAA) containing three unspecified intervening nucleotides (N3 sites), STAT6 can bind N3 sites as well as those containing an additional nucleotide in the central core (TTCNNNNGAA) (N4 sites). Despite this broad binding specificity, STAT6 transactivates only genes containing N4 sites (Schindler *et al.*, 1995; Seidel *et al.*, 1995; Ohmori *et al.*, 1996). The promoter of the secreted form of the IL-1Ra gene contains a tandem pair of N4 sites; while both bind STAT6, only the more distal site is required for the transcriptional response to IL-4 (Figure 2.3) (Ohmori *et al.*, 1996). As with other genes, the induction of sIL-1Ra expression is enhanced cooperatively by other transcription factors which function through interaction with their own cognate sites (Gravallese *et al.*, 1991). As IL-13 shares receptor components with IL-4 and is also a potent activator of STAT6, these two cytokines exhibit extensive overlap in the patterns of inducible gene expression (Cash *et al.*, 1994; D'Andrea *et al.*, 1995; Lefort *et al.*, 1995).

5.1.5 Mechanisms for positive and negative cooperativity

Functional cooperativity between IFN-γ and LPS, TNF or IL-1 is well recognized and is mediated at least in part through the modulation of gene transcription (Johnson and Pober, 1994; Ohmori and Hamilton, 1995; Marfaing-Koka *et al.*, 1995; Warfel *et al.*, 1995; Ohmori *et al.*, 1997). Indeed, the expression of a gene in response to either agent alone is often modest while the response to the combination may be enhanced 20–100 times over the additive effects. This synergistic phenomenon depends upon the presence of binding sites for both NF-kB and STAT1 within the gene promoter (Ohmori and Hamilton, 1995; Ohmori *et al.*, 1997). Indeed, the expression of both IP-10 and MIG involves such cooperativity between the IFN-responsive factor-bindings sites (either ISRE or gRE) and the NF-kB-binding sites (Ohmori and Hamilton, 1995; Ohmori *et al.*, 1997; T.A. Hamilton and Y. Ohmori, unpublished) (see Figure 2.3). It is clear, however, that the magnitude of the cooperative effect is influenced by the sequence environment in individual promoters, and how the basic transcription machinery responds differentially to these factors when encountered in these different settings is not understood.

IL-4 (and IL-13) not only induces new gene expression but also suppresses responses to type I signals such as IFN-γ (Fenton *et al.*, 1992; Gautam *et al.*, 1992; Donnelly *et al.*,

1993; Herbert *et al.*, 1993; Deng *et al.*, 1994; D'Andrea *et al.*, 1995; Kambayashi *et al.*, 1996; Ohmori and Hamilton, 1997). This does not result from IL-4-mediated interference with IFN-γ-stimulated activation of STAT1 (Ohmori and Hamilton, 1997; Goenka *et al.*, 1999). Both stimulatory and suppressive functions of IL-4 depend on STAT6 (Kaplan *et al.*, 1996; Ohmori and Hamilton, 1997; Takeda *et al.*, 1997; Goenka *et al.*, 1999). The inhibitory activity of STAT6 may be related to its ability to bind N3-type nucleotide sequences without transactivating activity (Ohmori and Hamilton, 1997, 1998). Thus the nature of the transcriptional modulatory activity exhibited by IL-4 is determined by the specific sequence motifs with which STAT6 binds. Interestingly, IFN-γ can also antagonize the responses to IL-4 and IL-13, though this appears to involve a distinct mechanism where IFN-γ induces the expression of genes (suppressors of cytokine signaling or SOCS) whose products can inhibit the IL-4/IL-13 signaling pathway leading to the activation of STAT6 (Dickensheets and Donnelly, 1997, 1999; Dickensheets *et al.*, 1999).

5.2 mRNA stability

The control of mature mRNA stability in the cytosol is now recognized as an important site for stimulus-specific control of gene expression (Ross, 1995; Liebhaber, 1997). Though the mechanisms involved in regulating the post-transcriptional processing and transport of mRNA have been the subject of extensive study and are, at least theoretically, attractive targets for regulation of gene expression, little is known currently about their contribution to macrophage activation. The importance of mRNA decay was first appreciated mechanistically with the identification of sequence motifs in the 3′-untranslated region (3′-UTR) of mRNAs encoding growth factors and cytokines which were expressed rapidly but transiently following stimulation (Caput *et al.*, 1986; Shaw and Kamen, 1986). These sequences, most often composed of reiterated pentameric AUUUA motifs, are now referred to as AU-rich elements (AREs) and confer instability to otherwise stable mRNAs (Chen and Shyu, 1995; Ross, 1995; Liebhaber, 1997). Interestingly, the same sites appear to contribute to translational control as well (see below) (Decker and Parker, 1995; Jacobson and Peltz, 1996; Mijatovic *et al.*, 1997). While the detailed mechanisms by which ARE-dependent mRNA destabilization occurs are not known, the initial step involves shortening of the poly(A) tail (Chen and Shyu, 1995; Ross, 1995). In some but not all circumstances, co-incident translation is also a component of the decay mechanism (Chen and Shyu, 1995; Chen *et al.*, 1995). There have been numerous efforts to identify proteins which can bind to ARE motifs with high specificity (Kiledjian *et al.*, 1997; Myer *et al.*, 1997; Peng *et al.*, 1998; Loflin *et al.*, 1999; Wilson and Brewer, 1999a,b). Though it is likely that more will be discovered, at present there are two major mRNA-binding proteins which exhibit specificity for AUUUA-containing motifs *and* have been functionally linked with mRNA decay. The *AUF1* gene, first described by Brewer and colleagues, encodes at least four isoforms which derive from a single gene by differential splicing (Wagner *et al.*, 1998). AUF1 expression and function correlate well with destabilization of mRNAs and have been linked in several cases with stimulus-dependent control of mRNA stability (De Maria and Brewer, 1996; Loflin *et al.*, 1999). The second protein is a member of the ELAV family (embryonic lethal abnormal visual) and is also known as HuA or HuR (Myer *et al.*, 1997; Peng *et al.*, 1998). This protein exhibits precise specificity for AUUUA motifs and has been shown in a variety of functional studies to stabilize ARE-containing mRNAs both *in vitro* and *in vivo* (Myer *et al.*, 1997; Ford *et al.*, 1999).

Recent evidence from a number of different laboratories has revealed an important role for one or more of the MAP kinase pathways in the modulation of mRNA stability (Chen *et al.*, 1998; Dean *et al.*, 1999; Winzen *et al.*, 1999). The availability of inhibitors which exhibit specificity for individual MAP kinase modules has implicated both the p38 and JNK kinases in controlling mRNA stability. These findings have been confirmed and extended by overexpression studies using plasmids encoding both constitutively active and dominant-negative forms of p38 or JNK kinase module components. At present, the final substrates of these pathways remain undefined.

In macrophages and monocytes, the control of mRNA stability has been demonstrated for a number of genes in response to several forms of stimulation. LPS, IL-1 and adhesion have all been reported to modulate the stability of specific mRNAs (Stoeckle, 1991; Ohmori and Hamilton, 1994a; Sirenko *et al.*, 1997; Dean *et al.*, 1999; Saklatvala *et al.*, 1999; Tebo *et al.*, 2000). These include the chemoattractant cytokine genes IL-8 and both human Gro-α and mouse KC. While all three stimuli have been shown to be potent inducers of transcription for these genes, mRNA stability also appears to play an essential role. Under conditions where stabilization is blocked either naturally or by experimental manipulation, mRNA accumulation is markedly reduced despite the frequent observation that transcriptional activities are high. Blocking the stabilization may indeed be a natural regulatory point. The control of both TNF-α and mouse KC mRNA levels following LPS stimulation are dependent upon ARE motifs in the 3'-UTR (Kim *et al.*, 1998; Kishore *et al.*, 1999). IL-10, a well-characterized anti-inflammatory cytokine which acts predominantly to block responses in macrophages and monocytes, is, in some cases, a poor inhibitor of gene transcription but instead appears to increase selective mRNA decay (Bogdan *et al.*, 1992; Kim *et al.*, 1998). While there have been some reports that IL-10 may function by blocking the activation of MAPK modules in response to the primary stimulus (e.g. LPS), there is not uniform agreement on this point in the literature (Isner and Dietz, 1988; Sato *et al.*, 1999; Song *et al.*, 1999; Suttles *et al.*, 1999).

5.3 Translational control

The mechanisms regulating both translational initiation and elongation have been studied intensively for many years and the mechanisms which control protein synthesisis in a global fashion (e.g. during virus infection) have been worked out in some detail (Sonenberg, 1994; Harford, 1995; Gray and Wickens, 1998; Preiss and Hentze, 1999). In contrast, examples of sequence-specific translational control are relatively few, and many are not well understood in mechanistic terms. In the case of macrophage activation, the best studied example is provided by LPS-stimulated TNF production (Han *et al.*,1990; Kruys and Huez, 1994; Kontoyiannis *et al.*, 1999). Beutler and his colleagues established that mRNA translation was an important regulatory site and showed that in most cells, TNF mRNA is poorly translated. This is determined by the presence of a cluster of AUUUA motifs in the 3'-UTR of TNF mRNA. In macrophages and other immune system cells, the translational blockade can be relieved in the presence of an appropriate stimulus (prototypically LPS) with an attendant increase in the rate of mRNA translation. Interestingly, while this AU motif is responsible for instability of the mRNA, LPS stimulation has been reported to have little effect on TNF-α mRNA stability (Han *et al.*, 1990; Kontoyiannis *et al.*, 1999). The p38 MAP kinase module may be an important signaling pathway mediating ARE-dependent regulation of TNF mRNA translation, suggesting further similarity with the control of mRNA decay (Lee and Young, 1996). As is the case for control of mRNA stability through AREs, the mechanism(s) and protein factors which are involved in stimulus-specific translational control are, at present, poorly understood (Gueydan *et al.*, 1996; Hel *et al.*, 1996; Lewis *et al.*, 1998).

6 Summary

Substantial progress in the understanding of macrophage activation has resulted largely from a number of achievements in molecular biology. First has been the ability to identify new proteins in functional cascades on the basis of protein–protein interactions. This has allowed, in particular, expanded appreciation of the complexity of receptor-initiated signaling pathways. Secondly, the ability to manipulate gene sequence has allowed rigorous evaluation of the linkage between protein structure and function and the development of reagents which can test the importance of candidate gene products in particular functional settings. Finally, the ability to characterize regulatory sequence in the genome through the use of reporter plasmid constructions has provided in-depth appreciation of transcriptional control of gene expression and will provide further characterization of post-transcriptional processes.

With this new information in hand and the further demonstration of macrophage functional heterogeneity *in vivo* and *in vitro*, it is possible to appreciate both the operational demonstration of diversity in macrophage activation and the conceptual and mechanistic bases for its generation. Interestingly, the potential for diversity is probably much larger than is actually utilized. While each gene can be shown to behave with some degree of independence from others, there are many regulatory features in common among genes which are expressed during an inflammatory response, and the control mechanisms for these are naturally overlapping.

The revolution in molecular biology will continue to make a substantial impact on functional dissection of the inflammatory response in macrophages and their regulation. This is likely to occur in several ways. First, we can expect to achieve more detailed appreciation of the basic mechanisms operant in control of classical pro-inflammatory responses. Secondly, it will be necessary to expand knowledge of important but under-studied macrophage phenotypes. Emerging methodologies and reagents should lead to molecular dissection of dendritic cell function and other macrophage functions which occur in physiological settings such as tissue remodeling and repair following injury. Such information will be necessary for ultimately defining the roles which macrophages play in the pathogenesis of chronic diseases including cancer and atherosclerosis.

References

Adams, D.O. and Hamilton, T.A. (1984). The cell biology of macrophage activation. *Annual Review of Immunology*, **2**, 283–318.

Adams, D.O. and Hamilton, T.A. (1992a). Molecular basis of macrophage activation: diversity and its origins. In Lewis, C.E. and O'D McGee, J. (ed.), *The Natural Immune System, Volume II: The Macrophage.* Oxford University Press, Oxford, p. 75–114..

Adams, D.O. and Hamilton, T.A. (1992b). Macrophages as destructive cells in host defense. In Gallin, J.I., Goldstein, I.M. and Snyderman, R. (ed.), *Inflammation: Basic Principles and Clinical Correlates.* Raven Press, New York, p. 637.

Askew, D., Havenith, C.E. and Walker,W.S. (1996). Heterogeneity of mouse brain macrophages in alloantigen presentation to naive CD8+ T cells as revealed by a panel of microglial cell lines. *Immunobiology*, **195**, 417.

Auron, P.E. (1998). The interleukin 1 receptor: ligand interactions and signal transduction, *Cytokine and Growth Factor Review*, **9**, 221.

Baggiolini, M. (1998). Chemokines and leukocyte traffic. *Nature*, **392**, 565.

Baichwal, V.R. and Baeuerle, P.A. (1997). Activate NF-kB or die? *Current Biology*, **7**, R94.

Baker, S.J. and Reddy, E.P. (1998). Modulation of life and death by the TNF receptor superfamily. *Oncogene*, **17**, 3261.

Baldwin, J.M. (1994). Structure and function of receptors coupled to G proteins. *Current Opinion in Cell Biology*, **6**, 180.

Barsig, J., Küsters, S., Vogt, K., Volk, H.D. Tiegs, G. and Wendel, A. (1995). Lipopolysaccharide-induced interleukin-10 in mice: role of endogenous tumor necrosis factor-α. *European Journal of Immunology*, **25**, 2888.

Bethea, J.R., Ohmori, Y. and Hamilton, T.A. (1997). A tandem GC box motif is necessary for lipopolysaccharide-induced transcription of the type II TNF receptor gene. *Journal of Immunology*, **158**, 5815.

Boehm, U., Klamp, T., Groot, M. and Howard, J.C. (1997). Cellular responses to interferon-γ. *Annual Review of Immunology*, **15**, 749.

Bogdan, C., Paik, J., Vodovotz,Y. and Nathan, C. (1992). Contrasting mechanisms for suppression of macrophage cytokine release by transforming growth factor-β and interleukin-10. *Journal of Biological Chemistry*, **267**, 23301.

Bosque, F., Belkaid, Y., Briend, E., Hevin, B., Lebastard, M., Soussi, N. and Milon, G. (1997). The biology of macrophages. *Pathologie et Biologie*, **45**, 103.

Brightbill, H.D., Plevy, S.E., Modlin, R.L. and Smale, S.T. (2000). A prominent role for Sp1 during lipopolysaccharide-mediated induction of the IL-10 promoter in macrophages, *Journal of Immunology*, **164**, 1940–51.

Camp, R., Fincham, N., Ross, J., Bird, C. and Gearing, A. (1990). Potent inflammatory properties in human skin of interleukin-1 α-like material isolated from normal skin. *Journal of Investigative Dermatology*, **94**, 735.

Caput, D., Beutler, B., Hartog, K., Thayer, R., Brown-Shimer, S. and Cerami, A. (1986). Identification of a common nucleotide sequence in the 3'-untranslated region of mRNA molecules specifying inflammatory mediators. *Proceedings of the National Academy of Sciences USA*, **83**, 1670.

Cash, E., Minty, A., Ferrara, P. Caput, D., Fradelizi, D. and Rott, O. (1994). Macrophage-inactivating IL-13 suppresses experimental autoimmune encephalomyelitis in rats. *Journal of Immunology*, **153**, 4258.

Chen, C.-Y.A. and Shyu, A.-B. (1995). AU-rich elements: characterization and importance in mRNA degradation. *Trends in Biochemical Science*, **20**, 465.

Chen, C.Y., Del Gatto-Konczak, F., Wu, Z. and Karin, M. (1998). Stabilization of interleukin-2 mRNA by the c-Jun NH$_2$-terminal kinase pathway. *Science*, **280**, 1945.

Chen, C.Y.A., Xu, N.H. and Shyu, A.B. (1995). mRNA decay mediated by two distinct AU-rich elements from c-*fos* and granulocyte–macrophage colony-stimulating factor transcripts: different deadenylation kinetics and uncoupling from translation. *Molecular and Cellular Biology*, **15**, 5777.

D'Andrea, A., Ma, X. Aste-Amezaga, M. Paganin, C. and Trinchieri, G. (1995). Stimulatory and inhibitory effects of interleukin (IL)-4 and IL-13 on the production of cytokines by human peripheral blood mononuclear cells: priming for IL-12 and tumor necrosis factor α production. *Journal of Experimental Medicine*, **181**, 537.

Darnay, B.G. and Aggarwal, B.B. (1997). Early events in TNF signaling: a story of associations and dissociations. *Journal of Leukocyte Biology*, **61**, 559.

Darnell, J.E., Jr (1997). STATs and gene regulation. *Science*, **277**, 1630.

Davie, J.R. and Spencer, V.A. (1999). Control of histone modifications. *Journal of Cell Biochemistry*, Suppl **32–33**, 141.

Davies, P. and MacIntyre, D.E. (1992). Prostaglandins and inflammation. In Gallin, J.I., Goldstein. I.M. and Snyderman, R. (ed.), *Inflammation: Basic Principles and Clinical Correlates*. Raven Press, New York, p. 123.

De Maria, C.T. and Brewer, G. (1996). AUF1 binding affinity to A+U-rich elements correlates with rapid mRNA degradation. *Journal of Biological Chemistry*, **271**, 12179.

Dean, J.L., Brook, M., Clark, A.R. and Saklatvala, J. (1999). p38 mitogen-activated protein kinase regulates cyclooxygenase-2 mRNA stability and transcription in lipopolysaccharide-treated human monocytes. *Journal of Biological Chemistry*, **274**, 264.

Decker, C.J. and Parker, R. (1995). Diversity of cytoplasmic functions for the 3' untranslated region of eukaryotic transcripts. *Current Opinion in Cell Biology*, **7**, 386.

Decker, T., Kovarik, P. and Meinke, A. (1997). GAS elements: a few nucleotides with a major impact on cytokine-induced gene expression. *Journal of Interferon and Cytokine Research*, **17**, 121.

Deng, W., Ohmori, Y. and Hamilton, T.A. (1994). Mechanisms of IL-4-mediated suppression of IP-10 gene expression in murine macrophages. *Journal of Immunology*, **153**, 2130.

Dickensheets, H.L. and Donnelly, R.P. (1997). IFN-γ and IL-10 inhibit induction of IL-1 receptor type I and type II gene expression by IL-4 and IL-13 in human monocytes. *Journal of Immunology*, **159**, 6226.

Dickensheets, H.L. and Donnelly, R.P. (1999). Inhibition of IL-4-inducible gene expression in human monocytes by type I and type II interferons. *Journal of Leukocyte Biology*, **65**, 307.

Dickensheets, H.L., Venkataraman, C., Schindler, U. and Donnelly, R.P. (1999). Interferons inhibit activation of STAT6 by interleukin 4 in human monocytes by inducing SOCS-1 gene expression. *Proceedings of the National Academy of Sciences USA*, **96**, 10800.

Dikic, I. and Blaukat, A. (1999). Protein tyrosine kinase-mediated pathways in G protein-coupled receptor signaling. *Cell Biochemistry and Biophysics*, **30**, 369.

Dinarello, C.A. (1998). Interleukin-1, interleukin-1 receptors and interleukin-1 receptor antagonist. *International Review of Immunology*, **16**, 457.

Donnelly, R.P., Crofford, L.J., Freeman, S.L., Buras, J., Remmers, E., Wilder, R.L. *et al.* (1993). Tissue-specific regulation of IL-6 production by IL-4: differential effects of IL-4 on nuclear factor-kB activity in monocytes and fibroblasts. *Journal of Immunology*, **151**, 5603.

Driggers, P.H., Ennist, D.L., Gleason, S.L., Mak, W.H., Marks, M.S., Levi, B.Z. *et al.* (1990). An interferon γ-regulated protein that binds the interferon-inducible enhancer element of major histocompatibility complex class I genes. *Proceedings of the National Academy of Sciences USA*, **87**, 3743.

Ernst, P. and Smale, S.T. (1995). Combinatorial regulation of transcription. I: general aspects of transcriptional control. *Immunity*, **2**, 311.

Farrar, M.A. and Schreiber, R.D. (1993). The molecular cell biology of interferon-γ and its receptor. *Annual Review of Immunology*, **11**, 571.

Fenton, M.J. and Golenbock, D.T. (1998). LPS-binding proteins and receptors. *Journal of Leukocyte Biology*, **64**, 25.

Fenton, M.J., Buras, J.A. and Donnelly, R.P. (1992). IL-4 reciprocally regulates IL-1 and IL-1 receptor antagonist expression in human monocytes. *Journal of Immunology*, **149**, 1283.

Finco, T.S. and Baldwin, A.S. (1995). Mechanistic aspects of NF-kB regulation: the emerging role of phosphorylation and proteolysis. *Immunity*, **3**, 263.

Ford, L.P., Watson, J., Keene, J.D. and Wilusz, J. (1999). ELAV proteins stabilize deadenylated intermediates in a novel *in vitro* mRNA deadenylation/degradation system. *Genes and Development*, **13**, 188.

Fraser, I.P., Koziel, H. and Ezekowitz, R.A. (1998). The serum mannose-binding protein and the macrophage mannose receptor are pattern recognition molecules that link innate and adaptive immunity. *Seminars in Immunology*, **10**, 363.

Gautam, S., Tebo, J.M. and Hamilton, T.A. (1992). IL-4 suppresses cytokine gene expression induced by IFN-γ and/or IL-2 in murine peritoneal macrophages. *Journal of Immunology*, **148**, 1725.

Gay, N.J. and Kubota, K. (1996). The signal transduction pathway leading from the Toll receptor to nuclear localization of Dorsal transcription factor. *Biochemical Society Transactions*, **24**, 35.

Ghosh, S., May, M.J. and Kopp, E.B. (1998). NF-kB and Rel proteins: evolutionarily conserved mediators of immune responses. *Annual Review of Immunology*, **16**, 225–60.

Gilman, A.G. (1995). Nobel Lecture. G proteins and regulation of adenylyl cyclase. *Bioscience Reports*, **15**, 65.

Goenka, S., Youn, J., Dzurek, L.M., Schindler, U., Yu-Lee, L.Y. and Boothby, M. (1999). Paired Stat6 C-terminal transcription activation domains required both for inhibition of an IFN-responsive promoter and trans-activation. *Journal of Immunology*, **163**, 4663.

Goerdt, S. and Orfanos, C.E. (1999). Other functions, other genes: alternative activation of antigen-presenting cells. *Immunity*, **10**, 137.

Goh, K.C., Haque, S.J. and Williams, B.R. (1999). p38 MAP kinase is required for STAT1 serine phosphorylation and transcriptional activation induced by interferons. *EMBO Journal*, **18**, 5601.

Goldstein, I.M. (1992). Complement: biologically active components. In Gallin, J.I., Goldstein. I.M. and Snyderman, R. (ed.), *Inflammation: Basic Principles and Clinical Correlates*. Raven Press, New York, p. 63.

Goodwin, R.G., Cerretti, D.P. and Smith, C.A. (1994). Cytokine receptors. In Ransohoff. R. and Benvensite E. (ed.), Cytokines and the CNS: Development, Defense, and Disease pp. 1–24. CRC, Boca Raton, FL.

Gordon, S. (1998). The role of the macrophage in immune regulation. *Research in Immunology*, **149**, 685.

Gordon, S., Clarke, S., Greaves. D. and Doyle, A. (1995). Molecular immunobiology of macrophages: recent progress. *Current Opinion in Immunology*, **7**, 24.

Gravallese, E.M., Darling, J.M., Glimcher, L.H. and Boothby, M. (1991). Role of lipopolysaccharide and IL-4 in control of transcription of the class II Aa gene. *Journal of Immunology*, **147**, 2377.

Gray, N.K. and Wickens, M. (1998). Control of translation initiation in animals. *Annual Review of Cell and Developmental Biology*, **14**, 399.

Grell, M., Zimmermann, G., Hülser, D., Pfizenmaier, K. and Scheurich, P. (1994). TNF receptors TR60 and TR80 can mediate apoptosis via induction of distinct signal pathways. *Journal of Immunology*, **153**, 1963.

Grunstein, M. (1997). Histone acetylation in chromatin structure and transcription. *Nature*, **389**, 349.

Gueydan, C., Houzet, L., Marchant, A., Sels, A., Huez, G. and Kruys, V. (1996). Engagement of tumor necrosis factor mRNA by an endotoxin-inducible cytoplasmic protein [published erratum appears in *Molecular Medicine* 1996 Nov;2(6):786]. *Molecular Medicine*, **2**, 479.

Hambleton, J., McMahon, M. and DeFranco, A.L. (1995). Activation of Raf-1 and mitogen-activated protein kinase in murine macrophages partially mimics lipopolysaccharide-induced signaling events. *Journal of Experimental Medicine*, **182**, 147.

Hambleton, J., Weinstein, S.L., Lem, L. and DeFranco, A.L. (1996). Activation of c-Jun N-terminal kinase in bacterial lipopolysaccharide-stimulated macrophages. *Proceedings of the National Academy of Sciences USA*, **93**, 2774.

Hamilton, T.A. (1988). Molecular mechanisms in the activation of mononuclear phagocytes. In Rogers, T.J. and Gilman, S.C. (ed.), *Immunopharmacology*. Telford Press, New Jersey, p. 213.

Hamilton, T.A. and Ohmori, Y. (1996). Intracellular signaling pathways regulating inflammatory gene expression in mononuclear phagocytes. In Lad, P.M., Kapstein,J.S. and Lin, C.K. (ed.), *Signal Transduction in Leukocytes: Role of G proteins and Other Pathways*. CRC Press, Boca Raton, FL, p. 325.

Hamilton, T.A., Ohmori, Y., Narumi, S. and Tannenbaum, C.S. (1992). Regulation of diversity in macrophage activation. In Lopez-Berestein, G. and Klostergaard, J. (ed.), *Mononuclear Phagocytes in Cell Biology*. CRC Press, New York, p. 47.

Hamilton, T.A., Ohmori, Y., Tebo, J.M. Narumi,S. and Tannenbaum, C.S. (1993). Transmembrane and intracellular signaling events in lipopolysaccharide-stimulated macrophages. In Zwilling, B.S. and Eisenstein, T.K. (ed.), *Macrophage–Pathogen Interactions*. Marcell Dekker, New York, p. 83.

Han, J., Brown, T. and Beutler, B. (1990). Endotoxin-responsive sequences control cachetin/tumor necrosis factor biosynthesis at the translation level. *Journal of Experimental Medicine*, **171**, 465.

Harford, J.B. (1995). Translation-targeted therapeutics for viral diseases. *Gene Expression*, **4**, 357.

Hattori, Y., Akimoto, K., Matsumura, M., Tseng, C.C., Kasai, K. and Shimoda, S.I. (1996). Effect of cycloheximide on the expression of LPS-inducible iNOS, IFN-β, and IRF-1 genes in J774 macrophages. *Biochemistry and Molecular Biology International*, **40**, 889.

Haziot, A., Lin, X.Y., Zhang, F. and Goyert, S.M. (1998). The induction of acute phase proteins by lipopolysaccharide uses a novel pathway that is CD14-independent. *Journal of Immunology*, **160**, 2570.

Hel, Z., Skamene, E. and Radzioch, D. (1996). Two distinct regions in the 3' untranslated region of tumor necrosis factor α mRNA form complexes with macrophage proteins. *Molecular and Cellular Biology*, **16**, 5579.

Herbert, J.M., Savi, P., Laplace, M.C., Lale, A., Dol, F., Dumas, A. *et al.* (1993). IL-4 and IL-13 exhibit comparable abilities to reduce pyrogen-induced expression of procoagulant activity in endothelial cells and monocytes. *FEBS Letters*, **328**, 268.

Horvath, C.M. and Darnell, J.E., Jr (1997). The state of the STATs: recent developments in the study of signal transduction to the nucleus. *Current Opinion in Cell Biology*, **9**, 233.

Hou, J., Schindler, U., Henzel, W.J., Ho, T.C., Brasseur, M. and McKnight, S.L. (1994). An interleukin-4-induced transcription factor: IL-4 Stat. *Science*, **265**, 1701.

Huang, L., Guan, R.J. and Pardee, A.B. (1999). Evolution of transcriptional control from prokaryotic beginnings to eukaryotic complexities. *Critical Reviews in Eukaryotic Gene Expression*, **9**, 175.

Ihle, J.N. (1996). STATs: signal transducers and activators of transcription. *Cell*, **84**, 331.

Ihle, J.N., Witthuhn, B.A., Quelle, F.W., Yamamoto, K. and Silvennoinen, O. (1995). Signaling through the hematopoietic cytokine receptors. *Annual Review of Immunology*, **13**, 369.

Ihle, J.N., Thierfelder, W., Teglund, S., Stravapodis, D., Wang, D., Feng, J. and Parganas, E. (1998). Signaling by the cytokine receptor superfamily. *Annals of the New York Academy of Sciences*, **865**, 1.

Isner, J.M. and Dietz, W.A. (1988). Cardiovascular consequences of recombinant DNA technology: interleukin-2. *Annals of Internal Medicine*, **109**, 933.

Jacobson, A. and Peltz, S.W. (1996). Interrelationships of the pathways of mRNA decay and translation in eukaryotic cells. *Annual Review of Biochemistry*, **65**, 693.

Johnson, D.R. and Pober, J.S. (1994). HLA class I heavy-chain gene promoter elements mediating synergy between tumor necrosis factor and interferons. *Molecular and Cellular Biology*, **14**, 1322.

Kambayashi, T., Jacob, C.O. and Strassmann, G. (1996). IL-4 and IL-13 modulate IL-10 release in endotoxin-stimulated murine peritoneal mononuclear phagocytes. *Cellular Immunology*, **171**, 153.

Kaplan, M.H., Schindler, U., Smiley, S.T. and Grusby, M.J. (1996). Stat6 is required for mediating responses to IL-4 and for development of Th2 cells. *Immunity*, **4**, 313.

Kielian, T.L. and Blecha, F. (1995). CD14 and other recognition molecules for lipopolysaccharide: a review. *Immunopharmacology*, **29**, 187.

Kiledjian, M., DeMaria, C.T., Brewer, G. and Novick, K. (1997). Identification of AUF1 (heterogeneous nuclear ribonucleoprotein D) as a component of the α-globin mRNA stability complex [published erratum appears in *Molecular and Cellular Biology* 1997 Oct;17(10):6202]. *Molecular and Cellular Biology*, **17**, 4870.

Kim, H.S., Armstrong, D., Hamilton, T.A. and Tebo, J.M. (1998). IL-10 suppresses LPS-induced KC mRNA expression via a translation-dependent decrease in mRNA stability, *Journal of Leukocyte Biology*, **64**, 33.

Kirschning, C.J., Wesche, H., Merrill Ayres, T. and Rothe, M. (1998). Human toll-like receptor 2 confers responsiveness to bacterial lipopolysaccharide. *Journal of Experimental Medicine*, **188**, 2091.

Kishore, R., Tebo, J.M., Kolosov, M. and Hamilton, T.A. (1999). Cutting edge: clustered AU-rich elements are the target of IL-10-mediated mRNA destabilization in mouse macrophages. *Journal of Immunology*, **162**, 2457.

Kontoyiannis, D., Pasparakis, M., Pizarro, T.T., Cominelli, F. and Kollias, G. (1999). Impaired on/off regulation of TNF biosynthesis in mice lacking TNF AU-rich elements: implications for joint and gut-associated immunopathologies. *Immunity*, **10**, 387.

Kotanides, H. and Reich, N.C. (1993). Requirement of tyrosine phosphorylation for rapid activation of a DNA binding factor by IL-4. *Science*, **262**, 1265.

Kovarik, P., Stoiber, D., Eyers, P.A., Menghini, R., Neininger, A., Gaestel, M. *et al.* (1999). Stress-induced phosphorylation of STAT1 at Ser727 requires p38 mitogen-activated protein kinase whereas IFN-γ uses a different signaling pathway. *Proceedings of the National Academy of Sciences USA*, **96**, 13956.

Krieger, M. (1997). The other side of scavenger receptors: pattern recognition for host defense, *Current Opinion in Lipidology*, **8**, 275.

Kruys, V. and Huez, G. (1994). Translational control of cytokine expression by 3' UA-rich sequences. *Biochimie*, **76**, 862.

Lam, B.K. and Austen, K.F. (1992). Leukotrienes: biosynthesis, release, and actions. In Gallin, J.I., Goldstein. I.M. and Snyderman, R. (ed.), *Inflammation: Basic Principles and Clinical Correlates.* Raven Press, New York, p. 139.

Lee, J.C. and Young, P.R. (1996). Role of CSBP/p38/RK stress response kinase in LPS and cytokine signaling mechanisms. *Journal of Leukocyte Biology*, **59**, 152.

Lefort, S., Vita, N., Reeb, R., Caput, D. and Ferrara, P. (1995). IL-13 and IL-4 share signal transduction elements as well as receptor components in TF-1 cells. *FEBS Letters*, **366**, 122.

Lewis, T., Gueydan, C., Huez, G., Toulme, J.J. and Kruys, V. (1998). Mapping of a minimal AU-rich sequence required for lipopolysaccharide-induced binding of a 55-kDa protein on tumor necrosis factor-α mRNA. *Journal of Biological Chemistry*, **273**, 13781.

Liebhaber, S.A. (1997). mRNA stability and the control of gene expression. *Nucleic Acids Research, Symposium Series*, **29**.

Lien, E., Sellati, T.J., Yoshimura, A., Flo, T.H., Rawadi, G., Finberg, R.W. *et al.* (1999). Toll-like receptor 2 functions as a pattern recognition receptor for diverse bacterial products. *Journal of Biological Chemistry*, **274**, 33419.

Loflin, P., Chen, C.Y. and Shyu, A.B. (1999). Unraveling a cytoplasmic role for hnRNP D in the *in vivo* mRNA destabilization directed by the AU-rich element. *Genes and Development*, **13**, 1884.

Lopez-Ilasaca, M. (1998). Signaling from G-protein-coupled receptors to mitogen-activated protein (MAP)-kinase cascades. *Biochemical Pharmacology*, **56**, 269.

Luster, A.D. (1998). Review articles: mechanisms of disease: chemokines—chemotactic cytokines that mediate inflammation. *New England Journal of Medicine*, **338**, 436.

Malek, N.P., Pluempe, J., Kubicka, S., Manns, M.P. and Trautwein, C. (1998). Molecular mechanisms of TNF receptor-mediated signaling. *Recent Results in Cancer Research*, **147**, 97.

Marfaing-Koka, A., Devergne, O., Gorgone, G., Portier, A., Schall, T.J., Galanaud, P. *et al.* (1995). Regulation of the production of the RANTES chemokine by endothelial cells: synergistic induction by IFN-γ plus TNF-α and inhibition by IL-4 and IL-13. *Journal of Immunology*, **154**, 1870.

May, M.J. and Ghosh, S. (1998). Signal transduction through NF-kB. *Immunology Today*, **19**, 80.

McCormack, J.M., Moore, S.C., Gatewood, J.W. and Walker, W.S. (1992). Mouse splenic macrophage cell lines with different antigen-presenting activities for CD4+ helper T cell subsets and allogeneic CD8+ T cells. *Cellular Immunology*, **145**, 359.

Medzhitov, R. and Janeway, C.A., Jr (1998). Innate immune recognition and control of adaptive immune responses. *Seminars in Immunology*, **10**, 351.

Mijatovic, T., Kruys, V., Caput, D., DeFrance, P. and Huez, G. (1997). Interleukin-4 and interleukin-13 inhibit tumor necrosis factor-α mRNA translational activation in lipopolysaccharide-induced mouse macrophages. *Journal of Biological Chemistry*, **272**, 14394.

Mikita, T., Campbell, D., Wu, P.G., Williamson, K. and Schindler, U. (1996). Requirements for interleukin-4-induced gene expression and functional characterization of Stat6. *Molecular and Cellular Biology*, **16**, 5811.

Morrison, D.C. and Ryan, J.L. (1979). Bacterial endotoxins and host immune responses. *Advances in Immunology*, **28**, 293.

Mosmann, T.R. and Sad, S. (1996). The expanding universe of T-cell subsets: Th1, Th2 and more. *Immunology Today*, **17**, 138.

Murphy, P.M. (1994). The molecular biology of leukocyte chemoattractant receptors. *Annual Review of Immunology*, **12**, 593.

Myer, V.E., Fan, X.C. and Steitz, J.A. (1997). Identification of HuR as a protein implicated in AUUUA-mediated mRNA decay. *EMBO Journal*, **16**, 2130.

Nakamura, S. (1996). Phosphatidylcholine hydrolysis and protein kinase C activation for intracellular signaling network. *Journal of Lipidid Mediated Cell Signaling*, **14**, 197.

Nathan, C.F. and Cohn, Z.A. (1995). Cellular components of inflammation: monocytes and macrophages. In Kelly, W., Harris, E., Ruddy S. and Hedge R. (ed.), *Textbook of Rheumatology*. W.B. Saunders, New York, p. 144.

Natoli, G., Costanzo, A., Guido, F., Moretti, F. and Levrero, M. (1998). Apoptotic, non-apoptotic, and anti-apoptotic pathways of tumor necrosis factor signalling. *Biochemical Pharmacology*, **56**, 915.

Nishizuka, Y. (1995). Protein kinase C and lipid signaling for sustained cellular responses, *FASEB Journal*, **9**, 484.

O'Garra, A. and Murphy, K. (1996). Role of cytokines in development of Th1 and Th2 cells. *Chemical Immunology*, **63**, 1.

Ogbourne, S. and Antalis, T.M. (1998). Transcriptional control and the role of silencers in transcriptional regulation in eukaryotes. *Biochemical Journal*, **331**, 1.

Ohmori, Y. and Hamilton, T.A. (1993). Cooperative interaction between interferon (IFN) stimulus response element and kB sequence motifs controls IFNg- and lipopolysaccharide-stimulated transcription from the murine IP-10 promoter. *Journal of Biological Chemistry*, 268, 6677.

Ohmori, Y. and Hamilton, T.A. (1994a). Cell type and stimulus specific regulation of chemokine gene expression. *Biochemical and Biophysical Research Communications*, **2**, 590.

Ohmori, Y. and Hamilton, T.A. (1994b). Regulation of macrophage gene expression by T cell derived lymphokines, *Pharmacology and Therapeutics*, **63**, 235.

Ohmori, Y. and Hamilton, T.A. (1995). The interferon stimulated response element and a kB site mediate synergistic induction of murine IP-10 gene transcription by IFNγ and TNFα. *Journal of Immunology*, **154**, 5235.

Ohmori, Y. and Hamilton, T.A. (1997). IL-4-induced STAT6 suppresses IFN-γ-stimulated STAT1-dependent transcription in mouse macrophages. *Journal of Immunology*, **159**, 5474.

Ohmori, Y. and Hamilton, T.A. (1998). STAT6 is required for the anti-inflammatory activity of interleukin-4 in mouse peritoneal macrophages. *Journal of Biological Chemistry*, **273**, 29202.

Ohmori, Y., Smith, M.F., Jr and Hamilton, T.A. (1996). IL-4-induced expression of the IL-1 receptor antagonist gene is mediated by STAT6. *Journal of Immunology*, **157**, 2058.

Ohmori, Y., Schreiber, R.D. and Hamilton, T.A. (1997). Synergy between interferon-γ and tumor necrosis factor-α in transcriptional activation is mediated by cooperation between signal transducer and activator of transcription 1 and nuclear factor kB. *Journal of Biological Chemistry*, **272**, 14899.

O'Neill, L.A. and Greene, C. (1998). Signal transduction pathways activated by the IL-1 receptor family: ancient signaling machinery in mammals, insects, and plants. *Journal of Leukocyte Biology*, **63**, 650.

Onishi, M., Nosaka, T. and Kitamura, T. (1998). Cytokine receptors: structures and signal transduction. *International Review of Immunology*, **16**, 617.

Pace, J.L., Russell, S.W., LeBlanc, P.A. and Murasko, D.M. (1985). Comparative effects of various classes of mouse interferons on macrophage activation for tumor cell killing. *Journal of Immunology*, **134**, 977.

Pahl, H.L. and Baeuerle, P.A. (1996). Control of gene expression by proteolysis. *Current Opinion in Cell Biology*, **8**, 340.

Peng, S.S., Chen, C.Y., Xu, N. and Shyu, A.B. (1998). RNA stabilization by the AU-rich element binding protein, HuR, an ELAV protein. *EMBO Journal*, **17**, 3461.

Piskurich, J.F., Linhoff, M.W., Wang, Y. and Ting, J.P. (1999). Two distinct γ interferon-inducible promoters of the major histocompatibility complex class II transactivator gene are differentially regulated by STAT1, interferon regulatory factor 1, and transforming growth factor β. *Molecular and Cellular Biology*, **19**, 431.

Politis, A.D., Ozato, K., Coligan, J.E. and Vogel, S.N. (1994). Regulation of IFN-γ-induced nuclear expression of IFN consensus sequence binding protein in murine peritoneal macrophages. *Journal of Immunology*, **152**, 2270.

Poltorak, A., He, X., Smirnova, I., Liu, M.Y., Huffel, C.V., Du, X. *et al.* (1998). Defective LPS signaling in C3H/HeJ and C57BL/10ScCr mice: mutations in *Tlr4* gene. *Science*, **282**, 2085.

Post, G.R. and Brown, J.H. (1996). G protein-coupled receptors and signaling pathways regulating growth responses. *FASEB Journal*, **10**, 741.

Preiss, T. and Hentze, M.W. (1999). From factors to mechanisms: translation and translational control in eukaryotes. *Current Opinion in Genetics and Development*, **9**, 515.

Qureshi, S.T., Lariviere, L., Leveque, G., Clermont, S., Moore, K.J., Gros, P. *et al.* (1999). Endotoxin-tolerant mice have mutations in Toll-like receptor 4 (Tlr4) [published erratum appears in *Journal of Experimental Medicine* 1999 May 3; 189(9):following 1518]. *Journal of Experimental Medicine*, **189**, 615.

Rock, F.L., Hardiman, G., Timans, J.C., Kastelein, R.A. and Bazan, J.F. (1998). A family of human receptors structurally related to *Drosophila* Toll. *Proceedings of the National Academy of Sciences USA*, **95**, 588.

Rollins, B.J. (1997). Chemokines. *Blood*, **90**, 909.

Romagnani, S. (1997). The Th1/Th2 paradigm. *Immunology Today*, **18**, 263.

Ross, J. (1995). mRNA stability in mammalian cells. *Microbiological Reviews*, **3**, 423.

Ruco, L.P. and Meltzer, M.S. (1978). Macrophage activation for tumor cytotoxicity: development of macrophage cytotoxic activity requires completion of a sequence of short lived intermediary reactions. *Journal of Immunology*, **121**, 2935.

Russell, S.W., Doe, W.F. and McIntosh, A.T. (1978). Functional characterization of a stable-non-cytolytic stage of macrophage activation in tumors. *Journal of Experimental Medicine*, **146**, 1511.

Saklatvala, J., Dean, J. and Finch, A. (1999). Protein kinase cascades in intracellular signalling by interleukin-I and tumour necrosis factor. *Biochemical Society Symposia*, **64**, 63.

Sato, K., Nagayama, H., Tadokoro, K., Juji, T. and Takahashi, T.A. (1999). Extracellular signal-regulated kinase, stress-activated protein kinase/c-Jun N-terminal kinase, and p38mapk are involved in IL-10-mediated selective repression of TNF-α-induced activation and maturation of human peripheral blood monocyte-derived dendritic cells. *Journal of Immunology*, **162**, 3865.

Scharton-Kersten, T., Contursi, C., Masumi, A., Sher, A. and Ozato, K. (1997). Interferon consensus sequence binding protein-deficient mice display impaired resistance to intracellular infection due to a primary defect in interleukin 12 p40 induction. *Journal of Experimental Medicine*, **186**, 1523.

Schindler, U., Wu, P., Rothe, M., Brasseur, M. and McKnight, S.L. (1995). Components of a Stat recognition code: evidence for two layers of molecular selectivity. *Immunity*, **2**, 689.

Schreiber, R.D., Pace, J.L., Russell, S.W., Altman, A. and Katz, D.H. (1983). Macrophage activating factor produced by a T-cell hybridoma: physicochemical and biosynthetic resemblance to γ interferon. *Journal of Immunology*, **131**, 283.

Schulze-Osthoff, K., Ferrari, D., Los, M., Wesselborg, S. and Peter, M.E. (1998). Apoptosis signaling by death receptors. *European Journal of Biochemistry*, **254**, 439.

Schwandner, R., Dziarski, R., Wesche, H., Rothe, M. and Kirschning, C.J. (1999). Peptidoglycan- and lipoteichoic acid-induced cell activation is mediated by toll-like receptor 2. *Journal of Biological Chemistry*, **274**, 17406.

Seidel, H.M., Milocco, L.H., Lamb, P., Darnell, J.E., Jr, Stein, R.B. and Rosen, J. (1995). Spacing of palindromic half sites as a determinant of selective STAT (signal transducers and activators of transcription) DNA binding and transcriptional activity. *Proceedings of the National Academy of Sciences USA*, **92**, 3041.

Shaw, G. and Kamen, R. (1986). A conserved AU sequence from the 3′ untranslated region of GM-CSF mRNA mediates selective mRNA degradation. *Cell*, **46**, 659.

Sims, S.H., Cha, Y., Romine, M.F., Gao, P.-Q., Gottleib, K. and Deisseroth, A.B. (1993). A novel interferon-inducible domain: structural and functional analysis of the human interferon regulatory factor 1 gene promoter. *Molecular and Cellular Biology*, **13**, 690.

Sirenko, O.I., Lofquist, A.K., De Maria, C.T., Morris, J.S., Brewer, G. and Haskill, J.S. (1997). Adhesion-dependent regulation of an A+U-rich element-binding activity associated with AUF1. *Molecular and Cellular Biology*, **17**, 3898.

Smith, C.A., Farrah, T. and Goodwin, R.G. (1994). The TNF receptor superfamily of cellular and viral proteins: activation, costimulation, and death. *Cell*, **76**, 959.

Snyderman, R. and Uhing, R.J. (1992). Chemoattractant stimulus–response coupling. In Gallin, J.I., Goldstein. I.M. and Snyderman, R. (ed.), *Inflammation: Basic Principles and Clinical Correlates*. Raven Press, New York, p. 421.

Sonenberg, N. (1994). mRNA translation: influence of the 5′ and 3′ untranslated regions. *Current Opinion in Genetics and Development*, **4**, 310.

Song, G.Y., Chung, C.S., Schwacha, M.G., Jarrar, D., Chaudry, I.H. and Ayala, A. (1999). Splenic immune suppression in sepsis: a role for IL-10-induced changes in P38 MAPK signaling. *Journal of Surgical Research*, **83**, 36.

Stancato, L.F., Sakatsume, M., David, M., Dent, P., Dong, F., Petricoin, E.F. *et al.* (1997). Beta interferon and oncostatin M activate Raf-1 and mitogen-activated protein kinase through a JAK1-dependent pathway. *Molecular and Cellular Biology*, **17**, 3833.

Stark, G.R., Kerr, I.M., Williams, B.R., Silverman, R.H. and Schreiber, R.D. (1998). How cells respond to interferons. *Annual Review of Biochemistry*, **67**, 227.

Stein, M., Keshav, S., Harris, N. and Gordon, S. (1992). Interleukin 4 potently enhances murine macrophage mannose receptor activity: a marker of alternative immunologic macrophage activation. *Journal of Experimental Medicine*, **176**, 287.

Stoeckle, M.Y. (1991). Post-transcriptional regulation of *gro*α, β, γ, and IL-8 mRNAs by IL-1b, *Nucleic Acids Research*, **19**, 917.

Strader, C.D., Fong, T.M., Graziano, M.P. and Tota, M.R. (1995). The family of G-protein-coupled receptors. *FASEB Journal*, **9**, 745.

Struhl, K. (1998). Histone acetylation and transcriptional regulatory mechanisms. *Genes and Development*, **12**, 599.

Suttles, J., Milhorn, D.M., Miller, R.W., Poe, J.C., Wahl, L.M. and Stout, R.D. (1999). CD40 signaling of monocyte inflammatory cytokine synthesis through an ERK1/2-dependent pathway. A target of interleukin (il)-4 and il-10 anti-inflammatory action. *Journal of Biological Chemistry*, **274**, 5835.

Sweet, M.J. and Hume, D.A. (1996). Endotoxin signal transduction in macrophages. *Journal of Leukocyte Biology*, **60**, 8.

Takeda, K., Kishimoto, T. and Akira, S. (1997). STAT6: its role in interleukin 4-mediated biological functions. *Journal of Molecular Medicine*, **75**, 317.

Takeuchi, O., Hoshino, K., Kawai, T., Sanjo, H., Takada, H., Ogawa, T. *et al.* (1999). Differential roles of TLR2 and TLR4 in recognition of gram-negative and gram-positive bacterial cell wall components. *Immunity*, **11**, 443.

Tannenbaum, C.S., Major, J.A. and Hamilton, T.A. (1993). IFN-γ and lipopolysaccharide differentially modulate expression of tumor necrosis factor receptor mRNA in murine peritoneal macrophages. *Journal of Immunology*, **12**, 6833.

Tapping, R.I., Gegner, J.A., Kravchenko, V.V. and Tobias, P.S. (1998). Roles for LBP and soluble CD14 in cellular uptake of LPS. *Progress in Clinical Biology Research*, **397**, 73.

Tartaglia, L.A., Weber, R.F., Figari, I.S., Reynolds, C., Palladino, M.A., Jr and Goeddel, D.V. (1991). The two different receptors for tumor necrosis factor mediate distinct cellular responses. *Proceedings of the National Academy of Sciences USA*, **88**, 9292.

Tebo, J.M., Kim, H.S., Gao, J. Armstrong, D.A. and Hamilton, T.A. (1998). Interleukin-10 suppresses IP-10 gene transcription by inhibiting the production of class I interferon. *Blood*, **92**, 4742.

Tebo, J., Datta, S., Kishore, R., Kolosov, M., Major, J.A., Ohmori, Y. *et al.* (2000). IL-1-mediated stabilization of mouse KC mRNA depends on sequences in both 5′ and 3′ untranslated regions. *Journal of Biological Chemistry*, **275**, 12987.

Ting, J.P. and Baldwin, A.S. (1993). Regulation of MHC gene expression. *Current Opinion in Immunology*, **5**, 8.

Tobias, P.S., Tapping, R.I. and Gegner, J.A. (1999). Endotoxin interactions with lipopolysaccharide-responsive cells. *Clinics in Infectious Diseases*, **28**, 476.

Tsuruta, L., Arai, N. and Arai, K. (1998). Transcriptional control of cytokine genes. *International Review of Immunology*, **16**, 581.

Uddin, S., Fish, E.N., Sher, D.A., Gardziola, C., White, M.F. and Platanias, L.C. (1997). Activation of the phosphatidylinositol 3-kinase serine kinase by IFN-α. *Journal of Immunology*, **158**, 2390.

Ulevitch, R.J. and Tobias, P.S. (1995). Receptor-dependent mechanisms of cell stimulation by bacterial endotoxin. *Annual Review of Immunology*, **13**, 437.

Ulevitch, R.J. and Tobias, P.S. (1999). Recognition of gram-negative bacteria and endotoxin by the innate immune system. *Current Opinion in Immunology*, **11**, 19.

Underhill, D.M., Ozinsky, A., Smith, K.D. and Aderem, A. (1999). Toll-like receptor-2 mediates mycobacteria-induced proinflammatory signaling in macrophages. *Proceedings of the National Academy of Sciences USA*, **96**, 14459.

Van Rooijen, N., Wijburg, O.L., van den Dobbelsteen, G.P. and Sanders, A. (1996). Macrophages in host defense mechanisms. *Current Topics in Microbiology and Immunology*, **210**, 159.

Vilcek, J., Gray, P.W., Rinderknect, E. and Sevastopoulos, C.G. (1985). Interferon g: a lymphokine for all seasons. *Lymphokines*, **11**, 1.

Vogel, S.N., Perera, P.Y., Detore, G.R., Bhat, N., Carboni, J.M., Haziot, A. *et al.* (1998). CD14 dependent and independent signaling pathways in murine macrophages from normal and CD14 'knockout' (CD14KO) mice stimulated with LPS or taxol. *Progress in Clinical and Biological Research*, **397**, 137.

Wagner, B.J., DeMaria, C.T., Sun, Y., Wilson, G.M. and Brewer, G. (1998). Structure and genomic organization of the human *AUF1* gene: alternative pre-mRNA splicing generates four protein isoforms. *Genomics*, **48**, 195.

Wajant, H., Grell, M. and Scheurich, P. (1999). TNF receptor associated factors in cytokine signaling. *Cytokine and Growth Factor Reviews*, **10**, 15.

Walker, W.S., Gatewood, J., Olivas, E., Askew, D. and Havenith,C.E. (1995). Mouse microglial cell lines differing in constitutive and interferon-γ-inducible antigen-presenting activities for naive and memory CD4⁺ and CD8⁺ T cells. *Journal of Neuroimmunology*, **63**, 163.

Warfel, A.H., Thorbecke, G.J. and Belsito, D.V. (1995). Synergism between interferon-γ and cytokines or lipopolysaccharide in the activation of the HIV-LTR in macrophages. *Journal of Leukocyte Biology*, **57**, 469.

Warzocha, K. and Salles, G. (1998). The tumor necrosis factor signaling complex: choosing a path toward cell death or cell proliferation. *Leukocytes and Lymphoma*, **29**, 81.

Weidemann, B., Schletter, J., Dziarski, R., Kusumoto, S., Stelter, F., Rietschel, E.T. *et al.* (1997). Specific binding of soluble peptidoglycan and muramyldipeptide to CD14 on human monocytes. *Infection and Immunity*, **65**, 858.

White, M.F. (1996). The IRS-signalling system in insulin and cytokine action. *Philosophical Transactions of the Royal Society of London Series B, Biological Sciences*, **351**, 181.

Wilson, G.M. and Brewer, G. (1999a). The search for *trans*-acting factors controlling messenger RNA decay. *Progress on Nucleic Acid Research and Molecular Biology*, **62**, 257.

Wilson, G.M. and Brewer, G. (1999b). Identification and characterization of proteins binding A + U-rich elements. *Methods*, 17, 74.

Winzen, R., Kracht, M., Ritter, B., Wilhelm, A., Chen, C.Y., Shyu, A.B. *et al.* (1999). The p38 MAP kinase pathway signals for cytokine-induced mRNA stabilization via MAP kinase-activated protein kinase 2 and an AU-rich region-targeted mechanism. *EMBO Journal*, **18**, 4969.

Wong, P., Severns, C.W., Guyer, N.B. and Wright, T.M. (1994). A unique palindromic element mediates g interferon induction of *mig* gene expression. *Molecular and Cellular Biology*, **14**, 914.

Wood, L.C., Elias, P.M., Calhoun, C., Tsai, J.C., Grunfeld, C. and Feingold, K.R. (1996). Barrier disruption stimulates interleukin-1 α expression and release from a pre-formed pool in murine epidermis. *Journal of Investigative Dermatology*, **106**, 397.

Wright, K.L., Chin, K.C., Linhoff, M., Skinner, C., Brown, J.A., Boss, J.M. *et al.* (1998). CIITA stimulation of transcription factor binding to major histocompatibility complex class II and associated promoters *in vivo*. *Proceedings of the National Academy of Sciences USA*, **95**, 6267.

Wurfel, M.M., Monks, B.G., Ingalls, R.R., Dedrick, R.L., Delude, R., Zhou, D. *et al.* (1997). Targeted deletion of the lipopolysaccharide (LPS)-binding protein gene leads to profound suppression of LPS responses *ex vivo*, whereas *in vivo* responses remain intact. *Journal of Experimental Medicine*, **186**, 2051.

Yoshimura, A., Lien, E., Ingalls, R.R., Tuomanen, E., Dziarski, R. and Golenbock, D. (1999). Cutting edge: recognition of Gram-positive bacterial cell wall components by the innate immune system occurs via Toll-like receptor 2. *Journal of Immunology*, **163**, 1.

Young, H.A. and Hardy, K.J. (1995). Role of interferon-γ in immune cell regulation. *Journal of Leukocyte Biology*, **58**, 373.

3 Macrophages as antigen-presenting cells: relationship to dendritic cells and use in vaccination studies

P. Paglia and M.P. Colombo

1 Introduction

Pioneering studies have demonstrated that only a very small proportion of an injected antigen (<1%) is involved in an immune response, the rest being rapidly degraded and excreted (Nossal, 1995). This suggests that antigen presentation is a rate-limiting step in an immune response and therefore needs to be handled in a highly specialized manner. A wide spectrum of cells can present antigens (Table 3.1) depending on how and where the antigen first encounters cells of the immune system and on the nature of the antigen itself. Antigen-presenting cells (APCs) have evolved in subtypes that have specialized features regarding the mechanism of antigen uptake, processing and transport to lymphoid organs, and interaction with lymphocytes. Many cells have the ability to capture pathogens and harmful cells and to process them somehow.

Immune responses are initiated when APCs present an antigen to T cells in the context of molecules of the major histocompatibility complex (MHC), class I or class II, and a second co-stimulatory signal(s) (Shimada *et al.*, 1987; Caux *et al.*, 1994a,b; Inaba *et al.*, 1994; Larsen *et al.*, 1994; Chang *et al.*, 1995; Sallusto *et al.*, 1995) is provided to activate T cells, inducing clonal expansion and production of the regulatory cytokines. Antigen presentation features direct the nature of the T cell-mediated responses (Banchereau and Steinman, 1998). Molecules involved in delivery of second signals from APCs to T cells have been defined (Shimada *et al.*, 1987; Caux *et al.*, 1994a,c; Inaba *et al.*, 1994; Larsen *et al.*, 1994; Chang *et al.*, 1995; Sallusto *et al.*, 1995); these include CD80/86 and CD40 which interact with CD28 and CD154, respectively, on T cells (Mackey *et al.*, 1998). Co-stimulatory signals are required to enhance cellular adhesion and signaling and promote maximal cross-talk between APCs and T cells.

Second signals might also regulate immunity through the selective activation of different subsets of T lymphocyte-mediated responses. A T-cell response can be of type 1 (mediated by Th1 and Tc1), that is involved primarily in cell-mediated immune responses against intracellular pathogens and tumors. A type 1 response is characterized by the production of interferon-γ (IFN-γ), tumor necrosis factor-α (TNF-α) and complement-fixing antibody (Lichtman and Abbas 1997). The type 2 response (mediated by Th2 and Tc2),

Table 3.1   Overview of antigen-presenting cells

	Phagocytosis	Cell type	Location	MHC II expression
Phagocytes (monocyte/ macrophage lineage)	+	Monocyte Macrophage MZ-macrophage Kupfer cells Microglia	Blood Tissue Spleen/lymph nodes Liver Brain	(–) to (++++) inducible
Non-phagocytic professional APCs	±	Langerhans cells Dendritic cells Follicular dendritic cells	Skin Tissue/lymph nodes Lymphoid tissue	+++ (constitutive) –
Lymphocytes	–	B and T lymphocytes	Lymphoid tissues and sites of immune reactions	(–) to (++++) inducible
Facultative APCs	+	Astrocytes Follicular cells	Brain Thyroid	Inducible Inducible
	–	Endothelium	Vascular and lymphoid tissue	(–) to (++++) inducible
		Fibroblast	Connective tissue	

conversely, is involved in regulating humoral immunity and is characterized by the production of interleukin-4 (IL-4), IL-5 and IL-13. These cytokines participate in immunoglobulin class switching and regulate the production of IgE and eosinophil-rich inflammatory infiltrates, which are particularly adapted to eliminate multicellular parasites (Moore *et al.*, 1993). An interesting hypothesis is that the nature of different stimuli provided by the environment, i.e. in the inflammatory context, makes the APCs able to regulate differently the 'type' of immune response to be issued. Therefore, the establishment of the role of different APCs in regulation of immune responses is a first essential step toward the generation of effective immunotherapeutic agents (Banchereau and Steinman, 1998). APCs serve as immunological windows to the outside world. In general, the different types of APCs can be subdivided into professional and non-professional cells. While the latter are found among non-lymphoid cells, professional APCs are an integral part of the immune system.

The APCs termed 'professional' are macrophages, Langerhans cells (LCs), myeloid dendritic cells and lymphoid dendritic cells, but B lymphocytes can also perform professional presentation of antigens (Bell *et al.*, 1999). Dendritic cells (DCs) and macrophages display extensive heterogeneity in phenotype and function, most probably due to the influence of the large number of cytokines and environmental factors that act on these cells during their differentiation/maturation pathway. The result is a network of APCs that range from immature progenitors to fully mature macrophages and DCs. This network is responsible for determining the type of T-cell response that will occur during an immune response. Phagocytosis and micropinocytosis are probably the most important functions by which cells can capture antigens for later processing and presentation to T lymphocytes. Phagocytosis is also important for clearing the body of microorganisms and damaged cells. The need to perform both antigen presentation and debris removal during a relatively short time span may explain in part the need for different subsets of APCs arising from a common intermediate, and might explain, at least to some extent, the observed *trans*-differentiation occurring between monocytes/macrophages and DCs (Randolph *et al.*, 1998, 1999; Palucka *et al.*, 1998; Banyer and Hapel, 1999). Basically, there are APCs with the ability to initiate a primary immune response by the presentation of antigens to naïve T cells, and there are APCs that will stimulate a secondary response by presenting the same antigens to already activated T cells. It has now become clear that it is only the DC system that has the former ability, while a number of different cells, including macrophages, may be engaged in secondary responses. However, it is probably obsolete to define DCs and macrophages as separate subtypes of APCs; rather it may be more appropriate to consider them as an interactive network, sensitive to intercellular cross-talk and extremely responsive to environmental factors. This network is able to discriminate dangerous entities from non-dangerous ones and to signal this danger appropriately to the armed branch of the immune system (Matzinger, 1994; Paglia and Guzman, 1998).

2 Origins of APCs: from the CD34⁺ hemopoietic multipotent progenitor to the myelodendritic precursors

The CD34 molecule belongs to the mucin membrane molecule family and is expressed on virtually all normal hematopoietic progenitors. Bone marrow-derived CD34$^+$ hemopoietic multipotent progenitors give rise to all cell types in the immune system (Figure 3.1).

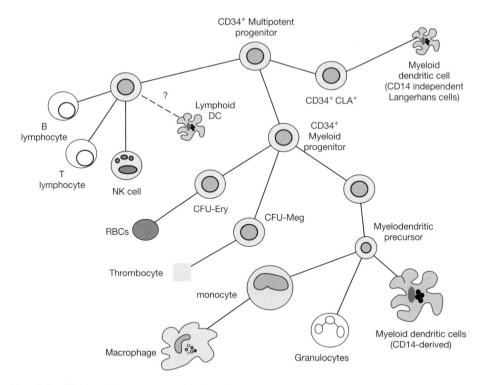

Fig. 3.1 CD34+ multipotent progenitor developmental pathways.

Macrophages originally were regarded as the principal APC population. This notion resulted from the initial work on APCs (Unanue, 1984) which found that accessory activity was lost on treatment with the phagotoxic agent L-leucine methyl ester (Thiele *et al.*, 1983). Phagocytic activity was considered as a hallmark of myeloid/monocytic descendants (van Furth, 1980). Cells lacking this classical monocyte/macrophage feature were, by definition, excluded from belonging to the mononuclear phagocyte system (MPS). As a consequence, DCs were long assumed to descend from a lineage distinct from that of monocytes/macrophages (Steinman and Cohn, 1973; Austyn, 1987). Although the real origin of the DC system is still not yet completely understood, it has been clearly demonstrated that DCs can differentiate from myeloid precursor and human peripheral blood monocytes. Moreover, the *in vitro* disruption of the classical DC differentiation pathway has been found to lead to an enhanced production of macrophages and neutrophils (Burkly *et al.*, 1995), thus indicating a compensatory mechanism and further supporting the concept of a common lineage for DCs and macrophages.

Although several questions remain concerning the descendants of so-called 'lymphoid DCs' and DCs arising from a CD14-independent pathway, as might be the case for LCs, it is now possible to define a single track, which starts from the myelodendritic precursor and has as its final outcome most professional APCs. This track would be better defined as a maturation than a differentiation pathway and the final APCs better considered as the product of sequential events depending on inflammatory signals, antigen-induced release of cytokines and release of innate immunity mediators which might influence this maturation differently. The myelodendritic progenitor is probably the cell progenitor most susceptible to environmental-dependent stimuli. Thus, cells with the properties of both macrophages and DCs can be derived from a single type of granulocyte–macrophage colony-stimulating factor (GM-CSF)-responsive progenitor cell. When differences in gene expression are analyzed as the cells mature along the DC and macrophage pathways, a distinctive pattern of differentially expressed cDNAs is observed. Macrophage-specific cDNAs are homologous to genes encoding cytoskeletal and cell surface proteins, whereas the DC-specific cDNAs are homologous to signaling-, chemokine- and IFN-γ-inducible genes. These data suggest that DCs and macrophages indeed have different characteristics that are somewhat interchangeable, depending on their surrounding environment.

Studies with multipotent CD34$^+$ progenitors and peripheral blood mononuclear cells (PBMCs) have discovered two other DC pathways, both associated with the myeloid lineage (Caux *et al.*, 1994b, 1997; Szabolics *et al.*, 1996; Cella *et al.*, 1997a; Hart, 1997; Reid, 1997; Shortman and Caux, 1997). One pathway is derived from a CD14$^+$ precursor and is represented by a CD14$^+$CD1a$^-$ intermediate; the other is derived from a CD14$^-$CD1a$^+$ precursor. Both lineages can produce mature DCs capable of stimulating strong naïve T-lymphocyte responses. The CD14-dependent (CD14-derived) DC pathway is closely related to the myelomonocytic pathway. Immature cells of this pathway exhibit non-specific esterase activity, complement receptors (CD11b), macrophage colony-stimulating factor receptors (M-CSFRs; CD115) and phagocytic potential, whereas the cells of the CD14-independent (CD1a-derived) pathway display low or undetectable levels of these markers (Caux *et al.*, 1996; Szabolics *et al.*, 1996). Mature DCs of both pathways express high levels of MHC I, MHC II and B7 molecules, but only mature CD14-derived DCs express CD68 and factor XIIIa (Caux 1998). Similarly, only mature CD1a-derived DCs exhibit intracellular Birbeck granules and E-cadherin (Caux 1998). TNF, GM-CSF and IL-4 modulate the maturation of CD14-derived DCs from CD34$^+$ progenitors or CD14$^+$ PBMCs (Caux, 1998; Cavanagh *et al.*, 1998). On the other hand, transforming growth factor-β (TGF-β) appears to be the principal factor required for CD1a-derived DC maturation (Geissmann *et al.*, 1998; Strobl *et al.*, 1998). TGF-β seems to act preferentially on a CD34$^+$CLA$^+$ (cutaneous leukocyte antigen) progenitor (Strunk *et al.*, 1997).

Myeloid DCs might be anatomically restricted: CD14-derived DCs most probably correspond to interstitial and/or circulating DCs, whereas CD1a-derived DCs are related to LCs (Caux, 1997; Shortman and Caux, 1997). Functional segregation within the myeloid DC lineage system can be identified. *In vitro* studies have shown that CD14-derived DCs prime T cells to activate preferentially Th1 responses and have implicated the release of IL-12 in this process (Hilkens *et al.*, 1997; McRae *et al.*, 1998). CD14-derived DCs but not CD1a-derived DCs activate naïve B cells to secrete IgM in the presence of CD40L and IL-2 (Shortman and Caux, 1997). Distinct DC subtypes activating either Th1 or Th2 responses have been observed in psoriasis and atopic asthma (Bellini *et al.*, 1993; Nestlé *et al.*, 1994). Additional observations indicate that CD14-derived DCs are increased in rheumatoid arthritis (Santiago-Schwarz *et al.*, 1998b), an autoimmune disorder predominantly associated with an inflammatory Th1 response (Dolhian *et al.*, 1996; Rocken *et al.*, 1996; Yin *et al.*, 1997). CD14$^+$CD1a$^-$ progenitor cells can differentiate into macrophages by three major pathways: respectively driven by M-CSF, GM-CSF or IL-3. Macrophages maintain the same M-CSF susceptibility as their precursors, they become strongly adherent phagocytic cells and express F4/80, Mac-1 and cell surface fms (a receptor tyrosine kinase for M-CSF). They originate directly from blood monocytes and reside in discrete sites as tissue macrophages. Monocytes are highly mobile cells that can be recruited steadily at sites of inflammation. Macrophages display the highest susceptibility to environmental stimuli and locally released cytokines [i.e. IL-1, IL-4, IFN-γ, IL-10, TNF-α, stem cell factor (SCF), leukemia inhibitory factor (LIF) and TGF-β]. These factors primarily modulate the functional maturation of locally recruited macrophages. These cells are particularly important for tissue remodeling, angiogenesis, removal of debris, and pathogen killing that is mediated by the release of toxic oxygen and nitrogen radicals (McKnight and Gordon, 1998).

The role of these macrophages in triggering immune response is contentious. They present antigens poorly and do not display mobility from the periphery towards lymphoid organs. Tissue macrophages might instead have a regulatory role; in fact they can display an immunosuppressive phenotype (Holt *et al.*, 1993). However, *trans*-differentiation between macrophages and DCs can occur, and this 'functional interchange' is well supported by an interesting *in vitro* model that uses Myb-transformed hematopoietic cells (MTHCs) (Banyer and Hapel, 1999). Enforced expression of Myb confers immortality to the transformed cells as long as these are maintained with a suitable cocktail of mitogenic cytokines. MTHCs retain the ability to respond to a wide variety of stimuli and maintain most of the properties of progenitor cells. Myb-transformed clones differentiate into macrophage-like cells in response to TNF-α plus IL-4 and into DCs if IFN-γ is substituted for IL-4. Mature DCs derived from MTHCs appear to *trans*-differentiate into macrophages when IL-4 is added, suggesting that morphological change induced by IL-4 is dominant over that induced by IFN-γ. Unstimulated MTHCs mostly resemble the bipotent CD14[+] cell derived from the fluorescence-activated cell sorting (FACS)-sorted CD34[+] myeloid cell pool (Cella *et al.*, 1997b). These CD14[+] cells mature into macrophages in the presence of M-CSF and into DCs in the presence of GM-CSF plus IL-4. MTHCs also respond to M-CSF, leading to macrophage differentiation. The combination of TNF-α with IL-4 is also a potent inducer of CD14[+] cell maturation to macrophage-like cells. Thus, TNF-α and IL-4 seem to provide powerful signals for macrophage differentiation. The relationship between M-CSF-, GM-CSF- or TNF-α- and IL-4-induced macrophages is not clear. The combination of GM-CSF, TNF-α and IL-4 induces the maturation of cells that by many conventional criteria would be considered macrophages but which are more closely related to DCs. When IFN-γ is substituted for IL-4 in this system, MTHCs develop into fully functional DCs.

3 Searching for the stimuli required for macrophage/DC differentiation: tuning immune responses

Although a DC-restricted cytokine does not appear to exist, several cytokines may act at different developmental stages to regulate myeloid DC ontogeny. CD14-dependent and -independent DC pathways develop simultaneously from CD34[+] cord blood progenitors on treatment with GM-CSF/TNF/SCF (GTS) (Caux *et al.*, 1996; Szabolcs *et al.*, 1996; Shortman and Caux, 1997; Santiago-Schwarz *et al.*, 1998a). Even though both differentiation pathways proceed in the presence of GTS, the CD1a[+] pathway eventually prevails (Szabolcs *et al.*, 1996). The early presence of TNF (within 48 h) is mandatory for DC hematopoiesis from CD34$^+$ progenitors to occur (Reid *et al.*, 1992; Santiago-Schwarz *et al.*, 1993). TNF up-regulates GM-CSF receptors on DC intermediates, inhibits the granulocytic pathway and induces specific apoptotic events of pro-myeloid progenitors (Reid *et al.*, 1992; Santiago-Schwarz *et al.*, 1993, 1997). If TNF activity is neutralized before 48 h of cytokine exposure, DC development is halted and granulocyte hematopoiesis is favored (Santiago-Schwarz *et al.*, 1993). The positive effect of TNF on DC generation from CD34$^+$ progenitors appears to be mediated exclusively by the type 1 TNF (p55) receptor (Lardon, 1997); however, other members of the TNF superfamily control DC differentiation and survival (Anderson *et al.*, 1997; Flores-Romo *et al.*, 1997; Pettitt *et al.*, 1997; Wong *et al.*, 1997). CD40L, a member of the TNFR family, drives a subset of CD34$^+$ progenitors to mature into DCs (Flores-Romo *et al.*, 1997). Because both TNF and CD40L activate NF-kB, there may be common mediators for distinct DC subtypes. RANK/TRANCE-R mediates the survival of mature DCs by preventing them undergoing apoptosis (Anderson *et al.*, 1997; Wong *et al.*, 1997). Other factors can prolong the survival of mature DCs via anti-apoptotic mechanisms: they include TNF, CD40L, IL-3 and GM-CSF (Hart, 1997; Shurin *et al.*, 1999). RelB, a member of the NF-B/Rel family of transcription factors, is stimulated by TNF and is expressed selectively by fully mature DCs (Pettitt *et al.*, 1997). SCF is not critical for the onset of DC hematopoiesis, but serves to amplify DC yield in GM-CSF/TNF-treated progenitor cell cultures by increasing the self-renewal and longevity of DC progenitors/precursors (Santiago-Scharwz *et al.*, 1995; Reid, 1996). A closely related, non-lineage-restricted cytokine, Flt3 ligand (FL), also acts at the progenitor/precursor level to increase cell proliferation within the myeloid DC lineage system *in vitro* (Strobl *et al.*, 1997; Rosenzwajg *et al.*, 1998). Gene knockout studies have helped to determine whose cytokines promote DC development *in vivo*. GM-CSF and GM-CSFR knockout mice exhibit almost normal numbers of DCs in lymphoid organs, suggesting the development of GM-CSF-independent DCs, including IL3-driven DC subtypes (Vremec *et al.*, 1997). TGF-β knockout mice have demonstrated the importance of this cytokine in the generation of CD1a-dependent (LC type) DCs (Borkowski *et al.*, 1996). In these animals, LCs, but not CD11c$^+$ DCs, are lacking. IL-6 is produced as an accessory secondary cytokine for DC development when CD34$^+$ progenitors are treated with GM-CSF and TNF (Borkowski *et al.*, 1996b). When combined with M-CSF, however, IL-6 treatment of CD34$^+$ progenitor cells down-regulates myeloid DC development and predominantly yields large macrophages with poor APC capabilities (Caux, 1998).

Conversely, what turns APCs off? Early studies have shown that IL-10 inhibits the antigen-presenting capacity of monocytes/macrophages (Moore, 1993). More recently, IL-10 was also shown to inhibit the APC functions of *in vitro* generated DCs (Caux, 1994b; Thomssen *et al.*, 1995). However, the precise mechanisms for this inhibition have not yet been precisely defined. Some studies indicate that IL-10 affects the expression of co-stimulatory molecules such as members of the 'B7 family' (Buelens *et al.*, 1995; Ozawa *et al.*, 1996; Steinbrink *et al.*, 1997). Moreover, other studies have never found any alterations in the expression of either the CD80/86 molecule or MHC–peptide complexes (Morel *et al.*, 1997). IL-10 may exert different effects depending on the maturation stage of DCs. CD83 and CD86 expression, as well as secretion of IL-8 and TNF, can be inhibited by IL-10 when DCs have been induced to mature fully with lipopolysaccharide (LPS). The same effects are not exerted by IL-10 when DCs have been exposed to CD40L as the maturation-inducing stimulus (Buelens *et al.*, 1997b). *In vitro*, IL-10-

treated DCs have been observed preferentially to induce the differentiation of naïve T cells toward the Th2 phenotype (Liu *et al.*, 1997; Allavena *et al.*, 1998). The most critical activity of IL-10 is exerted at the level of precursor differentiation: IL-10 inhibits the IL-4/GM-CSF-induced proliferation of monocytes into DCs (Buelens *et al.*, 1997a; Moore *et al.*, 1997), with the benefit of macrophage development (Allavena *et al.*, 1998). In addition, IL-10 can induce apoptosis of both DCs, by acting as an antagonist of TNF, and freshly isolated LCs (Ludewig *et al.*, 1995). Finally, the inhibitory role of IL-10 has been shown *in vivo*, where IL-10-expressing tumors blocked the GM-CSF-dependent recruitment of DCs within neoplasia (Qin *et al.*, 1997).

4 Inside the dendritic cell system

It would be unwise to construct an ideal profile for macrophages or DCs: no single characteristic, but rather a host of criteria that cover different features, either morphological or functional, must be carefully taken into account for a correct classification. All tissues, with the possible exception of brain and testis, contain immature DCs; these cells are capable of capturing antigens but do not yet possess the panel of accessory molecules that are required for potent stimulation of naïve T lymphocytes. Notably, antigens that are able to drive an immune response are those that initiate the maturation of DCs most efficiently.

DCs were characterized initially by the presence of veils, polarized lamellipodia and long spiny processes continuously extended and retracted, thus allowing these cells to be extremely motile and therefore named 'dendritic'. The shape and motility of DCs fit well with their functions, which are to capture antigens in peripheral tissues and select rare antigen-specific T cells once they have migrated into lymphoid organs. DCs have a peculiar morphology: they are large cells, irregularly shaped with long motile cytoplasmic processes or veils (about 10 μm) DCs have a lobulated nucleus, and a large Golgi apparatus required for intense synthesis of MHC, co-stimulatory molecules and cytokines. The multivesicular bodies are also extremely rich, and comprise endosomes, lysosome and MHC II-enriched compartments (MIICs), all structures involved in processing and presentation of antigens. Notably, in the absence of specific DC lineage markers, these morphological features have for a long time been considered essential in identifying DCs. Up to now, DCs have been defined more by the lack than by the presence of selectively expressed cell surface molecules. DCs can never be observed as a static population, but their phenotype, as defined by the expression of cell surface antigens, and their functions are changing continuously throughout the maturation stages they undergo. Two functional stages distinguish immature and mature DCs. The main function of immature or tissue DCs is to patrol peripheral tissues and capture antigens for processing and delivery to lymphoid organs. Mature DCs are specialized in presenting processed antigens to naïve T lymphocytes. The maturation stages of DCs are associated with peculiar patterns of both surface and intracellular molecule expression and functional properties (Figure 3.2). DCs are present in most tissues in an immature state, unable to stimulate T lymphocytes but fully equipped to capture and process antigens. Immature DCs can internalize efficiently a diverse array of antigens for processing and loading onto MHC molecules, as a consequence of high endocytic activity. Antigen uptake by immature DCs can occur via distinct mechanisms: (1) macropinocytosis; (2) receptor-mediated endocytosis through Fc receptors; (3) receptor-mediated endocytosis

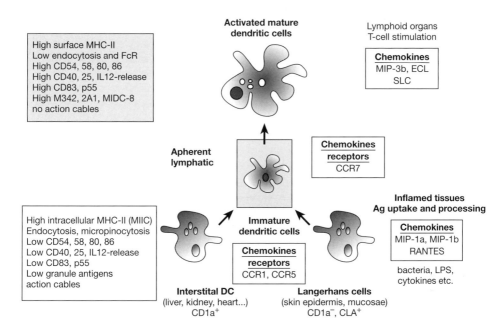

Fig. 3.2   Features of dendritic cells trafficking from peripheral tissues to lymphoid organs.

through the mannose receptor or the C-type lectin receptor DEC205; and (4) engulfment of apoptotic bodies through the vitronectin receptor α(v) β₃. (Bell *et al.*, 1999). Macropinocytosis and receptor-mediated antigen capture make antigen processing by DCs so efficient that only picomolar antigen concentrations are required, whereas micromolar levels are required by other types of APCs. Macropinocytosis is constitutive in immature DCs. This function allows DCs to sample a volume of extracellular fluid similar to half the volume of one DC every hour (Sallusto *et al.*, 1995).

LCs, the skin DCs and interstitial DCs are phagocytic, although to a lesser extent than macrophages. Human epidermal LCs, but not other epidermal cells, express FcεRI and use it to maximize antigen uptake via specific IgEs. DCs also use FcγR whose expression is down-regulated in response to maturation stimuli, showing again that antigen capture is reduced by maturation. DCs express high levels of both mannose receptor and DEC205, which are involved in the internalization of glycoproptein. While Fc receptors are degraded together with their cargo, the mannose receptor is equipped to release its ligand at endosomal pH and it is therefore recycled onto the cell surface. This allows the uptake and accumulation of many ligands by a relative small number of receptors. Mannose receptors have a critical role in phagocytosis of microbes (Reis e Sousa *et al.*, 1993). Such molecules are thought to play a key role in the first line of defense against infectious agents. Alveolar macrophages express relatively high levels of mannose receptor that have a precise role in innate immunity against airborne pathogens. In addition to phagocytosis, the engagement of the mannose receptor leads to the release of an array of inflammatory mediators such as reactive oxygen intermediates and neutral proteinases (McKnight *et al.*, 1998). DEC205 is an integral membrane protein homologous to the mannose receptor, and it is probably the most 'DC-restricted' molecule. DEC205 and its antigenic ligand on the surface of DCs are internalized rapidly by means of coated pits and vesicles, and then delivered to a multi-vescicular endosomal compartment that morphologically resembles MIIC vesicles, and is involved in antigen processing (Jiang *et al.*, 1995; Geuze, 1998).

Macrophages are extremely active in both endocytosis and phagocytosis, even in the absence of any inflammatory signals, but express low levels of co-stimulatory accessory molecules. Exposure of macrophages to a number of inflammatory cytokines triggers the increase of both endocytic activity and expression of co-stimulatory molecules. The process of phagocytosis *per se* is able to up-regulate co-stimulatory molecules (De Bruijin *et al.*, 1996), thus enabling the presentation of antigens at sites of antigen deposition within peripheral tissues. In this sense, macrophages might contribute in preventing primed T cells becoming tolerised in peripheral tissues or might locally amplify the response of primed T lymphocytes. A special feature of DCs is to capture and engulf apoptotic cells. DCs internalize apoptotic bodies by binding them preferentially through $\alpha_v \beta_5$, $\alpha_v \beta_3$ and the CD36/thrombospondin receptor (Albert *et al.*, 1998a; Bell *et al.*, 1999). The internalization of apoptotic bodies by this mechanism raises the intracellular concentration of free Ca^{2+}, which is essential for the engulfment (Rubartelli *et al.*, 1997). Macrophages also engulf apoptotic bodies using multiple surface receptors, CD14, CD36 and the phosphatidylserine receptor. Although macrophages internalize apoptotic cells very efficiently, they are unable to present apoptotic body-associated antigens, probably due to the lack of $\alpha_v \beta_5$ molecules which are responsible for the transport of apoptotic bodies to the processing compartment. Macrophages engulfing apoptotic cells are unable to stimulate specific cytotoxic T lymphocytes (CTLs); macrophages might display a regulatory role in this context, preventing DC-mediated CTL generation by locally sequestering the antigen.

Capture of antigens provides DCs with signals to mature. During migration towards lymphoid organs, immediately after antigen loading in peripheral tissues, DCs undergo changes in phenotype and function as part of their maturation program. Uptake receptors and phagocytic ability and all features related to antigen capture are progressively lost during DC maturation (Reis e Sousa *et al.*, 1993; Fanger *et al.*, 1996). It is clear that DC maturation is critical for the initiation of immunity. Maturation can be influenced by a variety of factors defined as 'danger signals' (Bevan, 1976a,b), notably microbial and inflammatory products. A variety of cytokines contribute to DCs maturation: these include IL-1 and TNF that can be released by a variety of cells, including locally recruited macrophages. Whole bacteria and some of their cell wall components such as LPS and teichoic acids stimulate DCs maturation (Rescigno *et al.*, 1998). In addition, signaling through the TNF receptor family (i.e. TNF-R, CD40 and TRANCE/RANK) activates the NF-kB cascade within DCs. Mature DCs express high levels of the NF-kB family of post-transcriptional control proteins (RelA/p65, RelB, RelC, p50 and p52) which regulate the expression of many genes encoding immune and inflammatory proteins (Granelli-Piperno *et al.*, 1995). In addition to efficient antigen capture, DCs fulfill other requirements for antigen presentation by synthesizing and expressing high levels of MHC molecules (Young *et al.*, 1992; Kleijmeer *et al.*, 1994). While in macrophages most of the protein substrate is concentrated in lysosomes where it is fully digested into amino acids, antigens captured by DCs are concentrated in the endocytic pathway, in MIICs, where large amounts of peptide–MHC complexes can be formed. MIICs are late endosomal compartment that contain HLA-DM or H-2M products, which enhance and control peptide binding to MHC II molecules. During maturation of DCs, MIICs convert to non-lysosomal vesicles that discharge their contents on the cell membrane allowing for high expression of MHC–peptide complexes on the outside cell surface (Cella *et al.*, 1997b; Pierre *et al.*, 1997). Considerable evidence indicates that the late endosomes, which develop from the vacuolar parts of the early endosome network, and their lysosomal derivatives, play a crucial role in MHC II-mediated antigen presenation. In DCs, the majority of intracellular class II molecules are found in late endocytic structures with numerous internal membrane vescicles and sheets, collectively named MIICs. A minor compartment is represented by early endosomes that contain mature MHC II molecules internalized directly from the cell surface and rapidly recycled. MIICs also contain newly synthesized MHC II molecules that are directed to this compartment by the Ii chain, together with DM molecules that are responsible for removing the Ii-derived class II-associated invariant chain peptide (CLIP) and promoting the formation of stable MHC–peptide complexes (Lanzavecchia, 1996).

During DC maturation, three sequential stages can be identified. In the early stage, MHC II and antigens are co-localized to lysosomal compartments. In the intermediate stage, DCs accumulate MHC II in distinctive non-lysosomal vescicles and, finally, in the mature DCs stage, peptide–MHC II complexes are present stably on the plasma membrane for long periods of time, thereby allowing the selection of even rare antigen-specific T cells (Cella *et al.*, 1997b; Pierre *et al.*, 1997). An important attribute of DCs is their mobility. This property allows DCs to move from the blood to peripheral tissues and from these tissues to lymphoid organs, where a pool of quiescent T cells recirculates. Following antigen capture and processing, DCs move towards lymphoid organs to meet antigen-specific T cells.

Migration is explained by the switch in expression of chemokine receptors, induced during DC maturation. Immature DCs express CCR1 and CCR5, whose ligands are the inflammatory cytokines MIP-1 α, MIP-1 β and RANTES. These receptors are down-regulated following signaling mediated by CD40L, TNF-α or LPS, thus allowing DCs to leave peripheral inflamed tissues through apherent lymphatics. At this stage of DCs maturation, expression of CCR7 is induced. MIP-3 β/EBI1 ligand (ELC) and secondary lymphoid tissue (SLC) chemokines, which are constitutively produced in lymphoid organs (Ward *et al.*, 1998), are the CCR7 receptors. In lymph nodes and spleen, DCs localize within T-dependent areas where they cluster with T lymphocytes. Several adhesion molecules (CD54, CD58 and CD102) that are abundantly expressed on the surface of mature DCs favor this interaction. The DC–T cell interaction is stabilized additionally by the specific recognition between MHC–peptide complex and the T-cell receptors (TCRs), which delivers the first activation signal to the T cells. A second co-stimulatory signal, which is absolutely required in order to avoid T-cell anergy and to promote T-cell proliferation, is therefore provided by mature DCs which have up-regulated the expression of the B7 molecules, CD80 and CD86, on their surface. Moreover, the CD40–CD40L-mediated interaction between T cells and DCs further enhances the expression of B7 molecules on DCs. The same interaction allows for the production of IL-12 by DCs. This cytokine promotes the development of the Th1 response, which is critical for induction of cellular immunity. *In vivo*, DCs initially activate CD4[+] T cells; these become CD40L[+] and in turn deliver a signal to DCs which is required for the activation of CD8[+] T cells, explaining why CD4[+] T help is required for DC-mediated priming of antigen-specific CD8[+] T lymphocytes. MHC I loading is critical for the activation of CD8[+] T lymphocytes. Professional APCs are the only cells capable of capturing exogenous antigens for presentation on MHC I molecules. In this way, professional APCs assure the efficient generation of cytotoxic T cells, which in turn are the principal mediators of the immune response against viruses, intracellular pathogens and tumors. This special mechanisms of antigen processing provides a unique mechanism of priming against antigens that are normally expressed only by non-professional APCs. This pathway is referred to as 'cross-priming' and it is probably the antigen processing and presentation pathway with the most important implications for the design of vaccines.

5 Cross-priming: processing and presentation of exogenous antigens mediated by dendritic cells *in vivo*

The term 'cross-priming' was first used by Bevan (1976a,b) to describe the ability of APCs to prime CTL responses against minor histocompatibility antigens captured from foreign donor cells *in vivo*. The term 'cross-presentation' has been used thereafter to describe the uptake and presentation of cell-associated antigens within the MHC class I pathway (Kurts *et al.*, 1996) but also more recently in association with class II-restricted presentation (Adler *et al.*, 1998). Cross-presentation has now been shown to be involved in a wide variety of CTL responses, both tolerogenic (cross-tolerance) and immunogenic (cross-priming), ranging from inducing tolerance to parenchymal antigens (Kurts *et al.*, 1997, 1998a; Adler *et al.*, 1998) to generating CTLs to tumors (Gooding and Edward, 1980; Huang *et al.*, 1994), grafts (Gordon *et al.*, 1976) or DNA-encoded antigens (Corr *et al.*, 1996). The study of cross-priming is essential to understand the mechanisms of tumor-associated antigen presentation and for the development of effective immunotherapeutic interventions in malignant diseases. Over the years, there have been many studies intended to understand the identity of APCs responsible for this phenomenon. Many cells have been identified as capable of *in vitro* cross-presentation, including macrophages (Norbury *et al.*, 1995) and B lymphocytes (Ke and Ka, 1996), but only DCs have been recognized as having a consistent *in vivo* role for both cross-presentation and priming (Pulaski *et al.*, 1996; Chiodoni *et al.*, 1999). Several reports describe how exogenous antigens can access the cross-presentation pathway (Norbury *et al.*, 1995, 1996). However, those pathways associated with presentation of cellular antigens are the most relevant for recognition of tumors, viruses and intracellular pathogens by the immune system.

   Class I MHC molecules do not generally become loaded with peptides following processing of exogenous antigens (Morrison *et al.*, 1986; Townsend and Bodmer, 1989). They are unstable on the cell surface unless already occupied by peptide (Ljunggren *et al.*, 1990) and are not found in the compartments where MHC II molecules become loaded (Peters *et al.*, 1991). Presumably this serves to prevent sensitization of cells that are not actually infected but may passively take up antigens recognizable by CD8[+] CTLs. On the other hand, it has been shown previously that CTLs can be induced *in vivo* by soluble (Staerz *et al.*, 1987; Wraith *et al.*, 1987) or particulate antigens (Harding and Song, 1994; Falo *et al.*, 1995) and by tumor cell-derived heat shock proteins (HSPs) (Udono and Shrivastava, 1993). In addition, the work of Kurts *et al.* provided the first evidence that tissue-associated 'self' antigens can be presented in the context of class I, via an exogenous processing pathway, offering the idea of a constitutive mechanism whereby

T cells can be primed to antigens that are present in non-lymphoid tissues, which are not normally surveyed by recirculating naive T cells (Kurts *et al.*, 1996). These apparently conflicting results have been partially explained by the *in vitro* molecular analysis of the pathways employed for presentation of exogenous antigens on MHC I molecules, which suggests that antigens taken up by phagocytosis or macropinocytosis may have enhanced access to MHC I molecules themselves. These endocytic pathways are particularly prominent in macrophages and DCs (Bevan, 1987).

Two distinct pathways have been described: the first involves unusual access to the conventional MHC I pathway, while the second utilizes an unusual post-Golgi loading of MHC I. Rock and colleagues have shown the presentation of exogenous soluble antigen on MHC I molecules (Rock *et al.*, 1990) and much more efficient presentation of antigen conjugated to latex beads by macrophages and macrophage cell lines (Kovacsoics *et al.*, 1993, 1995). Presentation was insensitive to leupeptin or chloroquine but sensitive to peptide aldehyde inhibitors of the proteasome, implying that cytosolic rather than phagosomal processing was required for MHC I loading. Consistent with this, presentation of particle-conjugated ovalbumin was dependent on a peptide transport system (transport-associated protein; TAP) and a functional secretory pathway (Kovasovics and Rock, 1995). However, in these and in other similar studies that use soluble antigen co-administered with particulates (Reis e Sousa and Germain, 1995), antigen might somehow gain access to the cytosol via phagosomes. Direct morphological evidence that macropinocytosed fluorescent tracers can gain access to the cytosol has been obtained in several cell types, including bone marrow-derived macrophages and DCs (Norbury *et al.*, 1995, 1996). In addition, the stimulation or the inhibition of macropinocytosis boosted and blocked, respectively, presentation of exogenous ovalbumin on MHC I molecules (Norbury *et al.*, 1995). As previously observed using bead-conjugated ovalbumin, presentation of exogenously supplied protein was unaffected by the presence of chloroquine but blocked by proteasomal inhibitors and was completely dependent on TAP (Norbury *et al.*, 1995, 1996). Bone marrow-derived DCs can present exogenous soluble protein constitutively on MHC I molecules, due to constitutive macropinocytosis in these cells, and are considerably more potent than bone marrow-derived macrophages (Norbury *et al.*, 1996; Paglia *et al.*, 1996). Since particulate material, including some bacteria, can be taken up by macropinocytic-like mechanisms (Alpuche *et al.*, 1995; Swanson and Baer, 1995), other forms of antigen can also use this processing pathway. Other studies have reported a distinct brefeldin A-resistant, TAP-independent pathway for MHC I-restricted loading of exogenous antigen, which may take place with (Pfeifer *et al.*, 1993; Schrimbeck *et al.*, 1995) or without (Bachmann *et al.*, 1995; De Bruijn *et al.*, 1995; Schrimbech *et al.*, 1995) the contribution of peptide regurgitation and recapture on surface MHC I molecules. Heat-inactivated Sendai virus can be presented via either brefeldin A-resistant or -sensitive pathways (Liu *et al.*, 1995). In these studies, the MHC molecules that become loaded with peptides may be those on the cell surface, those phagocytosed from the cell surface or those newly synthesized and targeted to the endocytic pathway in association with the Ii chain (Sugita and Brenner, 1995). Presentation of exogenous antigens in the context of MHC I molecules allows the immune system to respond to a broader range of viral or tumor antigens than that synthesized *de novo* within professional APCs. Such antigens might be presented following phagocytic or macropinocytic capture (Bachmann *et al.*, 1995; Bevan, 1995; Norbury *et al.*, 1995).

Antigen entry into the conventional class I presentation pathway may induce more useful effector CTLs because it seems unlikely that phagosomal processing would reproducibly generate the same profile of T-cell epitopes generated by the proteasome/TAP system. Cross-priming was shown recently to be a TAP-dependent process in a tumor model. This may mean that exogenous cellular material can gain access to the cytosol of professional APCs *in vivo*, and DCs isolated from tumor biopsies have been demonstrated to hold tumor-associated antigen (TAA) immunodominant peptides within MHC I molecules (Huang *et al.*, 1996; Chiodoni *et al.*, 1999). While all DCs seem to be equipped for cross-priming, only a subpopulation of macrophages appeared to present exogenous antigens on MHC I, based on both functional (Reis e Sousa and Germain, 1995; Suto and Shrivastava, 1995) and morphological data (Norbury *et al.*, 1995). However, this may in fact be advantageous because it would still permit CTL induction without rendering large numbers of APCs targets for killing. Cells harboring intracellular pathogens may also be eliminated via presentation of their determinants on MHC I molecules and activation of IFN-secreting CD8$^+$ T cells (Rock *et al.*, 1990). In this case, either the brefeldin A-sensitive or -insensitive routes would contribute to eliciting potentially useful CD8$^+$ cells.

With respect to induction of CTL responses to tumor antigens, several HSPs, particularly HSP70, HSP90 and gp96, have been shown to induce CTL responses that are specific for antigens derived from donor cells (Shrivastava *et al.*, 1986; Ullrich *et al.*, 1986; Udono and Shrivastava, 1993; Arnold *et al.*, 1995). These HSPs appear to perform chaperone functions, carrying precursors of cellular peptide antigens that are capable of presentation by any MHC haplotype on APCs. HSPs, such as gp96 isolated from tumor cells, can confer specific tumor immunity *in vivo* and could sensitize a fraction of macrophages *in vitro* in a brefeldin A-sensitive fashion (Suto and Shrivastava, 1995). How exogenous gp96 delivers its associated antigen to class I molecules is not known. One possibility is that it gains access to the cytosol by micropinocytosis and subsequently crosses the processing pathway for MHC I ligands at this level. Alternatively, gp96 may bind to one or more cell surface receptors and could conceivably be retrieved to the lumen of the endoplasmic reticulum where it normally resides.

HSPs may be ideal candidate immunogens for vaccination purposes, but it is questionable whether they represent the physiological mechanism by which cell-associated antigens cross-prime (Albert *et al.*, 1998b). Since the generation of CTL responses by cross-priming requires the cooperation of both CD4$^+$ and CD8$^+$ T cells, it is clear that APCs must present both class I- and class II-restricted determinants, and DCs have been shown to be able to cross-present phagocytosed cellular fragments in association with MHC II molecules too (Inaba *et al.*, 1998). Finally, antigens may physiologically access the cross-presentation pathway, provided they are expressed in relatively large amounts (Kurts *et al.*, 1998b). For effective CTL priming, the APCs must be signaled by a CD4$^+$ helper T cell. Studies involving bone marrow chimeras showed that CD8$^+$ T cells and their CD4$^+$ helpers needed to see antigen on the same APCs for effective cross-priming (Bennet *et al.*, 1997). This implied a three-cell cluster, for provision of short-range soluble signals such as IL-2, or a sequential interaction where the CD4$^+$ cell first modifies the APCs to a subsequent and effective CTL priming. While there is little evidence for the ability of soluble cytokines to substitute for CD4$^+$ T cell help *in vivo*, CD40 has been identified as the signaling molecule endowing APCs with the ability to prime CTLs potently (Cella *et al.*, 1996; Bennett *et al.*, 1998). Stimulation of CD40 on APCs has been

reported to up-regulate or induce the expression of several molecules required in the generation of CTLs including B7.1 and B7.2, CD44H, ICAM-I, IL-1 and IL-12; however, it
is still unclear which one of these molecules represents the most critical downstream
signal for CTL generation. IL-12 is the strongest candidate as mediator of soluble help
provision; however, other candidates such as 4-1BB ligand, acting through the 4-1BB
molecule expressed by activated CD8$^+$ T cells, need further investigation.

6 Recognition of death: immunological consequences of phagocytosis of apoptotic cells

It has been demonstrated recently that DCs have the ability to capture and cross-present
antigens from apoptotic cells (Albert *et al.*, 1998). Phagocytosis of apoptotic cells is an
extremely interesting mechanism of antigen uptake for cross-presentation, because this is
the antigen source most physiologically available to APCs *in vivo*.

Phagocytosis by neighboring cells is the normal fate of cells that die by apoptosis.
Recognition, uptake and degradation of dying cells by phagocytes occur extremely
rapidly, preventing inappropriate exposure of adjacent tissues to the intracellular contents
of the cell undergoing apoptosis (Savill *et al.*, 1993; Savill, 1997). The fact that 'free' or
'non-phagocytosed' dying cells are rarely observed *in vivo* because of their quick removal
partly explains why apoptosis has been identified only recently as a frequent physiological event. Aging and death of cells are widespread, but we still have a poor understanding
of where in the body these cells are cleared, the mechanisms through which they are recognized and the physiological and immunological consequences.

Although the biological events that occur in the cytoplasm and nucleus following the
induction of apoptosis are well understood, relatively little is known about the changes in
the plasma membrane of the dying cell. Moreover, an appropriate ligand on the surface of
the dying cell is clearly required for recognition, efficient binding and ingestion by the
phagocyte. Major recognizable changes on the surface of apoptotic cells could include
modifications in the glycosylation, charge and composition of surface lipids (Savill *et al.*,
1993; Hart *et al.*, 1996; Savill, 1997). The exposure on the outer surface of the plasma
membrane of phosphatidylserine (Zwaal and Schroit, 1997), which usually is retained on
the inner layer by healthy cells, is the major candidate for signaling of cell death.

On the other hand, the successful ingestion of dying cells requires the presence of
receptor(s) on the surface of the phagocyte that can mediate rapid recognition and uptake
of an apoptotic cell before the integrity of its membrane is lost. The nature of the receptors that can discriminate 'dying' (or 'altered self') cells from healthy cells is of particular
interest because of the possible implications on the mechanism of induction of self-toler-
ance. Binding of the dying cell to a phagocyte is the first requirement for its ingestion. A
major role for the $\alpha_v \beta_3$ vitronectin receptor has been shown in the recognition of apoptotic neutrophils by blood-derived macrophages (Savill *et al.*, 1993). Antibodies directed
against vitronectin receptor and peptides that include the Asp–Gly–Asp adhesion motif
can block uptake of dying neutrophils, eosinophils and lymphocytes by macrophages and
the phagocytosis of neutrophils by fibroblasts (Savill *et al.*, 1993; Hall *et al.*, 1994). More
recently, the molecule recognized by an antibody that could inhibit binding of apoptotic B
cells to human macrophages was shown to be CD14 (Devitt *et al.*, 1998), which is better
known as a receptor for bacterial LPS. This demonstration of dual activity for a single

receptor might be important in confirming evolutionary relationships as well as the differences between phagocytosis of either dying host cells or foreign cells.

Furthermore, several members of the scavenger receptor (SR) family have been implicated in the recognition of apoptotic cells (Krieger and Hertz , 1994). SR-positive cells are located in the spleen, both in the red pulp and in the marginal zone, in lymph nodes, peritoneum, thymic medulla, liver, lung and gut where SR is well recognized by the monoclonal antibody 2F8 (Fraser *et al.*, 1993). The expression of SRs is considered a maturation hallmark of macrophages; SRs are not expressed on circulating monocytes. The pattern of expression of this receptor family suggests their key role in the innate immune response, particularly at the cross-roads between the inner and the outer world: the lungs and the intestinal mucosa (Hughes *et al.*, 1995). SRs bind a very wide range of polyanionic ligands, including lipoteichoic acid, an outer cell wall component of Gram-positive bacteria, as well as LPS, further supporting their role in host defense through recognition and endocytosis of pathogens. In addition, SRs have been involved in the uptake of apoptotic thymocytes by peritoneal macrophages *in vitro* (Platt *et al.*, 1996). Another interesting SR is CD36 (Greenwalt *et al.*, 1992). Like other SRs, CD36 binds to several ligands, but its specificity differs from that of SR-A and might show species-specific variation (Pearson, 1996). Savill and co-workers have investigated CD36 and the clearance of apoptotic cells at sites of inflammation (Savill *et al.*, 1993; Savill, 1997), showing for the first time that SR is a phagocytic receptor for apoptotic cells. CD36 is found on a number of cell types, including platelets, endothelial cells and adipocytes (Greenwalt *et al.*, 1992) but, moreover, CD36 is expressed consistently on the surface of APCs. Following ingestion, the intracellular pathway(s) into which the apoptotic debris is directed might have significant implications for immune function. The ability of macrophages to present endogenous antigen from apoptotic cells via MHC II remains controversial; studies of negative selection in the thymus suggest that only DCs are involved (Zal *et al.*, 1994) and that apoptotic material taken up by macrophages is degraded extensively (Brazil *et al.*, 1997). Albert *et al.* have studied the capacity of HLA-A2.1$^+$ DCs to present antigens to MHC class I-restricted, autologous CD8$^+$ T cells (Albert *et al.*, 1998a). The indirect or antigen transfer pathway became apparent by placing the influenza matrix gene in an HLA-A2.1$^-$ cell that was either infected or transfected. The HLA-A2.1$^+$ DCs presented matrix peptide as long as the HLA-2.1$^-$ cell had undergone apoptosis (Albert *et al.*, 1998a), and the recipient DCs were of the immature phagocytic type expressing the $\alpha_V \beta_5$ integrin (Albert *et al.*, 1998b).

The indirect presentation of apoptosis-associated antigens was addressed similarly using the Y-Ae monoclonal antibody, which is directed to a defined MHC II–peptide complex, formed when an I-A^b class II product presents a peptide derived from another MHC II product, the I-E molecule (Inaba *et al.*, 1998). Apoptotic BALB/c B cells, rich in I-E but lacking I-A^b, were used to feed immature C57BL/6 DCs, lacking I-E but expressing I-A^b. In this assay, it was clear that immature DCs process the I-E peptide from donor B cells, when B cells were provided together with a stimulus for maturation of DCs. In contrast to the MHC class I presentation studies of Albert *et al.*, where apoptotic cells were processed exclusively (Albert *et al.*, 1998a), MHC II-restricted presentation occurred following uptake of both necrotic and apoptotic B cells. Most B-cell fragments were observed to localize within MIICs, and blocking studies indicated that phagocytosis necessarily preceded the formation of Y-Ae complexes. In this sytem, DCs were able to produce the same number, about 10^4, of MHC–peptide complexes as they normally do when they process the endogenous I-E molecule. Therefore, the availability of the Y-Ae antibody to the MHC–peptide complex, as well as antibodies to the peptide donor, the I-E protein, has made it possible to uncover two striking features of cellular antigen capture and processing by DCs (Inaba *et al.*, 1998). One is the efficiency. A concentration of 1 nM pre-processed I-E peptide is equivalent in efficacy to 0.3 μ M I-E protein in the B blasts. Therefore, the phagocytosed B-cell fragment is 3000 times more efficient in forming MHC–peptide complexes than pre-processed peptide. The difference is probably closer to 10 000-fold, considering that many B blasts are scavenged by macrophages. A second discovery comes from *in vivo* experiments in which BALB/c DCs were injected into the paws of C57BL/6 mice. Normally, DCs migrate through the afferent lymph into proximal nodes where they probably die, since DCs have never been found in efferent lymph. A few donor I-E$^+$ DCs are detected in the draining lymph nodes 1–2 days later, but more impressive is the expression of Y-Ae MHC–peptide complexes on recipient DCs. Most recipient I-A^b DCs have MHC–peptide complexes, identified by FACS or visualized by immunocytochemistry in tissue sections through the T-cell areas. Since lymph node DCs are not known to turn over in 1–2 days, it is unlikely that recipient, Y-Ae$^+$ DCs pick up I-E peptide in the periphery and migrate to the nodes. Likewise, if apoptotic DCs are injected, little Y-Ae labeling is seen on recipient lymph node DCs. Therefore, it is more likely that donor DCs, after reaching the T-cell area, undergo apoptosis and are phagocytosed and processed efficiently by recipient DCs there. Except for a study showing DCs in the T-cell area in the process of phagocytosing fragments of allogeneic leukocytes (Fossum and Rolstad, 1986), it has not been possible to prove that DCs, which are located abundantly in the T-cell area, are capable of capturing and processing exogenous substrates.

Antigen transfer from apoptotic cells may fundamentally contribute to immune responses observed during transplantation. Immature DCs are constantly trafficking through tissues and phagocytosing the cells undergoing apoptosis during tissue remodeling and turnover. If DCs from the recipient of a tissue graft pick up donor-derived cells or debris and also encounter a maturation stimulus, these DCs migrate to the lymph node and stimulate immunity to those donor-derived peptides generated by cross-priming. If the DCs do not encounter a maturation stimulus, as probably occurs when DCs traffic through tissues in the steady state, they die within the T-cell area and are probably processed by other DCs which are resident within the lymph node. DCs die in the absence of a maturation stimulus because they cannot up-regulate molecules such as CD40 and TRANCE receptor that are needed to maintain their viability (Caux *et al.*, 1994; Wong *et al.*, 1997). Lymphoid DCs may be responsible for processing immature DC trafficking through secondary lymphoid organs. These cells are bringing to the node antigens sampled in the periphery in the absence of 'danger signals'. Therefore, lymphoid DCs, processing migrating immature DCs, may be able to regulate the T-cell response indirectly in the periphery (Suss and Shortman, 1996). This explains the fact that marrow-derived APCs can induce peripheral tolerance to peptides derived from somatic cells: a phenomenon referred as 'cross-tolerance' observations (Forster and Lieberam, 1996; Kurts *et al.*, 1997). Another possibility is that immature DCs from the periphery induce T-cell tolerance directly rather than indirectly following antigen transfer to lymphoid DCs. Finally, cell death by necrosis, in contrast to apoptosis, typically is associated with inflammation. Immature DCs can take up apoptotic cells efficiently, but to act as potent APCs they must undergo changes termed maturation. Therefore, optimal cross-presentation of tumor antigens requires the fulfillment of these two essential steps. While apoptotic tumor cells provide antigenic material for MHC I-restricted presentation by DCs, a maturation signal is delivered to DCs by the exposure to necrotic tumor cells. In this way, DCs are able to distinguish between the two different types of cell death, with necrosis providing a signal critical for triggering the immune response.

7 Myeloid dendritic cells hold promise for development of immunotherapy

The possibility of obtaining large numbers of specialized antigen-specific DCs *in vitro* for subsequent *in vivo* administration has generated enormous clinical interest. This has a major impact in choosing DCs over macrophages. The latter are much more difficult to obtain, even if several methods to immortalize them have been described (Paglia *et al.*, 1992). Because CD14-derived DCs preferentially promote Th1 responses (Hilkens *et al.*, 1997; McRae *et al.*, 1998), this DC subtype is actively being sought for generating specific antitumor responses in a range of malignancies and for generating antiviral-specific responses in diseases such as AIDS (Lotze *et al.*, 1999). The ability of immature DCs to capture and present antigens from apoptotic cells has also revealed a potentially powerful approach to obtain physiologically relevant antigenic material, especially in clinical settings in which drug-induced apoptosis of malignant cells is easily achieved (Lotze *et al.*, 1999). Although promising, this approach suffers from the difficulties associated with generating sufficient numbers of antigen-specific DCs for repeated immunization (Lotze *et al.*, 1999). This limitation stems partly from the short life span of mature DCs and from the inability to obtain self-renewing progenitors for specific DC subtypes. Cautionary notes underline that tumor cells may promote apoptosis of DCs within tumor sites and produce substances that interfere with DC maturation (Ishida *et al.*, 1998; Shurin *et al.*, 1999). Thus, the success of DC-based immunotherapy may rest on achieving methods for generating large numbers of functionally specialized DC subtypes that will exhibit sustained survival *in vivo*.

8 Preclinical studies of tumor antigen presentation by dendritic cells

8.1 Dendritic cell vaccination in animal tumor model systems

The induction of antitumor immune responses by injection of antigen-loaded DCs has been studied extensively in animals. Initially, it was shown that administration of density gradient-purified splenic DCs pulsed with either soluble tumor antigen expressed by a B-cell lymphoma (Flamand *et al.*, 1994) or with a synthetic MHC class I-restricted peptide derived from a model tumor antigen (Ossevoort *et al.*, 1995) could induce protective anti-tumor immunity mediated by the induction of specific CTLs. Thus, it was clear that the *ex vivo* delivery of purified tumor antigen to a defined population of APCs could result in an effective tumor vaccine. The development of techniques for generating large numbers of DCs *in vitro* from murine bone marrow (Inaba *et al.*, 1992) has allowed this approach to be exploited adequately. Such bone marrow-derived DCs, when pulsed with MHC I-restricted peptides derived from model tumor antigens, can induce potent antitumor CTL responses, as well as protective tumor immunity in vaccinated mice (Mayordomo *et al.*, 1995; Porgador *et al.*, 1996). These responses are apparent after injection of as few as 10^5 cells and are dependent on CD8[+] T cells. Furthermore, administration of peptide-pulsed DCs was able to cure animals bearing established small tumors, demonstrating the striking potency of the vaccination approach. Importantly, comparable CTL activity and tumor protection have been elicited using protein-pulsed DCs (Paglia *et al.*, 1996). Although these results demonstrate *in vivo* activity of antigen-pulsed DC vaccines against tumors, the model systems employed are highly artificial; in fact, genes encoding foreign proteins are introduced into tumors to serve as model tumor antigens. Such tumors tend to be highly immunogenic and thus behave unlike most human cancers.

In order to study peptide-pulsed DC vaccination in a more clinically relevant setting, mice bearing established, poorly immunogenic tumors were used (Zitvogel *et al.*, 1996). Vaccination using DCs pulsed with unfractionated peptides acid-eluted from the MHC I molecules on the surface of tumor cells markedly suppressed tumor growth, even when initiated 7 days after tumor inoculation. Another clinically pertinent tumor model is the murine Meth A sarcoma, which, like many human malignancies, expresses mutant p53. Vaccination with DCs pulsed with a class I MHC-binding mutant p53 peptide has been found to induce both protective and therapeutic immunity against this tumor (Mayordomo *et al.*, 1996). These studies provided the proof-of-principle for antigen-pulsed DC vaccination against cancer.

Recent investigations have focused on discovering more effective methods of delivering tumor antigens to DCs *ex vivo*, in a manner that does not require knowledge of the relevant tumor peptide sequences and allows for co-presentation on both MHC I and MHC II molecules, as T-helper cell functions are required to facilitate the induction of CTL responses. Physical (i.e. electroporation) or chemical (e.g. cationic lipids or calcium phosphate precipitation) methods of DNA transfection have proven either ineffective or too toxic for delivery of genes into DCs (Arthur *et al.*, 1997). Conversely, vaccination with DCs pulsed with tumor antigen-encoding RNA or tumor cell-derived polyadenylated RNA can induce CTLs and protective tumor immunity (Boczkowski *et al.*, 1996). Recombinant viruses have proved to be a highly efficient means of introducing tumor antigen sequences into DCs. Adenovirus, poxvirus and retroviral vectors encoding model tumor antigens have been used to infect DCs and induce both protective and therapeutic tumor immunity (Song *et al.*, 1997; Specht *et al.*, 1997). An alternative approach to obtain a vaccine formulation featuring DC function and tumor antigen repertoire is the cell hybrid between DCs and tumor cells. Although not all co-stimulatory and functional molecules of DC and not all the possible tumor-associated antigens can be segregated together in such cell hybrids, their use induces protective immunity against hepatocarcinoma (Guo *et al.*, 1994) and adenocarcinoma (Gong *et al.*, 1997) in animals. Lastly, the presence of genetic abnormalities in myeloid hematological malignancies that may be recognized by the immune system prompted the idea of generating functional monocyte-derived DCs starting from such malignant cells. Taking advantage of the described differentiation pathways starting from CD34[+] cells, DCs carrying the specific genetic lesion have been obtained from acute myeloid and lymphoid leukemia (AML) (Choudhury *et al.*, 1999; Cignetti *et al.*, 1999) as well as from chronic myelogenous leukemia (CML)

(Choudhury *et al.*, 1997) and used to generate cellular cytotoxicity against Philadelphia chromosome-positive CML (Choudhury *et al.*, 1997).

8.2 Generation of human dendritic cells for cancer immunotherapy

Clinical trials of DC vaccination have been made possible by the development of methods for obtaining large numbers of human DCs. Two general approaches have been exploited: (1) the purification of immature DC precursors from peripheral blood; and (2) the *in vitro* differentiation of DCs from peripheral blood monocytes or CD34$^+$ hematopoietic progenitor cells. The former approach represents the most direct method of DCs isolation and the first utilized in clinical studies of DC vaccination. Circulating immature DC precursors, representing less than 0.5 per cent of PBMCs, can be isolated from T cell and monocyte-depleted peripheral blood cells after 1–2 days of *in vitro* culture (in the absence of cytokines). During this time, DC precursors undergo maturation and acquire a low buoyant density, which allows their purification by density gradient. Typically, 5×10^6 DCs are obtained from the PBMCs of a single leukapheresis. However, large numbers of DCs can be generated by *in vitro* culture of monocytes or CD34$^+$ progenitor cells in the presence of cytokines. Culture of adherent PBMCs with GM-CSF and IL-4 for 5–7 days results in the generation of DCs (Romani *et al.*, 1994). These cells arise largely through the differentiation of CD14$^+$ monocytes without substantial proliferation, and up to $3–8 \times 10^6$ of such cells can be obtained from 40 ml of blood. Notably, these DCs maintain the ability to take up and efficiently present protein antigen to T cells (Sallusto and Lanzavecchia, 1994). The continued presence of GM-CSF and IL-4 in these cultures is mandatory in order to avoid DCs reverting to adherent, monocyte-like cells since this would impair their ability to function to present tumor antigen once administered *in vivo*. Conditioned media, containing TNF-α or monocyte-derived factors, have been developed to achieve stable maturation of these DCs, and adapted for the generation of clinical grade DCs using culture media approved for human use and substituting bovine serum components with autologous plasma (Romani *et al.*, 1996). Human CD34$^+$ hematopoietic progenitor cells purified from bone marrow, umbilical cord blood or peripheral blood, and mobilized with cytokines such as granulocyte colony-stimulating factor (G-CSF) or GM-CSF can also serve as a source of precursors for the *in vitro* expansion of DCs. In the presence of GM-CSF and TNF-α, CD34$^+$ cells expressing SCGF and Flt3L expand 10- to 30-fold and differentiate into characteristic DCs that share the immunophenotypic and functional properties of monocyte-derived DCs (Shortman and Caux, 1997). The potential for human DCs to prime tumor antigen-specific T lymphocytes *in vitro* has been demonstrated repeatedly. CD34$^+$-derived DCs obtained from breast cancer patients can stimulate autologous peripheral blood CD4$^+$ T cells to proliferate in response to an MHC class II-restricted peptide derived from the HER-2/neu oncogene product (Bernhard *et al.*, 1995). DCs pulsed with tumor antigen peptides (Bakker *et al.*, 1995; Brossart *et al.*, 1998) or transduced with tumor antigen-encoding DNA (Reeves *et al.*, 1996) or RNA (Nair *et al.*, 1998) can stimulate the *in vitro* expansion and maturation of CTLs from autologous peripheral blood lymphocytes, and the resulting CTLs are able to lyse tumor cells. Although both monocyte and CD34$^+$-derived DCs can stimulate these *in vitro* CTL responses, CD34$^+$-derived DCs have been superior in their ability to stimulate rare, tumor antigen-specific CTL precursors derived from cancer patients (Mortarini *et al.*, 1997).

9 Clinical trials involving dendritic cell-based vaccination

There are few published studies of DC vaccinations for cancer immunotherapy (Mukherji *et al.*, 1995; Hu *et al.*, 1996; Nair, 1997; Nestle *et al.*, 1998). These early pilot trials have nonetheless established the general safety and feasibility of this approach, and reported some clinical activity against tumors of several types. These results, together with the preclinical results cited above, support the many ongoing clinical trials (Table 3.2). Although this new generation of studies will continue to address the safety and efficacy of DC vaccination, future studies should address several variables that are critical to optimizing this approach. First the source of DCs for clinical use should be considered, as well as the choice of tumor antigens and methods for antigen loading of DCs. The relationship between the number of DCs to be administered and the clinical outcome also needs to be investigated using individual cell preparation methods and, finally, the optimal route and frequency of administration should be determined.

10 *In vivo* targeting of APCs: strategies to improve antigen uptake and cross-presentation *in vivo*

Many developing immunotherapeutic strategies against cancer seek to exploit the powerful antigen-presenting properties of DCs. Although the vaccination approaches have demonstrated clinical activity and feasibility, techniques for targeting tumor antigens to DCs *in situ* are highly desirable in order to avoid their *ex vivo* manipulation. Major efforts have been devoted to targeting DCs *in vivo* in their physiological environment, either by directly providing antigens by means of bacterial carriers which have tropism for APCs (Paglia *et al.*, 1997, 1998; Medina *et al.*, 1999) or, alternatively, stimulating the uptake and cross-presentation of tumor antigens by providing cytokines and co-stimulatory signals *in situ* (Stoppacciaro *et al.*, 1997; Chiodoni *et al.*, 1999). *Salmonella*-based DNA immunization allows specific targeting of antigen expression *in vivo* to APCs, thus inducing MHC I- and II-restricted antitumor immune responses. Vaccine-mediated induction of the TAA-specific immune response, although required, could be insufficient to reject a tumor in the absence of appropriate inflammatory co-stimuli, and such co-stimulation may avoid tolerance or ignorance of the antigen. The bacterial carrier may function as a natural adjuvant since bacteria are known to induce release of TNF-α, IFN-γ, IL-12 and other pro-inflammatory mediators that enhance early innate immunity and thereafter create an inflammatory context which probably favors DC maturation to a high antigen-presenting phenotype. To favor the interaction of tumor cells with host DCs and therefore cross-priming, BALB/c-derived C-26 colon carcinoma cells have been transduced with GM-CSF and CD40L genes. Co-transduced cells showed reduced tumorigenicity, and tumor appearance was followed by regression in some mice. *In vivo* tumors were heavily infiltrated with DCs that were isolated, phenotyped and tested *in vitro* for stimulation of tumor-specific CTLs. BALB/c C-26 carcinoma cells express the endogenous MuLV *emv-1* gene as a tumor-associated antigen. This antigen is shared among solid tumors of BALB/c and C57BL6 mice and contains two epitopes, AH-1 and KSP, that are recognized in the context of MHC class I molecules H-2L^d and H-2K^b, respectively. DCs isolated from C-26/GM/CD40L tumors grown in BALB/c $\times$ C57BL/6 F$_1$ mice (H-2^{dxb})

Table 3.2   Clinical trials involving dendritic cell-based vaccination

Malignancy	Antigen(s)	Source of DC
Melanoma	Autologous tumor lysate	Monocyte-derived
	gp100, MART-1, MAGE-1	CD34+ cell-derived
	MAGE-3 and tyrosinase	CD36+ cell derived and G-CSF-mobilized
	peptides	
Prostate	Xenogeneic PAP	Peripheral blood
Carcinoma	PAP	Peripheral blood
	PSMA peptides	Monocyte-derived
Lung, breast,	CEA CAP-1 peptide	Monocyte-derived
colon, renal	CEA RNA	Monocyte-derived
carcinomas	HER-2/neu RNA	Monocyte-derived
	Total tumor RNA	Monocyte-derived
	Autologous tumor lysate	Monocyte-derived
	Mutant p53 and ras peptide	Monocyte-derived
	Wild-type p53 protein	Monocyte-derived
Multiple myeloma	Immunoglobulin idiotype	Peripheral blood
	Immunoglobulin idiotype	CD34+-cell derived
	protease digested	
B-cell lymphoma	Immunoglobulin idiotype	Peripheral blood

Abbreviations: CEA = carcinoembryonic antigen; PAP = prostatic alkaline phosphatase; PSMA = prostate-specific membrane antigen.

stimulated IFN-γ production by both anti-AH-1 and KSP CTLs, whereas tumor-infiltrating DCs (TIDCs) of BALB/c mice stimulated only anti-AH-1 CTLs. Furthermore, TIDCs primed naive mice for CTL activity as early as 2 days after injection into the footpad, whereas double-transduced tumor cells required at least 5 days for priming; this difference may reflect direct DC priming versus indirect tumor cell priming. Immunohistochemical staining indicated co-localization of DCs and apoptotic bodies in the tumors. These data indicate that DCs, which infiltrate tumors that produce GM-CSF and CD40L, can capture cellular antigens, probably through uptake of apoptotic bodies, and that they mature *in situ* to a stage suitable for antigen presentation. Thus, tumor cell-based vaccines engineered to favor the interaction with host DCs can be considered. The efficient isolation and preparation of both human and murine DCs are now possible, and applications for these cells in cancer immunotherapy are envisaged. DCs seem especially promising in this respect, since they can be loaded with an array of peptides or DNAs representing known and unknown tumor-associated antigens. A critical issue is whether *in vitro*-manipulated DCs retain all their physiological properties. Indeed, in one clinical study, they were injected directly into the lymph node. Attempt to target DCs directly *in vivo* may help to maintain their properties. Finally, priming and boosting might depend differently on APC functions: activated T cells can kill DCs carrying the antigen. This indicates the need for a tight control of the timing of sequential injection as well as the choice of different APCs for priming or boosting the immune response.

11 Summary

Macrophages and DCs in their wide range of habitats *in vivo* display extensive heterogeneity in phenotype and function. This heterogeneity appears to be due to the influence of the large number of cytokines and environmental factors that act on myeloid cells during their differentiation/maturation pathway. The result is a network of antigen-handling cells that ranges from immature progenitor cells to fully mature macrophages and DCs. This web of cells is responsible for determining the T-cell response to a particular antigenic stimulus.

Acknowledgments

Mrs Grazia Barp is acknowledged for editorial assistance. The authors are supported by Associazione Italiana per la Ricerca sul Cancro (AIRC), Telethon-Italy (grant nos A102 and A315), Consiglio Nazionale delle Ricerche (CNR) PF-Biotechnology and Istituto Superiore di Sanità (ISS)-National Program for AIDS Research (grant 40B.1.6).

References

Adler, A.J., Marsh, D.W., Yochum, G.S., Guzzo, J.L., Nigam, A. and Nelson, W.G. (1988). CD4$^+$ T cell tolerance to parenchymal self-antigens requires presentation by bone marrow-derived antigen-presenting cells. *Journal of Experimental Medicine*, **187**, 1555–64.

Albert, M.L., Pearce, S.F., Francisco, L.M., Sauter, B., Roy, P. and Silverstein, R.L. (1998a). Immature dendritic cells phagocytose apoptotic cells via $\alpha_v \beta_5$ and CD36, and cross-present antigens to cytotoxic T lymphocytes. *Journal of Experimental Medicine*, **188**, 1359–68.

Albert, M.L., Sauter, B. and Bhardwaj, N. (1998b). Dendritic cells acquire antigen from apoptotic cells and induce class I-restricted CTLs. *Nature*, **392**, 86–89.

Allavena, P., Piemonti, L., Longoni, D., Bernasconi, S., Stoppacciaro, A., Ruco, L. *et al.* (1988). IL-10 prevents the differentiation of monocytes to dendritic cells but promotes their maturation to macrophages. *European Journal of Immunology*, **28**, 359–69.

Alpuche Aranda, C.M., Berthiaume, E.P., Mock, B., Swanson, J.A. and Miller, S.I. (1995). Spacious phagosome formation within mouse macrophages correlates with *Salmonella* serotype pathogenicity and host susceptibility. *Infection and Immunity*, **63**, 4456–62.

Anderson, D.M., Maraskovsky, E., Billingsley, W.L., Dougall, W.C., Tometsko, M., Roux, E.R. *et al.* (1997). A homologue of the TNF receptor and its ligand enhance T cell growth and dendritic cell function. *Nature*, **390**, 175–9.

Arnold, D., Faath, S., Rammensee, H. and Schild, H. (1995). Cross-priming of minor histocompatibility antigen-specific cytotoxic T cells upon immunization with the heat shock protein gp96. *Journal of Experimental Medicine*, **182**, 885–9.

Arthur, J.F., Butterfield, L.H., Roth, M.D., Bui, L.A., Kiertscher, S.M. and Lau, R. (1997). A comparison of gene transfer methods in human dendritic cells. *Cancer Gene Therapy*, **4**, 17.

Austyn, J.M. (1987). Lymphoid dendritic cells. *Immunology*, **62**, 161–70.

Bachmann, M.F., Oxenius, A., Pircher, H., Hengartner, H., Ashton-Rickardt, P.A., Tonegawa, S. *et al.* (1995). TAP1-independent loading of class I molecules by exogenous viral proteins. *European Journal of Immunology*, **25**, 1739–43.

Bakker, A.B., Marland, G., de Boer, A.J., Huijbens, R.J., Danen, E.H. and Adema, G.J. (1995). Generation of antimelanoma cytotoxic T lymphocytes from healthy donors after presentation of melanoma-associated antigen-derived epitopes by dendritic cells *in vitro*. *Cancer Research*, **55**, 5330–4.

Banchereau, J. and Steinman, R.M. (1998). Dendritic cells and the control of immunity. *Nature*, **392**, 245–52.

Banyer, J.L. and Hapel, A.J. (1999). Myb-transformed hematopoietic cells as a model for monocyte differentiation into dendritic cells and macrophages. *Journal of Leukocyte Biology*, **66**, 217–23.

Bell, D., Young, J.W. and Banchereau, J. (1999). Dendritic cells. *Advances in Immunology*, **72**, 255–324.

Bellini, A., Vittori, E., Marini, M., Ackerman, V. and Mattoli, S. (1993). Intraepithelial dendritic cells and selective activation of Th2-like lymphocytes in patients with atopic asthma. *Chest*, **103**, 997–1005.

Bennett, S.R., Carbone, F.R., Karamalis, F., Miller, J.F. and Heath, W.R. (1997). Induction of a CD8+ cytotoxic T lymphocyte response by cross-priming requires cognate CD4+ T cell help. *Journal of Experimental Medicine*, **186**, 65–70.

Bennett, S.R., Carbone, F.R., Karamalis, F., Flavell, R.A., Miller, J.F. and Heath, W.R. (1998). Help for cytotoxic-T-cell responses is mediated by CD40 signalling. *Nature*, **393**, 478–80.

Bernhard, H., Disis, M.L., Heimfeld, S., Hand, S., Gralow, J.R. and Cheever, M.A. (1995). Generation of immunostimulatory dendritic cells from human CD34+ hematopoietic progenitor cells of the bone marrow and peripheral blood. *Cancer Research*, **55**, 1099–104.

Bevan, M.J. (1976a). Minor H antigens introduced on H-2 different stimulating cells cross-react at the cytotoxic T cell level during *in vivo* priming. *Journal of Immunology*, **117**, 2233–8.

Bevan, M.J. (1976b). Cross-priming for a secondary cytotoxic response to minor H antigens with H-2 congenic cells which do not cross-react in the cytotoxic assay. *Journal of Experimental Medicine*, **143**,1283–8.

Bevan, M.J. (1987). Class discrimination in the world of immunology. *Nature*, **325**, 192–4.

Bevan, M.J. (1995). Antigen presentation to cytotoxic T lymphocytes *in vivo*. *Journal of Experimental Medicine*, **182**, 639–41.

Boczkowski, D., Nair, S.K., Snyder, D. and Gilboa, E. (1996). Dendritic cells pulsed with RNA are potent antigen-presenting cells *in vitro* and *in vivo*. *Journal of Experimental Medicine*, **184**, 465–72.

Borkowski, T.A., Letterio, J.J., Farr, A.G. and Udey, M.C. (1996) A role for endogenous transforming growth factor β1 in Langerhans cell biology: the skin of transforming growth factor β1 null mice is devoid of epidermal Langerhans cells. *Journal of Experimental Medicine*, **184**, 2417–22.

Brazil, M.I., Weiss, S. and Stockinger, B. (1998). Excessive degradation of intracellular protein in macrophages prevents presentation in the context of major histocompatibility complex class II molecules. *European Journal of Immunology*, **27**, 1506–14.

Brossart, P., Stuhler, G., Flad, T., Stevanovic, S., Rammensee, H.G. and Kanz, L. (1998). Her-2/neu-derived peptides are tumor-associated antigens expressed by human renal cell and colon carcinoma lines and are recognized by *in vitro* induced specific cytotoxic T lymphocytes. *Cancer Research*, **58**, 732–6.

Buelens, C., Willems, F., Delvaux, A., Pierard, G., Delville, J.P., Velu, T. *et al.* (1995). Interleukin-10 differentially regulates B7-1 (CD80) and B7-2 (CD86) expression on human peripheral blood dendritic cells. *European Journal of Immunology*, **25**, 2668–72.

Buelens, C., Verhasselt, V., De Groote, D., Thielemans, K., Goldman, M. and Willems, F. (1997a). Interleukin-10 prevents the generation of dendritic cells from human peripheral blood mononuclear cells cultured with interleukin-4 and granulocyte/macrophage-colony-stimulating factor. *European Journal of Immunology*, **27**, 756–62.

Buelens, C., Verhasselt, V., De Groote, D., Thielemans, K., Goldman, M. and Willems, F. (1997b). Human dendritic cell responses to lipopolysaccharide and CD40 ligation are differentially regulated by interleukin-10. *European Journal of Immunology*, **27**, 1848–52.

Burkly, L., Hession, C., Ogata, L., Reilly, C., Marconi, L.A., Olson, D. *et al.* (1995). Expression of relB is required for the development of thymic medulla and dendritic cells. *Nature*, **73**, 531–6.

Caux, C. (1998). Pathways of development of human dendritic cells. *European Journal of Dermatology*, **8**, 375–84.

Caux, C., Massacrier, C., Vanbervliet, B., Barthelemy, C., Liu, Y.J. and Banchereau J. (1994a). Interleukin 10 inhibits T cell alloreaction induced by human dendritic cells. *International Immunology*, **6**, 1177–85.

Caux, C., Massacrier, C., Vanbervliet, B., Dubois, B., Van Kooten, C., Durand, I. *et al.* (1994b). Activation of human dendritic cells through CD40 cross-linking. *Journal of Experimental Medicine*, **180**, 1263–72.

Caux, C., Vanbervliet, B., Massacrier, C., Azuma, M., Okumura, K., Lanier, L.L. *et al.* (1994c). B70/B7-2 is identical to CD86 and is the major functional ligand for CD28 expressed on human dendritic cells. *Journal of Experimental Medicine*, **180**, 1841–7.

Caux, C., Vanbervliet, B., Massacrier, C., Dezutter-Dambuyant, C., de Saint-Vis, B., Jacquet, C. *et al.* (1996). CD34+ hematopoietic progenitors from human cord blood differentiate along two independent dendritic cell pathways in response to GM-CSF + TNF. *Journal of Experimental Medicine*, **184**, 695–706.

Caux, C., Massacrier, C., Vanbervliet, B., Dubois, B., Durand, I., Cella, M. *et al.* (1997). CD34+ hematopoietic progenitors from human cord blood differentiate along two independent dendritic cell pathways in response to granulocyte–macrophage colony-stimulating factor plus tumor necrosis factor: II. Functional analysis. *Blood*, **90**, 1458–70.

Cavanagh, L.L., Saal, R.J., Grimmett, K.L. and Thomas, R. (1998). Proliferation in monocyte-derived dendritic cell cultures is caused by progenitors cells capable of myeloid differentiation. *Blood*, **92**, 1598–607.

Cella, M., Scheidegger, D., Palmer-Lehmann, K., Lane, P., Lanzavecchia, A. and Alber, G. (1996). Ligation of CD40 on dendritic cells triggers production of high levels of interleukin-12 and enhances T cell stimulatory capacity: T–T help via APC activation. *Journal of Experimental Medicine*, **184**, 747–52.

Cella, M., Sallusto, F. and Lanzavecchia, A. (1997a). Origin, maturation and antigen presenting function of dendritic cells. *Current Opinion in Immunology*, **9**, 10–16.

Chang, C. H., Furue, M. and Tamaki, K. (1995). B7-1 expression of Langerhans cells is up-regulated by pro-inflammatory cytokines, and is down-regulated by interferon-γ or by interleukin-10. *European Journal of Immunology*, **25**, 394–8.

Chiodoni, C., Paglia, P., Stoppacciaro, A., Rodolfo, M., Parenza, M. and Colombo, M.P. (1999). Dendritic cells infiltrating tumors cotransduced with granulocyte/macrophage colony-stimulating factor (GM-CSF) and CD40 ligand genes take up and present endogenous tumor-associated antigens, and prime naive mice for a cytotoxic T lymphocyte response. *Journal of Experimental Medicine*, **190**, 125–33.

Choudhury, A., Gajewski, J.L., Liang, J.C., Popat, U., Claxton, D.F., Kliche, K.O. *et al.* (1997). Use of leukemic dendritic cells for the generation of antileukemic cellular cytotoxicity against Philadelphia chromosome-positive chronic myelogenous leukemia. *Blood*, **89**, 1133–42.

Choudhury, B.A., Liang, J.C., Thomas, E.K., Flores-Romo, L., Xie, Q.S., Agusala, K. *et al.* (1999). Dendritic cells derived *in vitro* from acute myelogenous leukemia cells stimulate autologous, antileukemic T-cell responses. *Blood*, **93**, 780–6.

Cignetti, A., Bryant, E., Allione, B., Vitale, A., Foa, R. and Cheever, M.A. (1999). CD34(+) acute myeloid and lymphoid leukemic blasts can be induced to differentiate into dendritic cells. *Blood*, **94**, 2048–55.

Corr, M., Lee, D.J., Carson, D.A. and Tighe, H. (1996). Gene vaccination with naked plasmid DNA: mechanism of CTL priming. *Journal of Experimental Medicine*, **184**, 1555–60.

De Bruijn, M.L., Jackson, M.R. and Peterson, P.A. (1995). Phagocyte-induced antigen-specific activation of unprimed CD8+ T cells *in vitro*. *European Journal of Immunology*, **25**, 1274–85.

De Bruijn, M.L., Peterson, P.A. and Jackson, M.R. (1996). Induction of heat-stable antigen expression by phagocytosis is involved in *in vitro* activation of unprimed CTL by macrophages. *Journal of Immunology*, **156**, 2686–92.

Devitt, A., Moffatt, O.D., Raykundalia, C., Capra, J.D., Simmons, D.L. and Gregory, C.D. (1998). Human CD14 mediates recognition and phagocytosis of apoptotic cells. *Nature*, **392**, 505–9.

Dolhain, R.J., van der Heiden, A.N., ter Haar, N.T., Breedveld, F.C. and Miltenburg, A.M. (1996). Shift toward T lymphocytes with a T helper 1 cytokine-secretion profile in the joints of patients with rheumatoid arthritis. *Arthritis and Rheumatology*, **39**, 1961–9.

Falo, L.D., Jr, Kovacsovisc-Bankowsik, M., Thompson, K. and Rock, K.L. (1995). Targeting antigen into the phagocytic pathway *in vivo* induces protective tumour immunity. *Nature Medicine*, **1**, 649–53

Fanger, N.A., Wardwell, K., Shen, L., Tedder, T.F. and Guyre, P.M. (1996). Type I (CD64) and type II (CD32) Fcg receptor-mediated phagocytosis by human blood dendritic cells. *Journal of Immunology*, **157**, 541–8.

Flamand, V., Sornasse, T., Thielemans, K., Demanet, C., Bakkus, M. and Bazin, H., (1994). Murine dendritic cells pulsed *in vitro* with tumor antigen induce tumor resistance *in vivo*. *European Journal of Immunology*, **24**, 605–10.

Flores-Romo, L., Bjorck, P., Duvert, V., van Kooten, C., Saeland, S. and Banchereau, J. (1997). CD40 ligation on human cord blood CD34+ hematopoietic progenitors induces their proliferation and differentiation into functional dendritic cells. *Journal of Experimental Medicine*, **185**, 341–9.

Forster, I. and Lieberam, I. (1996). Peripheral tolerance of CD4 T cells following local activation in adolescent mice. *European Journal of Immunology*, **26**, 3194–202.

Fossum, S. and Rolstad, B. (1986). The roles of interdigitating cells and natural killer cells in the rapid rejection of allogeneic lymphocytes. *European Journal of Immunology*, **16**, 440–50.

Fraser, I., Hughes, D. and Gordon, S. (1993). Divalent cation-independent macrophage adhesion inhibited by monoclonal antibody to murine scavenger receptor. *Nature*, **364**, 343–6.

Geissmann, F., Prost, C., Monnet, J.P., Dy, M., Brousse, N. and Hermine, O. (1998). Transforming growth factor β1, in the presence of granulocyte macrophage colony stimulating factor and interleukin 4, induces differentiation of human peripheral blood monocytes into dendritic Langerhans cells. *Journal of Experimental Medicine*, **187**, 961–6.

Geuze, H.J. (1998). The role of endosomes and lysosomes in MHC class II functioning. *Immunology Today*, **19**, 282–7.

Gong, J., Chen, D., Kashiwaba, M. and Kufe, D. (1997). Induction of antitumor activity by immunization with fusions of dendritic and carcinoma cells. *Nature Medicine*, **3**, 558–61.

Gooding, L.R. and Edwards, C.B. (1980). H-2 antigen requirements in the *in vitro* induction of SV40-specific cytotoxic T lymphocytes. *Journal of Immunology*, **24**, 1258–62.

Gordon, R.D., Mathieson, B.J., Samelson, L.E., Boyse, E.A. and Simpson, E. (1976). The effect of allogeneic presensitization on H-Y graft survival and *in vitro* cell-mediated responses to H-y antigen. *Journal of Experimental Medicine*, **144**, 810–20.

Granelli-Piperno, A., Pope, M., Inaba, K. and Steinman, R.M. (1995). Coexpression of NF-kB/Rel and Sp1 transcription factors in human immunodeficiency virus 1-induced, dendritic cell-T-cell syncytia. *Proceeding of the National Academy of Sciences USA*, **92**, 10944–8.

Greenwalt, D.E., Lipsky, R.H., Ockenhouse, C.F., Ikeda, H., Tandon, N.N. and Jamieson, G.A. (1992). Membrane glycoprotein CD36: a review of its roles in adherence, signal transduction, and transfusion medicine. *Blood*, **80**, 1105–15.

Guo, Y., Wu, M., Chen, H., Wang, X., Liu, G., Li, G. *et al.* (1994). Effective tumor vaccine generated by fusion of hepatoma cells with activated B cells. *Science*, **263**, 518–20.

Hall, S.E., Savill, J.S., Henson, P.M. and Haslett, C. (1994). Apoptotic neutrophils are phagocytosed by fibroblasts with participation of the fibroblast vitronectin receptor and involvement of a mannose/fucose-specific lectin. *Journal of Immunology*, **153**, 3218–27.

Harding, C.V. and Song, R. 1(994). Phagocytic processing of exogenous particulate antigens by macrophages for presentation by class I MHC molecules. *Journal of Immunology*, **153**, 4925–33.

Hart, D.N.J. (1997). Dendritic cells: unique leukocyte populations, which control the primary immune response. *Blood*, **90**, 3245–87.

Hart, S.P., Haslett, C. and Dransfield, I. (1996). Recognition of apoptotic cells by phagocytes. *Experientia*, **52**, 950–6.

Hilkens, C.M.U., Kalinski, P., de Boer, M. and Kapsenberg, M.L. (1997). Human dendritic cells require exogenous interleukin-12-inducing factors to direct the development of naive T-helper cells toward the Th1 phenotype. *Blood*, **90**, 1920–6.

Holt, P.G., Oliver, J., Bilyk, N., McMenamin, C., McMenamin, P.G., Kraal, G. *et al.* (1993). Downregulation of the antigen presenting cell function(s) of pulmonary dendritic cells *in vivo* by resident alveolar macrophages. *Journal of Experimental Medicine*, **177**, 397–407.

Hu, X., Chakraborty, N.G., Sporn, J.R., Kurtzman, S.H., Ergin, M.T. and Mukherji, B. (1996). Enhancement of cytolytic T lymphocyte precursor frequency in melanoma patients following immunization with the MAGE-1 peptide loaded antigen presenting cell-based vaccine. *Cancer Research*, **56**, 2479–83.

Huang, A.Y., Golumbek, P., Ahmadzadeh, M., Jaffee, E., Pardoll, D. and Levitsky, H. (1994). Role of bone marrow-derived cells in presenting MHC class I-restricted tumor antigens. *Science*, **264**, 961–5.

Huang, A.Y.C., Bruce, A.T., Pardoll, D.M. and Levitsky, H.I. (1996). *In vivo* cross-priming of MHC class I-restricted antigens requires the TAP transporter. *Immunity*, **4**, 349–55.

Hughues, D.A., Fraser, I. and Gordon, S. (1995). Murine macrophage scavenger receptor: *in vivo* expression and function as receptor for macrophage adhesion in lymphoid and non-lymphoid organs. *European Journal of Immunology*, **25**, 466–73.

Inaba, K., Inaba, M., Romani, N., Aya, H., Deguchi, M. and Ikehara, S. (1992). Generation of large numbers of dendritic cells from mouse bone marrow cultures supplemented with granulocyte/macrophage colony-stimulating factor. *Journal of Experimental Medicine*, **176**, 1693–702.

Inaba, K., Witmer-Pack, M., Inaba, M., Hathcock, K.S., Sakuta, H., Azuma, M. *et al.* (1994). The tissue distribution of the B7-2 co-stimulator in mice: abundant expression on dendritic cells *in situ* and during maturation *in vitro*. *Journal of Experimental Medicine*, **180**, 1849–60.

Inaba, K., Turley, S., Yamaide, F., Iyoda, T., Mahnke, K., Inaba, M. *et al.* (1998). Efficient presentation of phagocytosed cellular fragments on the MHC class II products of dendritic cells. *Journal of Experimental Medicine*, **188**, 2163–73.

Ishida, T., Oyama, T., Carbone, D.P. and Gabrilovich, D.I. (1998). Defective function of Langerhans cells in tumor-bearing animals is the result of defective maturation from hemopoietic progenitors. *Journal of Immunology*, **161**, 4842–51.

Jiang, W., Swiggard, W.J., Heufler, C. , Peng, M., Mirza, A., Steinman, R.M. *et al.* (1995). The receptor DEC-205 expressed by dendritic cells and thymic epithelial cells is involved in antigen processing. *Nature*, **375**, 151–5.

Ke, Y. and Ka, J.A. (1996). Exogenous antigens gain access to the major histocompatibility complex class I processing pathway in B-cells by receptor-mediated uptake. *Journal of Experimental Medicine*, **184**, 1179–84.

Kleijmeer, M.J., Oorschot, V.M. and Geuze, H.J. (1994). Human resident Langerhans cells display a lysosomal compartment enriched in MHC class II. *Journal of Investigative Dermatology*, **103**, 516–23.

Kovacsovics-Bankowski, M. and Rock, K.L. (1995). A phagosome-to-cytosol pathway for exogenous antigens presented on MHC class I molecules. *Science*, **267**, 243–6.

Kovacsovics-Bankowski, B.M., Clark, K., Benacerraf, B. and Rock, K.L. (1993). Efficient major histocompatibility complex class I presentation of exogenous antigen upon phagocytosis by macrophages. *Proceeding of the National Academy of Sciences USA*, **90**, 4942–6.

Krieger, M. and Herz, J. (1994). Structures and functions of multiligand lipoprotein receptors: macrophage scavenger receptors and LDL receptor-related protein (LRP). *Annual Review of Biochemestry*, **63**, 601–37.

Kurts, C., Heath, W.R., Carbone, F.R., Allison, J., Miller, J.F.A.P. and Kosaka, H. (1996). Constitutive class I-restricted presentation of self antigens *in vivo*. *Journal of Experimental Medicine*, **184**, 923–30.

Kurts, C., Kosaka, H., Carbone, F.R., Miller, J.F.A.P. and Heath, W.R. (1997). Class I-restricted cross-presentation of exogenous self antigens leads to deletion of autoreactive CD8⁺ T cells. *Journal of Experimental Medicine*, **186**, 239–45.

Kurts, C., Heath, W.R., Kosaka, H., Miller, J.F. and Carbone, F.R. (1998a). The peripheral deletion of autoreactive CD8⁺ T cells induced by cross-presentation of self-antigens involves signaling through CD95 (Fas, Apo-1). *Journal of Experimental Medicine*, **188**, 415–20.

Kurts, C., Miller, J.F., Subramaniam, R.M., Carbone, F.R. and Heath, W.R. (1998b). Major histocompatibility complex class I-restricted cross-presentation is biased towards high dose antigens and those released during cellular destruction. *Journal of Experimental Medicine*, **188**, 409–14.

Lanzavecchia, A. (1996). Mechanisms of antigen uptake for presentation. *Current Opinion in Immunology*, **8**, 348–54.

Lardon, F., Snoeck, H.W., Berneman, Z.N., Van Tendeloo, V.F., Nijs, G., Lenjou, M. *et al.* (1997). Generation of dendritic cells from bone marrow progenitors using GM-CSF, TNF-, and additional cytokines: antagonistic effects of IL-4 and IFN and selective involvement of the TNF receptor-1. *Immunology*, **91**, 553–9.

Larsen, C.P., Ritchie, S.C., Hendrix, R., Linsley, P.S., Hathcock, K.S., Hodes, R.J. *et al.* (1994). Regulation of immunostimulatory function and costimulatory molecule (B7-1 and B7-2) expression on murine dendritic cells. *Journal of Immunology*, **152**, 5208–19.

Lichtman, A.H. and Abbas, A.K. (1997). T-cell subsets: recruiting the right kind of help. *Current Biology*, **7**, R242–44.

Liu, T., Zhou, X., Orvell, C., Lederer, E., Ljunggren., H.-G. and Jondal, M. (1995). Heat-inactivated Sendai virus can enter multiple MHC class I processing pathways and generate cytotoxic T lymphocyte responses *in vivo*. *Journal of Immunology*, **154**, 3147–55.

Liu, Y. J., Xu, J., de Bouteiller, O., Parham, C.L., Grouard, G., Djossou, O. *et al*. (1997). Follicular dendritic cells specifically express the long CR2/CD21 isoform. *Journal of Experimental Medicine*, **185**, 165–70.

Ljunggren, H.G., Stam, N.J., Ohlen, C., Neffjes, J.J., Hoglund, P., Heemels, M.T. *et al*. (1990). Empty class I MHC molecules come out in the cold. *Nature*, **346**, 476–80.

Lotze, M., Farhood, H., Wilson, C.C. and Storkus, W. (1999). Dendritic cell therapy of cancer and HIV infection. In Lotze, M.T. and Thomson, A.W. (ed.), *Dendritic Cells*. Academic Press, San Diego, pp. 459–85.

Ludewig, B., Graf, D., Gelderblom, H.R., Becker, Y., Kroczek, R.A. and Pauli, G. (1995). Spontaneous apoptosis of dendritic cells is efficiently inhibited by TRAP (CD40-ligand) and TNF-α, but strongly enhanced by interleukin-10. *European Journal of Immunology*, **25**, 1943–50.

Mackey, M.F., Barth, R.J. and Noelle, R.J. (1998). The role of CD40/CD154 interactions in the priming, differentiation, and effector function of helper and cytotoxic T cells. *Journal of Leukocyte Biology*, **63**, 418–28.

Matzinger, P. (1994). Tolerance, danger, and the extended family. *Annual Review of Immunology*, **12**, 991–1045.

Mayordomo, J.I., Zorina, T., Storkus, W.J., Zitvogel, L., Celluzzi, C. and Falo, L.D. (1995). Bone marrow-derived dendritic cells pulsed with synthetic tumor peptides elicit protective and therapeutic antitumor immunity. *Nature Medicine*, **1**, 1297–302.

Mayordomo, J.I., Loftus, D.J., Sakamoto, H., De Cesare, C.M., Aasamy, P.M. and Lotze, M.T. (1996). Therapy of murine tumors with p53 wild-type and mutant sequence peptide-based vaccines. *Journal of Experimental Medicine*, **183**,1357–65.

McKnight, A.J. and Gordon, S. (1998). Membrane molecules as differentiation antigens of murine macrophages. *Advances in Immunology*, **68**, 271–314.

McRae, B.L., Semnani, R.T., Hayes, M.P. and van Seventer, G.A. (1998). Type 1 IFNs inhibit human dendritic cell IL-12 production and Th1 cell development. *Journal of Immunology*, **160**, 4298–304.

Medina, E., Guzman, C.A., Staendner, L.H., Colombo, M.P. and Paglia, P. (1999). *Salmonella* vaccine carrier strains: effective delivery system to trigger anti-tumor immunity by oral route. *European Journal of Immunology*, **29**, 693–9.

Moore, K.W., O'Garra, A., de Waal Malefyt, R., Vieira, P. and Mosmann, T.R. (1993). Interleukin-10. *Annual Review of Immunology*, **11**, 165–90.

Morel, A.S., Quaratino, S., Douek, D.C. and Londei, M. (1997). Split activity of interleukin-10 on antigen capture and antigen presentation by human dendritic cells: definition of a maturative step. *European Journal of Immunology*, **27**, 26–34.

Morrison, L.A., Lukacher, A.E., Braciale, V.L., Fan, D.P. and Braciale, T.J. (1986). Differences in antigen presentation to MHC class I- and class-II restricted influenza virus-specific cytolytic T lymphocyte clones. *Journal of Experimental Medicine*, **163**, 903–21.

Mortarini, R., Anichini, A., Di Nicola, M., Siena, S., Bregni, M. and Belli, F. (1997). Autologous dendritic cells derived from CD34+ progenitors and from monocytes are not functionally equivalent antigen-presenting cells in the induction of Melan-A/Mart-1(27–35)-specific CTLs from peripheral blood lymphocytes of melanoma patients with low frequency of CTL precursors. *Cancer Research*, **57**, 5534–41.

Mukherji, B., Chakraborty, N.G., Yamasaki, S., Okino, T., Yamase, H. and Sporn, J.R. (1995). Induction of antigen-specific cytolytic T cells i*n situ* in human melanoma by immunization with synthetic peptide-pulsed autologous antigen presenting cells. *Proceeding of the National Academy of Sciences USA*, **92**, 8078–82.

Nair, S.K. (1997). Immunotherapy of cancer with dendritic cell-based vaccines. *Gene Therapy*, **5**, 1445–6.

Nair, S.K., Boczkowski, D., Morse, M., Cumming, R.I., Lyerly, H.K. and Gilboa, E. (1998). Induction of primary carcinoembryonic antigen (CEA)-specific cytotoxic T lymphocytes *in vitro* using human dendritic cells transfected with RNA. *Nature Biotechnology*, **16**, 364–69.

Nestle, F.O., Turka, L.A. and Nickloff, B.J. (1994). Characterization of dermal dendritic cells in psoriasis: autostimulation of T lymphocytes and induction of Th1 type cytokines. *Journal of Clinical Investigation*, **94**, 202–9.

Nestle, F.O., Alijagic, S., Gilliet, M., Sun, Y., Grabbe S. and Dummer, R. (1998). Vaccination of melanoma patients with peptide- or tumor lysate-pulsed dendritic cells. *Nature Medicine*, **4**, 328–2.

Norbury, C.C., Hewlett, L.J., Prescott, A.R., Shastri, N. and Watts, C. (1995). Class I MHC presentation of exogenous soluble antigen via macropinocytosis in bone marrow macrophages. *Immunity*, **3**, 783–791.

Norbury, C.C., Chambers, B.J., Prescott, A.R., Ljunggren, H.-G. and Watts, C. (1996). Constitutive macropinocytosis allows TAP-dependent presentation of exogenous antigen on class I MHC molecules by bone marrow derived dendritic cells. *European Journal of Immunology*, **27**, 358–74.

Nossal, G.J. (1995). Choices following antigen entry: antibody formation or immunologic tolerance. *Annual Review of Immunology*, **3**, 1–27.

Ossevoort, M.A., Feltkamp, M.C., van Veen, K.J., Melief, C.J. and Kast, W.M. (1995). Dendritic cells as carriers for a cytotoxic T-lymphocyte epitope-based peptide vaccine in protection against a human papillomavirus type 16-induced tumor. *Journal of Immunotherapy with Emphasis in Tumor Immunology*, **18**, 86–94.

Ozawa, H., Aiba, S., Nakagawa, S. and Tagami, H. (1996). Interferon-γ and interleukin-10 inhibit antigen presentation by Langerhans cells for T helper type 1 cells by suppressing their CD80 (B7-1) expression. *European Journal of Immunology*, **26**, 648–52.

Paglia, P. and Guzman, C.A. (1998). Keeping the immune system alerted against cancer. *Cancer Immunology and Immunotherapy*, **46**, 88–92.

Paglia, P., Chiodoni, C., Rodolfo, M. and Colombo, M.P. (1996). Murine dendritic cells loaded *in vitro* with soluble protein prime cytotoxic T lymphocytes against tumor antigen *in vivo*. *Journal of Experimental Medicine*, **183**, 317–22.

Paglia, P., Arioli, I., Frahm, N., Chakraborty, T., Colombo, M.P. and Guzman, C.A. (1997). The defined attenuated *Listeria monocytogenes* delta mp12 mutant is an effective oral vaccine carrier to trigger a long-lasting immune response against a mouse fibrosarcoma. *European Journal of Immunology*, **27**, 1570–5.

Paglia, P., Medina, E., Arioli, I., Guzman, C.A. and Colombo, M.P. (1998). Gene transfer in dendritic cells, induced by oral DNA vaccination with *Salmonella typhimurium*, results in protective immunity against a murine fibrosarcoma. *Blood*, **92**, 3172–6.

Palucka, K.A., Taquet, N., Sanchez-Chapuis, F. and Gluckman, J.C. (1998). Dendritic cells as the terminal stage of monocyte differentiation. *Journal of Immunology*, **160**, 4587–95.

Pearson, A.M. (1996). Scavenger receptors in innate immunity. *Current Opinion in Immunology*, **8**, 20–8.

Peters, P.J., Neefjes, J.J., Oorschot, V., Ploegh, H.L. and Geuze, H.J. (1991). Segregation of MHC class II molecules from MHC class I molecules in the Golgi complex for transport to lysosomal compartments. *Nature*, **349**, 669–76 .

Pettit, A.R., Quinn, C., MacDonald, K.P., Cavanagh, L.L., Thomas, G., Townsend, W. *et al.* (1997). Nuclear localization of RelB is associated with effective antigen presenting cell function. *Journal of Immunology*, **159**, 3681–91.

Pfeifer, J.D., Wick, M.J., Roberts, R.L., Findlay, K., Normark, S.J. and Harding, C.V. (1993). Phagocytic processing of bacterial antigens for class I MHC presentation to T cells. *Nature*, **361**, 359–62.

Pierre, P., Turley, S.J., Gatti, E., Hull, M., Meltzer, J., Mirza, A. *et al.* (1997). Developmental regulation of MHC class II transport in mouse dendritic cells. *Nature*, **388**, 787–92.

Platt, N., Suzuki, H., Kurihara, Y., Kodama, T. and Gordon, S. (1996). Role for the class A macrophage scavenger receptor in the phagocytosis of apoptotic thymocytes *in vitro*. *Proceeding of the National Academy of Sciences USA*, **93**, 12456–60.

Porgador, A., Snyder, D. and Gilboa, E. (1996). Induction of antitumor immunity using bone marrow-γenerated dendritic cells. *Journal of Immunology*, **156**, 2918–26.

Pulaski, B.A., Yeh, K.Y., Shastri, N., Maltby, K.M., Penney, D.P. and Lord, E.M. (1996). Interleukin 3 enhances cytotoxic T lymphocyte development and class I major histocompatibility complex 're-presentation' of exogenous antigen by tumor-infiltrating antigen-presenting cells. *Proceeding of the National Academy of Sciences USA*, **93**, 3669–74.

Qin, Z., Noffz, G., Mohaupt, M. and Blankenstein, T. (1997). Interleukin-10 prevents dendritic cell accumulation and vaccination with granulocyte–macrophage colony-stimulating factor gene-modified tumor cells. *Journal of Immunology*, **159**, 770–6.

Randolph, G.J., Beaulieu, S., Lebecque, S., Steinman, R.M. and Muller, W.A. (1998). Differentiation of monocytes into dendritic cells in a model of transendothelial trafficking. *Science*, **282**, 480–3.

Randolph, G.J., Inaba, K., Robbiani, D.F., Steinman, R.M. and Muller, W.A. (1999). Differentiation of phagocytic monocytes into lymph node dendritic cells *in vivo*. *Immunity*, **11**, 753–61.

Reeves, M.E., Royal, R.E., Lam, J.S., Rosenberg, S.A. and Hwu, P. (1996). Retroviral transduction of human dendritic cells with a tumor-associated antigen gene. *Cancer Research*, **56**, 5672–7.

Reid, C. (1996). Stem cell factor and the regulation of dendritic cell production from CD34+ progenitors in bone marrow and cord blood. *British Journal of Haematology*, **93**, 258–64.

Reid, C.D.L. (1997). The dendritic cell lineage in haemopoiesis. *British Journal of Haematology*, **96**, 217–23.

Reid, C.D., Stackpoole, A., Meager, A. and Tikerpae, J. (1992). Interactions of tumor necrosis factor with granulocyte–macrophage colony-stimulating factor and other cytokines in the regulation of dendritic cell growth *in vitro* from early bipotent CD34+ progenitors in human bone marrow. *Journal of Immunology*, **149**, 2681–8.

Reis e Sousa, C. and Germain, R.N. (1995). Major histocompatibility complex class I presentation of peptides derived from soluble exogenous antigen by a subset of cells engaged in phagocytosis. *Journal of Experimental Medicine*, **182**, 841–51.

Reis e Sousa, C., Stahl, P.D. and Austyn, J.M. (1993). Phagocytosis of antigens by Langerhans cells *in vitro*. *Journal of Experimental Medicine*, **78**, 509–19.

Rescigno, M., Citterio, S., Thery, C., Rittig, M., Medaglini, D., Pozzi, G. *et al.* (1998). Bacteria-induced neo-biosynthesis, stabilization, and surface expression of functional class I molecules in mouse dendritic cells. *Proceeding of the National Academy of Sciences USA*, **95**, 5229–34.

Rock, K.L., Gamble, S. and Rothstein, L. (1990). Presentation of exogenous antigen with class I major histocompatibility complex molecules. *Science*, **249**, 918–21.

Rocken, M., Racke, M. and Shevach, E.M. (1996). IL-4-induced immune deviation as antigen-specific therapy for inflammatory autoimmune disease. *Immunology Today*, **17**, 225–31.

Romani, N., Gruner, S., Brang, D., Kampgen, E., Lenz A. and Trockenbacher B. (1994). Proliferating dendritic cell progenitors in human blood. *Journal of Experimental Medicine*, **180**, 83–93.

Romani, N., Reider, D., Heuer, M., Ebner, S., Kampgen, E. and Eibl, B. (1996). Generation of mature dendritic cells from human blood. An improved method with special regard to clinical applicability. *Journal of Immunology Methods*, **196**, 137–51.

Rosenzwajg, M., Camus, S., Guigon, M. and Gluckman, J.C. (1998). The influence of interleukin (IL)-4, IL-13, and Flt3 ligand on human dendritic cell differentiation from cord blood CD34⁺ progenitor cells. *Experimental Hematology*, **26**, 63–72.

Rubartelli, A., Poggi, A. and Zocchi, M.R. (1997). The selective engulfment of apoptotic bodies by dendritic cells is mediated by the $\alpha(v)$ $\beta3$ integrin and requires intracellular and extracellular calcium. *European Journal of Immunology*, **27**, 1893–900.

Sallusto, F. and Lanzavecchia, A. (1994). Efficient presentation of soluble antigen by cultured human dendritic cells is maintained by granulocyte/macrophage colony-stimulating factor plus interleukin 4 and downregulated by tumor necrosis factor α. *Journal of Experimental Medicine*, **179**, 1109–13.

Sallusto, F., Cella, M., Danieli, C. and Lanzavecchia, A. (1995). Dendritic cells use macropinocytosis and the mannose receptor to concentrate macromolecules in the major histocompatibility complex class II compartment: downregulation by cytokines and bacterial products. *Journal of Experimental Medicine*, **182**, 389–400.

Santiago-Schwarz, F., Borrero, M., Tucci, J., Palaia, T. and Carsons, S.E. (1997). *In vitro* expansion of CD13⁺CD33⁺ dendritic cell precursors from multipotent progenitors is regulated by a discrete fas-mediated apoptotic schedule. *Journal of Leukocyte Biology*, **62**, 493–502.

Santiago-Schwarz, F., Divaris, N., Kay, C. and Carsons, S.E. (1993). Mechanisms of tumor necrosis factor-granulocyte–macrophage colony-stimulating factor-induced dendritic cell development. *Blood*, **82**, 3019–28.

Santiago-Schwarz, F., Rappa, D., Laky, K. and Carsons, S.E. (1995). Stem cell factor augments TNF/GM-CSF mediated dendritic cell development. *Stem Cells*, **13**, 186–97.

Santiago-Schwarz, F., McCarthy, M., Tucci, J. and Carsons, S.E. (1998a). Neutralization of tumor necrosis factor activity shortly after the onset of dendritic cell hematopoiesis reveals a novel mechanism for the selective expansion of the CD14-dependent dendritic cell pathway. *Blood*, **92**, 745–55.

Santiago-Schwarz, F., Tucci, J. and Carsons, S.E. (1998b). Immature progenitors in rheumatoid arthritis peripheral blood and synovial fluid preferentially respond to cytokine combinations that yield CD14 dependent dendritic cells. *Arthritis and Rheumatology*, **41**, S36.

Savill, J. (1997). Recognition and phagocytosis of cells undergoing apoptosis. *British Medical Bulletin*, **53**, 491–508.

Savill, J., Fadok, V., Henson, P. and Haslett, C. (1993). Phagocyte recognition of cells undergoing apoptosis. *Immunology Today*, **14**, 131–6.

Schirmbeck, R., Bohm, W., Melber, K. and Reimann, J. (1995). Processing of exogenous heat-aggregated (denatured) and particulate (native) hepatitis B surface antigen for class I-restricted epitope presentation. *Journal of Immunology*, **155**, 4676–84.

Shimada, S., Caughman, S.W., Sharrow, S.O., Stephany, D. and Katz, S.I. (1987). Enhanced antigen-presenting capacity of cultured Langerhans' cells is associated with markedly increased expression of Ia antigen. *Journal of Immunology*, **139**, 2551–5.

Shortman, K. and Caux, C. (1997). Dendritic cell development: multiple pathways to nature's adjuvants. *Stem Cells*, **15**, 409–19.

Shrivastava, P.K., DeLeo, A.B. and Old, L.J. (1986). Tumor rejection antigens of chemically induced sarcomas of inbred mice. *Proceeding of the National Academy of Sciences USA*, **83**, 3407–11.

Shurin, M.R., Esche, C., Lokshin, A. and Lotze, M.T. (1999). Apoptosis in dendritic cells. In Lotze, M.T. and Thomson, A.W. (ed.), *Dendritic Cells,* Academic Press, San Diego, pp. 673–82.

Song, W., Kong, H.L., Carpenter, H., Torii, H., Granstein, R. and Rafii, S. (1997). Dendritic cells genetically modified with an adenovirus vector encoding the cDNA for a model antigen induce protective and therapeutic antitumor immunity. *Journal of Experimental Medicine*, **186**, 1247–56.

Specht, J.M., Wang, G., Do, M.T., Lam, J.S., Royal, R.E. and Reeves, M.E. (1997). Dendritic cells retrovirally transduced with a model antigen gene are therapeutically effective against established pulmonary metastases. *Journal of Experimental Medicine*, **186**, 1213–21.

Staerz, U.D., Karasuyama, H. and Garner, A.M. (1987). Cytotoxic T lymphocytes against a soluble protein. *Nature*, **329**, 449–51.

Steinbrink, K., Wolfl, M., Jonuleit, H., Knop, J. and Enk, A.H. (1997). Induction of tolerance by IL-10-treated dendritic cells. *Journal of Immunology*, **159**, 4772–80.

Steinman, R.M. and Cohn, Z.A. (1973). Identification of a novel cell type in peripheral lymphoid organs of mice. I. Morphology, quantitation, tissue distribution. *Journal of Experimental Medicine*, **137**, 1142–62.

Stoppacciaro, A., Paglia, P., Lombardi, L., Parmiani, G., Baroni C. and Colombo, M.P. (1997). Genetic modification of a carcinoma with the IL-4 gene increases the influx of dendritic cells relative to other cytokines. *European Journal of Immunology*, **27**, 2375–82.

Strobl, H., Bello-Fernandez, C., Riedl, E., Pickl, W.F., Majdic, O., Lyman, S.D. *et al.* (1997). Flt3 ligand in cooperation with transforming growth factor-1 potentiates *in vitro* development of Langerhans type dendritic cells and allows single cell dendritic cell cluster formation under serum free conditions. *Blood*, **90**, 1425–34.

Strobl, H., Riedl, E., Bello-Fernandez, C. and Knapp, W. (1998). Epidermal Langerhans cell development and differentiation. *Immunobiology*, **198**, 588–605.

Strunk, D., Egger, C., Leitner, G., Hanau, D. and Stingl, G. (1997). A skin homing molecule defines the Langerhans cell progenitor in human peripheral blood. *Journal of Experimental Medicine*, **185**, 1131–6.

Sugita, M. and Brenner, M.B. (1995). Association of the invariant chain with major histocompatibility complex class I molecules directs trafficking to endocytic compartments. *Journal of Biological Chemistry*, **270**, 1443–8.

Suss, G. and Shortman, K. (1996). A subclass of dendritic cells kills CD4 T cells via Fas/Fas-ligand induced apoptosis. *Journal of Experimental Medicine*, **183**, 1789–96.

Suto, R. and Srivastava, P.K. (1995). A mechanism for the specific immunogenicity of heat shock protein-chaperoned peptides. *Science*, **269**, 1585–8.

Swanson, J.A. and Baer, S.C. (1995). Phagocytosis by zippers and triggers. *Trends in Cell Biology*, **5**, 89–92.

Szabolics, P., Avigan, D., Gezelter, S., Ciocon, D.H., Moore, M.A.S., Steinman, R.M. *et al.* (1996). Dendritic cells and macrophages can mature independently from a human bone marrow-derived, post-colony-forming unit intermediate. *Blood*, **87**, 4520–30.

Thiele, D.L., Kurosaka, M. and Lipsky, P.E. (1983). Phenotype of the accessory cell necessary for mitogen-stimulated T and B cell responses in human peripheral blood: delineation by its sensitivity to the lysosomotropic agent, L-leucine methyl ester. *Journal of Immunology*, **131**, 2282–90.

Thomssen, H., Kahan, M. and Londei, M. (1995). Differential effects of interleukin-10 on the expression of HLA class II and CD1 molecules induced by granulocyte/macrophage colony-stimulating factor/interleukin-4. *European Journal of Immunology*, **25**, 2465–70.

Townsend, A.R.M. and Bodmer, H. (1989). Antigen recognition by class I MHC-restricted T lymphocytes. *Annual Review of Immunology*, **7**, 601–24.

Udono, H. and Srivastava, P.K. (1993). Heat shock protein 70-associated peptides elicit specific cancer immunity. *Journal of Experimental Medicine*, **178**, 1391–6 .

Ullrich, S.J., Robinson, E.A., Law, L.W., Willingham, M. and Appella, E. (1986). A mouse tumor-specific transplantation antigen is a heat shock-related protein. *Proceeding of the National Academy of Sciences USA*, **83**, 3121–5.

Unanue, E.R. (1984). Antigen-presenting function of the macrophage. *Annual Review of Immunology*, **2**, 395–428.

van Furth, R. (1980). The mononuclear phagocyte system. *Verhanglen der Deutschen Gesellschaft für Pathologie*, **4**, 1–11.

Vremec, D., Lieschke, G.J., Dunn, A.R., Robb, L., Metcalf, D. and Shortman, K. (1997). The influence of granulocyte macrophage colony stimulating factor on dendritic cell levels in mouse lymphoid organs. *European Journal of Immunology*, **1**, 40–4.

Ward, S.G., Bacon, K. and Westwick, J. (1998). Chemokines and T lymphocytes: more than an attraction. *Immunity*, **9**, 1–11.

Wong, B.R., Josien, R., Lee, S.Y., Sauter, B., Li, H., Steinman, R.M. and Choi, Y. (1997). TRANCE (tumor necrosis factor [TNF]-related activation-induced cytokine), a new TNF family member predominantly expressed in T cells, is a dendritic cell specific survival factor. *Journal of Experimental Medicine*, **186**, 2075–80.

Wraith, D.C., Vessey, A.E. and Askonas, B.A. (1987). Purified influenza virus nucleoprotein protects mice from lethal infection. *Journal of General Virology*, **68**, 433–40.

Yin, Z., Neure, L., Grolms, S., Eggens, U., Radbruch, A., Braun, J. and Sieper, J. (1997). Th1/Th2 cytokine pattern in the joint of rheumatoid arthritis and reactive arthritis patients: analysis at the single cell level. *Arthritis and Rheumatology*, **40**, S37.

Young, J.W., Koulova, L., Soergel, S.A., Clark, E.A., Steinman, R.M. and Dupont B. (1992). The B7/BB1 antigen provides one of several costimulatory signals for the activation of CD4+ T lymphocytes by human blood dendritic cells *in vitro*. *Journal of Clinical Investigation*, **90**, 229–37.

Zal, T., Volkmann, A. and Stockinger, B. (1994). Mechanisms of tolerance induction in major histo-compatibility complex class II-restricted T cells specific for a blood-borne self-antigen. *Journal of Experimental Medicine*, **180**, 2089–99.

Zitvogel, L., Mayordomo, J.I., Tjandrawan, T., DeLeo, A.B., Clarke, M.R. and Lotze, M.T. (1996). Therapy of murine tumors with tumor peptide-pulsed dendritic cells: dependence on T cells, B7 costimulation, and T helper cell-associated cytokines. *Journal of Experimental Medicine*, **183**, 87–97.

Zwaal, R.F. and Schroit, A.J. (1997). Pathophysiologic implications of membrane phospholipid asymmetry in blood cells. *Blood*, **89**, 1121–32.

4 *Macrophage–virus interactions*

W. Zink, L. Ryan and H.E. Gendelman

1 Introduction

Mononuclear phagocytes (MPs) (blood monocytes, tissue macrophages, connective tissue histiocytes, dendritic cells in lymph nodes and spleen, Langerhans cells of skin, Kupffer cells of liver and microglial cells of brain) comprise one of the principle elements in the clearance and inactivation of microbial pathogens including viruses. Paradoxically, these cells also represent a major target cell and infectious reservoir for a number of persistent viral infections. Alterations in MP function resulting from viral infection may lead to a number of pathological outcomes. Ultimately, the interaction between the virus and MPs is the net result of a complex series of intracellular events and can lead to the destruction or persistence of the pathogen and/or the precipitation of disease through alterations in immune responses.

MPs contribute to virus immunity in many ways.

(1)   A a central feature of macrophages is the ability to eliminate free or opsonized virus from the circulation following blood-borne infection (phagocytosis). This is mediated through phagosome–lysosome fusion (intracellular killing).

(2)   MPs express high levels of major histocompatibility complex (MHC) antigens and T lymphocyte co-stimulatory molecules. MPs present antigen to surveillance CD4$^+$ and CD8$^+$ T cells creating the initial communication between the innate and acquired arms of the immune system (antigen presentation).

(3)   Macrophage-secreted cytokines (secretory function) can induce an ensuing T-lymphocyte-mediated immune response which ultimately results in cellular cyto-toxic effector mechanisms (Th1) or B-cell activation (Th2) (effector function).

(4)   The macrophage is a potent source of chemotactic cytokines (chemokines) that can recruit nascent leukocytes to the site of an inflammatory lesion.

(5)   The macrophage can secrete soluble factors to restrict virus infection or replication in proximal cells, most notably interferons (innate immunity).

Although MP functions primarily serve to aid host survival, MPs also participate in tissue destructive processes during disease and notably during viral infections. In some cases, viruses can infect macrophages and in so doing circumvent macrophage-mediated immune defense mechanisms. Because MPs are terminally differentiated cells with migratory potential, they can be an important viral target, infectious reservoir and mech-anism for widespread dissemination within organisms. Viruses that infect macrophages are predisposed to establishing chronic infections. In other cases, virus-stimulated MP activation and soluble factor secretion contribute to destruction of host tissue. This chapter will discuss the various outcomes resulting from interactions between viruses and the macrophage.

2 Mononuclear phagocyte (MP) function

2.1 MP phagocytosis and intracellular killing

Macrophages internalize particles, viruses and microbes through receptor-independent or -dependent mechanisms. Receptor-independent endocytosis (pinocytosis) is a relatively inefficient mechanism for generating MHC II-associated foreign antigens. Virions and macromolecules ingested through pinocytosis frequently are not associated with a cell surface receptor. In contrast, phagocytosis is a receptor-mediated and highly efficient mechanism for degrading viral particles and generating antigens for immune presentation. A defining function of the macrophage, phagocytosis usually is described in the context of antibacterial defense. However, macrophages also can ingest and destroy viral particles (Van Strijp *et al.*, 1990). Complement and opsonizing antibody markedly increase viral uptake (Van Strijp *et al.*, 1989). In the case of viremia, phagocytosis of virus by splenic macrophages, liver Kupffer cells, alveolar, gut and perivascular macrophages (the so-called reticuloendothelial system) is a major mech-anism for viral clearance.

Viral attachment to macrophage surface glycoproteins initiates phagocytosis. Macrophages express Fc receptors (FcRs), complement receptors, integrins, mannose receptors (MRs), class A scavenger receptors (SR-A), macrosialin, low-density lipopro-tein (LDL) receptors and a plethora of other surface molecules that participate in phago-cytosis. Receptor–virus interaction stimulates clustering and cross-linking of phagocytic receptors, signal transduction events lead to protrusion of membrane pseudopodia around the virus and actin polymerization within the cytosol adjacent to the site of virus contact. Different phagocytosis receptors employ distinct signal transduction pathways to stimu-late phagocytosis. For example, phagocytosis via IgG FcRs depends on recruitment of multiple cytosolic tyrosine kinases (Greenberg and Silverstein, 1993), while phagocytosis via complement receptor 3 is not sensitive to tyrosine kinase inhibitors (Allen and Aderem, 1996).

Fusion of opposing plasma membrane surfaces is a costly in terms of free energy. Transmembrane proteins and soluble linkers provide docking sites for opposing mem-brane surfaces, coupling endocytic processes to biochemical energy consumption. The ability of macrophages to phagocytose viruses and other extracellular material necessi-tates internalization and recycling of the plasma membrane. Unlike other phagocytic cell types, macrophages lack a distinct peri-centriolar membrane recycling mechanism. Instead, the cells maintain membrane surface area through a system of tubules and vesi-cles that fuse with the plasma membrane in a coordinated fashion to balance membrane internalization during phagocytosis (Cox *et al.*, 2000).

After engulfing host cells, microbes or free antigen, MP phagosomes fuse with lyso-somes through interactions between *N*-ethylmaleimide-sensitive fusion (Nsf) proteins and Nsf attachment protein receptors (SNAREs) (Hackam, 1996; Ward *et al.*, 1997). The vesicle formed from phagosome–lysosome fusion is called a secondary lysosome. Unlike secondary lysosome fusion in neutrophils, phagosome–lysosome fusion in macrophages is not dependent on increases in cytosolic Ca^{2+}, although cytosolic Ca^{2+} rises concurrent with phagocytosis (Jaconi *et al.*, 1990; Zimmerli *et al.*, 1996). In the secondary lyso-some, ingested extracellular material is exposed to a pH of 4–5, oxygen free radicals, cation chelatases and scores of proteolytic enzymes (Mims, 1964; Oppenheim, 1989).

Viruses also use MP-expressed surface receptors to enter MPs thereby circumventing the phagocytic system. In some cases, the outcome of virus–MP interaction depends on the ability of virus to enter MPs by receptor-mediated mechanisms more rapidly than the phagocytic machinery can engulf the virus. For example, African swine fever virus (ASFV) entry into swine macrophages is mediated by saturable binding sites on the plasma membrane, whereas entry of this virus into non-permissive rabbit cells is medi-ated by non-saturable mechanisms (Alcami *et al.*, 1990). The outcome of this microbio-logical cell interaction has profound consequences for host survival. Because MPs are potent immune scavenger cells, the balance between MP-mediated viral destruction and permissivity in MPs frequently determines whether a virus will persist and cause disease in a host. For example, in murine cytomegalovirus (MCMV) infections, replication in monocytes and macrophages represents a major determinant of pathogenesis (Hanson *et al.*, 1999).

After establishing infection of MPs, viruses can retard phagocytosis and destruction of other viruses and microbes. Influenza virus infection of human alveolar macrophages reduces the phagocytic activity and correlates with decreased intrapulmonary killing of gram-positive bacteria (Nickerson and Jakab, 1990). Bovine viral diarrhea virus (BVDV) of calves causes decreased FcR and C3R expression, phagocytosis and microbicidal activity (Welsh and Adair, 1995). Human immunodeficiency virus type 1 (HIV-1) has been shown to cause impairment of phagosome–lysosme fusion, perhaps through CD4-dependent signal transduction (Ahn *et al.*, 1996).

2.2 Antigen presentation: class I and II MHC pathways

(See also Chapter 3 for a detailed discussion of the role of macrophages as antigen-presenting cells.)

MPs take up, process and present antigen for lymphocyte recognition involving both MHC class I and class II pathways. In general, antigens in the class I pathway originate from cytosolic proteins and antigens in the class II pathway originate in lysosomes.

Class I MHC molecules are expressed on the surface on most nucleated cells (neurons are a notable exception). Cytosolic proteins degraded in proteasomes are transported as 8–12 amino acid peptides into the endoplasmic reticulum (ER) by transport-associated protein (TAP). In the ER, class I MHC molecules associate with β_2-microglobulin and proteasome-generated peptides before traveling to the cell surface as trimers. After direct viral infection of MPs, viral antigens are processed in the cytosol, transported into the ER and presented on the surface of MPs in association with β_2-microglobulin and class I MHC. On the MP surface, CD8[+] T lymphocytes expressing antigen-specific T-cell receptors (TCRs) scan antigen presented in the class I MHC peptide-binding groove. When a TCR recognizes cognate antigen–MHC I– β_2-microglobulin in an appropriate milieu, MPs and CD8[+] lymphocytes engage in a complex dialog usually resulting in stimulation of cytotoxic effector mechanisms.

Unlike most cells, MPs express high levels of class II MHC molecules. Peptide loading into class II MHC heterodimers occurs in the secondary lysosome. The MHC II–antigen trimer is transported to the MP surface to be recognized by TCRs expressed on the surface of CD4[+] lymphocytes. MPs and CD4[+] lymphocytes also can engage, often resulting in stimulation of a Th response, B-cell activation, Ig secretion and, later, class switching. Following recognition of MHC-bound viral antigen by TCRs, multiple events are necessary for lymphocyte activation to occur. First, CD4 or CD8 also must interact with MP-expressed, antigen-bound MHC. Secondly, multiple adhesion molecules must interact to stabilize the T cell–MP interaction. Thirdly, co-stimulatory molecules expressed by MPs must bind receptors on the T cell to stimulate activation and proliferation. Two co-stimulatory molecules in particular appear crucial for T-cell activation, B7.1 (CD80) and B7.2 (CD86).

DNA viruses or retroviruses that establish chronic infection of MPs can interfere with cellular function, including antigen presentation in the context of cellular MHC (Yewdell and Bennick, 1999). Lytic infection with vaccinia viruses, herpesviruses and adenoviruses reduces expression of all surface molecules by non-specifically decreasing expression of host proteins. Specific mechanisms of interference with antigen presentation also exist. In immortal cell lines, human cytomegalovirus (HCMV) has been shown to down-regulate class I activity through viral genes *US3*, *US6* and *US11* (Kim *et al.*, 1995; Ahn *et al.*, 1996). US6 is a type I membrane glycoprotein that localizes to the ER and blocks import of antigens to class I (Hengel *et al.*, 1997). The MCMV protein gp40 catalyzes the retention of MHC class I molecules (Zeigler, 2000). HIV-1 proteins Vpu and Nef have been shown to mediate post-transcriptional inhibition of class I expression (Schwartz *et al.*, 1996; Kerkau, 1997). *In vivo*, MCMV infection of simian virus 40 (SV40) immune mice reduces the ability of macrophages to present SV40 and stimulate CD8$^+$ T-lymphocyte proliferation (Campbell *et al.*, 1992). Viral infection of MPs can also interfere with presentation of non-viral class II MHC-associated antigens. Friend leukemia virus decreases macrophage class II antigen presentation in murine macrophages (Jones *et al.*, 1992). In mice, a lethal herpes simplex virus-2 (HSV-2) strain (KOS) alters class II trafficking following intraocspular inoculation (Lewandowski *et al.*, 1993). KOS-infected microglia display a peculiar nuclear localization of class II molecules.

Virus modulation of MP co-stimulatory molecule expression may have devastating consequences for the host. For example, central nervous system (CNS) MP's isolated from mice inoculated intracerebrally with Theiler's murine encephalomyelitis virus (TMEV) express elevated levels of B7.1 and B7.2 (Pope *et al.*, 1998). Alteration of co-stimulatory factor expression probably contributes to amplification of the T-cell response against viral and host antigens, resulting in autoimmune demyelination through overstimulation of CD4$^+$ and CD8$^+$ lymphocyte effector pathways. Conversely, HIV-1 down-regulates B7 expression in infected MPs (Dudhane *et al.*, 1996; Kumar *et al.*, 1999). In the absence of appropriate co-stimulation, the MP–T lymphocyte interaction fails to stimulate interleukin (IL-2) secretion and ultimately results in T-cell apoptosis (Dudhane *et al.*, 1996; Kumar *et al.*, 1999). HIV-1-infected MPs may even destroy uninfected lymphocytes owing to defective B7 expression (Lewis *et al.*, 1999). MPs and T cells seem to have a dichotomous relationship in that effective antigen presentation in the presence of co-stimulatory recognition leads to lymphocyte proliferation and activation, but antigen presentation in the absence of T-cell stimulation leads to T-cell death.

2.3 Viral modulation of pro-inflammatory cytokine secretion

Viruses also can interfere with critical steps in cytokine-mediated inflammatory cascades. MP-secreted tumor necrosis factor-α (TNF-α), IL-1 and IL-12 contribute to innate immune responses early in viral infection and expansion of antigen-specific responses later in infection. IL-12 is a potential site for viral interference. MPs secrete heterodimeric IL-12 in response to viral infection or through CD40L–CD40 interactions. IL-12 induces interferon-γ (IFN-γ) expression by T lymphocytes and natural killer (NK) cells, leading to progression of a Th1 response, T_C cell stimulation and activities, potent antiviral IL-12 expression is highly sensitive to regulation through separate immune signaling pathways. In an example of negative feedback, cross-linking of MP complement receptors (Marth and Kelsall, 1997; Sutterwala *et al.*, 1997) or complement-regulatory molecules leads to down-regulation of IL-12. Measles virus infection leads to cross-linking of the complement regulatory molecule CD46 and a subsequent blockade of IL-

12 expression (Karp *et al.*, 1996). Other immunological pathways exist that lead to viral suppression of IL-12 secretion from MPs. IL-10 expression by lymphocytes usually results in reduced IL-12 secretion from neighboring MPs and represents a mechanism the cellular immune system uses to regulate the balance between Th1 and Th2 responses. HIV takes advantage of this relationship by up-regulating IL-10 secretion from infected CD4⁺ lymphocytes, leading to suppression of IL-12 *in vitro* and *in vivo* (Chehimi *et al.*, 1994; Chougnet *et al.*, 1996).

2.4 Viruses manipulate MP chemotactic machinery

Chemokines are soluble molecules secreted by multiple cell types for the purpose of recruiting immune cells to the site of inflammation. Chemokine gradients cause leukocytes to migrate through post-capillary venule endothelium into a discrete organs or the lymphatic circulation. Chemokines bind carbohydrates with high affinity (Lalani, 1997), a property that may account for their inability to survive in the circulation for long periods of time. More than 40 chemokines have been identified and can be divided into four groups based on the arrangement of cysteine residues within the receptor-binding domain. For CXC-(α-) chemokines, two cysteines are separated by a single amino acid (Baggiolini *et al.*, 1997). CC-(β-) chemokines have two adjacent cysteines. A single CX_3C-(γ-) chemokine called fractalkine or neurotactin and a C-(γ-) chemokine, lymphotactin are also operative CXC-chemokines principally recruit neutrophils but also can recruit lymphocytes. CC-chemokines principally recruit lymphocytes and monocytes.

Chemokine receptors are seven-pass transmembrane receptors coupled to GTP-binding clustered proteins (G-proteins). G-protein-coupled receptors are categorized in parallel with their ligand. So α-chemokine receptors (CXCRs) are characterized by binding to CXC-chemokines, and so on. Like all G-protein-coupled receptors, the extracellular domain contains three loops and the N-terminal tail. The extracellular domains are highly variable between the different receptors, probably confer ligand specificity and contain multiple potential *N*-linked glycosylation sites. All four extracellular domains contain conserved cysteine residues that probably form intramolecular disulfide bonds to maintain receptor structure. The cytosolic C-terminal region also has three loops and a C-terminal tail associated with a heterotrimeric G-protein involved in signal transduction.

Blood monocytes and tissue MPs express chemokine receptors. Among MPs, chemokine receptor expression varies greatly with their differentiation and activation state. Other cell types also express chemokine receptors, including granulocytes and lymphocytes in blood, marrow, lymphatics and secondary lymphoid tissue; and, curiously, resident neurons, astrocytes and microglia in brain. In addition to expressing chemokine receptors, MPs also secrete high levels of CXC- and CC-chemokines to recruit other inflammatory cells out of the circulation and into inflammatory lesions.

Viruses frequently manipulate the macrophage chemotactic machinery for their own benefit. In some infections, membrane-bound chemokine receptors allow viral entry. HIV illustrates this mechanism. HIV relies on CD4 as the principal docking site on macrophage and helper T-cell surfaces, but also requires chemokine receptor co-expression for entry and replication. CXCR4 and CCR5 have been identified as the principal co-receptors for T-cell tropic and macrophage-tropic (M-tropic) HIV-1 infection, respectively. Chemokine receptors are structurally necessary for initiation of membrane fusion events, but whether chemokine receptor-mediated signal transduction is necessary for permissivity of HIV-1 in macrophages remains disputed (Atchison *et al.*, 1996; Alfano *et al.*, 1999).

Large DNA viruses frequently encode chemokine homologs that function as full or partial receptor agonists that can augment leukocyte recruitment. Herpesviruses encode chemokine homologs that are expressed during lytic infection for the recruitment of additional viral target cells. For example, the HCMV gene *UL146* product, designated vCXC-1, can recruit neutrophils with potency approaching that of endogenous IL-8 (Penfold *et al.*, 1999). Soluble vCXC-1 binds cellular CXCR2. MCMV carries a CC-homolog whose products, MCK-1 and MCK-2, vigorously recruit monocytes to areas of viral infection. Both mutants induce reduced monocyte-associated viremia in infected mice (Saederup *et al.*, 1999). In contrast, poxviruses have two families of chemokine-binding proteins that retard immune recruitment, exemplified by rabbitpox M-T1 protein, rabbit myxoma virus M-T7 protein and the human poxvirus *Molluscum contagiosum* MC148 protein. In rabbits, infection with rabbitpox viruses lacking M-T1 displayed increased leukocyte infiltration (Graham, 1997). This effect is increased or diminished depending on allelic variation within the virus and/or host (Martinex-Pomares *et al.*, 1995). Both M-T1 and M-T7 interact with heparin-binding domains within the extracellular loops of multiple chemokine receptors (Lalani and McFadden, 1997). M-T1 and M-T7 interaction with heparin-binding domains may account for the ability of these soluble factors to bind chemokine receptor subtypes. In the case of MC148, *in vitro* competition binding, calcium mobilization and functional chemotaxis assays using human cell lines demonstrate that MC148 is a highly specific CCR8 antagonist (Luttichau *et al.*, 2000).

Viruses also can encode chemokine receptors. The HCMV gene *US28* encodes a seven-pass transmembrane receptor that binds a broad spectrum of CC chemokines with subnanomolar affinity and causes Ca^{2+} mobilization in target cells (Gao and Murphy, 1994). In cell lines expressing *US28*, HIV-1 has been shown to use the cytomegalovirus encoded chemokine receptor homolog as an entry cofactor (Pleskoff *et al.*, 1997). The open reading frames (ORFs) of multiple other herpesviruses encode chemokine receptor homologs such as the human herpesvirus-6 (HHV-6) gene *U12*, which encodes a functional CC chemokine receptor (Isegawa *et al.*, 1998).

In the same vein, viruses can regulate expression of cellular chemokines or chemokine receptors (Schmidtmayerova *et al.*, 1996; Cremer *et al.*, 1999). Future phylogenetic investigations may reveal that cellular chemokines (and other clustered immune genes) were originally derived from herpesviruses during genesis of the immune system. The interplay between host- and viral-encoded immune genes represents a molecular 'cat-and-mouse' game that has been played for as long as herpesviruses can infect leukocytes.

2.5 Type I interferons and potent antiviral defenses

Type I interferons are soluble immune molecules that are up-regulated and secreted by MPs in response to a variety of microbes, including viruses. Type I interferons include IFN-α and IFN-β. IFN-γ is considered a type II interferon and is secreted primarily by T cells. Small amounts of whole virus, viral nucleic acid or poly(I:C) can induce vigorous type I interferon secretion within hours of infection. The mechanisms through which viruses induce IFN-α/β expression involve activation and nuclear translocation of transcription enhancers including nuclear factor-κB (NF-κB) (Kirchhoff *et al.*, 1999) and interferon regulatory factor (IRF) family proteins (Schafer *et al.*, 1998). Both are constitutively expressed in MPs and a variety of other tissues. Upon encountering transcription elements in the MP cytosol, viral kinases phosphorylate and activate such elements (Hiscott *et al.*, 1999). Through this mechanism or perhaps others, MP phagocytosis of viral particles or viral infection stimulates MP transcription and secretion of type I interferons.

IFN-α/β plays a major role in restricting viral growth in cells expressing IFN-α/β receptors (IFNARs) *in vitro* and contributes to abortive infections *in vivo*. IFN-α/β stimulates multiple antiviral mechanisms in MPs (Gendelman *et al.*, 1990). MPs express IFNARs consisting of two tyrosine kinase-associated single-pass transmembrane subunits. Mice lacking IFNAR subunit expression show significant increases in susceptibility to viral infections (van den Broek *et al.*, 1995). IFNAR1 and IFNAR2 dimerize upon IFN-α/β binding. In the ligand-free state, the cytosolic domain of IFNAR1 is associated with the small kinase, Tyk. Ligand-free IFNAR2 is associated with signal transducers and activators of transcription (STATs) and Janus-family kinases (JAKs). Upon binding of IFN-α/β to IFNAR1 and IFNAR2, receptor dimerization occurs and multiple cross-phosphorylation events ensue, resulting in STAT dimerization through SH2 recognition of newly modified phosphotyrosine residues. STAT dimers then translocate to the nucleus and enhance gene transcription by sequence-specific DNA binding.

STAT family members are ubiquitous signaling molecules with diverse potential targets. In MPs, STAT-enhanced gene transcription is modulated by interaction with p48, a member of the IRF family of transcription factors. In the MP nucleus, p48 binds STAT dimers forming trimeric STAT–STAT–p48 complexes. The trimeric complex of STAT1, STAT2 and p48, collectively referred to as IFN-stimulated gene factor 3 (ISGF3), recognizes IFN-α/β-stimulated regulatory elements (ISREs) and enhances downstream gene transcription. Analysis of p48-null human cells (John *et al.*, 1991; Bluyssen *et al.*, 1995) and p48-knockout mice (Harada *et al.*, 1996) shows severe deficits in IFN-α/β induction of expression of IRSE-containing genes, emphasizing the crucial role of p48 in MP antiviral defense. Positive feedback loops exist at multiple levels for amplifying interferon antiviral responses. For example, IRF family proteins, known to enhance transcription of IFN-α/β, are up-regulated in MPs in response to interferon stimulation (Lehtonen *et al.*, 1997). As IFN-α/β levels increase, so does IRF. As IRF levels increase, transcription and secretion of IFN-α/β increases, IFN-α/β binds to MP-expressed IFNARs through autocrine and paracrine circuitry, IFNAR-dependent STAT activation increases and ISRE-mediated transcription escalates.

Multiple effector genes contain ISREs. The double-stranded RNA-dependent protein kinase (PKR) is encoded by a 50 kb gene regulated through an ISRE. PKR inhibits viral growth by binding to and inactivating eukaryotic initiation factor-2 (IF-2), leaving the infected cell unable to initiate protein synthesis. PKR-mediated protein synthesis deficits ultimately lead to apoptosis. Because of the dependence of PKR on the presence of double-stranded RNA for activation, only virus-infected cells suffer from inhibition of protein synthesis. In experimental systems, PKR expression and activity can be induced with low levels of poly(I:C). Not surprisingly, some viruses have evolved mechanisms to combat the antiviral effects of PKR. For example, adenovirus uses oligoribonucleotides as competitive inhibitors of PKR. Adenovirus contains virus-associated RNA (VA RNA) that is not involved directly in the viral life cycle, but instead binds and inhibits PKR (Kitajewski *et al.*, 1986). Mutant adenoviruses lacking VA RNA are more sensitive to IFN-mediated inhibition (Anderson and Fennie, 1987). Epstein–Barr virus (EBV)-encoded small non-polyadenylated RNAs (EBERs) may play a similar role in mediating EBV replication in the face of host interferon responses (Kitajewski *et al.*, 1986). The HIV Tat (McMillan, 1994; Brand *et al.*, 1997) and the hepatitis C NS5A proteins (Gale *et al.*, 1997) interact with PKR directly, allowing viral replication in spite of IFN-stimulated PKR expression. In poliovirus-infected cells, PKR is proteolytically cleaved (Black *et al.*, 1989), though whether this is due to altered host protease or expression of viral encoded enzyme(s) is not clear.

2–5 Oligoadenylate synthetases catalyze polymerization of ATP into $2',5'$-oligoadenylates (2–5A) and also are regulated through ISREs (Hannigan and Williams, 1991; Wang and Floyd-Smith 1997). 2–5A synthetases are encoded by multiple genes and exist in multiple cellular compartments. 2–5A binds to inactive, cellular RNase L monomers causing homodimerization and activation (Cole *et al.*, 1997). RNase L monomers are the product of a unique human gene mapped to human chromosome 1q25 (Squire *et al.*, 1994). In general, RNase L activity is defined as the ability to degrade single-stranded RNA through endonuclease hydrolysis of phosphodiester linkages. In the MP cytosol, high RNase L activity leads to preferential degradation of viral RNA. However, a cellular message is also affected, contributing to MP apoptosis. IFN-induced RNase L activity is reversible (Carroll *et al.*, 1997). Animal functional studies have confirmed the role of RNase L in IFN-mediated antiviral defense. Transfection of a dominant-negative 2–5A-dependent RNase L construct into murine cells failed to block replication of encephalomyocarditis virus (ECMV) compared with controls (Hassel *et al.*, 1993). RNase L-deficient mice are unresponsive to the antiviral effects of IFN-α and experience increased mortality due to ECMV infection (Silverman and Cirino, 1997; Zhou *et al.*, 1997).

Mx proteins, including MxA in humans and Mx1 in mice, are GTP hydrolases of the dynamin superfamily (Arnheiter *et al.*, 1996) that mediate resistance against influenza and other viruses. In human macrophages, MxA is up-regulated by low levels of interferon (Ronni *et al.*, 1998). The MxA regulatory element contains ISRE sequences (Nakade *et al.*, 1997), and ISGF-3 activity at the MxA gene is known to recruit transcription factors and enhance transcription following type I IFN stimulation (Schumacher *et al.*, 1994). Mx proteins interfere with viral replication by binding to the virus ribonucleoprotein complex, rendering the viral polymerase functionless (Stranden *et al.*, 1993). MxA has been shown to inhibit growth of influenza, vesicular stomatitis, measles, bunya, phlebo, hanta and influenza viruses *in vitro*. Conversely, overexpression of the influenza virus protein PB2 reduces Mx function (Stranden *et al.*, 1993).

Considering the strong evolutionary pressure exerted on viruses by IFN-induced defenses, other unidentified strategies are likely to exist for virus subversion of IFN-stimulated compromise of the viral protein synthesis machinery.

3 Viral infection of MPs

3.1 Target cells for viral infection

Attachment to MP surface determinants is the first step in receptor-mediated phagocytosis and also the first step in the viral life cycle. In many cases, the ability of a virus to cross the MP plasma membrane determines whether it will infect and replicate or will be exposed to the MP intracellular degradative pathway. Enveloped and non-enveloped viruses use different strategies to accomplish this task. Many enveloped viruses have their own membrane fusion machinery, proteins that share functional similarity with Nsf proteins and SNAPs. Some viruses rely on the same protein, or protein complex, for attachment and fusion. Others encode discrete fusion proteins. Lentiviruses employ the former strategy. The lentiviral Env protein is a multisubunit transmembrane glycoprotein that mediates attachment and fusion. Env has a transmembrane subunit (e.g. HIV gp41) and a non-covalently associated subunit (e.g. HIV gp120). The associated subunit interacts with surface receptor(s), exposing regions of the transmembrane subunit involved in fusion. Paramyxoviruses employ the latter strategy. Hemagglutinin (HA) and neuraminidase (NA) are paramyxoviral proteins that mediate attachment. F protein is a distinct, two-subunit type I integral glycoprotein necessary for fusion and replication competence of paramyxoviruses (Scheid and Choppin, 1977). Influenza virus is a special example of the two-protein model of viral fusion. HA binds MP surface determinants, but cannot immediately fuse and enter. At low pH in the late endosome, HA undergoes a conformation rearrangement, exposing the fusogenic F protein (Korte *et al.*, 1999).

Generally, MPs resist infection by unenveloped viruses. SV40 and hepatitis B viruses are notable exceptions. Unenveloped viruses are believed to insert pores into the plasma membrane or disrupt vesicle membranes within the endocytic pathway. For example, it has been proposed that during phagocytosis, SV40 recruits membrane-associated caveolar proteins to facilitate translocation across the plasma membrane (Parton and Lindsay, 1999). The molecular mechanisms involved in entry of naked viruses into MPs are not fully understood. Classes of viruses that infect MPs are shown in Table 4.1. Representative viruses are described for each class.

3.2 Viral infection and monocyte-macrophage differentation

After mobilization from bone marrow, monocytes circulate for 2–4 days before extravasating into tissue or being sequestered in the spleen. Monocytes that cross microvascular boundaries and enter tissues differentiate into mature MPs. Many tissues have resident MPs, including microglial cells in the brain, alveolar macrophages in the lung, Langerhans cells in the skin and promonocytes in the bone marrow. Perivascular macrophages in all tissues, Kupffer cells in the liver and splenic macrophages have been collectively called the reticuloendothelial system based on their functional ability to clear macromolecules, viruses and bacteria from the circulation. The process of monocyte differentiation involves differential expression of cellular structural and functional genes.

For *in vitro* experimentation, peripheral blood mononuclear cells (PBMCs) may be isolated by peripheral elutriation. Alternatively, PBMCs can be isolated from whole blood buffy coat cell extracts. Monocytes then can be separated from other mononuclear cells by counter-current centrifugation or preferential adhesion techniques. *In vitro*, monocytes can be forced to differentiate into resting (unactivated) macrophages in the presence of

Table 4.1   Representative classes of viruses and their major mechanisms of interaction with monocytes and macrophages

Class	Nucleic acid/virion structure	Viruses	Virus–macrophage interaction
Retroviridae Oncovirinae	ssRNA, enveloped, proviral DNA in replication cycle	Avian myeloblastoma virus (AMV), Avian myelocytomatosis virus (MC29), Murine spleen focus-forming virus (AF-1)	Macrophage transformation correlates with induction of tumors *in vivo*. Replication in bone marrow progenitor cells
Lentivirinae	ssRNA, enveloped, proviral DNA in replication cycle	Human immunodeficiency virus (HIV)	Latent, restricted and permissive infections of brain and spinal cord macrophages and microglia, pulmonary macrophages, follicular dendritic cells, blood monocytes and Langerhans cells (infrequently)
	ssRNA, enveloped, proviral DNA in replication cycle	Simian immunodeficiency virus (SIV)	Permissive. Tropism for macrophages in brain, lung, gut and lymph nodes. Similar macrophage–virus interactions to those described with HIV.
	ssRNA, enveloped, proviral DNA in replication cycle	Visna–maedi virus (VMV)	Latent, restricted and permissive. Near 'exclusive' tropism for cells of monocyte lineage. Bone marrow promonocytes, blood monocytes and macrophages in brain, lung and lymph node.
	ssRNA, enveloped, proviral DNA in replication cycle	Caprine arthritis–encephalitis virus (CAEV)	Latent, permissive and near-exclusive tropism for cells of monocyte lineage, including blood monocytes, brain and synovial macrophages
Togaviridae Pestivirus	ssRNA, enveloped (+)sense genome	Lactate dehydrogenase virus (LDV)	Replication restricted to class II (Ia⁺) macrophages, leading to increased incidence of autoimmunity. Association between expression of endogenous retroviruses and cytocidal replication of LDV.
Alphavirus/ Flavivirus	ssRNA, enveloped (+)sense genome	Murray valley encephalitis virus, Dengue virus, West Nile virus, Yellow fever virus	Associated with antibody-dependent enhancement (ADE) of viral infection of cells bearing Fc receptors.
Rubivirus	ssRNA, enveloped (+)sense genome	Rubella virus	Replication in monocytes and macrophages, level of virus replication dependent on cellular differentiation/activation.
Coronaviridae	ssRNA, enveloped (+)sense genome	Respiratory coronavirus (229E)	Productive infection of monocytes and macrophages.
	ssRNA, enveloped (+)sense genome ssRNA, enveloped (+)sense genome	Feline infectious peritonitis virus Transmissible gastroenteritis coronavirus (TGEV)	Monocytes are predominant target. ADE reported. Productive replication in swine alveolar macrophages.

Table 4.1 Continued

Class	Nucleic acid/virion structure	Viruses	Virus–macrophage interaction
Orthomyxoviridae	ssRNA, enveloped (−)sense genome	Influenza A	Restricted infection in monocytes and T cells. Macrophage infection linked to TNF-α production.
Arenaviridae	ssRNA, enveloped (−)sense genome	Junin, Lassa, Machupo, Rift valley fever	Permissive replication in cultured mouse peritoneal macrophages, limited cytopathicity
	ssRNA, enveloped (−)sense genome	Lympocytic choriomeningitis virus (LCV)	Permissive replication in cultured mouse peritoneal and splenic macrophages.
Hepadnaviridae	dsDNA, non-enveloped	Hepatitis B virus	Target monocytes, probably reservoir during subclinical infections, related to secondary hematological complications
Papovaviridae	dsDNA, non-enveloped	Simian virus 40 (SV40)	Macrophage transformation
Herpesviridae	dsDNA, enveloped	Cytomegalovirus (CMV)	Restricted replication at level of immediate-early gene expression. Virulence of murine CMV is associated with monocyte/macrophage susceptibility to infection.
	dsDNA, enveloped	Herpes simplex virus (HSV)	Restricted replication in promonocytes, monocytes and tissue macrophages at the level of DNA polymerase immediate-early gene expression. Viral replication dependent on animal strain, age and stage of cellular differentiation.
Iridoviridae	dsDNA, enveloped	African swine fever virus (AFSV)	Primary productive replication in monocytes and macrophages or restricted replication
Poxviridae	dsDNA, enveloped	Ectromelia virus	Permissive replication in lymph node and resident peritoneal macrophages.

macrophage colony-stimulating factor (MCSF) or phorbol esters. As monocytes differentiate, expression of surface proteins and functional capacity change. Functionally, macrophage vesicles are more acidified, more extracellular material enters the phagocytic pathway, intracellular killing is increased and the enzymes acid phosphatase and β-galactosidase show increased activity compared with blood monocytes (Basta *et al.*, 1999). Macrophages also express mannose receptor and complement 3 receptor (Mac-1), which blood monocytes do not. Differentiated human macrophages show increased expression of MHC class II antigens (Andreesen *et al.*, 1990). However, porcine macrophages express lower levels of class I and II MHC antigens, secrete reduced levels of IL-1 and have reduced lymphocyte proliferative potential compared with fresh monocytes (Basta *et al.*, 1999).

Differentiation into macrophages alters the ability of viruses to infect monocytic lineage cells and the expression of viral genes in previously infected cells. Direct infection of macrophages has four potential outcomes, illustrated in Figure 4.1. If the viral life cycle cannot be completed because of a defect in early stages of the life cycle, an 'abortive' infection occurs. In the case of DNA viruses or retroviruses, if the virus infects macrophages and proviral DNA is translocated to the nucleus but viral genes are not expressed, the infection is said to be 'latent'. If viral infection results in production of

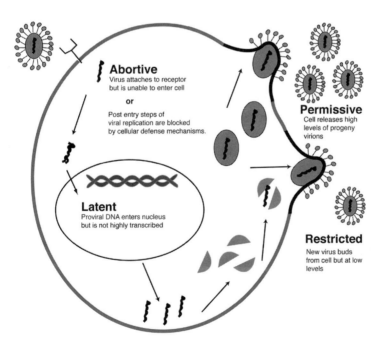

Abortive
Virus attaches to receptor but is unable to enter cell

or

Post entry steps of viral replication are blocked by cellular defense mechanisms.

Permissive
Cell releases high levels of progeny virions

Latent
Proviral DNA enters nucleus but is not highly transcribed

Restricted
New virus buds from cell but at low levels

Fig. 4.1 Virus–MP interactions may result in multiple outcomes. Abortive infection can occur if the virus fails to engage an appropriate cellular receptor or viral entry into the cell is blocked after binding to the MP membrane. Latent infection occurs if virus enters the cells, uncoats, enters the nucleus, but fails to express high levels of viral products. Latency is defined as genomic integration (retroviridae) or episome formation (herpesviridae) with little or no expression of viral genes. Production of low levels of virus is called a restrictive (chronic active) infection. Permissive infection proceeds if the viral life cycle reaches completion with formation of high levels of progeny virions.

constant low levels of progeny virions that are cleared by the immune system at the same rate at which they are produced, the infection is termed 'restricted'. If virus is produced in increasing quantities such that virus spreads among target cells, the infection is said to be 'permissive'. MPs sustain all four types of infection and all can contribute to clinical disease.

For visna–maedi virus (VMV) and caprine arthritis–encephalitis virus (CAEV), viral gene expression is closely linked to monocyte differentiation (Anderson *et al.*, 1983; Narayan *et al.*, 1983; Gendelman *et al.*, 1986). *In vivo*, VMV infection is closely linked to MP tissue specificity. Blood monocytes, alveolar macrophages, nodal dendritic cells and brain microglia are susceptible; Kuppfer cells and connective tissue histiocytes are not (Rodgers and Mims, 1981). Direct infection of macrophages has four potential outcomes. The close correlation between monocyte maturation and viral gene expression is linked in a causal fashion to the induction of specific cellular nucleic acid-binding proteins (Gabuzda *et al.*, 1989). HIV-1 infection of fresh monocytes results in an abortive infection with low viral titers and minimal cytopathic effect. However, after culturing monocytes for 7–10 days in the presence of MCSF, HIV-1 can establish a restricted infection characterized by a marked cytopathic effect (Meltzer and Gendelman, 1988; Orenstein *et al.*, 1988). Similarly, in most examples of HSV-infected monocyte lineage cells, phorbol ester-stimulated differentiation is associated with enhanced viral gene expression. In untreated macrophages infected with HSV, immediate-early and some early viral transcripts can be detected, but mRNAs for the viral polymerase, the major DNA-binding protein (ICP-8) and glycoprotein C are absent (Tenney and Morahan, 1991).

3.3 Viruses prime macrophages for subsequent immune activation

Cellular activation is characterized by the rapid increase in transcription of functional genes caused by stimulation of previously expressed signal transduction machinery, and by enhancers of transcription. Functional genes up-regulated in activated compared with resting MPs include inducible nitric oxide synthetase (iNOS), cyclooxygenase isozymes, mannose receptors, Rab 5a and other phagocytosis pathways, class II major histocompatibility antigens and other antigen presentation factors, pro-inflammatory cytokines (IL-1, IL-6, IL-12 and TNF-α) and cell surface determinants (CD54, CD80 and CD86). See also Chapter 2 for information on macrophage activation. Activation may represent a terminal step in differentiation.

In vitro, MPs can be activated by membrane-bound receptor-mediated pathways or by receptor-independent stimulation of cytosolic kinases. The gram-negative bacterial component lipopolysaccharide (LPS) is a potent receptor-mediated macrophage activator. CD14, a surface-associated protein linked to the external face of the MP plasma membrane by a prenyl tail, is the primary LPS receptor, although LPS has been shown to interact with other MP surface molecules such as the macrophage scavenger receptor (Dunne *et al.*, 1994) and members of the integrin superfamily of receptors (Aoki *et al.*, 1991; Ingalls and Golenbock, 1995). LPS treatment of macrophages results in increased transcription and expression of multiple cellular factors. Phorbol esters, like phorbol 12-myristate 13-acetate (PMA), activate macrophages through receptor-independent mechanisms. PMA stimulates protein kinases in the macrophage cytosol—protein kinase C in particular—leading to activation. Expression of macrophage activation genes is faster and more vigorous following exposure to LPS than PMA. The faster speed of LPS activation is due to the more rapid flow of information across the plasma membrane by receptor-mediated transduction. Phorbol esters require diffusion into the cytosol. The more vigorous response is also due to the promiscuity of LPS and CD14. LPS can bind multiple receptors and CD14 can stimulate multiple transduction pathways. PMA stimulates only protein kinases. Activation can be induced by a single stimulus, or through a two-step process of priming and subsequent activation. LPS is the most potent identified one-hit MP activator.

In addition to LPS and phorbol esters, soluble and membrane-bound CD40L, a TNF family member, has also been shown to activate macrophages by acting through its surface receptor, CD40, a typical member of the TNFR superfamily. Because CD40L is expressed on CD4$^+$ T lymphocytes, macrophages and other cells, the CD40L–CD40 response has been proposed as a physiological mechanism for MP activation in multiple disease states, including HIV-1-associated dementia (HAD) and Alzheimer's disease (AD) (Cotter *et al.*, 1999; Cotter *et al.* 2001).

Priming is the stimulus-dependent expression of signal transduction machinery above baseline levels. In the presence of elevated concentrations of cytosolic and nuclear signaling molecules, primed MPs respond more vigorously to activation stimuli. The delineation between priming and activation events is not perfectly distinct. Most transduction molecules are transcribed in an inactive form. For instance, many kinases themselves must be phosphorylated for activity; enzymes involved in second messenger formation require catalytic activation; and transcription factors frequently require dimerization and nuclear translocation. Regulated signaling elements exist in the cell in equilibrium between inactive and active forms. Transcription of signaling molecules causes increases in both the active and inactive forms, proportional to the equilibrium constant of the given molecule in the given milieu. In this way, priming events increase the total cellular activity of signaling constituents, creating downstream effects. However, the magnitude of the downstream events is small compared with post-transcriptional activation of signaling molecules.

Signal transduction-sensitive transcription factors frequently exist in the cytosol of MPs and other cells in an inactive form. For example, NF-κB interacts with an inhibitor of κB (IκB) in the cytosol of resting, inactivated macrophages. When free of IκB repression, NF-κB translocates to the nucleus and mediates expression of immune molecules in activated macrophages (Shakhov *et al.*, 1990; Drouet *et al.*, 1991; Xie *et al.*, 1994). Similarly, signal transducer and activator of transcription (STAT) family members are inactive in the cytosol until phosphorylated by tyrosine kinase-associated signal transduction. Transcription factors can be up-regulated by priming events, causing modest increases in transcription of target genes and, more importantly, preparing the cell for a vigorous response to receptor-mediated signals. Priming appears to cause increased expression of multiple transcription factors that subsequently increase expression of macrophage genes in response to activation stimuli. In addition to NF-κB, candidate transcription factors that may be up-regulated in response to priming events include myeloid differentiation transcriptional regulators (e.g. PU.1), interferon-responsive factors (e.g. p48 and STATs), cAMP response element-binding protein/activating transcription factor complex (CREB/ATF) and the fos/jun heterodimer (AP-1) (Wong *et al.*, 1998; Gupta *et al.*, 1999; Revy *et al.*, 1999).

In macrophages, mechanical disturbance, direct contact with other cell types, extracellular matrix (ECM) components, glass fibers, chitin and other carbohydrates, iron and other stimuli all can lead to MP priming (Formica *et al.*, 1994; Shibata *et al.*, 1997; Tsukamoto *et al.*, 1999; Ye *et al.*, 1999). Viral infection can also serve to prime MPs for activation. Flaviviruses, reoviruses, HSV-2, Newcastle disease virus (NDV) and BVDV have been shown to prime host macrophages upon infection (Ellermann-Eriksen, 1993; Kreil and Eibl, 1995; Pertile *et al.*, 1995; Bukrinsky *et al.*, 1996; Adler *et al.*, 1997; Rautenschlein and Sharma, 1999).

Molecular pathways through which viruses induce expression but not activity of enhancers of transcription are not well understood. It has been suggested that infected MPs secrete soluble factors such as IFNs or other cytokines that prime groups of cells (Adler *et al.*, 1997). In this paradigm, many MPs can be primed following infection of a single cell. A second paradigm proposes that viral infection of MPs leads to increases in available transduction/transcription machinery within the infected cell only. Some herpesviruses encode homologs of cellular signal transduction and/or transcriptional proteins that could up-regulate transcription factors after infection. In general, viral kinases may alter the phosphorylation of cellular proteins, leading to increased responsiveness of the signaling machinery. These mechanisms do not account for priming of uninfected neighboring cells, but predicate priming upon infection.

Unlike many viruses that prime macrophages for activation, CMV infection retards MP activation. During initial infection of MPs, MCMV up-regulates MP secretion of IL-10 (Redpath *et al.*, 1999), which in turn down-regulates expression of MHC class II antigens on macrophages and other neighboring antigen-presenting cells. MCMV and HCMV block the ability of IFN-γ to induce class II MHC expression (Heise and Virgin, 1995; Miller *et al.*, 2000).

3.4 Antibody-dependent enhancement (ADE) of viral infection

During productive viral infections, the host humoral immune response generates antibodies with a wide range of antigenic specificity, but only a fraction have antiviral activity. Some have no neutralizing activity and others enhance infection *in vitro*. Fc and complement receptors tightly grasp opsonized virus and initiate phagocytosis. However, there exists a temporal window of opportunity between the initiation of phagocytosis and endosome–lysosme fusion during which a virus may use these immune receptors for membrane fusion, entry and escape from MP degradative pathways. In some cases, antibody stabilization of the Fc receptor–virus interaction can enhance infectivity. Antibody-dependent enhancement (ADE) was first characterized with Flaviviridae. Murray Valley encephalitis virus yields were increased more than 5-fold in chick embryo monolayer cultures if virus was mixed with antiviral antibody, compared with viral inoculation without antibody (Kliks and Halstead, 1983). In the case of Dengue hemorrhagic fever virus, replication in PBMCs was enhanced 50- to 100-fold by subneutralizing concentrations of antiviral antibody (Halstead *et al.*, 1976). Alphaviridae, rhabdoviridae, bunyaviridae, coronaviridae, reoviridae, herpesviridae, poxviridae, lentivirinae and paramyxoviridae demonstrate ADE *in vitro* (Burstein *et al.*, 1983; Robinson *et al.*, 1988; Takeda *et al.*, 1988; Ochiai *et al.*, 1990). [In some cases, addition of anti-Fc antibody to viral inoculum reverses ADE (Peiris *et al.*, 1981).]

ADE is most likely to occur when viral inoculum is exposed to immune serum generated in related, yet slightly different viral strains. In order to enhance Fc-mediated entry, antibody must recognize and tightly bind viral surface determinants to facilitate interaction between viral proteins and the MP-expressed Fc receptor. Yet if antibody entirely coats the virus to the extent that fusogenic viral proteins are not exposed, entry cannot occur and virus enters into the phagocytic pathway. Viruses with rapidly mutable surface determinants are likely to display ADE. Antibodies that inhibit spread of a group of viral particles may not interact similarly with mutated progeny. Influenza A envelope glycoproteins NA and HA have high mutation rates. Anti-NA antibodies inhibit the spread of influenza among infected cells, but usually are not completely neutralizing. Influenza virus treated with homologous human immune serum shows increased infectivity *in vitro* (Tamura *et al.*, 1991). Repeat infections cross-react with sera generated from the initial infection and show still greater ADE.

Like influenza antigens HA and NA, HIV-1 gp120 is involved in viral attachment and entry into MP and is rapidly mutable. Immune sera generated against T-cell tropic syncytium-inducing (SI) variants increased infectivity of M-tropic non-syncytium-inducing (NSI) variants, *in vitro* (Schutten *et al.*, 1995). Further, it has been shown that virus neutralizing activity of antibody (257-D) generated against a specific epitope of HIV-1 gp120 in a SI variant is not a function of its relative affinity for HIV-1 gp120. 257-D has identical relative affinities for SI *env* cleavage products but possesses no neutralizing activity (Langedijk *et al.*, 1991; Gorny *et al.*, 1993). Therefore, a second property of antibody–HIV-1 gp120 interaction must exist to confer neutralizing capability. This property is probably the ability of antibody to obstruct the fusogenic region of HIV-1 gp41 after binding of antibody to the Fc receptor and depends on conformational interactions between immune sera and viral glycoproteins. Complement-associated HIV-1 particles have also demonstrated *in vitro* ADE of monocytes and macrophages through interaction with complement receptors CR1 (CD35) and CR3 (CD11b/CD18) (Thieblemont *et al.*, 1993).

Whether a variant escapes immune recognition and replicates in MPs may depend not on recognition of cognate viral antigen, but on conformational relationships between antibody and viral envelope glycoproteins. In light of the potential for ADE, a vigorous immune response may drive viral evolution toward an M-tropic, NSI phenotype by facilitating entry into MPs via Fc receptors and limiting entry into CD4$^+$ lymphocytes. This hypothesis has been the subject of mathematical and computer modeling and may explain why some individuals experience vigorous macrophage-mediated pathology in brain and other tissues late in disease. However, the role of ADE in the spread of virus during animal disease has not been substantiated with *in vivo* evidence.

4 Virus, MP and murine central nervous system diseases

4.1 Theiler's murine encephalomyelitis virus (TMEV)

Theiler's murine encephalomyelitis virus (TMEV) is a natural enteric pathogen that can cause demyelination when injected intracerebrally. TMEV belongs to the genus cardiovirus, family picornaviridae and is also referred to as the murine poliovirus. Its closest taxonomic relation, the only other member of the genus cardiovirus, is human encephalomyocarditis virus (EMCV), also called Mengo virus. Like all picornaviruses, TMEV is a single-stranded, positive-sense RNA virus, and has a genome of about 8000 bases in length. The genome is divided into the leader (L) and precursor protein (P1, P2 and P3) regions, flanked by untranslated regions (UTRs). Differences in interactions between the viral 5′-UTR and host factors may be involved in post-entry blocks or enhancement of replication. A small protein (VPg) is *O*-linked to the 5′ terminus of the viral message and the 3′ terminus is polyadenylated. Viral RNA molecules with shorter 3′ poly(A) tails show lower infectivity (Sarnow, 1989).

TMEV strains are divided into two subgroups, GDVII and Theiler's original (TO), based on the course of CNS pathogenesis following intracerebral inoculation (Lorch *et al.*, 1981). Within the GDVII subgroup, two discrete strains have been identified, GDVII and FA. Intracerebral inoculation with GDVII causes rapid demyelination and death. Four strains have been identified within the TO subgroup, Daniel's (DA), BeAn, WW and Yale (Lipton *et al.*, 1995). Intracerebral inoculation with TO strains causes a biphasic CNS disease in susceptible mice. An acute encephalitis lasts up to a week, followed by chronic demyelination lasting the lifetime of the mouse. Observable relapsing–remitting neuro-logical deficits emerge about 40 days after intracerebral inoculation. Inoculation of BeAn into SJL/J mice has been used as a model for human multiple sclerosis (MS) (Pope *et al.*, 1998). Non-susceptible mice show immune clearance of TO subgroup viruses following the acute phase (Rodriguez *et al.*, 1987).

In the acute encephalitic phase, TMEV antigens and transcripts are detected primarily in brain gray matter near the site of inoculation. During the first week of infection, neurons represent the major viral target (Pena Rossi *et al.*, 1997). As the disease progresses, from the acute to the chronic phase, shifts in regional and cellular viral tropism occur. Peripheral macrophages begin to infiltrate the CNS at 2–7 days. Two weeks post-infection, 25–45 per cent of TMEV-infected cells in the mouse spinal cord are macrophages (Pena Rossi *et al.*, 1997).

Histologically, chronic TMEV-induced demyelinating disease (TMEV-IDD) in spinal cord shows a perivascular mononuclear infiltrate, diffuse parenchymal astrocytosis, microglial activation and myelin destruction with conservation of axons. Animal and *in vitro* data correlate susceptibility to pathology with development of class II-dependent immune responses and not with peripheral antiviral antibody titers (Clatch *et al.*, 1985, 1986, 1987). Immunosuppressive (Lipton and Dal Canto, 1976; Lipton and Canto, 1977), anti-Ia (Rodriguez *et al.*, 1986; Friedmann *et al.*, 1987) and anti-CD4 (Welsh *et al.*, 1987) reduce incidence/severity of disease, suggesting that the demyelination and motor decline observed in TMEV-IDD is the consequence of a peripheral cellular inflammatory response rather than a direct cytopathic effect in neurons or oligodendrocytes. Interestingly, although CD8[+] T cells are crucial for TMEV clearance, these cells do not appear to mediate demyelination (Fiette *et al.*, 1993).

Macrophages and microglia represent the major viral reservoir fueling persistent infection throughout the course of chronic TMEV-IDD (Clatch *et al.*, 1990; Lipton *et al.*, 1995; Pope *et al.*, 1996). B lymphocytes, and CD4[+] and CD8[+] T lymphocytes are present, but are not infected (Cash *et al.*, 1989; Lindsley and Rodriguez, 1989). Viral RNA and/or antigens have been detected in astrocytes, oligodendrocytes, microglia and CNS macrophages (Brahic *et al.*, 1981; Aubert *et al.*, 1987). *In vitro* data show that fully differentiated macrophages are more susceptible than monocytes to TMEV infection (Jelachich *et al.*, 1995; Shaw-Jackson and Michiels, 1997). Within mature macrophage populations, activated cells, identified by morphology, adherence and TNF-α secretion, express more TMEV RNA and antigens than inactivated cells (Shaw-Jackson and Michiels, 1997). Entry factors expressed by the host affect replication among myeloid lineage cells (Shaw-Jackson and Michiels, 1997). Although differentiated macrophages represent an important target for infection, brain macrophages are still relatively restrictive hosts compared with highly permissive BHK-21 cells. The ability of TMEV to enter macrophages and remain dormant is a salient feature of TMEV persistence.

Restricted TMEV infection of macrophages causes apoptosis (Jelachich and Lipton, 1999; Tsunoda *et al.*, 1997). At first glance, TMEV-induced macrophage apoptosis may seem to contradict the idea that the macrophages are an important viral reservoir in the CNS, for how can a virus persist within a cell population that it destroys? The answer is that TMEV-induced macrophage apoptosis is lengthy, killing only a fraction of infected cells over a long time course. In contrast, the viral life cycle is rapid (7 h in BHK-21 cells). The constant influx of peripheral macrophages, the slow tempo of macrophage apoptosis and the ability of TMEV also to infect oligodendrocytes ensure persistence in the face of limited macrophage cell death. Cell to cell spread of virus appears necessary for tissue persistence. Further, TMEV-dependent macrophage apoptosis may help explain the relapsing–remitting course of the disease. During periods of high viral replication, inflammation and tissue damage occurs. However, viral replication is followed by macrophage apoptosis. Dying macrophages lead to reduced antigen presentation, chemokine secretion and remission of disease. This type of cellular negative feedback ensures that lulls in antigen presentation follow rapid viral growth. It is important to note that TMEV does not induce apoptosis in permissive BHK-21 cells (Jelachich and Lipton, 1996).

Viral antigen presentation by brain MPs elicits a specific immune response directed against oligodendrocytes. Two conflicting explanations have been used for the immunological basis of myelin damage following intracerebral inoculation of TMEV: mimicry and epitope spreading. In the mimicry model, viral epitopes with structural similarity to oligodendrocyte epitopes stimulate antigen-specific autoimmunity. Experimental data show that mice infected with TMEV generate antibodies against proteolipid protein (PLP) and myelin oligodendrocyte glycoprotein (MOG) (Vanderlugt *et al.*, 1998). However, immune recognition of viral and myelin antigens is temporally distinct, undermining the mimicry argument. Peripheral TMEV antigen recognition occurs during acute disease, while PLP and MOG recognition occurs late. *In vitro* evidence generated using T-cell lines and hybridomas shows further that there is no cross-reactivity between TMEV and myelin epitopes (Miller *et al.*, 1997).

More probaby, TMEV-IDD occurs when lymphocytes specific for epitopes structurally distinct from inciting (viral) epitopes become activated by brain MPs. Viral infection is known to prime MPs for activation. In the presence of a lymphocytic infiltrate, MP activation leads to increased antigen presentation and potentially the loss of anergy. As disease progresses, previously untolerized cellular epitopes are exposed and presented to CD4[+] T lymphocytes by the MP class II processing system. Autoantigens are uncovered as disease progresses, and new lymphocyte populations respond. In the scenario of TMEV-IDD, macrophages and microglia presenting TMEV antigens, and later myelin antigens, induce a pro-inflammatory CD4⁺ Th1 response (Gerety *et al.*, 1994; Karpus *et al.*, 1995; Pope *et al.*, 1996). Cytokines secreted from pro-inflammatory CD4⁺ Th1 cells and activ-ated macrophages recruit cytotoxic T lymphocytes. Whether MPs, CD4⁺ T lymphocytes, CD8⁺ T lymphocytes, or combinations of all three mediate tissue damage in TMEV lesions is not clear.

4.2 Mouse hepatitis virus (JHM-MHV)-induced demyelination

Mouse hepatitis virus (MHV) belongs to the coronavirus family of enveloped, single-stranded RNA viruses responsible for a wide range of human and animal disease. MHV envelope protein forms distinctive transmembrane studs that can be visualized by electron microscopy. The viral genome is the longest of any known RNA virus, ranging from 27.6 to 31 kb long, encodes 7–10 functional genes, has a 5′ methylguanine cap and a 3′ polyadenine tail, can function as mRNA and is infectious.

In susceptible mice, JHM-MHV strains cause biphasic neurological lesions (Bailey *et al.*, 1949; Cheever *et al.*, 1949; Kyuwa and Stohlman, 1990). Originally isolated from mice spontaneously developing hind limb paralysis, neurovirulent JHM-MHV strains cause rapid fatal encephalomyelitis through direct infection of neurons (Fishman *et al.*, 1985). Attenuated JHM-MHV isolates exist that preferentially infect murine glial cells after intracerebral inoculation and are not always fatal (Herndon *et al.*, 1975). Still, in attenuated virus models of demyelination, the majority of infected mice die from acute viral neurological disease. Alternatively, suckling mice infected intranasally are able to survive the acute disease phase when nursed with dams previously immunized with JHM-MHV (Perlman *et al.*, 1987). Passive maternal immunity attenuates acute viral infection and allows consistent survival. Within 10–12 days after intranasal infection, 40–90 per cent of mice display hind limb paralysis followed by histological evidence of demyelination within 3–8 weeks. These features usually persist for the life of the infected animal. Because the chronic central demyelinating histopathology observed in these murine paradigms pathologically resembles that of human multiple sclerosis (MS), JHM-MHV has been used as an experimental model for virus-induced demyelination.

Viral persistence appears to trigger chronic immune-mediated inflammatory demyelination. Virus can be detected in the CNS of mice with chronic demyelinating lesions, and in the absence of a persistent infection demyelination does not occur. Astrocytes appear to be the major CNS reservoir for JHM-MHV, and oligodendrocytes are also infected. Infected cells of both types are found in inflammatory demyelinating lesions in brain and spinal cord. Neurons appear uninfected and are not destroyed. However, virus alone is not responsible for the pathologies associated with JHM-MHV. Whole-body γ-irradiation abrogates chronic virus-induced demyelination (Wang *et al.*, 1990). Subsequent adoptive transfer of splenocytes partially restores demyelination. Based on these findings, direct viral cytolysis cannot be excluded as a mechanism, but does not appear to be the primary cause for JMH-MHV demyelination.

Experimental evidence suggests that, in contrast to TMEV-IDD, the peripheral macrophage is a bystander in JHM-MHV-mediated demyelination. JHM-MHV can infect and cause apoptosis in macrophages (Belyavsky *et al.*, 1998), and macrophage infiltration has a strong temporal correlation with demyelination (Wu and Perlman,

1999). However, MPs are not a reservoir for JHM-MHV, and depletion of peripheral macrophages by mannosylated liposomes encapsulating dichloromethylene diphosphonate (C1$_2$MDP) does not prevent demyelination (Xue *et al.*, 1999). Mannosylated liposomes effectively deplete peripheral macrophages but do not penetrate into brain perivascular or parenchymal spaces. In the CNS, antigen presentation and stimulation of antigen-specific immunity can be accomplished by brain microglia and perivascular macrophages independently of infiltrating peripheral macrophages. JHM-MHN demyelination may involve preferentially microglial activation rather than infiltration and activation of peripheral monocytes.

5 MPs and herpesviral infections

5.1 Overview

Herpesviridae family members consist of a core of linear double-stranded DNA in the form of a torus (Nazerian, 1974), an icosahedral protein capsid containing 162 capsomeres embedded in an amorphous tegument and a viral envelope derived from the host nuclear membrane (Roizmann *et al.*, 1992). The capsid diameter is about 100–125 nm and the diameter of the whole virus is about 215 nm (Schrag *et al.*, 1989). Herpesviruses all share the capacity to establish persistent and latent infections in nearly all host cells. Like other viruses, herpesviruses frequently rely on activation receptors such as integrins (Bergelson and Finberg, 1993) and tumor necrosis factor receptors (TNFRs) (Montgomery *et al.*, 1996; Marsters *et al.*, 1997), or immune molecules such as MHC class I α-chain (Wyllie *et al.*, 1980; Grundy *et al.*, 1987; Price *et al.*, 1995) for binding and entry. Heparin blocks viral attachment (Kimpton *et al.*, 1989), highlighting the importance of proteoglycans and carbohydrates in tropism and viral entry. Interaction between herpesvirus glycoproteins and cell surface receptors is the major determinant of tropism and, ultimately, biological outcome. Although most herpesviruses have multiple tropisms, cellular predilection is observed.

The family herpesviridae is divided into three groups (α, β and γ) based primarily on genomic structural homology, with some exceptions. Each subclass also tends to share common biological properties (Roizmann *et al.*, 1992). α-Herpesviridae are characterized by the ability to remain latent in sensory neuronal ganglia. Human α-herpesviridae members include HSV-1 and HSV-2 and varicella zoster virus (VZV, also called HHV-3). Although α-herpesviruses can infect MPs *in vitro*, MP infection generally does not contribute to α-herpesvirus pathology. In contrast, β-herpesviridae infect leukocytes, salivary glands and kidney, and include HCMV, HHV-6 and HHV-7. MPs represent an important target cell for β-herpesviruses. In CMV disease, replication in MPs is a major determinant of pathogenesis. MPs can support viral replication and harbor latent CMV DNA (Hanson *et al.*, 1999), contributing to disease progression in liver, kidney and bone marrow. γ-Herpesviridae include HHV-8 and EBV. Tropism of γ-herpesviridae is still poorly defined.

In MPs and other cells, upon entry and nuclear translocation, the herpesvirus genome quickly circularizes. During latency, viral DNA remains in the form of extrachromosomal episomes and only a small subset of viral genes is expressed (Mellerick and Fraser, 1987). Viral gene expression can be reactivated through multiple mechanisms *in vitro* and *in vivo*, including systemic immune compromise and pro-inflammatory cytokine stimulation. Reactivation usually involves transcription and expression of viral lytic stage genes, DNA synthesis mediated by viral-encoded polymerases and completion of the viral life cycle. Unlike lentiviruses, genomic integration is not an obligatory step in the life cycle of the typical herpesvirus. Herpesvirus DNA replication is mediated by viral polymerases. After reactivation, new DNA-containing capsids assemble in the nucleus. Progeny virions bud through the nuclear membrane and, in so doing, acquire the viral envelope. During lysis, the host plasma membrane ultimately ruptures, releasing progeny virions.

Two sets of evidence suggest that herpesviruses and host cells have engaged in bidirectional exchange of ORFs during evolution. First, genomes within the family herpesviridae contain a plethora of cellular homologs. Some gene-dense regions of the human genome such as the MHC may represent germline integration of herpesviruses. Given the propensity for herpesvirus latency, it is entirely possible that many animal gene-dense regions are genetic remnants of herpesviruses that integrated into the host germline long ago, lost replication competence through host recombination or other genetic events, and since have evolved within the host. Secondly, intron-replete ORFs within herpesviruses strongly suggest acquisition of cellular cDNA. Animal cells frequently have reverse transcriptase activity resulting from expression of retrotransposable elements. Herpesviruses generally do not encode reverse transcriptase. The common themes of viral/cellular homology reflect interdependent evolution of viral genes and animal cells.

At the functional level, molecular homologies between herpesviruses and cellular genes belie multiple viral mechanisms for immune evasion. Herpesvirus products potentially can mimic and/or antagonize MP soluble signaling molecules such as IFNs or chemokines, interfere with MP antigen presentation through MHC molecules and cause hyperplasia. These mechanisms, combined with the ability to remain latent for indefinite periods in MPs and other cells, help explain why many herpesviral infections are never cleared by the immune system.

5.2 CMV

Most adults harbor latent HCMV but display no signs of viral pathology (Ho, 1991). Fifty to eighty per cent of the immunocompetent Western adult population express antibodies to CMV (Huang *et al.*, 1976; Bale, 1984). Some areas of Africa and the Far East show seroprevalence close to 100 per cent (Ho, 1991). Vertical transmission can occur *in utero* through transplacental routes, during birth from an infected maternal cervix, or post-partum through breast milk. Blood transfusion represents a potential mechanism for horizontal transmission. Other mechanisms have not been clearly identified. Circumstantial evidence suggests that day-care, sexual and intimate oral exposures may contribute to community spread. There are no known non-human reservoirs for HCMV. In some infected immunocompetent humans, primary HCMV infection results in mononucleosis. Viremia is detected for weeks to months after resolution of symptoms and proviral DNA can be isolated from circulating and nodal monocytes and lymphocytes. Transplant patients on immunosuppressive regimens and HIV-1 patients frequently experience vigorous HCMV-dependent pathology including allograft atherosclerosis (chronic rejection). Active HCMV disease has been demonstrated in more than 95 per cent of homosexual men in late-stage HIV disease (Drew *et al.*, 1984) and is the most common pathogen observed within the first 6 month of post-transplant immuno-suppressive regimens.

Laboratory analyses have identified peripheral monocytes as the predominant infected blood cell in HCMV disease (Soderberg *et al.*, 1993; von Laer *et al.*, 1995; Link *et al.*, 1996) and in seropositive, asymptomatic individuals (Dankner *et al.*, 1990; Taylor-Wiedeman *et al.*, 1991). However, HCMV can infect many cell types, including epithelium, endothelium and connective tissue. It is not clear whether the predilection of HCMV for monocytes is caused by interactions between viral and cellular surface determinants or simply reflects the ubiquitous presence of monocytes and MPs in many tissues.

Molecular mechanisms for HCMV binding and entry are not exclusive to MPs. HCMV encodes a homolog of a class I MHC gene (CMV UL20) that interacts with soluble β_2-microglobulin secreted by host cells. β_2-Microglobulin forms a bridge between UL20 associated with the viral envelope or tegument and cellular transmembrane class I α-chains, facilitating entry into cells. Viral glycoproteins gB (UL55) and gH (UL75) are also involved in binding and entry (Yurochko *et al.*, 1997). In addition to the role of soluble proteins in viral entry, coating of MCMV helps virus evade opsonization and receptor-mediated phagocytosis by MPs and neutrophils.

Differentiated macrophages have a greater ability to phagocytose HCMV than blood monocytes, but are also more susceptible to HCMV infection (Weinshenker *et al.*, 1988). As in many other viral infections, mature macrophages have the dual roles of immune effector and cell target for HCMV. After entry, HCMV mediates multiple alterations in macrophage homeostasis including down-regulation of MHC class II, proto-oncogene induction, increase in Ca^{2+} influx, accelerated phospholipid turnover, altered kinase activity and increased expression of transcription factors (Boldogh *et al.*, 1990, 1993; Albrecht *et al.*, 1991; Sedmak *et al.*, 1994; Keay *et al.*, 1995; Yurochko *et al.*, 1997; Yurochko and Huang, 1999). Populations of fully differentiated tissue macrophages demonstrate the ability to sustain and spread infection *in vitro* (Weinshenker *et al.*, 1988; Ibanez *et al.*, 1991; Maciejewski *et al.*, 1993). Infected cells frequently display a characteristic nuclear inclusion originally described by Cowdry in multiple cell types (Cowdry, 1934). The presence of 'Cowdry bodies' is requisite for diagnosis of CMV inclusion disease (CID) in all tissues. Macrophages can have Cowdry-type inclusions and also frequently can be observed surrounding Cowdry body-containing endothelial cells.

In monocytes, HCMV rarely completes a full replication cycle. The processes of differentiation and activation, both of which involve transcriptional enhancement of cellular genes, can stimulate HCMV to emerge from latency and enter into productive infection (Taylor-Wiedeman *et al.*, 1994). HCMV expression in quiescent, immature or resting MPs is limited to immediate-early (IE) gene products. The IE gene products are important laboratory tools in the study of HCMV infection because they allow detection of HCMV transcription in MPs and other restricted cell lines. The two most abundantly expressed (IE1 and 2) are splice variants of the same gene. Enhanced IE1 and IE2 expression, above levels detected in latently infected cells, leads to *trans*-activation of many HCMV promoters, and reactivation of the viral life cycle. The IE1/2 promoter includes sequence-specific binding domains for multiple cellular factors including NF-κB, CREB and others (Mocarski 1993). In reciprocal fashion, IE1 binds to the promoter of the NF-κB gene (Mocarski *et al.*, 1990), representing a potential positive feedback loop. These binding sites may function like molecular switches during emergence from viral latency by linking increased cellular transcription to viral reactivation. Activation of macrophages is associated with expression of HCMV genes and viral DNA synthesis (Brautigam *et al.*, 1979).

MCMV serves as a useful animal model for disease pathogenesis because MCMV disease mimics many of the salient features of HCMV. Like HCMV, IE1 expression has been detected in asymptomatic mice recovered from acute MCMV infection (Henry and Hamilton, 1993; Yuhasz *et al.*, 1994; Yu *et al.*, 1995). Like HCMV disease, MCMV replication in monocytes represents a major determinant of pathogenesis (Hanson *et al.*, 1999). MCMV infection following adoptive transfer of blood elements into sublethally irradiated mice recapitulates HCMV disease in bone marrow transplant patients and can be fatal. In these studies, it has been proposed that increases in TNF-α from monocyte/macrophages leads to a vascular reaction similar to endotoxic shock (Pasternack *et al.*, 1990).

5.3 Human herpesvirus-8 (HHV-8) and Kaposi's sarcoma

γ-Herpesviridae genomes contain blocks of conserved genes containing major structural proteins, DNA synthetic enzymes, glycoproteins, and a viral protease and assembly protein (Schulz, 1998). Some γ-herpesviruses also contain genes outside of these blocks, such as cellular growth factor homologs (Neipel *et al.*, 1997b), chemokines (Moore *et al.*, 1996a; Nicholas *et al.*, 1997b) and pro-inflammatory cytokines homologs (Neipel *et al.*, 1997a); Nicholas *et al.*, 1997b), IRF's (Nicholas *et al.*, 1997a), G-protein-coupled receptors (Cesarman *et al.*, 1996), anti-apoptotic proteins (Sarid *et al.*, 1997) and homologs of cell cycle regulatory proteins (Sarid *et al.*, 1997; Thome *et al.*, 1997). Taxonomically, γ-herpesvivirdae are divided into γ1 and γ2 subgroups based on genomic homology to subgroup prototypes. EEBV, a common B-cell-tropic human virus shown to be associated with mononucleosis and Burkitt's lymphoma, is the prototypical g1 herpesvirus. Other g1 subgroup members include equine herpesvirus-2 (EHV-2), murine herpesvirus-68 (MHV-68), bovine herpesvirus-4 (BHV-4) and avian herpesvirus-1 (AHV-1). Members of the γ2 subgroup are collectively called rhadinoviruses. Herpesvirus samiri (HVS), a squirrel monkey T-cell lymphomavirus, is the rhadinovirus prototype. Other rhadinoviruses include herpesvirus ateles, herpesvirus sylvigus and some alcephaline, bovine, equine, murine and ovine herpesviruses (Neipel *et al.*, 1998).

HHV-8, also called Kaposi's sarcoma herpes virus (KSHV), is the only known human rhadinovirus and shares closest genomic structure and sequence homology with HVS. Other related mammalian rhadinovirues have been detected in captive macaques (Desrosiers *et al.*, 1997; Rose *et al.*, 1997). In addition to structural homology, rhadinoviruses share the trait of causing no apparent disease in the main host, but causing fulminate lymphoproliferative disease in related species (Neipel *et al.*, 1998). For example, squirrel monkeys infected with KSHV show no clinical signs of infection, but infected marmosets develop polyclonal T-cell lymphomas (Meinl *et al.*, 1996). Given that the human HHV-8-associated Kaposi's sarcoma (KS) lesion was characterized originally in the middle nineteenth century, and that HHV-8 infects multiple groups of humans distinct in geography, behavior, ethnicity and immune status, one wonders if a non-human reservoir for HHV-8 exists. The complete DNA sequence is available for γ1 herpesvirus EBV (Baer *et al.*, 1984), EHV-2 (Telford *et al.*, 1995) and MHV-68 (Virgin *et al.*,

1997), and for γ2 herpesviruses HVS (Albrecht *et al.*, 1992) and HHV-8 (Russo *et al.*, 1996).

The association between HHV-8-and KS must reconcile epidemiological and biological findings. Four independent populations of KS patients have been described. The first group is late-stage HIV-1 patients. KS occurs in 30 per cent of the HIV-1-infected, homosexual population. Its incidence is 10- to 20-fold greater in the male homosexual population than in other HIV-positive risk groups, although non-homosexual HIV-1 patients are also at greater risk of acquiring KS compared with the general population (Beral *et al.*, 1990; Biggar and Rabkin, 1996; Biggar *et al.*, 1996). Secondly, iatrogenic KS results in transplant recipients, secondary to immunosuppressive therapy. Thirdly, Jews of Mediterranean and eastern European descent, and equatorial Africans have increased risk for KS compared with populations in other parts of the world. HHV-8 is endemic among Mediterranean/ European Jews and sub-Saharan Africans although mechanisms of transmission are not well defined.

KS is a multifocal, angioproliferative disorder that usually manifests in the loose connective tissue of the dermis, but can also occur in visceral tissue or lymph nodes. In early-stage KS, dermal vessels are surrounded by multiple small endothelial-lined spaces accompanied by a mononuclear infiltrate. On the skin surface, this lesion appears as a red patch. Later, during the plaque stage, microvascular channels expand through the dermis, forming slit-like vessels that appear not to be fully closed. In the nodular stage, sheets of spindle cells surround newly formed microvasculature. Red blood cells can be observed outside vascular channels, and the dermal extracellular matrix is smattered with hemosiderin. HHV-8 antigens have been detected in monocyte-derived macrophages found in neovascularized human KS lesions with no apparent spindle morphology (Blasig *et al.*, 1997). The final stage is the KS nodule. Most KS nodules have three salient components: neovascularization, hyperplastic stroma (spindle cells) and an inflammatory infiltrate. KS lesions resemble granulation tissue, to an extent, and most, but not all KS lesions contain spindle cells. Cultured KS spindle cells have been shown to express HHV-8 sequences using differential display (Chang *et al.*, 1994) and can be infected with HHV-8 in *ex vivo* systems (Boshoff *et al.*, 1995). When transplanted into the dermis of immunodeficient mice, human spindle cells form neovascularized masses containing infiltrating mouse cells (Salahuddin *et al.*, 1988). Xenotransplanted experimental KS masses regress in about 10 days.

Active expression of HHV-8 is necessary for the formation of KS lesions. Serological analysis gathered from independent investigators shows that 89 per cent or more of KS-afflicted patients in each population have antibodies to latent or lytic stage HHV-8 antigens compared with 2–7 per cent of healthy patients (Simpson *et al.*, 1996; Boshoff and Weiss, 1998; Chatlynne *et al.*, 1998). HHV-8 sequences have been detected in PBMCs before KS onset (Lefrere *et al.*, 1996), and in KS lesions from HIV-1-infected individuals (Chang *et al.*, 1994; Moore *et al.*, 1996b). No major genomic differences have yet been discovered between different KS lesions in the same individual (Nicholas *et al.*, 1997a). HHV-8 expression is also associated with other proliferative skin lesions. An important epidemiological negative control, HHV-8 DNA, was isolated from 82 per cent of non-KS skin lesions from HIV-uninfected, immunocompromised transplant patients (Rady *et al.*, 1995). It is not understood whether HHV-8 is causative for proliferative inflammatory processes or simply has a predilection for rapidly dividing monocytic cells (see below), lymphocytes, fibroblasts and/or endothelium.

Tissue macrophages represent the major source of productive viral infection in human KS lesions. Simultaneous application of immunohistochemistry and *in situ* hybridization performed with strand-specific RNA probes complementary to the sequences coding for the minor capsid protein (VP23) of HHV-8 detects a strong hybridization only in a small subset of cells in KS lesions. The VP23 gene is expressed specifically during the lytic or replicative period of the virus life cycle, and therefore is a useful marker to detect productively infected cells. All double-positive cells are monocyte derived (Blasig *et al.*, 1997). The association between HHV-8 infection of tissue macrophages and KS lesions may represent simple causation or correlation of common antecedent. HHV-8-infected macrophages in tissue may cause or contribute to KS lesion formation. Alternatively, peripherally infected macrophages may be recruited preferentially to the site of dermal hyperplasia and neovascularization.

Whether KS spindle cells are derived from infiltrating macrophages, resident fibroblasts or endothelium is unclear. Spindle cell cultures derived from KS lesions shows heterogeneous subpopulations (Kaaya *et al.*, 1995). One group of spindle cells stains positive for TE7 and collagen types I and III antigens. These cells are likely derived from fibroblasts. Another discrete population reacts with CD45 and CD68, suggesting a marrow-derived monocytic origin. It is not known whether HHV-8-infected monocytes have proliferative potential. Monocyte macrophage lineage cells have been demonstrated in other lesions including peripheral infiltrate in and surrounding murine sarcomas (Bottazzi *et al.*, 1990) and foamy cells found in atherosclerotic plaques. Given that HHV-8 is a DNA virus that infects macrophages, many DNA viruses are transforming, and HHV-8 has been found in association with proliferating lesions in dermal and hematological sites [including multicentric Castleman's disease (MCD) and primary effusion lymphoma (PEL)], it is possible that macrophages contribute to the proliferative component of KS. Interestingly, spindle cell cultures do not react with endothelial immunohistochemical markers CD34, CD45, CD62, factor VIII, EN4 or PAL-E (Blasig *et al.*, 1997). In vascular endothelial growth factor (VEGF)-dependent human endothelial cultures derived from bone marrow (BMEC) and umbilical vein (HUVEC) microvascular endothelial cells, HHV-8 infection causes extensive cytopathicity and death. However, surviving endothelial cells displayed spindle morphology, increased telomerase expression and, in the case of HUVECs, increased proliferation (Flore *et al.*, 1998). Investigators working closely with KS cultures have suggested that HHV-8 infection transforms endothelial cells, causing loss of typical endothelial phenotype (morphology, protein expression and cell cycle resting state; Reitz *et al.*, 1999).

Perturbed cytokine secretion and cellular responses may represent the link connecting immune alteration, HHV-8 and proliferative skin lesions such as KS. In transplant patients, progression of KS remits or regresses following termination or reduction in immunosuppressive therapy. However, HIV-2-dependent immunodeficiency in areas of high HHV-8 seroprevalence is associated with a greatly reduced incidence of KS compared with HIV-1 immunodeficiency (Ariyoshi *et al.*, 1998), suggesting that abrogation of immune pressure does not account entirely for the high number of KS cases in the HIV-1 population. Systemic HIV-1 infection contributes to the progression of HHV-8-associated KS lesions in a way that HIV-2 does not. The finding that HIV-1 antigens or tran-

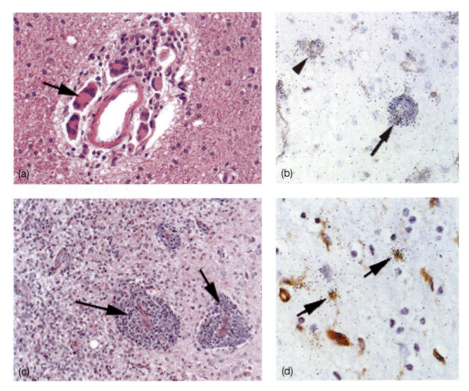

Plate 1 Central nervous system pathology induced by lentivirus-infected brain macrophages. (a) A microvessel in the brain of macaques with SIV encephalitis. A perivascular leukocyte aggregate (cuff) consists primarily of a monocyte-derived macrophage and multinucleated giant cells (arrowed) with few lymphocytes. (b) The brain pathology characteristic of SIV encephalitis. The tissue was immunostained with lectin RCA-1 to identify blood vessels and peripheral macrophages (brown). *In situ* hybridization was performed with a full-length recombinant DNA clone to SIV to identify viral RNA (black grains). The arrowheads identify a multinucleated giant cell expressing viral RNA trafficking into the brain. (c) A brain microvessel in sheep brain with visna–maedi virus (VMV) encephalitis. Dense perivascular cuffs (arrowed) include lymphocytes and macrophages. Surrounding parenchyma also shows an infiltrate of macrophages and lymphocytes. (D) Brain parenchyma in sheep infected with VMV encephalitis. RCA-1 staining (brown) identifies vessels and macrophages. *In situ* hybridization with a recombinant VMV (black grains) identifies lentiviral RNA. Courtesy of Christine Zink, PhD, The Johns Hopkins University School of Medicine.

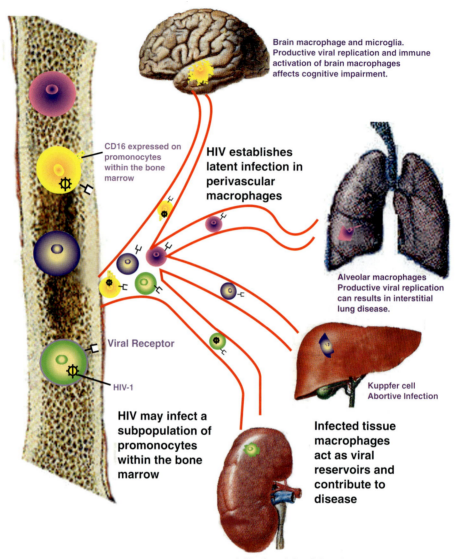

Brain macrophage and microglia. Productive viral replication and immune activation of brain macrophages affects cognitive impairment.

CD16 expressed on promonocytes within the bone marrow

HIV establishes latent infection in perivascular macrophages

Alveolar macrophages Productive viral replication can results in interstitial lung disease.

Viral Receptor

HIV-1

Kuppfer cell Abortive Infection

HIV may infect a subpopulation of promonocytes within the bone marrow

Infected tissue macrophages act as viral reservoirs and contribute to disease

Infiltration of virus-infected macrophages may induce nephropathy

Plate 2 Macrophages and HIV-1 disease. During primary HIV-1 infection, blood monocytes are infected with macrophage-tropic variants. Later in the course of viral infection and disease, infected and uninfected monocytes can become immune activated. Sites of macrophage activation include the bone marrow, blood, secondary lymphoid tissue and brain. Activation entails alteration of innate and acquired immune responses, up-regulation of adhesion factors and increased transendothelial migration into multiple tissues. In tissue, macrophages harbor and/or secrete low levels of progeny virus and can initiate a toxic secretory cascade. The ultimate result is alteration of tissue/cell function and clinical disease, the most common of which is HIV-1-associated dementia.

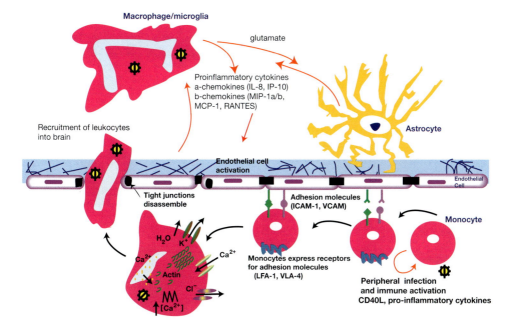

Plate 3 Model for the neuropathogenesis of HIV-1 infection. During HIV-1 infection, monocytes can become immune activated. Like the Trojan horse, infected monocytes can carry virus into the CNS. Infected and/or immune-activated macrophages may reside in and around the microvasculature or migrate into brain parenchyma and differentiate into macrophages and microglia, the brain's resident MPs. A key to monocyte transendothelial microglia is changes in ion channels (potassium, calcium, and chloride channels). Activated brain MPs secrete chemokines to attract more monocytes into tissue and amplify the immune cascade. Diffuse MP activation in brain disrupts neuronal homeostasis, leading to motor and cognitive dysfunction. These events may occur at all stages of disease, but are most prominent during advanced viral disease.

scripts are absent in the majority of KS lesions (Jahan *et al.*, 1989) supports the idea that HIV-1 does not play a direct role in KS progression. Interaction between HIV-1 disease and HHV-8-associated KS progression probably occurs through immune and cytokine circuitry. Increased levels of cytokines secreted from HIV-1-infected, immune-activated macrophages and lymphocytes may cause transcription of HHV-8 genes in infected cells. Consider the differential effects of TNF-α on uninfected and HHV-8-infected cells. In uninfected cells, MP-secreted TNF-α stimulates apoptosis by binding the TNFR expressed on target cells. TNF-α binding to TNFR stimulates the activity of 'death domains' on the cytoplasmic portion of the TNFR, leading to activation of caspases, apoptosis-inducing aspartic proteases associated with the mitochondrial membrane system (Boldin *et al.*, 1996). *In vitro*, TNF-α causes apoptosis of multiple cell types (Slowik *et al.*, 1997; Haas *et al.*, 1999; Kawakami *et al.*, 1999; Messmer *et al.*, 1999). However, administration of TNF-α in clinical trials is associated with vigorous expansion and spread of KS lesions (Kaplan *et al.*, 1989). The dichotomous effects of TNF-α may be reconciled by close analysis of HHV-8-encoded response elements and their corresponding ORFs.

Activation of HHV-8-infected cells has three consequences. First, infected cells become hyperplastic. Secondly, infected cells secrete pro-inflammatory cytokines and chemokines that recruit and perpetuate a mononuclear inflammatory response. Thirdly, infected cells secrete angiogenic factors that contribute to angiogenesis. During this process, transformation of a previously hyperplastic KS spindle cell clone may occur, but is not obligatory for KS to progress to the nodular form. HHV-8-expressed proteins conceivably could cause infected cells to enter a hyperplastic growth phase, home to a source of chemokine production, secrete chemokines to attract inflammatory cells and more HHV-8 infected cells, and stimulate angiogenesis of neighboring microvasculature.

At least 81 ORFs have been identified within the HHV-8 genome (Moore and Chang, 1998). Those lacking an HVS homolog are given the suffix 'K'. HHV-8 encodes at least 14 reading frames that are homologous to cellular genes (Neipel *et al.*, 1998), many of which are responsive to cellular enhancers of transcription. HHV-8 encodes a homolog (vIRF), an IL-8 receptor homolog (vIL-8R), MIP-1α, MIP-1β and IL-6 homologs (vMIP-1A, vMIP-IB, vIL-6), a D-type cyclin analog (v-cyc), an anti-apoptotic bcl family protein (v-bcl-2) and a G-protein-coupled chemokine receptor in ORF 74 that most closely resembles the human IL-8 receptor (Cesarman *et al.*, 1996; Moore *et al.*, 1996a; Guo *et al.*, 1997; Nicholas *et al.*, 1997b). Cytokine stimulation of HHV-8-infected cells could result in surface expression of chemokine receptors, secretion of chemokines, altered regulation of cell cycle check points and secretion of vasculogenic factors. The HHV-8 genome includes a new set of gene regulatory elements that may allow for different interpretation of autocrine or paracrine cytokine signals. Reactivation of HHV-8 by chemokine signals late in HIV-1 disease may drive progression of KS lesions.

6 Lentivirinae: an overview

Lentiviruses are a subfamily of retroviruses that have a prolonged disease progression ('lenti' is Latin for slow), are transmitted exclusively by exchange of bodily fluids, have a high mutation rate, cause pneumonia, arthritis, and encephalitis and cannot be eradicated from an infected host. Like other retroviruses, the lentivirus particle consists of a protein capsid surrounded by a proteolipid envelope. The enveloped particle is 80–120 nm in size. The electron-dense conical capsid contains diploid viral genomes held together by RNA-binding proteins and multiple complementary nucleic acid regions; a molecule of tRNA bound near the 5′ terminus of each genomic copy; Mg^{2+}-dependent reverse transcriptase, RNase H and integrase activities; and accessory proteins. Lentiviruses frequently rely on accessory protein function for temporal expression of gene products necessary for replication competence. Post-entry interference with accessory protein function can lead to abortive or restricted infections.

Upon attachment to MPs, lentiviruses are rapidly ingested by phagocytic vacuoles. Lentiviruses usually fuse with the MP plasma membrane and enter the cytosol before MPs can complete phagocytosis. In macrophages, virions bud from the host cytosol, through the plasma membrane, and into cytoplasmic vesicles (Orenstein *et al.*, 1988). In other cell types, lentiviruses bud directly into the extracellular space, presumably because the secretory compartment in non-myeloid cells is less developed than in MPs. Viral proteins expressed on the MP surface mediate cell–cell fusion and formation of multinucleated giant cells. Multinucleated giant cells are the hallmark of multiple lentiviral tissue pathologies.

The lentiviral genome is 7–10 kb long and encompasses four structural genes common to all retroviruses: *gag, pro, pol* and *env*. The order of these structural genes from 5′ to 3′ is *gag–pro–pol–env*. The *gag* gene encodes structural components of the viral capsid and matrix. The viral protease (*pro*) is encoded in between the *gag* and *pol* genes and frequently overlaps *pol*. Lentiviral genes are usually transcribed as polyproteins that require post-translational cleavage by the viral protease. The *pol* gene encodes viral enzymatic functions including RNA-dependent DNA polymerase (reverse transcriptase) activity. The *env* gene encodes viral glycoproteins that are embedded in the host plasma membrane and acquired during budding. Lentiviruses encode accessory products in addition to *gag–pro–pol–env* and therefore are called 'complex retroviruses.' Like all retroviruses, lentiviral genomes are flanked by long terminal repeats (LTRs) that can be hundreds of bases long. Transcription of lentivirus genes is driven by a single promoter, within the LTR U3, that can be regulated by cellular and viral elements. For example, the HIV-1 LTR includes binding sites for NF-κB, Sp1, EBP-1, UBP-1 and RNA polymerase II (Jones *et al.*, 1986; Garcia *et al.*, 1987; Nabel and Baltimore, 1987; Wu *et al.*, 1988). The viral protein Tat also enhances transcriptional activity through the HIV-1 promoter and is essential for permissive infection (Fisher *et al.*, 1986).

From a pathogenesis perspective, there are two types of lentiviruses: immunodeficiency viruses and ungulate lentiviruses. In both types, MPs are important for transmission, represent an important target cell early in infection and sustain a reservoir for latent lentivirus throughout disease. However, unlike ungulate lentiviruses, immunodeficiency viruses also infect lymphocytes, eventually resulting in host immunosuppression. In the absence of an effective Th (helper) lymphocyte compartment, opportunistic viral and fungal infections and cancers can lead to multisystem organ dysfunction and ultimately host demise. Immunodeficiency viruses have been isolated from humans (HIV-1 and HIV-2) (Barre-Sinoussi *et al.*, 1983; Clavel *et al.*, 1986), cats (FIV) (Pedersen *et al.*, 1987), Asian macaques (SIV_{mac}) (Daniel *et al.*, 1985) and several species of African monkeys (SIV_{agm}, SIV_{mnd}, SIV_{smn}, SIV_{syk}) (Kanki *et al.*, 1985; Murphey-Corb *et al.*,

1986; Ohta *et al.*, 1988; Tsujimoto *et al.*, 1988; Hirsch *et al.*, 1993). SIV is not indigenous in Asian macaques, and SIV$_{mac}$ strains probably represent intraspecies transfer from sooty mangabeys in captive environments in the USA (Gardner and Luciw, 1989).

7 MP infection: a hallmark of ungulate lentivirus infections

Ungulate lentiviruses include visna–maedi virus of sheep (VMV) (Icelandic: visna = paralysis and cachexia, maedi = labored breathing) (Nathanson *et al.*, 1985), caprine arthritis–encephalitis virus (CAEV) (Cork *et al.*, 1974), bovine immunodeficiency virus (BIV) (Gonda *et al.*, 1987) and the first identified retrovirus, equine infectious anemia virus (EIAV) (Valee and Carre, 1904). Lentivirus-infected ungulates display interstitial pneumonia, pulmonary lymphoid hyperplasia, lymphocytic mastitis, arthritis, vasculitis, glomerulonephropathy, autoimmune hemolytic anemia and encephalomyelitis. All of these pathologies revolve around infected MPs, including interstitial alveolar macrophages, lymph node macrophages, synovial macrophages, bone marrow monocytic progenitors and/or nurse cells, and brain microglia. Not all infected ungulates manifest disease. For example, nearly all BIV- and many VMV-infected animals show few clinical signs of disease.

In ungulate lentiviral infections, there exists a demonstrable correlation between productive viral infection in infiltrating macrophages and disruption of tissue architecture. Immune suppression is not part of ungulate lentiviral disease and opportunistic pathogens play no part in pathogenesis because lymphocytes are not infected and acquired immunity is not impaired. BIV is something of a misnomer. It was named for structural homology to HIV, SIV and FIV, but does not infect lymphocytes and causes little or no apparent immunodeficiency in cattle.

EIAV is the most important infectious disease of horses and has a world-wide distribution. EIAV can be transmitted by blood-suckling horse flies and, as such, is the only lentivirus known that can spread through an insect vector (Issel *et al.*, 1990). In most equidae, initial infection with EIAV is characterized by an early reaction within 1 month of inoculation that includes anorexia and cachexia, fever, labored breathing and acute-onset anemia (Narayan and Clements, 1989). The initial reaction can last days, during which time many animals succumb. Those that survive regain appetite and some muscle tone but display progressive anemia and lymphadenopathy. After weeks or months, acute wasting may recur and remit. EIAV cycles in this manner for months to years. Late-stage EIAV-infected individuals display glomerulonephropathy, autoimmune hemolytic anemia and encephalopathy manifest as perivascular mononuclear cuffing and gliosis (Narayan and Clements, 1989). EIAV establishes chronic MP reservoirs in liver, spleen, lymph node, kidney and lung (Sellon *et al.*, 1992). Unlike HIV-1, EIAV also appears to infect immature myeloid lineage progenitors in bone marrow explant culture systems (Swardson *et al.*, 1992), a tropism that may instigate the immune-mediated hemolytic anemia for which the virus is named. Some infected horses never develop clinical symptoms.

VMV spread rapidly among sheep in Iceland following introduction of latently infected rams from Europe in the 1930s (Sigurdsson, 1954). Natural spread of VMV peaked in the 1950s. Virus can be spread horizontally through exchange of bodily fluids. Vertical transmission can occur through transplacental routes, exposure to maternal blood during birth or through colostrum. In subclinical stages of infection, VMV replication is minimal and confined to the MP compartment (Gendelman *et al.*, 1985). In some animals, systemic viral loads and frequency of infected circulating cells rise later in the course of infection. Clinical VMV initially manifests as an interstitial pneumonia (Narayan and Cork 1985). Intravascular and alveolar macrophages are the only cells from these lesions that produce progeny virions, but viral RNA and proviral DNA can be detected in lung fibroblasts and alveolar epithelial cells (Brodie *et al.*, 1995). Later in the disease, a secondary neurological component frequently develops in which infected brain perivascular and parenchymal MPs are the main cell type involved in virus invasion and viral protein expression (Chebloune *et al.*, 1998). Figure 4.2 shows representative sections comparing infected brain tissue in an SIV-infected macaque (Figure 4.2a and b) and a VMV-infected sheep (Figure 4.2c and d). Ependymal cells also contain viral RNA and/or DNA (Staskus *et al.*, 1991). Arthritis is a variable finding mediated by infiltration of infected MPs. Although bone marrow progenitors can sustain a productive infection (Gendelman *et al.*, 1985), VMV-infected sheep fail to display gross hematological abnormalities, perhaps because slow progression of the viral life cycle does not interfere with formation of blood elements. The finding that VMV-infected macrophages can transmit virus to otherwise non-permissive neighboring cells through cell–cell contact (Singh *et al.*, 1999) has tremendous significance in the context of vertical transmission of all lentiviruses. Whether HIV-infected human MPs can cause infection of adjacent human trophoblast or cervical epithelial cells through a similar mechanism *in vivo* is not known.

CAEV is manifest by insidious onset synovitis that can progress into a debilitating radiocarpal arthritis. Mammary tissue, lungs and other joints may also display MP-mediated pathology (Cork and Narayan 1980; Crawford *et al.*, 1980). In young goats, slow-onset neurological impairment has been reported, similar to VMV in sheep (Clements *et al.*, 1994). Blood-derived macrophages represent the primary viral target *in vivo* (Klevjer-Anderson and Anderson, 1982). Like other lentiviruses, CAEV depends on accessory gene function for replication in MPs (Harmache *et al.*, 1996). Macrophages in colostrum represent an important source of transmission to kids (Kennedy-Stoskopf *et al.*, 1985). CAEV has multiple mechanisms for evasion of the host immune response. Like other lentiviruses, latency in MPs allows persistence and long-term survival. In addition, the CAEV envelope glycoprotein is more heavily glycosylated than most lentiviral surface proteins, which may aid in immune escape (Georgsson *et al.*, 1976).

8 HIV infection of macrophages and disease pathogenesis

Immunodeficiency viruses have two major cellular targets, MPs and Th lymphocytes. Like ungulate lentiviruses, HIV-1 infection of MPs disrupts organ architecture and function independently of opportunistic infection, including pancytopenia, glomerulonephropathy and encephalopathy. In addition, immunodeficiency virus infection of host Th lymphocytes precipitates depletion of CD4$^+$ lymphocytes, opportunistic infection and death. Although delineation of macrophage and CD4$^+$ lymphocyte components of HIV-1 disease is useful for the purpose of consideration, HIV-1 pathogenesis should not be thought of as two separate superimposed diseases. On the contrary, the macrophage and CD4$^+$ lymphocyte compartments interact at multiple stages in HIV-1 pathogenesis. For

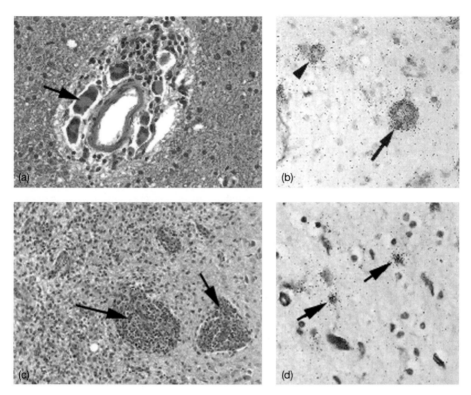

Fig. 4.2 Central Nervous system pathology induced by lentivirus-infected brain macrophages. (a) A microvessel in the brain of macaques with SIV encephalitis. A perivascular leukocyte aggregate (cuff) consists primarily of a monocyte-derived macrophage and multinucleated giant cells (arrowed) with few lymphocytes. (b) The brain pathology characteristic of SIV encephalitis. The tissue was immunostained with lectin RCA-1 to identify blood vessels and peripheral macrophages (brown). *In situ* hybridization was performed with a full-length recombinant DNA clone to SIV to identify viral RNA (black grains). The arrowheads identify a multinucleated giant cell expressing viral RNA trafficking into the brain. (c) A brain microvessel in sheep brain with visna–maedi virus (VMV) encephalitis. Dense perivascular cuffs (arrowed) include lymphocytes and macrophages. Surrounding parenchyma also shows an infiltrate of macrophages and lymphocytes. (d) Brain parenchyma in sheep infected with VMV encephalitis. RCA-1 staining (brown) identifies vessels and macrophages. *In situ* hybridization with a recombinant VMV (black grains) identifies lentiviral RNA. Courtesy of Christine Zink, PhD, The Johns Hopkins University School of Medicine. *See Plate 1.*

example, altered gene expression in HIV-1-infected macrophages may contribute to the shift from the predominant Th1–Th1-type cytokine response observed early in HIV-1 disease to a predominant Th2 response in late-stage disease. In the Th2 milieu, amplification of virus and progression of disease is favored. Conversely, expansion of viral load, decrease in number and function of peripheral CD4$^+$ lymphocytes and increases in circulating M-CSF observed in late-stage HIV-1 disease may activate bone marrow monocytes, predisposing them for attachment to post-capillary venule endothelium, transmigration into tissue and initiation of macrophage-mediated tissue destruction (Gartner, 2000). *In totem*, HIV-1-infected MPs and lymphocytes together cause synergistic immune alterations that allow viral persistence and cause tissue pathology, immune compromise and ultimately death in the infected human host.

8.1 HIV-1 tropism

By far the more prevalent and virulent human immunodeficiency virus, HIV-1, is responsible for the current pandemic. For taxonomic purposes, two groups of HIV-1 exist. Most HIV-1 isolates are included in group M and outliers are included in group O. Within group M, multiple clades (A–J) exist based on sequence variability in the *gag* and *env* genes (Vasil *et al.*, 1998). Among viral isolates, two general HIV-1 tropisms exist defined by *in vitro* properties. Laboratory M-tropic strains infect both immortalized monocytoid and T-lymphocytoid cells *in vitro*, but do not cause T-cell fusion and syncytia formation. Laboratory T-lymphocyte tropic (T-tropic) strains infect immortalized T-cell lineages *in vitro*, induce T-cell fusion and syncytia formation, and infect macrophages poorly, if at all. The inability of laboratory T-tropic strains to infect macrophages does not imply that T-tropic virus cannot infect macrophages *in vivo*. In fact, primary isolates that form T-cell syncytia frequently infect macrophages, suggesting that the ability of a viral strain to induce T-cell syncytia does not preclude macrophage infection. However, after multiple passages in T-cell lineages *in vitro*, laboratory strains of T-tropic isolates can accrue mutations in envelope genes that retard replication in macrophages.

In vivo, differences in the HIV-1 *env* gene are responsible for the different tropisms of HIV-1 isolates. The smaller cleavage product of the *env* gene, gp41, is expressed as a transmembrane protein in the host cell plasma membrane and ultimately in the viral envelope. The larger *env* cleavage product, gp120, is trafficked into the host cell secretory pathway and associates with gp41 through non-covalent interactions on the external face of the envelope. gp120 has six constant and five variable regions (C1–C6 and V1–V5). Viral attachment to host cells usually is mediated by binding of viral gp120 to cellular CD4, an invariant transmembrane accessory molecule. Based on shearing forces in blood and tissue that might strip a virion of associated gp120, it has been estimated that roughly 1 in 60 000 viral particles is infectious (Piatak *et al.*, 1993). CD4 expression alone is sufficient for viral attachment, but a second co-receptor is necessary for viral entry. Interaction between gp120 and seven transmembrane, G-protein-coupled chemokine receptors expressed on MPs and lymphocytes initiates viral fusion events (Dragic *et al.*, 1996). In MPs, CCR5 is the primary chemokine receptor involved in viral entry. In T cells, CXCR4 is the primary HIV-1 co-receptor. Domains within the V3 region of gp120 determine whether a particular virion can interact with CCR, CXCR or both receptors (Choe *et al.*, 1996; Cocchi *et al.*, 1996). After attachment to the MP surface, via gp120–CD4, gp120–Ig-Fc or gp120–Ig-C3a–Mac1 interactions, the viral particle must remain associated with the cell surface while lateral motion within the MP plasma membrane brings CCR5 in contact with gp120. After HIV-1 attachment, chemokine receptors interact with the gp120–CD4 complex causing conformational changes in gp120 and possibly in gp41, exposing fusogenic regions within gp41.

8.2 M-tropic virus in the transmission, persistence and progression of HIV-1 infection

In the USA, homosexual contact is the most common means of HIV-1 transmission, followed by sharing of intravenous drug paraphernalia. In less developed parts of the world, heterosexual contact is the most common route of transmission. Vertical transmission accounts for the vast majority of pediatric HIV-1 infections world-wide. Primary infection with HIV-1 is associated with non-specific clinical symptoms such as fever, malaise, lymphadenopathy, sore throat, headaches and, less commonly, aseptic meningitis, retroorbital pain, photophobia and headaches (Gabuzda and Hirsch, 1987; Clark *et al.*, 1991; Daar *et al.*, 1991; Tindall and Cooper, 1991). Viral strains that establish infection in the new host are M-tropic in over 95 per cent of early asymptomatic individuals (Schuitemaker *et al.*, 1991; Roos *et al.*, 1992). Failure of T-tropic virus to be transmitted to a new host and persist beyond primary infection may be a function of tropism-dependent transmission restrictions and/or virus–immune system interaction following transmission.

HIV-1-infected macrophages from an infected individual represent an important source of transmitted virus from fluids and tissues of transmitting hosts. Free virus or HIV-1-infected macrophages in semen or vaginal secretions are transferred to the new host (Phillips *et al.*, 1998). In vertical infections, placental (Kesson *et al.*, 1994; McGann *et al.*, 1994) cervical (Miller *et al.*, 1992b) or breast milk (Van de Perre and Cartoux, 1995; Van de Perre, 2000) macrophages mediate transmission.

Blood and mucosa are portals of entry for horizontal transmission of HIV. Because of the prominent role of tissue macrophages in non-specific immunity and the reticuloendothelial system in clearance of virus from circulation, macrophages represent an accessible target to free virus during primary infection. Following sexual contact, submucosal macrophages in the rectum, vagina and mouth may be infected. Reticuloendothelial macrophages represent an important early target for individuals infected intravenously.

After transmission, the ability of M-tropic virus to evade the host immune response allows chronic persistence. During the early viremic phase, infected MPs travel to or are infected in multiple organs. The HIV-1-infected MP is a vector for spread of virus through blood and lymphatic circulation. Blood-borne HIV-1-infected monocytes migrate through post-capillary venules, bringing virus into peripheral tissues much like the fabled wooden horse brought Spartan soldiers into the ancient city of Troy (Meltzer *et al.*, 1990). Figure 4.3 depicts this process. In lymphoid tissue, HIV-1 becomes trapped within the processes of follicular MPs in the germinal centers of lymph nodes and spleen (Pantaleo *et al.*, 1993). A vigorous immune response destroys infected CD4$^+$ lymphocytes and controls primary viremia (Tersmette and Miedema, 1990; Groenink *et al.*, 1991), but is unable to eliminate HIV-1 from MP reservoirs, particularly in lymphoid tissue. HIV-specific CD8$^+$ effector function emerges prior to neutralizing antibody and is a necessary component of controlling primary HIV-1 infection (Safrit *et al.*, 1994). CD8$^+$ lymphocytes destroy HIV-1-infected CD4$^+$ lymphocytes by secretion of perforin and granzyme and surface expression of Fas ligand. CD8$^+$ lymphocytes also interfere with HIV-1 replication by secretion of β-chemokines (Cocchi *et al.*, 1996). After primary HIV-1 inoculation, patients show major expansions of certain subsets of CD8$^+$ T cells (Musey *et al.*, 1997).

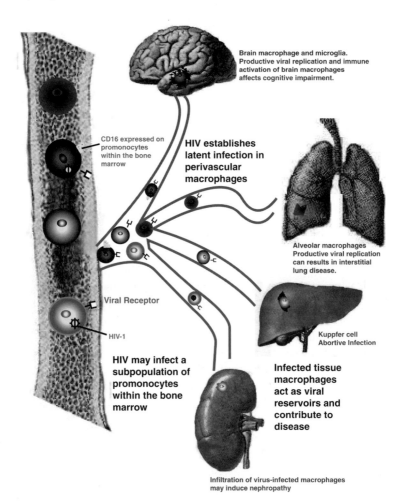

Brain macrophage and microglia. Productive viral replication and immune activation of brain macrophages affects cognitive impairment.

CD16 expressed on promonocytes within the bone marrow

HIV establishes latent infection in perivascular macrophages

Alveolar macrophages Productive viral replication can results in interstitial lung disease.

Viral Receptor

HIV-1

HIV may infect a subpopulation of promonocytes within the bone marrow

Kuppfer cell Abortive Infection

Infected tissue macrophages act as viral reservoirs and contribute to disease

Infiltration of virus-infected macrophages may induce nephropathy

Fig. 4.3 Macrophages and HIV-1 disease. During primary HIV-1 infection, blood monocytes are infected with macrophage-tropic variants. Later in the course of viral infection and disease, infected and uninfected monocytes can become immune activated. Sites of macrophage activation include the bone marrow, blood, secondary lymphoid tissue and brain. Activation entails alteration of innate and acquired immune responses, up-regulation of adhesion factors and increased transendothelial migration into multiple tissues. In tissue, macrophages harbor and/or secrete low levels of progeny virus and can initiate a toxic secretory cascade. The ultimate result is alteration of tissue/cell function and clinical disease, the most common of which is HIV-1-associated dementia. *See Plate 2.*

8.3 MP–HIV interactions

Lymphocytes are highly permissive to HIV-1 and synthesize orders of magnitude more virus per cell than HIV-1-infected macrophages. In contrast, HIV-1 can establish restricted infection of MPs. HIV-1 infection causes functional alterations in MPs, such as reduced phagocytosis (Crowe *et al.*, 1994), increased expression of adhesion molecules (Stent *et al.*, 1994) and increased expression of iNOS (Rostasy *et al.*, 1999). One or more copies of proviral DNA per MP are expressed at low levels, allowing secretion of progeny virions without stimulating a strong host immune response. MPs in spleen, lymphoid tissue, brain and lung represent important viral reservoirs throughout HIV-1 disease (Gendelman *et al.*, 1989). Unlike latent HCMV infections, in which infected MPs effectively eliminate transcription of viral genes for extended periods of time, HIV-1-infected MPs synthesize constant low levels of virus. During the asymptomatic period, HIV-1 is not in true latency from a molecular standpoint. Viral production and immune-mediated viral neutralization are in equilibrium, reflecting a chronic active disease process.

Tat or Rev proteins, UV light, phorbol esters, cytokines and other stimuli can up-regulate viral gene expression in latently infected MPs (Fauci, 1996; Vicenzi *et al.*, 1997; Houle *et al.*, 1999). Cytokines can also modulate expression of HIV-1 genes in MPs, creating autocrine/paracrine feedback loops in multiple *in vitro* systems (Poli *et al.*, 1990, 1994; Kinter *et al.*, 1995). For example, binding of TNF-α to MP-expressed TNFR induces transcription of HIV-1 genes through activation of NF-κB (Poli and Fauci, 1996).

From active MP reservoirs, T-tropic variants ultimately emerge and precipitate advanced disease progression. Chronic active viral replication within the macrophage compartment combined with the high mutation rate of the viral polymerase accounts for the emergence of T-tropic mutants that eventually predominate late in disease. However, the ability of the cytotoxic arm of the immune system to control primary infection effectively begs the question 'why can't CD8$^+$ effector function control emergence of T-tropic virus and spreading infection among CD4$^+$ lymphocytes later in disease?' Interestingly, in late-stage HIV-1 disease, re-emergence of T-tropic strains and progression to end-stage HIV-1 disease occurs in conjunction with a steady decline in overall CD8$^+$ T-cell function. As disease progresses, the HIV-1-infected host becomes less efficient at stimulating Th1-type immune responses, resulting in an overall shift of the CD4$^+$ T-cell population to a Th2 phenotype, and decreasing the ability of the HIV-1-infected host to mount an amplified CD8$^+$ response against virus-infected cells. Defective Th1 function manifests as subtle decreases in CD8$^+$ cell numbers, but becomes more conspicuous as HIV-1 spreads unabated among CD4$^+$ T cells, precipitating global immune decline and entry into late-stage HIV-1 disease. Viral alteration of MP co-stimulatory molecule expression (Dudhane *et al.*, 1996) or cytokine secretion (Millar *et al.*, 1991; Graziosi *et al.*, 1994; Poli and Fauci, 1996) represent potential mechanisms through which HIV-1–macrophage interactions could contribute to defects in the Th1-type response to virus.

8.4 Chemokine receptor polymorphisms and disease progression

CC chemokine receptor polymorphisms have been identified as host susceptibility factors for infection upon exposure and progression after infection. Up to 20 per cent of whites carry a CCR5 allele with a 32 bp deletion (D32) that introduces a premature stop codon (Huang *et al.*, 1996). CCR5 is encoded on chromosome 3p22. Transcribed, translated CCR5-Δ32 lacks an appropriate cellular targeting sequence and consequently is not expressed on the plasma membrane. CCR5-Δ32 homozygotes are substantially protected against HIV-1 infection and disease progression after infection (Dean *et al.*, 1996; Huang *et al.*, 1996).

A second, distinct chemokine polymorphism at the CCR2 locus located on chromosome 3p23 confers a similar effect. Substitution of valine for isoleucine at amino acid position 64 in the first transmembrane domain of a minor HIV co-receptor (CCR2) has also been associated with delayed progression of HIV-1 disease and death (Smith *et al.*, 1997). In contrast, individuals homozygous for a multisite haplotype of the CCR5 regulatory element CCR5-P1 experience accelerated progression of HIV-1 disease (Martin *et al.*, 1998). Ten CCR5 promoter haplotype alleles exist, CCR5-P1–P10. Four are common variants, including CCR5-P1, and six are rare. Rapid progression of HIV-1 disease in CCR5-P10 individuals does not necessarily reflect altered phenotype conferred through dysregulation of CCR5. Linkage analysis suggests that CCR5-P1 may be linked to the CCR2-641 allele and that accelerated HIV-1 disease is caused by a trait conferred through CCR2 expression (Martin *et al.*, 1998).

8.5 HIV-1 infection and pancytopenia

Lentiviral infections have a long incubation period associated with constant production of minimal quantities of virus in lymphatic tissue. Some investigators have failed to show evidence that HIV-1 infects human $CD34^+$ marrow cells in culture using polymerase chain reaction (PCR) and fluorescence-activated cell sorting (FACS) analysis (von Laer *et al.*, 1990). However, other investigators have detected HIV-1 mRNA expression in $CD34^+$ hematological progenitor cells *ex vivo* (Stanley *et al.*, 1992). HIV-1 has been shown to bind and enter early blood progenitors; however, it is not clear if such infections are productive. Clusters of HIV-1-infected cells can be observed around seroconversion and represent a reservoir for low-level productive infection during clinical latency. Interestingly, individuals expressing HIV-1 mRNA in bone marrow appear more likely to suffer from HIV-1 encephalitis late in the disease than those in whom no viral message could be found (Weiser *et al.*, 1996). MPs are the primary infected cell infected in marrow, kidney, lung and brain.

Marrow studies of HIV-1-infected individuals create no specific picture. Marrow cellularity may be increased, normal or decreased (Shenoy and Lin, 1986; Zon *et al.*, 1987). A slight myeloid hyperplasia has been reported (Zon *et al.*, 1987; O'Hara, 1989). Quantitative studies show increases in monocytes and giant metamyelocytes of 35 and 17.5 per cent, respectively (Kaloutsi *et al.*, 1994). Large numbers of denuded megakaryocyte nuclei are observed even in the absence of thrombocytopenia (Zucker-Franklin *et al.*, 1989). Macrophage iron stores (Costello, 1988) and marrow reticulin are frequently increased (Spivak *et al.*, 1984), particularly in HIV-1-infected individuals with concurrent viral or mycobacterial infection. High marrow macrophage iron grade has a strong inverse correlation with survival (de Monye *et al.*, 1999), probably because increased marrow iron usually reflects an opportunistic viral or mycobacterial infection. It seems that despite infection of common or myeloid-specific progenitors, HIV-1 infection of marrow has little effect on bone marrow histology.

Peripheral findings are strangely incongruent with marrow histology. HIV-1 patients commonly experience anemia, granulocytopenia with a left shift, lymphopenia and thrombocytopenia (Karpatkin, 1987; Folks *et al.*, 1988; Sun *et al.*, 1989). Components of HIV-1-associated pancytopenia can worsen with disease progression. For instance, as $CD4^+$ lymphocyte counts decline, anemia and thrombocytopenia emerge. Clinical evidence shows that between 5 and 16 per cent of asymptomatic HIV-1-infected individuals (Metroka *et al.*, 1983; Abrams, 1986) and 70–95 per cent of late-stage HIV-1 patients are anemic upon presentation (Spivak *et al.*, 1984; Zon *et al.*, 1987). HIV-1-associated anemia is associated with disproportionately low reticulocyte counts (Aboulafia and Mitsuyasu, 1991), suggesting ineffective erythropoiesis, yet marrow studies show no apparent defect in red cell maturation. The incidence of thrombocytopenia in asymptomatic HIV-1-infected individuals ranges between 5 and 12 per cent and can be as high as 30 per cent in end-stage HIV-1 patients. Many investigators have focused on the marrow and HIV-1 infection of CD34$^+$ as the precipitating event preceding HIV-1-associated pancytopenia (Schneider and Picker, 1985; Delacretaz *et al.*, 1987; Zon and Groopman, 1988). Although marrow infection represents a potent reservoir for virus during disease progression, HIV-1 infection of progenitor cells probably does not contribute to the abnormally low numbers of circulating peripheral blood elements. Instead, there may exist a peripheral mechanism for anergy or premature removal of otherwise healthy cells from the circulation (Abrams *et al.*, 1984).

8.6 HIV-associated nephropathy (HIVAN)

Overall, 40 per cent of HIV-1 patients exhibit proteinuria at some point in the disease (Bourgoignie, 1990). HIV-1-infected humans can suffer many different types of parenchymal kidney diseases secondary to systemic immune dysregulation or opportunistic infection, including acute tubular dysfunction, hemolytic–uremic syndrome, lupuslike syndrome and immune complex deposition diseases (Guerra *et al.*, 1987; Kim and Factor; 1987; Kenouch *et al.*, 1990; Beaufils *et al.*, 1995). Other patients develop a nonspecific progressive nephrotic syndrome in association with HIV-1 disease called HIV-1-associated nephropathy (HIVAN) (Gardenswartz *et al.*, 1984; Pardo *et al.*, 1984; Rao *et al.*, 1984; Cohen and Nast, 1988).

HIVAN is characterized by focal segmental and global glomerulosclerosis, mild to severe proliferation of mesangial cells (MCs), thickening of the mesangial matrix, vacuolation of glomerular epithelial cells (so-called urine microcysts) and eventual collapse of glomerular capillaries (Ray *et al.*, 1995; D'Agati and Appel, 1997). Tubular and interstitial tissue destruction is also observed (Cohen and Nast, 1988). This constellation is known as HIVAN, in America affects mostly blacks and may progress to end-stage renal disease in months (D'Agati and Appel, 1997).

Infiltration of monocytes and macrophages (Neumann *et al.*, 1995) has been observed in conjunction with HIVAN and may drive disease pathogenesis. Infection and proliferation of MCs also appear to be involved. MCs share some phenotypic traits with marrow-derived macrophages. For instance, MCs express Fc receptors and CD4 (Neuwirth *et al.*, 1988; Green *et al.*, 1992; Gomez-Guerrero *et al.*, 1993) and can be infected with HIV-1 *in vitro* (Green *et al.*, 1992). CCR chemokine receptors also have been detected in an immortal MC line *in vitro* (Banas *et al.*, 1999). However, MCs are not derived from bone marrow but rather from vascular smooth muscle cells (Schlondorff, 1987). HIV-1 genes have been detected in renal biopsy specimens from HIV-1-infected individuals (Kimmel *et al.*, 1993), though the predominant mechanism for viral entry in HIV-1-infected individuals remains unclear. MCs probably are infected by M-tropic HIV-1 strains during early stages of infection, before or around seroconversion. *In vitro*, supernatants from HIV-1-infected macrophages lead to MC proliferation and collagen synthesis (Mattana *et al.*, 1993). During the clinical latent period, infected kidney cells seem to produce little virus. In late-stage HIV-1 disease, viral replication may be reactivated. Spread of viral infection among MP populations in the glomerular microenvironment may prime kidney MPs for subsequent immune activation. Activated peripheral MPs and MCs create a destructive immune cascade leading to alteration of glomerular architecture, vacuolation and functional renal compromise (much like in the brain). MCs have the capability to secrete chemokines, attract leukocytes into kidney parenchyma and propagate immune-mediated damage.

The effector mechanisms for MP-mediated renal damage probably involve the fibrogenic cytokine, transforming growth factor-β (TGF-β) (Okuda *et al.*, 1990). TGF-β has been shown to increase MC production and deposition of basement membrane components such as type IV collagen, fibronectin and laminin in experimental models of glomerulonephritis (MacKay *et al.*, 1989; Okuda *et al.*, 1990; Wardle, 1991). In the kidney, TGF-β is secreted by activated macrophages and resident MCs. In HIV-1 patients, TGF-β is also elevated in serum (Allen *et al.*, 1991). Whether TGF-β from blood or from infiltrating monocytes stimulates MCs to synthesize matrix components *in vivo* is not clear. The HIV-1 early regulatory protein Tat also may play a role in glomerular pathogenesis. Tat has been detected in HIVAN kidneys but not in similar specimens taken from HIV-1-infected, HIVAN (–) individuals (Yamamoto *et al.*, 1999). These findings may indicate that pathogenesis depends on local viral replication, may implicate Tat as a stimulator of TGF-β secretion from mesangial and/or peripheral mononuclear cells, or may represent deposition of viral protein from peripheral blood.

8.7 HIV-1 and pulmonary interstitial pneumonitis

HIV-associated interstitial lung disease (HIV-ILD) affects predominantly vertically infected pediatric patients, but also can affect HIV-1-infected adults during late-stage disease (Chayt *et al.*, 1986). Both populations display a non-specific diffuse pulmonary infiltrate on chest X-ray. Afflicted children typically develop insidious cough, digital clubbing, salivary gland enlargement and lymphadenopathy despite normal auscultory exam (Pitt, 1991). Adults usually present with dyspnea (Griffiths *et al.*, 1995). Before the era of highly active antiretroviral therapy (HAART), an estimated 30–50 per cent of children perinatally infected with HIV-1 developed ILD (Jason *et al.*, 1988; Pizzo *et al.*, 1988). At least 59 per cent of HIV-1-positive adults displayed infiltrative alveolar lymphocytosis, independent of disease stage or clinical symptoms (Guillon *et al.*, 1988; Palange *et al.*, 1991). Biopsy is necessary for diagnosis. In both populations, alveolar and interlobular septae, and subpleural and peribronchial lymphatics become infiltrated with benign polyclonal B cells, plasma cells, and CD4+ and CD8+ T lymphocytes (Plata *et al.*, 1987; Moran *et al.*, 1994; Griffiths *et al.*, 1995), most of which have anti-HIV activity. The pattern of lymphocytic infiltration is usually diffuse with occasional nodules.

Alveolar macrophages (AMs) become infected at or around the time of the acute seroconversion reaction and then are primed for subsequent immune activation. Because AMs are the primary antigen-presenting cells in lung, HIV-1-infected, activated AMs recruit CD4+ T lymphocytes for MHC surveillance. Infected AMs preferentially stimulate the Th1 arm of the immune response and direct recruitment of CD8+ T lymphocytes into lung parenchyma. However, unlike CD8+ T lymphocyte responses to many other pulmonary viruses, the anti-HIV CD8+ response is greatly amplified by cytokine overexpression by AMs. AMs from HIV-1-infected patients secrete elevated levels of IL-8, MIP-1α, TNF-α, IL-12, granulocyte–macrophage colony-stimulating factor (GM-CSF) and IL-10 (Agostini *et al.*, 1992; Antinori *et al.*, 1992; Denis and Ghadirian, 1994a,b). The fact that infiltrating CD8+ cells have specific cytotoxic effects against HIV-1-infected cells suggests that presentation of HIV-1 antigens by AMs is necessary to initiate pathogenic events in HIV-1- ILD. However, there appears to be no strict quantitative correlation between increased HIV antigen expression and immune response in HIV-1-ILD (Denis and Ghadirian, 1994b), suggesting that the abnormally vigorous CD8⁺ lymphocyte infiltrate is a function of immune activation not absolute tissue virus burden.

8.8 HIV-1 neuropathogenesis

Virus enters CNS parenchyma and the highly vascularized meninges at or around the time of the acute HIV-1 seroconversion reaction (Davis *et al.*, 1992). Early neurological symptoms manifest as an aseptic meningoencephalitis complex including transient nuchal rigidity, retroorbital headaches and photophobia. HIV-1-infected peripheral monocytes and/or CD4⁺ T lymphocytes are the first infected cells to enter the brain. Lymphocytes may migrate in and out of brain parenchyma through the microvasculature, but do not play an appreciable role in HIV-1 neuropathogenesis. Terminally differentiated brain MPs harbor the majority of integrated virus in the brain. As peripheral viral loads decline during immune control of primary infection, trafficking of HIV-1-infected MPs in and out of perivascular regions of the brain also declines. Indeed, brains of asymptomatic individuals usually contain low levels of HIV-1 nucleic acids (RNA or proviral DNA) or none at all (Koenig *et al.*, 1986; Bell *et al.*, 1993; Donaldson *et al.*, 1994; Gosztonyi *et al.*, 1994; Teo *et al.*, 1997). HIV-1 infection primes MPs for a vigorous response to heterogeneous activation signals (Cotter *et al.*, 2000), but is not the major determinant of MP-mediated tissue destruction in brain.

In late-stage HIV-1 disease, patients can develop motor impairment and severe cognitive impairment, including distraction, forgetfulness, apathy, withdrawal, disinterest, emotional lability and florid dementia (Zink *et al.*, 1999b). Taken together, multiple lines of evidence suggest that clinical neurological symptoms observed late in HIV-1 disease result from re-colonization of brain by HIV-1-infected bone marrow-derived macrophages (Gartner, 2000). First, clinical neurological symptoms appear subsequent to the decline in blood CD4⁺ T lymphocyte counts. Secondly, symptoms correlate better with infiltration of peripheral macrophages in brain than with absolute virus in cerebrospinal fluid (CSF) or parenchyma (Glass *et al.*, 1995). Thirdly, molecular analysis of highly variable regions of the HIV-1 *env* gene shows that brain isolates from deep white matter of brain late in HIV-1 disease are more closely related to bone marrow isolates than those from any other tissue (Gartner, 2000). Fourthly, increases in CD16 (an activation marker) on circulating macrophages correlates with dementia (Pulliam *et al.*, 1997). Late in HIV-1 disease, peripheral macrophages become activated, predisposing them to adhesion to microvascular endothelium in brain, as shown in Figure 4.4, and other tissues. HIV-1 infection of monocytes and macrophages may not be a prerequisite for endothelial transmigration and entry into brain and other tissues.

Within the brain, immune activated perivascular MPs secrete soluble mediators that activate resident microglia, creating a self-sustaining immune cascade that diffuses into parenchyma and can lead to global brain MP activation and functional neurological impairments. Multinucleated giant cells formed from fusion of HIV-infected MPs are the pathological hallmark of HIV-1-associated neuropathology and can be found predominantly in subcortical white matter, deep white tracts and basal ganglia. Other histological features include microglial nodules, neuronal dropout, diffuse myelin pallor and reactive astrocytosis.

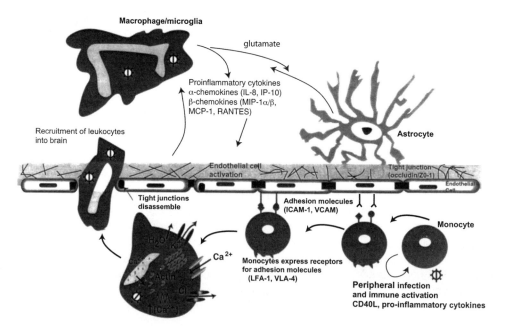

Fig. 4.4 Model for the neuropathogenesis of HIV-1 infection. During HIV-1 infection, monocytes can become immune activated. Like the Trojan horse, infected monocytes can carry virus into the CNS. Infected and/or immune-activated macrophages may reside in and around the microvasculature or migrate into brain parenchyma and differentiate into macrophages and microglia, the brain's resident MPs. A key to monocyte transendothelial microglia is changes in ion channels (potassium, calcium, and chloride channels). Activated brain MPs secrete chemokines to attract more monocytes into tissue and amplify the immune cascade. Diffuse MP activation in brain disrupts neuronal homeostasis, leading to motor and cognitive dysfunction. These events may occur at all stages of disease, but are most prominent during advanced viral disease. See Plate 3.

Activated brain MPs alter neuronal function and affect the induction of HIV-1 associated dementia or HAD through multiple mechanisms. First, the healthy CNS relies on microglia to produce neurotrophins. HIV hijacks constitutive protein synthesis machinery and prevents microglia-mediated neurotrophin synthesis. Secondly, MP secretory products disrupt neuron–astrocyte and/or neuron–oligodendrocyte interactions, leading to impaired neuronal function and ultimately cell death. Thirdly, activated MPs kill neurons directly through secretion of inflammatory factors. Candidate neurotoxins include small molecules such as nitric oxide (NO), lipids such as platelet-activating factor (PAF) and other arachidonic acid metabolites, kyneurine metabolites and pro-inflammatory cytokines. Fourthly, the MP compartment serves as a site of synthesis and export for viral products that are toxic to neurons. Tat and gp120 have both been shown to cause neuronal damage and destruction *in vitro*. In general, the pathogenesis of HIV encephalitis is not limited to single mechanisms, but rather represents multiple insults resulting from dysregulation of brain MP homeostasis.

8.9 HIV-2

HIV-2 is found primarily in western regions of Africa and its sequence is more homologous to that of SIVs isolated from indigenous primates than to HIV-1 (Marx *et al.*, 1991; Gao *et al.*, 1992). Analyses of genetic variation primarily within the envelope gene among a panel of HIV-2 isolates have revealed five subtypes (A–E) (Gao *et al.*, 1994), only two of which (A and B) appear to be widespread (Dietrich *et al.*, 1989; Sankale *et al.*, 1995).

HIV-1 and HIV-2 share some geographical overlap in central Africa, and co-infection of individuals with HIV-1 and -2 has been reported (Takehisa *et al.*, 1998). Routes of transmission appear to be identical to those of HIV-1. Clinical progression of HIV-2 patients is generally slower than that of HIV-1-infected patients, but few specific data describing the natural history of HIV-2 are available. It has been shown that HIV-2 patients display elevated neopterin and β_2-microglobulin levels compared with healthy controls (Kestens *et al.*, 1992), suggesting that the immune response in HIV-2 infection resembles that in HIV-1 patients.

Unlike in HIV infection, early HIV-2 isolates can infect both macrophages and T cells and generally do not cause syncytia in T-cell cultures. Non-syncytia-forming isolates are associated with a 'slow-low' clinical progression in which viral load is low (Essex and Kanki, 1999). During disease progression, syncytia-inducing strains can emerge and are associated with higher viral loads. Morphologically, HIV-2 can be distinguished from HIV-1 in some electron micrographs based on a lucent space surrounding the electron-dense capsid (Palmer *et al.*, 1988, 1985). This slight ultrastructural divergence may be due to the localization of Vpx, a single gene product unique to HIV-2, in the proteina-ceous matrix surrounding the capsid.

8.10 SIV

Experimental and naturally occurring SIV strains resemble HIV in genomic organiza-tion, cellular tropism and tissue distribution (Chakrabarti *et al.*, 1987; Narayan and Clements, 1989). SIV strains share greater sequence homology and morphology with HIV-2 than with HIV-1. HIV-1 expresses the accessory protein Vpu, not found in SIV or HIV-2. SIV and HIV-2 express the gene *vpx*, not found in HIV-1. Vpx seems to have an essential though unidentified role in replication in macrophages. Biologically, SIV and HIV-1 share many properties but differ in others. For instance, like HIV-1, M-tropic SIV strains use CD4 for attachment and CCR5 for entry into macrophages. However, unlike HIV-1, lymphotropic SIV strains also frequently rely on CCR5, but not CXCR4, for entry into lymphocytes (Edinger *et al.*, 1997). Despite the use of CCR5 for entry into both target cells, distinct cellular tropism exists among SIV variants. Site-directed mutagenesis studies within SIV *env* have shown that as few as three or four amino acid substitutions can shift cellular tropism (Mori *et al.*, 1992, 1993). Mutations within the V3 region of SIV *env* alter virus attachment and entry. However, *env* mutations in regions other than V3 also affect macrophage tropism, suggesting that *env* determinants possibly contribute to tropism through alterations of post-entry stages in the lentiviral life cycle (Mori *et al.*, 1993).

Simian models have provided highly relevant information describing immunological events surrounding primary infection. SIV infection of mucosal macrophages and CD1a$^+$ dendritic cells, both of which express CD4, is a crucial and reproducible component of primary infection in monkeys inoculated through oral and vaginal mucosa (Miller *et al.*, 1992a; Miller *et al.*, 1992b). However, some SIV strains that replicate well in simian macrophages *in vitro* do not initiate systemic infection after inoculation of the vaginal mucosa (Miller *et al.*, 1998). As in primary HIV-1 infection of humans, SIV-specific

CD8$^+$ T cells are crucial for reducing primary viremia and forcing the virus into a chronic active state within MP reservoirs (Matano *et al.*, 1998; Igarashi *et al.*, 1999; Schmitz *et al.*, 1999). Differences in the primary CD8$^+$ T-cell response may account for the differential infectivity of SIV strains *in vivo*.

At the functional level, AMs removed from an SIV-infected primate demonstrate reduced intracellular killing and O_2^- release (Brodie *et al.*, 1994). These effects probably result from *in vivo* alterations in the lymphocyte–macrophage interaction based on three lines of evidence (Brodie *et al.*, 1994). SIV infection of macrophages from uninfected primates does not cause functional defects in macrophage function *in vitro*; *ex vivo* analysis of alveolar macrophages from SIV-infected individuals showed no functional differences between p27$^+$ and p27$^-$ (SIV capsid protein) cells; and supernatants from stimulated PBMCs or CD4$^+$ T cells partially restore macrophage function *in vitro*.

Infected macrophages contribute to tissue degeneration in multiple organs, making the simian model attractive for studying macrophage-mediated tissue destruction. Late-stage SIV infection is associated with hematological abnormalities, including myelodysplasia, pancytopenia and autoimmune hemolytic anemia (Kitagawa *et al.*, 1991). SIV-infected macrophages contribute to suppression of hematopoietic progenitor colony formation in laboratory analysis. SIV infection alters secretion of cytokines and other factors from bone marrow macrophages (Leiderman *et al.*, 1987; Cannistra *et al.*, 1988). SIV may also infect early myelocytes or common hematopoietic progenitors (Folks *et al.*, 1988). In kidney, SIV infection causes focal and global glomerulosclerosis, mesangial proliferation, immune complex deposition and sometimes mild azotemia (Gattone *et al.*, 1998). CD68$^+$ peripheral macrophages deliver SIV to the mesangium and spread infection to mesangial cells and possibly tubular epithelial cells as detected by p27 immunohistochemistry. SIV-induced renal pathology differs from HIV-1-induced renal pathology in humans in that SIV seems to spare tubulointerstitial regions more than the human counterpart. Development of SIV renal pathology is associated with inoculation or generation of M-tropic variants (Stephens *et al.*, 1998). Some M-tropic variants, such as SIV$_{mac}$R71/17E, may cause greater glomerulosclerosis, while others, such as SIV$_{mac}$239, may have a greater effect on tubulointerstitial pathology (Stephens *et al.*, 1998). In lung, about 20–50 per cent of SIV-infected individuals develop infiltration of alveolar septa by CD8$^+$ lymphocytes and hyperplasia of peribronchial and perivascular lymphoid tissue (Baskerville *et al.*, 1992; Mankowski *et al.*, 1998). Infiltrating CD8$^+$ cells may represent an immunopathological response to M-tropic virus (Mankowski *et al.*, 1998).

Progression of SIV neurological disease also mimics that observed in HIV-1-infected humans. During primary infection, SIV-infected macrophages traverse the blood–brain-barrier and colonize tissue surrounding brain microvasculature (Chakrabarti *et al.*, 1991; Hurtrel *et al.*, 1993). Later in disease, SIV-infected macrophages again migrate into brain, re-establishing perivascular viral reservoirs. The presence of SIV correlates with increased density of perivascular macrophages and microglia in cerebral subcortical white matter and increased intrathecal levels of macrophage-produced quinolinic acid (Lane *et al.*, 1996). The number of perivascular macrophages, in turn, correlates with the severity of CNS lesions (Zink *et al.*, 1999a). Monocytic cuffing of brain microvasculature is observed in HIV-1-infected humans but is not as pronounced as similar lesions from lentiviruses-infected ungulates.

   The propensity of SIV infections to recapitulate features of tissue pathology in bone marrow, kidney, lung and brain (Kitagawa *et al.*, 1991; Baskerville *et al.*, 1992; Sharma *et al.*, 1992; Alpers *et al.*, 1997) makes SIV an invaluable model for studying temporal and cellular aspects of immunodeficiency virus disease. However, both HIV-2, which can infect baboons and cause immunodeficiency (Barnett *et al.*, 1994), and SIV have structural features within the *env* gene that distinguish them from HIV-1 and make them unsuitable for studying many molecular aspects of immune system–virus interaction. The ideal primate model for HIV-1 disease, then, would have three features. First, the macrophage component of the disease would mimic that observed in HIV-1 infection. Initial inoculation should be carried out with M-tropic virus directly into blood or at the oral, vaginal or rectal mucosa. Later in disease, macrophage-mediated pathology would be observed in multiple tissues. Secondly, the lymphocyte component of the disease would mimic that of HIV-1. Emergence of lymphocyte-tropic viral strains would correlate with a shift from a Th1 to Th2 phenotype, increased viral replication in lymphoid tissue and peripheral blood, increased viral load, decline in the number of circulating $CD4^+$ lymphocytes, clinical immune deficiency and opportunistic infections and/or tumors. Thirdly, the lentiviral strain used should express the HIV-1 *env* gene. Rapid and continued viral diversity is typical of lentiviruses, particularly within *env*. For this reason, animal studies elucidating the kinetics of HIV-1 *env* mutation are crucial for development of vaccines, therapeutics and neutralizing antibody targeted against the viral envelope. Although HIV-1 can infect chimpanzees, it causes neither immunodeficiency nor tissue pathology in this host (Spertzel 1989).

   The most relevant animal model for HIV-1 disease uses primates infected with SIV–HIV chimeras to recapitulate tissue, immune and molecular features of HIV-1 disease. So-called SHIV chimeras have been derived expressing HIV-1 *tat*, *rev*, *vpu* and *env* genes within an SIV background. Early SHIV isolates infect macaque PBMCs *in vitro* (Shibata *et al.*, 1991) and *in vivo* (Li *et al.*, 1992; Sakuragi *et al.*, 1992), but failed to recapitulate the lymphocyte and macrophage components of disease. Recently, an M-tropic clone, $SHIV_{KU-2}$, has been characterized that recapitulates many features of HIV-1 disease in macaques. (Liu *et al.*, 1999). $SHIV_{KU-2}$ was isolated from the CSF of a Rhesus macaque following inoculation with $SHIV_{KU-1}$, a chimeric virus originally isolated from a Pig-tailed macaque that developed severe $CD4^+$ lymphocyte loss and immunodeficiency (Joag *et al.*, 1994; Stephens *et al.*, 1997). Inoculation of oral and vaginal mucosa with $SHIV_{KU-2}$ can initiate disease. The clinical asymptomatic period between seroconversion and clinical progression is shorter and end-stage decline is more rapid in the chimeric model compared with HIV-1. $SHIV_{KU-2}$ rapidly replicates to high titers, causes a subsequent reduction in $CD4^+$ T lymphocytes, and is associated with histopathology in lymphoid tissue, spleen, kidney and brain resembling that of HIV-1 (Liu *et al.*, 1999). Because chimeric virions express HIV-1 *env*, the $SHIV_{KU-2}$ model provides means for studying effects of mutations within HIV-1 *env* on cellular tropism, immune response and disease pathogenesis *in vivo*; testing therapeutic and vaccine strategies; and evaluating temporal pathophysiological changes in marrow, brain, kidney and lung.

8.11 Murine HIV-1 infections

In the absence of an identified murine lentivirus, multiple approaches have been applied to generate small animal models for HIV-1 disease. Xenograft models have provided valuable information describing tissue-specific responses to HIV-1, but each represents only a single component of disease. For example, SCID mice reconstituted with human hematopoietic cells and infected with HIV-1 recapitulate some of the lymphocyte aspects of disease (McCune *et al.*, 1991), but do not develop multiorgan system disease. Engraftment of human tissue into the anterior chamber of the rat eye or into the interscapular fat pad of SCID mice (Cvetkovich *et al.*, 1992; Achim *et al.*, 1993), or inoculation of HIV-1-infected human macrophages into target organs (Tyor *et al.*, 1993; Persidsky *et al.*, 1996) have provided information on tissue-specific responses to HIV-1, but fail to describe interaction between organ degeneration and disease evolution in the periphery.

A transgenic mouse expressing human CD4 was constructed, but could not be infected by HIV-1 (Lores *et al.*, 1992). However, after discovery of chemokine receptors and their importance in the early stages if the HIV-1 life cycle, a transgenic model expressing human CD4 and human CCR5 was developed that is susceptible to HIV-1 infection (Browning *et al.*, 1997). Although HIV-1 DNA was detected in lymph nodes and splenocytes, macrophages from these tissues did not synthesize progeny virions, suggesting a block in post-integration stages of the viral life cycle. A different group created a transgenic mouse expressing the complete HIV-1 coding sequences under the control of a hCD4 promoter, so that only CD4$^+$ lymphocytes and MPs would become infected (Hanna *et al.*, 1998). These CD4C/HIV^{WT} mice developed severe immunosuppression, muscle wasting and characteristic HIV-1 tissue pathology in lymphoid organs, kidneys and lungs.

9 Summary

Several themes underlie virus–MP interactions.

(1) Macrophages have a dual role in viral pathogenesis. They can assist in both innate and acquired immune responses to eliminate virus through phagocytosis and entracellular of viral particles, presentation of viral antigen in the context of class I and class II MHC molecules and secretion of potent soluble antiviral factors such as IFNs and tissue toxins.

(2) Despite these functions, macrophages are commonly target cells for abortive, latent, restricted and permissive infections. Infected MPs can act as a reservoir during disease progression. Many herpesviruses establish latent infections in MPs in which viral genome remains in the nucleus in the form of a circularized episome. For lentiviruses, the viral genome integrates into host chromosomes and is transcribed at low levels. Murine polioviruses can infect brain MPs and persist in the face of immune pressure despite their inability to form episomes or integrate. In all cases, transcription of viral genes is determined by interplay among the MP, the virus and the exogenous environment (cytokines, chemokines and other immune factors).

(3) The infected MP may itself participate in disease pathogenesis. Alterations in effector functions and cytokine profiles can lead to altered MP phenotypes. Examples include hyperplasia as in the case of Kaposi's sarcoma or neurodegeneration in the case of HAD.

These ideas, taken together, reflect the diverse outcomes of MP–virus interactions.

Acknowledgements

We thank Ms. Robin Taylor for outstanding administrative and secretarial support. This work was supported, in part, by research grants (to H.E.G.) by the National Institutes of Health USA; Pol NS31492-01, Rol NS 34239-01, Rol NS342239-01, Rol NS361226-01, and Pol MH57556-01.

References

Aboulafia, D.M. and Mitsuyasu, R.T. (1991). Hematologic abnormalities in AIDS. *Hematology/Oncology Clinics of North America*, **5**, 195–214.

Abrams, D.I. (1986). Lymphadenopathy related to the acquired immunodeficiency syndrome in homosexual men. *Medical Clinics of North America*, **70**, 693–706.

Abrams, D.I., Chinn, E.K., Lewis, B.J., Volberding, P.A., Conant, M.A. and Townsend, R.M. (1984). Hematologic manifestations in homosexual men with Kaposi's sarcoma. *American Journal of Clinical Pathology*, **81**, 13–8.

Achim, C.L., Miners, D.K., Burrola, P.G., Martin, F.C. and Wiley, C.A. (1993). *In vivo* model of HIV infection of the human brain. *Developmental Neuroscience*, **15**, 423–32.

Adler, B., Adler, H., Pfister, H., Jungi, T.W. and Peterhans, E. (1997). Macrophages infected with cytopathic bovine viral diarrhea virus release a factor(s) capable of priming uninfected macrophages for activation-induced apoptosis. *Journal of Virology*, **71**, 3255–8.

Agostini, C., Trentin, L., Zambello, R., Bulian, P., Caenazzo, C., Cipriani, A. *et al.* (1992). Release of granulocyte–macrophage colony-stimulating factor by alveolar macrophages in the lung of HIV-1-infected patients. A mechanism accounting for macrophage and neutrophil accumulation. *Journal of Immunology*, **149**, 3379–85.

Ahn, K., Angulo, A., Ghazal, P., Peterson, P.A., Yang, Y. and Fruh, K. (1996). Human cytomegalovirus inhibits antigen presentation by a sequential multistep process. *Proceedings of the National Academy of Sciences USA*, **93**, 10990–5.

Albrecht, T., Fons, M.P., Boldogh, I., AbuBakar, S., Deng, C.Z. and Millinoff, D. (1991). Metabolic and cellular effects of human cytomegalovirus infection. *Transplantation Proceedings*, **23**, 48–54, discussion 54–5.

Albrecht, J.C., Nicholas, J., Biller, D., Cameron, K.R., Biesinger, B., Newman, C. *et al.* (1992). Primary structure of the herpesvirus saimiri genome. *Journal of Virology*, **66**, 5047–58.

Alcami, A., Carrascosa, A.L. and Vinuela, E. (1990). Interaction of African swine fever virus with macrophages. *Virus Research*, **17**, 93–104.

Alfano, M., Schmidtmayerova, H., Amella, C.A., Pushkarsky, T. and Bukrinsky, M. (1999). The B-oligomer of pertussis toxin deactivates CC chemokine receptor 5 and blocks entry of M-tropic HIV-1 strains. *Journal of Experimental Medicine*, **190**, 597–605.

Allen, J.B., Wong, H.L., Guyre, P.M., Simon, G.L. and Wahl, S.M. (1991). Association of circulating receptor FcγRIII-positive monocytes in AIDS patients with elevated levels of transforming growth factor-β. *Journal of Clinical Investigation*, **87**, 1773–9.

Allen, L.A. and Aderem, A. (1996). Molecular definition of distinct cytoskeletal structures involved in complement- and Fc receptor-mediated phagocytosis in macrophages. *Journal of Experimental Medicine*, **184**, 627–37.

Alpers, C.E., Tsai, C.C., Hudkins, K.L., Cui, Y., Kuller, L., Benveniste, R.E. *et al.* (1997). Focal segmental glomerulosclerosis in primates infected with a simian immunodeficiency virus. *AIDS Research and Human Retroviruses*, **13**, 413–24.

Anderson, K.P. and Fennie, E.H. (1987). Adenovirus early region 1A modulation of interferon antiviral activity. *Journal of Virology*, **61**, 787–95.

Anderson, L., Klevjer-Anderson, P. and Leggitt, H. (1983). Susceptibility of blood-derived monocytes and macrophages to caprine arthritis encephalitis virus. *Infection and Immunity*, **41**, 837–40.

Andreesen, R., Brugger, W., Scheibenbogen, C., Kreutz, M., Leser, H.G., Rehm, A. *et al.* (1990). Surface phenotype analysis of human monocyte to macrophage maturation. *Journal of Leukocyte Biology*, **47**, 490–7.

Antinori, A., Tamburrini, E., Pagliari, G., Maiuro, G., Pallavicini, F., De Luca, A. *et al.* (1992). Alveolar macrophages from AIDS patients spontaneously produce elevated levels of TNF-α *in vitro*. *Allergologia et Immunopathologia*, **20**, 249–54.

Aoki, E., Semba, R., Mikoshiba, K. and Kashiwamata, S. (1991). Predominant localization in glial cells of free L-arginine. Immunocytochemical evidence. *Brain Research*, **547**, 190–2.

Ariyoshi, K., Schim van der Loeff, M., Cook, P., Whitby, D., Corrah, T., Jaffar, S. *et al.* (1998). Kaposi's sarcoma in the Gambia, West Africa is less frequent in human immunodeficiency virus type 2 than in human immunodeficiency virus type 1 infection despite a high prevalence of human herpesvirus 8. *Journal of Human Virology*, **1**, 193–9.

Arnheiter, H., Frese, M., Kambadur, R., Meier, E. and Haller, O. (1996). Mx transgenic mice–animal models of health. *Current Topics in Microbiology and Immunology*, **206**, 119–47.

Atchison, R.E., Gosling, J., Monteclaro, F.S., Franci, C., Digilio, L., Charo, I.F. *et al.* (1996). Multiple extracellular elements of CCR5 and HIV-1 entry: dissociation from response to chemokines. *Science*, **274**, 1924–6.

Aubert, C., Chamorro, M. and Brahic, M. (1987). Identification of Theiler's virus infected cells in the central nervous system of the mouse during demyelinating disease. *Microbial Pathogenesis*, **3**, 319–26.

Baer, R., Bankier, A.T., Biggin, M.D., Deininger, P.L., Farrell, P.J., Gibson, T.J. *et al.* (1984). DNA sequence and expression of the B95-8 Epstein–Barr virus genome. *Nature*, **310**, 207–11.

Baggiolini, M., Dewald, B. and Moser, B. (1997). Human chemokines: an update. *Annual Review of Immunology*, **15**, 675–705.

Bailey, O.T., Pappenheimer, A.M., Cheever, F.S., Daniels, J.B. (1949). A murine virus (JHM) causing disseminated encephalomyelitis with extensive destruction of myelin. II. Pathology *Journal of Experimental Medicine*, **90**, 195–212.

Bale, J.F., Jr (1984). Human cytomegalovirus infection and disorders of the nervous system. *Archives of Neurology*, **41**, 310–20.

Banas, B., Luckow, B., Moller, M., Klier, C., Nelson, P.J., Schadde, E. *et al.* (1999). Chemokine and chemokine receptor expression in a novel human mesangial cell line. *Journal of the American Society for Nephrology*, **10**, 2314–22.

Barnett, S.W., Murthy, K.K., Herndier, B.G. and Levy, J.A. (1994). An AIDS-like condition induced in baboons by HIV-2. *Science*, **266**, 642–6.

Barre-Sinoussi, F., Chermann, J.C., Rey, F., Nugeyre, M.T., Chamaret, S., Gruest, J. *et al.* (1983). Isolation of a T-lymphotropic retrovirus from a patient at risk for acquired immune deficiency syndrome (AIDS). *Science*, **220**, 868–71.

Baskerville, A., Ramsay, A.D., Addis, B.J., Dennis, M.J., Cook, R.W., Cranage, M.P. *et al.* (1992). Interstitial pneumonia in simian immunodeficiency virus infection. *Journal of Pathology*, **167**, 241–7.

Basta, S., Knoetig, S.M., Spagnuolo-Weaver, M., Allan, G. and McCullough, K.C. (1999). Modulation of monocytic cell activity and virus susceptibility during differentiation into macrophages. *Journal of Immunology*, **162**, 3961–9.

Beaufils, H., Jouanneau, C., Katlama, C., Sazdovitch, V. and Hauw, J.J. (1995). HIV-associated IgA nephropathy—a post-mortem study. *Nephrology Dialysis Transplantation*, **10**, 35–8.

Bell, J.E., Busuttil, A., Ironside, J.W., Rebus, S., Donaldson, Y.K., Simmonds, P. *et al.* (1993). Human immunodeficiency virus and the brain: investigation of virus load and neuropathologic changes in pre-AIDS subjects. *Journal of Infectious Diseases*, **168**, 818–24.

Belyavsky, M., Belyavskaya, E., Levy, G.A. and Leibowitz, J.L. (1998). Coronavirus MHV-3 induced apoptosis in macrophages. *Virology*, **250**, 41–49.

Beral, V., Peterman, T.A., Berkelman, R.L. and Jaffe, H.W. (1990). Kaposi's sarcoma among persons with AIDS: a sexually transmitted infection? *Lancet*, **335**, 123–8.

Bergelson, J.M. and Finberg, R.W. (1993). Integrins as receptors for virus attachment and cell entry. *Trends in Microbiology*, **1**, 287–8.

Biggar, R.J. and Rabkin, C.S. (1996). The epidemiology of AIDS-related neoplasms. *Hematology/Oncology Clinics of North America*, **10**, 997–1010.

Biggar, R.J., Rosenberg, P.S. and Cote, T. (1996). Kaposi's sarcoma and non-Hodgkin's lymphoma following the diagnosis of AIDS. Multistate AIDS/Cancer Match Study Group [published erratum appears in *International Journal of Cancer* 1997 Mar 17;70(6):727]. *International Journal of Cancer*, **68**, 754–8.

Black, T.L., Safer, B., Hovanessian, A. and Katze, M.G. (1989). The cellular 68,000-Mr protein kinase is highly autophosphorylated and activated yet significantly degraded during poliovirus infection: implications for translational regulation. *Journal of Virology*, **63**, 2244–51.

Blasig, C., Zietz, C., Haar, B., Neipel, F., Esser, S., Brockmeyer, N.H. *et al.* (1997). Monocytes in Kaposi's sarcoma lesions are productively infected by human herpesvirus 8. *Journal of Virology*, **71**, 7963–8.

Bluyssen, H.A., Muzaffar, R., Vlietstra, R.J., van der Made, A.C., Leung, S., Stark, G.R. *et al.* (1995). Combinatorial association and abundance of components of interferon-stimulated gene factor 3 dictate the selectivity of interferon responses. *Proceedings of the National Academy of Sciences USA*, **92**, 5645–9.

Boldin, M.P., Goncharov, T.M., Goltsev, Y.V. and Wallach, D. (1996). Involvement of MACH, a novel MORT1/FADD-interacting protease, in Fas/APO-1- and TNF receptor-induced cell death. *Cell*, **85**, 803–15.

Boldogh, I., AbuBakar, S. and Albrecht, T. (1990). Activation of proto-oncogenes: an immediate early event in human cytomegalovirus infection. *Science*, **247**, 561–4.

Boldogh, I., Fons, M.P. and Albrecht, T. (1993). Increased levels of sequence-specific DNA-binding proteins in human cytomegalovirus-infected cells. *Biochemical and Biophysical Research Communications*, **197**, 1505–10.

Boshoff, C. and Weiss, R.A. (1998). Kaposi's sarcoma-associated herpesvirus. *Advances in Cancer Research*, **75**, 57–86.

Boshoff, C., Schulz, T.F., Kennedy, M.M., Graham, A.K., Fisher, C., Thomas, A. *et al.* (1995). Kaposi's sarcoma-associated herpesvirus infects endothelial and spindle cells. *Nature Medicine*, **1**, 1274–8.

Bottazzi, B., Erba, E., Nobili, N., Fazioli, F., Rambaldi, A. and Mantovani, A. (1990). A paracrine circuit in the regulation of the proliferation of macrophages infiltrating murine sarcomas. *Journal of Immunology*, **144**, 2409–12.

Bourgoignie, J.J. (1990). Renal complications of human immunodeficiency virus type 1. *Kidney International*, **37**, 1571–84.

Brahic, M., Stroop, W.G. and Baringer, J.R. (1981). Theiler's virus persists in glial cells during demyelinating disease. *Cell*, **26**, 123–8.

Brand, S.R., Kobayashi, R. and Mathews, M.B. (1997). The Tat protein of human immunodeficiency virus type 1 is a substrate and inhibitor of the interferon-induced, virally activated protein kinase, PKR. *Journal of Biological Chemistry*, **272**, 8388–95.

Brautigam, A.R., Dutko, F.J., Olding, L.B. and Oldstone, M.B. (1979). Pathogenesis of murine cytomegalovirus infection: the macrophage as a permissive cell for cytomegalovirus infection, replication and latency. *Journal of General Virology*, **44**, 349–59.

Brodie, S.J., Sasseville, V.G., Reimann, K.A., Simon, M.A., Sehgal, P.K. and Ringler, D.J. (1994). Macrophage function in simian AIDS. Killing defects *in vivo* are independent of macrophage infection, associated with alterations in Th phenotype, and reversible with IFN-γ. *Journal of Immunology*, **153**, 5790–801.

Brodie, S.J., Pearson, L.D., Zink, M.C., Bickle, H.M., Anderson, B.C., Marcom, K.A. *et al.* (1995). Ovine lentivirus expression and disease. Virus replication, but not entry, is restricted to macrophages of specific tissues. *American Journal of Pathology*, **146**, 250–63.

Browning, J., Horner, J.W., Pettoello-Mantovani, M., Raker, C., Yurasov, S., DePinho, R.A. *et al.* (1997). Mice transgenic for human CD4 and CCR5 are susceptible to HIV infection. *Proceedings of the National Academy of Sciences USA*, **94**, 14637–41.

Bukrinsky, M., Schmidtmayerova, H., Zybarth, G., Dubrovsky, L., Sherry, B. and Enikolopov, G. (1996). A critical role of nitric oxide in human immunodeficiency virus type 1-induced hyperresponsiveness of cultured monocytes. *Molecular Medicine*, **2**, 460–8.

Burstein, S., Brandriss, M. and Schlesinger, J. (1983). Infection of a macrophage cell line P388D1 with reovirus:effects on immune ascitic fluids and monoclonal antibodies on neutralization and on enhancement of viral growth. *Journal of Immunology*, **130**, 2915–9.

Campbell, A., Slater, J., Cavanaugh, V. and Stenberg, R. (1992). An early event in murine cytomegalovirus replication inhibits presentation of cellular antigens to cytotoxic T lymphocytes. *Journal of Virology*, **66**, 3011–7.

Cannistra, S.A., Groshek, P. and Griffin, J.D. (1988). Monocytes enhance γ-interferon-induced inhibition of myeloid progenitor cell growth through secretion of tumor necrosis factor. *Experimental Hematology*, **16**, 865–70.

Carroll, S.S., Cole, J.L., Viscount, T., Geib, J., Gehman, J. and Kuo, L.C. (1997). Activation of RNase L by 2′,5′-oligoadenylates. Kinetic characterization. *Journal of Biological Chemistry*, **272**, 19193–8.

Cash, E., Bandeira, A., Chirinian, S. and Brahic, M. (1989). Characterization of B lymphocytes present in the demyelinating lesions induced by Theiler's virus [published erratum appears in *Journal of Immunology* 1989 Sep 15;143(6):2081]. *Journal of Immunology*, **143**, 984–8.

Cesarman, E., Nador, R.G., Bai, F., Bohenzky, R.A., Russo, J.J., Moore, P.S. *et al.* (1996). Kaposi's sarcoma-associated herpesvirus contains G protein-coupled receptor and cyclin D homologs which are expressed in Kaposi's sarcoma and malignant lymphoma. *Journal of Virology*, **70**, 8218–23.

Chakrabarti, L., Guyader, M., Alizon, M., Daniel, M.D., Desrosiers, R.C., Tiollais, P. *et al.* (1987). Sequence of simian immunodeficiency virus from macaque and its relationship to other human and simian retroviruses. *Nature*, **328**, 543–7.

Chakrabarti, L., Hurtrel, M., Maire, M.A., Vazeux, R., Dormont, D., Montagnier, L. *et al.* (1991). Early viral replication in the brain of SIV-infected rhesus monkeys. *American Journal of Pathology*, **139**, 1273–80.

Chang, Y., Cesarman, E., Pessin, M.S., Lee, F., Culpepper, J., Knowles, D.M. *et al.* (1994). Identification of herpesvirus-like DNA sequences in AIDS-associated Kaposi's sarcoma. *Science*, **266**, 1865–9.

Chatlynne, L.G., Lapps, W., Handy, M., Huang, Y.Q., Masood, R., Hamilton, A.S. *et al.* (1998). Detection and titration of human herpesvirus-8-specific antibodies in sera from blood donors, acquired immunodeficiency syndrome patients, and Kaposi's sarcoma patients using a whole virus enzyme-linked immunosorbent assay. *Blood*, **92**, 53–8.

Chayt, K.J., Harper, M.E., Marselle, L.M., Lewin, E.B., Rose, R.M., Oleske, J.M. *et al.* (1986). Detection of HTLV-III RNA in lungs of patients with AIDS and pulmonary involvement [published erratum appears in *Journal of the American Medical Association* 1987 Jan 16;257(3):317]. *Journal of the American Medical Association*, **256**, 2356–9.

Chebloune, Y., Karr, B.M., Raghavan, R., Singh, D.K., Leung, K., Sheffer, D. *et al.* (1998). Neuroinvasion by ovine lentivirus in infected sheep mediated by inflammatory cells associated with experimental allergic encephalomyelitis. *Journal of Neurovirology*, **4**, 38–48.

Cheever, F., Daniels, J., Pappenheimer, A. and Bailey, O. (1949). A murine virus (JHM) causing disseminated encephalomyelitis and with extensive destruction of myelin. I. *Journal of Experimental Medicine*, **165**, 1539–51.

Chehimi, J., Starr, S.E., Frank, I., D'Andrea, A., Ma, X., MacGregor, R.R. *et al.* (1994). Impaired interleukin 12 production in human immunodeficiency virus-infected patients. *Journal of Experimental Medicine*, **179**, 1361–6.

Choe, H., Farzan, M., Sun, Y., Sullivan, N., Rollins, B., Ponath, P.D. *et al.* (1996). The β-chemokine receptor CCR3 and CCR5 facilitate infection by primary HIV-1 isolates. *Cell*, **85**, 1135–48.

Chougnet, C., Wynn, T.A., Clerici, M., Landay, A.L., Kessler, H.A., Rusnak, J. *et al.* (1996). Molecular analysis of decreased interleukin-12 production in persons infected with human immunodeficiency virus. *Journal of Infectious Diseases*, **174**, 46–53.

Clark, S.J., Saag, M.S., Decker, W.D., Campbell-Hill, S., Roberson, J.L., Veldkamp, P.J. *et al.* (1991). High titers of cytopathic virus in plasma of patients with symptomatic primary HIV-1 infection. *New England Journal of Medicine*, **324**, 954–60.

Clatch, R.J., Melvold, R.W., Miller, S.D. and Lipton, H.L. (1985). Theiler's murine encephalomyelitis virus (TMEV)-induced demyelinating disease in mice is influenced by the H-2D region: correlation with TEMV-specific delayed-type hypersensitivity. *Journal of Immunology*, **135**, 1408–14.

Clatch, R.J., Lipton, H.L. and Miller, S.D. (1986). Characterization of Theiler's murine encephalomyelitis virus (TMEV)-specific delayed-type hypersensitivity responses in TMEV-induced demyelinating disease: correlation with clinical signs. *Journal of Immunology*, **136**, 920–7.

Clatch, R.J., Melvold, R.W., Dal Canto, M.C., Miller, S.D. and Lipton, H.L. (1987). The Theiler's murine encephalomyelitis virus (TMEV) model for multiple sclerosis shows a strong influence of the murine equivalents of HLA-A, B, and C. *Journal of Neuroimmunology*, **15**, 121–35.

Clatch, R.J., Miller, S.D., Metzner, R., Dal Canto, M.C. and Lipton, H.L. (1990). Monocytes/macrophages isolated from the mouse central nervous system contain infectious Theiler's murine encephalomyelitis virus (TMEV). *Virology*, **176**, 244–54.

Clavel, F., Guetard, D., Brun-Vezinet, F., Chamaret, S., Rey, M.A., Santos-Ferreira, M.O. *et al.* (1986). Isolation of a new human retrovirus from West African patients with AIDS. *Science*, **233**, 343–6.

Clements, J.E., Zink, M.C., Narayan, O. and Gabuzda, D.H. (1994). Lentivirus infection of macrophages. *Immunology Series*, **60**, 589–600.

Cocchi, F., DeVico, A.L., Garzino-Demo, A., Cara, A., Gallo, R.C. and Lusso, P. (1996). The v3 domain of the HIV-1 gp120 envelope glycoprotein is critical for chemokine-mediated blockade of infection. *Nature Medicine*, **2**, 1244–1247.

Cohen, A.H. and Nast, C.C. (1988). HIV-associated nephropathy. A unique combined glomerular, tubular, and interstitial lesion. *Modern Pathology*, **1**, 87–97.

Cole, J.L., Carroll, S.S., Blue, E.S., Viscount, T. and Kuo, L.C. (1997). Activation of RNase L by 2′,5′-oligoadenylates. Biophysical characterization. *Journal of Biological Chemistry*, **272**, 19187–92.

Cork, L.C., Hadlow, W.J., Crawford, T.B., Gorham, J.R. and Piper, R.C. (1974). Infectious leukoen-cephalomyelitis of young goats. *Journal of Infectious Diseases*, **129**, 134–41.

Cork, L.C. and Narayan, O. (1980). The pathogenesis of viral leukoencephalomyelitis–arthritis of goats. I. Persistent viral infection with progressive pathologic changes. *Laboratory Investigation*, **42**, 596–602.

Costello, C. (1988). Haematological abnormalities in human immunodeficiency virus (HIV) disease. *Journal of Clinical Pathology*, **41**, 711–5.

Cotter, R., Burke, W., Thomas, V., Potter, J., Zheng, J. and Gendelman, H.E. (1999). Insights into the neurodegenerative process of Alzheimer's Disease: A role for mononuclear phagocyte-asso-ciated inflammation and Neurotoxicity. *Journal of Leukocyte Biology*, **65**, 416–27.

Cotter, R., Zheng, J., Bauer, M., Ryan, L., Niemann, D., Thomas, E. *et al.* (2001). Regulation of HIV-1 replication β-chemokines and β-chemokine receptors in CD40L-stimulated macrophages: Relevance for HIV-1-associated dementia. *Journal of Virology*, **75**, 6572–83.

Cowdry, E. (1934). The problem of intranuclear inclusion in virus disease. *Archives of Pathology*, **18**, 525–42.

Cox, D., Lee, D.J., Dale, B.M., Calafat, J. and Greenberg, S. (2000). A Rab11-containing rapidly recycling compartment in macrophages that promotes phagocytosis. *Proceedings of the National Academy of Sciences USA*, **97**, 680–5.

Crawford, T.B., Adams, D.S., Sande, R.D., Gorham, J.R. and Henson, J.B. (1980). The connective tissue component of the caprine arthritis–encephalitis syndrome. *American Journal of Pathology*, **100**, 443–54.

Cremer, I., Vieillard, V. and De Maeyer, E. (1999). Interferon-β-induced human immunodeficiency virus resistance in CD34(+) human hematopoietic progenitor cells: correlation with a down-regulation of CCR-5 expression. *Virology*, **253**, 241–9.

Crowe, S.M., Vardaxis, N.J., Kent, S.J., Maerz, A.L., Hewish, M.J., McGrath, M.S. *et al.* (1994). HIV infection of monocyte-derived macrophages *in vitro* reduces phagocytosis of *Candida albi-cans*. *Journal of Leukocyte Biology*, **56**, 318–27.

Cvetkovich, T.A., Lazar, E., Blumberg, B.M., Saito, Y., Eskin, T.A., Reichman, R. *et al.*, (1992). Human immunodeficiency virus type 1 infection of neural xenografts. *Proceedings of the National Academy of Sciences USA*, **89**, 5162–6.

D'Agati, V. and Appel, G. B. (1997). HIV infection and the kidney. *Journal of the American Society for Nephrology*, **8**, 138–52.

Daar, E.S., Moudgil, T., Meyer, R.D. and Ho, D.D. (1991). Transient high levels of viremia in patients with primary human immunodeficiency virus type 1 infection. *New England Journal of Medicine*, **324**, 961–4.

Daniel, M.D., Letvin, N.L., King, N.W., Kannagi, M., Sehgal, P.K., Hunt, R.D. *et al.* (1985). Isolation of T-cell tropic HTLV-III-like retrovirus from macaques. *Science*, **228**, 1201–4.

Dankner, W.M., McCutchan, J.A., Richman, D.D., Hirata, K. and Spector, S.A. (1990). Localization of human cytomegalovirus in peripheral blood leukocytes by *in situ* hybridization. *Journal of Infectious Diseases*, **161**, 31–6.

Davis, L.E., Hjelle, B.L., Miller, V.E. *et al.* (1992). Early viral brain invasion in iatrogenic human immunodeficiency virus infection. *Neurology*, **42**, 1736–1739.

Dean, M., Carrington, M., Winkler, C., Huttley, G.A., Smith, M.W., Allikmets, R. *et al.* (1996). Genetic restriction of HIV-1 infection and progression to AIDS by a deletion allele of the CKR5 structural gene. Hemophilia Growth and Development Study, Multicenter AIDS Cohort Study, Multicenter Hemophilia Cohort Study, San Francisco City Cohort, ALIVE Study [published erratum appears in *Science* 1996 Nov 15;274(5290):1069]. *Science*, **273**, 1856–62.

Delacretaz, F., Schmidt, P.M., Piguet, D., Bachmann, F. and Costa, J. (1987). Histopathology of myelodysplastic syndromes. The FAB classification (proposals) applied to bone marrow biopsy. *American Journal of Clinical Pathology*, **87**, 180–6.

de Monye, C., Karcher, D.S., Boelaert, J.R. and Gordeuk, V.R. (1999). Bone marrow macrophage iron grade and survival of HIV-seropositive patients. *AIDS*, **13**, 375–80.

Denis, M. and Ghadirian, E. (1994a). Alveolar macrophages from subjects infected with HIV-1 express macrophage inflammatory protein-1 α (MIP-1 α): contribution to the CD8$^+$ alveolitis. *Clinical and Experimental Immunology*, **96**, 187–92.

Denis, M. and Ghadirian, E. (1994b). Dysregulation of interleukin 8, interleukin 10, and interleukin 12 release by alveolar macrophages from HIV type 1-infected subjects. *AIDS Research and Human Retroviruses*, **10**, 1619–27.

Desrosiers, R.C., Sasseville, V.G., Czajak, S.C., Zhang, X., Mansfield, K.G., Kaur, A. *et al.* (1997). A herpesvirus of rhesus monkeys related to the human Kaposi's sarcoma-associated herpesvirus. *Journal of Virology*, **71**, 9764–9.

Dietrich, U., Adamski, M., Kreutz, R., Seipp, A., Kuhnel, H. and Rubsamen-Waigmann, H. (1989). A highly divergent HIV-2-related isolate. *Nature*, **342**, 948–50.

Donaldson, Y.K., Bell, J.E., Ironside, J.W., Brettle, R.P., Robertson, J.R., Busuttil, A. *et al.* (1994). Redistribution of HIV outside the lymphoid system with onset of AIDS. *Lancet*, **343**, 383–5.

Dragic, T., Litwin, V., Allaway, G.P., Martin, S.R., Huang, Y., Nagashima, K.A. *et al.* (1996). HIV-1 entry into CD4$^+$ cells is mediated by the chemokines receptor CC-CKR-5. *Nature*, **381**, 667–673.

Drew, W.L., Sweet, E.S., Miner, R.C. and Mocarski, E.S. (1984). Multiple infections by cytomegalovirus in patients with acquired immunodeficiency syndrome: documentation by Southern blot hybridization. *Journal of Infectious Diseases*, **150**, 952–3.

Drouet, C., Shakhov, A.N. and Jongeneel, C.V. (1991). Enhancers and transcription factors control-ling the inducibility of the tumor necrosis factor-α promoter in primary macrophages. *Journal of Immunology*, **147**, 1694–700.

Dudhane, A., Conti, B., Orlikowsky, T., Wang, Z.Q., Mangla, N., Gupta, A. *et al.* (1996). Monocytes in HIV type 1-infected individuals lose expression of costimulatory B7 molecules and acquire cytotoxic activity. *AIDS Research and Human Retroviruses*, **12**, 885–92.

Dunne, D.W., Resnick, D., Greenberg, J., Krieger, M. and Joiner, K.A. (1994). The type I macrophage scavenger receptor binds to gram-positive bacteria and recognizes lipoteichoic acid. *Proceedings of the National Academy of Sciences USA*, **91**, 1863–7.

Edinger, A.L., Amedee, A., Miller, K., Doranz, B.J., Endres, M., Sharron, M. *et al.* (1997). Differential utilization of CCR5 by macrophage and T cell tropic simian immunodeficiency virus strains. *Proceedings of the National Academy of Sciences USA*, **94**, 4005–10.

Ellermann-Eriksen, S. (1993). Autocrine secretion of interferon-α/β and tumour necrosis factor-α synergistically activates mouse macrophages after infection with herpes simplex virus type 2. *Journal of General Virology*, **74**, 2191–9.

Essex, M. and Kanki, P. (1999). Human immunodeficiency virus type 2 (HIV-2). In Merigan, T.C.Jr., Bartlett, J.G. and Bolognesi, D. (ed.), *Textbook of AIDS Medicine*. Williams and Wilkins, Baltimore, 985–1001.

Fauci, A.S. (1996). Host factors and the pathogenesis of HIV-induced disease. *Nature*, **384**, 529–34.

Fiette, L., Aubert, C., Brahic, M. and Rossi, C.P. (1993). Theiler's virus infection of β₂-microglobulin-deficient mice. *Journal of Virology*, **67**, 589–92.

Fisher, A.G., Feinberg, M.B., Josephs, S.F., Harper, M.E., Marselle, L.M., Reyes, G. *et al.* (1986). The trans-activator gene of HTLV-III is essential for virus replication. *Nature*, **320**, 367–71.

Fishman, P.S., Gass, J.S., Swoveland, P.T., Lavi, E., Highkin, M.K. and Weiss, S.R. (1985). Infection of the basal ganglia by a murine coronavirus. *Science*, **229**, 877–9.

Flore, O., Rafii, S., Ely, S., O'Leary, J.J., Hyjek, E.M. and Cesarman, E. (1998). Transformation of primary human endothelial cells by Kaposi's sarcoma-associated herpesvirus. *Nature*, **394**, 588–92.

Folks, T.M., Kessler, S.W., Orenstein, J.M., Justement, J.S., Jaffe, E.S. and Fauci, A.S. (1988). Infection and replication of HIV-1 in purified progenitor cells of normal human bone marrow. *Science*, **242**, 919–22.

Formica, S., Roach, T.I. and Blackwell, J.M. (1994). Interaction with extracellular matrix proteins influences Lsh/Ity/Bcg (candidate Nramp) gene regulation of macrophage priming/activation for tumor necrosis factor-α and nitrite release. *Immunology*, **82**, 42–50.

Friedmann, A., Frankel, G., Lorch, Y. and Steinman, L. (1987). Monoclonal anti-I-A antibody reverses chronic paralysis and demyelination in Theiler's virus-infected mice: critical importance of timing of treatment. *Journal of Virology*, **61**, 898–903.

Gabuzda, D., Hess, J., Small, J. and Clements, J. (1989). Regulation of the visna virus long terminal repeat in macrophages involves cellular factors that bind sequences containing AP-1 sites. *Molecular and Cellular Biology*, **9**, 2973–84.

Gabuzda, D.H. and Hirsch, M.S. (1987). Neurologic manifestations of infection with human immunodeficiency virus. Clinical features and pathogenesis. *Annals of Internal Medicine*, **107**, 383–91.

Gale, M.J., Jr, Korth, M.J., Tang, N.M., Tan, S.L., Hopkins, D.A., Dever, T.E. *et al.* (1997). Evidence that hepatitis C virus resistance to interferon is mediated through repression of the PKR protein kinase by the nonstructural 5A protein. *Virology*, **230**, 217–27.

Gao, F., Yue, L., White, A.T., Pappas, P.G., Barchue, J., Hanson, A.P. *et al.* (1992). Human infection by genetically diverse SIVSM-related HIV-2 in west Africa. *Nature*, **358**, 495–9.

Gao, F., Yue, L., Robertson, D.L., Hill, S.C., Hui, H., Biggar, R.J. *et al.* (1994). Genetic diversity of human immunodeficiency virus type 2: evidence for distinct sequence subtypes with differences in virus biology. *Journal of Virology*, **68**, 7433–47.

Gao, J.L. and Murphy, P.M. (1994). Human cytomegalovirus open reading frame US28 encodes a functional β chemokine receptor. *Journal of Biological Chemistry*, **269**, 28539–42.

Garcia, J.A., Wu, F.K., Mitsuyasu, R. and Gaynor, R.B. (1987). Interactions of cellular proteins involved in the transcriptional regulation of the human immunodeficiency virus. *EMBO Journal*, **6**, 3761–70.

Gardenswartz, M.H., Lerner, C.W., Seligson, G.R., Zabetakis, P.M., Rotterdam, H., Tapper, M.L. *et al.* (1984). Renal disease in patients with AIDS: a clinicopathologic study. *Clinical Nephrology*, **21**, 197–204.

Gardner, M.B. and Luciw, P.A. (1989). Animal models of AIDS. *FASEB Journal,* **3**, 2593–606.

Gartner, S. (2000). HIV infection and dementia. *Science*, **287**, 602–4.

Gattone, V.H., 2nd, Tian, C., Zhuge, W., Sahni, M., Narayan, O. and Stephens, E.B. (1998). SIV-associated nephropathy in rhesus macaques infected with lymphocyte-tropic SIVmac239. *AIDS Research and Human Retroviruses*, **14**, 1163–80.

Gendelman, H.E., Narayan, O., Molineaux, S., Clements, J.E. and Ghotbi, Z. (1985). Slow, persistent replication of lentiviruses: role of tissue macrophages and macrophage precursors in bone marrow. *Proceedings of the National Academy of Sciences USA*, **82**, 7086–90.

Gendelman, H.E., Narayan, O., Kennedy-Stoskopf, S., Kennedy, P.G., Ghotbi, Z., Clements, J.E. *et al.* (1986). Tropism of sheep lentiviruses for monocytes: susceptibility to infection and virus gene expression increase during maturation of monocytes to macrophages. *Journal of Virology*, **58**, 67–74.

Gendelman, H.E., Orenstein, J.M., Baca, L.M., Weiser, B., Burger, H., Kalter, D.C. *et al.* (1989). The macrophage in the persistence and pathogenesis of HIV infection. *AIDS*, **3**, 475–95.

Gendelman, H.E., Baca, L., Turpin, J.A., Kalter, D.C., Hansen, B.D., Orenstein, J.M. *et al.* (1990). Restriction of HIV replication in infected T cells and monocytes by interferon-α. *AIDS Research and Human Retroviruses*, **6**, 1045–9.

Georgsson, G., Nathanson, N., Palsson, P.A. and Petursson, G. (1976). The pathology of visna and maedi in sheep. *Frontiers in Biology*, **44**, 61–96.

Gerety, S.J., Karpus, W.J., Cubbon, A.R., Goswami, R.G., Rundell, M.K., Peterson, J.D. *et al.* (1994). Class II-restricted T cell responses in Theiler's murine encephalomyelitis virus-induced demyelinating disease. V. Mapping of a dominant immunopathologic VP2 T cell epitope in susceptible SJL/J mice. *Journal of Immunology*, **152**, 908–18.

Glass, J.D., Fedor, H., Wesselingh, S.L. and McArthur, J.C. (1995). Immunocytochemical quantitation of human immunodeficiency virus in the brain: correlation with dementia. *Annals of Neurology*, **38**, 755–762.

Gomez-Guerrero, C., Gonzalez, E. and Egido, J. (1993). Evidence for a specific IgA receptor in rat and human mesangial cells. *Journal of Immunology*, **151**, 7172–81.

Gonda, M.A., Braun, M.J., Carter, S.G., Kost, T.A., Bess, J.W., Jr, Arthur, L.O. *et al.* (1987). Characterization and molecular cloning of a bovine lentivirus related to human immunodeficiency virus. *Nature*, **330**, 388–91.

Gorny, M.K., Xu, J.Y., Karwowska, S., Buchbinder, A. and Zolla-Pazner, S. (1993). Repertoire of neutralizing human monoclonal antibodies specific for the V3 domain of HIV-1 gp120. *Journal of Immunology*, **150**, 635–43.

Gosztonyi, G., Artigas, J., Lamperth, L. and Webster, H.D. (1994). Human immunodeficiency virus (HIV) distribution in HIV encephalitis: study of 19 cases with combined use of *in situ* hybridization and immunocytochemistry. *Journal of Neuropathology and Experimental Neurology*, **53**, 521–34.

Graham, K. (1997). The T1/35kDa family of poxvirus secreted proteins bind chemokines and modulate leukocyte influx into virus infected tissues. *Virology*, **229**, 12–24.

Graziosi, C., Pantaleo, G. and Fauci, A.S. (1994). Comparative analysis of constitutive cytokine expression in peripheral blood and lymph nodes of HIV-infected individuals. *Research in Immunology*, **145**, 602–5; discussion 605–7.

Greber, U.F., Willetts, M., Webster, P. and Helenius, A. (1993). Stepwise dismantling of adenovirus 2 during entry into cells. *Cell*, **75**, 477–86.

Green, D.F., Resnick, L. and Bourgoignie, J.J. (1992). HIV infects glomerular endothelial and mesangial but not epithelial cells *in vitro*. *Kidney International*, **41**, 956–60.

Greenberg, S., Chang, P. and Silverstein, S.C. (1993). Tyrosine phosphorylation is required for Fc receptor-mediated phagocytosis in mouse macrophages. *Journal of Experimental Medicine*, **177**, 529–33.

Griffiths, M.H., Miller, R.F. and Semple, S.J. (1995). Interstitial pneumonitis in patients infected with the human immunodeficiency virus. *Thorax*, **50**, 1141–6.

Groenink, M., Fouchier, R.A., de Goede, R.E., de Wolf, F., Gruters, R.A., Cuypers, H.T. *et al.* (1991). Phenotypic heterogeneity in a panel of infectious molecular human immunodeficiency virus type 1 clones derived from a single individual. *Journal of Virology*, **65**, 1968–75.

Grundy, J.E., McKeating, J.A., Ward, P.J., Sanderson, A.R. and Griffiths, P.D. (1987). β_2 microglobulin enhances the infectivity of cytomegalovirus and when bound to the virus enables class I HLA molecules to be used as a virus receptor. *Journal of General Virology*, **68**, 793–803.

Guerra, I.L., Abraham, A.A., Kimmel, P.L., Sabnis, S.G. and Antonovych, T.T. (1987). Nephrotic syndrome associated with chronic persistent hepatitis B in an HIV antibody positive patient. *American Journal of Kidney Disease*, **10**, 385–8.

Guillon, J.M., Autran, B., Denis, M., Fouret, P., Plata, F., Mayaud, C.M. *et al.* (1988). Human immunodeficiency virus-related lymphocytic alveolitis. *Chest*, **94**, 1264–70.

Guo, H.G., Browning, P., Nicholas, J., Hayward, G.S., Tschachler, E., Jiang, Y.W. *et al.* (1997). Characterization of a chemokine receptor-related gene in human herpesvirus 8 and its expression in Kaposi's sarcoma. *Virology*, **228**, 371–8.

Gupta, D., Wang, Q., Vinson, C. and Dziarski, R. (1999). Bacterial peptidoglycan induces CD14-dependent activation of transcription factors CREB/ATF and AP-1. *Journal of Biological Chemistry*, **274**, 14012–20.

Haas, E., Grell, M., Wajant, H. and Scheurich, P. (1999). Continuous autotropic signaling by membrane-expressed tumor necrosis factor. *Journal of Biological Chemistry*, **274**, 18107–12.

Hackam, E.A. (1996). Characterization and subcellular localization of target membrane soluble NSF attachment protein receptors (t-SNARE) in macrophages. Syntaxins 2, 3, and 4 are present on phagosomal membranes. *Journal of Immunology*, **156**, 4377–83.

Halstead, S., Marchette, N., Chow, J. and Lolekha, S. (1976). Dengue virus replication enhancement in peripheral blood leukocytes from immune human beings. *Proceedings of the Society for Experimental Biology and Medicine*, **5**, 136–139.

Hanna, Z., Kay, D.G., Cool, M., Jothy, S., Rebai, N. and Jolicoeur, P. (1998). Transgenic mice expressing human immunodeficiency virus type 1 in immune cells develop a severe AIDS-like disease. *Journal of Virology*, **72**, 121–32.

Hannigan, G. and Williams, B. (1991). Induced factor binding to the interferon-stimulated response element. Interferon-α and platelet derived growth factor utilize distinct signaling pathways. *Journal of Biological Chemistry*, **266**, 8765–70.

Hanson, L.K., Slater, J.S., Karabekian, Z., Virgin, H.W.T., Biron, C.A., Ruzek, M.C. *et al.* (1999). Replication of murine cytomegalovirus in differentiated macrophages as a determinant of viral pathogenesis. *Journal of Virology*, **73**, 5970–80.

Harada, H., Matsumoto, M., Sato, M., Kashiwazaki, Y., Kimura, T., Kitagawa, M. *et al.* (1996). Regulation of IFN-α/β genes: evidence for a dual function of the transcription factor complex ISGF3 in the production and action of IFN-α/β. *Genes to Cells*, **1**, 995–1005.

Harmache, A., Russo, P., Guiguen, F., Vitu, C., Vignoni, M., Bouyac, M. *et al.* (1996). Requirement of caprine arthritis encephalitis virus *vif* gene for *in vivo* replication. *Virology*, **224**, 246–55.

Hassel, B., Zhou, A., Sotomayor, C., Maran, A. and Silverman, R. (1993). A dominant negative mutant of 2–5A dependent RNase suppresses antiproliferative and antiviral effects of interferon. *EMBO Journal*, **12**, 3297–304.

Heise, M.T. and Virgin, H.W.T. (1995). The T-cell-independent role of g interferon and tumor necrosis factor α in macrophage activation during murine cytomegalovirus and herpes simplex virus infections. *Journal of Virology*, **69**, 904–9.

Hengel, H., Koopmann, J.O., Flohr, T., Muranyi, W., Goulmy, E., Hammerling, G.J. *et al.* (1997). A viral ER-resident glycoprotein inactivates the MHC-encoded peptide transporter. *Immunity*, **6**, 623–32.

Henry, S.C. and Hamilton, J.D. (1993). Detection of murine cytomegalovirus immediate early 1 transcripts in the spleens of latently infected mice. *Journal of Infectious Diseases*, **167**, 950–4.

Herndon, R.M., Griffin, D.E., McCormick, U. and Weiner, L.P. (1975). Mouse hepatitis virus-induced recurrent demyelination. A preliminary report. *Archives of Neurology*, **32**, 32–5.

Hirsch, V.M., Dapolito, G.A., Goldstein, S., McClure, H., Emau, P., Fultz, P.N. *et al.* (1993). A distinct African lentivirus from Sykes' monkeys. *Journal of Virology*, **67**, 1517–28.

Hiscott, J., Pitha, P., Genin, P., Nguyen, H., Heylbroeck, C., Mamane, Y. *et al.* (1999). Triggering the interferon response: the role of IRF-3 transcription factor. *Journal of Interferon and Cytokine Research*, **19**, 1–13.

Ho, M. (1991). Epidemiology of CMV in man. In M.H. (ed.) *Cytomegalovirus: Biology and Infection*. Plenum Publishing, New York, pp. 155–87.

Houle, M., Thivierge, M., Le Gouill, C., Stankova, J. and Rola-Pleszczynski, M. (1999). IL-10 up-regulates CCR5 gene expression in human monocytes. *Inflammation*, **23**, 241–51.

Huang, E.S., Kilpatrick, B.A., Huang, Y.T. and Pagano, J.S. (1976). Detection of human cytomegalovirus and analysis of strain variation. *Yale Journal of Biological Medicine*, **49**, 29–43.

Huang, Y., Paxton, W.A., Wolinsky, S.M., Neumann, A.U., Zhang, L., He, T. *et al.* (1996). The role of a mutant CCR5 allele in HIV-1 transmission and disease progression. *Nature Medicine*, **2**, 1240–3.

Hurtrel, B., Chakrabarti, L., Hurtrel, M. and Montagnier, L. (1993). Target cells during early SIV encephalopathy. *Research in Virology*, **144**, 41–6.

Ibanez, C.E., Schrier, R., Ghazal, P., Wiley, C. and Nelson, J.A. (1991). Human cytomegalovirus productively infects primary differentiated macrophages. *Journal of Virology*, **65**, 6581–8.

Igarashi, T., Endo, Y., Englund, G., Sadjadpour, R., Matano, T., Buckler, C. *et al.* (1999). Emergence of a highly pathogenic simian/human immunodeficiency virus in a rhesus macaque treated with anti-CD8 mAb during a primary infection with a nonpathogenic virus. *Proceedings of the National Academy of Sciences USA*, **96**, 14049–54.

Ingalls, R.R. and Golenbock, D.T. (1995). CD11c/CD18, a transmembrane signaling receptor for lipopolysaccharide. *Journal of Experimental Medicine*, **181**, 1473–9.

Isegawa, Y., Ping, Z., Nakano, K., Sugimoto, N. and Yamanishi, K. (1998). Human herpesvirus 6 open reading frame U12 encodes a functional β-chemokine receptor. *Journal of Virology*, **72**, 6104–12.

Issel, C.J., McManus, J.M., Hagius, S.D., Foil, L.D., Adams, W.V., Jr and Montelaro, R.C. (1990). Equine infectious anemia: prospects for control. *Developmental Biology Standards*, **72**, 49–57.

Jaconi, M.E., Lew, D.P., Carpentier, J.L., Magnusson, K.E., Sjogren, M. and Stendahl, O. (1990). Cytosolic free calcium elevation mediates the phagosome–lysosome fusion during phagocytosis in human neutrophils. *Journal of Cell Biology*, **110**, 1555–64.

Jahan, N., Razzaque, A., Greenspan, J., Conant, M.A., Josephs, S.F., Nakamura, S. *et al.* (1989). Analysis of human KS biopsies and cloned cell lines for cytomegalovirus, HIV-1, and other selected DNA virus sequences. *AIDS Research and Human Retroviruses*, **5**, 225–31.

Jason, J.M., Stehr-Green, J., Holman, R.C. and Evatt, B.L. (1988). Human immunodeficiency virus infection in hemophilic children. *Pediatrics*, **82**, 565–70.

Jelachich, M.L., Bandyopadhyay, P., Blum, K. and Lipton, H.L. (1995). Theiler's virus growth in murine macrophage cell lines depends on the state of differentiation. *Virology*, **209**, 437–44.

Jelachich, M.L. and Lipton, H.L. (1999). Restricted Theiler's murine encephalomyelitis virus infection in murine macrophages induces apoptosis. *Journal of General Virology*, **80**, 1701–5.

Jelachich, M.L. and Lipton, H.L. (1996). Theiler's murine encephalomyelitis virus kills restrictive but not permissive cells by apoptosis. *Journal of Virology*, **70**, 6856–61.

Joag, S.V., Stephens, E.B., Adams, R.J., Foresman, L. and Narayan, O. (1994). Pathogenesis of SIV_{mac} infection in Chinese and Indian rhesus macaques: effects of splenectomy on virus burden. *Virology*, **200**, 436–46.

John, J., McKendry, R., Pellegrini, S., Flavell, D., Kerr, I.M. and Stark, G.R. (1991). Isolation and characterization of a new mutant human cell line unresponsive to α and β interferons. *Molecular and Cellular Biology*, **11**, 4189–95.

Jones, K.A., Kadonaga, J.T., Luciw, P.A. and Tjian, R. (1986). Activation of the AIDS retrovirus promoter by the cellular transcription factor, Sp1. *Science*, **232**, 755–9.

Jones, S.M., Moors, M.A., Ryan, Q., Klyczek, K.K. and Blank, K.J. (1992). Altered macrophage antigen-presenting cell function following Friend leukemia virus infection. *Viral Immunology*, **5**, 201–11.

Kaaya, E.E., Parravicini, C., Ordonez, C., Gendelman, R., Berti, E., Gallo, R.C. *et al.* (1995). Heterogeneity of spindle cells in Kaposi's sarcoma: comparison of cells in lesions and in culture. *Journal of AIDS and Human Retrovirology*, **10**, 295–305.

Kaloutsi, V., Kohlmeyer, U., Maschek, H., Nafe, R., Choritz, H., Amor, A. *et al.* (1994). Comparison of bone marrow and hematologic findings in patients with human immunodeficiency virus infection and those with myelodysplastic syndromes and infectious diseases. *American Journal of Clinical Pathology*, **101**, 123–9.

Kanki, P.J., Alroy, J. and Essex, M. (1985). Isolation of T-lymphotropic retrovirus related to HTLV-III/LAV from wild-caught African green monkeys. *Science*, **230**, 951–4.

Kaplan, L.D., Abrams, D.I., Sherwin, S.A., Kahn, J. and Volberding, P.A. (1989). A phase I/II study of recombinant tumor necrosis factor and recombinant interferon g in patients with AIDS-related complex. *Biotechnological Therapy*, **1**, 229–36.

Karp, C.L., Wysocka, M., Wahl, L.M., Ahearn, J.M., Cuomo, P.J., Sherry, B. *et al.* (1996). Mechanism of suppression of cell-mediated immunity by measles virus [published erratum appears in *Science* 1997 Feb 21;275(5303):1053]. *Science*, **273**, 228–31.

Karpatkin, S. (1987). Immunologic thrombocytopenic purpura in patients at risk for AIDS. *Blood Reviews*, **1**, 119–25.

Karpus, W.J., Pope, J.G., Peterson, J.D., Dal Canto, M.C. and Miller, S.D. (1995). Inhibition of Theiler's virus-mediated demyelination by peripheral immune tolerance induction [published erratum appears in *Journal of Immunology* 1996 Apr 15;156(8):following 3088]. *Journal of Immunology*, **155**, 947–57.

Kawakami, A., Nakashima, T., Sakai, H., Hida, A., Urayama, S., Yamasaki, S. *et al.* (1999). Regulation of synovial cell apoptosis by proteasome inhibitor. *Arthritis and Rheumatism*, **42**, 2440–8.

Keay, S., Baldwin, B.R., Smith, M.W., Wasserman, S.S. and Goldman, W.F. (1995). Increases in [Ca2+]i mediated by the 92.5-kDa putative cell membrane receptor for HCMV gp86. *American Journal of Physiology*, **269**, C11–21.

Kennedy-Stoskopf, S., Narayan, O. and Strandberg, J.D. (1985). The mammary gland as a target organ for infection with caprine arthritis–encephalitis virus. *Journal of Comparative Pathology*, **95**, 609–17.

Kenouch, S., Delahousse, M., Mery, J.P. and Nochy, D. (1990). Mesangial IgA deposits in two patients with AIDS-related complex. *Nephron*, **54**, 338–40.

Kerkau, T., Bacik, I., Bennink, J.R., Yewdell, J.W., Hurig, T., Schimpl, A. and Schubert, U. (1997). The human immunodeficiency virus type-1 (HIV-1) Vpu protein interferes with an early step in the biosynthesis of MHC class I molecules. *Journal of Experimental Medicine*, **185**, 1295–305.

Kesson, A.M., Fear, W.R., Williams, L., Chang, J., King, N.J. and Cunningham, A.L. (1994). HIV infection of placental macrophages: their potential role in vertical transmission. *Journal of Leukocyte Biology*, **56**, 241–6.

Kestens, L., Brattegaard, K., Adjorlolo, G., Ekpini, E., Sibailly, T., Diallo, K. *et al.* (1992). Immunological comparison of HIV-1-, HIV-2- and dually-reactive women delivering in Abidjan, Cote d'Ivoire. *AIDS*, **6**, 803–7.

Kim, H.-J., Gatz, C., Hillen, W. and Jones, T. (1995). Tetracycline repressor-regulated gene repression in recombinant human cytomegalovirus. *Journal of Virology*, **69**, 2565–73.

Kim, K.K. and Factor, S.M. (1987). Membranoproliferative glomerulonephritis and plexogenic pulmonary arteriopathy in a homosexual man with acquired immunodeficiency syndrome. *Human Pathology*, **18**, 1293–6.

Kimmel, P.L., Phillips, T.M., Ferreira-Centeno, A., Farkas-Szallasi, T., Abraham, A.A. and Garrett, C.T. (1993). HIV-associated immune-mediated renal disease. *Kidney International*, **44**, 1327–40.

Kimpton, C.P., Morris, D.J. and Corbitt, G. (1989). Inhibitory effects of various anticoagulants on the infectivity of human cytomegalovirus. *Journal of Virological Methods*, **24**, 301–6.

Kinter, A.L., Poli, G., Fox, L., Hardy, E. and Fauci, A.S. (1995). HIV replication in IL-2-stimulated peripheral blood mononuclear cells is driven in an autocrine/paracrine manner by endogenous cytokines. *Journal of Immunology*, **154**, 2448–59.

Kirchhoff, S., Wilhelm, D., Angel, P. and Hauser, H. (1999). NFκB activation is required for interferon regulatory factor-1-mediated interferon β induction. *European Journal of Biochemistry*, **261**, 546–54.

Kitagawa, M., Lackner, A.A., Martfeld, D.J., Gardner, M.B. and Dandekar, S. (1991). Simian immunodeficiency virus infection of macaque bone marrow macrophages correlates with disease progression *in vivo*. *American Journal of Pathology*, **138**, 921–30.

Kitajewski, J., Schneider, R.J., Safer, B., Munemitsu, S.M., Samuel, C.E., Thimmappaya, B. *et al.* (1986). Adenovirus VAI RNA antagonizes the antiviral action of interferon by preventing activation of the interferon-induced eIF-2 α kinase. *Cell*, **45**, 195–200.

Klevjer-Anderson, P. and Anderson, L.W. (1982). Caprine arthritis–encephalitis virus infection of caprine monocytes. *Journal of General Virology*, **58**, 195–8.

Kliks, S.C. and Halstead, S.B. (1983). Role of antibodies and host cells in plaque enhancement of Murray Valley encephalitis virus. *Journal of Virology*, **46**, 394–404.

Koenig, S., Gendelman, H.E., Orenstein, J.M., Canto, M.C.D., Pezeshkpour, G.H., Yungbluth, M. *et al.* (1986). Detection of AIDS virus in macrophages in brain tissue from AIDS patients with encephalopathy. *Science*, **233**, 1089–93.

Korte, T., Ludwig, K., Booy, F.P., Blumenthal, R. and Herrmann, A. (1999). Conformational inter-mediates and fusion activity of influenza virus hemagglutinin. *Journal of Virology*, **73**, 4567–74.

Kreil, T.R. and Eibl, M.M. (1995). Viral infection of macrophages profoundly alters requirements for induction of nitric oxide synthesis. *Virology*, **212**, 174–8.

Kumar, A., Angel, J.B., Aucoin, S., Creery, W.D., Daftarian, M.P., Cameron, D.W. *et al*. (1999). Dysregulation of B7.2 (CD86) expression on monocytes of HIV-infected individuals is associ-ated with altered production of IL-2. *Clinical and Experimental Immunology*, **117**, 84–91.

Kyuwa, S. and Stohlman, S. (1990). Pathogensis of a neurotropic murine coronavirus, strain JHM in the central nervous system of mice. *Seminars in Virology*, **1**, 273–80.

Lalani, A. (1997). The purified myxoma virus g interferon receptor homolog M-T7 interacts with the heparin binding domains of chemokines. *Journal of Virology*, **71**, 4356–63.

Lalani, A.S. and McFadden, G. (1997). Secreted poxvirus chemokine binding proteins. *Journal of Leukocyte Biology*, **62**, 570–6.

Lane, J., Sasseville, V., Smith, M., Vogel, P., Pauley, D., Heyes, M. *et al*. (1996). Neuroinvasion by simian immunodeficiency virus coincides with increased numbers of perivascular macrophages/microglia and intrathecal immune activation. *Journal of Neurovirology*, **2**, 423–432.

Langedijk, J.P., Back, N.K., Durda, P.J., Goudsmit, J. and Meloen, R.H. (1991). Neutralizing activ-ity of anti-peptide antibodies against the principal neutralization domain of human immun-odeficiency virus type 1. *Journal of General Virology*, **72**, 2519–26.

Lefrere, J.J., Meyohas, M.C., Mariotti, M., Meynard, J.L., Thauvin, M. and Frottier, J. (1996). Detection of human herpesvirus 8 DNA sequences before the appearance of Kaposi's sarcoma in human immunodeficiency virus (HIV)-positive subjects with a known date of HIV seroconver-sion. *Journal of Infectious Diseases*, **174**, 283–7.

Lehtonen, A., Matikainen, S. and Julkunen, I. (1997). Interferons upregulate STAT1, STAT2 and IRF family transcription factor gene expression in human peripheral blood mononuclear cells and macrophages. *Journal of Immunology*, **159**, 794–803.

Leiderman, I.Z., Greenberg, M.L., Adelsberg, B.R. and Siegal, F.P. (1987). A glycoprotein inhibitor of *in vitro* granulopoiesis associated with AIDS. *Blood*, **70**, 1267–72.

Lewandowski, G., Lo, D. and Bloom, F. (1993). Interference with major histocombatibility complex class II-restricted antigen presentation in the brain by herpes simplex virus type I: a possible mechanism of evasion of the immune response. *Proceedings of the National Academy of Sciences USA*, **90**, 2005–9.

Lewis, D., Ng-Tang, D., Wang, X. and Kozinetz, C. (1999). Costimulatory pathways mediate monocyte-dependent lymphocyte apoptosis in HIV. *Clinical Immunology*, **90**, 302–12.

Li, J., Lord, C.I., Haseltine, W., Letvin, N.L. and Sodroski, J. (1992). Infection of cynomolgus monkeys with a chimeric HIV-1/SIV$_{mac}$ virus that expresses the HIV-1 envelope glycoproteins. *Journal of AIDS*, **5**, 639–46.

Lindsley, M.D. and Rodriguez, M. (1989). Characterization of the inflammatory response in the central nervous system of mice susceptible or resistant to demyelination by Theiler's virus. *Journal of Immunology*, **142**, 2677–82.

Link, R.E., Desai, K., Hein, L., Stevens, M.E., Chruscinski, A., Bernstein, D. *et al*. (1996). Cardiovascular regulation in mice lacking α2-adrenergic receptor subtypes b and c. *Science*, **273**, 803–805.

Lipton, H.L. and Canto, C.D. (1977). Contrasting effects of immunosuppression on Theiler's virus infection in mice. *Infection and Immunity*, **15**, 903–9.

Lipton, H.L. and Dal Canto, M.C. (1976). Theiler's virus-induced demyelination: prevention by immunosuppression. *Science*, **192**, 62–4.

Lipton, H.L., Twaddle, G. and Jelachich, M.L. (1995). The predominant virus antigen burden is present in macrophages in Theiler's murine encephalomyelitis virus-induced demyelinating disease. *Journal of Virology*, **69**, 2525–33.

Liu, Z.Q., Muhkerjee, S., Sahni, M., McCormick-Davis, C., Leung, K., Li, Z. *et al.* (1999). Derivation and biological characterization of a molecular clone of SHIV(KU-2) that causes AIDS, neurological disease, and renal disease in rhesus macaques. *Virology*, **260**, 295–307.

Lorch, Y., Friedmann, A., Lipton, H.L. and Kotler, M. (1981). Theiler's murine encephalomyelitis virus group includes two distinct genetic subgroups that differ pathologically and biologically. *Journal of Virology*, **40**, 560–7.

Lores, P., Boucher, V., Mackay, C., Pla, M., Von Boehmer, H., Jami, J. *et al.* (1992). Expression of human CD4 in transgenic mice does not confer sensitivity to human immunodeficiency virus infection. *AIDS Research and Human Retroviruses*, **8**, 2063–71.

Luttichau, B.H., Stine, J., Boesen, T.P., Johnsen, A.H., Chantry, D., Gerstoft, J. *et al.* (2000). A highly selective CC chemokine receptor (CCR)8 antagonist encoded by the poxvirus molluscum contagiosum. *Journal of Experimental Medicine*, **191**, 171–80.

Maciejewski, J.P., Bruening, E.E., Donahue, R.E., Sellers, S.E., Carter, C., Young, N.S. *et al.* (1993). Infection of mononucleated phagocytes with human cytomegalovirus. *Virology*, **195**, 327–36.

MacKay, K., Striker, L.J., Stauffer, J.W., Doi, T., Agodoa, L.Y. and Striker, G.E. (1989). Transforming growth factor-β. Murine glomerular receptors and responses of isolated glomerular cells. *Journal of Clinical Investigation*, **83**, 1160–7.

Mankowski, J.L., Carter, D.L., Spelman, J.., Nealen, M.L., Maughan, K.R., Kirstein, L.M. *et al* (1998). Pathogenesis of simian immunodeficiency virus pneumonia: an immunopathological response to virus. *American Journal of Pathology*, **153**, 1123–30.

Marsters, S.A., Ayres, T.M., Skubatch, M., Gray, C.L., Rothe, M. and Ashkenazi, A. (1997). Herpesvirus entry mediator, a member of the tumor necrosis factor receptor (TNFR) family, interacts with members of the TNFR-associated factor family and activates the transcription factors NF-κB and AP-1. *Journal of Biological Chemistry*, **272**, 14029–32.

Marth, T. and Kelsall, B.L. (1997). Regulation of interleukin-12 by complement receptor 3 signaling. *Journal of Experimental Medicine*, **185**, 1987–95.

Martin, M.P., Dean, M., Smith, M.W., Winkler, C., Gerrard, B., Michael, N.L. *et al.* (1998). Genetic acceleration of AIDS progression by a promoter variant of CCR5. *Science*, **282**, 1907–11.

Martinex-Pomares, L., Thompson, J. and Moyer, R. (1995). Mapping and investigation of the role in pathogenesis of the major unique secreted 35-kDa protein of rabbitpox virus. *Virology*, **206**, 591–600.

Marx, P.A., Li, Y., Lerche, N.W., Sutjipto, S., Gettie, A., Yee, J.A. *et al.* (1991). Isolation of a simian immunodeficiency virus related to human immunodeficiency virus type 2 from a west African pet sooty mangabey. *Journal of Virology*, **65**, 4480–5.

Matano, T., Shibata, R., Siemon, C., Connors, M., Lane, H.C. and Martin, M.A. (1998). Administration of an anti-CD8 monoclonal antibody interferes with the clearance of chimeric simian/human immunodeficiency virus during primary infections of rhesus macaques. *Journal of Virology*, **72**, 164–9.

Mattana, J., Abramovici, M. and Singhal, P.C. (1993). Effects of human immunodeficiency virus sera and macrophage supernatants on mesangial cell proliferation and matrix synthesis. *American Journal of Pathology*, **143**, 814–22.

McCune, J., Kaneshima, H., Krowka, J., Namikawa, R., Outzen, H., Peault, B. *et al.* (1991). The SCID-hu mouse: a small animal model for HIV infection and pathogenesis. *Annual Review of Immunology*, **9**, 399–429.

McGann, K.A., Collman, R., Kolson, D.L., Gonzalez-Scarano, F., Coukos, G., Coutifaris, C. *et al.* (1994). Human immunodeficiency virus type 1 causes productive infection of macrophages in primary placental cell cultures. *Journal of Infectious Diseases*, **169**, 746–53.

McMillan, N. (1994). Tat directly interacts with the interferon-induced, double-stranded RNA-dependent kinase, PKR. *Virology*, **213**, 413–24.

Meinl, E., Fickenscher, H. and Fleckenstein, B. (1996). Chemokine receptors and chemokine-inducing molecules of lymphotropic herpesviruses. *Immunology Today*, **17**, 199.

Mellerick, D.M. and Fraser, N.W. (1987). Physical state of the latent herpes simplex virus genome in a mouse model system: evidence suggesting an episomal state. *Virology*, **158**, 265–75.

Meltzer, M.S. and Gendelman, H.E. (1988). Effects of colony stimulating factors on the interaction of monocytes and the human immunodeficiency virus. *Immunology Letters*, **19**, 193–8.

Meltzer, M.S., Skillman, D.R., Gomatos, P.J., Kalter, D.C. and Gendelman, H.E. (1990). Role of mononuclear phagocytes in the pathogenesis of human immunodeficiency virus infection. *Annual Review of Immunology*, **8**, 169–94.

Messmer, U.K., Briner, V.A. and Pfeilschifter, J. (1999). Tumor necrosis factor-α and lipopolysac-charide induce apoptotic cell death in bovine glomerular endothelial cells. *Kidney International*, **55**, 2322–37.

Metroka, C.E., Cunningham-Rundles, S., Pollack, M.S., Sonnabend, J.A., Davis, J.M., Gordon, B. *et al.* (1983). Generalized lymphadenopathy in homosexual men. *Annals of Internal Medicine*, **99**, 585–91.

Millar, A.B., Miller, R.F., Foley, N.M., Meager, A., Semple, S.J. and Rook, G.A. (1991). Production of tumor necrosis factor-α by blood and lung mononuclear phagocytes from patients with human immunodeficiency virus-related lung disease. *American Journal of Respiratory Cell and Molecular Biology*, **5**, 144–8.

Miller, C.J., Alexander, N.J., Vogel, P., Anderson, J. and Marx, P.A. (1992a). Mechanism of genital transmission of SIV: a hypothesis based on transmission studies and the location of SIV in the genital tract of chronically infected female rhesus macaques. *Journal of Medical Primatology*, **21**, 64–8.

Miller, C.J., McChesney, M. and Moore, P.F. (1992b). Langerhans cells, macrophages and lympho-cyte subsets in the cervix and vagina of rhesus macaques. *Laboratory Investigation*, **67**, 628–34.

Miller, C.J., Marthas, M., Greenier, J., Lu, D., Dailey, P.J. and Lu, Y. (1998). *In vivo* replication capacity rather than *in vitro* macrophage tropism predicts efficiency of vaginal transmission of simian immunodeficiency virus or simian/human immunodeficiency virus in rhesus macaques [published erratum appears in *Journal of Virology* 1998 Jul;72(7):6277]. *Journal of Virology*, **72**, 3248–58.

Miller, D.M., Zhang, Y., Rahill, B.M., Kazor, K., Rofagha, S., Eckel, J.J. *et al.* (2000). Human cytomegalovirus blocks interferon-γ stimulated up-regulation of major histocompatibility complex class I expression and the class I antigen processing machinery. *Transplantation*, **69**, 687–90.

Miller, S.D., Vanderlugt, C.L., Begolka, W.S., Pao, W., Yauch, R.L., Neville, K.L. *et al.* (1997). Persistent infection with Theiler's virus leads to CNS autoimmunity via epitope spreading. *Nature Medicine*, **3**, 1133–6.

Mims, C. (1964). Aspects of the pathogenesis of viral disease. *Bacteriological Reviews*, **28**, 30–71.

Mocarski, E. (1993). Cytomegalovirus biology and replication. In Roizman, B., Whitley, R. and Lopez, C. (ed.), *The Human Herpesviruses*. Raven Press, New York, pp. 173–226.

Mocarski, E.S., Jr, Abenes, G.B., Manning, W.C., Sambucetti, L.C. and Cherrington, J.M. (1990). Molecular genetic analysis of cytomegalovirus gene regulation in growth, persistence and latency. *Current Topics in Microbiology and Immunology*, **154**, 47–74.

Montgomery, R.I., Warner, M.S., Lum, B.J. and Spear, P.G. (1996). Herpes simplex virus-1 entry into cells mediated by a novel member of the TNF/NGF receptor family. *Cell*, **87**, 427–36.

Moore, P.S., Boshoff, C., Weiss, R.A. and Chang, Y. (1996a). Molecular mimicry of human cytokine and cytokine response pathway genes by KSHV. *Science*, **274**, 1739–44.

Moore, P.S., Gao, S.J., Dominguez, G., Cesarman, E., Lungu, O., Knowles, D.M. *et al.* (1996b). Primary characterization of a herpesvirus agent associated with Kaposi's sarcomae [published erratum appears in *Journal of Virology* 1996 Dec;70(12):9083]. *Journal of Virology*, **70**, 549–58.

Moore, P.S. and Chang, Y. (1998). Kaposi's sarcoma-associated herpesvirus-encoded oncogenes and oncogenesis. *Journal of the National Cancer Institute Monograph*, **23**, 65–71.

Moran, C.A., Suster, S., Pavlova, Z., Mullick, F.G. and Koss, M.N. (1994). The spectrum of pathological changes in the lung in children with the acquired immunodeficiency syndrome: an autopsy study of 36 cases. *Human Pathology*, **25**, 877–82.

Mori, K., Ringler, D.J. and Desrosiers, R.C. (1993). Restricted replication of simian immunodeficiency virus strain 239 in macrophages is determined by *env* but is not due to restricted entry. *Journal of Virology*, **67**, 2807–14.

Mori, K., Ringler, D.J., Kodama, T. and Desrosiers, R.C. (1992). Complex determinants of macrophage tropism in *env* of simian immunodeficiency virus. *Journal of Virology*, **66**, 2067–75.

Murphey-Corb, M., Martin, L.N., Rangan, S.R., Baskin, G.B., Gormus, B.J., Wolf, R.H. *et al.* (1986). Isolation of an HTLV-III-related retrovirus from macaques with simian AIDS and its possible origin in asymptomatic mangabeys. *Nature*, **321**, 435–7.

Musey, L., Hughes, J., Schacker, T., Shea, T., Corey, L. and McElrath, M.J. (1997). Cytotoxic-T-cell responses, viral load, and disease progression in early human immunodeficiency virus type 1 infection. *New England Journal of Medicine*, **337**, 1267–74.

Nabel, G. and Baltimore, D. (1987). An inducible transcription factor activates expression of human immunodeficiency virus in T cells [published erratum appears in *Nature* 1990 Mar 8;344(6262):178]. *Nature*, **326**, 711–3.

Nakade, K., Hande, H. and Nagata, K. (1997). Promoter structure of the MxA gene that confers resistance to influenza virus. *FEBS Letters*, **418**, 315–8.

Narayan, O. and Clements, J.E. (1989). Biology and pathogenesis of lentiviruses. *Journal of General Virology*, **70**, 1617–39.

Narayan, O. and Cork, L.C. (1985). Lentiviral diseases of sheep and goats: chronic pneumonia leukoencephalomyelitis and arthritis. *Reviews of Infectious Diseases*, **7**, 89–98.

Narayan, O., Kennedy-Stotskopf, S., Sheffer, D., Griffin, D. and Clements, J. (1983). Activation of caprine arthritis–encephalitis virus expression during maturation of monocytes to macrophages. *Infection and Immunity*, **41**, 67–73.

Nathanson, N., Georgsson, G., Palsson, P.A., Najjar, J.A., Lutley, R. and Petursson, G. (1985). Experimental visna in Icelandic sheep: the prototype lentiviral infection. *Reviews of Infectious Diseases*, **7**, 75–82.

Nazerian, K. (1974). DNA configuration in the core of Marek's disease virus. *Journal of Virology*, **13**, 1148–50.

Neipel, F., Albrecht, J.C., Ensser, A., Huang, Y.Q., Li, J.J., Friedman-Kien, A.E. *et al.* (1997a). Human herpesvirus 8 encodes a homolog of interleukin-6. *Journal of Virology*, **71**, 839–42.

Neipel, F., Albrecht, J.C. and Fleckenstein, B. (1997b). Cell-homologous genes in the Kaposi's sarcoma-associated rhadinovirus human herpesvirus 8: determinants of its pathogenicity? *Journal of Virology*, **71**, 4187–92.

Neipel, F., Albrecht, J.C. and Fleckenstein, B. (1998). Human herpesvirus 8—the first human Rhadinovirus. *Journal of the National Cancer Institute Monograph*, **23**, 73–7.

Neumann, M., Felber, B.K., Kleinschmidt, A., Froese, B., Erfle, V., Pavlakis, G.N. *et al.* (1995). Restriction of human immunodeficiency virus type 1 production in a human astrocytoma cell line is associated with a cellular block in Rev function. *Journal of Virology*, **69**, 2159–67.

Neuwirth, R., Singhal, P., Diamond, B., Hays, R.M., Lobmeyer, L., Clay, K. *et al.* (1988). Evidence for immunoglobulin Fc receptor-mediated prostaglandin2 and platelet-activating factor formation by cultured rat mesangial cells. *Journal of Clinical Investigation*, **82**, 936–44.

Nicholas, J., Ruvolo, V., Zong, J., Ciufo, D., Guo, H.G., Reitz, M.S. *et al.* (1997a). A single 13-kilobase divergent locus in the Kaposi sarcoma-associated herpesvirus (human herpesvirus 8) genome contains nine open reading frames that are homologous to or related to cellular proteins. *Journal of Virology*, **71**, 1963–74.

Nicholas, J., Ruvolo, V.R., Burns, W.H., Sandford, G., Wan, X., Ciufo, D. *et al.* (1997b). Kaposi's sarcoma-associated human herpesvirus-8 encodes homologues of macrophage inflammatory protein-1 and interleukin-6. *Nature Medicine*, **3**, 287–92.

Nickerson, C.L. and Jakab, G.J. (1990). Pulmonary antibacterial defenses during mild and severe influenza virus infection. *Infection and Immunity*, **58**, 2809–14.

O'Hara, C. (1989). The lymphoid and hematopoietic systems. In Harawi, S. and O'Hara, C. (ed.), *Pathology and Physiology of AIDS*. Mosby, St. Louis, pp. 135–99.

Ochiai, H., Kurokawa, M., Kuroki, Y. and Niwayama, S. (1990). Infection enhancement of influenza A H1 subtype viruses in macrophage-like P388D1 cells by cross-reactive antibodies. *Journal of Medical Virology*, **30**, 258–65.

Ohta, Y., Masuda, T., Tsujimoto, H., Ishikawa, K., Kodama, T., Morikawa, S. *et al.* (1988). Isolation of simian immunodeficiency virus from African green monkeys and seroepidemiologic survey of the virus in various non-human primates. *International Journal of Cancer*, **41**, 115–22.

Okuda, S., Languino, L.R., Ruoslahti, E. and Border, W.A. (1990). Elevated expression of transforming growth factor-β and proteoglycan production in experimental glomerulonephritis. Possible role in expansion of the mesangial extracellular matrix [published erratum appears in *Journal of Clinical Investigation* 1990 Dec;86(6):2175]. *Journal of Clinical Investigation*, **86**, 453–62.

Oppenheim, J. and Leonard, E.J. (1989). Introduction to human monocytes. In Zembala, M. and Asherson, G.L. (ed.), *Human Monocytes*. Academic Press, New York.

Orenstein, J.M., Meltzer, M.S., Phipps, T. and Gendelman, H.E. (1988). Cytoplasmic assembly and accumulation of human immunodeficiency virus types 1 and 2 in recombinant human colony-stimulating factor-1-treated human monocytes: an ultrastructural study. *Journal of Virology*, **62**, 2578–86.

Palange, P., Carlone, S., Venditti, M., Antony, V.B., Angelici, E., Forte, S. *et al.* (1991). Alveolar cell population in HIV infected patients. *European Respiratory Journal*, **4**, 639–42.

Palmer, E., Sporborg, C., Harrison, A., Martin, M.L. and Feorino, P. (1985). Morphology and immunoelectron microscopy of AIDS virus. *Archives of Virology*, **85**, 189–96.

Palmer, E., Martin, M.L., Goldsmith, C. and Switzer, W. (1988). Ultrastructure of human immun-odeficiency virus type 2. *Journal of General Virology*, **69**, 1425–9.

Pantaleo, G., Graziosi, C. and Fauci, A. (1993). New concepts in the immunopathogenesis of human immunodeficiency virus infection. *New England Journal of Medicine*, **328**, 327–335.

Pardo, V., Aldana, M., Colton, R.M., Fischl, M.A., Jaffe, D., Moskowitz, L. *et al.* (1984). Glomerular lesions in the acquired immunodeficiency syndrome. *Annals of Internal Medicine*, **101**, 429–34.

Parton, R.G. and Lindsay, M. (1999). Exploitation of major histocompatibility complex class I molecules and caveolae by simian virus 40. *Immunological Reviews*, **168**, 23–31.

Pasternack, M.S., Medearis, D.N., Jr and Rubin, R.H. (1990). Cell-mediated immunity in experimental cytomegalovirus infections: a perspective. *Reviews of Infectious Diseases*, **12** Supplement 7, S720–6.

Pedersen, N.C., Ho, E.W., Brown, M.L. and Yamamoto, J.K. (1987). Isolation of a T-lymphotropic virus from domestic cats with an immunodeficiency-like syndrome. *Science*, **235**, 790–3.

Peiris, J.S., Gordon, S., Unkeless, J.C. and Porterfield, J.S. (1981). Monoclonal anti-Fc receptor IgG blocks antibody enhancement of viral replication in macrophages. *Nature*, **289**, 189–91.

Pena Rossi, C., Delcroix, M., Huitinga, I., McAllister, A., Van Rooijen, N., Claassen, M. *et al.* (1997). Role of macrophages during Theiler's virus infection. *Journal of Virology*, **71**, 3336–3340.

Penfold, M.E., Dairaghi, D.J., Duke, G.M., Saederup, N., Mocarski, E.S., Kemble, G.W. *et al.* (1999). Cytomegalovirus encodes a potent α chemokine. *Proceedings of the National Academy of Sciences USA*, **96**, 9839–44.

Perlman, S., Schelper, R., Bolger, E. and Ries, D. (1987). Late onset, symptomatic, demyelinating encephalomyelitis in mice infected with MHV-JHM in the presence of maternal antibody. *Microbial Pathogenesis*, **2**, 185–94.

Persidsky, Y., Limoges, J., McComb, R., Bock, P., Baldwin, T., Tyor, W. *et al.* (1996). Human immunodeficiency virus encephalitis in SCID mice. *American Journal of Pathology*, **149**, 1027–1053.

Pertile, T.L., Sharma, J.M. and Walser, M.M. (1995). Reovirus infection in chickens primes splenic adherent macrophages to produce nitric oxide in response to T cell-produced factors. *Cellular Immunology*, **164**, 207–16.

Phillips, D.M., Tan, X., Perotti, M.E. and Zacharopoulos, V.R. (1998). Mechanism of monocyte–macrophage-mediated transmission of HIV. *AIDS Research and Human Retroviruses*, **14** Supplement 1, S67–70.

Piatak, M., Jr, Saag, M.S., Yang, L.C., Clark, S.J., Kappes, J.C., Luk, K.C. *et al.* (1993). High levels of HIV-1 in plasma during all stages of infection determined by competitive PCR. *Science*, **259**, 1749–54.

Pitt, J. (1991). Lymphocytic interstitial pneumonia. *Pediatric Clinics of North America*, **38**, 89–95.

Pizzo, P.A., Eddy, J. and Faloon, J. (1988). Acquired immune deficiency syndrome in children. Current problems and therapeutic considerations. *American Journal of Medicine*, **85**, 195–202.

Plata, F., Autran, B., Martins, L.P., Wain-Hobson, S., Raphael, M., Mayaud, C. *et al.* (1987). AIDS virus-specific cytotoxic T lymphocytes in lung disorders. *Nature*, **328**, 348–51.

Pleskoff, O., Treboute, C., Brelot, A., Heveker, N., Seman, M. and Alizon, M. (1997). Identification of a chemokine receptor encoded by human cytomegalovirus as a cofactor for HIV-1 entry. *Science*, **276**, 1874–1878.

Poli, G. and Fauci, A. (1996). Cytokine cascades in HIV infection. In Gupta, S. (ed.), *Immunology of HIV Infection*. Plenum Press, New York, 285–301.

Poli, G., Bressler, P., Kinter, A., Duh, E., Timmer, W.C., Rabson, A. *et al.* (1990). Interleukin 6 induces human immunodeficiency virus expression in infected monocytic cells alone and in synergy with tumor necrosis factor α by transcriptional and post-transcriptional mechanisms. *Journal of Experimental Medicine*, **172**, 151–8.

Poli, G., Kinter, A.L. and Fauci, A.S. (1994). Interleukin 1 induces expression of the human immunodeficiency virus alone and in synergy with interleukin 6 in chronically infected U1 cells: inhibition of inductive effects by the interleukin 1 receptor antagonist. *Proceedings of the National Academy of Sciences USA*, **91**, 108–12.

Pope, J.G., Karpus, W.J., VanderLugt, C. and Miller, S.D. (1996). Flow cytometric and functional analyses of central nervous system-infiltrating cells in SJL/J mice with Theiler's virus-induced demyelinating disease. Evidence for a CD4$^+$ T cell-mediated pathology. *Journal of Immunology*, **156**, 4050–8.

Pope, J.G., Vanderlugt, C.L., Rahbe, S.M., Lipton, H.L. and Miller, S.D. (1998). Characterization of and functional antigen presentation by central nervous system mononuclear cells from mice infected with Theiler's murine encephalomyelitis virus. *Journal of Virology*, **72**, 7762–71.

Price, P., Allcock, R.J., Coombe, D.R., Shellam, G.R. and McCluskey, J. (1995). MHC proteins and heparan sulphate proteoglycans regulate murine cytomegalovirus infection. *Immunology and Cell Biology*, **73**, 308–15.

Pulliam, L., Gascon, R., Stubblebine, M., Mcguire, D. and McGrath, M.S. (1997). Unique monocyte subset in patients with AIDS dementia. *Lancet*, **349**, 692–695.

Rady, P.L., Yen, A., Rollefson, J.L., Orengo, I., Bruce, S., Hughes, T.K. *et al.* (1995). Herpesvirus-like DNA sequences in non-Kaposi's sarcoma skin lesions of transplant patients. *Lancet*, **345**, 1339–40.

Rao, T.K., Filippone, E.J., Nicastri, A.D., Landesman, S.H., Frank, E., Chen, C.K. *et al.* (1984). Associated focal and segmental glomerulosclerosis in the acquired immunodeficiency syndrome. *New England Journal of Medicine*, **310**, 669–73.

Rautenschlein, S. and Sharma, J.M. (1999). Response of turkeys to simultaneous vaccination with hemorrhagic enteritis and Newcastle disease viruses. *Avian Diseases*, **43**, 286–92.

Ray, N.B., Ewalt, L.C. and Lodmell, D.L. (1995). Rabies virus replication in primary murine bone marrow macrophages and in human and murine macrophage-like cell lines: implications for viral persistence. *Journal of Virology*, **69**, 764–772.

Redpath, S., Angulo, A., Gascoigne, N.R. and Ghazal, P. (1999). Murine cytomegalovirus infection down-regulates MHC class II expression on macrophages by induction of IL-10. *Journal of Immunology*, **162**, 6701–7.

Reitz, M. S., Jr, Nerurkar, L.S. and Gallo, R.C. (1999). Perspective on Kaposi's sarcoma: facts, concepts, and conjectures. *Journal of the National Cancer Institute*, **91**, 1453–8.

Revy, P., Hivroz, C., Andreu, G., Graber, P., Martinache, C., Fischer, A. *et al.* (1999). Activation of the Janus kinase 3–STAT5a pathway after CD40 triggering of human monocytes but not of resting B cells. *Journal of Immunology*, **163**, 787–93.

Robinson, W.E., Jr, Montefiori, D.C. and Mitchell, W.M. (1988). Antibody-dependent enhancement of human immunodeficiency virus type 1 infection. *Lancet*, **1**, 790–4.

Rodgers, B. and Mims, C.A. (1981). Interaction of influenza virus with mouse macrophages. *Infection and Immunity*, **31**, 751–7.

Rodriguez, M., Lafuse, W.P., Leibowitz, J. and David, C.S. (1986). Partial suppression of Theiler's virus-induced demyelination *in vivo* by administration of monoclonal antibodies to immune-response gene products (Ia antigens). *Neurology*, **36**, 964–70.

Rodriguez, M., Oleszak, E. and Leibowitz, J. (1987). Theiler's murine encephalomyelitis: a model of demyelination and persistence of virus. *Critical Reviews in Immunology*, **7**, 325–65.

Roizmann, B., Desrosiers, R.C., Fleckenstein, B., Lopez, C., Minson, A.C. and Studdert, M.J. (1992). The family Herpesviridae: an update. The Herpesvirus Study Group of the International Committee on Taxonomy of Viruses. *Archives of Virology*, **123**, 425–49.

Ronni, T., Matikainen, S., Lehtonen, A., Palvimo, J., Dellis, J., Van Eylen, F. *et al.* (1998). The proximal interferon-stimulated response elements are essential for interferon responsiveness: a promoter analysis of the antiviral MxA gene. *Journal of Interferon and Cytokine Research*, **18**, 773–81.

Roos, M.T., Lange, J.M., de Goede, R.E., Coutinho, R.A., Schellekens, P.T., Miedema, F. *et al.* (1992). Viral phenotype and immune response in primary human immunodeficiency virus type 1 infection. *Journal of Infectious Diseases*, **165**, 427–32.

Rose, T.M., Strand, K.B., Schultz, E.R., Schaefer, G., Rankin, G.W., Jr, Thouless, M.E. *et al.* (1997). Identification of two homologs of the Kaposi's sarcoma-associated herpesvirus (human herpesvirus 8) in retroperitoneal fibromatosis of different macaque species. *Journal of Virology*, **71**, 4138–44.

Rostasy, K., Monti, L., Yiannoutsos, C., Kneissl, M., Bell, J., Kemper, T.L. *et al.* (1999). Human immunodeficiency virus infection, inducible nitric oxide synthase expression, and microglial activation: pathogenetic relationship to the acquired immunodeficiency syndrome dementia complex. *Annals of Neurology*, **46**, 207–16.

Russo, J.J., Bohenzky, R.A., Chien, M.C., Chen, J., Yan, M., Maddalena, D. *et al.* (1996). Nucleotide sequence of the Kaposi sarcoma-associated herpesvirus (HHV8). *Proceedings of the National Academy of Sciences USA*, **93**, 14862–7.

Saederup, N., Lin, Y.C., Dairaghi, D.J., Schall, T.J. and Mocarski, E.S. (1999). Cytomegalovirus-encoded β chemokine promotes monocyte-associated viremia in the host. *Proceedings of the National Academy of Sciences USA*, **96**, 10881–6.

Safrit, J.T., Andrews, C.A., Zhu, T., Ho, D.D. and Koup, R.A. (1994). Characterization of human immunodeficiency virus type 1-specific cytotoxic T lymphocyte clones isolated during acute seroconversion: recognition of autologous virus sequences within a conserved immunodominant epitope. *Journal of Experimental Medicine*, **179**, 463–72.

Sakuragi, S., Shibata, R., Mukai, R., Komatsu, T., Fukasawa, M., Sakai, H. *et al.* (1992). Infection of macaque monkeys with a chimeric human and simian immunodeficiency virus. *Journal of General Virology*, **73**, 2983–7.

Salahuddin, S.Z., Nakamura, S., Biberfeld, P., Kaplan, M.H., Markham, P.D., Larsson, L. *et al.* (1988). Angiogenic properties of Kaposi's sarcoma-derived cells after long-term culture *in vitro*. *Science*, **242**, 430–3.

Sankale, J.L., de la Tour, R.S., Renjifo, B., Siby, T., Mboup, S., Marlink, R.G. *et al.* (1995). Intrapatient variability of the human immunodeficiency virus type 2 envelope V3 loop. *AIDS Research and Human Retroviruses*, **11**, 617–23.

Sarid, R., Sato, T., Bohenzky, R.A., Russo, J.J. and Chang, Y. (1997). Kaposi's sarcoma-associated herpesvirus encodes a functional bcl-2 homologue. *Nature Medicine*, **3**, 293–8.

Sarnow, P. (1989). Role of 3'-end sequences in infectivity of poliovirus transcripts made *in vitro*. *Journal of Virology*, **63**, 467–70.

Schafer, S.L., Lin, R., Moore, P.A., Hiscott, J. and Pitha, P.M. (1998). Regulation of type I interferon gene expression by interferon regulatory factor-3. *Journal of Biological Chemistry*, **273**, 2714–20.

Scheid, A. and Choppin, P.W. (1977). Two disulfide-linked polypeptide chains constitute the active F protein of paramyxoviruses. *Virology*, **80**, 54–66.

Schlondorff, D. (1987). The glomerular mesangial cell: an expanding role for a specialized pericyte. *FASEB Journal*, **1**, 272–81.

Schmidtmayerova, H., Nottet, H., Nuovo, G., Raabe, T., Flanagan, C., Dubrovsky, L. *et al.* (1996). Human immunodeficiency virus type 1 infection alters chemokine β peptide expression in human monocytes: implications for recruitment of leukocytes into brain and lymph nodes. *Proceedings of the National Academy of Sciences USA*, **93**, 700–704.

Schmitz, J.E., Kuroda, M.J., Santra, S., Sasseville, V.G., Simon, M.A., Lifton, M.A. *et al.* (1999). Control of viremia in simian immunodeficiency virus infection by CD8+ lymphocytes. *Science*, **283**, 857–60.

Schneider, D.R. and Picker, L.J. (1985). Myelodysplasia in the acquired immune deficiency syndrome. *American Journal of Clinical Pathology*, **84**, 144–52.

Schrag, J.D., Prasad, B.V., Rixon, F.J. and Chiu, W. (1989). Three-dimensional structure of the HSV1 nucleocapsid. *Cell*, **56**, 651–60.

Schuitemaker, H., Kootstra, N.A., de Goede, R.E., de Wolf, F., Miedema, F. and Tersmette, M. (1991). Monocytotropic human immunodeficiency virus type 1 (HIV-1) variants detectable in all stages of HIV-1 infection lack T-cell line tropism and syncytium-inducing ability in primary T-cell culture. *Journal of Virology*, **65**, 356–63.

Schulz, T.F. (1998). Kaposi's sarcoma-associated herpesvirus (human herpesvirus-8). *Journal of General Virology*, **79**, 1573–91.

Schumacher, B., Bernasconi, D., Schultz, U. and Staeheli, P. (1994). The chicken Mx promoter contains an ISRE motif and confers interferon inducibility to a reporter gene in chick and monkey cells. *Virology*, **203**, 144–8.

Schutten, M., Andeweg, A.C., Bosch, M.L. and Osterhaus, A.D. (1995). Enhancement of infectivity of a non-syncytium inducing HIV-1 by sCD4 and by human antibodies that neutralize syncytium inducing HIV-1. *Scandinavian Journal of Immunology*, **41**, 18–22.

Schwartz, O., Marechal, V., Le Gall, S., Lemonnier, F. and Heard, J.M. (1996). Endocytosis of major histocompatibility complex class I molecules is induced by the HIV-1 Nef protein. *Nature Medicine*, **2**, 338–42.

Sedmak, D.D., Guglielmo, A.M., Knight, D.A., Birmingham, D.J., Huang, E.H. and Waldman, W.J. (1994). Cytomegalovirus inhibits major histocompatibility class II expression on infected endothelial cells. *American Journal of Pathology*, **144**, 683–92.

Sellon, D.C., Perry, S.T., Coggins, L. and Fuller, F.J. (1992). Wild-type equine infectious anemia virus replicates *in vivo* predominantly in tissue macrophages, not in peripheral blood monocytes. *Journal of Virology*, **66**, 5906–13.

Shakhov, A.N., Collart, M.A., Vassalli, P., Nedospasov, S. and Jongeneel, C.V. (1990). Kappa B-type enhancers are involved in lipopolysaccharide-mediated transcriptional activation of the tumor necrosis factor α gene in primary macrophages. *Journal of Experimental Medicine*, **171**, 35–47.

Sharma, D.P., Zink, M.C., Anderson, M., Adams, R., Clements, J.E., Joag, S.V. *et al.* (1992). Derivation of neurotropic simian immunodeficiency virus from exclusively lymphocytetropic parental virus: pathogenesis of infection in macaques. *Journal of Virology*, **66**, 3550–6.

Shaw-Jackson, C. and Michiels, T. (1997). Infection of macrophages by Theiler's murine encephalomyelitis virus is highly dependent on their activation or differentiation state. *Journal of Virology*, **71**, 8864–7.

Shenoy, C.M. and Lin, J.H. (1986). Bone marrow findings in acquired immunodeficiency syndrome (AIDS). *American Journal of Medical Science*, **292**, 372–5.

Shibata, R., Kawamura, M., Sakai, H., Hayami, M., Ishimoto, A. and Adachi, A. (1991). Generation of a chimeric human and simian immunodeficiency virus infectious to monkey peripheral blood mononuclear cells. *Journal of Virology*, **65**, 3514–20.

Shibata, Y., Foster, L.A., Metzger, W.J. and Myrvik, Q.N. (1997). Alveolar macrophage priming by intravenous administration of chitin particles, polymers of *N*-acetyl-D-glucosamine, in mice. *Infection and Immunity*, **65**, 1734–41.

Sigurdsson, B. (1954). Maedi, a slow progressive pneumonia of sheep: an epizoological and pathological study. *British Journal of Veterinary Research*, **110**, 255–70.

Silverman, R. and Cirino, N. (1997). RNA decay by the interferon-regulated 2-5A system as a host defense against viruses. In Morris, D. and Harford T (ed.), *mRNA Metabolism and Post-transcriptional Gene Regulation*. Wiley-Liss, Inc. New York. pp. 295–309.

Simpson, G.R., Schulz, T.F., Whitby, D., Cook, P.M., Boshoff, C., Rainbow, L. *et al.* (1996). Prevalence of Kaposi's sarcoma associated herpesvirus infection measured by antibodies to recombinant capsid protein and latent immunofluorescence antigen. *Lancet*, **348**, 1133–8.

Singh, D.K., Chebloune, Y., Mselli-Lakhal, L., Karr, B.M. and Narayan, O. (1999). Ovine lentivirus-infected macrophages mediate productive infection in cell types that are not susceptible to infection with cell-free virus. *Journal of General Virology*, **80**, 1437–44.

Slowik, M.R., Min, W., Ardito, T., Karsan, A., Kashgarian, M. and Pober, J.S. (1997). Evidence that tumor necrosis factor triggers apoptosis in human endothelial cells by interleukin-1-converting enzyme-like protease-dependent and -independent pathways. *Laboratory Investigation*, **77**, 257–67.

Smith, M.W., Dean, M., Carrington, M., Winkler, C., Huttley, G.A., Lomb, D.A. *et al.* (1997). Contrasting genetic influence of CCR2 and CCR5 variants on HIV-1 infection and disease progression. Hemophilia Growth and Development Study (HGDS), Multicenter AIDS Cohort Study (MACS), Multicenter Hemophilia Cohort Study (MHCS), San Francisco City Cohort (SFCC), ALIVE Study. *Science*, **277**, 959–65.

Soderberg, C., Larsson, S., Bergstedt-Lindqvist, S. and Moller, E. (1993). Definition of a subset of human peripheral blood mononuclear cells that are permissive to human cytomegalovirus infection. *Journal of Virology*, **67**, 3166–75.

Spertzel, R.O. (1989). Animal models of human immunodeficiency virus infection. Public Health Service Animal Models Committee. *Antiviral Research*, **12**, 223–30.

Spivak, J.L., Bender, B.S. and Quinn, T.C. (1984). Hematologic abnormalities in the acquired immune deficiency syndrome. *American Journal of Medicine*, **77**, 224–8.

Squire, J., Zhou, A., Sotomayor, C., Maran, A. and Silverman, R. (1994). Localization of the interferon induced 2–5A dependent RNAse gene (RNS4) to human chromosome Iq25. *Genomics*, **19**, 174–5.

Stanley, S.K., Kessler, S.W., Justement, J.S., Schnittman, S.M., Greenhouse, J.J., Brown, C.C. *et al.* (1992). CD34⁺ bone marrow cells are infected with HIV in a subset of seropositive individuals. *Journal of Immunology*, **149**, 689–97.

Staskus, K.A., Couch, L., Bitterman, P., Retzel, E.F., Zupancic, M., List, J. *et al.* (1991). *In situ* amplification of visna virus DNA in tissue sections reveals a reservoir of latently infected cells. *Microbial Pathogenesis*, **11**, 67–76.

Stent, G., Cameron, P.U. and Crowe, S.M. (1994). Expression of CD11/CD18 and ICAM-1 on monocytes and lymphocytes of HIV-1-infected individuals. *Journal of Leukocyte Biology*, **56**, 304–9.

Stephens, E.B., Mukherjee, S., Sahni, M., Zhuge, W., Raghavan, R., Singh, D.K. *et al.* (1997). A cell-free stock of simian-human immunodeficiency virus that causes AIDS in pig-tailed macaques has a limited number of amino acid substitutions in both SIVmac and HIV-1 regions of the genome and has offered cytotropism. *Virology*, **231**, 313–21.

Stephens, E.B., Tian, C., Li, Z., Narayan, O. and Gattone, V.H., 2nd (1998). Rhesus macaques infected with macrophage-tropic simian immunodeficiency virus (SIVmacR71/17E) exhibit extensive focal segmental and global glomerulosclerosis. *Journal of Virology*, **72**, 8820–32.

Stranden, A.M., Staeheli, P. and Pavlovic, J. (1993). Function of the mouse Mx1 protein is inhibited by overexpression of the PB2 protein of influenza virus. *Virology*, **197**, 642–51.

Sun, N.C., Shapshak, P., Lachant, N.A., Hsu, M.Y., Sieger, L., Schmid, P. *et al.* (1989). Bone marrow examination in patients with AIDS and AIDS-related complex (ARC). Morphologic and *in situ* hybridization studies. *American Journal of Clinical Pathology*, **92**, 589–94.

Sutterwala, F.S., Noel, G.J., Clynes, R. and Mosser, D.M. (1997). Selective suppression of inter-leukin-12 induction after macrophage receptor ligation. *Journal of Experimental Medicine*, **185**, 1977–85.

Swardson, C.J., Kociba, G.J. and Perryman, L.E. (1992). Effects of equine infectious anemia virus on hematopoietic progenitors *in vitro*. *American Journal of Veterinary Research*, **53**, 1176–9.

Takeda, A., Tuazon, C.U. and Ennis, F.A. (1988). Antibody-enhanced infection by HIV-1 via Fc receptor-mediated entry. *Science*, **242**, 580–3.

Takehisa, J., Zekeng, L., Ido, E., Mboudjeka, I., Moriyama, H., Miura, T. *et al.* (1998). Various types of HIV mixed infections in Cameroon. *Virology*, **245**, 1–10.

Tamura, M., Webster, R.G. and Ennis, F.A. (1991). Antibodies to HA and NA augment uptake of influenza A viruses into cells via Fc receptor entry. *Virology*, **182**, 211–9.

Taylor-Wiedeman, J., Sissons, J.G., Borysiewicz, L.K. and Sinclair, J.H. (1991). Monocytes are a major site of persistence of human cytomegalovirus in peripheral blood mononuclear cells. *Journal of General Virology*, **72**, 2059–64.

Taylor-Wiedeman, J., Sissons, P. and Sinclair, J. (1994). Induction of endogenous human cytomegalovirus gene expression after differentiation of monocytes from healthy carriers. *Journal of Virology*, **68**, 1597–604.

Telford, E.A., Watson, M.S., Aird, H.C., Perry, J. and Davison, A.J. (1995). The DNA sequence of equine herpesvirus 2. *Journal of Molecular Biology*, **249**, 520–8.

Tenney, D. and Morahan, P. (1991). Differentiation of the U937 macrophage cell line removes an early block of HSV-1 infection. *Viral Immunology,* Vol. 4, pp. 91–102.

Teo, I., Veryard, C., Barnes, H., An, S.F., Jones, M., Lantos, P.L. *et al.* (1997). Circular forms of unintegrated human immunodeficiency virus type 1 DNA and high levels of viral protein expression: association with dementia and multinucleated giant cells in the brains of patients with AIDS. *Journal of Virology*, **71**, 2928–33.

Tersmette, M. and Miedema, F. (1990). Interactions between HIV and the host immune system in the pathogenesis of AIDS. *AIDS*. **4**, S57–66.

Thieblemont, N., Haeffner-Cavaillon, N., Ledur, A., L'Age-Stehr, J., Ziegler-Heitbrock, H.W. and Kazatchkine, M.D. (1993). CR1 (CD35) and CR3 (CD11b/CD18) mediate infection of human monocytes and monocytic cell lines with complement-opsonized HIV independently of CD4. *Clinical and Experimental Immunology*, **92**, 106–13.

Thome, M., Schneider, P., Hofmann, K., Fickenscher, H., Meinl, E., Neipel, F. *et al.* (1997). Viral FLICE-inhibitory proteins (FLIPs) prevent apoptosis induced by death receptors. *Nature*, **386**, 517–21.

Tindall, B. and Cooper, D.A. (1991). Primary HIV infection: host responses and intervention strategies. *AIDS*, **5**, 1–14.

Tsujimoto, H., Cooper, R.W., Kodama, T., Fukasawa, M., Miura, T., Ohta, Y. *et al.* (1988). Isolation and characterization of simian immunodeficiency virus from mandrills in Africa and its relationship to other human and simian immunodeficiency viruses. *Journal of Virology*, **62**, 4044–50.

Tsukamoto, H., Lin, M., Ohata, M., Giulivi, C., French, S.W. and Brittenham, G. (1999). Iron primes hepatic macrophages for NF-κB activation in alcoholic liver injury. *American Journal of Physiology*, **277**, G1240–50.

Tsunoda, I., Kurtz, C.I. and Fujinami, R.S. (1997). Apoptosis in acute and chronic central nervous system disease induced by Theiler's murine encephalomyelitis virus. *Virology*, **228**, 388–93.

Tyor, W.R., Power, C., Gendelman, H.E. and Markham, R.B. (1993). A model of human immunodeficiency virus encephalitis in scid mice. *Proceedings of the National Academy of Sciences USA*, **90**, 8658–62.

Valee, H. and Carre, H. (1904). Sur la nature infectieuse de l'anemie du cheval. *Compte Rendu de l'Academie des Sciences*, **139**, 331–3.

van den Broek, M.F., Muller, U., Huang, S., Aguet, M. and Zinkernagel, R.M. (1995). Antiviral defense in mice lacking both α/β and γ interferon receptors. *Journal of Virology*, **69**, 4792–6.

Van Strijp, J.A., Van Kessel, K.P., van der Tol, M.E., Fluit, A.C., Snippe, H. and Verhoef, J. (1989). Phagocytosis of herpes simplex virus by human granulocytes and monocytes. *Archives of Virology*, **104**, 287–98.

Van Strijp, J.A., Miltenburg, L.A., van der Tol, M.E., Van Kessel, K.P., Fluit, A.C. and Verhoef, J. (1990). Degradation of herpes simplex virions by human polymorphonuclear leukocytes and monocytes. *Journal of General Virology*, **71**, 1205–9.

Van de Perre, P. and Cartoux, M. (1995). Retroviral Transmission and Breast-feeding. Clinical Microbiology & Infection, **1**, 6–12.

Van de Perre P. (2000). Breast milk transmission of HIV-1. Laboratory and clinical studies. Annals of the NY Academy of Science, **918**, 122–7.

Vanderlugt, C.L., Begolka, W.S., Neville, K.L., Katz-Levy, Y., Howard, L.M., Eagar, T.N. *et al.* (1998). The functional significance of epitope spreading and its regulation by co-stimulatory molecules. *Immunological Reviews*, **164**, 63–72.

Vasil, S., Thakallpally, R., Korber, B. and Foley, B. (1998). Global variation in the HIV-1 V3 region. In Korber, B. *et al.* (ed.), *Human Retroviruses and AIDS*. Los Alamos National Laboratory, Los Alamos, pp. III118–265.

Vicenzi, E., Biswas, P., Mengozzi, M. and Poli, G. (1997). Role of pro-inflammatory cytokines and β-chemokines in controlling HIV replication. *Journal of Leukocyte Biology*, **62**, 34–40.

Virgin, H.W.T., Latreille, P., Wamsley, P., Hallsworth, K., Weck, K.E., Dal Canto, A.J. *et al.* (1997). Complete sequence and genomic analysis of murine gammaherpesvirus 68. *Journal of Virology*, **71**, 5894–904.

von Laer, D., Hufert, F.T., Fenner, T.E., Schwander, S., Dietrich, M., Schmitz, H. *et al.* (1990). CD34$^+$ hematopoietic progenitor cells are not a major reservoir of the human immunodeficiency virus. *Blood*, **76**, 1281–6.

von Laer, D., Serr, A., Meyer-Konig, U., Kirste, G., Hufert, F.T. and Haller, O. (1995). Human cytomegalovirus immediate early and late transcripts are expressed in all major leukocyte populations *in vivo*. *Journal of Infectious Diseases*, **172**, 365–70.

Wang, F.I., Stohlman, S.A. and Fleming, J.O. (1990). Demyelination induced by murine hepatitis virus JHM strain (MHV-4) is immunologically mediated. *Journal of Neuroimmunology*, **30**, 31–41.

Wang, Q. and Floyd-Smith, G. (1997). The p69/71 2–5A synthetase promoter contains multiple regulatory elements required for interferon-α-induced expression. *DNA Cell Biology*, **16**, 1385–94.

Ward, D.M., Leslie, J.D. and Kaplan, J. (1997). Homotypic lysosome fusion in macrophages: analysis using an *in vitro* assay. *Journal of Cell Biology*, **139**, 665–73.

Wardle, E.N. (1991). Cytokine growth factors and glomerulonephritis. *Nephron*, **57**, 257–61.

Weinshenker, B.G., Wilton, S. and Rice, G.P. (1988). Phorbol ester-induced differentiation permits productive human cytomegalovirus infection in a monocytic cell line. *Journal of Immunology*, **140**, 1625–31.

Weiser, B., Burger, H., Campbell, P., Donelan, S. and Mladenovic, J. (1996). HIV type 1 RNA expression in bone marrows of patients with a spectrum of disease. *AIDS Research and Human Retroviruses*, **12**, 1551–8.

Welsh, C.J., Tonks, P., Nash, A.A. and Blakemore, W.F. (1987). The effect of L3T4 T cell depletion on the pathogenesis of Theiler's murine encephalomyelitis virus infection in CBA mice. *Journal of General Virology*, **68**, 1659–67.

Welsh, M. and Adair, B. (1995). Effect of BVD virus on alveolar macrophage function. *Immuno Immunopathology*, **46**, 195–210.

Wong, L.H., Hatzinisiriou, I., Devenish, R.J. and Ralph, S.J. (1998). IFN-γ priming up-regulates IFN-stimulated gene factor 3 (ISGF3) components, augmenting responsiveness of IFN-resistant melanoma cells to type I IFNs. *Journal of Immunology*, **160**, 5475–84.

Wu, F.K., Garcia, J.A., Harrich, D. and Gaynor, R.B. (1988). Purification of the human immunodeficiency virus type 1 enhancer and TAR binding proteins EBP-1 and UBP-1. *EMBO Journal*, **7**, 2117–30.

Wu, G.F. and Perlman, S. (1999). Macrophage infiltration but not apoptosis is correlated with immune mediated demyelination following murine infection with a neurotropic coronavirus. *Journal of Virology*, **73**, 8771–80.

Wyllie, A.H., Kerr, J.F.R. and Currie, A.R. (1980). Cell death: the significance of apoptosis. *International Review of Cytology*, **68**, 251–301.

Xie, Q.W., Kashiwabara, Y. and Nathan, C. (1994). Role of transcription factor NF-κB/Rel in induction of nitric oxide synthase. *Journal of Biological Chemistry*, **269**, 4705–8.

Xue, S., Sun, N., Rooijen, N.V. and Perlman, S. (1999). Depletion of blood-borne macrophages does not reduce demyelination in mice infected with a neurotropic coronavirus. *Journal of Virology*, **73**, 6327–6334.

Yamamoto, T., Noble, N.A., Miller, D.E., Gold, L.I., Hishida, A., Nagase, M. *et al.* (1999). Increased levels of transforming growth factor-β in HIV-associated nephropathy. *Kidney International*, **55**, 579–92.

Ye, J., Shi, X., Jones, W., Rojanasakul, Y., Cheng, N., Schwegler-Berry, D. *et al.* (1999). Critical role of glass fiber length in TNF-α production and transcription factor activation in macrophages. *American Journal of Physiology*, **276**, L426–34.

Yewdell, J. and Bennick, J. (1999). Mechanisms of viral interference with MHC class I antigen processing and presentation. *Annual Review of Cell and Developmental Biology*, **15**, 579–606.

Yu, Y., Henry, S.C., Xu, F. and Hamilton, J.D. (1995). Expression of a murine cytomegalovirus early-late protein in 'latently' infected mice. *Journal of Infectious Diseases*, **172**, 371–9.

Yuhasz, S.A., Dissette, V.B., Cook, M.L. and Stevens, J.G. (1994). Murine cytomegalovirus is present in both chronic active and latent states in persistently infected mice. V*irology*, **202**, 272–80.

Yurochko, A.D. and Huang, E.S. (1999). Human cytomegalovirus binding to human monocytes induces immunoregulatory gene expression. *Journal of Immunology*, **162**, 4806–16.

Yurochko, A.D., Hwang, E.S., Rasmussen, L., Keay, S., Pereira, L. and Huang, E.S. (1997). The human cytomegalovirus UL55 (gB) and UL75 (gH) glycoprotein ligands initiate the rapid activation of Sp1 and NF-κB during infection. *Journal of Virology*, **71**, 5051–9.

Zeigler, H. (2000). The luminal part of the murine ctomegalovirus glycoprotein gp40 catalyzes the retention of MHC class I molecules. *EMBO Journal*, **19**, 870–881.

Zhou, A., Paranjape, J., Brown, T.L., Nie, H., Naik, S., Dong, B. *et al.* (1997). Interferon action and apoptosis are defective in mice devoid of 2′,5′-oligoadenylate-dependent RNase L. *EMBO Journal*, **16**, 6355–63.

Zimmerli, S., Majeed, M., Gustavsson, M., Stendahl, O., Sanan, D.A. and Ernst, J.D. (1996). Phagosome–lysosome fusion is a calcium-independent event in macrophages. *Journal of Cell Biology*, **132**, 49–61.

Zink, M.C., Suryanarayana, K., Mankowski, J.L., Shen, A., Piatak, M., Jr, Spelman, J.P. *et al.* (1999a). High viral load in the cerebrospinal fluid and brain correlates with severity of simian immunodeficiency virus encephalitis. *Journal of Virology*, **73**, 10480–8.

Zink, W.E., Zheng, J., Persidsky, Y., Poluektova, L. and Gendelman, H.E. (1999b). The neuropathogenesis of HIV-1 infection. *FEMS Immunology and Medical Microbiology*, **26**, 233–241.

Zon, L.I., Arkin, C. and Groopman, J.E. (1987). Haematologic manifestations of the human immune deficiency virus (HIV). *British Journal of Haematology*, **66**, 251–6.

Zon, L.I. and Groopman, J.E. (1988). Hematologic manifestations of the human immune deficiency virus (HIV). *Seminars in Hematology*, **25**, 208–18.

Zucker-Franklin, D., Termin, C.S. and Cooper, M.C. (1989). Structural changes in the megakaryocytes of patients infected with the human immune deficiency virus (HIV-1). *American Journal of Pathology*, **134**, 1295–303.

5 *Macrophages in bacterial infection*

J.-P. Heale and D.P. Speert

1 Introduction

1.1 Role of macrophages in defense against infection

Bacterial pathogens must breach normal host defenses to establish invasive infections. The macrophage stands guard at potential portals of entry to discourage such intruders and to maintain sterility of deep tissues. Despite the rich panoply of antimicrobial devices available to the macrophage, many bacterial species have developed means of resisting these normal *cidal* mechanisms. Some bacteria are able to persist within macrophages and some are even dependent upon this intracellular haven for their survival. This chapter will provide an overview of the macrophage's antibacterial activities and will describe some of the strategies used by intra- and extracellular pathogens to overcome these normal host defense mechanisms.

Macrophages are poised to exert their antibacterial activity at mucosal surfaces and as filtering agents within the lymphoid organs (reticuloendothelial system). The lungs are protected against inhaled infectious microorganisms by the pulmonary alveolar macrophages. These cells are unique among macrophages in their phenotypic characteristics that may derive from their oxygen-rich environment. Therefore, generalizations from the pulmonary alveolar macrophage to other macrophage phenotypes should be made with caution. Other 'free' macrophages can be found in the pleural spaces, synovial fluid, peritoneum and at inflammatory sites.

Fixed macrophages within the liver (Kupffer cells) and the spleen provide a robust form of protection against blood-borne bacterial infection (Rogers, 1960). Whereas the pulmonary alveolar macrophage must be prepared at times to phagocytose bacteria in the absence of opsonins, splenic and hepatic macrophages can be assisted by circulating complement and immunoglobulin (Ig). Fixed tissue macrophages are also found in the bone marrow, lamina propria of the gastrointestinal tract, lymph nodes, brain (microglia), skin (Langerhans cells), kidney, endocrine organs and perivascular space.

Macrophages can be viewed as a dispersed secretory organ capable of augmenting the antibacterial activities of the other types of leukocytes. In addition to producing interleukin (IL)-1, IL-6 and tumor necrosis factor-α (TNF-α), pulmonary alveolar macrophages secrete cytokines that recruit and activate neutrophils (e.g. IL-8). These and other secretory products with defined antibacterial roles will be discussed.

1.2 The macrophage as a safe haven for intracellular parasites

Pathogenic bacteria have evolved many creative means of evading normal host defenses. As macrophages and neutrophils play such a critical role in protecting the host against infection, many bacterial virulence mechanisms are directed at subjugating normal phagocytic processes. Extracellular pathogens are virulent by avoiding phagocytic recognition and/or ingestion. Intracellular pathogens, on the other hand, are able to survive within phagocytic cells and may even depend upon the environment within the macrophage for persistence and growth. Facultative intracellular parasites (such as *Salmonella typhimurium*) are those which are able to grow within or without eukaryotic cells and can be cultivated on artificial laboratory media. Obligate intracellular parasites (such as *Mycobacterium leprae*) are those which are absolutely dependent upon the intracellular niche for their growth.

Intracellular parasites may exploit other features of macrophages to enhance their virulence. The blood–brain barrier is quite effective in limiting the spread of bacteria to the central nervous system (CNS). Under certain circumstances, however, bacteria gain access to the CNS after being phagocytosed by monocytes (Williams and Blakemore, 1990). This 'Trojan horse' phenomenon has been shown for *Streptococcus suis* (Williams and Blakemore, 1990) and also plays a role in the spread of other bacteria and viruses, such as the human immunodeficiency virus (Vitkovicn *et al.*, 1995).

To understand the nature of intracellular parasitism within macrophages, it is essential to recognize that there is a dynamic interplay between prokaryote and eukaryote. Study of bacterial features is not informative unless their effects upon the host cell are understood. Similarly, the effects of bacterial products on macrophage function are meaningful only in so far as they influence the fate of the microorganism. An example of this dynamic interaction is seen when *Salmonella cholerasuis* and epithelial cells are co-cultivated. Contact with the host causes a change in bacterial phenotype, marked by activation and expression of a type III secretion system that mediates invasion (Galan and Collmer, 1999). Other examples of this sort of dynamic interplay will be discussed later.

2 Phenotypic and genotypic differences among macrophages

2.1 Phenotypic differences among macrophages

As discussed in Chapter 1, macrophages have a wide tissue distribution. In studies using a highly specific monoclonal antibody, the relative density of macrophages has been estimated in different murine tissues (Lee *et al.*, 1985; Gordon *et al.*, 1988). The organs with the highest density of macrophage-specific antigen are the liver, large and small bowel, bone marrow, spleen, lymph nodes and kidney (Lee *et al.*, 1985). The bulk of tissue macrophages appear to have developed from circulating blood monocytes under the influence of the local environment in which they have come to reside (Gordon *et al.*, 1988). The marked differences among conditions within these various tissues may be largely responsible for the phenotypic diversity among macrophages. In addition to those macrophages found imbedded deep within tissues are classes of macrophages associated with vascular endothelium, pulmonary alveoli and serosal surfaces. It is in these locations that macrophages are poised to exert their function as scavengers of microbial pathogens. Each macrophage phenotype has unique characteristics which may serve to arm it for battle with microbes under the special conditions in which it must function.

In addition to the resident tissue macrophages, additional monocytic cells are recruited by inflammatory stimuli, such as thioglycollate broth or bacterial infection (North, 1970, 1978; Cohn, 1978). These recruited cells are phenotypically different from resident cells: they have alterations in expression and function of surface antigens and receptors (Cohn, 1978), and an enhanced capacity to produce reactive oxygen and nitrogen intermediates (Cohn, 1978, Kaplan *et al.*, 1996) and kill intracellular pathogens (North, 1970).

Macrophage phenotypic characteristics can also be modulated by other local factors. Cytokines, such as interferon-γ (IFN-γ), have profound effects upon expression of receptors and other surface molecules (Basham and Merrigan, 1983; Becker, 1984). The effects are specific, with up-regulation of certain receptors and the suppression of others (Guyre *et al.*, 1983; Perussia *et al.*, 1983; Mokoena and Gordon, 1985; Wright *et al.*, 1986). Multiple effector functions of macrophages are enhanced by IFN-γ, chief among which is the generation of reactive oxygen and nitrogen intermediates (Nathan *et al.*, 1983; Nathan and Xie, 1994). Dexamethasone counters many of the effects of IFN-γ, including expression of mannose receptors (Mokoena and Gordon, 1985) and Fc receptors (Warren and Vogel, 1985) (see Section 3.1).

2.1.1 Phagocytic and bacteriocidal activity of different macrophage phenotypes

Evidence that circulating monocytes have an enhanced capacity to kill bacteria as compared with fixed tissue macrophages comes from studies of *Listeria monocytogenes* infections in mice (Lepay *et al.*, 1985a,b). Shortly after intravenous infection, monocytes are recruited from the peripheral blood to the liver where they appear to be critically important in eliminating infective foci. Upon resolution of the infection, new monocytes are no longer recruited. As the inflammation subsides, many bacteria-laden leukocytes apoptose and subsequently are ingested by tissue macrophages (Hilbi *et al.*, 1997; Mecklenburgh *et al.*, 1999). Observations such as this have suggested that there are intrinsic differences in the capacity of mononuclear phagocytes of different phenotype to phagocytose and kill bacteria.

Comparisons of phagocytic activity *in vitro* have been made among different cell types, and for the same type between different animal species. Human peripheral blood monocytes are capable of killing a diverse range of bacterial species, but they do so less efficiently than polymorphonuclear leukocytes (PMNs) (Steigbigel *et al.*, 1974; Peterson *et al.*, 1977a). The difference between these two cell types appears to be due to intrinsic differences in phagocytic rather than bacteriocidal capacity. Studies on peritoneal and pulmonary alveolar macrophages from humans, rabbits, guinea pigs, hamsters, rats and mice demonstrate intact oxygen-dependent and -independent bacteriocidal mechanisms (Nguyen *et al.*, 1982; Verbrugh *et al.*, 1983; Peterson *et al.*, 1985; Catterall *et al.*, 1987; Kemmerich *et al.*, 1987). Notable differences are observed among species (Nguyen *et al.*, 1982; Catterall *et al.*, 1987) and between cells obtained from different sites (Catterall *et al.*, 1987; Kemmerich *et al.*, 1987). Whereas murine macrophages can produce nitric oxide (NO) efficiently, human macrophages appear to be attenuated in their capacity to produce reactive nitrogen intermediates (ROIs) (Albina, 1995).

Human pulmonary alveolar macrophages generate greater quantities of ROIs than do monocytes upon stimulation. This difference is reflected in their superior capacity to kill *Pseudomonas aeruginosa* and *L.monocytogenes* (Kemmerich *et al.*, 1987). However, under the influence of IFN-γ, the respiratory burst and microbicidal capacity of monocytes, but not alveolar macrophages, are enhanced (Kemmerich *et al.*, 1987). Pulmonary alveolar macrophages also depend upon high oxygen tension (Cohen and Cline, 1971) and oxidative phosphorylation for metabolic energy to a greater extent than do monocytes or PMNs. The resting respiratory rate of human pulmonary alveolar macrophages is three times greater than that of the monocyte (Fels and Cohn, 1986).

Human and murine peritoneal macrophages have notable similarities. Resident (unelicited) cells generate a feeble respiratory burst upon stimulation as compared with elicited (with thioglycollate in mice; by chronic peritoneal dialysis in humans) cells (Peterson *et al.*, 1985). These elicited human peritoneal cells kill opsonized *Staphylococcus epidermidis*, *Staphylococcus aureus* and *Escherichia coli* as efficiently as do PMNs (Verbrugh *et al.*, 1983).

Some functional differences have been described between human umbilical cord blood monocyte-derived macrophages and those from the peripheral blood of healthy adults

(Marodi *et al.*, 1984). Significant differences in susceptibility to phagocytosis have been noted among various bacterial species. Phagocytosis of *S.aureus, E.coli* and Group A streptococci by cord blood monocyte-derived macrophages is normal when compared with adult cells. However, killing of *S.aureus*, and both phagocytosis and killing of Group B streptococci are impaired (Marodi *et al.*, 1984).

2.1.2 Pulmonary alveolar macrophages and protection of the lungs against inhaled bacteria

The respiratory tract is exposed to an enormous quantity of bacteria and other inhaled particles, some of which gain access to the lower airways. Pulmonary macrophages play a critically important role in protecting the lung against infection by these inhaled microorganisms and stand guard as the resident phagocytic cells (Goldstein *et al.*, 1974; Hocking and Golde, 1979; Rehm *et al.*, 1980; Fels and Cohn, 1986; Coonrod, 1989). Neutrophils are recruited as 'professional' phagocytes when pulmonary alveolar macrophages release TNF-α in response to bacterial lipopolysaccharide (LPS) (Hachicha *et al.*, 1998). Pulmonary macrophages are found in the alveoli, small and large airways, interstitium of the lung and lining the pulmonary vessels (Sibille and Reynolds, 1990). The best characterized of these cells are those which can be lavaged from the lung, generally referred to as pulmonary alveolar macrophages.

The normal human tracheobronchial secretions have relatively low levels of complement and IgM, but IgG and IgA are generally present (Reynolds and Thompson, 1973; Reynolds and Newball, 1974). The pulmonary alveolar macrophage has greatly reduced levels of receptors for complement and the Fc portion of IgG (Stokes *et al.*, 1998). It is reasonable to assume that pulmonary alveolar macrophages may rely upon non-opsonic phagocytosis more than other tissue macrophages which benefit from the full array of serum opsonins.

Receptors for a wide array of ligands are found on pulmonary alveolar macrophages, permitting ingestion of a disparate range of particulate and soluble substances (Fels and Cohn, 1986). The human pulmonary alveolar macrophage is also armed with surface-exposed 'cytophilic' IgG (Verbrugh *et al.*, 1982). Strains of *S.aureus* which express protein A bind IgG in a non-immunological fashion and are phagocytosed non-opsonically by pulmonary alveolar macrophages. In general, pulmonary alveolar macrophages phagocytose and clear Gram-positive bacteria better than Gram-negatives in the absence of serum opsonins (Sibille and Reynolds, 1990). Strains of *Haemophilus influenzae* type B and encapsulated *Streptococcus pneumoniae*, which are pathogenic for humans, are relatively resistant to opsonization by normal human serum (Jonsson *et al.*, 1985), a factor which may aid their virulence in pulmonary infections. Non-pathogenic bacteria, such as unencapsulated *H.influenzae*, are susceptible to phagocytosis and killing by pulmonary alveolar macrophages after opsonization with normal human serum (Jonsson *et al.*, 1985). Pulmonary alveolar macrophages are unique among human phagocytic cells in their dependence upon oxygen for optimum phagocytosis (Cohen and Cline, 1971).

Pulmonary alveolar macrophages elaborate an impressive array of secretory products and enzymes with potential antibacterial properties. In addition to lysozyme, which constitutes 25 per cent of the total protein released, these cells produce lysosomal acid hydrolases and neutral proteases (Fels and Cohn, 1986; Sibille and Reynolds, 1990). They also secrete a wide array of cytokines, biologically active lipids, reactive oxygen and nitrogen radicals, complement components, and free fatty acids, all with potential antibacterial activity (Sibille and Reynolds, 1990; Kaplan *et al.*, 1996).

2.1.3 Kupffer cells and protection against blood-borne infection

Transient bacteremia is probably a common daily occurrence, but septicemia is a relatively rare event. Macrophages of the reticuloendothelial system serve to filter bacteria from the blood and prevent infection except by those species of bacteria that are able to resist this normal host defense (Frank, 1989). The resident macrophage of the liver, the Kupffer cell, is located in the hepatic sinusoids where it is exposed to the constant flow of blood. It is thus poised to remove potential pathogens from the circulation. Splenic macrophages also play a critical role in bloodstream clearance but they have not been studied as thoroughly *in vitro* as Kupffer cells. Pulmonary intravascular macrophages probably also play an important role in removing certain bacteria, after intravenous injection (Bowdy *et al.*, 1990). The critical role of Kupffer cells is demonstrated in individuals with reticuloendothelial system blockade (Frank *et al.*, 1979) or in animals whose Kupffer cells have been damaged artificially (Frieman and Moon, 1977). Hepatic phagocytic cells have an enormous capacity to phagocytose bacteria and other particulate debris non-opsonically (Wardle, 1987), a feature largely due to the presence of lectins of different specificities (Hubbard and Stukenbrok, 1979; Leunk and Moon, 1982; Perry and Ofek, 1984; Rumelt *et al.*, 1988). Opsonins also play a critical role in augmenting reticuloendothelial clearance of blood-borne bacteria; disabling the complement system drastically lowers the lethal dose (LD_{50}) for some bacteria species (Frank *et al.*, 1979). Opsonizing antibody also enhances the phagocytic capacity of Kupffer cells and permits the elimination of the more virulent species of bacteria (Rogers, 1960). Kupffer cells and splenic macrophages appear to complement each other; the former clear complement-coated particles predominantly whereas the latter phagocytose those opsonized with IgG (Frank *et al.*, 1979).

Upon activation, Kupffer cells have an enhanced capacity to phagocytose IgG-coated particles (Wardle, 1987), and are able to produce reactive oxygen radicals (Kausalya *et al.*, 1996; Spolarics, 1996). In addition to Kupffer cells that are activated by exposure to various cytokines, monocytes are recruited to the liver upon bacterial infection. These monocytes are also capable of generating reactive oxygen radicals and killing intracellular parasites (Lepay *et al.*, 1985b).

2.2 Genetic influences on macrophage antibacterial activities

Genetic differences in susceptibility to infection are suggested by the observation that particular infectious diseases occur more frequently in certain ethnic groups. Furthermore, differences in permissiveness to infection with intracellular parasites imply a genetic influence on macrophage bacteriocidal capacity. Skamene and co-workers have explored the reasons for differences in susceptibility to infection among different inbred strains of mice. Intracellular pathogens studied include *S.typhimurium*, *Leishmania donovani* and *Mycobacterium bovis* (Gros *et al.*, 1981; Skamene *et al.*, 1982; Denis *et al.*, 1988; Buschman *et al.*, 1989; Schurr *et al.*, 1989, 1990). They found that strains segregated into groups on the basis of susceptibility or resistance to all three of these pathogens, suggesting that the inheritance is under monogenic dominant control (Skamene *et al.*, 1982). The genes controlling susceptibility to each of these pathogens have been designated *Ity* (for *S.typhimurium*), *Lsh* (for *L.donovani*) and *Bcg* (for *M.bovis*). These genes are in fact one autosomal dominant gene termed *Nramp* for natural resistance-associated macrophage protein (Vidal *et al.*, 1995a). The gene encodes a 2.4 kb mRNA product found exclusively in the reticuloendothelial organs, and greatly enriched in mature tissue macrophages (Vidal *et al.*, 1995a), whose expression can be dramatically induced by IFN-γ and LPS (Govoni *et al.*, 1995). *Nramp1* has structural similarities to a variety of bacterial and eukaryotic transport proteins and it has been hypothesized to be involved in the transport of oxidized nitrogen radicals (Vidal *et al.*, 1995a). Targeted disruption of *Nramp1* abrogates natural resistance to infection with intracellular parasites, such as *M.bovis*, *L.donovani* and lethal *S.typhimurium* infection (Vidal *et al.*, 1995b).

3 Phagocytosis of microorganisms

3.1 Macrophage receptors

Phagocytosis is a dynamic process in which bacteria are first bound to the macrophage membrane in preparation for ingestion. This attachment step is mediated by specific macrophage receptors and is dependent upon the nature of the bacterial surface. A list of macrophage phagocytic receptors is given in Table 5.1. Opsonization of bacteria with complement and/or Ig permits macrophages and other phagocytic cells to recognize, by a limited number of receptors, a wide array of bacterial species with broad heterogeneity in surface characteristics. The principal macrophage phagocytic receptors recognize the breakdown products of complement component 3 (C3b and C3bi) and the Fc portion of IgG (Silverstein *et al.*, 1989; Carroll, 1998). The role(s) in antibacterial defense played by the receptors for the Fc portion of IgA (FcαR, CD89) (Richards and Gauldie, 1985; Morton *et al.*, 1986) is less well defined although it has a limited role in phagocytosis of IgA-opsonized bacteria and triggering the macrophage respiratory burst. The macrophage receptors for fibronectin, Vla-4 and 5, are members of the β₁ integrin family which bind fibronectin, present in extracellular matrices (Lobb and Hemler, 1994). Binding of fibronectin induces activation of cytoplasmic protein tyrosine kinases, which in turn up-regulates complement receptor 3 (CR3) and phagocytosis of complement-coated particles (Berton and Lowell, 1999). In addition to phagocytosis via opsonic receptors, macrophages are well equipped for non-opsonic phagocytosis (Ofek *et al.*, 1995; Stahl and Ezekowitz, 1998; van der Laan *et al.*, 1999). Although described as 'non-specific' phagocytosis, the involvement of specific receptors in the process has been demonstrated, among them the multifunctional CR3 molecule (Ross and Vetvicka, 1993; Dunne *et al.*, 1994; Palecanda *et al.*, 1999). The mannose receptor is perhaps the best characterized of the non-opsonic receptors. In addition to its role in recycling mannosylated macromolecules from the circulation (Stahl and Ezekowitz, 1998), it appears to be involved in the ingestion of certain bacteria, fungi and parasites (Blackwell *et al.*, 1985; Kan and Bennett, 1998; Ofek *et al.*, 1995). CD14 is also a non-opsonic receptor involved in macrophage phagocytosis, in particular the ingestion of Gram-negative bacteria (Schiff *et al.*, 1998). Other lectin-like interactions have been described (Hansen and Holmskov, 1998); an example is phagocytosis of FimH-expressing enterobacteria by macrophages expressing a FimH receptor (CD48) (Baorto *et al.*, 1997).

Table 5.1   Human macrophage receptors for phagocytosis of bacteria

Receptor	Ligand	References
Opsonic receptors		
Fcγ-RI (CD64)	IgG1 > IgG3 > IgG4 > > IgG2	[Ravetch, 1994], [Ravetch, 1997]
Fcγ-RII (CD32)	IgG1 > IgG2 = IgG4 > > IgG3	[Ravetch, 1994], [Ravetch, 1997]
Fcγ-RIII (CD16)	IgG1 and IgG3	[Ravetch, 1994], [Ravetch, 1997]
Fcα-R (CD89)	IgA	[Morton, 1996]
CR1 (CD35)	C3b	[Brown, 1991]
CR3 (CD11b/CD18)	C3bi	[Sengelov, 1995]
CR4 (CD11c/CD18)	C3bi	[Sengelov, 1995]
C1q receptor	Mannose-binding protein	[Tenner, 1995]
SPR210	Lung surfactant protein A	[Weikert, 1997], [Epstein, 1996]
CD14	LPS-binding protein	[Wright, 1990]
Non-opsonic receptors		
CR3 (CD11b/CD18)	β-glucan, LPS	[Ross, 1993]
Mannose receptor	Mannosylated	
	macromolecules	[Stahl, 1998]
CD14	LPS	[Schiff, 1997]

3.1.1 Heterogeneity of macrophage receptors

The expression and function of macrophage phagocytic receptors are influenced pro-foundly by local conditions. For instance, the presence of IFN-γ causes the quantity of Fc receptors to be increased, but their capacity to mediate ingestion is greatly diminished (Wright *et al.*, 1986). Similarly, IFN-γ down-regulates the phagocytic capacity of CR3 (Speert and Thorson, 1991). Mannose receptor function is also grossly inhibited under the same conditions (Mokoena and Gordon, 1985). Similar marked differences in macrophage phenotype are found between resident and recruited peritoneal macrophages (Gordon *et al.*, 1988). Murine Kupffer cells lack detectable CR3, as opposed to circulat-ing monocytes and those that are freshly recruited to the liver (Gordon *et al.*, 1988). Human Fcγ receptors also display considerable heterogeneity (Unkeless, 1989). For instance, FcγRIII is found on neutrophils and tissue macrophages but not on circulating monocytes. This heterogeneity in macrophage phagocytic receptors emphasizes the unique antibacterial potential among the different phenotypes.

3.2 Opsonization

The immune system is able to eliminate potential pathogens by opsonizing them with specific IgG and phagocytosing them via Fcγ receptors. Complement acts synergistically with Ig, enhancing the efficiency of Fc receptor-mediated phagocytosis. In the absence of specific opsonizing antibody, some strains of bacteria fix and activate complement; this process results in the deposition of C3 breakdown products (C3b and C3bi) for which receptors exist on macrophages (complement receptors 1 and 3, respectively). Bacteria can activate complement via the classical or alternative pathway in an antibody-dependent or -independent fashion. The characteristics of the bacterial surface determine the nature of complement activation, and the deposition and accessibility for ligation by macrophage receptors. For instance, the carbohydrate composition of *S.typhimurium* LPS determines the degree of complement deposition, susceptibility to phagocytosis and virulence among various strains (Liang-Takasaki *et al.*, 1982). Although encapsulated *S.aureus* activates and fixes complement to its surface, the bacteria may be resistant to *in vitro* phagocytosis;

the activated complement components are deposited below the capsule, and therefore not available for ligation to complement receptors (Wilkinson *et al.*, 1979). In general, encapsulated bacteria are virulent by virtue of their resistance to phagocytosis. Specific opsonizing antibodies are elicited during the immune response; these antibodies are deposited on the capsule, rendering the bacteria susceptible to phagocytosis.

There are other components which opsonize bacteria prior to ingestion via a phagocytic receptor; these include the mannose-binding protein, aptly named as it binds mannan and is internalized subsequently by the C1q receptor, and lung surfactant protein A, which binds carbohydrates and is recognized by the receptor SPR210 (Tenner *et al.*, 1995; Epstein *et al.*, 1996; Weikert *et al.*, 1997).

3.3 The process of phagocytosis

The phagocytic process has been characterized with the aid of particles coated by mono-specific ligands. This has permitted the detailed characterization of individual phagocytic receptors. Sheep erythrocytes can be coated with IgG, IgM, C3b or C3bi. Using this system, investigators have made seminal observations about the functions of the receptors for Fcγ and complement (Griffin *et al.*, 1975). Macrophage receptors which mediate phagocytosis of Fc-opsonized bacteria are FcγRI, FcγRIIA and FcγRIII (Ravetch, 1997). Upon ligation with Ig, FcγRIIA receptors cross-link with other FcγRIIA receptors, initiating tyrosine phosphorylation of an ITAM motif in the cytoplasmic tail (Ravetch, 1994). FcγRI and FcγRIII, whose cytoplasmic tails lack an ITAM motif, interact with dimers of transmembrane proteins containing ITAM motifs and, upon antibody ligation, cross-linking occurs with subsequent tyrosine phosphorylation (Takai *et al.*, 1994). Tyrosine phosphorylation of the ITAM motif is necessary for induction of the signaling cascade which triggers phagocytosis.

Macrophages have three main receptors responsible for binding and/or internalization of complement-coated bacteria: CR1 (CD35), CR3 (CD11b/CD18) and CR4 (CD11c/CD18) (Carroll, 1998). CR1 binds C3b, C4b and C3bi, but by itself does not promote internalization (Brown, 1991). CR3 and CR4 are members of the β_2 integrin family (Sengelov, 1995). Both receptors bind bacteria coated with C3bi and, upon macrophage activation, internalize the opsonized bacteria (Wright *et al.*, 1993). It appears that particles must be coated circumferentially with a phagocytosis-promoting ligand in order for ingestion to occur. If an opsonin is only deposited on one pole of a particle, attachment to the macrophage membrane without subsequent ingestion is observed.

Bacteria opsonized by IgG and subsequently ingested by Fcγ receptors are internalized by mechanisms different from complement-coated bacteria (Allen and Aderem, 1996a). Both methods of phagocytosis require actin polymerization (Allen and Aderem, 1996b), but electron microscopy has revealed different macrophage membrane interactions with the particle to be engulfed. FcγR-mediated phagocytosis results in the membrane of the macrophage erupting from the cell surface to engulf the IgG-coated particle, and subsequently draw it into the macrophage (Allen and Aderem, 1996a). Early studies termed this process the 'zipper hypothesis', as the macrophage membrane progressed along the opsonized particle, finally 'zippering' it shut (Griffin *et al.*, 1975). Complement receptor (CR) phagocytosis occurs as a variation of the 'zipper hypothesis', as complement-coated particles sink into the cell without any evidence of pseudopodia extending outwards to engulf the particle (Figure 5.1) (Allen and Aderem, 1996a).

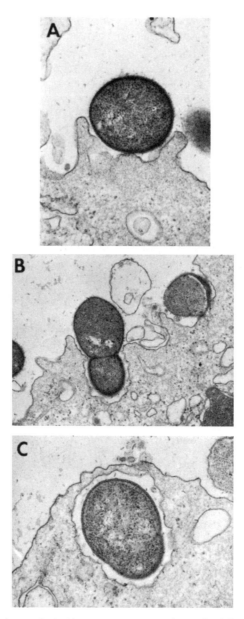

Fig. 5.1 'Conventional' phagocytosis. Human monocytes and a strain of *Streptococcus pneumoniae* were co-incubated, fixed, and examined by electron microscopy. A bacterium is shown entering the monocyte by the conventional process: pseudopodia extend around the bacterium (A and B), fuse, and engulf it within a phagosome (C). (Reproduced from Cell (1984), **36**, 27–33, with permission from Dr Marcus Horwitz and Cell Press.)

FcγR- and CR-mediated phagocytosis also differ in that FcγR- (but not CR-mediated) phagocytosis is coupled with an inflammatory response which includes the production of cytokines and chemokines, as well as an increased respiratory burst and production of arachidonic acid metabolites (Wright and Silverstein, 1983; Aderem *et al.*, 1985). A molecular basis for these differences has been suggested. The Rho family of GTPases are involved in the reorganization of filamentous actin structures in response to external stimuli, i.e. receptor ligation. Rac and Cdc42 (Rho GTPases) regulate actin polymerization into membrane protrusions, gene transcription mediated by NF-κB and p38 mitogen-activated protein (MAP) kinase, as well as the reduction of NADPH oxidase that is responsible for the macrophage respiratory burst (Caron and Hall, 1998). FcγR cross-linking activates the Cdc42–Rac–Rho cascade, thereby eliciting the inflammatory response (Caron and Hall, 1998). CR ligation activates only Rho, and thus CR-mediated phagocytosis does not provoke an inflammatory response (Caron and Hall, 1998).

3.4 Phagocytosis of specific bacterial species

The mechanism of bacterial entry into phagocytic cells is of great interest, as the specific receptor ligated may determine the ultimate fate of the ingested microbe. For instance, when *Toxoplasma gondii* is ingested non-opsonically, it fails to trigger an oxidative burst and survives, whereas when opsonized with IgG, it is killed by ROIs (Wilson *et al.*, 1980). Similar events have been described for bacteria. For some pathogens, establishment of intracellular parasitism requires that they be ingested without triggering fusion of phagosome and lysosome. Such is the case when unopsonized *Chlamydia psittaci* (Wyrick and Brownridge, 1978) and *Mycobacterium tuberculosis* (Armstrong and Hart, 1975) are ingested by macrophages. However, when they are opsonized by IgG, and subsequently ingested, phagosome–lysosome fusion occurs, exposing the ingested bacteria to the toxic effects of lysosomal antibacterial products (Armstrong and Hart, 1975; Wyrick and Brownridge, 1978).

Certain intracellular pathogens, such as *Legionella pneumophila*, enter macrophages via a process called 'coiling phagocytosis' (Horwitz, 1984) (Figure 5.2). This mode of ingestion is mediated by complement receptors and is common to human monocytes, pulmonary alveolar macrophages and PMNs (Payne and Horwitz, 1987), but it is not seen if bacteria are opsonized with specific IgGs (Horwitz, 1984). The mechanism underlying coiling phagocytosis is incompletely understood.

Salmonella typhimurium is an intracellular pathogen of macrophages (Finlay and Cossart, 1997). Virulent strains of *S.typhimurium* bind to macrophages, which leads to membrane ruffling and internalization into a 'spacious' phagosome resembling a macropinosome (Alpuche-Aranda *et al.*, 1995). The receptor responsible for mediating this ingestion is unknown. *Salmonella typhimurium* possesses a type III secretion system which can inject a host cell with a protein termed SopE that has GDP/GTP exchange activity specific for Rac and Cdc42 (Hardt *et al.*, 1998). The specific nature of the SopE interaction with Rho GTPases has yet to be elucidated.

4 Bacteriocidal mechanisms of macrophages

Macrophages are equipped for killing ingested prey by both oxygen-dependent and oxygen-independent mechanisms (Table 5.2) (Andrew *et al.*, 1985; Lowrie and Andrew, 1988; Rooik, 1989). Macrophage bacteriocidal power varies among different phenotypes and is clearly inferior to that of circulating PMNs. Indeed, the somewhat effete microbicidal potential of macrophages makes them an attractive niche for survival of intracellular pathogens. Much of what is known about leukocyte microbicidal action is derived from studies on PMNs. Nonetheless, some notable differences exist between

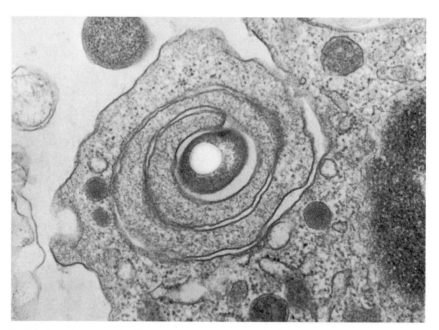

Fig. 5.2 *Coiling phagocytosis.* Human monocytes and *Legionella pneumophila* were co-incubated, fixed and examined by electron microscopy. A single *L.pneumophila* bacterium is seen within a coiled monocyte pseudopod. This process of coiling phagocytosis is also seen when human alveolar macrophages and neutrophils ingest *L.pneumophila.* The process is not observed when the bacteria are opsonized with specific antibody to *L.pneumophila*, but phagocytosis occurs by conventional phagocytosis. [Reproduced from *Cell* (1984), **36**, 27–33, with the permission of Dr Marcus Horwitz and Cell Press.]

Table 5.2   Macrophage antimicrobial mechanisms

Mechanism	Product	References
Oxygen dependent		
	hydrogen peroxide	[Smith, 1991]
	hydroxyl radical	[Hampton, 1998]
	singlet oxygen	[Rosen, 1995]
	hypochlorite	[Albrich, 1982], [Harrison, 1976]
	aromatic radicals	[Hampton, 1998]
Oxygen-independent		
	nitric oxide	[Kaplan, 1996]
	antibacterial peptides	[Lehrer, 1991]
	nutritional immunity	[Carlin, 1987]

macrophages and PMNs, particularly with respect to their oxidative and nitrogen-based microbicidal activity.

4.1 Oxygen-dependent microbicidal mechanisms

When macrophages are activated by bacterial LPS (Johnston *et al.*, 1978) or IFN-γ (Nathan *et al.*, 1983), their capacity to produce ROIs dramatically increases. Activated macrophages undergo a respiratory burst during which macrophages oxidize glucose by means of the hexose monophosphate shunt, ultimately resulting in the reduction of NADP to NADPH. NADPH oxidase is a transmembrane enzyme which resides in the phagosomal membrane and, upon oxidation of NADPH, electrons are transferred to molecular oxygen. The resultant superoxide (O_2^-) can dismutate to form hydrogen peroxide (H_2O_2) (Smith and Curnutte, 1991; Segal and Abo, 1993). ROIs are microbicidal by virtue of the damage they cause to bacterial DNA and membranes (Hampton *et al.*, 1998).

4.1.1 Hydroxyl radical production

Macrophages can generate hydroxyl radicals (OH·) as bactericidal components by means of a superoxide-driven Fenton reaction. Using a transition metal catalyst, interaction of superoxide and hydrogen peroxide yields highly reactive oxygen intermediates such as hydroxyl radicals and singlet oxygen (Rosen *et al.*, 1995). Hydroxyl radicals are extremely reactive, although their resultant duration of action is very short (Hampton *et al.*, 1998). There is some controversy as to whether hydroxyl radicals themselves are effective bactericidal components, or if they merely serve to generate secondary radicals from bicarbonate and chloride (Hampton *et al.*, 1998).

4.1.2 Myeloperoxidase production of ROIs

Hydrogen peroxide produced in neutrophils and monocytes is degraded by myeloperoxidase in order to oxidize aromatic compounds and chloride ions (Harrison and Schultz, 1976; Hurst, 1991; Marquez *et al.*, 1996). Oxidized aromatic compounds, such as phenylalanine and tyrosine, yield substrate radicals, while oxidation of chloride ions produces HOCl, a strong non-radical oxidant (Klebanoff, 1968). HOCl is bactericidal to many species (Albrich and Hurst, 1982) as it inactivates bacterial iron–sulfur proteins, membrane transport proteins (Albrich *et al.*, 1986) and ATP-generating systems (Barrette *et al.*, 1989). The principal site of HOCl-mediated action is the bacterial origin of replication, knocking out bacterial DNA synthesis (McKenna and Davies, 1988; Rosen and Michel, 1997). Myeloperoxidase also oxidizes iodide, bromide, thiocyanate and nitrite to produce reactive components of varying bactericidal capabilities (Thomas and Fishman, 1986; van Dalen *et al.*, 1997; van der Vliet *et al.*, 1997).

4.2 Oxygen-independent microbicidal mechanisms

Reactive nitrogen intermediates have been identified as macrophage effectors in killing internalized bacteria (Brunelli *et al.*, 1995; Kaplan *et al.*, 1996). Nitric oxide synthase (NOS) generates NO from consumption of L-arginine. The resultant NO is rapidly converted to NO_2^- and NO_3^- by oxidation (Baumler and Heffron, 1995). NOS levels, and thus the NO produced by it, respond to stimulation by bacterial LPS and IFN-γ (Nathan and Hibbs, 1991). Myeloperoxidase and HOCl can also oxidize nitrite to produce NO (Klebanoff, 1993; van der Vliet *et al.*, 1997). NO is toxic to bacteria as it inactivates DNA and proteins, as well as provoking membrane damage (Kaplan *et al.*, 1996).

4.2.1 Macrophage antibacterial peptides

Antibacterial peptides, termed defensins, are produced by macrophages and are present in the early phagosome (Geisow *et al.*, 1981; Ganz *et al.*, 1986). These peptides form pores in artificial membranes, and may result in permeabilization of bacterial inner and outer membranes, with subsequent bacterial death (Sawyer *et al.*, 1988; Lehrer *et al.*, 1989,

1991). Defensins function best between pH 7 and 8, conditions which exist in the phago-some immediately after phagocytosis (Geisow *et al.*, 1981).

4.2.2 Lysosome contents

Lysosomes contain many degradative enzymes that function optimally upon acidification of the phago-lysosome (Andrew *et al.*, 1985). There is no conclusive evidence to suggest that lysosomal enzymes kill ingested bacteria. Their principal role may be digestive rather than bactericidal (Andrew *et al.*, 1985.

4.2.3 Nutritional immunity

Nutritional immunity describes a macrophage defense system in which essential nutrients are made unavailable to ingested bacteria. Within IFN-γ-activated macrophages, trypto-phan is metabolized, and thus unavailable to internalized bacteria (Carlin *et al.*, 1987). This immunity remains theoretical as bacteria can synthesize tryptophan, therefore imply-ing that bacterial multiplication would be hindered, but not eliminated.

Hypoferremia is another form of nutritional immunity, and describes a physiological response to infection during which serum iron is reduced by approximately 30 per cent. Macrophages are the major cell involved in iron recirculation by means of senescent red blood cell clearance (Kay, 1989). Upon infection, macrophages decrease iron release and increase intracellular synthesis of the iron storage protein ferritin (Byrd and Horwitz, 1989). While iron deprivation in the serum may aid in the prevention of bacteremia, it sets the stage for macrophage intracellular parasitism by providing ingested bacteria with an ample supply of iron.

5 Antibacterial secretory activities of macrophages

Macrophages produce over 100 substances with wide-ranging effects upon bacteria as well as on other organs and tissues (Nathan, 1987). Many of the antimicrobial substances elaborated (such as reactive oxygen and nitrogen intermediates) are secreted and exert their effects outside the confines of the lysosomal compartment (Table 5.3). Lysozyme is secreted from macrophages constitutively, and comprises 2.5 per cent of the total

Table 5.3 Antibacterial secretory products of macrophages

Product	Function	References
IL-1	Stimulates proliferation and differentiation of T and B cells, promotes IL-2, -8, -9, and CSF production, endotoxic shock	[Dinarello, 1996]
TNFα	Stimulates IL-6, -8, -9, and CSF, promotes endotoxic shock, upregulates CR3	[Baumler, 1995]
IL-6	Blocks LPS induction of IL-1 and TNFα	[Schindler, 1990]
IL-8	Stimulates neutrophil, monocyte activation and chemotaxis	[Richman-Eisenstat, 1996]
Reactive oxygen species	Both reactive species kill bacteria by	[Hampton, 1998]
Reactive nitrogen species	Altering lipids, DNA, and proteins	[Kaplan, 1996]
Lysozyme	Lyses bacteria with specific LPS linkages	[Gordon, 1974]
Complement	Opsonizes bacteria to facilitate phagocytosis	[Nathan, 1987]

macrophage cellular protein produced (Gordon *et al.*, 1974). Lysozyme has the ability to lyse bacteria in which the LPS has a specific glucosidic linkage (Gordon *et al.*, 1974).

5.1 Macrophage activation and antibacterial activities

The concept of the activated macrophage evolved from studies on animals with acquired resistance to infection (Mackaness, 1964). In these classical studies, it was demonstrated that non-specific antibacterial activity developed in animals after infection with specific pathogens. Subsequent studies demonstrated that this state of activation was derived from the effect of lymphocyte products (Mackaness, 1969), ultimately shown to be IFN-γ (Nathan *et al.*, 1983). Activated macrophages are larger in size, have pronounced plasma membrane ruffling, an enhanced capacity for spreading and attaching to solid surfaces, and increased secretion of neutral proteases (Cohn, 1978; North, 1978). In addition, these cells gain the capacity to ingest complement-coated particles via CR3 (Ross and Vetvika, 1993), and to secrete superoxide anion and NO in nanomolar concentrations, equivalent to PMNs (Cohn, 1978; Nathan and Hibbs, 1991). Activated macrophages also secrete increased quantities of lysosomal enzymes including plasminogen activators, collagenase and elastase (Cohn, 1978).

With enhanced secretion of reactive oxygen and nitrogen intermediates, as well as lysosomal enzymes, a wide range of pathogens fall prey to the antibacterial arsenal of the activated macrophage (Nathan, 1982; Beckman and Crow, 1993). Activation appears to be primarily effective in enhancing the bacteriocidal capacity of macrophages for intracellular pathogens. This has been demonstrated with macrophages incubated in the presence of recombinant IFN-γ (Section 6.1). While enhancing reactive oxygen and nitrogen intermediate production, IFN-γ impairs the capacity of human-derived macrophages to ingest particles via Fc and complement receptors (Wright *et al.*, 1986; Speert and Thorson, 1991). It also impairs phagocytosis via the mannose receptor (Mokoena and Gordon, 1985).

5.2 Cytokine production

Macrophages secrete cytokines when activated or stimulated by other leukocyte products or bacterial LPS. Cytokines have multiple activities, both pro- and anti-inflammatory, some of which influence the ability of the host to respond to infections (Bendtzen, 1988; Groopman *et al.*, 1989). Production of TNF-α and IL-1 constitutes an immediate response to infection and induces inflammation (Dinarello, 1996).

5.2.1 Interleukin-1 (IL-1)

IL-1 is an endogenous pyrogen that can raise body temperature through induction of prostaglandins (Dinarello, 1996). The elevation of body temperature is associated with the acute phase response and modulation of the immune system (Dinarello *et al.*, 1988). IL-1 is produced by macrophages after stimulation by almost all infectious agents (Dinarello *et al.*, 1988), in particular LPS of Gram-negative bacteria. IL-1 affects immunity by stimulating proliferation and differentiation of T and B cells, as well as T-cell production of IL-2. The production of IL-1 is tightly controlled, as the level between therapeutic benefit and toxicity to humans is quite narrow (Dinarello, 1996). When infused into rabbits, recombinant IL-1β acts synergistically with TNF-α to induce shock (Okusawa *et al.*, 1988), a manifestation of Gram-negative bacterial septicemia. Severe sepsis is marked by a rise in both IL-1 and TNF-α which occurs in proportion to the degree of hypotension and organ failure (Calandra *et al.*, 1990; Cannon *et al.*, 1990).

5.2.2 Tumor necrosis factor-α

TNF-α has many redundant functions with IL-1. TNF-α and IL-1 act synergistically to induce inflammation and fever, and both are produced as a macrophage response to Gram-negative LPS exposure (Michie *et al.*, 1988). TNF-α mediates the macrophage response to LPS by triggering a respiratory burst and production of reactive nitrogen intermediates in macrophages and neutrophils (Baumler and Heffron, 1995). The level of secreted TNF-α within a given mouse strain will determine its innate resistance to bacterial infection, while depletion of TNF-α will lead to an increased susceptibility to bacterial infection (Michie *et al.*, 1988). In neutropenic mice with *P.aeruginosa* pneumonia, combination therapy with TNF-α and IL-1β synergistically reduces mortality rates (Shirai *et al.*, 1997). The therapeutic benefit of TNF-α is realized only at low levels, as LPS-activated macrophage release of TNF-α is a critical mediator of septic shock reactions. Animals with high TNF-α serum levels rapidly succumbed to septic shock (Fruh *et al.*, 1995). TNF-α causes an increase in CR3 expression and function on both neutrophils and macrophages, which in turn leads to increased rates of phagocytosis, both opsonically and non-opsonically (Ross and Vetvika, 1993). TNF-α release induces the production of an anti-inflammatory cytokine, IL-6, by many different cell types, including monocytes, which in turn inhibits expression of both TNF-α and IL-1 (Schindler *et al.*, 1990).

5.3 Macrophage products with direct effects on neutrophils

TNF-α and IL-1 stimulate the production of IL-8 by monocytes and macrophages, and IL-9 by T cells, both of which have chemotactic and activating properties primarily for neutrophils (McElvaney *et al.*, 1992; Richman-Eisenstat, 1996), but also for monocytes. The activation of neutrophils enhances exocytosis of vesicles and granules, expression of receptors and release of reactive oxygen and, possibly, nitrogen intermediates.

6 Augmentation of macrophage antibacterial function

Although macrophages are able to ingest and kill certain bacterial species unaided by opsonins or cytokines, optimum antibacterial activity depends upon the involvement of a diverse range of substances (Table 5.4). These substances are either distributed widely (complement) or restricted to specific organs (pulmonary surfactant). Their enhancing activity is either non-specific (complement) or limited to specific bacterial species (mannose-binding protein, LPS-binding protein).

6.1 Interferon-γ

T cells and natural killer (NK) cells respond to infection, in particular to bacterial LPS, by releasing IFN-γ (Hill *et al.*, 1991). In response to IFN-γ, macrophages rapidly up-regulate production of reactive oxygen and nitrogen intermediates (Nathan *et al.*, 1983; Stuehr and Marletta, 1987), as well as catabolism of intracellular tryptophan (Carli *et al.*, 1987) and scavenging available intracellular iron (Byrd and Horwitz, 1989; Alford *et al.*, 1991). These enhanced macrophage effector functions have translated into augmented

Table 5.4   Factors that enhance macrophage antibacterial activity

Product	Function	Reference
IFNγ	Activates monocytes, macrophages, and neutrophils, produced by T-cells and natural killer cells	[Hill, 1991]
Colony stimulating factors	Increases the production and antibacterial function of macrophages and neutrophils	[Metcalf, 1987; Shirai, 1997]
Complement	Chemotaxis, opsonization, bacterial killing	[Snyderman, 1981;
1,25(OH)	in the presence of autologous serum,	Rautemaa, 1998]
Vitamin D_3	Aids in the killing of *M. tuberculosis*	[Crowle, 1987]
Surfactant protein A	Opsonize and facilitate phagocytosis of	[Tenner, 1989]
Mannose binding protein, LPS binding protein	bacteria	[Tenner, 1989] [Kuhlman, 1989]

bactericidal activity against a wide range of intracellular pathogens (Murray, 1988). It therefore seems likely that IFN-γ plays a pivotal role in controlling intracellular infection. IFN-γ has been shown to enhance the superoxide production of neutrophils and mono-cytes from patients with variant forms of chronic granulomatous disease (Ezekowitz *et al.*, 1987, 1988). Although most of these patients demonstrate a capacity to generate ROIs while receiving IFN-γ, their enhanced microbicidal activity may be out of propor-tion to a modest respiratory burst.

The macrophage enzyme responsible for NO production is NOS and, unlike other forms of NOS which are constitutive, macrophage NOS is inducible, particularly by IFN-γ (Nathan and Xie, 1994). IFN-γ causes an increase in iNOS transcription and stabil-ity (Nathan and Xie, 1994). Many studies have shown a high level of NO production by murine macrophages in response to IFN-γ and LPS; however, similar evidence for human macrophages is elusive. A few reports have described human macrophage production of NO; however, these levels have been low in comparison with that of murine macrophages (Albina, 1995; Weinberg, 1995).

Macrophages that have been cultured in the presence of IFN-γ have an enhanced capac-ity to kill certain bacterial intracellular pathogens. When treated with recombinant human IFN-γ, human monocytes and pulmonary alveolar macrophages gain the capacity to inhibit the multiplication of *L.pneumophila* (Nash *et al.*, 1984; Jensen *et al.*, 1987; Byrd and Horwitz, 1989). Studies with human monocytes (Byrd and Horwitz, 1989) have demonstrated that *L.pneumophila* is dependent upon iron for growth, and that IFN-γ enhances monocyte antibacterial activity by down-regulating transferrin receptors and limiting access of intracellular bacteria to iron (Byrd and Horwitz, 1989; Alford *et al.*, 1991).

The effect of IFN-γ on bacteriocidal activity against *Mycobacteria* is determined largely by the animal species from which the macrophages are obtained (Rook *et al.*, 1986). Whereas recombinant IFN-γ enhances the cidal capacity of murine bone marrow-derived macrophages for *M.tuberculosis* (Flesh and Kaufmann, 1987, 1988), human monocyte-derived macrophages become less microbicidal after maturation in the pres-ence of IFN-γ (Douvas *et al.*, 1985). This is perhaps a result of the failure of human macrophages to elicit production of reactive nitrogen intermediates.

6.2 Colony-stimulating factors

Colony-stimulating factors are cytokines that increase the production and antibacterial function of macrophages and neutrophils. Colony-stimulating factors were discovered due to their effects on cultured bone marrow cells. Macrophage colony-stimulating factor (M-CSF) and granulocyte–macrophage colony-stimulating factor (GM-CSF) induce production of peripheral blood monocytes and neutrophils from bone marrow as the respective names would suggest. Both colony-stimulating factors are secreted constitutively, but their levels are increased after bacterial infection or exposure to LPS as mediated by TNF-α (Metcalf, 1987; Shirai *et al.*, 1997). They are both produced by fibroblasts, whereas GM-CSF is also elaborated by endothelial cells and T cells, and M-CSF by monocytes and endothelial cells (Clark and Kamen, 1987; Metcalf, 1987). Although their principal function may be that of increasing macrophage proliferation, they also can enhance secretion of other inflammatory mediators, such as superoxide anion, protaglandin E, arachidonic acid, IL-1, plasminogen activator, IFN-γ, TNF-α and other colony-stimulating factors (Metcalf, 1987). Furthermore, these colony-stimulating factors enhance the phagocytic and cidal activities of macrophages (Metcalf, 1987; Cheers *et al.*, 1989; Ruef and Coleman, 1990).

6.3 Complement

Complement profoundly enhances the antibacterial activity of macrophages. The critical role of complement in the clearance of bacteria from the bloodstream has been demonstrated in animals depleted of serum complement by treatment with cobra venom factor (to remove C3–C9), as well as in animals with a congenital deficiency of specific complement components (C3 and C4) (Hosea *et al.*, 1980; Noel *et al.*, 1990). Clearance of *S.pneumoniae* is optimum in the presence of an intact classical complement pathway; the alternative pathway is of critical importance in enhancing clearance in the non-immune animal (Hosea *et al.*, 19809). Despite the presence of circulating specific antibody, depletion of complement by cobra venom factor produces a lethal defect in these animals.

Complement also plays an important role in enhancing clearance of certain bacterial species from the lung (Gross *et al.*, 1978; Heidbrink *et al.*, 1982). After depletion of complement with cobra venom factor, clearance of *S.pneumoniae* and *P.aeruginosa* from the murine lung was compromised, but clearance of *S.aureus* was unaffected (Gross *et al.*, 1978). The normal clearance of *S.aureus* in the complement-deficient animal could be mediated by macrophages armed with cytophilic antibody (Verbrugh *et al.*, 1982).

Complement may enhance bacterial clearance by any of several mechanisms. C5a, produced in response to complement activation, is a potent chemotactic factor for macrophages (Snyderman and Goetzl, 1981). Complement provides the necessary opsonins for enhancing phagocytosis; C3 activation products may be deposited on the bacterial surface via the classical or alternative pathway. Complement also facilitates the lysis of certain Gram-negative bacterial species (Frank *et al.*, 1987; Rautemaa *et al.*, 1998). Finally, acting in concert with Ig, complement has been shown to be necessary for intracellular killing of staphylococci (Leijh *et al.*, 1979).

6.4 Other factors capable of enhancing the microbicidal activity of macrophages

Fibronectin is a glycoprotein with a wide tissue distribution and with diverse effects upon phagocytic cells (Proctor, 1987). Of particular importance in antibacterial defenses, fibronectin enhances the capacity of human monocyte-derived macrophages to ingest complement-coated particles (Wright *et al.*, 1983) and to kill ingested bacteria (Proctor *et al.*, 1985; Proctor, 1987).

6.4.1 Surfactant

Pulmonary alveolar macrophages function in an environment with very low levels of complement and Ig, concentrations too low to provide optimal opsonization of bacteria for phagocytosis. The alveolar spaces are bathed in surfactant that serves primarily to maintain their patency. Surfactant protein A is a component of pulmonary surfactant that can function as an opsonin and has striking similarities to both complement subunit C1q and mannose-binding protein (Tenner *et al.*, 1989). Surfactant protein A has a long collagen-like domain that mediates binding to the C1q receptor of mononuclear phago-cytes (Malhotra *et al.*, 1990) and can enhance phagocytosis (Tenner *et al.*, 1989). Although surfactant protein A enhances phagocytosis by both Fc and complement receptors, it cannot substitute for C1q in forming hemolytically active C1 (Tenner *et al.*, 1989). Phagocytosis but not killing of *S.aureus* by pulmonary alveolar macrophages is enhanced by surfactant protein A, and the effect is additive to that of serum (O'Neill *et al.*, 1984).

6.4.2 Vitamin D

1,25(OH)-vitamin D_3 has been shown to enhance the antituberculous activity of human monocyte-derived macrophages (Crowle *et al.*, 1987). These studies were performed in order to explain the observation that sunlight bolsters natural resistance to infection with *M.tuberculosis* (Crowle *et al.*, 1987). The enhancing effect of the vitamin D metabolite was demonstrated best in the presence of autologous serum and less so with heterologous serum or an artificial substitute.

6.4.3 Mannose-binding protein

As described above, there is considerable structural homology between surfactant protein A, C1q and the human mannose-binding protein (Tenner *et al.*, 1989). The humman mannose-binding protein, like the other two substances, acts as an opsonin; it binds to the C1q receptor (Malhotra *et al.*, 1990) and enhances the phagocytosis of bacteria rich in surface mannose residues, such as *Salmonella montevideo* (Kuhlman *et al.*, 1989). Mutations within the mannose-binding protein gene have been shown to lead to immun-odeficiencies (Amoroso *et al.*, 1999; Neonato *et al.*, 1999; Wallis *et al.*, 1999).

6.4.4 Lipopolysaccharide-binding protein

LPS-binding protein (Kuhlman *et al.*, 1989) acts in an analogous fashion to the mannose-binding protein. It is an acute phase reactant that binds to LPS of Gram-negative bacteria. Subsequent ligation by macrophage CD14 results in internalization of the opsonized bacteria (Wright *et al.*, 1990; Schiff *et al.*, 1998).

7 Defects in macrophage antibacterial activity

Inborn errors of bacteriocidal or phagocytic functions that are restricted to the mono-cyte/macrophage system have not been identified (Johnston, 1988). Nonetheless, several disease states, both inherited and acquired, have an associated impairment or enhance-ment of macrophage function (Douglas and Musson, 1986; Johnston, 1988). As these disease states are associated with widespread pathophysiological abnormalities, it has been difficult to gain new insights into the normal functions of the macrophage from these conditions.

7.1 Chronic granulomatous disease (CGD)

CGD is a syndrome characterized by an inability of leukocytes to mount an oxidative burst upon membrane stimulation (Curnutte and Babior, 1987). The disease is predomi-nantly of X-linked recessive inheritance and is due to an absence of a specific membrane-bound cytochrome, necessary for single electron transfer. Approximately one-third of patients have normal levels of cytochrome but lack one of several cytosolic factors essen-tial for generating an oxidative burst. CGD is a defect of both granulocytes and mononucelar phagocytes (Douglas and Musson, 1986). Bacteria that are killed predomi-nantly by ROIs and make catalase (to protect themselves against the toxic effects of bac-terial hydrogen peroxide) are particularly virulent in these patients. A wide range of bacteria can infect CGD patients, but *S.aureus*, *Serratia marcescens*, other Gram-negative bacteria and several different fungal species are particularly problematical. IFN-γ has been shown partially to correct the bacteriocidal defect in these patients (Ezekowitz *et al.*, 1988), but the mechanism remains to be elucidated fully.

7.2 Leukocyte adhesion deficiency (LAD)

Like CGD, this is a disease that effects both granulocytes and mononuclear phagocytes but, unlike CGD, oxidative metabolism of cells from affected individuals is normal. Leukocytes from patients with LAD lack the three glycoproteins which comprise the β_2 integrins (LFA-1, CR3 and CR4) due to subnormal expression of the common β-chain, CD18 (Anderson *et al.*, 1985; Johnston *et al.*, 1988), and are unable to marginate to the site of infection. These patients are prone to recurrent soft tissue infections, most com-monly *S.aureus* and *P.aeruginosa* (Schmalstieg, 1988). Patients with LAD may be severely or moderately affected depending upon the concentration of adhesion-promoting glycoproteins on their leukocytes (Anderson *et al.*, 1985).

7.3 Secondary or acquired abnormalities of macrophage function

Abnormalities of mononuclear phagocytic bactericidal or phagocytic function may accompany an acquired non-infectious disease or may be seen during an acute viral infec-tion.

7.3.1 Systemic lupus erythematosus (SLE)

Patients with SLE have a defect in reticuloendothelial clearance (Frank *et al.*, 1979). Such a defect is not unexpected since these patients have elevated levels of circulating immune complexes. Clearance of sensitized erythrocytes by splenic Fc receptors is impaired in SLE; the degree of impairment is correlated with disease severity and with the level of circulating immune complexes (Frank *et al.*, 1979). Blockade of the reticuloendothelial system by immune complexes may also interfere with clearance of bacteria opsonized with IgG and put these patients at increased risk for infection.

7.3.2 End-stage renal disease

Abnormalities similar to SLE in reticuloendothelial system Fc receptor-mediated clearance of sensitized erythrocytes can occur in patients with end-stage renal disease (Ruiz *et al.*, 1990). These patients are at increased risk for sepsis or pneumonia by encapsulated bacteria. Patients with markedly impaired Fc receptor-mediated clearance of IgG-sensitized erythrocytes are at greatest risk for sepsis and pneumonia (Ruiz *et al.*, 1990). Pathogens in these patients are encapsulated, and include *S.pneumoniae*, *S.aureus*, *H.influenzae*, *P.aeruginosa* and *E.coli*. This underscores the critical role played by fixed tissue macrophages in maintaining sterility of the bloodstream.

7.3.3 Corticosteroid therapy

Patients receiving prednisone develop monocytopenia and a transient defect in monocyte bacteriocidal and fungicidal activity (Rinehart *et al.*, 1975).

7.3.4 Acute viral infection

Patients with acute viral infections often develop bacterial superinfection, raising the possibility of transient immunosuppression. Among macrophage antibacterial activities impaired by viral infection are chemotaxis, attachment of particles to phagocytic receptors, receptor-mediated phagocytosis and bacterial killing mediated by phagosome–lysosome fusion (Rouse and Horohov, 1986).

8 Bacterial strategies for subversion of macrophage defenses

In order for bacteria to cause disease, they must be able to circumvent the formidable array of antibacterial defenses elaborated and displayed by the normal host. As the macrophage stands guard as gatekeeper, bacteria have had to develop strategies for breaching this first line of defense. With the aid of modern microbial molecular biological techniques, much has been learned in the past two decades about the means by which pathogenic bacteria achieve their goal of persisting and causing disease in a hostile environment. This section provides an overview of the means by which bacteria survive, in spite of, or partly because of the presence of macrophages. However, these descriptions are brief and are meant to provide examples that exemplify different bacterial pathogenic strategies. More thorough overviews of bacterial virulence determinants and mechanisms of intracellular survival are provided in other articles (Peterson *et al.*, 1977a; Heinzen *et al.*, 1996; Ruckdeschel *et al.*, 1997; Schorey *et al.*, 1997; Gardner *et al.*, 1998; Heinzen *et al.*, 1998).

8.1 Bacterial antiphagocytic strategies

Bacteria are able to survive and cause disease by evading one or more of the steps in the normal phagocytic/bacteriocidal process. Both intracellular and extracellular pathogens have developed a clever array of methods to avoid phagocytosis or to subvert normal processes once they have been phagocytosed. Extracellular pathogens often depend upon characteristics of their cell surface to avoid opsonization and phagocytosis. Intracellular pathogens, on the other hand, may require the intra-macrophage environment for their survival, thereby depending upon phagocytosis for expression of virulence. Strategies deployed by bacteria to avoid normal defences are outlined in Table 5.5 and briefly described and illustrated with examples below. Although much has been discovered about bacterial virulence mechanisms, a great deal remains to be learned. The observations described below represent possible explanations for bacterial survival in the face of macrophage antibacterial activities. No doubt many bacterial species use multiple mechanisms to evade host phagocytic defenses and may employ strategies yet to be defined.

8.2 Avoidance of phagocytosis

Pyogenic extracellular pathogens are generally resistant to phagocytosis in the absence of serum opsonins. These bacterial species are often encapsulated (e.g. *H.influenzae*, *S.pneumoniae*, *S.aureus* and *E.coli*) and require specific anticapsular antibody for phagocytosis by neutrophils and macrophages (Wilkinson *et al.*, 1979; Horwitz and Silverstein, 1980; Whitnack *et al.*, 1981; Cross, 1990). They generally do not activate or fix complement to their surfaces in the absence of specific IgG or IgM. Streptococci become coated with

Table 5.5 Bacterial strategies to subvert macrophage defences

Strategy	Bacterial species (examples)	References
Avoidance of phagocytosis antiphagocytic capsule	*Haemophilus influenzae*	[Cross, 1990]
	Streptococcus pneumoniae	[Cross, 1990]
	Staphylococcal aureus	[Wilkinson, 1979]
	Escherichia coli	[Horwitz, 1980]
antiphagocytic slime	*Pseudomonas aeruginosa*	[Cabral, 1987], [Krieg, 1988]
IgG improperly bound	*Staphylococcus aureus*	[Peterson, 1977]
Inhibition of chemotaxis	*Bordetella pertussis*	[Spangrude, 1985]
Escape from phagosome	*Shigella flexneri*	[Sansonetti, 1986]
	Listeria monocytogenes	[Marquis, 1997]
Prevention of phagosome/ lysosome fusion	*Mycobacterium tuberculosis*	[Sturgill-Koszycki, 1994]
	Chlamydia trachomatis	[Hackstadt, 1995]
Lysosome tolerance	*Coxiella burnetti*	[Heinzen, 1996]
Resistance to oxidative		
	Mycobacterium laprae	[Learn, 1987], [Wheeler, 1980]
	Mycobacterium tuberculosis	[Storz, 1990], [Chan, 1991]
	Pseudomonas aeruginosa	[Learn, 1987]
Resistance to non- oxidative killing	*Escherichia coli*	[Gardner, 1998]
	Salmonella typhimurium	[Crawford, 1998], [Groisman, 1990]
Failure to trigger respiratory burst	*Mycobacterium tuberculosis*	[Schorey, 1997]
Inhibits macrophage activation	*Mycobacterium leprae*	[Roach, 1993]
Macrophage killing apoptosis)	*Yersinia enterocolitica*	[Ruckdeschel, 1997]
Inhibition of antigen presentation	*Mycobacterium tuberculosis*	[Pancholi, 1993], [Clemens, 1995]

IgA which serves to inhibit complement from binding through steric hinderance (Mims *et al.*, 1998). Some bacterial species, such as encapsulated *S.aureus*, may fix complement in a cryptic subcapsular location inaccessible for ligation by complement receptors (Wilkinson *et al.*, 1979).

In addition to capsules, some bacteria elaborate an antiphagocytic slime substance. This material is loosely affixed to the bacterial surface and may interfere with different macrophage antibacterial activities. Mucoid strains of *P.aeruginosa* from patients with cystic fibrosis elaborate a polyuronic acid polysaccaharide which is highly viscous and interferes with leukocyte chemotaxis (Stiver *et al.*, 1988) and phagocytosis (Cabral *et al.*, 1987; Krieg *et al.*, 1988). Mucoid exopolysaccharide forms a biofilm around *Pseudomonas* microcolonies and renders them antiphagocytic in the presence of opsonic antibodies (Hatano *et al.*, 1995; Meluleni *et al.*, 1995). The antiphagocytic properties of the mucoid exopolysaccharide can be overridden by specific opsonizing antibodies (Pier, 1997). Macrophage-mediated anti-*Pseudomonas* activity is compromised further in patients with cystic fibrosis by virtue of fragmented immunoglobulin present in serum and bronchopulmonary secretions (Fick *et al.*, 1981, 1984). Although phagocytosis of *P.aeruginosa* is enhanced by specific opsonizing antibody (Reynolds and Thompson, 1973; Reynolds, 1974; Reynolds *et al.*, 1975; Murphey *et al.*, 1979), IgG from patients with cystic fibrosis may lack the Fc portion, rendering it antiphagocytic; it binds to the bacterial surface but is unable to ligate Fc receptors on the macrophage (Fick *et al.*, 1981, 1984). Furthermore, complement product iC3b (which opsonizes *P.aeruginosa* to facilitate ingestion by CR3) and phagocyte receptor CR1 (which recognizes C3b) are susceptible to proteolytic cleavage within the cystic fibrosis lung (Berger *et al.*, 1989; Tosi *et al.*, 1990; Speert, 1993). *Pseudomonas aeruginosa* also produces low levels of rhamnolipids which have been shown to inhibit phagocytosis of *P.aeruginosa* by macrophages and interfere with phagosome/lysosome fusion (McClure and Schiller, 1996).

As described previously, many strains of *S.aureus* possess surface-exposed protein A, which is capable of directly binding IgG via its Fc domain. This characteristic makes the organism susceptible to phagocytosis by macrophages possessing cytophilic IgG (Verbrugh *et al.*, 1983). However, the same bacterial feature provides an antiphagocytic defense by binding IgG in the incorrect orientation to the bacterial surface (with the Fc domain buried), rendering the bacteria resistant to phagocytosis by macrophages and neutrophils lacking cytophilic antibody (Peterson *et al.*, 1977b). A direct correlation exists between the level of protein A expressed on the bacterial surface and the resistance to opsonic phagocytosis (Peterson *et al.*, 1977b).

8.3 Inhibition of chemotaxis

Bordetella pertussis, the agent of whooping cough, elaborates a number of extracellular products with profound effects on the host (Weiss and Hewlett, 1986). Chief among these toxins is lymphocytosis-promoting factor (pertussis toxin), a protein that impairs macrophage chemotaxis (Meade *et al.*, 1984; Sprangude *et al.*, 1985) by disabling pertussis-sensitive G-proteins within monocyte cell membranes (Badolato *et al.*, 1995). The disease is characterized by destruction of respiratory ciliated epithelial cells without evidence of bacterial invasion. The microbial virulence is probably enhanced by its ability to inhibit the recruitment of phagocytic cells. Macrophage bacterioicidal capacity is impaired further by a bacterial adenylate cyclase that interferes with superoxide generation by both alveolar macrophages and neutrophils (Confer and Eaton, 1982; Friedman *et al.*, 1987).

8.4 Escape from the phagosome

Once ingestion has occurred, microbicidal substances must be delivered to the phagosome in order for the bacteria to be killed. *Listeria monocytogenes* is able to survive within macrophages by escaping from the phagosome into the cytoplasm (Tilney and Portnoy, 1989). This phenomenon is mediated by a secreted hemolysin, listeriolysin O, as well as two separate phospholipase C enzymes (Kuhn *et al.*, 1988; Portnoy *et al.*, 1988; Marquis *et al.*, 1997). Once free within the cytoplasm, *Listeria* is immediately covered by host actin filaments which facilitate bacterial spread from cell to cell (Tilney and Portnoy, 1989; Ireton *et al.*, 1997). This process is mediated by polymerization of host actin filaments; when cytochalasin D is added to the system, the bacteria fail to spread (Tilney and Portnoy, 1989). The key role played by the hemolysin in intracellular parasitism was demonstrated when the hemolysin gene was transformed into *Bacillus subtilis*; the recipient bacteria are able to survive and grow in macrophages (Bielecki *et al.*, 1990). *Shigella flexneri* is also able to escape from the phagosome of macrophages and spread to other cells via actin filaments (Sansonetti *et al.*, 1986; Hackstadt, 1998).

8.5 Prevention of phagosome–lysosome fusion

The contents of macrophage granules are delivered to bacteria-containing phagosomes by the process of phagosome–lysosome fusion. This process is initiated immediately following ingestion of most bacteria, but some species survive because they prevent fusion. The capacity of ingested organisms to inhibit phagosome–lysosome fusion was shown in classic studies by Jones and Hirsh with *Toxoplasma gondii* (Jones and Hirsh, 1972). The viability of ingested microbes, and the state of opsonization, largely determines whether fusion occurs. For instance, unopsonized *Chlamydia psittaci* enter macrophages and survive without evidence of phagosome–lysosome fusion. On the other hand, if the *Chlamydia* is opsonized with specific antiserum, fusion occurs shortly after ingestion (Wyrick and Brownridge, 1978). A similar sequence of events is seen with *L.pneumophila*, where opsonization determines whether phagosome–lysosome fusion occurs (Horwitz, 1983).

When *M.tuberculosis* is ingested by a macrophage, the resultant phagosome does not acidify. Although the phagosome does acquire lysosomal markers such as LAMP-1, it does not fuse with ATPase⁺-containing vesicles (Sturgill-Koszycki *et al.*, 1994). It is the proton-adenosine triphosphatase (ATPase) that is responsible for phagosomal acidification (Sturgill-Koszycki *et al.*, 1994). *Chlamydia trachomatis* also evades phagosome–lysosome fusion, although by a different method; *Chlamydia* undergo their life cycle within a membrane-limited parasitophorous vacuole, termed an inclusion (Moulder, 1991). Such inclusions lack lysosomal markers such as LAMP-1, LAMP-2, cathespin D or ATPase (Heinzen *et al.*, 1996). The *Chlamydia* inclusion incorporates host sphingomyelin (Hackstadt *et al.*, 1995), and occupies a site distal to the Golgi apparatus (Hackstadt *et al.*, 1996).

8.6 Lysosome tolerance

The bacteria *Coxiella burnetii*, the cause of Q fever, is considered very stable (aerosol transmission) and infectious (Hackstadt, 1998). *Coxiella* has a life cycle contained within a mature lysosome in which it not only avoids digestion but requires the extreme acidic conditions for growth (Heinzen *et al.*, 1996). Optimal pH for *Coxiella* metabolism is between 4.7 and 4.8, and without such conditions, replication will not occur (Hackstadt and Williams, 1981). Whereas *Chlamydia*-containing vacuoles lack lysosomal markers, *Coxiella* vacuoles contain the lysosomal markers LAMP-1, LAMP-2, cathepsin D and vacuolar ATPase (Heinzen *et al.*, 1996).

8.7 Resistance to oxidative killing

Once within the phagolysosome, bacteria are exposed to the full brunt of the macrophage's oxidative attack. Some bacteria are intrinsically resistant to killing by ROIs, while others are able to detoxify oxygen radicals. For instance, *M.leprae* elaborates superoxide dismutase that may interfere with bacteriocidal effects of O_2^- (Wheeler and Gregory, 1980). The glycolipid lipoarabinomannan, produced in large amounts by *M.tuberculosis* and *M.leprae*, is capable of scavenging free oxygen radicals within the macrophage. As such, the cytocidal activity of the macrophage is greatly hampered and may facilitate *Mycobacterium* survival within the macrophage (Neill and Klebanoff, 1988; Chan *et al.*, 1991). The mucoid exopolysaccharide from *P.aeruginosa* is also able to scavenge hypochlorite, thereby protecting the bacteria from its potent toxic effects (Learn *et al.*, 1987).

8.8 Resistance to non-oxidative killing

Salmonella typhimurium is a facultative intracellular pathogen. After macrophage phagocytosis, phagosome–lysosome fusion occurs, but the bacteria are able to survive. Digestion of killed but not live bacteria occurs, suggesting that the viable bacteria are resistant to the effects of lysosomal enzymes (Carroll *et al.*, 1979). *Burkholderia* (formely *Pseudomonas*) *cepacia* is an important evolving pathogen in both cystic fibrosis and CGD. It is highly resistant to non-reactive killing by virtue of an unusual outer membrane, a factor which is probably responsible for its prototypic virulence (Speert *et al.*, 1994). *Salmonella typhimurium* strains harboring a deletion in the flavohemoglobin gene are sensitive to NO (Crawford and Goldberg, 1998). *Escherichia coli* produces a nitric oxide dioxygenase with high homology to flavohemoglobin, and is also capable of detoxifying NO (Gardner *et al.*, 1998). Flavohemoglobin/nitric oxide dioxygenase *E.coli* mutants are sensitive to growth inhibition by gaseous NO (Gardner *et al.*, 1998). Transcription of these genes is increased as levels of NO are elevated (Groisman and Saier, 1990; Gardner *et al.*, 1998).

8.9 Failure to trigger a respiratory burst

The receptor-mediated process by which bacteria enter macrophages appears to be critical in determining their intracellular fate, as the ligation of certain receptors, but not others, initiates the generation of ROIs (Wright and Griffin, 1985). Entry via the macrophage Fc receptor, but not via CR3, has been shown to stimulate a respiratory burst resulting in reactive oxygen and nitrogen intermediates (Wilson *et al.*, 1980). Mycobacteria associate with a complement cleavage product, C2a, which in turn cleaves C3, resulting in C3b opsonization of the mycobacteria. The macrophages in turn ingest the mycobacteria via CR3, thereby avoiding the respiratory burst (Schorey *et al.*, 1997).

8.10 Inhibition of macrophage activation

As previously mentioned, *M.leprae* exhibit multiple mechanisms for evasion of normal macrophage bacteriocidal defenses. A key factor in its survival is its capacity to prevent macrophage activation, even after stimulation with IFN-γ (Sibley and Krahenbuhl, 1987). IFN-γ is the main primary signal for induction of NOS, the resultant NO being a bacterio-cidal component within macrophages (Drapier *et al.*, 1988; Denis, 1991; James, 1993). One of the hallmarks of lepromatous leprosy is the presence within dermal lesions of macrophages laden with a large mycobacterial load, with few infiltrating lymphocytes (Birdi and Antia, 1989; Kaplan and Hancock, 1989). The immunological defect in patients with lepromatous leprosy is an inability to activate macrophages for mycobacter-ial killing (Bloom and Mehra, 1984). This appears not to be a secondary rather than a primary macrophage abnormality, with suboptimal production of macrophage-activating factor/cytokines, such as IL-2 (Kaplan and Cohn, 1985). IL-1 production from peripheral blood mononuclear cells of lepromatous leprosy patients is also deficient (Watson *et al.*, 1984). Certain strains of mycobacteria produce lipoarabinomannan, which can scavenge cytotoxic oxygen free radicals and inhibit protein kinase C activity, thereby impairing macrophage activation (Chan *et al.*, 1991).

The dermal lesions in patients with lepromatous leprosy respond to local immunother-apy (Kaplan *et al.*, 1989). Shortly after IL-2 is injected intradermally into the lesions, there is an influx of lymphocytes. This is followed by liberation of the mycobacteria from disintegrating macrophages and immigration of blood monocytes with mycobacteriocidal capacity. This clearly demonstrates the importance of macrophage activation and the role of cytokines in the effective eradication of intracellular parasites.

8.11 Macrophage killing (apoptosis)

During the course of infection, *Yersinae* remain extracellular to the macrophage but, due to contact-dependent secretion of proteins encoded by a type III secretion system, apop-tosis is induced (Mecsas and Strauss, 1996). The effector proteins responsible for apopto-sis are from the Yop family, whose only function is to destroy macrophages and lymphocytes (Ruckdeschel *et al.*, 1997; Monack *et al.*, 1998). Proteins are released by a type III secretion mechanism upon contact between the bacteria and macrophage. Pores are formed in the macrophage membrane through which bacterial molecules are injected (Mecsas and Strauss, 1996). In particular, YopJ appears essential for persistence of *Yersinae* within the host (Monack *et al.*, 1998). YopJ induces apoptosis of macrophages, and is believed to reduce host inflammatory responses by removing many of the cells involved in TNF-α production, allowing the infection to persist (Palmer *et al.*, 1998; Schesser *et al.*, 1998).

Salmonella species also use a type III secretion system to deliver an invasin termed SipB. SipB associates with the pro-apoptotic protease caspase-1, resulting in activation of caspase-1 and hence apoptosis (Hersh *et al.*, 1999). An analogous system functions in *Shigella* (Hersh *et al.*, 1999).

8.12 Inhibition of antigen presentation

As mycobacteria grow within macrophage phagosomes, they are able to escape major histocompatibility complex class I and II processing pathways for antigen presentation. *Mycobacterium tuberculosis* is able to down-regulate the surface expression of class I and II molecules by sequestering them within the phagosomal membrane, or specifically blocking antigen processing via MHC class II (Pancholi *et al.*, 1993; Clemens and Horwitz, 1995). Thus CD4+ helper T cells are unable to mediate immunity to tuberculosis, a phenomenon which may contribute to mycobacterial virulence (Pancholi *et al.*, 1993).

9 Summary

Macrophages play a critically important role in host defense against bacterial infection. They exert their antibacterial activities at mucosal surfaces and as filtering agents within the reticuloendothelial system. The phenotypic diversity among macrophages attests to their adaptation to a wide range of environmental conditions and the special requirements for function in these diverse arenas.

Phagocytosis and bacterial killing are functions for which macrophages are well suited. They ingest potential pathogens via an array of non-opsonic and opsonic receptors and kill their prey with the aid of reactive oxygen and nitrogen intermediates and non-oxidative factors. The capacity to ingest and kill bacteria is enhanced by an assortment of opsonins, cytokines and other immunomodulators. Despite the impressive antibacterial armaments with which macrophages are fortified, they are impotent in the eradication of certain bacterial strains and species.

Many bacterial species are virulent because of their resistance to normal phagocytic defenses. Extracellular pathogens generally resist phagocytosis except when opsonized with specific Ig. Intracellular pathogens thrive within eukaryotic cells and are able to withstand the macrophage's bacteriocidal assault. Bacteria utilize a clever array of survival strategies: avoidance of phagocytosis, failure to trigger respiratory burst, escape from the phagosome, prevention of phagosome–lysosome fusion, resistance to oxidative or non-oxidative killing and directed apoptosis of macrophages. New therapeutic strategies are being developed to augment natural antibacterial defenses and prevent these intracellular pathogens from parasitizing macrophages.

References

Aderem, A.A. *et al.* (1985). Ligated complement receptors do not activate the arachidonic acid cascade in resident peritoneal macrophages. *Journal of Experimental Medicine*, **161**, 617–22.

Albina, J.E. (1995). On the expression of nitric oxide synthase by human macrophages. Why no NO? *Journal of Leukocyte Biology*, **58**, 643–9.

Albrich, J.M. and Hurst, J.K. (1982). Oxidative inactivation of *Escherichia coli* by hypochlorous acid. Rates and differentiation of respiratory from other reaction sites. *FEBS Letters*, **144**, 157–61.

Albrich, J.M. *et al.* (1986). Effects of the putative neutrophil-generated toxin, hypochlorous acid, on membrane permeability and transport systems of *Escherichia coli*. *Journal of Clinical Investigation*, **78**, 177–84.

Alford, C.E., King, T.E., Jr and Campbell, P.A. (1991). Role of transferrin, transferrin receptors, and iron in macrophage listericidal activity. *Journal of Experimental Medicine*, **174**, 459–66.

Allen, L.A. and Aderem, A. (1996a). Molecular definition of distinct cytoskeletal structures involved in complement- and Fc receptor-mediated phagocytosis in macrophages. *Journal of Experimental Medicine*, **184**, 627–37.

Allen, L.A. and Aderem, A. (1996b). Mechanisms of phagocytosis. *Current Opinion in Immunology*, **8**, 36–40.

Alpuche-Aranda, C.M. *et al.* (1995). Spacious phagosome formation within mouse macrophages correlates with *Salmonella* serotype pathogenicity and host susceptibility. *Infection and Immunity*, **63**, 4456–62.

Amoroso, A. *et al.* (1999). Polymorphism at codon 54 of mannose-binding protein gene influences AIDS progression but not HIV infection in exposed children. *AIDS*, **13**, 863–4.

Anderson, D.C. *et al.* (1985). The severe and moderate phenotypes of heritable Mac-1, LFA-1 deficiency: their quantitative definition and relation to leukocyte dysfunction and clinical features. *Journal of Infectious Diseases*, **152**, 668–89.

Andrew, P.W., Jackett, P.S. and Lowrie, D.B. (1985). Killing and degradation of microorganisms in macrophages. In Dean, R.T. and Jessup, W. (ed.), *Mononuclear Phagocytes: Physiology and Pathology*. Elsevier, New York.

Armstrong, J.A. and Hart, P.D. (1975). Phagosome–lysosome interactions in cultured macrophages infected with virulent tubercle bacilli. Reversal of the usual nonfusion pattern and observations on bacterial survival. *Journal of Experimental Medicine*, **142**, 1–16.

Badolato, R. *et al.* (1995). Serum amyloid A induces calcium mobilization and chemotaxis of human monocytes by activating a pertussis toxin-sensitive signaling pathway. *Journal of Immunology*, **155**, 4004–10.

Baorto, D.M. *et al.* (1997). Survival of FimH-expressing enterobacteria in macrophages relies on glycolipid traffic. *Nature*, **389**, 636–9.

Barrette, W.C., Jr *et al.* (1989). General mechanism for the bacterial toxicity of hypochlorous acid: abolition of ATP production. *Biochemistry*, **28**, 9172–8.

Basham, T.Y. and Merigan, T.C. (1983). Recombinant interferon-γ increases HLA-DR synthesis and expression. *Journal of Immunology*, **130**, 1492–4.

Baumler, A.J. and Heffron, F. (1995). Microbial resistance to macrophage effector functions: stratagies for evading microbicidal mechanisms and scavenging nutrients within mononuclear phagocytes. In Roth, J.A. (ed.), *Virulence Mechanisms of Bacterial Pathogens*, 2nd edn. American Society for Microbiology, Washington, DC.

Becker, S. (1984). Interferons as modulators of human monocyte–macrophage differentiation. I. Interferon-γ increases HLA-DR expression and inhibits phagocytosis of zymosan. *Journal of Immunology*, **132**, 1249–54.

Beckman, J.S. and Crow, J.P. (1993). Pathological implications of nitric oxide, superoxide and peroxynitrite formation. *Biochemical Society Transactions*, **21**, 330–4.

Bendtzen, K. (1988). Interleukin 1, interleukin 6 and tumor necrosis factor in infection, inflammation and immunity. *Immunology Letters*, **19**, 183–91.

Berger, M. *et al.* (1989). Complement receptor expression on neutrophils at an inflammatory site, the *Pseudomonas*-infected lung in cystic fibrosis. *Journal of Clinical Investigation*, **84**, 1302–13.

Berton, G. and Lowell, C.A. (1999). Integrin signalling in neutrophils and macrophages. *Cell Signaling*, **11**, 621–35.

Bielecki, J., Youngman, P., Connelly, P. and Portnoy, D.A. (1990). *Bacillus subtilis* expressing a haemolysin gene from *Listeria monocytogenes* can grow in mammalian cells. *Nature*, **345**, 175–6.

Birdi, T.J. and Antia, N.H. (1989). The macrophage in leprosy: a review on the current status. *International Journal of Leprosy and Other Mycobacterial Diseases*, **57**, 511–25.

Blackwell, J.M., Ezekowitz, R.A.B., Roberts, M.B., Channon, J.Y., Sim, R.B. and Gordon, S. (1985). Macrophage complement and lectin-like receptors bind *Leishmania* in the absence of serum. *Journal of Experimental Medicine*, **162**, 324–31.

Bloom, B.R. and Mehra, V. (1984). Immunological unresponsiveness in leprosy. *Immunological Reviews*, **80**, 5–28.

Bowdy, B.D. *et al.* (1990). Organ-specific disposition of group B streptococci in piglets: evidence for a direct interaction with target cells in the pulmonary circulation. *Pediatric Research*, 1990. **27**, 344–8.

Brown, E.J. (1991). Complement receptors and phagocytosis. *Current Opinion in Immunology*, **3**, 76–82.

Brunelli, L., Crow, J.P. and Beckman, J.S. (1995). The comparative toxicity of nitric oxide and per-oxynitrite to *Escherichia coli*. *Archives of Biochemistry and Biophysics*, **316**, 327–34.

Buschman, E., Taniyama, T., Nakamura, R. and Skamene, E. (1989). Functional expression of the Bcg gene in macrophages. *Research in Immunology*, **140**, 793–7.

Byrd, T.F. and Horwitz, M.A. (19789). Interferon γ-activated human monocytes downregulate transferrin receptors and inhibit the intracellular multiplication of *Legionella pneumophila* by limiting the availability of iron. *Journal of Clinical Investigation*, **83**, 1457–65.

Cabral, D.A., Loh, B.A. and Speert, D.P. (1987). Mucoid *Pseudomonas aeruginosa* resists nonopsonic phagocytosis by human neutrophils and macrophages. *Pediatric Research*, **22**, 429–31.

Calandra T. *et al.* (1990). Prognostic values of tumor necrosis factor/cachectin, interleukin-1, interferon-α, and interferon-γ in the serum of patients with septic shock. Swiss–Dutch J5 Immunoglobulin Study Group. *Journal of Infectious Diseases*, **161**, 982–7.

Cannon, J.G. *et al.* (1990). Circulating interleukin-1 and tumor necrosis factor in septic shock and experimental endotoxin fever. *Journal of Infectious Diseases*, **161**, 79–84.

Carlin, J.M. *et al.* (1987). Biologic-response-modifier-induced indoleamine 2,3-dioxygenase activity in human peripheral blood mononuclear cell cultures. *Journal of Immunology*, **139**, 2414–8.

Caron, E. and Hall, A. (1998). Identification of two distinct mechanisms of phagocytosis controlled by different Rho GTPases. *Science*, **282**, 1717–21.

Carrol, M.E., Jackett, P.S., Aber, V.R. and Lowrie, D.B. (1979). Phagolysosome formation, cyclic adenosine 3′:5′-monophosphate and the fate of *Salmonella typhimurium* within mouse peritoneal macrophages. *Journal of General Microbiology*, **110**, 421–9.

Carroll, M.C. (1998). The role of complement and complement receptors in induction and regulation of immunity. *Annual Review of Immunology*, **16**, 545–68.

Catterall, J.R., Black, C.M., Leventhal, J.P., Rizk, N.W., Wachtel, J.S. and Remington, J.S. (19867). Nonoxidative microbicidal activity in normal human alveolar and peritoneal macrophages. *Infection and Immunity*, **55**, 1635–40.

Chan, J. *et al.* (1991). Lipoarabinomannan, a possible virulence factor involved in persistence of *Mycobacterium tuberculosis* within macrophages. *Infection and Immunity*, **59**, 1755–61.

Cheers, C., Hill, M., Haigh, A.M. and Stanley, E.R. (1989). Stimulation of macrophage phagocytic but not bactericidal activity by colony-stimulating factor 1. *Infection and Immunity*, **57**, 1512–6.

Clark, S.C. and Kamen, R. (1987). The human hematopoietic colony-stimulating factors. *Science,* **236**, 1229–37.

Clemens, D.L. and Horwitz, M.A. (1995). Characterization of the *Mycobacterium tuberculosis* phagosome and evidence that phagosomal maturation is inhibited. *Journal of Experimental Medicine,* **181**, 257–70.

Cohen, A.B. and Cline, M.J. (1971). The human alveolar macrophage: isolation, cultivation *in vitro,* and studies of morphologic and functional characteristics. *Journal of Clinical Investigation,* **50**, 1390–8.

Cohn, Z.A. (1978). Activation of mononuclear phagocytes: fact, fancy, and future. *Journal of Immunology,* **121**, 813–6.

Confer, D.L. and Eaton, J.W. (1982). Phagocyte impotence caused by an invasive bacterial adenylate cyclase. *Science,* **217**, 948–50.

Coonrod, J.D. (1989). Role of leukocytes in lung defenses. *Respiration,* **55** (Supplement 1), 9–13.

Crawford, M.J. and Goldberg, D.E. (1998). Role for the *Salmonella* flavohemoglobin in protection from nitric oxide. *Journal of Biological Chemistry,* **273**, 12543–7.

Cross, A.S. (1990). The biologic significance of bacterial encapsulation. *Current Topics in Microbiology and Immunology,* **150**, 87–95.

Crowle, A.J., Ross, E.J. and May, M.H. (1987). Inhibition by 1,25(OH)2-vitamin D3 of the multiplication of virulent tubercle bacilli in cultured human macrophages. *Infection and Immunity,* **55**, 2945–50.

Curnutte, J.T. and Babior, B.M. (1987). Chronic granulomatous disease. *Advances in Human Genetics,* **16**, 229–97.

Denis, M. (1991). Interferon-γ-treated murine macrophages inhibit growth of tubercle bacilli via the generation of reactive nitrogen intermediates. *Cellular Immunology,* **132**, 150–7.

Denis, M., Forget,A., Pelletier, M. and Skamene, E. (1988). Pleiotropic effects of the Bcg gene: III. Respiratory burst in Bcg-congenic macrophages. *Clinical and Experimental Immunology,* **73**, 370–5.

Dinarello, C.A. (1996). Biologic basis for interleukin-1 in disease. *Blood,* **87**, 2095–147.

Dinarello, C.A., Cannon, J.G. and Wolff, S.M. (1988). New concepts on the pathogenesis of fever. *Reviews of Infectious Diseases,* **10**, 168–89.

Douglas, S.D. and Musson, R.A. (1986). Phagocytic defects—monocytes/macrophages. *Clinical Immunology and Immunopathology,* **40**, 62–8.

Douvas, G.S., Looker, D.L., Vatter, A.E. and Crowle, A.J. (1985). Gamma interferon activates human macrophages to become tumoricidal and leishmanicidal but enhances replication of macrophage-associated mycobacteria. *Infection and Immunity,* **50**, 1–8.

Drapier, J.C., Wietzerbin, J. and Hibbs, J.B., Jr (1988). Interferon-γ and tumor necrosis factor induce the L-arginine-dependent cytotoxic effector mechanism in murine macrophages. *European Journal of Immunology,* **18**, 1587–92.

Dunne, D.W. *et al.* (1994). The type I macrophage scavenger receptor binds to Gram-positive bacteria and recognizes lipoteichoic acid. *Proceedings of the National Academy of Sciences USA,* **91**, 1863–7.

Epstein, J. *et al.* (1996). The collectins in innate immunity. *Current Opinion in Immunology,* **8**, 29–35.

Ezekowitz, R.A., Orkin, S.H. and Newburger, P.E. (1987). Recombinant interferon γ augments phagocyte superoxide production and X-chronic granulomatous disease gene expression in X-linked variant chronic granulomatous disease. *Journal of Clinical Investigation,* **80**, 1009–16.

Ezekowitz, R.A., Dinauer, M.C., Jaffe, H.S., Orkin, S.H. and Newburger, P.E. (1988). Partial correction of the phagocyte defect in patients with X-linked chronic granulomatous disease by subcutaneous interferon γ. *New England Journal of Medicine*, **319**, 146–51.

Fels, A.O. and Cohn, Z.A. (1986). The alveolar macrophage. *Journal of Applied Physiology*, **60**, 353–69.

Fick, R.B., Jr, Naegel, G.P., Matthay, R.A. and Reynolds, H.Y. (1981). Cystic fibrosis *Pseudomonas* opsonins. Inhibitory nature in an *in vitro* phagocytic assay. *Journal of Clinical Investigation*, **68**, 899–914.

Fick, R.B., Jr, Naegel, G.P., Squier, S.U., Wood, R.E., Gee, J.B.L. and Reynolds, H.Y. (1984). Proteins of the cystic fibrosis respiratory tract. Fragmented immunoglobulin G opsonic antibody causing defective opsonophagocytosis. *Journal of Clinical Investigation*, **74**, 236–48.

Finlay, B.B. and Cossart, P. (1997). Exploitation of mammalian host cell functions by bacterial pathogens [published erratum appears in *Science* 1997 Oct 17;278(5337):373] *Science*, **276**, 718–25.

Flesch, I. and Kaufmann, S.H. (1987). Mycobacterial growth inhibition by interferon-g-activated bone marrow macrophages and differential susceptibility among strains of *Mycobacterium tuberculosis*. *Journal of Immunology*, **138**, 4408–13.

Flesch, I. and Kaufmann, S.H. (1988). Attempts to characterize the mechanisms involved in mycobacterial growth inhibition by γ-interferon-activated bone marrow macrophages. *Infection and Immunity*, **56**, 1464–9.

Frank, M.M. (1989) The role of macrophages in blood stream clearance. In Zembala, M. and Asherson, G.L. (ed.), *Human Monocytes*. Academic Press, London.

Frank, M.M., Hamburger, M.I., Lawley, T.J., Kimberly, R.P. and Plotz, P.H. (1979). Defective reticuloendothelial system Fc-receptor function in systemic lupus erythematosus. *New England Journal of Medicine*, **300**, 518–23.

Frank, M.M., Joiner, K. and Hammer, C. (1987). The function of antibody and complement in the lysis of bacteria. *Reviews of Infectious Diseases*, **9** (Supplement 5), S537–45.

Friedman, R.L. and Moon, R.J. (1977). Hepatic clearance of *Salmonella typhimurium* in silica-treated mice. *Infection and Immunity*, **16**, 1005–12.

Friedman, R.L. *et al.* (1987). *Bordetella pertussis* adenylate cyclase: effects of affinity-purified adenylate cyclase on human polymorphonuclear leukocyte functions. *Infection and Immunity*, **55**, 135–40.

Fruh, R. *et al.* (1995). TH1 cells trigger tumor necrosis factor α-mediated hypersensitivity to *Pseudomonas aeruginosa* after adoptive transfer into SCID mice. *Infection and Immunity*, **63**, 1107–12.

Galan, J.E. and Collmer, A. (1999). Type III secretion machines: bacterial devices for protein delivery into host cells. *Science*, **284**, 1322–8.

Ganz, T., Selsted, M.E. and Lehrer, R.I. (1986). Antimicrobial activity of phagocyte granule proteins. *Seminars in Respiratory Infections*, **1**, 107–17.

Gardner, P.R. *et al.* (1998). Nitric oxide dioxygenase: an enzymic function for flavohemoglobin. *Proceedings of the National Academy of Sciences USA*, **95**, 10378–83.

Geisow, M.J., D'Arcy Hart, P. and Young, M.R. (1981). Temporal changes of lysosome and phagosome pH during phagolysosome formation in macrophages: studies by fluorescence spectroscopy. *Journal of Cell Biology*, **89**, 645–52.

Goldstein, E., Lippert, W. and Warshauer, D. (1974). Pulmonary alveolar macrophage. Defender against bacterial infection of the lung. *Journal of Clinical Investigation*, **54**, 519–28.

Gordon, S., Todd, J. and Cohn, Z.A. (1974). *In vitro* synthesis and secretion of lysozyme by mononuclear phagocytes. *Journal of Experimental Medicine*, **139**, 1228–48.

Gordon, S., Perry, V.H., Rabinowitz, S., Chung, L. and Rosen, H. (1988). Plasma membrane receptors of the mononuclear phagocyte system. *Journal of Cell Science* (Supplement), **9**, 1–26.

Govoni, G. *et al.* (1995). Genomic structure, promoter sequence, and induction of expression of the mouse *Nramp1* gene in macrophages. *Genomics*, **27**, 9–19.

Griffin, F.M., Jr, Griffin, J.A., Leider, J.E. and Siverstein, S.C. (1975). Studies on the mechanism of phagocytosis. I. Requirements for circumferential attachment of particle-bound ligands to specific receptors on the macrophage plasma membrane. *Journal of Experimental Medicine*, **142**, 1263–82.

Groisman, E.A. and Saier, M.H., Jr (1990). *Salmonella* virulence: new clues to intramacrophage survival. *Trends in Biochemical Sciences*, **15**, 30–3.

Groopman, J.E., Molina, J.M. and Scadden, D.T. (1989). Hematopoietic growth factors. Biology and clinical applications. *New England Journal of Medicine*, **321**, 1449–59.

Gros, P., Skamene, E. and Forget, A. (1981). Genetic control of natural resistance to *Mycobacterium bovis* (BCG) in mice. *Journal of Immunology*, **127**, 2417–21.

Gross, G.N., Rehm, S.R. and Pierce, A.K. (1978). The effect of complement depletion on lung clearance of bacteria. *Journal of Clinical Investigation*, **62**, 373–8.

Guyre, P.M., Morganelli, P.M. and Miller, R. (1983). Recombinant immune interferon increases immunoglobulin G Fc receptors on cultured human mononuclear phagocytes. *Journal of Clinical Investigation*, **72**, 393–7.

Hachicha, M. *et al.* (1998). Regulation of chemokine gene expression in human peripheral blood neutrophils phagocytosing microbial pathogens. *Journal of Immunology*, **160**, 449–54.

Hackstadt, T. (1998). The diverse habitats of obligate intracellular parasites. *Current Opinion in Microbiology*, **1**, 82–7.

Hackstadt, T. and Williams, J.C. (1981). Biochemical stratagem for obligate parasitism of eukaryotic cells by *Coxiella burnetii*. *Proceedings of the National Academy of Sciences USA*, **78**, 3240–4.

Hackstadt, T., Scidmore, M.A. and Rockey, D.D. (1995). Lipid metabolism in *Chlamydia trachomatis*-infected cells: directed trafficking of Golgi-derived sphingolipids to the chlamydial inclusion. *Proceedings of the National Academy of Sciences USA*, **92**, 4877–81.

Hackstadt, T. *et al.* (1996). *Chlamydia trachomatis* interrupts an exocytic pathway to acquire endogenously synthesized sphingomyelin in transit from the Golgi apparatus to the plasma membrane. *EMBO Journal*, **15**, 964–77.

Hampton, M.B., Kettle, A.J. and Winterbourn, C.C. (1998). Inside the neutrophil phagosome: oxidants, myeloperoxidase, and bacterial killing. *Blood*, **92**, 3007–17.

Hansen, S. and Holmskov, U. (1998). Structural aspects of collectins and receptors for collectins. *Immunobiology*, **199**, 165–89.

Hardt, W.D. *et al.* (1998). *S.typhimurium* encodes an activator of Rho GTPases that induces membrane ruffling and nuclear responses in host cells. *Cell*, **93**, 815–26.

Harrison, J.E. and Schultz, J. (1976). Studies on the chlorinating activity of myeloperoxidase. *Journal of Biological Chemistry*, **251**, 1371–4.

Hatano, K., Goldberg, J.B. and Pier, G.B. (1995). Biologic activities of antibodies to the neutral-polysaccharide component of the *Pseudomonas aeruginosa* lipopolysaccharide are blocked by *O* side chains and mucoid exopolysaccharide (alginate). *Infection and Immunity*, **63**, 21–6.

Heidbrink, P.J., Toews, G.B., Gross, G.N. and Pierce, A.K. (1982). Mechanisms of complement-mediated clearance of bacteria from the murine lung. *American Review of Respiratory Diseases*, **125**, 517–20.

Heinzen, R.A. *et al.* (1996). Differential interaction with endocytic and exocytic pathways distinguish parasitophorous vacuoles of *Coxiella burnetii* and *Chlamydia trachomatis*. *Infection and Immunity*, **64**, 796–809.

Hersh, D. *et al.* (1999). *The Salmonella* invasin SipB induces macrophage apoptosis by binding to caspase-1. *Proceedings of the National Academy of Sciences USA*, **96**, 2396–401.

Hilbi, H., Zychlinsky, A. and Sansonetti, P.J. (1997). Macrophage apoptosis in microbial infections. *Parasitology*, **115** Supplement S79–87.

Hill, H.R., Augustine, N.H. and Jaffe, H.S. (1991). Human recombinant interferon γ enhances neonatal polymorphonuclear leukocyte activation and movement, and increases free intracellular calcium. *Journal of Experimental Medicine*, **173**, 767–70.

Hocking, W.G. and Golde, D.W. (1979). The pulmonary-alveolar macrophage (first of two parts). *New England Journal of Medicine*, **301**, 580–7.

Horwitz, M.A. (1983). The Legionnaires' disease bacterium (*Legionella pneumophila*) inhibits phagosome–lysosome fusion in human monocytes. *Journal of Experimental Medicine*, **158**, 2108–26.

Horwitz, M.A. (1984). Phagocytosis of the Legionnaires' disease bacterium (*Legionella pneumophila*) occurs by a novel mechanism: engulfment within a pseudopod coil. *Cell*, **36**, 27–33.

Horwitz, M.A. and Silverstein, S.C. (1980). Influence of the *Escherichia coli* capsule on complement fixation and on phagocytosis and killing by human phagocytes. *Journal of Clinical Investigation*, **65**, 82–94.

Hosea, S.W., Brown, E.J. and Frank, M.M. (1980). The critical role of complement in experimental pneumococcal sepsis. *Journal of Infectious Diseases*, **142**, 903–9.

Hubbard, A.L. and Stukenbrok, H. (1979). An electron microscope autoradiographic study of the carbohydrate recognition systems in rat liver. II. Intracellular fates of the ^{125}I-ligands. *Journal of Cell Biology*, **83**, 65–81.

Hurst, J.K. (1991). Myleperoxidase: active site structure and catalytic mechanisms. In Everse, J., Everse, K.E. and Grisham, M.B. (ed.), *Peroxidases in Chemistry and Biology*. CRC Press, Boca Raton.

Ireton, K. and Cossart, P. (1997). Host–pathogen interactions during entry and actin-based movement of *Listeria monocytogenes*. *Annual Review of Genetics*, **31**, 113–38.

James, S.L. (1995). Role of nitric oxide in parasitic infections. *Microbiological Reviews*, **59**, 533–47.

Jensen, W.A., Rose, R.M., Wasserman, A.S., Kalb, T.H., Anton, K. and Remold, H.G. (1987). *In vitro* activation of the antibacterial activity of human pulmonary macrophages by recombinant γ interferon. *Journal of Infectious Diseases*, **155**, 574–7.

Johnston, R.B., Jr (1988). Current concepts: immunology. Monocytes and macrophages. *New England Journal of Medicine*, **318**, 747–52.

Johnston, R.B., Jr, Godzik, C.A. and Cohn, Z.A. (1978). Increased superoxide anion production by immunologically activated and chemically elicited macrophages. *Journal of Experimental Medicine*, **148**, 115–27.

Jones, T.C. and Hirsch, J.G. (1972). The interaction between *Toxoplasma gondii* and mammalian cells. II. The absence of lysosomal fusion with phagocytic vacuoles containing living parasites. *Journal of Experimental Medicine*, **136**, 1173–94.

Jonsson, S., Musher , D.M., Chapman, A., Goree, A. and Lawrence, E.C. (1985). Phagocytosis and killing of common bacterial pathogens of the lung by human alveolar macrophages. *Journal of Infectious Diseases*, **152**, 4–13.

Kan, V.L. and Bennett, J.E. (1988). Lectin-like attachment sites on murine pulmonary alveolar macrophages bind *Aspergillus fumigatus* conidia. *Journal of Infectious Diseases*, **158**, 407–14.

Kaplan, G. and Cohn, Z.A. (1985). Cell-mediated immunity in lepromatous and tuberculoid leprosy. In van Furth, R. (ed.), *Mononuclear Phagocytes: Characteristics, Physiology and Function*. Martinus Nijhoff, Boston.

Kaplan, G. and Hancock, G.E.(1989). Macrophages in leprosy. In Zembala, M. and Asherson, G.L. (ed.), *Human Monocytes*. Academic Press, London.

Kaplan, G. *et al.* (1989). The reconstitution of cell-mediated immunity in the cutaneous lesions of leprmatous leprosy by recombinant interleukin 2. *Journal of Experimental Medicine*, **169**, 893–907.

Kaplan, S.S. *et al.* (1996). Effect of nitric oxide on staphylococcal killing and interactive effect with superoxide. *Infection and Immunity*, **64**, 69–76.

Kausalya, S. *et al.* (1996). Microbicidal mechanisms of liver macrophages in experimental visceral leishmaniasis. *Apmis*, **104**, 171–5.

Kay, M.M.B. (1989). Recognition and removal of senescent cells. In Sousa, M.D. and Brock, J.H. (ed.), *Iron in Immunity, Cancer and Inflammation*. John Wiley and Sons, New York.

Kemmerich, B., Rossing, T.H. and Pennington, J.E. (1987). Comparative oxidative microbicidal activity of human blood monocytes and alveolar macrophages and activation by recombinant γ interferon. *American Review of Respiratory Disease*, **136**, 266–70.

Klebanoff, S.J. (1968). Myeloperoxidase–halide–hydrogen peroxide antibacterial system. *Journal of Bacteriology*, **95**, 2131–8.

Klebanoff, S.J. (1993). Reactive nitrogen intermediates and antimicrobial activity: role of nitrite. *Free Radical Biology and Medicine*, **14**, 351–60.

Krieg, D.P., Helmke, R.J., German, V.F. and Mangos, J.A. (1988). Resistance of mucoid *Pseudomonas aeruginosa* to nonopsonic phagocytosis by alveolar macrophages *in vitro*. *Infection and Immunity*, **56**, 3173–9.

Kuhlman, M., Joiner, K. and Ezekowitz, R.A. (1989). The human mannose-binding protein functions as an opsonin. *Journal of Experimental Medicine*, **169**, 1733–45.

Kuhn, M., Kathariou, S. and Goebel, W. (1988). Hemolysin supports survival but not entry of the intracellular bacterium *Listeria monocytogenes*. *Infection and Immunity*, **56**, 79–82.

Learn, D.B., Brestel, E.P. and Seetharama, S. (1987). Hypochlorite scavenging by *Pseudomonas aeruginosa* alginate. *Infection and Immunity*, **55**, 1813–8.

Lee, S.H., Starkey, P.M. and Gordon, S. (1985). Quantitative analysis of total macrophage content in adult mouse tissues. Immunochemical studies with monoclonal antibody F4/80. *Journal of Experimental Medicine*, **161**, 475–89.

Lehrer, R.I., Barton, A., Daher, K.A., Harwig, S.S., Ganz, T. and Selsted, M.E. (1989). Interaction of human defensins with *Escherichia coli*. Mechanism of bactericidal activity. *Journal of Clinical Investigation*, **84**, 553–61.

Lehrer, R.I., Ganz, T. and Selsted, M.E. (1991). Defensins: endogenous antibiotic peptides of animal cells. *Cell*, **64**, 229–30.

Leijh, P.C., van den Barselaar, M.T., van Zwet, T.L., Daha, M.R. and van Furth, R. (1979). Requirement of extracellular complement and immunoglobulin for intracellular killing of microorganisms by human monocytes. *Journal of Clinical Investigation*, **63**, 772–84.

Lepay, D.A., Nathan, C.F., Steinman, R.M., Murray, H.W. and Cohn, Z.A. (1985a). Murine Kupffer cells. Mononuclear phagocytes deficient in the generation of reactive oxygen intermediates. *Journal of Experimental Medicine*, **161**, 1079–96.

Lepay, D.A., Steinman, R.M., Nathan, C.F., Murray, H.W. and Cohn, Z.A. (1985b). Liver macrophages in murine listeriosis. Cell-mediated immunity is correlated with an influx of macrophages capable of generating reactive oxygen intermediates. *Journal of Experimental Medicine*, **161**, 1503–12.

Leunk, R.D. and Moon, R.J. (1982). Association of type 1 pili with the ability of livers to clear *Salmonella typhimurium*. *Infection and Immunity*, **36**, 1168–74.

Liang-Takasaki, C.J., Makela, P.H. and Leive, L. (1982). Phagocytosis of bacteria by macrophages: changing the carbohydrate of lipopolysaccharide alters interaction with complement and macrophages. *Journal of Immunology*, **128**, 1229–35.

Lobb, R.R. and Hemler, M.E. (1994). The pathophysiologic role of α4 integrins *in vivo*. *Journal of Clinical Investigation*, **94**, 1722–8.

Lowrie, D.B. and Andrew, P.W. (1988). Macrophage antimycobacterial mechanisms. *British Medical Bulletin*, **44**, 624–34.

Mackaness, G.B. (1964). The immunological basis of acquired cellular resistance. *Journal of Experimental Medicine*, **120**, 105–20.

Mackaness, G.B. (1969). The influence of immunologically committed lymphoid cells on macrophage activity *in vivo*. *Journal of Experimental Medicine*, **129**, 973–92.

Malhotra, R., Thiel, S., Reid, K.B.M. and Sim, R.B. (1990). Human leukocyte C1q receptor binds other soluble proteins with collagen domains. *Journal of Experimental Medicine*, **172**, 955–9.

Marodi, L., Leijh, P.C. and van Furth, R. (1984). Characteristics and functional capacities of human cord blood granulocytes and monocytes. *Pediatric Research*, **18**, 1127–31.

Marquez, L.A. *et al.* (1996). Kinetic and spectral properties of pea cytosolic ascorbate peroxidase. *FEBS Letters*, **389**, 153–6.

Marquis, H., Goldfine, H. and Portnoy, D.A. (1997). Proteolytic pathways of activation and degradation of a bacterial phospholipase C during intracellular infection by *Listeria monocytogenes*. *Journal of Cell Biology*, **137**, 1381–92.

McClure, C.D. and Schiller, N.L. (1996). Inhibition of macrophage phagocytosis by *Pseudomonas aeruginosa* rhamnolipids *in vitro* and *in vivo*. *Current Microbiology*, **33**, 109–17.

McElvaney, N.G. *et al.* (1992). Modulation of airway inflammation in cystic fibrosis. *In vivo* suppression of interleukin-8 levels on the respiratory epithelial surface by aerosolization of recombinant secretory leukoprotease inhibitor. *Journal of Clinical Investigation*, **90**, 1296–301.

McKenna, S.M. and Davies, K.J. (1988). The inhibition of bacterial growth by hypochlorous acid. Possible role in the bactericidal activity of phagocytes. *Biochemical Journal*, **254**, 685–92.

Meade, B.D., Kind, P.D., Ewell, J.B., McGrath, P.P. and Manclark, C.R. (1984). *In vitro* inhibition of murine macrophage migration by *Bordetella pertussis* lymphocytosis-promoting factor. *Infection and Immunity*, **45**, 718–25.

Mecklenburgh, K. *et al.* (1999). Role of neutrophil apoptosis in the resolution of pulmonary inflammation. *Monaldi Archives for Chest Disease*, **54**, 345–9.

Mecsas, J.J. and Strauss, E.J. (1996). Molecular mechanisms of bacterial virulence: type III secretion and pathogenicity islands. *Emerging Infectious Diseases*, **2**, 270–88.

Meluleni, G.J. *et al.* (1995). Mucoid *Pseudomonas aeruginosa* growing in a biofilm *in vitro* are killed by opsonic antibodies to the mucoid exopolysaccharide capsule but not by antibodies produced during chronic lung infection in cystic fibrosis patients. *Journal of Immunology*, **155**, 2029–38.

Metcalf, D. (1987). The role of the colony-stimulating factors in resistance to acute infections. *Immunology and Cell Biology*, **65**, 35–43.

Michie, H.R., *et al.* (1988). Detection of circulating tumor necrosis factor after endotoxin administration. *New England Journal of Medicine*, **318**, 1481–6.

Mims, C. *et al.* (1998). *Natural Defences in Action*. Mosby International Ltd, London. pp. 111–118.

Mokoena, T. and Gordon, S. (1985). Human macrophage activation. Modulation of mannosyl, fucosyl receptor activity *in vitro* by lymphokines, γ and α interferons, and dexamethasone. *Journal of Clinical Investigation*, **75**, 624–31.

Monack, D.M. *et al.* (1998). *Yersinia*-induced apoptosis *in vivo* aids in the establishment of a systemic infection of mice. *Journal of Experimental Medicine*, **188**, 2127–37.

Morissette, C. *et al.* (1996). Lung phagocyte bactericidal function in strains of mice resistant and susceptible to *Pseudomonas aeruginosa*. *Infection and Immunity*, **64**, 4984–92.

Morton, H.C., van Egmond, M. and van de Winkel, J.G. (1996). Structure and function of human IgA Fc receptors (Fc αR). *Critical Reviews in Immunology*, **16**, 423–40.

Moulder, J.W. (1991). Interaction of chlamydiae and host cells *in vitro*. *Microbiological Reviews*, **55**, 143–90.

Murphey, S.A., Root, R.K. and Schreiber, A.D. (1979). The role of antibody and complement in phagocytosis by rabbit alveolar macrophages. *Journal of Infectious Diseases*, **140**, 896–903.

Murray, H.W. (1988). Interferon-γ, the activated macrophage, and host defense against microbial challenge. *Annals of Internal Medicine*, **108**, 595–608.

Nash, T.W., Libby, D.M. and Horwitz, M.A. (1984). Interaction between the legionnaires' disease bacterium (*Legionella pneumophila*) and human alveolar macrophages. Influence of antibody, lymphokines, and hydrocortisone. *Journal of Clinical Investigation*, **74**, 771–82.

Nathan, C.F. (1982). Secretion of oxygen intermediates: role in effector functions of activated macrophages. *Federation Proceedings*, **41**, 2206–11.

Nathan, C.F. (1987). Secretory products of macrophages. *Journal of Clinical Investigation*, **79**, 319–26.

Nathan, C.F. and Hibbs, J.B., Jr. (1991). Role of nitric oxide synthesis in macrophage antimicrobial activity. *Current Opinion in Immunology*, **3**, 65–70.

Nathan, C. and Xie, Q.W. (1994). Regulation of biosynthesis of nitric oxide. *Journal of Biological Chemistry*, **269**, 13725–8.

Nathan, C.F. Murray, H.W., Wiebe, M.E. and Rubin, B.Y. (1983). Identification of interferon-γ as the lymphokine that activates human macrophage oxidative metabolism and antimicrobial activity. *Journal of Experimental Medicine*, **158**, 670–89.

Neill, M.A. and Klebanoff, S.J. (1988). The effect of phenolic glycolipid-1 from *Mycobacterium leprae* on the antimicrobial activity of human macrophages. *Journal of Experimental Medicine*, **167**, 30–42.

Neonato, M.G. *et al.* (1999). Genetic polymorphism of the mannose-binding protein gene in children with sickle cell disease: identification of three new variant alleles and relationship to infections. *European Journal of Human Genetics*, **7**, 679–86.

Nguyen, B.Y., Peterson, P.K., Verbrugh, H.A., Quie, P.G., and Hoidal, J.R. (1982). Differences in phagocytosis and killing by alveolar macrophages from humans, rabbits, rats, and hamsters. *Infection and Immunity*, **36**, 504–9.

Noel, G.J., Mosser, D.M. and Edelson, P.J. (1990). Role of complement in mouse macrophage binding of *Haemophilus influenzae* type b. *Journal of Clinical Investigation*, **85**, 208–18.

North, R.J. (1970). The relative importance of blood monocytes and fixed macrophages to the expression of cell-mediated immunity to infection. *Journal of Experimental Medicine*, **132**, 521–34.

North, R.J. (1978). The concept of the activated macrophage. *Journal of Immunology*, **121**, 806–9.

O'Neill, S.J., Lesperance, E. and Klass, D.J. (1984). Human lung lavage surfactant enhances staphylococcal phagocytosis by alveolar macrophages. *American Review of Respiratory Diseases*, **130**, 1177–9.

Ofek, I. *et al.* (1995). Nonopsonic phagocytosis of microorganisms. *Annual Review of Microbiology*, **49**, 239–76.

Okusawa, S., Gelfand, J.A., Ikejima, T., Connolly, R.J. and Dinarello, C.A. (1988). Interleukin 1 induces a shock-like state in rabbits. Synergism with tumor necrosis factor and the effect of cyclooxygenase inhibition. *Journal of Clinical Investigation*, **81**, 1162–72.

Palecanda, A. *et al.* (1999). Role of the scavenger receptor MARCO in alveolar macrophage binding of unopsonized environmental particles. *Journal of Experimental Medicine*, **189**, 1497–506.

Palmer, L.E. *et al.* (1998). YopJ of *Yersinia pseudotuberculosis* is required for the inhibition of macrophage TNF-α production and downregulation of the MAP kinases p38 and JNK. *Molecular Microbiology*, **27**, 953–65.

Pancholi, P. *et al.* (1993). Sequestration from immune CD4$^+$ T cells of mycobacteria growing in human macrophages. *Science*, **260**, 984–6.

Payne, N.R. and Horwitz, M.A. (1987). Phagocytosis of *Legionella pneumophila* is mediated by human monocyte complement receptors. *Journal of Experimental Medicine*, **166**, 1377–89.

Perry, A. and Ofek, I. (1984). Inhibition of blood clearance and hepatic tissue binding of *Escherichia coli* by liver lectin-specific sugars and glycoproteins. *Infection and Immunity*, **43** 257–62.

Perussia, B. Dayton, E.T., Lazarus, R., Fanning, V. and Trinchieri, G. (1983). Immune interferon induces the receptor for monomeric IgG1 on human monocytic and myeloid cells. *Journal of Experimental Medicine*, **158**, 1092–113.

Peterson, P.K., Verhoef, J., Schmeling, D. and Quie, P.G. (1977a). Kinetics of phagocytosis and bacterial killing by human polymorphonuclear leukocytes and monocytes. *Journal of Infectious Diseases*, **136**, 502–9.

Peterson, P.K., Verhoef, J., Sabath, L.D. and Quie, P.G. (1977b). Effect of protein A on staphylococcal opsonization. *Infection and Immunity*, **15**, 760–4.

Peterson, P.K., Graziano, E., Suh, H.J., Devalon, M., Peterson, L. and Keane, W.F. (1985). Antimicrobial activities of dialysate-elicited and resident human peritoneal macrophages. *Infection and Immunity*, **49**, 212–8.

Pier, G.B. (1997). Rationale for development of immunotherapies that target mucoid *Pseudomonas aeruginosa* infection in cystic fibrosis patients. *Behring Institute Mitteilungen*, **98**, 350–60.

Portnoy, D.A., Jacks, P.S. and Hinrichs, D.J. (1988). Role of hemolysin for the intracellular growth of *Listeria monocytogenes*. *Journal of Experimental Medicine*, **167**, 1459–71.

Proctor, R.A. (1987). Fibronectin: an enhancer of phagocyte function. *Reviews of Infectious Diseases*, **9** (Supplement 4), S412–9.

Proctor, R.A., Textor, J.A., Vann, J.M. and Mosher, D.F. (1985). Role of fibronectin in human monocyte and macrophage bactericidal activity. *Infection and Immunity*, **47**, 629–37.

Rautemaa, R. *et al.* (1998). Acquired resistance of *Escherichia coli* to complement lysis by binding of glycophosphoinositol-anchored protectin (CD59). *Infection and Immunity*, **66**, 1928–33.

Ravetch, J.V. (1994). Fc receptors: rubor redux. *Cell*, **78**, 553–60.

Ravetch, J.V. (1997). Fc receptors. *Current Opinion in Immunology*, **9**, 121–5.

Rehm, S.R., Gross, G.N. and Pierce, A.K. (1980). Early bacterial clearance from murine lungs. Species-dependent phagocyte response. *Journal of Clinical Investigation*, **66**, 194–9.

Reynolds, H.Y. (1974). Pulmonary host defenses in rabbits after immunization with *Pseudomonas antigens*: the interaction of bacteria, antibodies, macrophages, and lymphocytes. *Journal of Infectious Diseases*, **130** (Supplement), S134–42.

Reynolds, H.Y. and Newball, H.H. (1974). Analysis of proteins and respiratory cells obtained from human lungs by bronchial lavage. *Journal of Laboratory and Clinical Medicine*, **84**, 559–73.

Reynolds, H.Y. and Thompson, R.E. (1973). Pulmonary host defenses. I. Analysis of protein and lipids in bronchial secretions and antibody responses after vaccination with *Pseudomonas aeruginosa*. *Journal of Immunology*, **111**, 358–68.

Reynolds, H.Y., Atkinson, J.P., Newball, H.H. and Frank, M.M. (1975). Receptors for immunoglobulin and complement on human alveolar macrophages. *Journal of Immunology*, **114**, 1813–9.

Richards, C.D. and Gauldie, J. (1985). IgA-mediated phagocytosis by mouse alveolar macrophages. *American Review of Respiratory Diseases*, **132**, 82–5.

Richman-Eisenstat, J. (1996). Cytokine soup: making sense of inflammation in cystic fibrosis. *Pediatric Pulmonology*, **21**, 3–5.

Rinehart, J.J., Sagone, A.L., Balcerzak, S.P., Ackerman, G.A. and LoBuglio, A.F. (1975). Effects of corticosteroid therapy on human monocyte function. *New England Journal of Medicine*, **292**, 236–41.

Rogers, D.E. (1960). Host mechanisms which act to remove bacteria from the blood stream. *Bacteriology Reviews*, **24**, 50–66.

Rook, G.A.W. (1989). Intracellular killing of microorganisms. In Zembala, M. and Asherson, G.L. (ed.), *Human Monocytes*. Academic Press, London.

Rook, G.A., Steele, J., Ainsworth, M. and Champion, B.R. (1986). Activation of macrophages to inhibit proliferation of *Mycobacterium tuberculosis*: comparison of the effects of recombinant γ-interferon on human monocytes and murine peritoneal macrophages. *Immunology*, **59**, 333–8.

Rosen, G.M. *et al.* (1995). Free radicals and phagocytic cells. *FASEB Journal*, **9**, 200–9.

Rosen, H. and Michel, B.R. (1997). Redundant contribution of myeloperoxidase-dependent systems to neutrophil-mediated killing of *Escherichia coli*. *Infection and Immunity*, **65**, 4173–8.

Ross, G.D. and Vetvicka, V. (1993). CR3 (CD11b, CD18): a phagocyte and NK cell membrane receptor with multiple ligand specificities and functions. *Clinical and Experimental Immunology*, **92**, 181–4.

Rouse, B.T. and Horohov, D.W. (1986). Immunosuppression in viral infections. *Reviews of Infectious Diseases*, **8**, 850–73.

Ruckdeschel, K. *et al.* (1997). Interaction of *Yersinia enterocolitica* with macrophages leads to macrophage cell death through apoptosis. *Infection and Immunity*, **65**, 4813–21.

Ruef, C. and Coleman, D.L. (1990). Granulocyte–macrophage colony-stimulating factor: pleiotropic cytokine with potential clinical usefulness. *Reviews of Infectious Diseases*, **12**, 41–62.

Ruiz, P., Gomez, F. and Schreiber, A.D. (1990). Impaired function of macrophage Fcγ receptors in end-stage renal disease. *New England Journal of Medicine*, **322**, 717–22.

Rumelt, S., Metzger, Z., Kariv, N. and Rosenberg, M (1988). Clearance of *Serratia marcescens* from blood in mice: role of hydrophobic versus mannose-sensitive interactions. *Infection and Immunity*, **56**, 1167–70.

Sansonetti, P.J. *et al.* (1986). Multiplication of *Shigella flexneri* within HeLa cells: lysis of the phagocytic vacuole and plasmid-mediated contact hemolysis. *Infection and Immunity*, **51**, 461–9.

Sawyer, J.G., Martin, N.L. and Hancock, R.E. (1988). Interaction of macrophage cationic proteins with the outer membrane of *Pseudomonas aeruginosa*. *Infection and Immunity*, **56**, 693–8.

Schesser, K. *et al.* (1998). The *yopJ* locus is required for *Yersinia*-mediated inhibition of NF-κB activation and cytokine expression: YopJ contains a eukaryotic SH2-like domain that is essential for its repressive activity. *Molecular Microbiology*, **28**, 1067–79.

Schiff, D.E. *et al.* (1997). Phagocytosis of Gram-negative bacteria by a unique CD14-dependent mechanism. *Journal of Leukocyte Biology*, **62**, 786–94.

Schindler, R. *et al.* (1990). Correlations and interactions in the production of interleukin-6 (IL-6), IL-1, and tumor necrosis factor (TNF) in human blood mononuclear cells: IL-6 suppresses IL-1 and TNF. *Blood*, **75**, 40–7.

Schmalstieg, F.C. (1988). Leukocyte adherence defect. *Pediatric Infectious Disease Journal*, **7**, 867–72.

Schorey, J.S., Carroll, M.C. and Brown, E.J. (1997). A macrophage invasion mechanism of pathogenic mycobacteria. *Science*, **277**, 1091–3.

Schurr, E., Skamene, E., Forget, A. and Gros, P. (1989). Linkage analysis of the *Bcg* gene on mouse chromosome 1. Identification of a tightly linked marker. *Journal of Immunology*, **142**, 4507–13.

Schurr, E., Buschman, E., Malo, D., Gros, P. and Skamene, E. (1990). Immunogenetics of mycobacterial infections: mouse–human homologies. *Journal of Infectious Diseases*, **161**, 634–9.

Segal, A.W. and Abo, A. (1993). The biochemical basis of the NADPH oxidase of phagocytes. *Trends in Biochemical Sciences*, **18**, 43–7.

Sengelov, H. (1995). Complement receptors in neutrophils. *Critical Reviews in Immunology*, **15**, 107–31.

Shirai, R. *et al.* (1997). Protective effect of granulocyte colony-stimulating factor (G-CSF) in a granulocytopenic mouse model of *Pseudomonas aeruginosa* lung infection through enhanced phagocytosis and killing by alveolar macrophages through priming tumour necrosis factor-α (TNF-α) production. *Clinical and Experimental Immunology*, **109** 73–9.

Sibille, Y. and Reynolds, H.Y. (1990). Macrophages and polymorphonuclear neutrophils in lung defense and injury. *American Review of Respiratory Diseases*, **141**, 471–501.

Sibley, L.D. and Krahenbuhl, J.L. (1987). *Mycobacterium leprae*-burdened macrophages are refractory to activation by γ interferon. *Infection and Immunity*, **55**, 446–50.

Silverstein, S.C., Greenberg, S., Di Virgilio, F. and Steinberg, T.H. (1989). Phagocytosis. In Paul, W.E. (ed.), *Fundamental Immunology*. Raven Press, New York.

Skamene, E., Gros, P., Forget, A., Kongshavn, P.A.L., St Charles, C. and Taylor, B.A. (1982). Genetic regulation of resistance to intracellular pathogens. *Nature*, **297**, 506–9.

Smith, R.M. and Curnutte, J.T. (1991). Molecular basis of chronic granulomatous disease. *Blood*, **77**, 673–86.

Snyderman, R. and Goetzl, E.J. (1981). Molecular and cellular mechanisms of leukocyte chemotaxis. *Science*, **213**, 830–7.

Spangrude, G.J. *et al.* (1985). Inhibition of lymphocyte and neutrophil chemotaxis by pertussis toxin. *Journal of Immunology*, **135**, 4135–43.

Speert, D.P. (1993). Phagocytosis of *Pseudomonas aeruginosa* by macrophages: receptor–ligand interactions. *Trends in Microbiology*, **1**, 217–21.

Speert, D.P. and Thorson, L. (1991). Suppression by human recombinant γ interferon of *in vitro* macrophage nonopsonic and opsonic phagocytosis and killing. *Infection and Immunity*, **59**, 1893–8.

Speert, D.P. *et al.* (1994). Infection with *Pseudomonas cepacia* in chronic granulomatous disease: role of nonoxidative killing by neutrophils in host defense. *Journal of Infectious Diseases*, **170**, 1524–31.

Spolarics, Z. (1996). Endotoxin stimulates gene expression of ROS-eliminating pathways in rat hepatic endothelial and Kupffer cells. *American Journal of Physiology*, **270**, G660–6.

Stahl, P.D. and Ezekowitz, R.A. (1998). The mannose receptor is a pattern recognition receptor involved in host defense. *Current Opinion in Immunology*, **10**, 50–5.

Steigbigel, R.T., Lambert, L.H., Jr and Remington, J.S. (1974). Phagocytic and bacterial properties of normal human monocytes. *Journal of Clinical Investigation*, **53**, 131–42.

Stiver, H.G., Zachidniak, K. and Speert, D.P. (1988). Inhibition of polymorphonuclear leukocyte chemotaxis by the mucoid exopolysaccharide of *Pseudomonas aeruginosa*. *Clinical and Investigative Medicine*, **11**, 247–52.

Stokes, R.W., Thorson, L.M. and Speert, D.P. (1998). Nonopsonic and opsonic association of *Mycobacterium tuberculosis* with resident alveolar macrophages is inefficient. *Journal of Immunology*, **160**, 5514–21.

Stuehr, D.J. and Marletta, M.A. (1987). Induction of nitrite/nitrate synthesis in murine macrophages by BCG infection, lymphokines, or interferon-γ. *Journal of Immunology*, **139**, 518–25.

Sturgill-Koszycki, S. *et al.* (1994). Lack of acidification in *Mycobacterium* phagosomes produced by exclusion of the vesicular proton-ATPase [published erratum appears in *Science* 1994 Mar 11;263(5152):1359]. *Science*, **263**, 678–81.

Takai, T. *et al.* (1994). FcR γ chain deletion results in pleiotrophic effector cell defects. *Cell*, **76**, 519–29.

Tenner, A.J., Robinson, S.L., Borchelt, J. and Wright, J.R. (1989). Human pulmonary surfactant protein (SP-A), a protein structurally homologous to C1q, can enhance FcR- and CR1-mediated phagocytosis. *Journal of Biological Chemistry*, **264**, 13923–8.

Tenner, A.J., Robinson, S.L. and Ezekowitz, R.A. (1995). Mannose binding protein (MBP) enhances mononuclear phagocyte function via a receptor that contains the 126,000 M(r) component of the C1q receptor. *Immunity*, **3**, 485–93.

Thomas, E.L. and Fishman, M. (1986). Oxidation of chloride and thiocyanate by isolated leukocytes. *Journal of Biological Chemistry*, **261**, 9694–702.

Tilney, L.G. and Portnoy, D.A. (1989). Actin filaments and the growth, movement, and spread of the intracellular bacterial parasite, *Listeria monocytogenes*. *Journal of Cell Biology*, **109**, 1597–608.

Tosi, M.F., Zakem, H. and Berger, M. (1990). Neutrophil elastase cleaves C3bi on opsonized *Pseudomonas* as well as CR1 on neutrophils to create a functionally important opsonin receptor mismatch. *Journal of Clinical Investigation*, **86**, 300–8.

Unkeless, J.C. (1989). Function and heterogeneity of human Fc receptors for immunoglobulin G. *Journal of Clinical Investigation*, **83**, 355–61.

van Dalen, C.J. *et al.* (1997). Thiocyanate and chloride as competing substrates for myeloperoxidase. *Biochemical Journal*, **327**, 487–92.

van der Laan, L.J. *et al.* (1999). Regulation and functional involvement of macrophage scavenger receptor MARCO in clearance of bacteria *in vivo*. *Journal of Immunology*, **162**, 939–47.

van der Vliet, A. *et al.* (1997). Formation of reactive nitrogen species during peroxidase-catalyzed oxidation of nitrite. A potential additional mechanism of nitric oxide-dependent toxicity. *Journal of Biological Chemistry*, **272**, 7617–25.

Verbrugh, H.A., Hoidal, J.R., Nguyen, B.T., Verhoef, J., Quie, P.G. and Peterson, P.K. (1982). Human alveolar macrophage cytophilic immunoglobulin G-mediated phagocytosis of protein A-positive staphylococci. *Journal of Clinical Investigation*, **69**, 63–74.

Verbrugh, H.A., Keane, W.F., Hoidal, J.R., Freiburg, M.R., Elliott, G.R. and Peterson, P.K. (1983). Peritoneal macrophages and opsonins: antibacterial defense in patients undergoing chronic peritoneal dialysis. *Journal of Infectious Diseases*, **147**, 1018–29.

Vidal, S., Gros, P. and Skamene, E. (1995a). Natural resistance to infection with intracellular parasites: molecular genetics identifies Nramp1 as the Bcg/Ity/Lsh locus. *Journal of Leukocyte Biology*, **58**, 382–90.

Vidal, S. *et al.* (1995b). The Ity/Lsh/Bcg locus: natural resistance to infection with intracellular parasites is abrogated by disruption of the *Nramp1* gene. *Journal of Experimental Medicine*, **182**, 655–66.

Vitkovic, L., Stover, E. and Koslow, S.H. (1995). Animal models recapitulate aspects of HIV/CNS disease. *AIDS Research and Human Retroviruses*, **11**, 753–9.

Wallis, R. and Cheng, J.Y. (1999). Molecular defects in variant forms of mannose-binding protein associated with immunodeficiency. *Journal of Immunology*, **163**, 4953–9.

Wardle, E.N. (1987). Kupffer cells and their function. *Liver*, **7**, 63–75.

Warren, M.K. and Vogel, S.N. (1985). Opposing effects of glucocorticoids on interferon-γ-induced murine macrophage Fc receptor and Ia antigen expression. *Journal of Immunology*, **134**, 2462–9.

Watson, S., Bullock, W., Nelson, K., Schauf, V., Gelber, R. and Jacobson, R. (1984). Interleukin 1 production by peripheral blood mononuclear cells from leprosy patients. *Infection and Immunity*, **45**, 787–9.

Weikert, L.F. *et al.* (1997). SP-A enhances uptake of bacillus Calmette–Guerin by macrophages through a specific SP-A receptor. *American Journal of Physiology*, **272**, L989–95.

Weinberg, J.B. *et al.* (1995). Human mononuclear phagocyte inducible nitric oxide synthase (iNOS): analysis of iNOS mRNA, iNOS protein, biopterin, and nitric oxide production by blood monocytes and peritoneal macrophages. *Blood*, **86**, 1184–95.

Weiss, A.A. and Hewlett, E.L. (1986). Virulence factors of *Bordetella pertussis*. *Annual Review of Microbiology*, **40**, 661–86.

Wheeler, P.R. and Gregory, D. (1980). Superoxide dismutase, peroxidatic activity and catalase in *Mycobacterium leprae* purified from armadillo liver. *Journal of General Microbiology*, **121**, 457–64.

Whitnack, E., Bisno, A.L. and Beachey, E.H. (1981). Hyaluronate capsule prevents attachment of group A streptococci to mouse peritoneal macrophages. *Infection and Immunity*, **31**, 985–91.

Wilkinson, B.J., Peterson, P.K. and Quie, P.G. (1979). Cryptic peptidoglycan and the antiphagocytic effect of the *Staphylococcus aureus* capsule: model for the antiphagocytic effect of bacterial cell surface polymers. *Infection and Immunity*, **23**, 502–8.

Williams, A.E. and Blakemore, W.F. (1990). Pathogenesis of meningitis caused by *Streptococcus suis* type 2. *Journal of Infectious Diseases*, **162**, 474–81.

Wilson, C.B., Tsai, V. and Remington, J.S. (1980). Failure to trigger the oxidative metabolic burst by normal macrophages: possible mechanism for survival of intracellular pathogens. *Journal of Experimental Medicine*, **151**, 328–46.

Wright, S.D. and Griffin, F.M., Jr (1985). Activation of phagocytic cells' C3 receptors for phagocytosis. *Journal of Leukocyte Biology*, **38**, 327–39.

Wright, S.D. and Silverstein, S.C. (1983). Receptors for C3b and C3bi promote phagocytosis but not the release of toxic oxygen from human phagocytes. *Journal of Experimental Medicine*, **158**, 2016–23.

Wright, S.D., Craigmyle, L.S. and Silverstein, S.C. (1983). Fibronectin and serum amyloid P component stimulate C3b- and C3bi-mediated phagocytosis in cultured human monocytes. *Journal of Experimental Medicine*, **158**, 1338–43.

Wright, S.D., Detmers, P.A., Jong, M.T.C. and Meyer, C. (1986). Interferon-γ depresses binding of ligand by C3b and C3bi receptors on cultured human monocytes, an effect reversed by fibronectin. *Journal of Experimental Medicine*, **163**, 1245–59.

Wright, S.D., Ramos, R.A., Tobias, P.S., Ulevitch, R.J. and Mathison, J.C. (1990). CD14, a receptor for complexes of lipopolysaccharide (LPS) and LPS binding protein. *Science*, **249**, 1431–3.

Wyrick, P.B. and Brownridge, E.A.(1978). Growth of *Chlamydia psittaci* in macrophages. *Infection and Immunity*, **19**, 1054–60.

6 *Macrophages in parasitic infection*

B. Vray

1 Introduction

1.1 Macrophages as host cells of parasitic microorganisms

Due to their widespread distribution in vertebrate host tissues and cavities, macrophages are among the first cells to encounter and then to combat invading microorganisms. However, in their non-activated (or resting state) and also in their primed state, they can act as 'host cells' of these microorganisms. Various ligand–receptor systems are involved in recognition/adhesion systems. For instance, fibronectin (FN) is a plasmatic dimeric multifunctional glycoprotein binding many microorganisms to their host cells. Macrophages and some parasites express both receptors for carbohydrate residues and glycoconjugates which serve as ligands so that double receptor–ligand systems modulate parasite–macrophage binding as shown by various *in vitro* experiments using lectins or sugars. In addition, opsonins [complement (C) or specific antibodies] also contribute to recognition/adhesion systems. As a result, protozoan parasites can invade macrophages through various parasite and macrophage molecules.

1.2 Macrophages as effector cells

Upon appropriate activation, macrophages become 'effector cells'. In addition to various stimuli [i.e. bacterial components (lipopolysaccharide or LPS)], and non specific activators (phorbol myristate acetate), phagocytosis of microorganisms can activate macrophages. Furthermore, dendritic cells (DCs) also interact with microorganisms and they induce the release of interferon-γ (IFN-γ) by natural killer (NK) cells so that macrophages are activated further. These events constitute the starting point of innate immunity. Later on, 'classically' or 'alternatively' activated macrophages are induced by Th1 or Th2 stimulation, respectively (Munder *et al.*, 1999; Goerdt *et al.*, 1999; Mills, Kincaid *et al.*, 2000). As a result, at least two potent transient processes producing reactive oxygen intermediates (ROIs) and reactive nitrogen intermediates (RNIs) are triggered (Bogdan *et al.*, 2000a). The respiratory burst leads to synthesis of ROIs such as superoxides produced via activation of the membrane NADPH oxidase, hydrogen peroxide via a superoxide dismutase, and hydroxyl radicals via the Haber–Weiss reaction (Gutteridge *et al.*, 1998).

RNI-generating processes involve CD40 which is a cell surface receptor expressed by various cells including macrophages. Interaction of CD40 with its CD40 ligand (CD40L or CD154) triggers a pleiotropic pathway involved in both humoral and cellular immunity. By exerting potent biological activities, this RNI-dependent pathway plays a major role in anti-infective host defense, resulting in the secretion of multiple cytokines such as interleukin (IL)-1, IL-6, IL-8, IL-10, IL-12, IFN-γ and tumor necrosis factor-α (TNF-α) by immunocompetent cells. In particular, IL-12 (Trinchieri and Scott, 1999) is produced by some macrophages activated through CD40 (Kato *et al.*, 1997) and has emerged as a potent immunoregulatory cytokine involved in the control of infections (Grewal and Flavell, 1998). IL-12 triggers NK cells and T cells to produce IFN-γ. In addition, IFN-γ synthesis and secretion by macrophages themselves is also reported (Puddu *et al.*, 1997). IFN-γ is a key mediator in the control of parasitic infections because it stimulates the synthesis of inducible nitric oxide synthase (iNOS or NOS2) and the release of nitric oxide (NO) from murine and human macrophages (Liew, 1993). However, IFN-γ does not act on its own since IFN-γ-induced TNF-α is a prerequisite for *in vitro* production of NO by murine macrophages (Frankova and Zidek, 1998). Finally, the sequence of macrophage activation includes CD40–CD40L interaction, IL-12, IFN-γ and TNF-α release, and NO production. NO is an important mediator in various physiological processes (vasodilatation, smooth muscle regulation, neurotransmission and apoptosis) and in antiparasitic immune responses where it plays the role of modulator in both innate and adaptative immunity (Bogdan *et al.*, 2000a,b). It is involved in several inflammatory diseases and is cytotoxic or cytostatic in a wide range of infections (Lowenstein *et al.*, 1994). NO is synthesized from the oxidation of the terminal guanido-nitrogen atom of L-arginine by NADPH-dependent NOS. Three isoforms of NOS have been identified. They differ in their tissue distributions and regulation. Neuronal NOS (nNOS or NOS1) and endothelial NOS (eNOS or NOS3) types are constitutively present in neurons and endothelial cells, respectively, and are calcium dependent (MacMicking *et al.*, 1997). The third NOS isoform (iNOS or NOS2) is synthesized in response to specific signals by cells such as hepatocytes, fibroblasts and macrophages and is calcium independent (Nathan and Xie, 1994). Its synthesis is induced mainly by IFN-γ and leads to the rapid production of large amounts of NO that protect the host organism against many infections. NO-mediated toxicity for intracellular parasites depends on its rapid diffusion into infected cells and it acts by inhibiting some of their key enzymes. Oxidoreductases (mitochondrial electron transport system), aconitase (a citric acid cycle enzyme) and enzymes essential for DNA synthesis contain catalytically active Fe–S groups which are inactivated by NO as a result of formation of nitrosyl–iron–sulfur complexes (James, 1995). On the other hand, NO reacts with ROIs to form peroxynitrites and it circulates in plasma mainly as *S*-nitroso-albumin which is responsible for the long-distance effects of NO such as apoptosis and antiparasite control (Gobert *et al.*, 1998).

Other macrophage-activating pathways currently are under investigation. Members of the chemokine family [i.e. macrophage inflammatory protein 1 (MIP-1) and monocyte chemoattractant protein 1 (MCP-1)] are closely related to cytokines. These small polypeptides are synthesized by various cells (endothelial cells, keratinocytes and fibroblasts), in particular NK cells and macrophages. In response to infection, immunocompetent cells are recruited, attracted and activated in the inflammation site via the chemokine pathway. Some recent reports underline the importance of chemokines in macrophage activation and infection control but their place in the cascade of macrophage activation is still unclear (Moll, 1997; Villalta *et al.*, 1998a; Aliberti *et al.*, 1999a).

On the whole, when they are suitably activated, macrophages participate as effector cells in infection control.

1.3 Macrophages as antigen-presenting cells

Macrophages are also 'antigen-presenting cells' (APCs). Indeed, macrophages constitutively express major histocompatibility complex (MHC) class I. Some of them also express MHC class II molecules constitutively (Küpffer cells) and, upon activation, they all express MHC class II, adhesion and co-stimulatory molecules. They process endogenous and exogenous proteins and they display the derived peptides in association with MHC class I or II molecules at their membrane, a subcellular process which results in T-lymphocyte reactivation of primed CD8 and CD4 T lymphocytes, respectively. Indeed, they cannot prime naive T lymphocytes. This is the cardinal function of DCs. Development of a specific immune response first depends on interactions between microorganisms and DCs, which act as sentinels of the immune system (Fearon and Locksley, 1996; Banchereau and Steinman, 1998; Bell *et al.*, 1999; Rescigno *et al.*, 1999; Sousa *et al.*, 1999a; Banchereau *et al.*, 2000). Residing in most tissues and organs, immature DCs (i.e. Langerhans cells in the epidermis) first interact with microorganisms and actively capture and process microorganisms and/or microorganism-derived antigenic molecules. Then, upon activation by microbial components (i.e. LPS) or cytokines [IL-1 β, granulocyte–macrophage colony-stimulating factor (GM-CSF), TNF-α], DCs migrate to lymph nodes draining the site of invasion and to the spleen. During their migration, they undergo a process of maturation, losing their capacity to capture and process antigens, but increasing their membrane expression of MHC class II, co-stimulatory (CD40, B7.1 or CD80, B7.2 or CD86) and adhesion molecules (ICAM-1 or CD54). They also upregulate their production of cytokines (IL-6, IL-10 and IL-12). In particular, IL-12 induces the production of IFN-γ from NK cells and initiates macrophage activation and innate immunity. Finally, DCs differentiate into fully potent APCs. In lymphoid organs, they prime rare naive T cells expressing the relevant T-cell receptors (TCRs) (Lanzavecchia and Sallusto, 2000), induce their proliferation and produce IL-12 which activates Th1 cells and IFN-γ production, NK cells and macrophages, a sequential process underlying the so-called adaptive immune response. On the other hand, IL-4 and IL-10 are thought to drive Th2 cells. In addition to signal 1 (TCR triggering) and signal 2 (co-stimulation), the existence of a third signal (polarization) involving IL-12 and CD8 α+ DCs has been proposed (Ley *et al.*, 1990; Hall and Joiner, 1993; Kalinski *et al.*, 1999; Sousa *et al.*, 1999a). The Th1/Th2 polarization of the immune response is thought to be important in the control of intracellular parasites (Th1 response), extracellular parasites (Th0 response) or metazoan parasites (Th2 response). In fact, in many cases, the immune response is not totally dominated by one of these Th1- or Th2-mediated responses (Allen and Maizels, 1997; Romagnani, 1997).

Differentiation and proliferation of CD4+ and CD8+ T lymphocytes are major steps in eliciting an immune adaptive response capable of interfering with the life cycle of the intracellular microorganisms and of destroying infected cells. Antigen-specific T lymphocytes do not interact with infected but non-activated macrophages. However, IFN-γ-primed macrophages enhance their expression of MHC class II molecules and interact with T cells, inducing their mutual activation and the production of IFN-γ and TNF-α, so that most often macrophages are finally fully activated and armed to kill extra- and intracellular parasites (Overath and Aebischer, 1999). On the other hand, B lymphocytes are stimulated to produce specific antibodies which will act as opsonins and favor antibody-dependent phagocytosis together with neutralization of extracellular parasites.

On the whole, DCs and macrophages are involved in both innate and adaptive immune responses and in particular macrophages constitute a basic element of these immune responses. They also represent an important line of defense against parasites despite the fact that they can act as host cells in many cases. Protozoan parasites with intramacrophage multiplication (i.e. *Trypanosoma cruzi*, *Leishmania* spp. and *Toxoplasma gondii*) (Bogdan and Rollinghoff, 1999), those with extracellular multiplication (i.e. *Trypanosoma brucei*) and parasitic metazoan helminths (i.e. *Schistosoma mansoni*) interact with macrophages in various ways. Some examples of these complex interactions will be discussed in this chapter.

2 *Trypanosoma cruzi*

Trypanosoma cruzi is an obligate intracellular protozoan parasite. It belongs to the family Trypanosomatidae, order Kinetoplastida, phylum Sarcomastigophora. It is the etiological agent of Chagas'disease, a major public health problem in South and Central America (Schofield and Dias, 1999). This hemoflagellate parasite infects humans as well as domestic and wild mammals (Tanowitz *et al.*, 1992). Transmission occurs after the bite of an infected blood-sucking bug (family Reduvidae) which harbors epimastigote forms in its gut and which releases metacyclic (infective) trypomastigotes in its feces or urine. Infective trypomastigotes enter mammalian hosts through skin abrasion or locally disrupted mucosal epithelia. In the vertebrate host, the parasite exists in two forms. The trypomastigote is the circulating blood form that infects several cells (macrophages, fibroblasts, nerve cells and muscle cells). It also infects human DCs, at least *in vitro* (Van Overtvelt *et al.*, 1999). The amastigotes replicate in the host cell cytosol (Burleigh and Andrews, 1998). Cell invasion and intracellular replication are essential for the initiation of the disease and the continuation of the parasite life cycle. In human infection, most patients survive the initial acute phase, but some develop the chronic manifestations of the disease characterized by long-lasting inflammatory lesions within smooth muscle and heart, and immune disorders years after the initial infection (Tarleton and Zhang, 1999). Experimental infection of mice mimics the human disease. It displays an acute phase with high parasitemia and mortality in susceptible mice, followed by a chronic phase during which parasites become undetectable in peripheral blood while persisting in tissues and inducing pathological manifestations (DosReis, 1997).

2.1 Recognition/adhesion systems

2.1.1 Fibronectin and laminin

By bridging FN receptors (FNRs) present on both *T.cruzi* and macrophage plasmic membranes, FN participates in *T.cruzi*–macrophage adhesion and enhances the percentage of infected murine macrophages and human monocytes. FNR recognizes a peptidic sequence (RGD or Arg–Gly–Asp) present on each FN monomer (Wirth and Kierszenbaum, 1984; Ouaissi *et al.*, 1986; Noisin and Villalta, 1989). At the begining of experimental *T.cruzi* infection in mice (acute phase), the plasma level of FN first increases. Four weeks after inoculation (chronic phase), the level of circulating FN decreases while a significant increase in RGD-reactive antibodies is detected, indicating that both FN and anti-FN antibodies are involved in the course of *T.cruzi* infection in mice (Truyens *et al.*, 1995) (Table 6.1).

Laminin-like protein is present on *T.cruzi* trypomastigote membranes and is involved in attachment to macrophages (Bretana *et al.*, 1986; Hynes, 1992). In addition, a glycoprotein belonging to the gp85 family is expressed on the membrane of *T.cruzi* trypomastigotes and binds *in vitro* to laminin present on the macrophage membrane, but not to FN (Giordano *et al.*, 1999).

2.1.2 Carbohydrate residues

Galactosyl-α-(1–3)-galactose epitopes are present on trypomastigotes of pathogenic strains of *T.cruzi* and interact with the D-galactose/*N*-acetyl-galactosamine membrane receptor of mouse peritoneal macrophages; the addition of galactose or *N*-acetyl-D-galac-

Table 6.1 Interactions between macrophages and intracellular parasitic protozoa

	Trypanosoma cruzi	*Leishmania* spp.	*Toxoplasma gondii*
Host cells	Macrophages, dendritic cells, muscle cells, nerve cells, fibroblasts (Tardieux *et al.*, 1992; Burleigh and Andrews, 1998; Van Overtvelt *et al.*, 1999)	Monocytes, macrophages, dendritic cells (Handman, 1999) and other cells (Rittig and Bogdan, 2000)	Phagocytic and non-phagocytic nucleated cells (Joiner and Dubremetz, 1993; Beaman *et al.*, 1994; Hunter and Remington, 1994; Channon *et al.*, 2000)
Recognition/ adhesion systems	**Fibronectin** (Wirth and Kierszenbaum, 1984; Ouaissi *et al.*, 1986; Noisin and Villalta, 1989; Truyens *et al.*, 1995; **Laminin** (Bretana, *et al.*, 1986; Giordano *et al.*, 1999) **Carbohydrate residues** (Araujo-Jorge and De Souza, 1988; Avila *et al.*, 1989; Bretana *et al.*, 1992; Bonay and Fresno, 1995) ***Trans*-sialidases** (Schenkman *et al.*, 1994; Pereira *et al.*, 1996; Villalta *et al.*, 1998a; Araujo-Jorge *et al.*, 1993; Krautz *et al.*, 2000) **Antibody** (Lages-Silva *et al.*, 1987; Araujo-Jorge, 1989; Hall and Joiner, 1993; Tomlinson *et al.*, 1994; Norris, 1998) **Complement** (Araujo-Jorge,	**Fibronectin** (Vannier-Santos *et al.*, 1992; **LPG, gp63** (Schneider *et al.*, 1990; Turco and Descoteaux, 1992; Joshi *et al.*, 1998; Handman, 1999) **Carbohydrate residues** (Avila *et al.*, 1989; Palatnik *et al.*, 1990; Bretana *et al.*, 1992) **Heparin-binding protein** (Butcher *et al.*, 1992; Love *et al.*, 1993) **CR1, CR3** (Puentes *et al.*, 1988; Da Silva *et al.*, 1989; Talamas-Rohana *et al.*, 1990; Bogdan and Rollinghoff, 1998)	**Laminin** (Furtado *et al.*, 1992) **SAG-1, SAG-2 and SAG-3** (Mineo *et al.*, 1993; Cesbron-Delauw *et al.*, 1994; Channon and Kasper, 1996; Grimwood and Smith, 1996; Grimwood *et al.*, 1996) **Lectins** (Ortega-Barria and Boothroyd, 1999) **Microneme-derived proteins** (Carruthers and Sibley, 1997)
Host cell invasion	**Phagocytosis** (Araujo-Jorge, 1989) **Induced phagocytosis** (Burleigh and Andrews, 1998)	**Phagocytosis** (Strauss *et al.*, 1993) **Coiling phagocytosis** (Rittig *et al.*, 1998)	**Active process** (Morisaki *et al.*, 1995; Dobrowolski *et al.*, 1997)
Parasitophorous vacuole	Parasites stay a short time in the PV and leave it to invade and to multiply into the cytosol (Andrews and Whitlow, 1989; Ley *et al.*, 1990; Burleigh and Andrews, 1998)	Parasites survive and multiply in the PV despite the lysosome–phagosome fusion (Talamas-Rohana *et al.*, 1990; Antoine *et al.*, 1998; Puentes *et al.*, 1988; Alexander *et al.*, 1999)	Parasites survive and multiply in the PV after modification of the membrane components leading to the inhibition of the lysosome–phagosome fusion (Mordue and Sibley, 1997)

tosamine to the culture medium inhibits the uptake of this parasite by macrophages. Binding to trypomastigotes of both anti-galactose antibodies and the lectin extracted from *Bandeiraea simplicifolia* is also inhibited in the presence of galactose (Araujo-Jorge and De Souza, 1988; Araujo-Jorge, 1989; Avila *et al.*, 1989; Bretana, 1992).

On the other hand, a family of carbohydrate-binding proteins has been identified on try-pomastigote and epimastigote forms of *T.cruzi*. These proteins are specific for mannose and galactose residues and bind to human and murine macrophages, suggesting their possible involvement in the recognition/adhesion systems between the parasite and its target cell (Bonay and Fresno, 1995).

2.1.3 *Trans*-sialidases

Trypanosoma cruzi trypomastigotes synthesize *trans*-sialidases and acquire sialic acid from their environment (Schenkman *et al.*, 1994). The *T.cruzi* membrane is covered mainly by glycosylinositolphospholipids (GIPLs) and glycosylphosphatidylinositol (GPI)-anchored mucin-like molecules (Ferguson, 1999) which are sialic acid acceptors (Previato *et al.*, 1995). Murine macrophages are probably not invaded through a *trans*-sialidase-dependent mechanism. The sialylation of the parasites impairs their invading ability. This occurs probably by masking parasite determinants interacting with macrophage receptors such as β-galactosyl residues (Araujo-Jorge, 1989; Schenkman *et al.*, 1994). In contrast, gp83 *trans*-sialidase facilitates parasite invasion of human monocyte-derived macrophages by inducing tyrosine phosphorylation of mitogen-activated protein (MAP) kinase (Villalta *et al.*, 1998a). Furthermore, parasite *trans*-sialidase is involved in *T.cruzi* invasion of non-phagocytic cells. Indeed, Chinese hamster ovary cells deficient in sialic acid are poorly infected, while re-sialylation of these cells restores *T.cruzi* adhesion and invasion (Ming *et al.*, 1993). In addition, 20–30 per cent of trypo-mastigotes express *trans*-sialidase activity and are infectious in comparison with the majority of parasites that do not express this enzyme (Pereira *et al.*, 1996). Mice highly susceptible to *T.cruzi* infection are protected when they are immunized previously with a *trans*-sialidase gene delivered as naked DNA or with recombinant *trans*-sialidase (Costa *et al.*, 1999).

2.1.4 Antibody- and complement-mediated opsonization

Internalization of *T.cruzi* trypomastigotes by mouse peritoneal macrophages occurs via opsonic antibodies (Lages-Silva *et al.*, 1987). Indeed, in the course of *T.cruzi* murine infection, a polyisotypic hypergammaglobulinemia and a stable polyisotypic parasite-specific response appear (el Bouhdidi *et al.*, 1994), and specific anti-*T.cruzi* antibodies have a protective effect, as shown by injecting immune serum prepared from immunized mice into *T.cruzi*-infected mice (Kierszenbaum and Howard, 1976). This antibody-mediated immune clearance depends on three mechanisms: (1) FcR-mediated macrophage phagocytosis; (2) antibody-dependent cell cytotoxicity (ADCC); and (3) appearance of antibodies that render the trypomastigotes sensitive to lysis through the alternative complement pathway (Krautz *et al.*, 2000). In addition, repeated injections of an anti-FcγRII, FcγRIII-reactive monoclonal antibody to *T.cruzi*-infected mice, in the early phase of infection, reduce both parasitemia and mortality of treated mice. Though the mechanism(s) of such an effect is still unclear, it can be hypothesized that soluble immune complexes could bridge FcγRs present on both macrophages and the parasite itself, and thus favor adhesion and internalization (Rodriguez *et al.*, 1991). Such a ligation would be inhibited by specific anti-FcγR antibodies (Araujo-Jorge *et al.*, 1993).

Trypanosoma cruzi metacyclic and blood circulating trypomastigotes, but not epimastigotes (the vector form), activate the alternative pathway of complement but they are not lysed. Tissue culture-derived trypomastigotes resist complement-mediated lysis at least partially through parasite membrane-bound sialic acid (Tomlinson *et al.*, 1994). In addition, the parasite expresses a complement regulatory protein which binds human complement C3b and C4b and inhibits C3 convertase formation. This contributes to the resistance of trypomastigotes not only to complement-mediated lysis but also to complement-mediated phagocytosis (Araujo-Jorge, 1989; Hall and Joiner, 1993; Norris, 1996).

2.2 Macrophage invasion

When interacting with macrophages, *T.cruzi* stimulates the phosphorylation of several tyrosine residues and this signal could be involved in the survival and multiplication as well as the pathogenicity of the parasite. Indeed, tyrosine phosphorylation plays a major role in macrophage functions and is catalyzed by protein tyrosine kinases (Ruta *et al.*, 1996). Human macrophages treated with recombinant gp83 *trans*-sialidase are heavily infected by *T.cruzi* trypomastigotes and this treatment induces tyrosine phosphorylation of several macrophage proteins. The inhibitor of MAP kinase phosphorylation, PD 98059, or genistein (a tyrosine kinase inhibitor) inhibits this enhancement (Villalta *et al.*, 1998a). In short, parasites or some of their components may modulate tyrosine phosphorylation to facilitate entering and surviving in the macrophages and/or may also impair cytotoxic mechanisms so that this pathway may be a part of a parasite escape strategy.

Trypanosoma cruzi trypomastigotes are taken up by macrophages and engulfed in a phagosome, probably by the phagocytic process known as the 'zippering mechanism' (Griffin *et al.*, 1975). Afterwards, parasite-containing phagosomes fuse with lysosomes to form a phagolysosome or parasitophorous vacuole (PV). Another type of phagocytosis, called 'coiling phagocytosis' (see Section 3.2), is very rare with *T.cruzi* trypomastigotes (Rittig *et al.*, 1998b). In a third process of engulfment, *T.cruzi* invades non-'professional' phagocytic cells. In this case, an 'induced phagocytosis' has been described for fibroblasts, epithelial cells and myoblasts. It involves the recruitment of host cell lysosomes which fuse with the plasma membrane at the site of parasite entry and contribute to the formation of the PV (Tardieux *et al.*, 1992; Burleigh and Andrews, 1998). The mobilization of Ca^{2+} from intracellular stores and the activity of an oligopeptidase (a *T.cruzi* serine peptidase) have been described recently for non-phagocytic cells but not for macrophages (Caler *et al.*, 2000). The invasion of non-phagocytic cells also depends on the activation of bradykinin β_2 receptors and the kinin-releasing activity of cruzipain (Scharfstein *et al.*, 2000).

Transforming growth factor-β (TGF-β) is a multipotent homodimeric protein (25 kDa) produced by various cells (T and B cells, NK cells) including macrophages. Host cell invasion by *T.cruzi* also depends on the activation of the TGF-β signaling pathway. Epithelial cells lacking TGF-βR-I or R-II allowed the attachment but not the penetration of *T.cruzi* trypomastigotes. On the other hand, priming of TGF-βR-positive target cells with recombinant TGF-β drastically enhanced the infection by *T.cruzi* (Ming *et al.*, 1995). A similar involvement of TGF-β could exist for macrophage invasion (see Section 2.5) (Reed, 1999).

2.3 Escape from the parasitophorous vacuole

In the PV, trypomastigotes differentiate into amastigotes. The internal face of the PV is covered with sialylated lysosomal glycoproteins that probably have a protecting effect against lysosomal enzymes and are potential targets for parasite *trans*-sialidases (Hall and Joiner, 1993). Parasites release neuraminidase and hemolysin which are activated at the acidic pH of the vacuolar medium. The de-sialylation of lysosomal membrane glyco-proteins by the parasites and the rupture of the PV membrane by a pore-forming protein (Tc-tox) facilitate parasite invasion of host cell cytoplasm (Andrews and Whitlow, 1989; Ley *et al.*, 1990). In the cytosol, amastigotes multiply in a safe shelter and, a few days later, they differentiate into trypomastigotes. This transformation depends on proteasomes found in *T.cruzi* as shown by inhibition of proteasome function with lactacystin (Gonzalez *et al.*, 1996). In addition, parasite cysteine proteases are involved in virulence, immune modulation and parasite differentiation (Mottram *et al.*, 1998). Indeed, their inhibition with fluoro-methyl ketone-derivatized inhibitors abruptly stops the transformation of trypomastigote to amastigote, and also from amastigote to trypomastigote in infected macrophages, indicating that these enzymes may also play a role in intracellular protein degradation and in remodeling of the parasites during transformation between stages (Harth *et al.*, 1993). Trypomastigotes are finally released in the bloodstream, probably through GIPL-parasite-induced apoptosis (Freire-de-Lima *et al.*, 1998).

2.4 Mechanisms of infection control

Trypanosoma cruzi does not trigger the respiratory burst in mouse peritoneal macrophages (McCabe and Mullins, 1990). It also fails to induce a chemiluminescent signal in a macrophage hybridoma cell line, despite various types of opsonization and IFN-γ exposure of macrophages (Vray *et al.*, 1991). This suggests that the parasite bypasses activation of the membrane NADPH oxydase by an as yet unknown mechanism.

Supernatants of murine spleen cells stimulated by 3T3 fibroblasts transfected with CD40L prevent the infection of mouse peritoneal macrophages by *T.cruzi*. This phenomenon depends on *de novo* production of NO as it is prevented by the addition of *N*-nitro-L-arginine methyl ester (NAME), a NOS2 inhibitor, and requires IL-12-mediated IFN-γ and TNF-α synthesis. A single intravenous injection of 3T3-CD40L-fibroblasts also protects mice against *T.cruzi* infection (Chaussabel *et al.*, 1999). In line with this, it has been shown that endogenous and exogenous IL-12 mediate resistance to *T.cruzi* infection in mice in association with IFN-γ and TNF-α (Aliberti *et al.*, 1996). Interestingly, *in vitro*, the platelet-activating factor (PAF) induces NOS2 and NO production by macrophages, allowing the control of infection. This control was inhibited by WEB 2170, an antagonist of the PAF, and by *N*-monomethyl-L-arginine (NMMA), a competitive inhibitor of NOS2 (Aliberti *et al.*, 1999b). *Trypanosoma cruzi* infection as well as a GPI-anchored mucin (Ag C10) purified from *T. cruzi* membrane inhibit IL-12 and TNF-α (but not IL-1 β) production by LPS-stimulated human monocytes and a J774 macrophage cell line (de Diego *et al.*, 1997). Surprisingly, live *T.cruzi*, UV- or γ-irradiated trypanomastigotes, but not heat-killed parasites or lysates, induce IL-12 production by spleen cells and bone marrow-derived macrophages (Frosch *et al.*, 1996).

The involvement of endogenous as well as exogenous IFN-γ in the control of *T.cruzi* infection is well documented (Reed, 1988; Torrico *et al.*, 1991). Furthermore, mice deficient in IFN-γR or NOS2 are extremely susceptible to *T.cruzi* infection (Holscher *et al.*, 1998). However, IFN-γ priming needs to be followed by TNF-α triggering. Large amounts of TNF-α are produced during the acute phase of infection (Tarleton, 1988) and this cytokine is known to potentiate the IFN-γ-mediated production of NO and thus has a central role in the control of infection (Silva *et al.*, 1995; Lima *et al.*, 1997). As compared with IFN-γ-primed mature murine macrophages, IFN-γ-primed immature murine macrophages are more susceptible to *T.cruzi* infection because of their lower production of TNF-α and NO (Plasman *et al.*, 1994).

NO-mediated control of *T.cruzi* infection has been studied extensively (Munoz-Fernandez *et al.*, 1992a). It is dependent on L-arginine supply (Norris *et al.*, 1995). It is inhibitable by competitive inhibitors of NOS2 such as NMMA or NAME. Addition of ROI inhibitors (superoxide dismutase and/or catalase) has no effect either on infection or on NO release by IFN-γ-pre-activated and infected mouse peritoneal macrophages (Metz *et al.*, 1993). *In vitro*, CD4 clones of the Th1 type generated from immunized mice effectively activate macrophages to kill intracellular *T.cruzi* amastigotes, while CD4 Th2-like clones do not. The protective activity of these Th1 cells is abolished in the presence of NOS2 inhibitors or anti-IFN-γ neutralizing antibodies (Rodrigues *et al.*, 2000). In accordance with this, in CD4+ T cells from infected mice, the onset of activation-induced cell death decreases IFN-γ production and favors parasite replication in murine macrophages (Nunes *et al.*, 1998).

When *T. cruzi* trypomastigotes are added to IFN-γ-activated macrophages, they become spherical and the macrophages are only weakly infected, suggesting that NO released in the cell vicinity is responsible for morphological alterations and extracellular killing of trypomastigotes (B. Vray, unpublished data).

Peritoneal or spleen macrophages harvested from mice in the acute phase of *T.cruzi* infection release large amounts of NO in the absence of any further stimuli and accumulate high levels of iNOS mRNA. Susceptibility of mice to *T.cruzi* infection is increased by *in vivo* administration of NMMA, demonstrating the protective role of NO released by activated macrophages (Vespa *et al.*, 1994; Petray *et al.*, 1995). Interestingly, *T.cruzi* on its own up-regulates the NO production of activated macrophages (Metz *et al.*, 1993). This is probably related to a parasite-released molecule (Tc52) which is able to synergize with IFN-γ to stimulate IL-12 and NOS2 gene expression together with NO production by macrophages (Fernandez-Gomez *et al.*, 1998). The overproduction of NO observed *in vitro* as well as *in vivo* could be responsible, at least partially, for the immunosuppression observed during the acute phase of infection (Abrahamsohn and Coffman, 1995; Fernandez-Gomez *et al.*, 1998). Indeed, suppressor macrophages have been identified previously (Cerrone *et al.*, 1992) and their anti-proliferative effect on T cells has been attributed to their NO production (Denham and Rowland, 1992; Munoz-Fernandez *et al.*, 1992b; Corradin *et al.*, 1993; Plasman *et al.*, 1994; Petray *et al.*, 1995).

Among other cells (hepatocytes and fibroblasts), macrophages produce α_2-macroglobulin (α_2-M), a high-affinity, non-specific proteinase inhibitor which bind to all four classes of proteinases. It is found abundantly in plasma and interstitial fluids. Concentrations of α_2-M and proteinase– α_2-M complexes are most elevated in patients with inflammatory diseases and in chagasic patients. *In vitro*, treatment of murine macrophages with α_2-M increases uptake and killing of trypomastigotes. In addition, an α_2-M receptor, expressed by the parasite, binds proteinase-complexed α_2-M (Coutinho *et al.*, 1998). *In vivo*, high levels of α_2-M correlate with the resistance of BALB/c mice to acute infection (Araujo-

Jorges *et al.*, 1990, 1992; Plasman *et al.*, 1994). This protective effect is probably linked to the production of NO by α_2-M-treated macrophages (Lysiak *et al.*, 1995).

A new activation mechanism is related to cysteine–cysteine chemokines (MIP-1 α and MIP-1 β). These chemokines enhance *T.cruzi* uptake by murine macrophages and induce NO production in a dose-dependent manner so that infection is inhibited. As expected, the addition of NMMA blocks the chemokine-induced production of NO (Aliberti *et al.*, 1999a). Similar results are obtained with human macrophages (Villalta *et al.*, 1998b).

2.5 Role of TGF-β and IL-10

In addition to its role in epithelial cell invasion (see Section 2.2), TGF-β is a potent inhibitor of macrophage-activating cytokines *in vivo* and *in vitro* and may play a role in regulating infection as shown by TGF-β treatment that markedly aggravates *T.cruzi* infection in both susceptible and resistant mice (Silva *et al.*, 1991; for a review, see Omer *et al.*, 2000). Furthermore, an interesting recent report indicates that a new pathway triggers TGF-β production and inhibits NO production. When interacting with apoptotic T cells, but not with necrotic or live T cells, *T.cruzi*-infected murine macrophages release increased amounts of both TGF-β and prostaglandin E$_2$ (PGE$_2$) and enhance their ornithine decarboxylase activity. This is due to engagement of the vitronectin receptor involved in phagocytosis of apoptotic cells by macrophages. As a consequence, IFN-γ-induced NO production is inhibited and macrophage infection is sharply enhanced (Freire-de-Lima *et al.*, 1998, 2000).

IL-10 is constitutively produced by several cell types (T cells, certain B cells and monocytes) including macrophages, and plays a complex role. It can act as a deactivating cytokine on macrophages: in *T.cruzi*-infected and IFN-γ-activated murine macrophages, IL-10 inhibits TNF-α and NO production (Gazzinelli *et al.*, 1992a,b). The injection of anti-IL-10 neutralizing antibody to infected susceptible mice has a protective effect (Reed *et al.*, 1994). In contrast, IL-10, in combination with IFN-γ and TNF-α, stimulates the NO production *in vitro* by murine macrophages (Zidek and Frankova, 1999). However, IL-10 decreases TNF-α release but enhances NO synthesis by LPS-activated mouse macrophages (Jacobs *et al.*, 1998a). *Trypanosoma cruzi*-infected IL-10–/– mice have higher levels of IL-12, IFN-γ and TNF-α but earlier mortality. This is reversed by injection of either exogenous IL-10 or anti-IL-12 neutralizing antibodies, indicating that overproduction of IL-12 (as shown with SCID IL-10–/– mice) can have pathological effects (Hunter *et al.*, 1997).

2.6 GM-CSF/TNF-α-mediated lysis of *T.cruzi*

GM-CSF is a multipotent cytokine released from different cell types including macrophages. GM-CSF induces the proliferation and the differentiation of hematopoietic progenitor cells and increases the effector functions of macrophages (Gasson, 1991). The protective role of GM-CSF is demonstrated in *T.cruzi*-infected mice (Olivares Fontt *et al.*, 1996). *In vitro*, GM-CSF-activated mouse peritoneal macrophages control the infection even in the absence of IFN-γ activation and NO production (Olivares Fontt and Vray, 1995), suggesting a parasiticidal effect for GM-CSF as previously shown for TNF-α on *T.brucei brucei*, an African trypanosome (Lucas *et al.*, 1994; Magez *et al.*, 1997) (see

Section 5.3). Indeed, in a cell-free system, GM-CSF-treated trypomastigotes are less infectious for mouse peritoneal macrophages. In addition, some trypomastigotes become spherical while other are lysed. When incubated with TNF-α or with a combination of both GM-CSF and TNF-α, parasites are lysed, following a lectin-like mediated mechanism similar to the one described for *T.brucei*. In this way, both GM-CSF and TNF-α might impair the infectivity of the parasites and participate in the *in vivo* control of infection (Olivares Fontt *et al.*, 1998).

2.7 Deficiency of macrophage-mediated antigen presentation

A possible deficiency of APC function in *T.cruzi*-infected macrophages could be part of a parasite strategy to evade host immune response. An experimental model, first used with *Leishmania amazonensis*-infected macrophages (Prina *et al.*, 1993) (see also Section 3.5), has been tested on *T.cruzi*-infected macrophages. The capacity of infected macrophages to capture and to catabolize exogenous non-parasitic antigen (bacteriophage λ repressor cI protein) is reduced. Stimulation of various specific I-A^d- or I-E^d-restricted CD4$^+$ T-cell hybridomas is lowered and binding of immunogenic cI(12–26) peptides to the plasma membrane Ia molecules of infected and paraformaldehyde-fixed macrophages is also reduced. Furthermore, the percentages of MHC class II- and IL-2R-positive macrophages are reduced after *T.cruzi* infection. Thus, *T.cruzi* infection *in vitro* results in deficient antigen processing and presentation of the derived immunogenic peptides to specific CD4$^+$ Th1 cell hybridomas (Plasman *et al.*, 1995).

In line with these data, *T.cruzi*-infected macrophages do not present antigen (surface antigen of *T.cruzi* trypomastigote or ovalbumin) to the relevant CD4$^+$ T-cell hybridomas. As a consequence, IL-2 production is reduced. Specific T-cell hybridoma cells also produce less IL-2 when incubated in the presence of infected and paraformaldehyde-fixed macrophages pulsed with ovalbumin peptide. In contrast to a previous report (Plasman, *et al.*, 1995), the expression of MHC class II molecules and class II–peptide complexes is not altered in *T.cruzi*-infected macrophages. The reason for such a discrepancy is unclear. It remains that, in this model, the APC defect is not due to reduced cell viability, or defective peptide loading or the absence of CD28 co-stimulation. However, a low level of adherence between T cells and infected macrophages is observed, so that the APC defect is due rather to a reduced expression of other adhesion molecules by infected macrophages (La Flamme *et al.*, 1997).

On the other hand, macrophages infected with transfected *T.cruzi* trypomastigotes expressing β-galactosidase do not stimulate specific cytotoxic T-cell hybridomas, suggesting a sequestration of this antigen (Buckner *et al.*, 1997). In contrast, fibroblasts infected with *T.cruzi* transfectants that secrete or release antigen (ovalbumin and ovalbumin-derived peptide 139–385) process and present this peptide via the MHC class I pathway and stimulate antigen-specific CD8$^+$ T-cell hybridomas and the cytolysis of infected cells. However, this is not the case with *T.cruzi* transfectants producing cytoplasmic or transmembrane forms of this antigen. These data indicate that antigen release is necessary to stimulate the MHC class I pathway (Garg *et al.*, 1997). Interestingly, expression of MHC class I molecules is not lowered in *T.cruzi*-infected macrophages which are able to present a β-galactosidase-derived peptide to a specific murine cytotoxic CD8$^+$ T-cell line through the MHC class I pathway, and a greater CD8$^+$-mediated cell lysis is obtained with infected macrophages versus uninfected ones (Buckner *et al.*,

1997). In addition, mice infected with ovalbumin-secreting parasites elicit ovalbumin-specific cytotoxic T lymphocytes (Garg *et al.*, 1997). These data suggest that parasite persistance in the host is not linked to an impairment of the MHC class I pathway, since *T.cruzi* infection does not impair the MHC class I route for secreted or released proteins.

In addition, bone marrow-derived macrophages infected with *T.cruzi* sharply up-regulate the expression of B7.2 molecules but not other co-stimulatory molecules. Consequently, Th1 cells stimulated with anti-CD3 antibodies or with specific antigen strongly proliferate in the presence of infected macrophages that become potent co-stimulatory cells (Frosch *et al.*, 1997).

Amastigote-infected macrophages are able to present parasite peptides associated with MHC I and II molecules and to activate *T.cruzi*-specific immune CD4$^+$ T cells in lymph nodes and spleen CD8$^+$ T cells which proliferate and produce cytokines (Caulada-Benedetti *et al.*, 1998). These data should be considered along with those of Nickell *et al.* (1993) showing that chronically infected mice produce CD8$^+$ T cells specific for parasite antigens, and those of Wizel *et al.* (1998) reporting that CD8$^+$ T cells specific for *trans*-sialidase-derived peptides are elicited in *T.cruzi* human infection. Similarly, chagasic patients develop both humoral and cellular immune responses against cruzipain, and human monocytes present cruzipain peptides to CD4$^+$ T cells from chagasic patients (Morrot *et al.*, 1997) (Table 6.2).

Taken together, these results suggest that *T.cruzi*-infected macrophages can process and present parasite antigens via both MHC class I and II pathways. This would not be the case for exogenous non-parasitic antigens or non-secreted parasitic antigens. Parasite persistence and chronic aspects of the disease may be found in other deficiencies of immune response such as (among others) alteration of DC–APC functions, parasite-induced immunosuppression, autoimmune responses and/or T- and B-cell polyclonal activation.

3 *Leishmania* spp.

Leishmania are obligate intracellular protozoan parasites. They are related to *T.cruzi* as they also belong to the family Trypanosomatidae, order Kinetoplastida, phylum Sarcomastigophora. The free-living and motile flagellated promastigotes multiply in the intestinal tract of blood-sucking vectors of the genus *Phlebotomus* (Old World) and *Lutzomyia* (New World). It becomes a metacyclic promastigote which is the infective form present in the anterior part of the digestive tract. When inoculated by the vector's bite to a suitable mammalian host, metacyclic promastigotes invade cells belonging to the monocyte/macrophage lineage but other cell types can also be invaded (Rittig and Bogdan, 2000). Once engulfed in phagosomes, they differentiate into non-motile amastigote forms which multiply in a PV. However, the existence of 'cytosolic' amastigotes, thus outside the PV, is proposed (Rittig and Bogdan, 2000). The lysis of infected macrophages releases amastigotes which, in turn, infect other macrophages. In addition to cells of the monocyte/macrophage lineage, mouse DCs internalize a small number of promastigotes which are degraded without switching to the amastigote stage (Konecny *et al.*, 1999). The parasites infect humans as well as domestic and wild mammals. Numerous species and subspecies of *Leishmania* have been described. In humans, some of them are responsible for various forms of *Leishmania*sis: cutaneous (*L.major*, *L.tropica*, *L.aethiopica*,

Table 6.2 Deficiencies of macrophage-mediated antigen presentation

	Trypanosoma cruzi	Leishmania spp	Toxoplasma gondii	Trypanosoma brucei
Antigen uptake and catabolism	Reduced (Plasman et al., 1995)	Not affected (Fruth et al., 1993)		Not affected (Namangala et al., 2000a)
Adhesion and co-stimulatory molecules	Macrophage–T cell adhesion reduced (La Flamme et al., 1997); up-regulation of B7.2 (Frosch et al., 1997)		CD40 enhanced (Subauste et al., 1999)	ICAM-1 not affected (Namangala et al., 2000a)
Expression of MHC class II	Reduced (Plasman et al., 1995) or not (La Flamme et al., 1997)	Not affected (Fruth et al., 1993)	Reduced (Luder et al., 1998)	Ia not affected (Namangala et al., 2000a) Ia enhanced (Grosskinsky et al., 1983)
Expression of MHC class I	Not affected (Buckner et al., 1997; Garg et al., 1997)	Reduced (Fruth et al., 1993) Reduced (Prina et al., 1993) Reduced for L.major (Frosch et al., 1996) and L.amazonensis (Prina et al., 1993), reduced when macrophages contain live amastigotes of L.mexicana (Wolfram et al., 1995, 1996) reduced for macrophages infected with amastigotes (not promastigotes) of L.amazonensis (Courret et al., 1999), L.major, L.mexicana (Kima et al., 1996), L.major, L.amazonensis (Prina et al., 1996)	Reduced (Luder, et al., 1998)	Not affected (Namangala et al., 2000a) Reduced (Namangala et al., 2000a)
Peptide binding to Ia molecules	Reduced (Plasman et al., 1995) or not (La Flamme et al., 1997)			
Stimulation of antigen-specific CD4+ T cell	Reduced (Plasman et al., 1995; La Flamme et al., 1997) or not affected for parasite peptides (Caulada-Benedetti et al., 1998)			
Stimulation of antigen-specific CD8+ T cell	Reduced (La Flamme et al., 1997) or not (Buckner et al., 1997; Caulada-Benedetti et al., 1998)			

Old World; *L.mexicana*, *L.amazonensis*, *L.panamensis*, *L.guyanensis*, New World), diffuse cutaneous (*L.pifanoï*, *L.amazonensis*, New World), muco-cutaneous (*L.brazilien-sis*, New World) and visceral (*L.donovani*, *L.infantum*, Old World, and *L.chagasi*, New World). As a consequence, leishmaniasis constitutes a public health problem, especially in tropical and subtropical developing countries; for a review, see Handman (1999).

3.1 Recognition/adhesion systems

Promastigotes of all known *Leishmania* species possess two major surface molecules [lipophosphoglycan (LPG) and glycoprotein 63 kDa (gp63)] (Ferguson, 1999) in addition to other binding systems ressembling those involved in *T.cruzi*–macrophage cross-talk at the entry stage (Table 6.1).

3.1.1 Lipophosphoglycan

Lipophosphoglycan (LPG) is a glycolipid with a GPI anchor (for reviews, see Turco and Descoteaux, 1992; Handman, 1999). It belongs to the phosphoglycan family including glycolipids and glycoproteins characterized by repeat units. LPG is present on the promastigote membrane of all *Leishmania* species.

The crucial role of LPG in the leishmanial infection is indicated by experiments showing that mice immunized with LPG are protected against a subsequent infection (Turco and Descoteaux, 1992). In addition, LPG-deficient *L.mexicana* promastigotes are avirulent although they also induce a protective immunity indicating the existence of other protective antigens (Kimsey *et al.*, 1993).

During the logarithmic growth phase, *L.major* promastigotes are not infective for macrophages. They are lysed by the alternate complement pathway and they express a LPG which is responsible for the promastigote agglutination by a lectin: the peanut agglutinin. At the end of the growing phase, the promastigotes undergo metacyclogenesis and become infective (metacyclic) promastigotes for the macrophages. They are no longer lysed by complement nor agglutinated by this lectin. This is due to the expression of a highly modified LPG involved in promastigote phagocytosis by macrophages (Puentes *et al.*, 1990; McConville *et al.*, 1992; Sacks, 1992).

CR3 also binds to C3bi and bacterial LPS. LPG interacts directly in a lectin-like car-bohydrate recognition mechanism with the 'LPS'-binding site of CR3 (Talamas-Rohana *et al.*, 1990). LPG interacts indirectly with CR1 and CR3 by opsonization with C3b and C3bi (Puentes *et al.*, 1988; Da Silva *et al.*, 1989). In addition, LPG binds to the mannose–fucose receptor and it also binds directly to C-reactive protein which in turn binds to C-reactive protein receptor (Culley *et al.*, 1996; Bogdan and Rollinghoff, 1998).

3.1.2 gp63

gp63 (or leishmanolysin or promastigote surface protease) is a glycoprotein with a GPI anchor (Schneider *et al.*, 1990; Joshi *et al.*, 1998; Voth *et al.*, 1998). A soluble intracellular leishmanolysin is also present in amastigotes of certain *Leishmania* species. gp63 is present on promastigote membranes of all *Leishmania* species but, as for LPG, in very small amounts on amastigotes. It exists as a heterogeneous family of proteins with sequences highly conserved despite their diverse geographical distribution (Medina-Acosta *et al.*, 1993). It is a zinc metalloprotease involved in *Leishmania*–macrophage binding in various ways. It contains a Ser–Arg–Tyr–Asp (SRYD) sequence which mimics the cell attachment sequence of FN and thus can bind to the RGDS domain of CR3 and the FNR (Soteriadou *et al.*, 1992). In addition, gp63 has mannose residues enhancing parasite–macrophage binding through mannose–fucose receptors. gp63 also protects the parasite against complement-mediated lysis. It inactivates C3b in C3bi which binds to CR3, its receptor on the macrophage membrane, and thus contributes to parasite–macrophage adhesion (Russell and Talamas-Rohana, 1989; Brittingham *et al.*, 1995, 1999; Mosser and Brittingham, 1997; Bogdan and Rollinghoff, 1998).

3.1.3 Other recognition/adhesion systems

As for *T.cruzi*, FN is implicated in the adherence of *L.amazonensis* promastigotes to macrophages through an FNR. However, this binding may result in enhanced killing of intracellular infective promastigotes upon FN addition to the macrophage cultures. Immunocytochemical observations show that promastigotes release bound FN by membrane shedding to evade intracellular killing (Vannier-Santos *et al.*, 1992).

Once again, as for *T.cruzi*, carbohydrate residues also modulate the binding of *Leishmania* to macrophages. The mannose/*N*-acetyl-D-glucosamine/fucose, the galactose/N-acetyl-D-galactosamine and the mannose-6-phosphate receptor participate in the *Leishmania*–macrophage interactions (Araujo-Jorge, 1989). Galactosyl-α-(1–3)-galactose epitopes present on *Leishmania* are recognized by galectin-3 (Gabius, 1997). Binding of both anti-galactose antibodies (see Section 2.1.3) and the lectin extracted from *B.simplicifolia* to promastigotes and amastigotes of different *Leishmania* species is also inhibited in the presence of galactose (Araujo-Jorge and De Souza, 1988; Araujo-Jorge, 1989; Bretana *et al.*, 1992).

Two glycoconjugates, the fucose–mannose glycoprotein ligand and the phosphate mannogalactan ligand, purified from *L.donovani* promastigotes, are potent inhibitors of parasite uptake by mouse peritoneal macrophages (Palatnik *et al.*, 1990).

A heparin-binding activity has been identified on the surface of *L.donovani* promastigotes and is recognized as an adhesion molecule. The expression of the heparin-binding activity coincides with the differentiation of the non-infective form into the infective metacyclic form of promastigotes (Butcher *et al.*, 1992; Kock *et al.*, 1997). *Leishmania major* amastigotes express LPG which is involved in macrophage adhesion as for promastigotes. For *L.amazonensis* amastigotes devoid of this important ligand, other molecules are proposed such as a heparin-binding activity (Love *et al.*, 1993) or glycosphingolipids (Straus *et al.*, 1997) or via FcR–antibody interaction for *L.mexicana mexicana* (Peters *et al.*, 1995). Proteophosphoglycans with a GPI anchor are present on *L.major* promastigotes and could be involved in macrophage binding. However, such a role remains to be determined precisely (Handman, 1999; Ilg, 2000).

3.2 Macrophage invasion

3.2.1 Metacyclic promastigotes

Leishmania spp. are taken up by macrophages by a classical phagocytic process mediated by the many molecules of LPG expressed on *Leishmania* spp. and the corresponding macrophage receptor (Kelleher *et al.*, 1995). As shown by scanning and transmission electron microscopy with *L.mexicana* and other *Leishmania* spp., morphological differences are seen between phagocytosis of promastigotes surrounded by long and prominent projections from mouse peritoneal macrophages while amastigotes lay on cup-shaped extensions. In both cases, parasites are progressively and completely engulfed in a PV (Strauss *et al.*, 1993).

Another type of phagocytosis, called coiling phagocytosis, also occurs. In this case, pseudopods arise from the membrane of human monocytes and murine macrophages and wrap around *L.major*, *L.donovani* and *L.aethiopica* promastigotes in multiple turns. Coiling phagocytosis probably derives from the classical phagocytic process and the so-called 'zippering mechanism' mediated by progressive receptor/opsonin binding of macrophage pseudopods around the particle to be ingested (Griffin *et al.*, 1975). *Leishmania major* and *L.donovani* promastigotes are taken up by macrophages via inter-actions with CR1 and CR3 (see Section 3.1.1.). It is hypothesized that an initial weak interaction between CR1- and C3b-opsonized promastigotes is replaced, in a second step, by a stronger interaction between CR3- and C3bi-opsonized promastigotes. Due to steric hindrance, there would be an asymmetric CR3 clustering, formation of a unilateral pseudopod and, finally, asymmetric engulfment (Rittig *et al.*, 1998a). However, coiling phagocytosis of *L.aethiopica* promastigotes is not affected by the inactivation of comple-ment, indicating that receptors (see Section 3.1.3.) other than CR1 and CR3 are probably involved, depending on the *Leishmania* species (Rittig *et al.*, 1998b).

A recent report brings an original and surprising insight into *Leishmania*–macrophage infection. *Leishmania* promastigotes bind natural anti-*Leishmania* IgM, which then acti-vates the classical complement pathway and opsonization by C3. The opsonized pro-mastigotes undergo an immune adherence reaction and bind quantitatively to erythrocytes through CR1. This implies promastigote transfer from erythrocytes to acceptor blood leukocytes. After 10 minutes of *ex vivo* infection, 25 per cent of all leukocytes contain intracellular parasites, indicating that blood cells are the early targets for the invading promastigotes (Dominguez and Torano, 1999).

3.2.2 Amastigotes

Leishmanial infection starts with metacyclic promastigotes that invade host cells. However, in the course of the infection, intracellular amastigotes multiply and, upon host cell disruption, they are released and, in turn, they have to encounter a new suitable host cell so that infection is maintained for a long time. In contrast to promastigote–macrophage interactions, little is known about amastigote interactions. Tyrosine phosphorylation occurs during macrophage infection with *L.amazonensis* amastigotes, and protein tyrosine kinase antagonists enhance the intracellular survival of the parasites (see Section 2.2). In addition, LPS-induced tyrosine phosphorylation of target host proteins is inhibited or reversed by living amastigotes. Such a reversion is contact dependent. Vanadate treatment of amastigotes prior to infection significantly decreases parasite intracellular survival. The mechanism is still unclear though the action of a putative leishmanial ecto-protein phosphatase is suspected (Martiny *et al.*, 1999).

3.3 Resistance to the phagosome–lysosome fusion

In the phagocytic vacuole, promastigotes differentiate into amastigotes. The vacuole fuses with lysosomes to form the PVs containing various hydrolases including proteases that cannot eliminate the parasites (Antoine *et al.*, 1998), and amastigotes produce several protective enzymes (superoxide dismutase, catalase, etc.), so that they can survive and multiply in this hostile environment (Russell *et al.*, 1992; Alexander *et al.*, 1999). Interestingly, striking morphological differences are seen between PVs induced by different species of *Leishmania*. Amastigotes of *L.amazonensis* and *L.mexicana* are tightly bound to the membrane of large PVs, while *L.donovani* and *L.major* amastigotes are tightly encircled in small PVs (Antoine *et al.*, 1998; Handman, 1999).

Among many other functions (Turco and Descoteaux, 1992) and in addition to its protective effect against the deleterious actions of host cell enzymes, LPG also has the capacity to slow down the phagosome–lysosome fusion. Indeed, only 50 per cent of vacuoles containing *L.donovani* promastigotes interact with endosomes or lysosomes, so that 'susceptible' promastigotes can differentiate into 'resistant' amastigotes. In contrast, vacuoles formed around *L.donovani* mutants lacking LPG fuse extensively with endosomes and lysosomes (Desjardins and Descoteaux, 1997). In the PV, amastigotes of many *Leishmania* species are devoid of LPG and gp63 molecules but it is thought that they are protected against enzymatic degradation by GIPLs which are related to LPG (Turco and Descoteaux, 1992; Kelleher *et al.*, 1995). Complement-mediated opsonization of promastigotes increases the intracellular survival of *L.major* (Mosser and Brittingham, 1997).

Cysteine proteases produced by *Leishmania* could play a major role in intracellular survival and could constitute parasite virulence factors (Mottram *et al.*, 1998a; Brooks *et al.*, 2000). *Leishmania mexicana* mutants lacking cysteine proteinase genes induce an attenuated infection in mice and a reduced rate of macrophage infection probably because these enzymes are necessary for their promastigote/amastigote transformation and for their survival into the macrophage PV. Furthermore, these parasites deficient in cysteine proteases induce a shift from a Th2 towards a protective Th1 immune response when compared with control mice infected with wild-type *L.mexicana* (Galvao-Quintao *et al.*, 1990; Ilg *et al.*, 1994; Alexander *et al.*, 1998). As shown below (see Section 3.5), cysteine proteases could also interfere with antigen presentation.

3.4 Mechanisms of infection control

3.4.1 Murine macrophages

The antiprotozoal effect of IFN-γ activation of mouse peritoneal macrophages *in vitro* and *in vivo* was at first attributed to ROI-dependent mechanisms. Addition of neutralizing anti-IFN-γ antibodies to activated macrophages inhibits H_2O_2 release and anti-*L.donovani* activity (Murray *et al.*, 1985b). However, intact *Leishmania* and *Leishmania* LPG have an inhibitory effect on ROI production (for reviews, see Mauel, 1996; Bogdan and Rollinghoff, 1998). These data suggested the existence of an ROI-independent control mechanism and, indeed, the role of NO is now evidenced by numerous reports (Green *et al.*, 1990; Mauel *et al.*, 1991; Roach *et al.*, 1991; Liew, 1993; Assreuy *et al.*, 1994; Stenger *et al.*, 1994; Reiner and Locksley, 1995).

Evidence of NO-mediated control of infection is demonstrated by the high susceptibility of mice deficient in the NOS2 gene to *L.major* infection (Wei *et al.*, 1995). In addition, results obtained with *L.donovani*-infected mice genetically deficient in ROI (X-CGD–/–) or in RNI (NOS2–/–) metabolism indicate that both deficient mice are more susceptible than control mice, at least during the early stage of infection. However, later on, NOS2–/– mice die while X-CGD–/– control the infection (Murray and Nathan, 1999).

In contrast, *L.major*-infected mice, deficient in Fas ligand (FasL–/–), can mount a protective CD4+ Th1 response and their macrophages can be activated by IFN-γ, but these mice do not control the infection. Injection of exogenous recombinant FasL to these deficient mice results in the healing of cutaneous lesions. These results suggest that NO production is probably not the major feature of the immune response with regard of Fas–FasL interactions which seem to play a central role in the anti-*L.major* immune response (Conceicao-Silva *et al.*, 1998; Huang *et al.*, 1998; Trinchieri and Scott, 1999).

It remains likely that this NO production depends on the CD40–CD40L/IL-12/IFN-γ/TNF-α cascade. Activated CD4+ T cells express CD40L and they interact with CD40-bearing cells, inducing the production of IL-12 (Soong *et al.*, 1996; Ferlin *et al.*, 1998). However, IL-12 production by mouse bone marrow-derived macrophages is inhibited by metacyclic promastigotes of *L.major* and *L.donovani* while production of other cytokines (IL-1 α, IL-1 β and TNF-α) and NOS2 expression are only weakly reduced (Carrera *et al.*, 1996). Phosphoglycan of *L.major* could be a good candidate as inhibitor of IL-12 synthesis since it was shown that this molecule inhibits the synthesis of IL-12 by activated murine macrophages in a dose-dependent manner (Piedrafita *et al.*, 1999). However, DCs are stimulated to produce IL-12 upon internalization of a small number of promastigotes which are finally degraded (Konecny *et al.*, 1999) so that these cells constitute an important source of IL-12 and thus induce IFN-γ production (Vieira *et al.*, 1994; Reiner and Locksley, 1995; Flohe *et al.*, 1998).

IL-12 induces a protective effect while the injection of anti-IL-12 antibody decreases endogenous IFN-γ production and exacerbates the infection (Murray, 1997). In addition, vaccination of mice with plasmid DNA encoding a leishmanial protein plus IL-12 DNA produces a long-lasting immunity against *L.major* infection, underlining that the persistence of IL-12 production plays a central role in cell-mediated immune responses against intracellular parasitic infection (Gurunathan *et al.*, 1998). Furthermore, this potent protective effect of IL-12 is confirmed by using mice injected with *L.major* antigen-pulsed and GM-CSF-treated macrophages. In these experiments, protection is antigen specific, and correlates with high levels of IL-12 and IFN-γ. IL-12 is synthesized by macrophages, and macrophages deficient in IL-12 production do not induce protection (Doherty and Coffman, 1999).

In addition to IL-12, IFN-γ is once again the pivotal cytokine of this NO pathway together with TNF-α which has a triggering effect in murine and human leishmaniasis (Green *et al.*, 1990; Barral-Netto *et al.*, 1991; Norris, 1998), except that this cytokine is probably not absolutely essential since mice deficient in TNF-αR p55 control *L major* infection and, *in vitro*, IFN-γ-activated macrophages from these mice produced NO and killed *L.major*. However, this TNF-α-independent production of NO requires the presence of the parasites, indicating that other signals and/or parasite-derived molecules are involved in this process (Vieira *et al.*, 1996).

As for *T.cruzi*, TGF-β favors leishmanial infections (cf. Section 2.6 and Omer *et al.*, 2000). A protective effect mediated by an enhanced NO production is obtained in *L.major*-infected mice when they are treated with anti-TGF-β neutralizing antibodies (Li *et al.*, 1999). TGF-β not only inhibits NO production (see above) but it also alters the antigen-presenting function of macrophages and induces a generalized immunosuppression as shown in *L.amazonensis*-infected mice (Barral-Netto *et al.*, 1992) and in *L.donovani*-infected hamsters (Rodrigues *et al.*, 1998).

Host antibodies and IL-10 also play a crucial role in murine leishmaniasis. Surface IgGs on amastigotes induce the production of IL-10 by macrophages and favor parasite intracellular survival. This correlates with a diminished production of IL-12 and TNF-α by activated macrophages together with control of disease progression in IL-10–/– BALB/c mice (Kane and Mosser, 2001).

Other molecules may also play a role in the control of infection. As in *T.cruzi* infection, chemokines exert a protective role in leishmanial infection. Indeed, the expression of the chemokine MCP-1 is associated with macrophage infiltration into the lesion and stimulation of leishmanicidal activity (Moll, 1997). BALB/c mice are susceptible to *L.major* infection while C57BL/6 are more resistant. Among other factors, this is probably due to a lower expression of three chemokines (MCP-1, IFN-γ-inducible protein 10 and lymphotactin) which are potent activators of NK cells. It remains to be determined if there is chemokine-dependent NO production (Vester *et al.*, 1999). In *L.donovani*-infected macrophages, phosphotyrosine phosphatases are activated so that MAP kinase signaling, NF-κB activation and NOS2 expression are reduced. This could also be another mechanism allowing the parasite to avoid the macrophage-mediated control of infection (Nandan *et al.*, 2000; Prive and Descoteaux, 2000).

3.4.2 Human macrophages

Monocytes and macrophages harvested from patients with granulomatous disease and activated by IFN-γ are able to control *L.donovani* infection. In addition, *Leishmania* antigens induce immune responses from CD4+ and CD8+ T cells, with the release of IFN-γ and/or TNF-α, and they can enhance *in vitro* leishmanicidal activity. These data suggest the existence of NO-mediated control of leishmanial infection as shown with activated murine macrophages (for reviews, see Reiner and Locksley, 1995; Mauel, 1996; Milon *et al.*, 1996; Bogdan and Rollinghoff, 1998; see also Section 3.4.1). Such a mechanism is now demonstrated with activated human macrophages. Furthermore, a completely different means of activation has also been discovered so that two independent pathways of leishmanicidal activity of human macrophages are now known.

Killing of *L.major* or *L.infantum* in human macrophages is mediated by IFN-γ, TNF-α and NO. Indeed, IFN-γ activation allows macrophages to exert a relative control of *L major* infection but it does not protect uninfected macrophages against a subsequent infection with this parasite (Mossalayi *et al.*, 1999). Human macrophages produce TGF-β after infection by *L.amazonensis*, *L.chagasi* or *L.braziliensis*. Addition of TGF-β to cultures of human macrophages infected with *L.braziliensis* increases the parasite burden and reverses the protective effect of IFN-γ, while TNF-α is able to counteract its suppressive effect (Barral-Netto *et al.*, 1991; Barral *et al.*, 1995).

Beside the IFN-γ/NO-mediated control of infection, a recently described mechanism is based on the FcϵRII (CD23) ligation by IgE. The b isoform of the CD23 molecule belongs to the C-type lectin family and is expressed by human, monkey and rat macrophages but not mouse macrophages. The CD23–IgE cross-linking also triggers NO production but is a more potent mechanism than IFN-γ activation of human macrophages. IgE synthesis is promoted by IL-4 and IL-13 while expression of CD23 is induced by CD40 ligation, IFN-γ, IL-4 and IL-13 (Mossalayi *et al.*, 1999). As for the IFN-γ-mediated pathway, CD23–IgE cross-linking induces a pro-inflammatory response in human and rat macrophages with TNF-α, IL-1, IL-6, thromboxane B$_2$, NO and ROI synthesis (Dugas *et al.*, 1995). CD23 ligation by IgE immune complexes or anti-CD23 monoclonal antibody results in a cure of macrophages infected with *L.major*, *L.infantum* or *L.braziliensis* (Vouldoukis *et al.*, 1995). Involvement of NO production by human macrophages activated by the CD23–IgE-mediated pathway is supported by: (1) the inhibitory effect of NMMA; (2) the correlation between the protective effect of CD23 ligation and NO production; (3) the killing of extra- and intracellular forms of *Leishmania* by NO donors; and (4) the increased expression of NO-inhibiting cytokines (IL-4, IL-10 and TGF-β) during disease progression. However, the inhibiting role of IL-4 and IL-10 on NO is complex. Indeed, it seems that when macrophages are activated by only one of these two pathways (either by IFN-γ or by CD23 ligation), IL-4 or IL-10 have a deactivating effect, reducing the leishmanicidal activity. However, when macrophages are activated by both IFN-γ and CD23 ligation, IL-4 and IL-10, alone or in combination, are unable to inhibit the leishmanicidal activity. This feature correlates with observations made on cytokines found in human skin lesions (Vouldoukis *et al.*, 1997).

As for murine macrophages, other molecules are probably involved in the control of infection. For instance, MCP-1 seems to play a protective role in *Leishmania*-infected human monocytes through the activating and deactivating role of IFN-γ and IL-4, respectively (Ritter and Moll, 2000).

3.5 Deficiency of macrophage-mediated antigen presention

Deficiency of macrophage-mediated antigen presention is thought to be an important escape mechanism. Consequently, this is the subject of many reports using various experimental models showing that this escape mechanism is dependent on various parameters (Antoine *et al.*, 1998; Overath and Aebischer, 1999). Macrophages infected with *Leishmania* parasites are probably good candidates to present antigens to parasite-specific $CD4^+$ and $CD8^+$ T lymphocytes, so expression and localization of both MHC class I and class II molecules are crucial points. In bone marrow-derived macrophages infected with *L.amazonensis*, *L.mexicana*, *L.major* or *L.donovani*, MHC class I molecules are expressed at the macrophage membrane but not in the PV. In contrast, MHC class II and H-2M molecules (known to favor the binding of peptides to MHC class II and to select stable MHC class II–peptide complexes) are found in the PV. However, despite the presence of all the molecules necessary for the formation of parasite antigen–MHC class II complexes, the formation of these complexes probably does not occur. In addition, as MHC class II molecules, H-2M molecules are internalized and degraded in the amastigotes of *L.amazonensis* and *L.mexicana* and found in megasomes. Interestingly, in the presence of cysteine protease inhibitor, such a degradation does not occur, indicating that cysteine protease participates in the down-regulation of molecules involved in antigen presentation (Antoine *et al.*, 1999).

Macrophage resistance to intracellular microorganisms is mediated by the natural resistance-associated macrophage protein-1 (Nramp-1) which is a divalent cation (Fe^{2+}, Zn^{2+} and Mn^{2+}) transporter, localized to late endosomes/lysosomes (Gruenheid and Gros, 2000; Blackwell *et al.* 2000; Jabado *et al.*, 2000). In addition, expression of MHC class II molecules is regulated by Nramp1 probably because Mn^{2+} could be important for metalloprotease activity in the endosomal compartment. The role of Nramp1 has been shown using the LACK (*Leishmania* homolog of receptors for activated C kinase) antigen model. LACK is a cytosolic protein expressed by both promastigote and amastigote forms of various *Leishmania* species such as *L.amazonensis*, *L.chagasi*, *L.donovani* and *L.major*. It is an immunodominant parasite antigen known to confer a protective immunity to IL-12-treated mice subsequently infected with metacyclic *L.major* promastigotes. Processing and efficient presentation of antigen to specific T cells occur with macrophages transfected with the wild-type allele of Nramp1, and MHC class II molecules are up-regulated in response to IFN-γ and LPS (Lang *et al.*, 1997).

Evidence of antigen presentation deficiency is reported in two studies showing that bone marrow-derived macrophages infected with *L.major* promastigotes (Fruth *et al.*, 1993) or with *L.amazonensis* amastigotes (Prina *et al.*, 1993) have a reduced capacity to present antigens to specific T-cell hybridomas. However, infected macrophages fixed with paraformaldehyde and pulsed with exogenously added antigenic peptides have a normal antigen-presenting capacity so that the failure to present native antigen is attributed to reduced intracellular loading of MHC class II molecules with antigenic peptides or to a defect in the formation of MHC class II–peptide complexes or to a competition for binding of these peptides and parasite molecules to MHC class II molecules (see Section 2.7).

In bone marrow-derived macrophages infected with *L.mexicana*, presentation of parasitic antigens (acid phosphatase molecules expressed on amastigote intracellular membrane and cysteine proteases located in amastigote lysosomes) and stimulation of specific T cells do not occur with live amastigotes, except when intramacrophage amastigotes are killed by drug treatment or IFN-γ/TNF-α activation. This indicates a possible traffic between the PV and the macrophage membrane. The amount of released antigens and duration of antigen exposure are two others parameters which influence the efficiency of antigen presentation (Wolfram *et al.*, 1995, 1996). In *L.amazonensis*-infected macrophages, cysteine proteases and LACK antigen are not presented. In contrast, in the case of amastigote killing, cysteine proteases, but not LACK antigen, are presented. These data also suggest that the stability of the antigens, and/or their resistance to enzymes present in the PV, could also be important parameters (Wolfram *et al.*, 1995; Courret *et al.*, 1999).

Absence of antigen presentation is also dependent on the infective stage of the parasite as shown in a model using the LACK antigen. Macrophages infected with promastigotes, but not with amastigotes, are able to present LACK antigen and to activate a LACK-specific T-cell hybridoma (Prina *et al.*, 1996). The mechanism of such an absence of antigen presentation has been documented further recently. Amastigotes and, to a lesser extent, metacyclic promastigotes are very efficient in altering APC function of macrophages while log-phase and stationary-phase promastigotes are unable to do so. Drug treatment of amastigote-infected macrophages does not improve the antigen presentation, indicating that the partial or total destruction of amastigotes is not sufficient to reverse the absence of antigen presentation. Nevertheless, these macrophages remain capable of presenting the epitope LACK (158–173) after addition of the recombinant form of LACK to the culture medium (Courret *et al.*, 1999). Similar conclusions on the importance of infective stages are reached using other *Leishmanial* antigens (Kima *et al.*, 1996) (Table 6.2).

On the other hand, immune responses are initiated by DC–microorganism interactions. Indeed, Langerhans cells (immature DCs of the skin) transport *L.major* from the infected skin to the draining lymph nodes, they mature in DCs and initiate antigen-specific T-cell immune responses, and they maintain persistent infection and sustain stimulation of para-site-specific T cells, insuring protection against reinfection in resistant mice (Flohe *et al.*, 1997, 1998; Moll and Flohe, 1997). Furthermore, murine DCs isolated from the spleen can internalize and degrade promastigotes (Flohe, 1997, 1998; Konecny *et al.*, 1999). In addition, *L.major*-infected human DCs release IL-12 upon CD40–CD40L interaction and are thought to have a protective role via IFN-γ production (Marovich *et al.*, 2000). However, cardinal functions of DCs can be impaired by *Leishmania* parasites as shown with splenic DCs harvested from *L.donovani*-infected mice (Basu *et al.*, 2000). On the whole, it is likely that specific T lymphocytes are not primed optimally by DCs and are not stimulated further by infected macrophages. As a consequence, deficiency of macrophage-mediated antigen presentation would be a potent strategy that allows *Leishmania* to decrease the host immune response efficiency.

4 *Toxoplasma gondii*

Toxoplasma gondii belongs to the class Coccidea, phylum Sporozoa. This obligate intra-cellular protozoan parasite has a cosmopolitan distribution and infects a large host range of warm-blooded vertebrates (Joiner and Dubremetz, 1993; Smith, 1995). Human infec-tion (toxoplasmosis) usually occurs by: (1) ingestion of oocysts issued from the sexual reproduction of the parasite in intestinal cells and released in cat feces; (2) ingestion of meat from infected animals containing long-lived tissue cysts; (3) in the case of an acquired toxoplasmosis by a non-immune mother in the course of her pregnancy and who transmits the parasites to her fœtus; or (4) in the case of transplantation, transfu-sion and laboratory accidents (Wong and Remington, 1994; Sibley *et al.*, 1999; Smith, 1999).

Infection of humans is common. It is most often benign and/or asymptomatic and confers a stable immunity for life. However, *T.gondii* is a major cause of morbidity and mortality in neonates and immunocompromised hosts in congenital toxoplasmosis and toxoplasmic encephalitis, respectively (Fagard *et al.*, 1999). Both acute invasion and reac-tivation of latent infection result in an inflammatory process with lymphocytes, macrophages and neutrophils. This latent infection may turn into a fatal disease in the case of immunodeficiencies such as those seen in transplantation, malignancies or acquired immune deficiency syndrome (AIDS; Minkoff *et al.*, 1997).

Acute toxoplasmosis is characterized by the fast intracellular multiplication of the tachyzoite forms in various nucleated cell types, including macrophages (Channon *et al.*, 2000). Afterwards, when the immune system controls the infection, some tachyzoites enter a dormant stage, become bradyzoites, with a slow multiplication rate, and remain encysted in muscle cells and brain cells for life (Hunter and Remington, 1994).

Successful invasion of macrophages by *T.gondii* and its intracellular survival are highly dependent on the origin of the macrophages. It has been shown that resident (non-activated) mouse peritoneal macrophages harbor intracellular multiplication of *T.gondii*. However, conflicting results have been reported using mouse alveolar macrophages. In contrast, peritoneal and alveolar macrophages from adult rats, but not from newborn rats, are highly resistant to *T.gondii*. Resident human alveolar and peri-toneal macrophages at least inhibit the *T.gondii* infection, and human monocyte-derived macrophages also control the infection except if they are cultured for seven or more days (for reviews, see Joiner and Dubremetz, 1993; Beaman *et al.*, 1994; Black and Boothroyd, 2000).

4.1 Recognition/adhesion systems

Toxoplasma gondii invades most of the phagocytic and non-phagocytic nucleated cells, but the molecules which participate in the recognition/adhesion systems are not yet well known (Table 6.1).

Toxoplasma gondii tachyzoites bear surface laminin which binds to multiple laminin receptors present on various cell types. This laminin is involved in attachment of tachyzoites to J774 cells, a mouse macrophage cell line, and a laminin-derived peptide (YIGSR or Tyr–Ile–Gly–Ser–Arg) inhibits macrophage invasion by blocking the laminin receptor (Furtado *et al.*, 1992).

SAG-1, a major surface antigen specifically expressed by the proliferative tachyzoites, has been shown to play such a role in human monocytes using inhibitory specific antibodies. Other related antigens (SAG-2 and SAG-3) are also probably involved (Cesbron-Delauw *et al.*, 1994; Channon and Kasper, 1996). SAG-1 is also implicated in adherence and invasion of various non-macrophagic cells. Indeed, anti-SAG1 antibodies inhibit infection of bovine kidney cells, human fibroblasts and murine enterocytes (Mineo *et al.*, 1993; Grimwood and Smith, 1996). However, SAG-1-deficient tachyzoites are still able to invade fibroblasts. Tachyzoite lectins are also involved in the attachment of the parasites to human fibroblasts. Sulfated sugars of host cells may function as a key parasite receptor (Ortega-Barria and Boothroyd, 1999).

Micronemes are small apical organelles of *T.gondii* that contain at least three specific proteins. All of them contain adhesin motifs (MICs). Human fibroblast binding triggers apical release of the micronemal protein MIC2 and the attachment zone that forms between the parasite and the membrane of the host cells. The protein MIC2 and the other micronemal proteins are probably responsible for the early interaction between the parasite and host cell, either in binding alone or in binding and motility, including invasion (Carruthers and Sibley, 1997).

In addition, other factors (host cell cycle which regulates expression of surface receptors, membrane fluidity, chemical composition and properties of the cytoskeleton) could also play a role in recognition of macrophagic and non-macrophagic cells (Grimwood and Smith, 1996; Grimwood *et al.*, 1996; Dubremetz, 1998).

4.2 Macrophage invasion

Toxoplasma gondii invades a large array of cell types, and both macrophagic and non-macrophagic cells seem to be actively invaded by the parasite. *Toxoplasma gondii* glides on the host cell membrane and the contact between its apical end and the host cell membrane initiates a progressive internalization into a PV. A ring-shaped junction appears between parasite membrane and host cell membrane. Within 25–40 s, the parasite penetrates into a tight-fitting vacuole formed by invagination of the plasma membrane. When the parasite is fully internalized, the vacuole is closed behind and the junction disappears. This invasion process does not induce either host cell membrane ruffling, actin filament reorganization or tyrosine phosphorylation of host proteins. Invasion is powered actively by an actin-based contractile system in the parasite (Dobrowolski *et al.*, 1997; Poupel *et al.*, 2000). In contrast, antibody-coated, live parasites are engulfed in a phagosome by extensive membrane ruffling (Morisaki *et al.*, 1995).

4.3 Inhibition of the phagosome–lysosome fusion

Toxoplasma gondii tachyzoites actively invade macrophages by squeezing through a moving junction that forms between the host cell plasma membrane and the parasites. *Toxoplasma gondii* selectively excludes host cell transmembrane proteins at the moving junction by a mechanism that depends on their anchoring in the membrane, thereby creating a non-fusogenic compartment (Sibley *et al.* 2000). They irreversibly modify the constituents of the PV avoiding its acidification and allowing the parasite to survive and to multiply. MHC class II molecules and FcRs are excluded from the PV. Such modifications of the PV membrane are related to the release of the parasite proteins contained in the conoids.

In contrast, antibody-opsonized and dead parasites are phagocytosed. Together with the parasite, MHC class II molecules and FcRs expressed on the macrophage membrane are internalized into the phagosome and then they are gradually lost. *Toxoplasma gondii*-containing phagosomes rapidly fuse with early endosomes, late endosomes and lysosomes (Mordue and Sibley, 1997).

4.4 Mechanisms of infection control

As with *T.cruzi* and *Leishmania*, *T.gondii* may be eliminated by macrophages activated by cytokines. When incubating mouse peritoneal macrophages with a monoclonal anti-murine IFN-γ antibody, the capacity of mitogen-induced lymphokines to enhance either H_2O_2 release or anti-*T.gondii* activity is abolished (Murray *et al.*, 1985b). Macrophages from healthy mice release very little H_2O_2 so that they allow multiplication of intracellular parasites. In contrast, macrophages from infected mice release a large amount of H_2O_2 and rapidly kill infecting parasites. The role of ROI metabolism in *T.gondii* infection *in vitro* is also demonstrated when using human monocytes, human IFN-γ-activated monocyte-derived macrophages and monocytes from patients with chronic granulomatous disease. Anti-toxoplasma activity is sharply reduced in the presence of ROI inhibitors such as superoxide dismutase and catalase (Murray *et al.*, 1985a). However, if macrophage activation by IFN-γ and TNF-α leads to the control of infection, other factors act in addition to or in parallel with the ROI-mediated control of infection, as shown by monocytes from patients with chronic granulomatous disease (Murray and Nathan, 1999).

A microbiostatic role for NO was first suspected in *T.gondii*-infected murine macrophages activated by IFN-γ and LPS. This microbiostatic effect is inhibited by NMMA while the addition of L-arginine reverses this inhibition (Adams *et al.*, 1990). A role for NO in the control of *T.gondii* infection of macrophages is also found in murine but not in human mononuclear phagocytes (Murray and Teitelbaum, 1992).

The protective effect of the CD40–CD40L/IL-12/FN-γ/TNF-α cascade is confirmed further by other reports (Chang *et al.*, 1990; Langermans *et al.*, 1992a; Subauste *et al.*, 1999; Reichmann *et al.*, 2000; Yap *et al.*, 2000). In particular, the importance of IFN-γ is underlined by its role in reactivation or recurrence of *T.gondii* infection in patients suffering from AIDS, which is related to its down-regulation (Langermans *et al.*, 1992b; Torre *et al.*, 1999). The protective effect of up-regulation of CD8⁺ T cells by IFN-γ indicates that a NOS2-independent mechanism(s) also exists, in addition to the NOS2-dependent metabolism (Khan *et al.*, 1998; Ely *et al.*, 1999; Yap and Sher, 1999).

Finally, as with *T.cruzi* and *Leishmania* spp., TGF-β and IL-10 control overproduction of IL-12, IFN-γ and TNF-α, avoiding immunopathology (Hunter *et al.*, 1995; Gazzinelli *et al.*, 1996; Villegas *et al.*, 2000).

4.5 Deficiency of macrophage-mediated antigen presentation

In comparison with leishmanial infection, deficiency of macrophage-mediated antigen presentation is poorly documented. However, in *T.gondii*-infected macrophages, the IFN-γ-induced expression of MHC class I and II molecules is significantly decreased compared with uninfected controls. However, the constitutive expression of MHC class I antigens is not altered. In IFN-γ-pre-activated macrophages, *T.gondii* infection is also able to reduce the already established expression of MHC class II molecules. Furthermore, supernatants from *T.gondii*-infected macrophage cultures contain factors that inhibit the expression of MHC class II molecules in uninfected macrophages. This inhibitory effect is not mediated by an increased production of PGE₂, IL-10, TGF-β or NO by infected macrophages (Luder *et al.* 1998). On the other hand, infection of human monocytes with viable (but not killed) tachyzoites of *T.gondii* induces the up-regulation of CD80 and CD86 molecules. This is an important point because early production of IFN-γ by T cells from *T.gondii*-seronegative individuals is dependent on this increased expression of CD80 and CD86 (Subauste *et al.*, 1999) (Table 6.2).

As already mentioned for leishmanial infection, control of *T.gondii* infection is also primarily dependent on DCs (Subauste and Wessendarp, 2000). A partial resistance is induced in *T.gondii*-infected mice by injecting DCs pulsed with *T.gondii*-sonicated antigens (Bourguin *et al.*, 1998). IL-12 production by DCs plays also a pivotal role. Human DCs derived from GM-CSF/IL-4-treated monocytes produce IL-12 when they are co-cultured with lymphocytes from *T.gondii*-positive donors (Seguin and Kasper, 1999). However, despite its well known protective effect, IL-12 also induces deleterious consequences when overproduced (Sousa *et al.*, 1999a,b). On the other hand, CD4⁺ T cells from *T.gondii*-infected susceptible mice show (1) DNA fragmentation (suggesting apoptosis) and (2) impaired expression or up-regulation of CTLA-4 or CD28 molecules (Khan *et al.*, 1996).

On the whole, these data indicate that immune responses to *T.gondii* depend on a fragile balance between DCs and their IL-12 production, CD4⁺ T cells and impaired expression of MHC class I and class II by infected macrophages.

5 *Trypanosoma brucei*

The *Trypanosoma brucei* species (genus *Trypanosoma*, order Kinetoplastida) contains three subspecies of protozoan hemoflagellates which are of human and animal importance. *Trypanosoma brucei gambiense* and *T.brucei rhodesiense* are the etiological agents of the human African trypanosomiasis, a debilitating infection always fatal when not treated. *Trypanosoma brucei brucei* infects wild animals which serve as a reservoir, as well as domestic animals (including pigs, cattle, camels and goats) causing a severe infection called 'nagana'. All three parasites are transmitted by the bites of blood-sucking tsetse flies (genus *Glossina*). In contrast to *T.cruzi*, the rapidly dividing long slender forms of *T.brucei* have extracellular multiplication in the bloodstream and in the lymph. They escape from the host immune response by continuously switching and exposing variant surface glycoproteins (VSGs) (Pays and Nolan, 1998; Ferguson, 1999). In addition to the VSG-mediated escape mechanisms, *T.brucei* induces a profound immunosuppression by modulating the secretion of IL-2 and IFN-γ (Darji *et al.*, 1996). Finally, invasion of the central nervous system is responsible for the many disorders such as paralysis and cachexia, giving to the disease the common name of 'sleeping sickness'.

5.1 Macrophage–*T.brucei* interactions

In contrast to *T.cruzi*, macrophages are not infected by African trypanosomes and they play their usual role in parasite clearance. Classical and coiling phagocytosis occur (Stevens and Moulton, 1978; Rittig *et al.*, 1998b) followed by degradation of *T.brucei*, by mouse peritoneal macrophages. Degradation is maximal, *in vitro* and *in vivo*, in the presence of specific antiserum and complement, and upon macrophage activation as shown by transmission electron microscopy (Stevens and Moulton, 1978). Bone marrow-derived macrophages from relatively resistant mice produce IL-12 and TNF-α in the presence of IFN-γ while those from susceptible mice produce more IL-6 and IL-10 following challenge with *T.brucei* (Kaushik *et al.*, 2000). Peritoneal macrophages from *T.brucei*-infected mice have characteristics of activated macrophages. Among others, they produce large amounts of ROIs and NO (Grosskinsky *et al.*, 1983; Mabbott *et al.*, 1995). Interactions between *T.brucei* trypomastigotes and an IFN-γ-activated macrophage cell line also induce the production of ROIs, while this production is inhibited by *T.cruzi* (Vray *et al.*, 1991). As a result, there is formation of nitrosylated albumin that is responsible for the death of extracellular parasites (Gobert *et al.*, 1998). Antibody-dependent phagocytosis is not altered during the course of *T.rhodesiense* murine infection. In mice infected with ^{75}Se-labeled trypomastigotes, parasite clearance occurs 5 days post-inoculation, mainly in the liver and correlated with the appearance of VSG-specific IgM and IgG antibodies (Dempsey and Mansfield, 1983). However, despite their obvious protective role, macrophages are also involved in many parasitic and pathological aspects of the disease.

5.2 Nitric oxide-mediated immunosuppression

Trypanosoma brucei infection induces immunosuppression through suppressor macrophages which produce high levels of NO and subsequent unresponsiveness in lymphocytes (Mabbott *et al.*, 1995). These data are documented further in a study showing that mice with a disrupted IFN-γR gene and infected with *T.b. rhodesiense* have a low macrophage activation and NO synthesis so that they only exert a poor control on parasitemia. However, anemia is reduced and spleen T-cell responsiveness is improved (Mabbott *et al.*, 1998). Similarly, in murine *T.b. brucei* infection, NO contributes to the suppressive activity of spleen and lymph node cells but only during early-stage infection. During late-stage infection, an IFN-γ-independent suppressive mechanism is elicited in the spleen from IFN-γ (–/–)-infected mice which do not produce NO but exert significant suppressive activity during the whole course of infection (Beschin *et al.*, 1998).

The role of suppressive cells and Th1–Th2 cytokine balance in resistance of mice to *T.b.brucei* infection is documented further in experiments showing that mice infected with an attenuated strain of *T.b.brucei* lacking the phospholipase C gene present a lower parasitemia and a longer survival. This resistance correlates with the absence of cells suppressing concanavalin A-induced T-cell proliferation in the lymph node compartment and a decreased production of the macrophage-activating cytokines (IFN-γ and TNF-α) together with an increased production of IL-4, IL-10 and anti-VSG IgG1 antibodies (Namangala *et al.*, 2000b).

5.3 Contrasting effects of TNF-α production by macrophages

IFN-γ-activated macrophages produce large amounts of TNF-α. Interestingly, soluble extracts from *T.b.brucei*, *T.evansi* and *T.congolense* (but not *T.cruzi*) are able to induce murine TNF-α secretion (Magez *et al.*, 1993). The GPI moiety of soluble VSG is a potent inducer of macrophage-dependent TNF-α synthesis upon IFN-γ activation (Magez *et al.*, 1997, 1998). This macrophage-dependent production of TNF-α could participate, at least partially, in the growth control of *T.brucei*. Indeed, in TNF-α–/– mice, parasitemia is strongly increased compared with the peak levels recorded in wild-type mice (Magez *et al.*, 1999). This cytokine exerts a trypanolytic effect which was first shown with *T.brucei*, and later on with *T.cruzi* (see Section 2.6). This TNF-α-mediated trypanolysis is dose dependent and is linked to the so-called TIP domain which has a lectin-like activity. As evidenced with TNF-α labeled with gold particles, the cytokine binds to a trypanosomal glycoprotein present in the flagellar pocket of the parasite, is endocytosed via coated pits and directed towards lysosome-like organelles resulting in a loss of osmoregulation and finally lysis. Anti-TNF-α treatment of *T.brucei*-infected mice increases parasitemia, indicating that TNF-α is involved in the growth control of *T.brucei* (Lucas *et al.*, 1994; Magez *et al.*, 1997; Beschin *et al.*, 1999).

However, TNF-α production is also linked to immunopathological features, such as immunosuppression and LPS hypersensitivity, which are sharply reduced in infected TNF-α–/– mice. These data indicate that TNF-α is a double-edged mediator, involved in both parasitemia control and pathological aspects of the infection (Magez *et al.*, 1999).

5.4 Deficiency of macrophage-mediated antigen presentation

While deficiency of macrophage-mediated antigen presentation is documented in the case of other parasitic protozoa, few data are available on macrophages from *T.brucei*-infected mice except that they present an enhanced expression of Ia antigen (Grosskinsky *et al.*, 1983). However, a recent report (Namangala *et al.*, 2000a) shows that macrophages harvested from *T.brucei*-infected mice have a reduced capacity to present hen egg lysozyme or a derived immunogenic peptide to Ia-restricted CD4+ T-cell hybridoma cells. Using an experimental model related to those previously used with *L.amazonensis* (Prina *et al.*, 1993; see also Section 3.5) and *T.cruzi* (Plasman, *et al.*, 1995; see also Section 2.7), the authors conclude that this can be due to an deficiency of co-expression of processed antigens and Ia molecules together with parasite-derived factors, including IL-10, which contribute to inhibit T-cell activation (Table 6.2).

6 *Schistosoma mansoni*

Many different parasitic worms affect humans all over the world. Among them, the so-called blood flukes, *Schistosoma mansoni*, *S.haematobium* and *S japonicum*, are the etiological agents of schistosomiasis, a tropical disease affecting 200 million people. They are members of the family Schistosomatidae, class Trematoda. The life cycle involves small snails living in fresh water (intermediate host) and humans (definitive host). Cercariae are the larval and infective forms released by infected snails. They swim and penetrate the skin of humans through water contact. After invasion, cercariae differentiate into schistosomula which migrate via the blood and lymphatics into the lung then to the liver, differentiate into male and female adult worms, and live for years attached to mesenteric veins. In particular, *S.mansoni* infects humans and primates, and hundreds of eggs are released daily by females, half of which pass through the intestinal wall, enter the lumen and are eliminated with feces (Nyindo and Farah, 1999). When reaching fresh water, eggs hatch and release their embryo (miracidium), a free-swimming larval form which will penetrate the snails and reproduce asexually in them. Eggs that are not eliminated with feces remain within the intestinal wall or are carried by the blood into the liver where they provoke a granulomatous focus with inflammatory reaction and fibrosis that is responsible for the pathological aspects of schistosomiasis.

The immune protective response is directed against schistosomulae and involves the complement system, the humoral response with the production of specific IgE and IgG antibodies, and the cellular response with a variety of effector cells such as eosinophils, macrophages and platelets (Capron *et al.*, 1999). Macrophage-mediated protective effects are closely related to those already described for protozoan parasites.

6.1 Nitric oxide and infection control

IFN-γ-activated murine macrophages are able to kill schitosomulae *in vitro* via TNF-α endogenous synthesis and subsequent production of NO (James and Glaven, 1989; Oswald *et al.*, 1992b; James *et al.*, 1998). Enzymes containing catalytically active Fe–S groups are the main targets of NO (see Section 2.5) (James and Hibbs, 1990). Indeed, killing of schistosomulae by activated macrophages is inhibited by the addition of iron in excess, or inhibitors of NO synthesis or anti-TNF-α neutralizing antibodies (James and Glaven, 1989). Furthermore, cytokines such as IL-4, IL-10 and TGF-β also inhibit the protective effect of NO, while IL-12 promotes this effect (Wynn *et al.*, 1996). Similar conclusions are reached when studying the immune response in murine models of infection using mice vaccinated or not with irradiated cercariae (James *et al.*, 1984, 1998; Gazzinelli *et al.*, 1992a; Oswald *et al.*, 1992a,b, 1998; Williams *et al.*, 1995). Similarly, human monocyte-derived macrophages can kill schistosomulae when activated with IFN-γ (Cottrell *et al.*, 1989; James *et al.*, 1990).

6.2 Antibody-dependent cell-mediated cytotoxicity (ADCC)

Macrophages exert a cytotoxic action against schistosomulae mainly through ADCC (Capron *et al.*, 1975; Vignali *et al.*, 1990). However, in addition to antibody–FcR interaction, receptor–ligand (lectin–sugar) interactions are also involved in ADCC. Macrophages interact with *S.mansoni* larvae through adhesion molecules [the β_2 integrin Mac-1 (CD11b/CD18), L-selectin (CD62-L) and the carbohydrate determinant sialyl Lewis(x) (sLe(x); sCD15)]. From the schistosomula surface, counter-receptors sharing common motifs with the mammalian selectin-carbohydrate families are also involved in ADCC (Trottein *et al.*, 1997) .

6.3 The many functions of granuloma macrophages

In the course of human and murine *S.mansoni* infection, egg deposition in organs (liver and intestines) and the release of egg antigens induce the formation of granulomas that trigger an inflammatory and a T cell-mediated immune response (Clark *et al.*, 1988). Granulomas are made of eosinophils, fibroblasts, monocytes that differentiate into multi-nucleated giant cells (Silva-Teixeira *et al.*, 1996) and macrophages. Granuloma macrophages not only participate in the building of a barrier, isolating eggs from the surrounding tissues, but they also synthesize various pro-inflammatory cytokines such as TNF-α (Joseph and Boros, 1993). In particular, IL-12 production by LPS-activated macrophages is enhanced by IFN-γ and TNF-α and down-regulated by IL-4 and IL-10 (Chensue *et al.*, 1995). In addition, various effector molecules are also implicated in granuloma formation: adhesion molecules (Jacobs *et al.*, 1998b), and chemokines MIP-1 α (Gao *et al.*, 1997) and MCP-1 (Lu *et al.*, 1998). In particular, a recent report indicates that peripheral blood mononuclear cells from schistosomiasis patients react with beads covered with *S.mansoni* antigens. In this *in vitro* granuloma model, NO production decreases the granuloma formation index while this index is augmented in the presence of NAME. At least one chemokine (MIP-1 α) seems to be involved in this process since its level is increased when NO production is inhibited with L-NAME. On the other hand, IL-10 secretion is decreased in the presence of NAME (Oliveira *et al.*, 1999).

Finally, the granuloma macrophages synthesize somatostatin, which decreases IFN-γ secretion. Somatostatin synthesis is down-regulated by substance P. LPS-, IFN-γ- or IL-10-activated splenic macrophages express somatostatin mRNA, but fail to do so in the presence of substance P in dispersed granuloma cells. IL-4 antagonized the SP effect in the spleen (Blum *et al.*, 1998).

7 Summary

Macrophages play a central role in parasitic infections. Parasitic protozoa take advantage of various molecules to recognize and invade macrophages which become host cells. Many recognition/adhesion systems, steps of cell invasion and escape mechanisms from the phagosome–lysome fusion are now known. These features are potential targets for new chemotherapeutic agents. For instance, inhibition of cysteine proteases could stop the transformation of trypomastigote to amastigote, and also from amastigote to trypomastigote in infected macrophages (Harth *et al.*, 1993; Bromme *et al.*, 1996). A successful treatment of an experimental infection with cruzipain inhibitors indicates that this protease is a target for the development of new chemotherapy (Meirelles *et al.*, 1992; Franke de Cazzulo *et al.*, 1994; Engel *et al.*, 1998; McKerrow *et al.*, 1999). Interestingly, similar observations have been made with *Leishmania* (Mottram *et al.*, 1998b; Barrett *et al.*, 1999). However, cysteine proteases are highly conserved molecules and special attention must be paid to avoid inhibition of host cysteine proteases.

Macrophages are also immunocompetent cells. When suitably activated, they are able to kill parasites or, at least, to limit their spreading. For this, cytokines produced by other immunocompetent cells (T lymphocytes, NK cells) in addition to those produced by DCs and macrophages themselves are of the greatest importance. In particular, cytokines such as IL-10, IL-12, IFN-γ, TNF-α, TGF-β and GM-CSF have emerged and play important roles in various effector mechanisms. New strategies based on immunostimulation have to be tested extensively to improve the effector function of macrophages in correlation with reinforcement of other immunocompetent cells such as DCs and production of potent cytokines as shown in recent studies (Gurunathan *et al.*, 1998; Chaussabel *et al.*, 1999). Macrophages also act as APCs and may reactivate primed CD4 and CD8 T cells. However, parasitic protozoa are able to interfere with this process, and a better understanding of these mechanisms is necessary in order to try to circumvent them.

Parasitic diseases represent a large array of complex public health problems in most developing countries. To combat these debilitating and/or deadly infections, it is essential to act from different starting points but towards converging goals. In addition to the improvement of social and economic status (including information, school attendance, nutrition, housing and drinking water distribution) of exposed people, it is necessary to develop further fundamental research, particularly in the field of immunoparasitology, to develop new tools against these diseases.

Acknowledgments

The author thanks the following colleagues for their interest and for providing encouragement, useful suggestions and critiques during the preparation of this chapter: G. Milon and J.-C. Antoine (Unité d'Immunophysiologie et Parasitisme Intracellulaire, Institut Pasteur, Paris, France); D. Bout (Immunologie des Maladies Infectieuses, UFR Sciences Pharmaceutiques, Tours, France); P. De Baetselier (Laboratory of Cellular Immunology, Vrije Universiteit Brussel, Brussels, Belgium); J. Hoebeke (Immunochimie des Peptides et des Virus, Institut de Biologie Moléculaire et Cellulaire, Strasbourg, France); G. Lalmanach (Enzymologie et Chimie des Protéines, Université F. Rabelais, Tours, France); E. Pays (Parasitologie Moléculaire, Institut de Biologie et de Médecine Moléculaire, Université Libre de Bruxelles, Gosselies, Belgium); and L. Van Overtvelt (Laboratoire d'Immunologie Expérimentale, Faculté de Médecine, Université Libre de Bruxelles, Brussels, Belgium). The help of Iolanda Mazza was greatly appreciated in preparing the manuscript. This work was supported, in part, by a grant 'Action de Recherche Concertée' from Communauté française de Belgique.

References

Abrahamsohn, I.A. and Coffman, R.L. (1995). Cytokine and nitric oxide regulation of the immunosuppression in *Trypanosoma cruzi* infection. *Journal of Immunology*, **155**, 3955–63.

Adams, L.B., Hibbs, J.B., Jr, Taintor, R.R. and Krahenbuhl, J.L. (1990). Microbiostatic effect of murine-activated macrophages for *Toxoplasma gondii*. Role for synthesis of inorganic nitrogen oxides from L-arginine. *Journal of Immunology*, **144**, 2725–9.

Alexander, J., Coombs, G.H. and Mottram, J.C. (1998). *Leishmania mexicana* cysteine proteinase-deficient mutants have attenuated virulence for mice and potentiate a Th1 response. *Journal of Immunology*, **161**, 6794–801.

Alexander, J., Satoskar, A.R. and Russell, D.G. (1999). *Leishmania* species: models of intracellular parasitism. *Journal of Cell Science*, **112**, 2993–3002.

Aliberti, J.C., Cardoso, M.A., Martins, G.A., Gazzinelli, R.T., Vieira, L.Q. and Silva, J.S. (1996). Interleukin-12 mediates resistance to *Trypanosoma cruzi* in mice and is produced by murine macrophages in response to live trypomastigotes. *Infection and Immunity*, **64**, 1961–7.

Aliberti, J.C., Machado, F.S., Souto, J.T., Campanelli, A.P., Teixeira, M.M., Gazzinelli, R.T. *et al.* (1999a). β-Chemokines enhance parasite uptake and promote nitric oxide-dependent microbiostatic activity in murine inflammatory macrophages infected with *Trypanosoma cruzi*. *Infection and Immunity*, **67**, 4819–26.

Aliberti, J.C., Machado, F.S., Gazzinelli, R.T., Teixeira, M.M. and Silva, J.S. (1999b). Platelet-activating factor induces nitric oxide synthesis in *Trypanosoma cruzi*-infected macrophages and mediates resistance to parasite infection in mice. *Infection and Immunity*, **67**, 2810–4.

Allen, J.E. and Maizels, R.M. (1997). Th1–Th2: reliable paradigm or dangerous dogma? *Immunology Today*, **18**, 387–92.

Andrews, N.W. and Whitlow, M.B. (1989). Secretion by *Trypanosoma cruzi* of a hemolysin active at low pH. *Molecular and Biochemical Parasitology*, **33**, 249–56.

Antoine, J.C., Prina, E., Lang, T. and Courret, N. (1998). The biogenesis and properties of the parasitophorous vacuoles that harbour *Leishmania* in murine macrophages. *Trends in Microbiology*, **6**, 392–401.

Antoine, J.C., Lang, T., Prina, E., Courret, N. and Hellio, R. (1999). H-2M molecules, like MHC class II molecules, are targeted to parasitophorous vacuoles of *Leishmania*-infected macrophages and internalized by amastigotes of *L. amazonensis* and *L. mexicana*. *Journal of Cell Science*, **112**, 2559–70.

Araujo-Jorge, T.C. (1989). The biology of *Trypanosoma cruzi*–macrophage interaction. *Memorial Institute Oswaldo Cruz*, **84**, 441–62.

Araujo-Jorge, T.C. and De Souza, W. (1988). Interaction of *Trypanosoma cruzi* with macrophages. Involvement of surface galactose and *N*-acetyl-D-galactosamine residues on the recognition process. *Acta Tropica*, **45**, 127–36.

Araujo-Jorge, T.C., de Meirelles, M.D. and Isaac, L. (1990). *Trypanosoma cruzi*: killing and enhanced uptake by resident peritoneal macrophages treated with α-2-macroglobulin. *Parasitology Research*, **76**, 545–52.

Araujo-Jorge, T.C., Lage, M.J., Rivera, M.T., Carlier, Y. and Van Leuven, F. (1992). *Trypanosoma cruzi*: enhanced α-macroglobulin levels correlate with the resistance of BALB/cj mice to acute infection. *Parasitology Research*, **78**, 215–21.

Araujo-Jorge, T., Rivera, M.T., el Bouhdidi, A., Daeron, M. and Carlier, Y. (1993). An FcγRII, FcγRIII-specific monoclonal antibody (2.4G2) decreases acute *Trypanosoma cruzi* infection in mice. *Infection and Immunity*, **61**, 4925–8.

Assreuy, J., Cunha, F.Q., Epperlein, M., Noronha-Dutra, A., O'Donnell, C.A. and Liew, F.Y. *et al.* (1994). Production of nitric oxide and superoxide by activated macrophages and killing of *Leishmania major*. *European Journal of Immunology*, **24**, 672–6.

Avila, J.L., Rojas, M. and Galili, U. (1989). Immunogenic Gal α1–3Gal carbohydrate epitopes are present on pathogenic American *Trypanosoma* and *Leishmania*. *Journal of Immunology*, **142**, 2828–34.

Banchereau, J. and Steinman, R.M. (1998). Dendritic cells and the control of immunity. *Nature*, **392**, 245–52.

Banchereau, J., Pulendran, B., Steinman, R. and Palucka, K. (2000). Will the making of plasmacytoid dendritic cells *in vitro* help unravel their mysteries? *Journal of Experimental Medicine*, **192**, F39–44.

Barral, A., Teixeira, M., Reis, P., Vinhas, V., Costa, J., Lessa, H. *et al.* (1995). Transforming growth factor-β in human cutaneous *leishmaniasis*. *American Journal of Pathology*, **147**, 947–54.

Barral-Netto, M., Badaro, R., Barral, A., Almeida, R.P., Santos, S.B., Badaro, F. *et al.* (1991). Tumor necrosis factor (cachectin) in human visceral *leishmaniasis*. *Journal of Infectious Diseases*, **163**, 853–7.

Barral-Netto, M., Barral, A., Brownell, C.E., Skeiky, Y.A., Ellingsworth, L.R., Twardzik, D.R. *et al.* (1992). Transforming growth factor-β in *leishmanial* infection: a parasite escape mechanism. *Science*, **257**, 545–8.

Barrett, M.P., Mottram, J.C. and Coombs, G.H. (1999). Recent advances in identifying and validating drug targets in trypanosomes and *leishmanias*. *Trends in Microbiology*, **7**, 82–8.

Basu, A., Chakrabarti, G., Saha, A. and Bandyopadhyay, S. (2000). Modulation of CD11C⁺ splenic dendritic cell functions in murine visceral *leishmaniasis*: correlation with parasite replication in the spleen. *Immunology*, **99**, 305–13.

Beaman, M.H., Subauste, C.S., Wong, S.Y. and Remington, J.S. (1994). *Toxoplasma*–macrophage interactions. *Immunology Series*, **60**, 475–93.

Bell, D., Young, J.W. and Banchereau, J. (1999). Dendritic cells. *Advances in Immunology*, **72**, 255–324.

Beschin, A., Brys, L., Magez, S., Radwanska, M. and De Baetselier, P. (1998). *Trypanosoma brucei* infection elicits nitric oxide-dependent and nitric oxide-independent suppressive mechanisms. *Journal of Leukocyte Biology*, **63**, 429–39.

Black, M.W. and Boothroyd, J.C. (2000). Lytic cycle of *Toxoplasma gondii*. *Microbiology and Molecular Biology Reviews*, **64**, 607–23.

Beschin, A., Bilej, M., Brys, L., Torreele, E., Lucas, R., Magez, S. *et al.* (1999). Convergent evolution of cytokines. *Nature*, **400**, 627–8.

Blackwell, J.M., Searle, S., Goswami, T. and Miller, E.N. (2000) Understanding the multiple functions of Nramp1. *Microbes and Infections*, **2**, 1–5.

Blum, A.M., Elliott, D.E., Metwali, A., Li, J., Qadir, K. and Weinstock, J.V. (1998). Substance P regulates somatostatin expression in inflammation. *Journal of Immunology*, **161**, 6316–22.

Bogdan, C. and Rollinghoff, M. (1998). The immune response to *Leishmania*: mechanisms of parasite control and evasion. *International Journal of Parasitology*, **28**, 121–34.

Bogdan, C. and Rollinghoff, M. (1999). How do protozoan parasites survive inside macrophages? *Parasitology Today*, **15**, 22–8.

Bogdan, C., Rollinghoff, M. and Diefenbach, A. (2000a). Reactive oxygen and reactive nitrogen intermediates in innate and specific immunity. *Current Opinion in Microbiology*, **12**, 64–76.

Bogdan, C., Rollinghoff, M. and Diefenbach, A. (2000b). The role of nitric oxide in innate immunity. *Immunology Reviews*, **173**, 17–26.

Bonay, P. and Fresno, M. (1995). Characterization of carbohydrate binding proteins in *Trypanosoma cruzi*. *Journal of Biological Chemistry*, **270**, 11062–70.

Bourguin, I., Moser, M., Buzoni-Gatel, D., Tielemans, F., Bout, D., Urbain, J. *et al.* (1998). Murine dendritic cells pulsed *in vitro* with *Toxoplasma gondii* antigens induce protective immunity *in vivo*. *Infection and Immunity*, **66**, 4867–74.

Bretana, A., Avila, J.L., Arias-Flores, M., Contreras, M. and Tapia, F.J. (1986). *Trypanosoma cruzi* and American *Leishmania* spp: immunocytochemical localization of a laminin-like protein in the plasma membrane. *Experimental Parasitology*, **61**, 168–175.

Bretana, A., Avila, J.L., Contreras-Bretana, M. and Tapia, F.J. (1992). American *Leishmania* spp. and *Trypanosoma cruzi*: galactosyl α(1–3) galactose epitope localization by colloidal gold immunocytochemistry and lectin cytochemistry. *Experimental Parasitology*, **74**, 27–37.

Brittingham, A., Morrison, C.J., McMaster, W.R., McGwire, B.S., Chang, K.P. and Mosser, D.M. (1995). Role of the *Leishmania* surface protease gp63 in complement fixation, cell adhesion, and resistance to complement-mediated lysis. *Journal of Immunology*, **155**, 3102–111.

Brittingham, A., Chen, G., McGwire, B.S., Chang, K.P. and Mosser,D.M. (1999). Interaction of *Leishmania* gp63 with cellular receptors for fibronectin. *Infection and Immunity*, **67**, 4477–84.

Bromme, D., Klaus, J.L., Okamoto, K., Rasnick, D. and Palmer, J.T. (1996). Peptidyl vinyl sulphones: a new class of potent and selective cysteine protease inhibitors: S2P2 specificity of human cathepsin O2 in comparison with cathepsins S and L. *Biochemical Journal*, **315**, 85–9.

Brooks, D.R., Tetley, L., Coombs, G.H. and Mottram, J.C. (2000). Processing and trafficking of cysteine proteases in *Leishmania mexicana*. *Journal of Cell Science*, **113**, 4035–41.

Buckner, F.S., Wipke, B.T. and Van Voorhis, W.C. (1997). *Trypanosoma cruzi* infection does not impair major histocompatibility complex class I presentation of antigen to cytotoxic T lymphocytes. *European Journal of Immunology*, **27**, 2541–8.

Burleigh, B.A. and Andrews, N.W. (1998). Signaling and host cell invasion by *Trypanosoma cruzi*. *Current Opinion in Microbiology*, **1**, 461–5.

Butcher, B.A., Sklar, L.A., Seamer, L.C. and Glew, R.H. (1992). Heparin enhances the interaction of infective *Leishmania donovani* promastigotes with mouse peritoneal macrophages. A fluorescence flow cytometric analysis. *Journal of Immunology*, **148**, 2879–86.

Caler, E.V., Morty, R.E., Burleigh, B.A. and Andrews, N.W. (2000). Dual role of signaling pathways leading to Ca(2+) and cyclic AMP elevation in host cell invasion by *Trypanosoma cruzi*. *Infection and Immunity*, **68**, 6602–10.

Capron, A., Dessaint, J.P., Capron, M. and Bazin, H. (1975). Specific IgE antibodies in immune adherence of normal macrophages to *Schistosoma mansoni* schistosomules. *Nature*, **253**, 474–5.

Capron, A., Dombrowicz, D. and Capron, M. (1999). Regulation of the immune response in experimental and human schistosomiasis: the limits of an attractive paradigm. *Microbes and Infection*, **1**, 485–490.

Carrera, L., Gazzinelli, R.T., Badolato, R., Hieny, S., Muller, W., Kuhn, R. *et al.* (1996). *Leishmania* promastigotes selectively inhibit interleukin 12 induction in bone marrow-derived macrophages from susceptible and resistant mice. *Journal of Experimental Medicine*, **183**, 515–26.

Carruthers, V.B. and Sibley, L.D. (1997). Sequential protein secretion from three distinct organelles of *Toxoplasma gondii* accompanies invasion of human fibroblasts. *European Journal of Cell Biology*, **73**, 114–23.

Caulada-Benedetti, Z., Vecchio, L.C., Pardi, C.C., Massironi, S.M., D'Imperio Lima, M.R. and Abrahamsohn, I.A. (1998). Activation of CD4+ and CD8+ parasite-specific T-cells by macrophages infected with live *T. cruzi* amastigotes. *Immunology Letters*, **63**, 97–105.

Cerrone, M.C., Ritter, D.M. and Kuhn, R.E. (1992). Effect of antigen-specific T helper cells or interleukin-2 on suppressive ability of macrophage subsets detected in spleens of *Trypanosoma cruzi*-infected mice as determined by limiting dilution–partition analysis. *Infection and Immunity*, **60**, 1489–98.

Cesbron-Delauw, M.F., Tomavo, S., Beauchamps, P., Fourmaux, M.P., Camus, D., Capron, A. *et al.* (1994). Similarities between the primary structures of two distinct major surface proteins of *Toxoplasma gondii*. *Journal of Biological Chemistry*, **269**, 16217–22.

Chang, H.R., Grau, G.E. and Pechere, J.C. (1990). Role of TNF and IL-1 in infections with *Toxoplasma gondii*. *Immunology*, **69**, 33–37.

Channon, J.Y. and Kasper, L.H. (1996). *Toxoplasma gondii*-induced immune suppression by human peripheral blood monocytes: role of γ interferon. *Infection and Immunity*, **64**, 1181–9.

Channon, J.Y., Seguin, R.M. and Kasper, L.H. (2000). Differential infectivity and division of *Toxoplasma gondii* in human peripheral blood leukocytes. *Infection and Immunity*, **68**, 4822–6.

Chaussabel, D., Jacobs, F., de Jonge, J., de Veerman, M., Carlier, Y., Thielemans, K. *et al.* (1999). CD40 ligation prevents *Trypanosoma cruzi* infection through interleukin-12 upregulation. *Infection and Immunity*, **67**, 1929–1934.

Chensue, S.W., Ruth, J.H., Warmington, K., Lincoln, P. and Kunkel, S.L. (1995). *In vivo* regulation of macrophage IL-12 production during type 1 and type 2 cytokine-mediated granuloma formation. *Journal of Immunology*, **155**, 3546–51.

Clark, C.R., Chen, B.D. and Boros, D.L. (1988). Macrophage progenitor cell and colony-stimulating factor production during granulomatous schistosomiasis mansoni in mice. *Infection and Immunity*, **56**, 2680–5.

Conceicao-Silva, F., Hahne, M., Schroter, M., Louis, J. and Tschopp, J. (1998). The resolution of lesions induced by *Leishmania major* in mice requires a functional Fas (APO-1, CD95) pathway of cytotoxicity. *European Journal of Immunology*, **28**, 237–45.

Corradin, S.B., Fasel, N., Buchmuller-Rouiller, Y., Ransijn, A., Smith, J. and Mauel, J. (1993). Induction of macrophage nitric oxide production by interferon-γ and tumor necrosis factor-α is enhanced by interleukin-10. *European Journal of Immunology*, **23**, 2045–8.

Costa, F., Pereira-Chioccola, V.L., Ribeirao, M., Schenkman, S. and Rodrigues, M.M. (1999). *Trans*-sialidase delivered as a naked DNA vaccine elicits an immunological response similar to a *Trypanosoma cruzi* infection. *Brazilian Journal of Medical and Biological Research*, **32**, 235–9.

Cottrell, B.J., Pye, C., Glauert, A.M. and Butterworth, A.E. (1989). Human macrophage-mediated cytotoxicity of *Schistosoma mansoni*. Functional and structural features of the effector cells. *Journal of Cell Science*, **94**, 733–41.

Courret, N., Prina, E., Mougneau, E., Saraiva, E.M., Sacks, D.L., Glaichenhaus, N. *et al.* (1999). Presentation of the *Leishmania* antigen LACK by infected macrophages is dependent upon the virulence of the phagocytosed parasites. *European Journal of Immunology*, **29**, 762–73.

Coutinho, C.M., Cavalcanti, G., DaMatta, .A., Van Leuven, F. and Araujo-Jorge, T.C. (1998). α-2-Macroglobulin receptor is differently expressed in peritoneal macrophages from C3H and C57/B16 mice and up-regulated during *Trypanosoma cruzi* infection. *Tissue and Cell*, **30**, 407–15.

Culley, F.J., Harris, R.A., Kaye, P.M., McAdam, K.P. and Raynes, J.G. (1996). C-reactive protein binds to a novel ligand on *Leishmania donovani* and increases uptake into human macrophages. *Journal of Immunology*, **156**, 4691–6.

Da Silva, R.P., Hall, B.F., Joiner, K.A. and Sacks, D.L. (1989). CR1, the C3b receptor, mediates binding of infective *Leishmania major* metacyclic promastigotes to human macrophages. *Journal of Immunology*, **143**, 617–22.

Darji, A., Beschin, A., Sileghem, M., Heremans, H., Brys, L. and De Baetselier, P. (1996). *In vitro* simulation of immunosuppression caused by *Trypanosoma brucei*: active involvement of γ interferon and tumor necrosis factor in the pathway of suppression. *Infection and Immunity*, **64**, 1937–43.

de Diego, J., Punzon, C., Duarte, M. and Fresno, M. (1997). Alteration of macrophage function by a *Trypanosoma cruzi* membrane mucin. *Journal of Immunology*, **159**, 4983–9.

Dempsey, W.L. and Mansfield, J.M. (1983). Lymphocyte function in experimental African try-panosomiasis. V. Role of antibody and the mononuclear phagocyte system in variant-specific immunity. *Journal of Immunology*, **130**, 405–411.

Denham, S. and Rowland, I.J. (1992). Inhibition of the reactive proliferation of lymphocytes by activated macrophages: the role of nitric oxide. *Clinical and Experimental Immunology*, **87**, 157–162.

Desjardins, M. and Descoteaux, A. (1997). Inhibition of phagolysosomal biogenesis by the *Leishmania* lipophosphoglycan. *Journal of Experimental Medicine*, **185**, 2061–8.

Dobrowolski, J.M., Carruthers, V.B. and Sibley, L.D. (1997). Participation of myosin in gliding motility and host cell invasion by *Toxoplasma gondii*. *Molecular Microbiology*, **26**, 163–73.

Doherty, T.M. and Coffman, R.L. (1999). Ability of macrophage subsets to transfer resistance to murine *Leishmania*sis is dependent on IL-12 production. *European Journal of Immunology*, **29**, 522–9.

Dominguez, M. and Torano, A. (1999). Immune adherence-mediated opsonophagocytosis: the mechanism of *Leishmania* infection. *Journal of Experimental Medicine*, **189**, 25–35.

DosReis, G.A. (1997). Cell-mediated immunity in experimental *Trypanosoma cruzi* infection. *Parasitology Today*, **13**, 335–42.

Dubremetz, J.F. (1998). Host cell invasion by *Toxoplasma gondii*. *Trends in Microbiology*, **6**, 27–30.

Dugas, B., Mossalayi, M.D., Damais, C. and Kolb, J.P. (1995). Nitric oxide production by human monocytes: evidence for a role of CD23. *Immunology Today*, **16**, 574–80.

el Bouhdidi, A., Truyens, C., Rivera, M.T., Bazin, H. and Carlier, Y. (1994). *Trypanosoma cruzi* infection in mice induces a polyisotypic hypergammaglobulinaemia and parasite-specific response involving high IgG2a concentrations and highly avid IgG1 antibodies. *Parasite Immunology*, **16**, 69–76.

Ely, K.H., Kasper, L.H. and Khan, I.A. (1999). Augmentation of the CD8⁺ T cell response by IFN-γ in IL-12-deficient mice during *Toxoplasma gondii* infection. *Journal of Immunology*, **162**, 5449–54.

Engel, J.C., Doyle, P.S., Hsieh, I. and McKerrow, J.H. (1998). Cysteine protease inhibitors cure an experimental *Trypanosoma cruzi* infection. *Journal of Experimental Medicine*, **188**, 725–34.

Fagard, R., Van Tan, H., Creuzet, C. and Pelloux, H. (1999). Differential development of *Toxoplasma gondii* in neural cells. *Parasitology Today*, **15**, 504–507.

Fearon, D.T. and Locksley, R.M. (1996). The instructive role of innate immunity in the acquired immune response. *Science*, **272**, 50–3.

Ferguson, M.A. (1999). The structure, biosynthesis and functions of glycosylphosphatidylinositol anchors, and the contributions of trypanosome research. *Journal of Cell Science*, **112**, 2799–809.

Ferlin, W.G., von der Weid, T., Cottrez, F., Ferrick, D.A., Coffman, R.L. and Howard, M.C. (1998). The induction of a protective response in *Leishmania major*-infected BALB/c mice with anti-CD40 mAb. *European Journal of Immunology*, **28**, 525–31.

Fernandez-Gomez, R., Esteban, S., Gomez-Corvera, R., Zoulika, K. and Ouaissi, A. (1998). *Trypanosoma cruzi*: Tc52 released protein-induced increased expression of nitric oxide synthase and nitric oxide production by macrophages. *Journal of Immunology*, **160**, 3471–9.

Flohe, S., Lang, T. and Moll, H. (1997). Synthesis, stability, and subcellular distribution of major histocompatibility complex class II molecules in Langerhans cells infected with *Leishmania major*. *Infection and Immunity*, **65**, 3444–50.

Flohe, S.B., Bauer, C., Flohe, S. and Moll, H. (1998). Antigen-pulsed epidermal Langerhans cells protect susceptible mice from infection with the intracellular parasite *Leishmania major*. *European Journal of Immunology*, **28**, 3800–11.

Franke de Cazzulo, B.M., Martinez, J., North, M.J., Coombs, G.H. and Cazzulo, J.J. (1994). Effects of proteinase inhibitors on the growth and differentiation of *Trypanosoma cruzi*. *FEMS Microbiology Letters*, **124**, 81–6.

Frankova, D. and Zidek, Z. (1998). IFN-γ-induced TNF-α is a prerequisite for *in vitro* production of nitric oxide generated in murine peritoneal macrophages by IFN-γ. *European Journal of Immunology*, **28**, 838–43.

Freire-de-Lima, C.G., Nunes, M.P., Corte-Real, S., Soares, M.P., Previato, J.O., Mendonca-Previato, L. *et al.* (1998). Proapoptotic activity of a *Trypanosoma cruzi* ceramide-containing glycolipid turned on in host macrophages by IFN-γ. *Journal of Immunology*, **161**, 4909–16.

Freire-de-Lima, C.G., Nascimento, D.O., Soares, M.B., Bozza, P.T., Castro-Faria-Neto, H.C., de Mello, F.G. *et al.* (2000). Uptake of apoptotic cells drives the growth of a pathogenic trypanosome in macrophages. *Nature*, **403**, 199–203.

Frosch, S., Kraus, S. and Fleischer, B. (1996). *Trypanosoma cruzi* is a potent inducer of interleukin-12 production in macrophages. *Medical Microbiology and Immunology*, **185**, 189–93.

Frosch, S., Kuntzlin, D. and Fleischer, B. (1997). Infection with *Trypanosoma cruzi* selectively upregulates B7-2 molecules on macrophages and enhances their costimulatory activity. *Infection and Immunity*, **65**, 971–7.

Fruth, U., Solioz, N. and Louis, J.A. (1993). *Leishmania major* interferes with antigen presentation by infected macrophages. *Journal of Immunology*, **150**, 1857–64.

Furtado, G.C., Slowik, M., Kleinman, H.K. and Joiner, K.A. (1992). Laminin enhances binding of *Toxoplasma gondii* tachyzoites to J774 murine macrophage cells. *Infection and Immunity*, **60**, 2337–2342.

Gabius, H.J. (1997). Animal lectins. *European Journal of Biochemistry*, **243**, 543–76.

Galvao-Quintao, L., Alfieri, S.C., Ryter, A. and Rabinovitch, M. (1990). Intracellular differentiation of *Leishmania amazonensis* promastigotes to amastigotes: presence of megasomes, cysteine proteinase activity and susceptibility to leucine-methyl ester. *Parasitology*, **101**, 7–13.

Gao, J.L., Wynn, T.A., Chang, Y., Lee, E.J., Broxmeyer, H.E., Cooper, S. *et al.* (1997). Impaired host defense, hematopoiesis, granulomatous inflammation and type 1–type 2 cytokine balance in mice lacking CC chemokine receptor 1. *Journal of Experimental Medicine*, **185**, 1959–68.

Garg, N., Nunes, M.P. and Tarleton, R.L. (1997). Delivery by *Trypanosoma cruzi* of proteins into the MHC class I antigen processing and presentation pathway. *Journal of Immunology*, **158**, 3293–302.

Gasson, J.C. (1991). Molecular physiology of granulocyte–macrophage colony-stimulating factor. *Blood*, **77**, 1131–45.

Gazzinelli, R.T., Oswald, I.P., James, S.L. and Sher, A. (1992a). IL-10 inhibits parasite killing and nitrogen oxide production by IFN-γ-activated macrophages. *Journal of Immunology*, **148**, 1792–6.

Gazzinelli, R.T., Oswald, I.P., Hieny, S., James, S.L. and Sher, A. (1992b). The microbicidal activity of interferon-γ-treated macrophages against *Trypanosoma cruzi* involves an L-arginine-dependent, nitrogen oxide-mediated mechanism inhibitable by interleukin-10 and transforming growth factor-β. *European Journal of Immunology*, **22**, 2501–6.

Gazzinelli, R.T., Wysocka, M., Hieny, S., Scharton-Kersten, T., Cheever, A., Kuhn, R. *et al.* (1996). In the absence of endogenous IL-10, mice acutely infected with *Toxoplasma gondii* succumb to a lethal immune response dependent on CD4+ T cells and accompanied by overproduction of IL-12, IFN-γ and TNF-α. *Journal of Immunology*, **157**, 798–805.

Giordano, R., Fouts, D.L., Tewari, D., Colli, W., Manning, J.E. and Alves, M.J. (1999). Cloning of a surface membrane glycoprotein specific for the infective form of *Trypanosoma cruzi* having adhesive properties to laminin. *Journal of Biological Chemistry*, **274**, 3461–8.

Gobert, A.P., Semballa, S., Daulouede, S., Lesthelle, S., Taxile, M., Veyret, B. *et al.* (1998). Murine macrophages use ox. *Infection and Immunity*, **66**, 4068–72.

Goerdt, S., Politz, O., Schledzewski, K., Birk, R., Gratchev, A., Guillot, P. *et al.* (1999). Alternative versus classical activation of macrophages. *Pathobiology*, **67**, 222–6.

Gonzalez, J., Ramalho-Pinto, F.J., Frevert, U., Ghiso, J., Tomlinson, S., Scharfstein, J. *et al.* (1996). Proteasome activity is required for the stage-specific transformation of a protozoan parasite. *Journal of Experimental Medicine*, **184**, 1909–18.

Green, S.J., Crawford, R.M., Hockmeyer, J.T., Meltzer, M.S. and Nacy, C.A. (1990). *Leishmania major* amastigotes initiate the L-arginine-dependent killing mechanism in IFN-γ-stimulated macrophages by induction of tumor necrosis factor-α. *Journal of Immunology*, **145**, 4290–7.

Grewal, I.S. and Flavell, R.A. (1998). CD40 and CD154 in cell-mediated immunity. *Annual Review of Immunology*, **16**, 111–35.

Griffin, F.M., Jr, Griffin, J.A., Leider, J.E. and Silverstein, S.C. (1975). Studies on the mechanism of phagocytosis. I. Requirements for circumferential attachment of particle-bound ligands to specific receptors on the macrophage plasma membrane. *Journal of Experimental Medicine*, **142**, 1263–82.

Grimwood, J. and Smith, J.E. (1996). *Toxoplasma gondii*: the role of parasite surface and secreted proteins in host cell invasion. *International Journal of Parasitology*, **26**, 169–73.

Grimwood, J., Mineo, J.R. and Kasper, L.H. (1996). Attachment of *Toxoplasma gondii* to host cells is host cell cycle dependent. *Infection and Immunity*, **64**, 4099–104.

Grosskinsky, C.M., Ezekowitz, R.A., Berton, G., Gordon, S. and Askonas, B.A. (1983). Macrophage activation in murine African trypanosomiasis. *Infection and Immunity*, **39**, 1080–6.

Gruenheid, S. and Gros, P. (2000). Genetic susceptibility to intracellular infections: Nramp1, macrophage function and divalent cations transport. *Current Opinion in Microbiology*, **3**, 43–8.

Gurunathan, S., Prussin, C., Sacks, D.L. and Seder, R.A. (1998). Vaccine requirements for sustained cellular immunity to an intracellular parasitic infection. *Nature Medicine*, **4**, 1409–15.

Gutteridge, J.M., Quinlan, G.J. and Kovacic, P. (1998). Phagomimetic action of antimicrobial agents. *Free Radical Research*, **28**, 1–14.

Hall, B.F. and Joiner, K.A. (1993). Developmentally-regulated virulence factors of *Trypanosoma cruzi* and their relationship to evasion of host defences. *Journal of Eukaryote Microbiology*, **40**, 207–13.

Handman, E. (1999). Cell biology of *Leishmania*. *Advances in Parasitology*, **44**, 1–39.

Harth, G., Andrews, N., Mills, A.A., Engel, J.C., Smith, R. and McKerrow, J.H. (1993). Peptide-fluoromethyl ketones arrest intracellular replication and intercellular transmission of *Trypanosoma cruzi*. *Molecular and Biochemical Parasitology*, **58**, 17–24.

Holscher, C., Kohler, G., Muller, U., Mossmann, H., Schaub, G.A. and Brombacher, F. (1998). Defective nitric oxide effector functions lead to extreme susceptibility of *Trypanosoma cruzi*-infected mice deficient in γ interferon receptor or inducible nitric oxide synthase. *Infection and Immunity*, **66**, 1208–15.

Huang, F.P., Xu, D., Esfandiari, E.O., Sands, W., Wei, X.Q. and Liew, F.Y. (1998). Mice defective in Fas are highly susceptible to *Leishmania major* infection despite elevated IL-12 synthesis, strong Th1 responses, and enhanced nitric oxide production. *Journal of Immunology*, **160**, 4143–7.

Hunter, C.A., Bermudez, L., Beernink, H., Waegell, W. and Remington, J.S. (1995). Transforming growth factor-β inhibits interleukin-12-induced production of interferon-γ by natural killer cells: a role for transforming growth factor-β in the regulation of T cell-independent resistance to *Toxoplasma gondii*. *European Journal of Immunology*, **25**, 994–1000.

Hunter, C.A. and Remington, J.S. (1994). Immunopathogenesis of toxoplasmic encephalitis. *Journal of Infectious Diseases*, **170**, 1057–67.

Hunter, C.A., Ellis-Neyes, L.A., Slifer, T., Kanaly, S., Grunig, G., Fort, M. *et al.* (1997). IL-10 is required to prevent immune hyperactivity during infection with *Trypanosoma cruzi*. *Journal of Immunology*, **158**, 3311–6.

Hynes, R.O. (1992). Integrins: versatility, modulation, and signaling in cell adhesion. *Cell*, 69, 11–25.

Ilg, T. (2000). Proteophosphoglycans of *Leishmania*. *Parasitology Today*, **16**, 489–97.

Ilg, T., Fuchs, M., Gnau, V., Wolfram, M., Harbecke, D. and Overath, P. (1994). Distribution of parasite cysteine proteinases in lesions of mice infected with *Leishmania mexicana* amastigotes. *Molecular and Biochemical Parasitology*, **67**, 193–203.

Jabado, N., Jankowski, A., Dougaparsad, S., Picard, V., Grinstein, S. and Gros, P. (2000). Natural resistance to intracellular infections. Natural resistance-associated macrophage protein 1 (nramp1) functions as a pH-dependent manganese transporter at the phagosomal membrane. *Journal of Experimental Medicine*, **192**, 1237–48.

Jacobs, F., Chaussabel, D., Truyens, C., Leclerq, V., Carlier, Y., Goldman, M. *et al.* (1998a). IL-10 up-regulates nitric oxide (NO) synthesis by lipopolysaccharide (LPS)-activated macrophages: improved control of *Trypanosoma cruzi* infection. *Clinical and Experimental Immunology*, **113**, 59–64.

Jacobs, W., Bogers, J.J., Timmermans, J.P., Deelder, A.M. and Van Marck, E.A. (1998b). Adhesion molecules in intestinal *Schistosoma mansoni* infection. *Parasitology Research*, **84**, 276–80.

James, S.L. (1995). Role of nitric oxide in parasitic infections. *Microbiological Reviews*, **59**, 533–47.

James, S.L. and Glaven, J. (1989). Macrophage cytotoxicity against schistosomula of *Schistosoma mansoni* involves arginine-dependent production of reactive nitrogen intermediates. *Journal of Immunology*, **143**, 4208–12.

James, S.L. and Hibbs, J.B., Jr (1990). The role of nitrogen oxides as effector molecules of parasite killing. *Parasitology Today*, **6**, 303–5.

James, S.L., Natovitz, P.C., Farrar, W.L. and Leonard, E.J. (1984). Macrophages as effector cells of protective immunity in murine schistosomiasis: macrophage activation in mice vaccinated with radiation-attenuated cercariae. *Infection and Immunity*, **44**, 569–75.

James, S.L., Cook, K.W. and Lazdins, J.K. (1990). Activation of human monocyte-derived macrophages to kill schistosomula of *Schistosoma mansoni in vitro*. *Journal of Immunology*, **145**, 2686–2690.

James, S.L., Cheever, A.W., Caspar, P. and Wynn, T.A. (1998). Inducible nitric oxide synthase-deficient mice develop enhanced type 1 cytokine-associated cellular and humoral immune responses after vaccination with attenuated *Schistosoma mansoni* cercariae but display partially reduced resistance. *Infection and Immunity*, **66**, 3510–8.

Joiner, K.A. and Dubremetz, J.F. (1993). *Toxoplasma gondii*: a protozoan for the nineties. *Infection and Immunity*, **61**, 1169–72.

Joseph, A.L. and Boros, D.L. (1993). Tumor necrosis factor plays a role in *Schistosoma mansoni* egg-induced granulomatous inflammation. *Journal of Immunology*, **151**, 5461–71.

Joshi, P.B., Sacks, D.L., Modi, G. and McMaster, W.R. (1998). Targeted gene deletion of *Leishmania major* genes encoding developmental stage-specific leishmanolysin (GP63). *Molecular Microbiology*, **27**, 519–30.

Kalinski, P., Hilkens, C.M., Wierenga, E.A. and Kapsenberg, M.L. (1999). T-cell priming by type-1 and type-2 polarized dendritic cells: the concept of a third signal. *Immunology Today*, **20**, 561–567.

Kane, M.M. and Mosser, D.M. (2001). The role of IL-10 in promoting disease progression in *leishmaniasis. Journal of Immunology*, **166**, 1141–7.

Kato, T., Yamane, H. and Nariuchi, H. (1997). Differential effects of LPS and CD40 ligand stimulations on the induction of IL-12 production by dendritic cells and macrophages. *Cell Immunology*, **181**, 59–67.

Kaushik, R.S., Uzonna, J.E., Zhang, Y., Gordon, J.R. and Tabel, H. (2000). Innate resistance to experimental African trypanosomiasis: differences in cytokine (TNF-α, IL-6, IL-10 and IL-12) production by bone marrow-derived macrophages from resistant and susceptible mice. *Cytokine*, **12**, 1024–34.

Kelleher, M., Moody, S.F., Mirabile, P., Osborn, A.H., Bacic, A. and Handman, E. (1995). Lipophosphoglycan blocks attachment of *Leishmania major* amastigotes to macrophages. *Infection and Immunity*, **63**, 43–50.

Khan, I.A., Matsuura, T. and Kasper, L.H. (1996). Activation-mediated CD4+ T cell unresponsiveness during acute *Toxoplasma gondii* infection in mice. *International Immunology*, **8**, 887–96.

Khan, I.A., Matsuura, T. and Kasper, L.H. (1998). Inducible nitric oxide synthase is not required for long-term vaccine-based immunity against *Toxoplasma gondii. Journal of Immunology*, **161**, 2994–3000.

Kierszenbaum, F. and Howard, J.G. (1976). Mechanisms of resistance against experimental *Trypanosoma cruzi* infection: the importance of antibodies and antibody-forming capacity in the Biozzi high and low responder mice. *Journal of Immunology*, **116**, 1208–11.

Kima, P.E., Soong, L., Chicharro, C., Ruddle, N.H. and McMahon-Pratt, D. (1996). *Leishmania*-infected macrophages sequester endogenously synthesized parasite antigens from presentation to CD4+ T cells. *European Journal of Immunology*, **26**, 3163–9.

Kimsey, P.B., Theodos, C.M., Mitchen, T.K., Turco, S.J. and Titus, R.G. (1993). An avirulent lipophosphoglycan-deficient *Leishmania major* clone induces CD4+ T cells which protect susceptible BALB/c mice against infection with virulent *L.major. Infection and Immunity*, **61**, 5205–13.

Kock, N.P., Gabius, H.J., Schmitz, J. and Schottelius, J. (1997). Receptors for carbohydrate ligands including heparin on the cell surface of *Leishmania* and other trypanosomatids. *Tropical Medicine and International Health*, **2**, 863–74.

Konecny, P., Stagg, A.J., Jebbari, H., English, N., Davidson, R.N. and Knight, S.C. (1999). Murine dendritic cells internalize *Leishmania major* promastigotes, produce IL-12 p40 and stimulate primary T cell proliferation *in vitro. European Journal of Immunology*, **29**, 1803–11.

Krautz, G.M., Kissinger, J.C. and Krettli, A.U. (2000). The targets of the lytic antibody response against *Trypanosoma cruzi. Parasitology Today*, **16**, 31–4.

La Flamme, A.C., Kahn, S.J., Rudensky, A.Y. and Van Voorhis, W.C. (1997). *Trypanosoma cruzi*-infected macrophages are defective in major histocompatibility complex class II antigen presentation. *European Journal of Immunology*, **27**, 3085–94.

Lages-Silva, E., Ramirez, L.E., Krettli, A.U. and Brener, Z. (1987). Effect of protective and non-protective antibodies in the phagocytosis rate of *Trypanosoma cruzi* blood forms by mouse peritoneal macrophages. *Parasite Immunology*, **9**, 21–30.

Lang, T., Prina, E., Sibthorpe, D. and Blackwell, J.M. (1997). Nramp1 transfection transfers Ity/Lsh/Bcg-related pleiotropic effects on macrophage activation: influence on antigen processing and presentation. *Infection and Immunity*, **65**, 380–386.

Langermans, J.A., van der Hulst, M.E., Nibbering, .H. and van Furth, R. (1992a). Endogenous tumor necrosis factor α is required for enhanced antimicrobial activity against *Toxoplasma gondii* and *Listeria monocytogenes* in recombinant γ interferon-treated mice. *Infection and Immunity*, **60**, 5107–12.

Langermans, J.A., van der Hulst, M.E., Nibbering, P.H., Hiemstra, P.S., Fransen, L. and van Furth, R. (1992b). IFN-γ-induced L-arginine-dependent toxoplasmastatic activity in murine peritoneal macrophages is mediated by endogenous tumor necrosis factor-α. *Journal of Immunology*, **148**, 568–74.

Lanzavecchia, A. and Sallusto, F. (2000). Dynamics of T lymphocyte responses: intermediates, effectors, and memory cells. *Science*, **290**, 92–7.

Ley, V., Robbins, E.S., Nussenzweig, V. and Andrews, N.W. (1990). The exit of *Trypanosoma cruzi* from the phagosome is inhibited by raising the pH of acidic compartments. *Journal of Experimental Medicine*, **171**, 401–13.

Li, J., Hunter, C.A. and Farrell, J.P. (1999). Anti-TGF-β treatment promotes rapid healing of *Leishmania major* infection in mice by enhancing *in vivo* nitric oxide production. *Journal of Immunology*, **162**, 974–9.

Liew, F.Y. (1993). The role of nitric oxide in parasitic diseases. *Annals of Tropical Medicine and Parasitology*, **87**, 637–42.

Lima, E.C., Garcia, I., Vicentelli, M.H., Vassalli, P. and Minoprio, P. (1997). Evidence for a protective role of tumor necrosis factor in the acute phase of *Trypanosoma cruzi* infection in mice. *Infection and Immunity*, **65**, 457–65.

Love, D.C., Esko, J.D. and Mosser, D.M. (1993). A heparin-binding activity on *Leishmania* amastigotes which mediates adhesion to cellular proteoglycans. *Journal of Cell Biology*, **123**, 759–66.

Lowenstein, C.J., Dinerman, J.L. and Snyder, S.H. (1994). Nitric oxide: a physiologic messenger. *Annals of Internal Medicine*, **120**, 227–37.

Lu, B., Rutledge, B.J., Gu, L., Fiorillo, J., Lukacs, N.W., Kunkel, S.L. *et al.* (1998). Abnormalities in monocyte recruitment and cytokine expression in monocyte chemoattractant protein 1-deficient mice. *Journal of Experimental Medicine*, **187**, 601–8.

Lucas, R., Magez, S., De Leys, R., Fransen, L., Scheerlinck, J.P., Rampelberg, M. *et al.* (1994). Mapping the lectin-like activity of tumor necrosis factor. *Science*, **263**, 814–7.

Luder, C.G., Lang, T., Beuerle, B. and Gross, U. (1998). Down regulation of MHC class II molecules and inability to upregulate class I molecules in murine macrophages after infection with *Toxoplasma gondii*. *Clinical and Experimental Immunology*, **112**, 308–16.

Lysiak, J.J., Hussaini, I.M., Webb, D.J., Glass, W.F., Allietta, M. and Gonias, S.L. (1995). α2-macroglobulin functions as a cytokine carrier to induce nitric oxide synthesis and cause nitric oxide-dependent cytotoxicity in the RAW 264.7 macrophage cell line. *Journal of Biological Chemistry*, **270**, 21919–27.

Mabbott, N.A., Sutherland, I.A. and Sternberg, J.M. (1995). Suppressor macrophages in *Trypanosoma brucei* infection: nitric oxide is related to both suppressive activity and lifespan *in vivo*. *Parasite Immunology*, **17**, 143–50.

Mabbott, N.A., Coulson, P.S., Smythies, L.E., Wilson, R.A. and Sternberg, J.M. (1998). African trypanosome infections in mice that lack the interferon-γ receptor gene: nitric oxide-dependent and -independent suppression of T-cell proliferative responses and the development of anaemia. *Immunology*, **94**, 476–80.

MacMicking, J., Xie, Q.W. and Nathan, C. (1997). Nitric oxide and macrophage function. *Annual Review of Immunology*, **15**, 323–50.

Magez, S., Lucas, R., Darji, A., Songa, E.B., Hamers, R. and De Baetselier, P. (1993). Murine tumour necrosis factor plays a protective role during the initial phase of the experimental infection with *Trypanosoma brucei brucei*. *Parasite Immunology*, **15**, 635–41.

Magez, S., Geuskens, M., Beschin, A., del Favero, H., Verschueren, H., Lucas, R. *et al.* (1997). Specific uptake of tumor necrosis factor-α is involved in growth control of *Trypanosoma brucei*. *Journal of Cell Biology*, **137**, 715–27.

Magez, S., Stijlemans, B., Radwanska, M., Pays, E., Ferguson, M.A. and De Baetselier, P. (1998). The glycosyl-inositol-phosphate and dimyristoylglycerol moieties of the glycosylphosphatidyli-nositol anchor of the trypanosome variant-specific surface glycoprotein are distinct macrophage-activating factors. *Journal of Immunology*, **160**, 1949–56.

Magez, S., Radwanska, M., Beschin, A., Sekikawa, K. and De Baetselier, P. (1999). Tumor necrosis factor α is a key mediator in the regulation of experimental *Trypanosoma brucei* infections. *Infection and Immunity*, **67**, 3128–32.

Marovich, M.A., McDowell, M.A., Thomas, E.K. and Nutman, T.B. (2000). IL-12p70 production by *Leishmania major*-harboring human dendritic cells is a CD40/CD40 ligand-dependent process. *Journal of Immunology*, **164**, 5858–65.

Martiny, A., Meyer-Fernandes, J.R., De Souza, W. and Vannier-Santos, M.A. (1999). Altered tyrosine phosphorylation of ERK1 MAP kinase and other macrophage molecules caused by *Leishmania* amastigotes. *Molecular and Biochemical Parasitology*, **102**, 1–12.

Mauel, J. (1996). Intracellular survival of protozoan parasites with special reference to *Leishmania* spp., *Toxoplasma gondii* and *Trypanosoma cruzi*. *Advances in Parasitology*, **38**, 1–51.

Mauel, J., Ransijn, A. and Buchmuller-Rouiller, Y. (1991). Killing of *Leishmania* parasites in activated murine macrophages is based on an L-arginine-dependent process that produces nitrogen derivatives. *Journal of Leukocyte Biology*, **49**, 73–82.

McCabe, R.E. and Mullins, B.T. (1990). Failure of *Trypanosoma cruzi* to trigger the respiratory burst of activated macrophages. Mechanism for immune evasion and importance of oxygen-independent killing. *Journal of Immunology*, **144**, 2384–8.

McConville, M.J., Turco, S.J., Ferguson, M.A. and Sacks, D.L. (1992). Developmental modification of lipophosphoglycan during the differentiation of *Leishmania major* promastigotes to an infectious stage. *EMBO Journal*, **11**, 3593–600.

McKerrow, J.H., Engel, J.C. and Caffrey, C.R. (1999). Cysteine protease inhibitors as chemotherapy for parasitic infections. *Bioorganic Medical Chemistry*, **7**, 639–44.

Medina-Acosta, E., Karess, R.E. and Russell, D.G. (1993). Structurally distinct genes for the surface protease of *Leishmania mexicana* are developmentally regulated. *Molecular and Biochemical Parasitology*, **57**, 31–45.

Meirelles,M.N., Juliano, L., Carmona, E., Silva, S.G., Costa, E.M., Murta, A.C. *et al.* (1992). Inhibitors of the major cysteinyl proteinase (GP57/51) impair host cell invasion and arrest the intracellular development of *Trypanosoma cruzi in vitro*. *Molecular and Biochemical Parasitology*, **52**, 175–84.

Metz, G., Carlier, Y. and Vray, B. (1993). *Trypanosoma cruzi* upregulates nitric oxide release by IFN-γ-preactivated macrophages, limiting cell infection independently of the respiratory burst. *Parasite Immunology*, **15**, 693–699.

Mills, C.D., Kincaid, K., Alt, J.M., Heilman, M.J. and Hill, A.M. (2000). M-1/M-2 macrophages and the Th1/Th2 paradigm. *Journal of Immunology*, **164**, 6166–73.

Milon, G., Belkaid, Y., Moufqia, J., Bosque, F., Colle, J.H. and Lebastard, M. (1996). Mononuclear phagocytes and dendritic leukocytes in the skin. *Clinical Dermatology*, **14**, 465–70.

Mineo, J.R., McLeod, R., Mack, D., Smith, J., Khan, I.A., Ely, K.H. *et al.* (1993). Antibodies to *Toxoplasma gondii* major surface protein (SAG-1, P30) inhibit infection of host cells and are produced in murine intestine after peroral infection. *Journal of Immunology*, **150**, 3951–64.

Ming, M., Chuenkova, M., Ortega-Barria, E. and Pereira, M.E. (1993). Mediation of *Trypanosoma cruzi* invasion by sialic acid on the host cell and *trans*-sialidase on the trypanosome. *Molecular and Biochemical Parasitology*, **59**, 243–52.

Ming, M., Ewen, M.E. and Pereira, M.E. (1995). Trypanosome invasion of mammalian cells requires activation of the TGF β signaling pathway. *Cell*, **82**, 287–96.

Minkoff, H., Remington, J.S., Holman, S., Ramirez, R., Goodwin, S. and Landesman, S. (1997). Vertical transmission of toxoplasma by human immunodeficiency virus-infected women. *American Journal of Obstetrics and Gynecology*, **176**, 555–9.

Moll, H. (1997). The role of chemokines and accessory cells in the immunoregulation of cutaneous leishmaniasis. *Behring Institut Mitteilungen*, 73–8.

Moll, H. and Flohe, S. (1997). Dendritic cells induce immunity to cutaneous *leishmaniasis* in mice. *Advances in Experimental Medicine and Biology*, **417**, 541–5.

Mordue, D.G. and Sibley, L.D. (1997). Intracellular fate of vacuoles containing *Toxoplasma gondii* is determined at the time of formation and depends on the mechanism of entry. *Journal of Immunology*, **159**, 4452–9.

Morisaki, J.H., Heuser, J.E. and Sibley, L.D. (1995). Invasion of *Toxoplasma gondii* occurs by active penetration of the host cell. *Journal of Cell Science*, **108**, 2457–64.

Morrot, A., Strickland, D.K., Higuchi, M.D., Reis, M., Pedrosa, R. and Scharfstein, J. (1997). Human T cell responses against the major cysteine proteinase (cruzipain) of *Trypanosoma cruzi*: role of the multifunctional α2-macroglobulin receptor in antigen presentation by monocytes. *International Immunology*, **9**, 825–34.

Mossalayi, M.D., Arock, M., Mazier, D., Vincendeau, P. and Vouldoukis, I. (1999). The human immune response during cutaneous *leishmaniasis*: NO problem. *Parasitology Today*, **15**, 342–5.

Mosser, D.M. and Brittingham, A. (1997). *Leishmania*, macrophages and complement: a tale of subversion and exploitation. *Parasitology*, **115** Supplement, S9–23.

Mottram, J.C., Brooks, D.R. and Coombs, G.H. (1998a). Roles of cysteine proteinases of trypanosomes and *Leishmania* in host–parasite interactions. *Current Opinion in Microbiology*, **1**, 455–60.

Munder, M., Eichmann, K., Moran, J.M., Centeno, F., Soler, G. and Modolell, M. (1999). Th1/Th2-regulated expression of arginase isoforms in murine macrophages and dendritic cells. *Journal of Immunology*, **163**, 3771–7.

Munoz-Fernandez, M.A., Fernandez, M.A. and Fresno, M. (1992a). Activation of human macrophages for the killing of intracellular *Trypanosoma cruzi* by TNF-α and IFN-γ through a nitric oxide-dependent mechanism. *Immunology Letters*, **33**, 35–40.

Munoz-Fernandez, M.A., Fernandez, M.A. and Fresno, M. (1992b). Synergism between tumor necrosis factor-α and interferon-γ on macrophage activation for the killing of intracellular *Trypanosoma cruzi* through a nitric oxide-dependent mechanism. *European Journal of Immunology*, **22**, 301–7.

Murray, H.W. (1997). Endogenous interleukin-12 regulates acquired resistance in experimental visceral *leishmaniasis*. *Journal of Infectious Diseases*, **175**, 1477–9.

Murray, H.W. and Nathan, C.F. (1999). Macrophage microbicidal mechanisms *in vivo*: reactive nitrogen versus oxygen intermediates in the killing of intracellular visceral *Leishmania donovani*. *Journal of Experimental Medicine*, **189**, 741–6.

Murray, H.W. and Teitelbaum, R.F. (1992). L-Arginine-dependent reactive nitrogen intermediates and the antimicrobial effect of activated human mononuclear phagocytes. *Journal of Infectious Diseases*, **165**, 513–7.

Murray, H.W., Rubin, B.Y., Carriero, S.M., Harris, A.M. and Jaffee, E.A. (1985a). Human mononuclear phagocyte antiprotozoal mechanisms: oxygen-dependent vs oxygen-independent activity against intracellular *Toxoplasma gondii*. *Journal of Immunology*, **134**, 1982–8.

Murray, H.W., Spitalny, G.L. and Nathan, C.F. (1985b). Activation of mouse peritoneal macrophages *in vitro* and *in vivo* by interferon-γ. *Journal of Immunology*, **134**, 1619–22.

Namangala, B., Brys, L., Magez, S., De Baetselier, P. and Beschin, A. (2000a). *Trypanosoma brucei brucei* infection impairs MHC class II antigen presentation capacity of macrophages. *Parasite Immunology*, **22**, 361–70.

Namangala, B., De Baetselier, P., Brijs, L., Stijlemans, B., Noel, W., Pays, E. *et al.* (2000b). Attenuation of *Trypanosoma brucei* is associated with reduced immunosuppression and concomitant production of Th2 lymphokines. *Journal of Infectious Diseases*, **181**, 1110–20.

Nandan, D., Knutson, K.L., Lo, R. and Reiner, N.E. (2000). Exploitation of host cell signaling machinery: activation of macrophage phosphotyrosine phosphatases as a novel mechanism of molecular microbial pathogenesis. *Journal of Leukocyte Biology*, **67**, 464–70.

Nathan, C. and Xie, Q.W. (1994). Nitric oxide synthases: roles, tolls, and controls. *Cell*, **78**, 915–8.

Nickell, S.P., Keane, M. and So, M. (1993). Further characterization of protective *Trypanosoma cruzi*-specific CD4+ T-cell clones: T helper type 1-like phenotype and reactivity with shed trypomastigote antigens. *Infection and Immunity*, **61**, 3250–8.

Noisin, E.L. and Villalta, F. (1989). Fibronectin increases *Trypanosoma cruzi* amastigote binding to and uptake by murine macrophages and human monocytes. *Infection and Immunity*, **57**, 1030–4.

Norris, K.A. (1996). Ligand-binding renders the 160 kDa *Trypanosoma cruzi* complement regulatory protein susceptible to proteolytic cleavage. *Microbial Pathogenesis*, **21**, 235–48.

Norris, K.A. (1998). Stable transfection of *Trypanosoma cruzi* epimastigotes with the trypomastigote-specific complement regulatory protein cDNA confers complement resistance. *Infection and Immunity*, **66**, 2460–5.

Norris, K.A., Schrimpf, J.E., Flynn, J.L. and Morris, S.M., Jr (1995). Enhancement of macrophage microbicidal activity: supplemental arginine and citrulline augment nitric oxide production in murine peritoneal macrophages and promote intracellular killing of *Trypanosoma cruzi*. *Infection and Immunity*, **63**, 2793–6.

Nunes, M.P., Andrade, R.M., Lopes, M.F. and DosReis, G.A. (1998). Activation-induced T cell death exacerbates *Trypanosoma cruzi* replication in macrophages cocultured with CD4+ T lymphocytes from infected hosts. *Journal of Immunology*, **160**, 1313–9.

Nyindo, M. and Farah, I.O. (1999). The baboon as a non-human primate model of human schistosome infection. *Parasitology Today*, **15**, 478–82.

Olivares Fontt, E.O. and Vray, B. (1995). Relationship between granulocyte macrophage-colony stimulating factor, tumour necrosis factor-α and *Trypanosoma cruzi* infection of murine macrophages. *Parasite Immunology*, **17**, 135–41.

Olivares Fontt, E.O., Heirman, C., Thielemans, K. and Vray, B. (1996). Granulocyte–macrophage colony-stimulating factor: involvement in control of *Trypanosoma cruzi* infection in mice. *Infection and Immunity*, **64**, 3429–34.

Olivares Fontt, E.O., De Baetselier, P., Heirman, C., Thielemans, K., Lucas, R. and Vray, B. (1998). Effects of granulocyte–macrophage colony-stimulating factor and tumor necrosis factor α on *Trypanosoma cruzi* trypomastigotes. *Infection and Immunity*, **66**, 2722–7.

Oliveira, D.M., Silva-Teixeira, D.N. and Goes, A.M. (1999). Evidence for nitric oxide action on *in vitro* granuloma formation through pivotal changes in MIP-1 α and IL-10 release in human schistosomiasis. *Nitric Oxide*, **3**, 162–71.

Omer, F.M., Kurtzhals, J.A. and Riley, E.M. (2000). Maintaining the immunological balance in parasitic infections: a role for TGF-β? *Parasitology Today*, **16**, 18–23.

Ortega-Barria, E. and Boothroyd, J.C. (1999). A *Toxoplasma* lectin-like activity specific for sulfated polysaccharides is involved in host cell infection. *Journal of Biological Chemistry*, **274**, 1267–76.

Oswald, I.P., Gazzinelli, R.T., Sher, A. and James, S.L. (1992). IL-10 synergizes with IL-4 and transforming growth factor-β to inhibit macrophage cytotoxic activity. *Journal of Immunology*, **148**, 3578–82.

Oswald, I.P., Wynn, T.A., Sher, A. and James, S.L. (1992). Interleukin 10 inhibits macrophage microbicidal activity by blocking the endogenous production of tumor necrosis factor α required as a costimulatory factor for interferon γ-induced activation. *Proceedings of the National Academy of Sciences USA*, **89**, 8676–80.

Oswald, I.P., Caspar, P., Wynn, T.A., Scharton-Kersten, T., Williams, M.E., Hieny, S.A., *et al.* (1998). Failure of P strain mice to respond to vaccination against schistosomiasis correlates with impaired production of IL-12 and up-regulation of Th2 cytokines that inhibit macrophage activation. *European Journal of Immunology*, **28**, 1762–72.

Ouaissi, M.A., Cornette, J., Afchain, D., Capron, A., Gras-Masse, H. and Tartar, A. (1986). *Trypanosoma cruzi* infection inhibited by peptides modeled from a fibronectin cell attachment domain. *Science*, **234**, 603–7.

Overath, P. and Aebischer, T. (1999). Antigen presentation by macrophages harboring intravesicular pathogens. *Parasitology Today*, **15**, 325–32.

Palatnik, C.B., Previato, J.O., Mendonca-Previato, L. and Borojevic, R. (1990). A new approach to the phylogeny of *Leishmania*: species specificity of glycoconjugate ligands for promastigote internalization into murine macrophages. *Parasitology Research*, **76**, 289–93.

Pays, E. and Nolan, D.P. (1998). Expression and function of surface proteins in *Trypanosoma brucei*. *Molecular and Biochemical Parasitology*, **91**, 3–36.

Pereira, M.E., Zhang, K., Gong, Y., Herrera, E.M. and Ming, M. (1996). Invasive phenotype of *Trypanosoma cruzi* restricted to a population expressing *trans*-sialidase. *Infection and Immunity*, **64**, 3884–92.

Peters, C., Aebischer, T., Stierhof, Y.D., Fuchs, M. and Overath, P. (1995). The role of macrophage receptors in adhesion and uptake of *Leishmania mexicana* amastigotes. *Journal of Cell Science*, **108**, 3715–24.

Petray, P., Castanos-Velez, E., Grinstein, S., Orn, A. and Rottenberg, M.E. (1995). Role of nitric oxide in resistance and histopathology during experimental infection with *Trypanosoma cruzi*. *Immunology Letters*, **47**, 121–6.

Piedrafita, D., Proudfoot, L., Nikolaev, A.V., Xu, D., Sands, W., Feng, G.J. *et al.* (1999). Regulation of macrophage IL-12 synthesis by *Leishmania* phosphoglycans. *European Journal of Immunology*, **29**, 235–44.

Plasman, N., Metz, G. and Vray, B. (1994). Interferon-γ-activated immature macrophages exhibit a high *Trypanosoma cruzi* infection rate associated with a low production of both nitric oxide and tumor necrosis factor-α. *Parasitology Research*, **80**, 554–8.

Plasman, N., Guillet, J.G. and Vray, B. (1995). Impaired protein catabolism in *Trypanosoma cruzi*-infected macrophages: possible involvement in antigen presentation. *Immunology*, **86**, 636–45.

Poupel, O., Boleti, H., Axisa, S., Couture-Tosi, E. and Tardieux, I. (2000). Toxofilin, a novel actin-binding protein from *Toxoplasma gondii*, sequesters actin monomers and caps actin filaments. *Molecular Biology of the Cell*, **11**, 355–68.

Previato, J.O., Jones, C., Xavier, M.T., Wait, R., Travassos, L.R., Parodi, A.J. *et al.* (1995). Structural characterization of the major glycosylphosphatidylinositol membrane-anchored glycoprotein from epimastigote forms of *Trypanosoma cruzi* Y-strain. *Journal of Biological Chemistry*, **270**, 7241–50.

Prina, E., Jouanne, C., de Souza, L.S., Szabo, A., Guillet, J.G. and Antoine, J.C. (1993). Antigen presentation capacity of murine macrophages infected with *Leishmania amazonensis* amastigotes. *Journal of Immunology*, **151**, 2050–61.

Prina, E., Lang, T., Glaichenhaus, N. and Antoine, J.C. (1996). Presentation of the protective parasite antigen LACK by *Leishmania*-infected macrophages. *Journal of Immunology*, **156**, 4318–27.

Prive, C. and Descoteaux, A. (2000). *Leishmania donovani* promastigotes evade the activation of mitogen-activated protein kinases p38, c-Jun N-terminal kinase, and extracellular signal-regulated kinase-1/2 during infection of naive macrophages. *European Journal of Immunology*, **30**, 2235–44.

Puddu, P., Fantuzzi, L., Borghi, P., Varano, B., Rainaldi, G., Guillemard, E. *et al.* (1997). IL-12 induces IFN-γ expression and secretion in mouse peritoneal macrophages. *Journal of Immunology*, **159**, 3490–7.

Puentes, S.M., Sacks, D.L., Da Silva, R.P. and Joiner, K.A. (1988). Complement binding by two developmental stages of *Leishmania major* promastigotes varying in expression of a surface lipophosphoglycan. *Journal of Experimental Medicine*, **167**, 887–902.

Puentes, S.M., Da Silva, R.P., Sacks, D.L., Hammer, C.H. and Joiner, K.A. (1990). Serum resistance of metacyclic stage *Leishmania major* promastigotes is due to release of C5b-9. *Journal of Immunology*, **145**, 4311–6.

Reed, S.G. (1988). *In vivo* administration of recombinant IFN-γ induces macrophage activation, and prevents acute disease, immune suppression, and death in experimental *Trypanosoma cruzi* infections. *Journal of Immunology*, **140**, 4342–7.

Reed, S.G. (1999). TGF-β in infections and infectious diseases. *Microbes and Infection*, **1**, 1313–25.

Reed, S.G., Brownell, C.E., Russo, D.M., Silva, J.S., Grabstein, K.H. and Morrissey, P.J. (1994). IL-10 mediates susceptibility to *Trypanosoma cruzi* infection. *Journal of Immunology*, **153**, 3135–40.

Reichmann, G., Walker, W., Villegas, E.N., Craig, L., Cai, G., Alexander, J. *et al.* (2000). The CD40/CD40 ligand interaction is required for resistance to toxoplasmic encephalitis. *Infection and Immunity*, **68**, 1312–8.

Reiner, S.L. and Locksley, R.M. (1995). The regulation of immunity to *Leishmania major*. *Annual Review of Immunology*, **13**, 151–77.

Rescigno, M., Granucci, F. and Ricciardi-Castagnoli, P. (1999). Dendritic cells at the end of the millennium. *Immunology and Cell Biology*, **77**, 404–410.

Ritter, U. and Moll, H. (2000). Monocyte chemotactic protein-1 stimulates the killing of *Leishmania major* by human monocytes, acts synergistically with IFN-γ and is antagonized by IL-4. *European Journal of Immunology*, **30**, 3111–20.

Rittig, M.G. and Bogdan, C. (2000). *Leishmania*-host–cell interaction: complexities and alternative views. *Parasitology Today*, **16**, 292–7.

Rittig, M.G., Burmester, G.R. and Krause, A. (1998). Coiling phagocytosis: when the zipper jams, the cup is deformed. *Trends in Microbiology*, **6**, 384–8.

Rittig, M.G., Schroppel, K., Seack, K.H., Sander, U., N'Diaye, E.N., Maridonneau-Parini, I. *et al.* (1998). Coiling phagocytosis of trypanosomatids and fungal cells. *Infection and Immunity*, **66**, 4331–9.

Roach, T.I., Kiderlen, A.F. and Blackwell, J.M. (1991). Role of inorganic nitrogen oxides and tumor necrosis factor α in killing *Leishmania donovani* amastigotes in γ interferon-lipopolysaccharide-activated macrophages from Lshs and Lshr congenic mouse strains. *Infection and Immunity*, **59**, 3935–44.

Rodrigues, M.M., Ribeirao, M. and Boscardin, S.B. (2000). CD4 Th1 but not Th2 clones efficiently activate macrophages to eliminate *Trypanosoma cruzi* through a nitric oxide dependent mechanism. *Immunology Letters*, **73**, 43–50.

Rodrigues, V., Jr, Santana,d. S. and Campos-Neto, A. (1998). Transforming growth factor β and immunosuppression in experimental visceral *Leishmania*sis. *Infection and Immunity*, **66**, 1233–6.

Rodriguez, D.C., Kierszenbaum, F. and Wirth, J.J. (1991). Binding of the specific ligand to Fc receptors on *Trypanosoma cruzi* increases the infective capacity of the parasite. *Immunology*, **72**, 114–20.

Romagnani, S. (1997). The Th1/Th2 paradigm. *Immunology Today*, **18**, 263–6.

Russell, D.G. and Talamas-Rohana, P. (1989). *Leishmania* and the macrophage: a marriage of inconvenience. *Immunology Today*, **10**, 328–33.

Russell, D.G., Xu, S. and Chakraborty, P. (1992). Intracellular trafficking and the parasitophorous vacuole of *Leishmania mexicana*-infected macrophages. *Journal of Cell Science*, **103**, 1193–210.

Ruta, S., Plasman, N., Zaffran, Y., Capo, C., Mege, J.L. and Vray, B. (1996). *Trypanosoma cruzi*-induced tyrosine phosphorylation in murine peritoneal macrophages. *Parasitology Research*, **82**, 481–4.

Sacks, D.L. (1992). The structure and function of the surface lipophosphoglycan on different developmental stages of *Leishmania* promastigotes. *Infectious Agents and Disease*, **1**, 200–6.

Scharfstein, J., Schmitz, V., Morandi, V., Capella, M.M., Lima, A.P., Morrot, A. *et al.* (2000). Host cell invasion by *Trypanosoma cruzi* is potentiated by activation of bradykinin B_2 receptors. *Journal of Experimental Medicine*, **192**, 1289–300.

Schenkman, S., Eichinger, D., Pereira, M.E. and Nussenzweig, V. (1994). Structural and functional properties of *Trypanosoma trans*-sialidase. *Annual Review of Microbiology*, **48**, 499–523.

Schneider, P., Ferguson, M.A., McConville, M.J., Mehlert, A., Homans, S.W. and Bordier, C. (1990). Structure of the glycosyl-phosphatidylinositol membrane anchor of the *Leishmania major* promastigote surface protease. *Journal of Biological Chemistry*, **265**, 16955–64.

Schofield, C.J. and Dias, J.C. (1999). The Southern Cone Initiative against Chagas disease. *Advances in Parasitology*, **42**, 1–27.

Seguin, R. and Kasper, L.H. (1999). Sensitized lymphocytes and CD40 ligation augment interleukin-12 production by human dendritic cells in response to *Toxoplasma gondii*. *Journal of Infectious Diseases*, **179**, 467–74.

Sibley, L.D., Mordue, D. and Howe, D.K. (1999). Experimental approaches to understanding virulence in toxoplasmosis. *Immunobiology*, **201**, 210–24.

Silva-Teixeira, D.N., Doughty, B.L. and Goes, A.M. (1996). Human schistosomiasis: modulation of *in vitro* granulomatous hypersensitivity and lymphocyte proliferative response by macrophages undergoing differentiation. *Scandinavian Journal of Immunology*, **44**, 522–9.

Silva, J.S., Twardzik, D.R. and Reed,S.G. (1991). Regulation of *Trypanosoma cruzi* infections *in vitro* and *in vivo* by transforming growth factor β (TGF-β). *Journal of Experimental Medicine*, **174**, 539–45.

Silva, J.S., Vespa, G.N., Cardoso, M.A., Aliberti, J.C. and Cunha, F.Q. (1995). Tumor necrosis factor α mediates resistance to *Trypanosoma cruzi* infection in mice by inducing nitric oxide production in infected γ interferon-activated macrophages. *Infection and Immunity*, **63**, 4862–7.

Smith, J.E. (1995). A ubiquitous intracellular parasite: the cellular biology of *Toxoplasma gondii*. *International Journal of Parasitology*, **25**, 1301–9.

Smith, J.L. (1999). Foodborne infections during pregnancy. *Journal of Food Protection*, **62**, 818–29.

Soong, L., Xu, J.C., Grewal, I.S., Kima, P., Sun, J., Longley, B.J. *et al.* (1996). Disruption of CD40–CD40 ligand interactions results in an enhanced susceptibility to *Leishmania amazonensis* infection. *Immunity*, **4**, 263–73.

Soteriadou, K.P., Remoundos, M.S., Katsikas, M.C., Tzinia, A.K., Tsikaris, V., Sakarellos, C. *et al.* (1992). The Ser–Arg–Tyr–Asp region of the major surface glycoprotein of *Leishmania* mimics the Arg–Gly–Asp–Ser cell attachment region of fibronectin. *Journal of Biological Chemistry*, **267**, 13980–5.

Sousa, C., Sher, A. and Kaye, P. (1999). The role of dendritic cells in the induction and regulation of immunity to microbial infection. *Current Opinion in Microbiology*, **11**, 392–9.

Sousa, C., Yap, G., Schulz, O., Rogers, N., Schito, M., Aliberti, J. *et al.* (1999). Paralysis of dendritic cell IL-12 production by microbial products prevents infection-induced immunopathology. *Immunity*, **11**, 637–47.

Stenger, S., Thuring, H., Rollinghoff, M. and Bogdan, C. (1994). Tissue expression of inducible nitric oxide synthase is closely associated with resistance to *Leishmania major*. *Journal of Experimental Medicine*, **180**, 783–93.

Stevens, D.R. and Moulton, J.E. (1978). Ultrastructural and immunological aspects of the phagocytosis of *Trypanosoma brucei* by mouse peritoneal macrophages. *Infection and Immunity*, **19**, 972–82.

Straus, A.H., Valero, V.B., Takizawa, C.M., Levery, S.B., Toledo, M.S., Suzuki, E. *et al.* (1997). Glycosphingolipid antigens from *Leishmania (L.) amazonensis* amastigotes. Binding of anti-glycosphingolipid monoclonal antibodies *in vitro* and *in vivo*. *Brazilian Journal of Medical and Biological Research*, **30**, 395–9.

Strauss, M., Tejero, F. and Arguello, C. (1993). *Leishmania braziliensis* promastigotes and amastigotes interact differently with host macrophages. *Journal of Submicroscopic Cytology and Pathology*, **25**, 449–54.

Subauste, C.S. and Wessendarp, M. (2000). Human dendritic cells discriminate between viable and killed *Toxoplasma gondii* tachyzoites: dendritic cell activation after infection with viable parasites results in CD28 and CD40 ligand signaling that controls IL-12-dependent and -independent T cell production of IFN-γ. *Journal of Immunology*, **165**, 1498–505.

Subauste, C.S., Wessendarp, M., Sorensen, R.U. and Leiva, L.E. (1999). CD40–CD40 ligand interaction is central to cell-mediated immunity against *Toxoplasma gondii*: patients with hyper IgM syndrome have a defective type 1 immune response that can be restored by soluble CD40 ligand trimer. *Journal of Immunology*, **162**, 6690–700.

Talamas-Rohana, P., Wright, S.D., Lennartz, M.R. and Russell, D.G. (1990). Lipophosphoglycan from *Leishmania mexicana* promastigotes binds to members of the CR3, p150,95 and LFA-1 family of leukocyte integrins. *Journal of Immunology*, **144**, 4817–24.

Tanowitz, H.B., Kirchhoff, L.V., Simon, D., Morris, S.A., Weiss, L.M. and Wittner, M. (1992). Chagas' disease. *Clinical Microbiological Reviews*, **5**, 400–419.

Tardieux, I., Webster, P., Ravesloot, J., Boron, W., Lunn, J.A., Heuser, J.E. *et al.* (1992). Lysosome recruitment and fusion are early events required for trypanosome invasion of mammalian cells. *Cell*, **71**, 1117–30.

Tarleton, R.L. (1988). *Trypanosoma cruzi*-induced suppression of IL-2 production. II. Evidence for a role for suppressor cells. *Journal of Immunology*, **140**, 2769–73.

Tarleton, R.L. and Zhang, L. (1999). Chagas disease etiology: autoimmunity or parasite persistence? *Parasitology Today*, **15**, 94–9.

Tomlinson, S., Pontes de Carvalho, L.C., Vandekerckhove, F. and Nussenzweig, V. (1994). Role of sialic acid in the resistance of *Trypanosoma cruzi* trypomastigotes to complement. *Journal of Immunology*, **153**, 3141–7.

Torre, D., Zeroli, C., Ferrario, G., Pugliese, A., Speranza, F., Orani, A. *et al.* (1999). Levels of nitric oxide, γ interferon and interleukin-12 in AIDS patients with toxoplasmic encephalitis. *Infection*, **27**, 218–220.

Torrico, F., Heremans, H., Rivera, M.T., Van Marck, E., Billiau, A. and Carlier, Y. (1991). Endogenous IFN-γ is required for resistance to acute *Trypanosoma cruzi* infection in mice. *Journal of Immunology*, **146**, 3626–3632.

Trinchieri, G. and Scott, P. (1999). Interleukin-12: basic principles and clinical applications. *Current Topics in Microbiology and Immunology*, **238**, 57–78.

Trottein, F., Nutten, S., Papin, J.P., Leportier, C., Poulain-Godefroy, O., Capron, A. *et al.* (1997). Role of adhesion molecules of the selectin-carbohydrate families in antibody-dependent cell-mediated cytoxicity to schistosome targets. *Journal of Immunology*, **159**, 804–11.

Truyens, C., Rivera, M.T., Ouaissi, A. and Carlier, Y. (1995). High circulating levels of fibronectin and antibodies against its RGD adhesion site during mouse *Trypanosoma cruzi* infection: relation to survival. *Experimental Parasitology*, **80**, 499–506.

Turco, S.J. and Descoteaux, A. (1992). The lipophosphoglycan of *Leishmania* parasites. *Annual Review of Microbiology*, **46**, 65–94.

Van Overtvelt, L., Vanderheyde, N., Verhasselt, V., Ismaili, J., De Vos, L., Goldman, M. *et al.* (1999). *Trypanosoma cruzi* infects human dendritic cells and prevents their maturation: inhibition of cytokines, HLA-DR, and costimulatory molecules. *Infection and Immunity*, **67**, 4033–40.

Vannier-Santos, M.A., Saraiva, E.M., Martiny, A., Neves, A. and De Souza, W. (1992). Fibronectin shedding by *Leishmania* may influence the parasite–macrophage interaction. *European Journal of Cell Biology*, **59**, 389–97.

Vespa, G.N., Cunha, F.Q. and Silva, J.S. (1994). Nitric oxide is involved in control of *Trypanosoma cruzi*-induced parasitemia and directly kills the parasite *in vitro*. *Infection and Immunity*, **62**, 5177–82.

Vester, B., Muller, K., Solbach, W. and Laskay, T. (1999). Early gene expression of NK cell-activating chemokines in mice resistant to *Leishmania major*. *Infection and Immunity*, **67**, 3155–9.

Vieira, L.Q., Hondowicz, B.D., Afonso, L.C., Wysocka, M., Trinchieri, G. and Scott, P. (1994). Infection with *Leishmania major* induces interleukin-12 production *in vivo*. *Immunology Letters*, **40**, 157–61.

Vieira, L.Q., Goldschmidt, M., Nashleanas, M., Pfeffer, K., Mak, T. and Scott, P. (1996). Mice lacking the TNF receptor p55 fail to resolve lesions caused by infection with *Leishmania major*, but control parasite replication. *Journal of Immunology*, **157**, 827–35.

Vignali, D.A., Bickle, Q.D., Crocker, P. and Taylor, M.G. (1990). Antibody-dependent killing of *Schistosoma mansoni* schistosomula *in vitro* by starch-elicited murine macrophages. Critical role of the cell surface integrin Mac-1 in killing mediated by the anti-Mr 16,000 mAb B3A. *Journal of Immunology*, **144**, 4030–7.

Villalta, F., Zhang, Y., Bibb, K.E., Burns, J.M., Jr and Lima, M.F. (1998a). Signal transduction in human macrophages by gp83 ligand of *Trypanosoma cruzi*: trypomastigote gp83 ligand up-regulates trypanosome entry through the MAP kinase pathway. *Biochemical and Biophysical Research Communications*, **249**, 247–52.

Villalta, F., Zhang, Y., Bibb, K.E., Kappes, J.C. and Lima, M.F. (1998b). The cysteine–cysteine family of chemokines RANTES, MIP-1 α, and MIP-1 β induce trypanocidal activity in human macrophages via nitric oxide. *Infection and Immunity*, **66**, 4690–5.

Villegas, E.N., Wille, U., Craig, L., Linsley, P.S., Rennick, D.M., Peach, R. *et al.* (2000). Blockade of costimulation prevents infection-induced immunopathology in interleukin-10-deficient mice. *Infection and Immunity*, **68**, 2837–44.

Voth, B.R., Kelly, B.L., Joshi, P.B., Ivens, A.C. and McMaster, W.R. (1998). Differentially expressed *Leishmania major* gp63 genes encode cell surface leishmanolysin with distinct signals for glycosylphosphatidylinositol attachment. *Molecular and Biochemical Parasitology*, **93**, 31–41.

Vouldoukis, I., Riveros-Moreno, V., Dugas, B., Ouaaz, F., Becherel, P., Debre, P. *et al.* (1995). The killing of *Leishmania major* by human macrophages is mediated by nitric oxide induced after ligation of the FcεRII/CD23 surface antigen. *Proceedings of the National Academy of Sciences USA*, **92**, 7804–8.

Vouldoukis, I., Becherel, P.A., Riveros-Moreno, V., Arock, M., da Silva, O., Debre, P. *et al.* (1997). Interleukin-10 and interleukin-4 inhibit intracellular killing of *Leishmania infantum* and *Leishmania major* by human macrophages by decreasing nitric oxide generation. *European Journal of Immunology*, **27**, 860–5.

Vray, B., De Baetselier, P., Ouaissi, A. and Carlier,Y. (1991). *Trypanosoma cruzi* but not *Trypanosoma brucei* fails to induce a chemiluminescent signal in a macrophage hybridoma cell line. *Infection and Immunity*, **59**, 3303–8.

Wei, X.Q., Charles, I.G., Smith, A., Ure, J., Feng, G.J., Huang, F.P. *et al.* (1995). Altered immune responses in mice lacking inducible nitric oxide synthase. *Nature*, **375**, 408–11.

Williams, M.E., Caspar, P., Oswald, I., Sharma, H.K., Pankewycz, O., Sher, A. *et al.* (1995). Vaccination routes that fail to elicit protective immunity against *Schistosoma mansoni* induce the production of TGF-β, which down-regulates macrophage antiparasitic activity. *Journal of Immunology*, **154**, 4693–700.

Wirth, J.J. and Kierszenbaum, F. (1984). Fibronectin enhances macrophage association with invasive forms of *Trypanosoma cruzi*. *Journal of Immunology*, **133**, 460–4.

Wizel, B., Palmieri, M., Mendoza, C., Arana, B., Sidney, J., Sette, A. *et al.* (1998). Human infection with *Trypanosoma cruzi* induces parasite antigen-specific cytotoxic T lymphocyte responses. *Journal of Clinical Investigation*, **102**, 1062–71.

Wolfram, M., Ilg, T., Mottram, J.C. and Overath, P. (1995). Antigen presentation by *Leishmania mexicana*-infected macrophages: activation of helper T cells specific for amastigote cysteine proteinases requires intracellular killing of the parasites. *European Journal of Immunology*, **25**, 1094–100.

Wolfram, M., Fuchs, M., Wiese, M., Stierhof, Y.D. and Overath, P. (1996). Antigen presentation by *Leishmania mexicana*-infected macrophages: activation of helper T cells by a model parasite antigen secreted into the parasitophorous vacuole or expressed on the amastigote surface. *European Journal of Immunology*, **26**, 3153–62.

Wong, S.Y. and Remington, J.S. (1994). Toxoplasmosis in pregnancy. *Clinics in Infectious Diseases*, **18**, 853–61.

Wynn, T.A., Reynolds, A., James, S., Cheever, A.W., Caspar, P., Hieny, S. *et al.* (1996). IL-12 enhances vaccine-induced immunity to schistosomes by augmenting both humoral and cell-mediated immune responses against the parasite. *Journal of Immunology*, **157**, 4068–78.

Yap, G.S. and Sher, A. (1999). Cell-mediated immunity to *Toxoplasma gondii*: initiation, regulation and effector function. *Immunobiology*, **201**, 240–7

Yap, G., Pesin, M. and Sher, A. (2000). Cutting edge: IL-12 is required for the maintenance of IFN-γ production in T cells mediating chronic resistance to the intracellular pathogen, *Toxoplasma gondii*. *Journal of Immunology*, **165**, 628–31.

Zidek, Z. and Frankova, D. (1999). Interleukin-10 in combination with interferon-γ and tumor necrosis factor-α enhances *in vitro* production of nitric oxide by murine resident paritoneal macrophage. *European Cytokine Network*, **10**, 25–32.

7 *Macrophages and Alzheimer's disease*

K.A. Carlson*, R.L. Cotter*, C.E. Williams,
C.E. Branecki, J. Zheng and H.E. Gendelman

*K.A.C and R.L.C contributed equally to this typescript

1 Introduction

Alzheimer's disease (AD) is a progressive, age-related, neurological disorder character-ized by impairments in memory, learning and behavior. As the most common cause of mental decline and loss of intellectual functioning (dementia) in elderly adults, AD affects over 4 million people in the USA (Martin, 1999) and nearly 14 million people world-wide. The onset of AD occurs often within the seventh to ninth decades of life and eventually leads to dementia. AD-associated complications usually result in death within 10 years of onset (Das and Lal, 1997), leading to approximately 100, 000 deaths per year (Martin, 1999). Although aging is the most significant risk factor for AD, genetic, immune, neurochemical, environmental and other as yet unidentified factors may also play a role in disease onset and progression.

Pathologically, AD is characterized by the presence of amyloid beta (Aβ) deposits, neuritic plaques (NPs), neurofibrillary tangles (NFTs) and neuronal loss in areas of the brain involved in cognition and memory, such as the hippocampus (Lombardi *et al.*, 1998). NPs occur extracellularly and feature a fibrillar amyloid core composed of Aβ, a 39–43 amino acid peptide fragment derived from the amyloid precursor protein (APP) (Iqbal and Grundke-Iqbal, 1991). In contrast, NFTs are intracellular pathological abnormalities that arise when the microtubule-associated protein, tau, becomes hyper-phosphorylated and thereby unable to bind properly to tubulin. Such events lead to the destabilization of microtubules within the neuron and result in the formation of intra-cellular cytoskeletal tangles. In addition to NPs and NFTs, AD is also associated with an immune-mediated inflammatory response that induces the recruitment and activation of mononuclear phagocytes (MPs)—which include perivascular and brain macrophages and microglia recruitment and activation, cytokine production, complement deposition and chronic inflammation. Although the sequence of cellular and molecular events that lead to synaptic loss and neuronal death remain to be elucidated, two distinct, but not mutually exclusive, theories for AD pathogenesis have emerged. The first proposes that neuronal damage is a direct consequence of the insoluble peptide fragment, $A\beta_{1-42}$. The second suggests that neuronal damage is driven indirectly by neurotoxic factors released from immune-activated MPs. This theory proposes that Aβ-containing NPs initiate a cascade of cellular reactions that result in MP activation and trigger an intense inflammatory response. Such activation, when sustained, can lead to the enhanced pro-duction of pro-inflammatory cytokines, chemokines and neurotoxins that affect neural function and survival.

Regardless of the mechanism(s) involved in AD neuropathogenesis—whether elicited directly by the Aβ-containing NPs or indirectly through MP activation and neurotoxin production—pathological examination, as well as *in vitro* biochemical studies, suggest that an inflammatory component is involved in perpetuating the disease process (Haga *et al.*, 1989). Therefore, this review examines the role of MPs in immune-mediated neuro-inflammatory events and the potential impact of such events on the initiation, progression and pathogenesis of AD. First, the genetic and pathological determinants of disease will be discussed. Next, the factors that induce MP secretory products, which result from cell activation, will be discussed relative to disease. Lastly, we will review current laboratory and animal models for AD and propose a unifying hypothesis that describes the potential role of MPs in disease pathogenesis.

2 Alzheimer's disease pathogenesis

AD pathogenesis involves a series of cellular and molecular events that lead to synaptic loss and neuronal death within regions of the brain involved in cognition and memory, such as the hippocampus (Lombardi *et al.*, 1998). Other neuropathological features of the disease include deposition of fibrillar amyloid beta (fAβ), formation of NPs and NFTs, the recruitment and activation of MPs and chronic brain inflammation (Arvin *et al.*, 1996; Markesbery and Mira, 1996). Many of the pathological hallmarks of disease are linked to specific genotypes or mutations associated with AD-related genes. These include: *APP* (chromosome 21), tau (chromosome 17), *presenilin 1* and *2* (*PS1* and *PS2*, chromosomes 14 and 1, respectively), and the apolipoprotein E alleles (*ApoE*, chromosome 19) (Jordan-Sciutto and Bowser, 1998).

2.1 APP, Aβ and neuritic plaques formation

The most widely studied AD-related gene resides on chromosome 21 and encodes APP. A developmentally regulated gene, APP is highly expressed in fetal neurons, yet also remains a transcript in the adult brain (LeBlanc *et al.*, 1991; Sandbrink *et al.*, 1991). While neurons are the primary source (Goedert, 1987), APP is also produced and metabolized to a lesser extent by other cells (microglia, astrocytes and macrophages) and tissues (LeBlanc *et al.*, 1991, 1996; Fuller *et al.*, 1995; Tienari *et al.*, 1997). Involved in the regulation of neuronal–cell or cell–matrix interactions, APP helps modulate neurite and synaptic growth, as well as synaptic plasticity and neuronal survival (Saitoh *et al.*, 1989; Schubert *et al.*, 1989; Milward *et al.*, 1992; Roch *et al.*, 1992; Mucke *et al.*, 1995; Furukawa *et al.*, 1996).

APP processing is mediated through the proteolytic activity of α, β and γ secretases. Currently, there are at least 18 known amyloid peptides, both soluble and insoluble, produced from the differential processing of APP (Citron *et al.*, 1996; Kisilevsky, 1998). Interestingly, at low concentrations, APP has been shown to be neuroprotective (Simon *et al.*, 1989). In contrast, certain mutations in the *APP* gene lead to the increased production of insoluble forms, such as $A\beta_{1-42}$, which are believed to be neurotoxic. Such mutations have been shown to correlate with the rare, early-onset form of AD, known as familial AD (FAD) (Goate *et al.*, 1991; Murrell *et al.*, 1991; Mullan *et al.*, 1992a; Borchelt *et al.*, 1996; Scheuner *et al.*, 1996).

Under abnormal conditions, APP is cleaved at the N-terminus by β-secretase or at the C-terminus by γ-secretase to produce amyloidogenic forms of the Aβ peptide (Haass and Selkow, 1993). Unlike the β- and γ-secretases, α-secretase prevents the formation of Aβ (Esch *et al.*, 1990; Sisodia *et al.*, 1990) by cleaving within the region of APP that contains the Aβ peptide sequence (Lendon and Goate, 1998). This suggests that production of amyloidogenic forms of Aβ could be suppressed by regulating α-, β- and γ-secretase-mediated cleavage of APP.

Importantly, Aβ is believed to contribute to disease pathology in AD through the formation of two distinct types of amyloid plaques, neuritic and diffuse (Sheng *et al.*, 1997; Lendon and Goate, 1998). Found in both normal aging and AD brains, diffuse plaques consist primarily of a non-fibrillar form of amyloid (Haga *et al.*, 1989; Wisniewski *et al.*, 1989). In contrast, NPs consist of an insoluble amyloid core, surrounded by neuronal processes and reactive glial cells (Iqbal and Grundke-Iqbal, 1991). While $A\beta_{1-40}$ is the predominant form of cerebrovascular amyloid (Castano *et al.*, 1996; Citron *et al.*, 1996), and accounts for approximately 90 per cent of the Aβ peptides released from cells in culture (Iwatsubo *et al.*, 1994; Lemere *et al.*, 1996), it is the fibrillar Aβ$_{1-42}$ fragment that comprises 70 per cent of the NP core (Burdick *et al.*, 1992; Jarrett *et al.*, 1993). A major difference between neuritic and diffuse plaques is the presence of reactive astrocytes and activated microglial cells. Although found around and within the neuritic shell of NPs, these cells have not been shown to associate with diffuse plaques (Mrak *et al.*, 1995). As phagocytic cells, MPs may accumulate around developing plaques in an attempt to process or remove Aβ. Unable to phagocytose or digest the insoluble amyloid fibrils associated with the NPs, MPs may become chronically activated, inducing a strong and potentially damaging, neuro-inflammatory response. Such pathological evidence suggests that MPs may play a critical role in AD pathogenesis (Haga *et al.*, 1989).

2.2 Tau, presenilins and neurofibrillary tangles formation

Another gene believed to be involved in the neuropathological abnormalities associated with AD is the *tau* gene. Located on chromosome 17, this gene encodes the microtubule associated protein, tau. Selectively expressed in the nervous system (Andreadis *et al.*, 1996; Thurston *et al.*, 1996), tau normally acts to stabilize microtubules by binding to tubulin. However, when tau becomes hyperphosphorylated, as is the case in AD, it loses its ability to bind to microtubules. This leads to the formation of paired helical filaments (PHFs), which are highly insoluble aggregates of cytoskeletal protein (Alonso *et al.*, 1996). Accumulation of these PHFs leads to the formation of intracellular NFTs and disruption of the neuronal cytoskeleton. Interestingly, the severity of AD correlates more strongly with the number of NFTs than with the number of NPs in the brain (Lendon and Goate, 1998). Unfortunately, the mechanisms underlying tau accumulation and abnormal phosphorylation in AD are not known. Le *et al.* (1997) proposed that tau phosphorylation and cell toxicity could be induced by amyloidogenic forms of Aβ. Recent studies have shown that fAβ is responsible for abnormal phosphorylation of tau. As demonstrated in studies by Geula *et al.* (1998), fAβ injected intracerebrally into Rhesus monkeys induces neuronal cell loss and tau hyperphosphorylation, leading to NFT-like molecules and microglial accumulation. Further support for Aβ-mediated hyperphosphorylation of tau is provided by *in vivo* studies using *APP* transgenic mouse models. In one study, increased tau phosphorylation was observed around NPs associated with dystrophic neurites (Sturchler-Pierrat *et al.*, 1997).

Another set of AD-related genes, *PS1* and *PS2*, may also contribute to NP and NFT formation. Approximately 30 per cent of early-onset FAD pedigrees co-segregate with mutations in *PS1* (Schellenberg, 1995) located on chromosome 14 (Mullan *et al.*, 1992b) and to a much lesser extent with *PS2* located on chromosome 1 (Levy-Lahad *et al.*, 1995). Due to the presence of PS1 staining in NFTs, it has been postulated that PS1 may play a role in tau phosphorylation (Yamada and Takashima, 1997). It appears that PS mutations may also alter APP metabolism and accelerate the production and deposition of fAβ (Borchelt *et al.*, 1996; Duff *et al.*, 1996; Scheuner *et al.*, 1996).

2.3 ApoE and neuronal maintenance

Genetic and epidemiological evidence suggests that the *ApoE* gene plays an important role in determining genetic susceptibility for AD (Saunders *et al.*, 1993; Weisgraber and

Mahley, 1996). Localized on the long arm of chromosome 19 (Pericak-Vance *et al.*, 1991), the *ApoE* gene expresses five different alleles. Three of these allelic variants (ε2, ε3 and ε4) have been shown to differentially affect the age of onset and risk for developing sporadic AD (Lendon and Goate, 1998). Studies have shown that heterozygosity for the *ApoE-ε4* allele leads to a 4-fold increase in the risk for developing AD, while homozygosity for this allele increases the risk by nearly 10-fold. In contrast, the risk for disease is lowered and the age of onset for disease is increased in individuals with the *Apo-ε2* allele (reviewed in Martin, 1999).

Interestingly, differences in the way these allelic variants interact with the neuronal proteins tau and Aβ (Roses, 1997) may explain why individuals with the *ApoE-ε4* allele are more susceptible to disease. For example, it has been demonstrated that hetero- or homozygosity for the apoE-ε4 variant, which is unable to properly bind to tau, correlates strongly with the development of NFTs. In contrast, the apoE-ε3 variant binds strongly to and prevents the hyperphosphorylation of tau. This, in turn, prevents the generation of PHFs, which serve as the primary component of NFTs (Nathan *et al.*, 1994) (Figure 7.1).

Long known for its role in cholesterol transport and lipoprotein metabolism in the periphery, apoE has been shown to have similar functions in the central nervous system (CNS), where it is expressed primarily by astrocytes, microglia and macrophages, and to a lesser extent by cortical and hippocampal neurons (Ji *et al.*, 1993; Fagan *et al.*, 1996; Das and Lal, 1997; Xu *et al.*, 1999). In the brain, apoE plays an important role in neuronal maintenance through its ability to regulate lipid metabolism and cytoskeletal stability (Xu *et al.*, 1999). Part of its role in regulating cholesterol and phospholipid metabolism is to bind to and transfer lipoproteins to the low-density lipoprotein receptors (LDL-Rs) expressed on macrophages, microglia and neurons. In addition to binding lipoproteins, *in vitro* studies have shown that apoE can also bind to or interact with Aβ (Montine *et al.*, 1999) to form apoE–Aβ complexes. Such complexes have been found to accumulate extracellularly in NPs and cerebral vascular amyloid deposits as well as intracellularly in NFTs (Bales *et al.*, 1997). This suggests that apoE may contribute to disease pathogenesis in AD through its interactions with Aβ. In support of this hypothesis, the apoE-ε4 isoform has been shown to enhance both the rate and density of fibril formation when incubated with Aβ *in vitro*. Through such activities, apoE may modulate the onset and/or rate of Aβ deposition and NP formation (Cole *et al.*, 1999). This suggests that apoE-ε4 may act as a 'pathological chaperone' that binds to soluble Aβ, enhances β-pleated sheet formation and leads to Aβ fibril stability (Lendon and Goate 1998).

apoE–Aβ interactions may affect the receptor-mediated reuptake of Aβ by neurons or clearance by macrophages and microglia (Winkler *et al.*, 1999). Support for this theory is provided by studies which demonstrate that lipoprotein carriers, such as apoE, and their receptors on macrophages and microglia help facilitate the accumulation or degradation of Aβ (Cole *et al.*, 1999; Krieger and Herz, 1994; Lucas and Mazzone, 1996). Indeed, both the *ApoE-ε2* and -*ε3* alleles have been shown to be highly effective in clearing Aβ (LaDu *et al.*, 1994).

During CNS injury or disease, deleterious apoE variants may contribute to neuronal injury by disrupting neuronal lipid transport and cytoskeletal stability. For example, Aβ fibrils attached to apoE may form Aβ–apoE complexes that compete with lipid–apoE complexes for binding to the neuronal LDL-R (Roses, 1997, 1998; Roses and Saunders, 1997; Selkoe, 1997; Xu *et al.*, 1999). Such activity could lead to a reduction in intracellu-

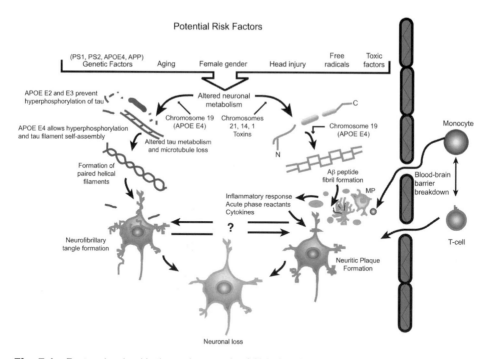

Fig. 7.1 Factors involved in the pathogenesis of Alzheimer's disease (AD). Mutations in the major AD-related genes (*PS1, PS2, ApoE-ε4* allele and *APP*), age, gender, head injury or exposure to abnormal levels of free radicals can predispose individuals to AD. Each of these factors, either alone or in combination, has the potential to alter neuronal metabolism and function. For example, apoE-ε4 can alter neuronal tau metabolism (shown in the counter-clockwise pathway). In healthy neurons, tau forms a complex with microtubules, leading to the stabilization of axons. However, when tau is hyperphosphorylated, it does not bind properly to microtubules. Instead, the hyper-phosphorylated form of tau assembles into PHFs, causing NFT formation and neuronal injury. The apoE-ε2 or -ε3 isoforms bind to dissociated tau and prevent abnormal phosphorylation. However, the apoE-ε4 isoform does not bind dissociated tau, thus allowing the hyperphosphorylation of tau and formation of NFTs. Acting in conjunction with other risk factors for AD, such as mutated *PS1, PS2* or *APP* gene products, the *ApoE-ε4* allele can also cause abnormal APP processing, leading to increased production of the neurotoxic peptide fragment, A β_{1-42} (shown in the clockwise pathway). In turn, the overproduction of this peptide primes resident and peripherally derived MPs for secondary immune activation, leading to the subsequent release of pro-inflammatory cytokines, chemokines and other acute phase reactants that can cause neuronal injury or death. This figure was adapted from Pendlebury and Solomon (1996) *with permission.*

lar neuronal cholesterol levels (Ma *et al.*, 1996) and, in turn, result in impaired neuronal function or death. Interestingly, certain forms of apoE are produced in excess by astrocytes in response to neuronal injury (Roses, 1997). This suggests that in contrast to the deleterious apoE-ε4 variant, other forms of apoE (apoE-ε2 and -ε3) may exert protective effects and support neuronal repair and remodeling (Benjamin *et al.*, 1994; Smith *et al.*, 1994; Talbot *et al.*, 1994; Weisgraber and Mahley, 1996).

As described in the previous sections, APP, Aβ, PS1, PS2, tau and apoE can elicit both direct and indirect effects on AD neuropathogenesis. While the genetic makeup of an individual plays a critical role in determining genetic susceptibility for disease, other factors, including the body's ability to respond to or repair injury caused by such genetic and pathological abnormalities, may also be involved in regulating disease onset and progression. Therefore, the following section examines the role of the immune system in this process and discusses how the recruitment and activation of MP may contribute to the neuro-inflammatory events associated with AD.

3 Immunity and AD: an overview

3.1 AD as an inflammatory disease

Although a variety of genetic, neurochemical (metabolic) and environmental factors appear to be related to AD pathogenesis, pathological examination and *in vitro* biochemical studies suggest that chronic immune activation and brain inflammation play a primary role in perpetuating the disease process (Arvin *et al.*, 1996). As the body's principle defense mechanism against infection or injury, inflammation is important in preventing or repairing damage to the CNS. Such inflammatory processes involve the release of inflammatory mediators, such as chemotactic cytokines and complement components (C5a), which lead to increased blood–brain barrier (BBB) permeability and the recruitment of immune effector cells to sites of tissue injury. These cells, in turn, secrete factors and enzymes that act to eliminate foreign pathogens or repair tissue injury. However, these events may also elicit non-specific injury to surrounding tissue. It has been proposed that such inflammatory processes may underlie or enhance neuropathogenesis in AD. Providing support for this hypothesis, immunohistochemical examination of post-mortem AD brain tissue, as well as *ex vivo* and *in vitro* studies, have shown that a variety of activation markers and inflammatory molecules are significantly elevated in AD brains (Haga *et al.*, 1989; Khachaturian *et al.*, 1994). Included in this list of inflammatory markers are: pro-inflammatory cytokines, complement components, acute phase reactants such as α1-antichymotrypsin (ACT), cell surface activation markers such as the major histocompatibility complex II (MHC II) and the presence of activated macrophages, microglia and lymphocytic infiltrates (Khachaturian *et al.*, 1994; Kalaria *et al.*, 1996a; Aisen, 1997). Interestingly, these inflammatory factors are found in regions of the brain featuring dense NPs and severe neuronal dysfunction (Itagaki *et al.*, 1989). This suggests that immune activation and inflammation play a critical role in the events underlying AD neuropathogenesis. However, the question arises, are these inflammatory molecules present to retard neuronal damage or are they effectors of injury themselves?

3.2 MP recruitment and activation

Found in close association with Aβ-containing NPs, MPs appear to be primary mediators of the inflammatory events involved in AD. However, whether activation of MPs is a primary event in neuronal injury or a reaction to the pathological process remains uncertain. Recruited in response to trauma- (Imamoto and Leblond, 1977), infection, autoimmune reactions (Huitinga *et al.*, 1990) and neurotoxin (metabolic)-related injury (Marty *et al.*, 1991), MPs play a major role in the inflammatory process by phagocytosing cellular debris that results from injury and by secreting growth factors and enzymes involved in repair. Whereas microglia are the resident brain representative of the MP system, monocyte-derived macrophages (MDMs) originate outside of the brain and migrate across the BBB in response to infection or injury. Such recruitment may be mediated through chemokines or other inflammatory factors that promote cellular adhesion and increase BBB permeability, allowing additional immune cells and soluble factors to migrate into the brain *en masse* (Rosenberg *et al.*, 1995). Through interactions between these cells, both infiltrating macrophages and endogenous microglia become immune activated. Activated MPs undergo changes in the expression of a large number of surface and secretory proteins (Eddleston and Mucke, 1993), which enable them to recruit additional leukocytes to sites of tissue injury and engage in a wide range of secretory activities. Unfortunately, as MDM and microglia are acting to defend the brain, they release toxic factors, including reactive oxygen species (ROS), complement proteins and excitotoxins (glutamate), which can cause or intensify neural damage (Akiyama, 1994; Arvin *et al.*, 1996; Chen *et al.*, 1996; Aisen, 1997; McGeer and McGeer, 1998; Xiao and Link, 1998). If not regulated properly, these MP-mediated immune events can contribute to the very pathogenic events they were mobilized to defend against.

Although MP-mediated inflammatory responses are not likely to be the primary cause of AD, they appear to play an important secondary role in disease. Therefore, the mechanisms by which MPs become primed and immune activated, the effects of these immunological events on MP function and the ultimate consequences of these events on neuronal survival will be addressed in the following sections.

4 Mechanisms for MP priming and activation in AD

While NPs and NFTs are both dominant features of AD pathology, they alone are not sufficient to induce the profound neuronal loss and cognitive dysfunction seen in AD. Accumulating evidence suggests that it is the interaction between Aβ and surrounding brain macrophages and microglia that leads to chronic inflammation and neural injury (Haga *et al.*, 1989). However, the mechanisms by which Aβ elicits such effects are unknown. Therefore, the following sections describe potential mechanisms by which Aβ can affect the intracellular signaling events that regulate MP activation and function.

4.1 Aβ primes MP

It has been demonstrated that Aβ can interact with MP receptors, such as the receptor for advanced glycation endproducts (RAGE) or the class A scavenger receptor (SR) (Paresce *et al.*, 1996; Yan *et al.*, 1996). Although RAGE is normally involved in the uptake of advanced glycation endproducts (AGEs), which are formed from the non-enzymatic glycation of lipids and extracellular matrix proteins (Neeper *et al.*, 1992; Schmidt *et al.*, 1992; Brett *et al.*, 1993; Huttunen *et al.*, 1999), this receptor may also aid in the clearance of Aβ in both neurons and MP (Yan *et al.*, 1996, 1997), or play a role in regulating cellular migration and activation in MP (Schmidt *et al.*, 1993; Yan *et al.*, 1996; Mackic *et al.*, 1998). In addition to RAGE, MPs also express other receptors, such as the SRs, which can aid in the clearance of Aβ-containing plaques (Paresce *et al.*, 1996) or transduce signals involved in Aβ-mediated priming and activation.

Presumably, upon engagement of these receptors, Aβ can induce intracellular signaling events that alter the threshold required for cellular activation (Christie *et al.*, 1996; El Khoury *et al.*, 1996, 1998; Paresce *et al.*, 1996; Yan *et al.*, 1996). These signaling events can initiate the accumulation of signal transduction machinery and/or transcriptional factors involved in regulating MP secretory factor production, thus conditioning or 'priming' the MP to respond more strongly to a subsequent immune stimulus (Yan *et al.*, 1996, 1997). Pro-inflammatory cytokines [interleukin (IL)-1 β, tumor necrosis factor-α (TNF-α) and IL-6] released by neighboring glial cells, or interferon-γ (IFN-γ) and CD40L produced by astriaites or lymphocytes traversing the BBB, can stimulate the primed MP to produce inflammatory factors or neurotoxins (Koh *et al.*, 1990; Mattson *et al.*, 1993a; Cotter *et al.*, 1999; Calingasan *et al.*, 2002). Such processes may alter or amplify the normal protective functions of the MP, leading to chronic inflammation, complement deposition, oxidative stress and neuronal injury (Figure 7.2) (Chen *et al.*, 1996; Yan *et al.*, 1996).

4.2 Factors involved in MP activation

By interacting with trafficking immune cells (T cells and peripheral macrophages) or resident brain cells (neurons, astrocytes and endothelial cells), MPs can become immune activated (Figure 7.2). Such activation may be induced by contact with cell surface molecules (CD40L), interaction with inflammatory cytokines (such as IFN-γ) and chemokines, or exposure to abnormal host proteins (Aβ) and other activating agents, such as bacterial lipopolysaccharide (LPS). Although MPs can be activated by such a wide variety of endogenous and/or exogenous stimuli, it is our hypothesis that such activation is mediated primarily through interactions between lymphocytes and other immune cells that traffic in and out of the brain during the course of an immune response. While in normal brain there is only minimal T cell trafficking, during CNS disease the number of T cells traversing the BBB increases in response to infection or injury. Providing support for this hypothesis, activated T cells and their cell-associated antigens have been found to co-localize with reactive microglia in AD brains (Rogers *et al.*, 1988; McGeer *et al.*, 1994; Singh, 1996; Oleana *et al.*, 1998). Such observations suggest that activated T cells or T-cell produced factors may be involved in the immune activation of brain cells during AD (Chabot *et al.*, 1997; Suttles *et al.*, 1999).

A pleiotropic cytokine, IFN-γ plays an important role in immune activation and regulation. Predominantly made by CD4+ and CD8+ T cells and natural killer cells (Young and Hardy 1995), IFN-γ is also produced to a lesser extent by macrophages (Fultz *et al.*, 1993), astrocytes and microglia (De Simone *et al.*, 1998). Important in regulating MP activity, IFN-γ has been shown to induce immune activation, increase MHC and Fc receptor expression, and up-regulate expression of genes for inflammatory cytokines, such as IL-1 α and TNF-α in MPs. In addition, IFN-γ has been shown to enhance the antimicrobial and cytotoxic activity of MPs by stimulating production of ROS, such as nitric oxide (NO) and hydrogen peroxide (H_2O_2). Through such activities, IFN-γ plays an important role in regulating the host immune response to injury or infection. However, if not regulated, the potent stimulatory actions of this cytokine may also elicit adverse effects. For example, IFN-γ may contribute to disease by facilitating BBB breakdown through the up-regulation of adhesion molecule expression (ICAM-1) on endothelial cells. Such IFN-γ-induced events may lead to the recruitment and activation of additional immune cells and trigger a cascade of inflammatory reactions that further damage the surrounding tissue. When used in conjunction with other immune agents, such as Aβ or the inflammatory cytokines TNF-α and IL-1β, IFN-γ can intensify the effects of these factors. For example, IFN-γ greatly enhances Aβ-, TNF-α- and IL-1 β-induced production of NO from microglia and astrocytes (Chao

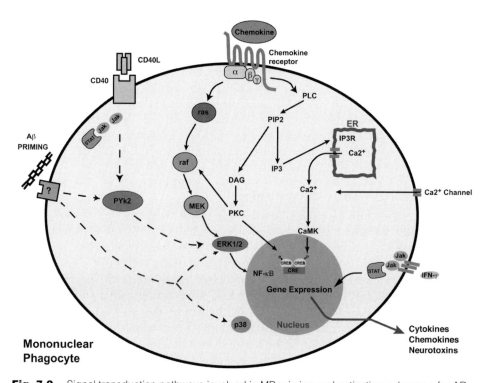

Fig. 7.2   Signal transduction pathways involved in MP priming and activation: relevance for AD. MPs may be primed by A β and secondarily activated by immune stimuli such as CD40L, IFN-γ or other inflammatory cytokines and chemokines. Upon binding to MP receptors (RAGE, SR, CD40 or G-protein-coupled receptors), these factors can initiate a cascade of intracellular signaling events, which result in the accumulation of cytosolic free Ca^{2+} or the activation of protein kinases, such as calcium calmodulin kinase (CaMK), protein kinase C (PKC) or mitogen-activated protein (MAP) kinases. These factors, in turn, can activate transcription factors, such as nuclear factor-κB (NF-κB) or signal transducers and activators of transcription (STATs), which are involved in enhancing or repressing expression of MP genes. For example, A β can activate tyrosine kinase-dependent signaling pathways, including those which involve PKC and the calcium-sensitive protein tyrosine kinase 2 (PYK2). A β-induced signaling can also induce activation of the MAP kinases, ERK1/ERK2 and p38, as well as transcription factors, such as the cAMP response element-binding protein (CREB). Immune activators, such as CD40L, can also initiate MP signaling pathways that lead to the activation of ERK1/2 and NF-κB. In addition, both IFN-γ and CD40L can induce tyrosine phosphorylation of Jaks and the subsequent induction of STATs. Upon activation, STAT proteins translocate to the nucleus where they bind to specific DNA sequences (response elements) and induce transcription of cellular genes involved in secretory factor production. MPs can also be activated by other factors, such as chemokines, which bind to G-protein-coupled receptors and induce a series of serine/threonine kinase events that result in the activation of MAP kinases. By altering or amplifying signaling pathways involved in the modification of enzymes, ion channels and transcriptional activators, A β and other immune activators, such as CD40L, can induce the production of factors involved in inflammatory responses or induce neuronal injury.

et al., 1995a,b; Meda *et al.*, 1995a). Moreover, treatment with IFN-γ in the presence of IL-1β has been shown to potentiate *N*-methyl-D-aspartate (NMDA) receptor-mediated neurotoxicity in murine neuronal cell cultures (Hewett *et al.*, 1994). Thus, as a potent immune activator and regulator, IFN-γ may be involved in initiating MP-mediated inflammation during AD.

Similarly, interactions between CD40L and its membrane-bound receptor, CD40, may also serve as a mechanism for activation of brain MPs during AD. A member of the TNF receptor superfamily, CD40 is expressed on numerous cell types including monocytes, dendritic cells and endothelial cells (Alderson *et al.*, 1993; Caux *et al.*, 1994; Wagner *et al.*, 1994; Mach *et al.*, 1997; Suttles *et al.*, 1999). The ligand for this receptor (CD40L) is expressed in both cell membrane-bound and secreted forms (sCD40L) (Graf *et al.*, 1995), allowing it to participate in both contact dependent and independent signaling events during an immune response (Alderson *et al.*, 1993; Wagner *et al.*, 1994; Kiener *et al.*, 1995; Shu *et al.*, 1995; Kooten and Banchereau, 1996). Although activated T cells are the primary source of CD40L (Lane *et al.*, 1993; Ranheim and Kipps, 1993), other cells, astrocytes (Calingasan *et al.*, 2002) including activated platelets and brain microvascular endothelial cells, constitutively express CD40L at low levels (Li *et al.*, 1994; Mach *et al.*, 1997; Henn *et al.*, 1998). Therefore, it is possible that activation of perivascular and brain MPs may result from interactions with CD40L-expressing astrocytes or endothelial cells. Importantly, CD40L-mediated activ-ation has been shown to increase the expression of pro-inflammatory cytokines, chemokines and other soluble mediators involved in regulating autocrine and paracrine immune responses. These factors include IL-1 β, IL-6, IL-10, IL-12, TNF-α, macrophage inflammatory protein (MIP)-1 α/ β, regulated on activation, normal T cell-expressed and secreted (RANTES), monocyte chemotactic protein-1 (MCP-1), as well as ICAM-1, and the matrix metalloproteinases (MMPs)-1, -2, -3 and -9 (Wagner *et al.*, 1994; Kiener *et al.*, 1995; Shu *et al.*, 1995; Tian *et al.*, 1995; Stout and Suttles, 1996; Malik *et al.*, 1996; Stout *et al.*, 1996).

While individual immune agents such CD40L, IFN-γ or Aβ can activate MPs, it is likely that combinations of these factors may be responsible for inducing MP responses during the course of an immune reaction. Acting simultaneously or sequentially, these factors may prime MP for subsequent immune responses through the up-regulation or activation of transcription factors involved in gene expression. Upon secondary activation, signaling pathways within the MP may become stimulated, leading to the potentiated production of cytokines, chemokines and other inflammatory mediators important in disease. The potential signal transduction pathways involved in mediating such events are discussed in the following section.

4.3 Signal transduction pathways

Signal transduction pathways play a critical role in the regulation of cellular function and survival. Interactions between extracellular stimuli (e.g. cytokines, chemokines or Aβ) and receptors expressed on MPs (e.g. RAGE, SR or CD40) can initiate a cascade of signaling pathways, that alter biochemical events within the cell. Importantly, these signaling pathways may act via intracellular second messengers such as Ca^{2+} to mediate their effects.

Upon stimulation of these receptors, the accumulation of cytosolic free Ca^{2+} and the activation of protein kinases can be induced. These protein kinases include calcium calmodulin kinase (CaMK), protein kinase C (PKC), phosphatidylinositol 3-kinase (PI3K) or the mitogen-activated protein (MAP) kinases. While all of these kinases are certainly involved in the regulation of MP function and activation, many of the signaling events reported involve MAP kinases. These kinases are important in coupling extracellular stimuli with intracellular signaling events, such as those involved in the activation of transcriptional enhancers or repressors. Signaling through the MAP kinase pathway stimulates cell growth and differentiation by regulating gene transcription and expression (Lopez-Ilasaca *et al.*, 1997; Lopez-Ilasaca, 1998). There are three distinct MAP kinase cascades: c-Jun N-terminal kinase/stress-activated protein kinase (JNK/SAPK), p38 (Lopez-Ilasaca, 1998) and the extracellular signal-regulated kinases (ERK1/ERK2, p42/p44). The JNK/SAPK pathway is induced by exposure to environmental stresses, such as UV radiation, heat shock or inflammatory cytokines, while the p38 pathway is activated in response to inflammatory cytokines, endotoxins and osmotic stress. ERK pathways are induced in response to growth factor stimulation or activation of high-affinity IgG receptors, the crystallizable fragment-γ receptors I and II (FcγRI and II) (Lopez-Ilasaca, 1998).

Induction of these signaling pathways can result in the downstream activation of transcription factors, involved in enhancing or repressing expression of MP genes. Transcription factors such as nuclear factor-κB (NF-κB) (Berberich *et al.*, 1994), c-Jun, c-Fos or signal transducers and activators of transcription (STATs) (Karras *et al.*, 1997) may provide the link between early membrane signaling events and altered gene expression. A pre-formed transcriptional factor, NF-κB, leads to transcriptional activation of genes important in immunity and inflammation, such as TNF-α, IL-6, IL-8, granulocyte–macrophage colony-stimulating factor (GM-CSF), acute phase proteins such as serum amyloid A (SAA), inducible nitric oxide synthase (iNOS), cyclooxygenase (COX-1, -2), MHC I and MHC II, MCP-1 and vascular cell adhesion molecule-1 (VCAM1) (Kaltschmidt *et al.*, 1993; O'Neill and Kaltschmidt, 1997).

4.3.1 Aβ signaling pathways

Several groups have shown that fibrillar forms of Aβ can activate tyrosine kinase-dependent signaling pathways in MPs. Specifically, fAβ has been shown to activate the tyrosine kinases, Lyn and Syk, which, in turn, induce signaling events that trigger the transient release of intracellular Ca^{2+}. Such events have also been shown to activate PKC (Klegeris *et al.*, 1997) and the calcium-sensitive protein tyrosine kinase 2 (PTK2) (Combs *et al.*, 1999). The downstream effects of such Aβ-induced signaling include activation of the MAP kinases, ERK1/ERK2 and p38 (McDonald *et al.*, 1998; Combs *et al.*, 1999), as well as transcription factors, such as the cAMP response element-binding protein (CREB). Activation of these effectors leads to altered MP gene expression and the production of superoxide radicals and cytokines, which can further stimulate inflammatory responses or induce neuronal injury (McDonald *et al.*, 1998). Interestingly, while both RAGEs and SRs have been shown to interact with Aβ, there currently is no evidence that these receptors are linked to the tyrosine kinase-dependent signaling pathways described above. This suggests that Aβ may act through a variety of receptors or signaling pathways to alter MP function (Figure 7.2).

4.3.2 CD40L and IFN-γ signaling pathways

Like many other cytokines, IFN-γ elicits its effects on cellular immune function through activation of the intracellular Jak–STAT pathway. This pathway involves a cascade of phosphorylation events mediated by tyrosine kinases from the Janus family of kinases (Jaks), Activation of these kinases leads to the phosphorylation of latent cytoplasmic proteins or STATs. Upon activation, these STAT proteins translocate to the nucleus, where they bind to specific DNA sequences (response elements) and induce transcription of cellular genes involved in secretory factor production.

While the signaling pathways activated in MPs upon engagement of CD40 remain to be fully elucidated, CD40L-mediated signaling in MPs may occur via pathways similar to those active in B cells. Such pathways may involve activation of src family protein tyrosine kinases (PTKs), serine/threonine kinases, Jak3, the MAP kinase family (JNK, p38 and ERK1/2) or phospholipase-γ2 (Faris *et al.*, 1994; Aagaard-Tillery and Jelinek, 1996; Hanissian and Geha, 1997). Indeed, in monocytes, CD40L-induced signaling events have been shown to involve tyrosine phosphorylation of Jak3 and the subsequent induction of STAT5a (Revy *et al.*, 1999). In addition, the MAP kinase family members, ERK1/2, also appear to be involved in CD40L-mediated signaling in MPs (Suttles *et al.*, 1999; Tan *et al.*, 1999). Several groups (Suttles *et al.*, 1999; Tan *et al.*, 1999) suggest that CD40L-mediated signaling events in human monocytes and macrophages, such as those involved in the production of cytokines and chemokines, occur through the activation of ERK1/2, and lead to the induction of transcription factors, such as NF-κB (Revy *et al.*, 1999). Moreover, activation of the ERK1/2-associated signal transduction pathway has been shown to be involved in the CD40L-mediated signaling events in murine microglia (Tan *et al.*, 1999). Interestingly, anti-inflammatory cytokines, such as transforming growth factor-1 β (TGF-1 β) and IL-10, have been shown to inhibit these CD40L-induced signaling events (Xiao *et al.*, 1996; Tan *et al.*, 1999). While some reports suggest that p38 and JNK/SAP may not be involved in CD40L-mediated signaling, further investigation into the role of these MAP kinases in such events is required.

Although multiple protein kinases may be involved in the production of putative neurotoxins from activated MPs, it is likely that signal transduction pathways involving MAP kinase family members link the priming responses induced by Aβ to the enhanced activation responses elicited by CD40L and IFN-γ. Thus, by altering or amplifying signaling pathways involved in the modification of enzymes, ion channels and transcriptional activators/regulators, Aβ and CD40L can affect MP function and survival. Moreover, disruption or inappropriate activation of these intracellular signaling pathways could elicit adverse effects, not only on the target cell but on surrounding cells as well (Saitoh *et al.*, 1993). Therefore, the effects of priming and activation on MP function are examined in the following section.

5 MP function and its relevance to AD pathogenesis

Brain macrophages and microglia appear to be primary mediators of the immuno-inflammatory events underlying AD pathogenesis (Lassmann *et al.*, 1993; Akiyama, 1994; Gehrmann *et al.*, 1995; Kreutzberg, 1996). As part of their normal, immunoregulatory functions, MPs are involved in removing foreign pathogens and cellular debris (phagocytosis), processing and presenting antigens via the MHCs (Frei *et al.*, 1987; Gehrmann *et al.*, 1995; Kalaria *et al.*, 1996a,b), releasing inflammatory factors which induce immune responses (secretory factor production) (Streit and Kincaid-Colton, 1995) as well as destroying invading pathogens (microbial killing) (Banati *et al.*, 1993; Gordon, 1995). Through these activities, MPs help maintain homeostasis within the CNS microenvironment (Elkabes *et al.*, 1996; Heese *et al.*, 1998). However, during disease, these functions can be altered or disrupted, leading to the dysregulated production of inflammatory cytokine and other factors capable of inducing CNS damage, including

proteases, excitatory amino acids (Dickson *et al.*, 1993; Gehrmann *et al.*, 1995), complement factors and NO (Banati *et al.*, 1993; Gordon, 1995).

5.1 Antigen presentation

MPs serve as the major antigen-presenting cells (APCs) of the brain. Whereas some MP
surface proteins are constitutively expressed, others are induced in response to injury,
infection or inflammation within the CNS (Rogers *et al.*, 1988; Akiyama and McGeer,
1990; Mattiace *et al.*, 1990; Tooyama *et al.*, 1990; DeNagel and Pierce, 1992; Benveniste,
1997a; McRae *et al.*, 1997). Activated MP express surface proteins, such as FcγRI and
FcγRII, and MHC antigens such as the human leukocyte antigen DR (HLA-DR) (Rogers
et al., 1988; McGeer *et al.*, 1989, 1994; Akiyama and McGeer, 1990; Mattiace *et al.*,
1990; Tooyama *et al.*, 1990; DeNagel and Pierce, 1992; Kalaria *et al.*, 1996b; McRae *et
al.*, 1997). *In vivo*, HLA-DR-positive microglia have been shown to accumulate around
NPs (Aisen, 1996; Pazmany *et al.*, 1999). Interestingly, individuals with the *ApoE-ε2/3*
genotype have normal MHC I and II expression, as compared with controls, while individuals with the *ApoE-ε3/4* and *-ε4/4* genotypes display increased levels of MHC II
expression (Lombardi *et al.*, 1998).

  In vitro, MPs can be induced, upon treatment with IFN-γ, to up-regulate expression of
MHC II antigens and other molecules, such as the leukocyte functional antigen-3 (LFA-3)
and ICAM-1, which are critical for effective antigen presentation (Frei *et al.*, 1987;
Amaldi *et al.*, 1989; Perlmutter *et al.*, 1992; Abdulkadir and Ono, 1995; De Simone *et al.*,
1995; Panek and Benveniste, 1995; Satoh *et al.*, 1995; Shrikant *et al.*, 1995; Hellendall
and Ting, 1997). Activated MPs also express the co-stimulatory factors, B7.1 and B7.2,
which are important in T-cell activation (Hofman *et al.*, 1986; De Simone *et al.*, 1995;
Gehrmann *et al.*, 1995; Windhagen *et al.*, 1995).

5.2 Phagocytosis

As scavenger cells, MPs act to eliminate foreign (viral, bacterial or parasitic) material and
cellular debris through phagocytosis. In AD, MPs may aid in the removal of Aβ and cellular
debris resulting from neuronal injury (Kalaria *et al.*, 1996b). In support of this, reactive
MPs have been shown to phagocytose complement-opsonized Aβ fibrils in vitro (Akiyama,
1994; McGeer *et al.*, 1994; Kalaria *et al.*, 1996b; Morelli *et al.*, 1999). Over time, the accumulation of these Aβ fibrils may create a 'phagocytolytic burden' too great for the MPs to
clear. Frustrated in their attempts to internalize and degrade the aggregated peptides, the
MPs may become chronically activated, producing increased levels of factors that help
perpetuate and sustain inflammation within the brain (McGeer and McGeer, 1995). It has
been proposed that MP receptors, such as RAGE or class A SR (see Section 4.1), may be
involved in such processes (Paresce *et al.*, 1996; Yan *et al.*, 1996).

  Constitutively expressed in both peripheral and brain macrophages and microglia (El
Khoury *et al.*, 1996; Yamada *et al.*, 1998), SRs are primarily involved in mediating the
uptake of macromolecules, such as the acetylated LDLs (Naito *et al.*, 1991, 1992; El
Khoury *et al.*, 1996). However, SRs can also participate in the uptake of matrix proteins
digested by metalloproteases during MP transmigration (Yamada *et al.*, 1998), or aid in
the phagocytosis of apoptotic cells. Interestingly, MPs that are deficient in SRs have
reduced phagocytic capacity. SR expression is increased in response to differentiation or

treatment with factors such as macrophage colony-stimulating factor (M-CSF) (Gough *et al.*, 1999), but is down-regulated in response to IFN-γ, TNF-α, TGF-β and IL-10 (Geng and Hansson, 1992; de Villiers *et al.*, 1994a,b). Aβ has been shown to bind to SRs expressed on macrophages and microglia (El Khoury *et al.*, 1996; Paresce *et al.*, 1996), suggesting that these receptors may play a role in the clearance of Aβ (Paresce *et al.*, 1996; Morelli *et al.*, 1999). Alternatively, binding of Aβ to these receptors may trigger a cascade of intracellular signaling events (Yamada *et al.*, 1998) that lead to the production of factors involved in sustaining inflammation or eliciting neural injury (Christie *et al.*, 1996; El Khoury *et al.*, 1996). However, whether SRs function alone, or with other receptors to initiate such responses remains to be clarified (El Khoury *et al.*, 1996).

5.3 Secretory activities

In addition to antigen presentation and phagocytosis, MPs also contribute to immune responses through the production of inflammatory or chemotactic factors. Upon immune activation, MPs release and respond to several cytokines that are instrumental in regulating their proliferation and differentiation, as well as their response to injury or immunological challenge (Gehrmann *et al.*, 1995; Xiao and Link, 1998). Such factors include inflammatory cytokines, proteases, excitatory amino acids, complement components and oxidative radicals such as NO (Heyes *et al.*, 1991; Banati *et al.*, 1993; Dickson *et al.*, 1993; Gehrmann *et al.*, 1995; Kerr *et al.*, 1998). Several lines of evidence suggest that when dysregulated, these factors can amplify and sustain inflammatory responses that affect neural function and survival (Benveniste, 1992). Therefore, the following sections examines several of these factors and their role in CNS inflammation and neurodegeneration.

5.3.1 Chemotactic factors

Secreted by macrophages, microglia, astrocytes, oligodendrocytes and other cells (Griffin, 1997) in response to tissue damage or immunological challenge (Kuby 1994), chemoattractant cytokines (chemokines) induce the recruitment of leukocytes and other immune cells to regions of brain injury and inflammation (Luster, 1998). Chemokine receptor expression and chemokine production has been found in many different types of cells, including endothelial cells, astrocytes, neurons and microglia. While chemokines, such as MIP-1 α, MIP-1 α, MCP-1, IL-8 and IL-10, and chemokine receptors, such as CXCR2, CXCR3, CXCR4, CCR3 and CCR5, have been shown to be expressed in the AD brain, the exact role of these factors in the disease process is not known (Ishizuka *et al.*, 1997; Mennicken *et al.*, 1999). A further indication of chemokine involvement in AD has been provided by *in vitro* studies, demonstrate that Aβ can induce production of MIP-1 β, MCP-1 and RANTES in both MPs and astrocytes (Johnstone *et al.*, 1999). Interestingly, MCP-1, itself, (Fuentes *et al.*, 1995; Bell *et al.*, 1996) has been shown to increase expression of other immune factors, such as IL-1 β, IL-6 and arachidonate (Sozzani *et al.*, 1994; Johnstone *et al.*, 1999). Thus, it has been proposed that MCP-1 and other chemotactic factors may contribute to neuronal injury in AD by recruiting additional immune cells to sites of Aβ plaque formation, where they are induced to secrete inflammatory factors and other neurotoxins (Johnstone *et al.*, 1999). Alternatively, it has been suggested that upon binding to their receptors on neurons, chemokines can induce the activation of MAP kinase pathways, leading to the hyperphosphorylation of tau and the subsequent formation of NFTs (Xia and Hyman, 1999).

5.3.2 Neurotrophins

Molecular and cellular analyses indicate that neurotoxic behavior is not a constitutive activity of MPs (Mallat and Chamak, 1994). Under normal homeostatic conditions, MP assume a supportive role within the CNS environment (Chao *et al.*, 1995d), producing trophic growth factors and cytokines that support normal development and CNS function. Derived from the Greek word meaning food, 'trophins' are factors involved in nourishing and sustaining neural and glial cells within the CNS (Tuszynski and Gage, 1994). Importantly, withdrawal or absence of these and other essential growth factors may inhibit growth and cause neuronal death (Martin *et al.*, 1988). A number of neurotrophins are secreted by MPs (Barnea *et al.*, 1996; Elkabes *et al.*, 1996), including brain-derived neurotrophic factor (BDNF) (Miwa *et al.*, 1997; Kerschensteiner *et al.*, 1999), TGF-β (Chao *et al.*, 1995e), neurotrophin-3 (NT3) (Mallat *et al.*, 1989; Saad *et al.*, 1991; Loy *et al.*, 1994; Rocamora *et al.*, 1996; Kullander *et al.*, 1997), glial-derived neurotrophic factor (GDNF) (Batchelor *et al.*, 1999), basic fibroblast growth factor (bFGF) (Rappolee *et al.*, 1988; Shimojo *et al.*, 1991; Elkabes *et al.*, 1996) and nerve growth factor (NGF) (Barnea *et al.*, 1996; Elkabes *et al.*, 1996). Many of these factors have been shown to enhance neuronal survival and neurite outgrowth (Mallat *et al.*, 1989; Shimojo *et al.*, 1991; Araujo and Cotman, 1992a) by stabilizing Ca^{2+} homeostasis, suppressing free radical accumulation and maintaining normal mitochondrial function (Mattson *et al.*, 1993a). For example, bFGF has been shown to suppress production of an NMDA receptor protein known to cause cytotoxic damage to hippocampal neurons (Mattson *et al.*, 1993b), and TGF-β has been shown to protect neurons from Aβ-induced damage (Flanders *et al.*, 1998). Interestingly, NGF can induce synthesis of c-Fos, a transcription factor involved in long-term memory (Taylor *et al.*, 1993). s100 β is another glial-derived neurotrophin, known to play a role in the development and maintenance of the nervous system. Overexpression of this factor can induce NO production and release from astrocytes, leading to neuronal injury (Hu *et al.*, 1997).

5.3.3 Cytokines and neurotoxins

Inflammatory cytokines, such as IL-1 β, IL-6 and TNF-α (Griffin *et al.*, 1989; Dickson *et al.*, 1993; Wood *et al.*, 1993; Cacabelos *et al.*, 1994; Walker *et al.*, 1995), are up-regulated in regions of the AD brain that contain Aβ-containing NPs (Fontana *et al.*, 1984; Giulian *et al.*, 1986; Lee *et al.*, 1993b). These factors (TNF-α and IL-1 β) have been shown to inhibit synaptic transmission, as well as long-term potentiation (LTP), within the hippocampus (Bellinger *et al.*, 1993) and amygdala (Tancredi *et al.*, 1992). *In vitro*, Aβ induces expression of IL-1 β, IL-1Ra, IL-8, MIP-1 α and other inflammatory factors in both macrophages and microglia (Lorton *et al.*, 1996; Meda *et al.*, 1999). Interestingly, Aβ does not affect production of factors such as TGF-β or IL-10, which are known to be important in down-regulating the immune response (Araujo and Cotman, 1992b; Santambrogio *et al.*, 1993; Kiefer *et al.*, 1995; Meda *et al.*, 1995b).

Produced primarily by microglia, macrophages and endothelial cells, IL-1 β is an inflammatory cytokine that has been shown to be important in CNS disease (Merrill *et al.*, 1989; Yamato *et al.*, 1990; Genis *et al.*, 1992). Within the brain, expression of IL-1 β has been shown to induce astrogliosis, resulting in the increased production of neurotrophic factors such as NGF and bFGF (Frei *et al.*, 1989; Bandtlow *et al.*, 1990; Araujo and Cotman, 1992a), and inflammatory mediators, such as the acute phase protease inhibitor, ACT (Lieb *et al.*, 1996), which prevents proteolytic digestion of Aβ fibrils, allowing for plaque formation to occur (Rozemuller *et al.*, 1991; Fraser *et al.*, 1993; Cacabelos *et al.*, 1994; Ma *et al.*, 1994). *In vitro*, IL-1 β has also been shown to increase production and secretion of neuronal APP (Blume and Vitek, 1989; Buxbaum *et al.*, 1992; Dash and Moore, 1995). Together, these observations suggest that IL-1 β may be involved in the formation of dense NPs (Sheng *et al.*, 1995).

IL-6 is another inflammatory cytokine produced by reactive macrophages and microglia (Strauss *et al.*, 1992; Gehrmann *et al.*, 1995). A pleiotropic cytokine, IL-6, is involved in cell–cell signaling, coordination of neuroimmune responses, as well as neuronal protection, differentiation, growth and survival (Gruol and Nelson, 1997). Up-regulated in NP regions within the AD brain, IL-6 has been shown to increase expression of *APP*, leading to the formation of Aβ fibrils (Goldgaber *et al.*, 1989; Abraham *et al.*, 1990; Donnelly *et al.*, 1990; Altstiel and Sperber, 1991; Akiyama *et al.*, 1992, 1993; Forloni *et al.*, 1992). This, in addition to its ability to induce elements of the acute phase response (Abraham *et al.*, 1990; Akiyama *et al.*, 1992, 1993; Gruol and Nelson, 1997), such as ACT, suggest that IL-6 may also play a key role in the inflammatory responses underlying AD. Although its specific role in disease is not yet known, IL-6 may contribute to neuronal injury by enhancing NMDA-mediated neurotoxicity (Poli *et al.*, 1990; Kolson and Pomerantz, 1996).

A potent proinflammatory cytokine, TNF-α is secreted by macrophages and microglia in response to a variety of immune stimuli (Benveniste, 1997b). In addition, TNF-α can also be produced by IL-1-stimulated astrocytes (Lee *et al.*, 1993a; Chao *et al.*, 1995d). TNF-α has been shown to contribute to immune activation by inducing MHC II expression and cytokine secretion. Interestingly, TNF-α can exert both neuroprotective and neurotoxic effects (Tracey and Cerami, 1993). Although involved in neural protection at low levels, increased levels of TNF-α can be neurotoxic in culture (Gelbard *et al.*, 1993; Blasko *et al.*, 1997). Moreover, TNF-α, when used in conjunction with IL-1 β, has been shown to induce neuronal injury by stimulating NO release (Chao *et al.*, 1995a) or by inhibiting glutamate reuptake activity in astroctyes. Such activity can lead to oxidative stress-related injury or glutamate receptor-mediated neurotoxicity. TNF-α may also contribute to neurotoxicity by inhibiting receptor signaling events mediated by survival peptides, such as the insulin-like growth factor 1 (IGF-1). In the presence of IFN-γ, TNF-α has been shown to induce the production of Aβ (Blasko *et al.*, 1999). In addition, TNF-α has been shown to contribute to the breakdown of the BBB by altering vascular endothelial cell function and enhancing the adhesion of lymphocytes and macrophages. Despite its potential role in cell injury, TNF-α has also been shown to have neuroprotective effects. These effects may be mediated through the induction of cytokines, such as TGF-β (Chao *et al.*, 1995a), which act to 'shut down' the immune response (Meucci and Miller, 1996; Prehn *et al.*, 1993, 1996) and protect neurons.

In response to inflammation, MPs, astrocytes and other neural cells produce increased levels of complement proteins (Chen *et al.*, 1996). It has been proposed that early complement activation factors may play a critical role in mediating Aβ deposition and inflammation (Eikelenboom and Veerhuis, 1996). In support of this, such factors have been shown to be associated with dense NPs and NFTs in the AD brain (Eikelenboom and Stam, 1982; McGeer *et al.*, 1989). Binding of Aβ to components of the classical complement cascade, such as C1q, leads to activation of the classical complement pathway (Painter, 1984; Rogers *et al.*, 1992; Jiang *et al.*, 1994; McGeer *et al.*, 1994; Webster and Rogers, 1996). Activation of the classical complement cascade can initiate an immune attack by providing signals for scavenger cell activation (anaphylotoxins C4a, C3a and C5a) and migration, by opsonizing specific targets (C3b, CR3, CR4) for destruction, or by directly lysing cells (C5b-9), permitting a massive influx of Ca^{2+} (Kuby, 1994). Such events can result in the formation of membrane attack complexes (MACs) (Chen *et al.*, 1996; Aisen, 1997; McGeer and McGeer, 1997) that in turn can induce neuronal injury. Alternatively, complement components, such as CR3 (Mac-1), can activate MPs or surrounding glial cells (Akiyama *et al.*, 1994). When not properly regulated, these factors can cause the indiscriminate destruction of innocent 'bystander' tissue, leading to a vicious cycle of inflammation, complement activation and injury within affected brain regions.

In addition to synthesizing inflammatory cytokines and complement factors, MPs also release other substances with the potential to induce damage (Kalaria *et al.*, 1996b). Included in this list of cytotoxic products are proteases (Cammer *et al.*, 1978; Beezhold and Personius, 1992; Colton *et al.*, 1993; Gehrmann *et al.*, 1995; Gottschall *et al.*, 1995), NO (Chao *et al.*, 1992; McGeer *et al.*, 1994; Gehrmann *et al.*, 1995; Kalaria *et al.*, 1996b), excess glutamate (Klegeris and McGeer, 1997), superoxide anions (Colton and Gilbert, 1987), H_2O_2 (Colton and Gilbert, 1987; Thery *et al.*, 1991), platelet-activating factor (PAF) (Gelbard *et al.*, 1994) and neurotoxins which act by way of NMDA receptors (Mallat and Chamak, 1994). These products have the potential to stimulate neurotransmitters, alter neuronal signaling and function, and induce neuronal death (Giulian, 1990; Pulliam *et al.*, 1991; Genis *et al.*, 1992; Giulian *et al.*, 1993). These factors are described in more detail in Section 6.

6 Mechanisms for MP-induced neuronal demise

Many of the neurological and behavioral symptoms of AD result from neural dysfunction or death. However, the pathogenic mechanisms underlying synaptic loss and neuronal death in AD (and the role of Aβ deposition and MP activation in such processes) remain unclear (Khachaturian *et al.*, 1994). It has been proposed that Aβ may contribute directly to neurotoxicity through oxidative stress, excitotoxicity or disruption of neuronal signaling and lipid transport. Alternatively, it has been suggested that Aβ may contribute indirectly to neuronal injury by activating brain MP, which in turn elicit neurotoxic effects. Therefore, the following section examines potential mechanisms by which Aβ and brain MP may induce or enhance neuronal injury. The extracellular events and the intracellular signaling pathways, that may ultimately lead to neuronal demise are discussed.

6.1 Neuronal signaling

Neurons express a wide variety of receptors, that enable them to respond to changes in their environment and communicate with other cells. Upon binding to these receptors, secretory factors from activated MPs and other neural cells can trigger intracellular signaling cascades, that affect gene expression, neuronal function and cell survival (Krammer *et al.*, 1994; Nagata and Golstein, 1995; Clement and Stamenkovic, 1996). For example, neurons express several GTP-binding protein (G protein)-coupled receptors, including the dopamine, chemokine and metabotropic glutamate receptors, which are involved in regulating normal cell functions (Gupta *et al.*, 1998). Depending on the type of receptor bound, such G-protein-linked signaling can elicit either inhibitory or stimulatory effects on the target cell. In the case of G_s-linked G-protein receptors, such binding activates adenylyl cyclase (AC). An intracellular enzyme involved in the formation of cAMP, AC is regulated by a wide range of factors, including extracellular neurotransmitter receptors, intracellular free Ca^{2+} levels and calmodulin. Stimulation of AC leads to formation of cAMP, which in turn can activate protein kinase A (PKA). Upon activation, PKA phosphorylates select proteins within the cell, leading to modifications in enzymes, ion channels, transcriptional activators and transcriptional regulators (Iismaa *et al.*, 1995).

Activating a different signal transduction cascade, binding to the G_q family of G-protein-coupled receptors results in increased phospholipase C (PLC) activity. Activated PLC leads to hydrolysis of the membrane-bound phosphatidylinositol-4,5-bisphosphate (PIP2) to produce diacylglycerol (DAG) and inositol trisphosphate (IP3) (Kelly *et al.*, 1996) (Figure 7.2). DAG activates PKC, an enzyme involved in regulating cell growth and differentiation. PKC also plays a role in the molecular events underlying associated learning and memory (Olds and Alkon, 1991). PKC activation has been shown to inhibit cellular production of Aβ from APP (Hung *et al.*, 1993). In AD, this signaling pathway is impaired and results in altered APP processing (Jope *et al.*, 1997), leading to the formation of amyloidgenic APP. Moreover, hyperactivation of PKC can lead to increased phosphorylation of tau and, subsequently, increased PHF formation (Boyce and Shea, 1997). The other product of PIP2 cleavage, IP3, is released into the cytoplasm upon cleavage, where it binds to IP3 receptors on the endoplasmic reticulum (ER) (Figure 7.2). This triggers the release of intracellular Ca^{2+}, which may act as a 'third messenger' exerting its own biochemical effects upon the cell. In AD, phosphoinositide signaling is disrupted at the IP3 receptor level (Young *et al.*, 1988) via calpain-mediated destruction of IP3-binding sites (Magnusson *et al.*, 1993; Saito *et al.*, 1993).

Maintaining intracellular Ca^{2+} homeostasis is vital for neuronal cell function and interneuronal communication (Hartmann *et al.*, 1994). Overactivation of IP3 and increased production of Ca^{2+} can activate kinases, such as CaMK-II and CaMK-IV, which are involved in mediating transcriptional activation of gene expression (Ghosh and Greenberg, 1995). For example, the CaMKs have been shown to play a role in regulating the formation of a complex between c-Fos and c-Jun (Figure 7.3). Transcription factors induced by CREB, c-Jun and c-Fos are involved in regulating several neural processes within the CNS. These include neuronal differentiation and regeneration, as well as apoptosis. Reported to be up-regulated in a variety of neurodegenerative diseases, including AD (MacGibbon *et al.*, 1997a), c-Jun acts as a master switch, determining whether cells will elicit neuroprotective or destructive effects. Involved in long-term memory, c-Fos has also been implicated in AD, where its activation has been shown to contribute to Aβ-induced neurotoxicity (Gillardon *et al.*, 1996).

During disease these signaling pathway(s) may be disrupted or amplified, leading to changes in membrane potential and resistance, disruption of ion flow, altered synaptic function, aberrant protein phosphorylation and defective neuronal metabolism (Saitoh *et al.*, 1993; Cowburn *et al.*, 1996; Pacheco and Jope, 1996) (Figure 7.3). Such events, in turn, can affect voltage-gated calcium channels and lead to additional Ca^{2+} influx. Excess levels of Ca^{2+} can disrupt mitochondrial function or activate lipases, proteases and

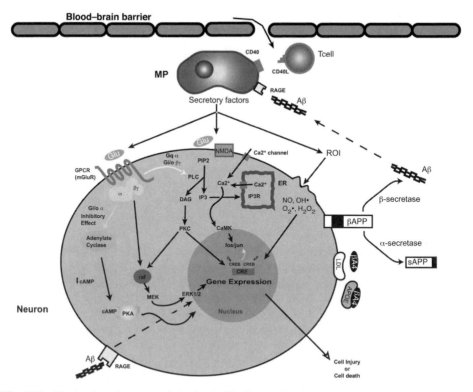

Fig. 7.3 Mechanisms for neuronal demise in AD. The mechanisms by which MP secretory factors lead to altered signaling, synaptic loss and neural injury have not yet been resolved. We propose the following model for MP-associated neuronal dysfunction in AD. Aβ may induce neuronal injury either directly, through binding to RAGE or LDL receptors expressed on neurons, or indirectly, by altering MP secretory functions. MP secretory factors can cause excitotoxic and oxidative stress-related damage, or alter signaling pathways that regulate neuronal function and survival. Upon binding to NMDA receptors on the plasma membrane, these factors may induce excitotoxic damage by increasing levels of intracellular calcium. Alternatively, MP may produce and release ROI, which can damage neuronal membranes or proteins. In addition, MP factors can alter neuronal signaling and function by binding to G-protein-coupled receptors, such as the metabotropic glutamate receptors (mGluRs). Such events can induce aberrant phosphorylation of nuclear proteins, such as the cAMP response element-binding protein (CREB), and alter gene expression. This, in turn, can affect transcription of factors, such as Fos/Jun, which are involved in regulating neuronal differentiation, regeneration or apoptosis. If not regulated or controlled, these events can disrupt neuronal lipid metabolism or alter APP processing, leading to the deposition of A β and formation of NPs. Likewise, increased kinase activity can cause abnormal phosphorylation of cytoskeletal proteins and lead to the formation of paired helical filaments and neurofibrillary tangles. This, in turn, can cause a breakdown in the cytoskeleton and lead to neuronal death.

endonucleases that aid in the destruction of cell membranes and the cytoskeleton. This, in turn, can lead to NFT formation, aberrant amyloid deposition and ultimately neuronal death (Mattson *et al.*, 1993a,b). Dysregulation of Ca^{2+} homeostasis has been implicated in a number of cellular associated with the aging brain and AD (Landfield *et al.*, 1992). For example, Aβ, generated through abnormal APP processing, can disrupt intracellular Ca^{2+} levels (Mattson *et al.*, 1992). In a healthy neuron, APP plays a protective role by regulating cytosolic Ca^{2+} and protecting neurons from glutamate-mediated neurotoxicity (Khachaturian, 1989; Khachaturian *et al.*, 1994). However, in AD, abnormal processing of APP leads to $A\beta$ formation. Unlike its neuroprotective precursor, $A\beta$ can generate free radicals that increase intracellular Ca^{2+} levels via voltage-sensitive calcium channels (VSCCs) (Ueda *et al.*, 1997).

6.2 Oxidative stress

Implicated as a major cause of neuronal cell injury in a wide range of neurological diseases, including AD (Mecocci *et al.*, 1994; Smith *et al.*, 1995, 1996; Vitek *et al.*, 1997), oxidative stress results from the accumulation of deleterious reactive oxygen and nitrogen byproducts formed during cellular metabolic processes, such as oxidative phosphorylation (Lipton *et al.*, 1994). Although typically produced by MPs and other inflammatory cells to destroy invading microorganisms, reactive oxygen (H_2O_2, superoxide and hydroxyl free radicals) and nitrogen intermediates (NO and peroxynitrite) may also cause damage to host cells if not properly regulated (Halliwell and Gutteridge, 1985; Buttke and Sandstrom, 1994). These factors can induce cellular damage by oxidatively modifying or cross-linking cellular proteins, lipid membranes and deoxynucleic acids within the targeted cell. In AD, oxidative stress may alter proteins, such as $A\beta$ and tau, making them insoluble or resistant to proteolytic degradation. Such modifications can affect the function of these proteins, and thereby contribute to $A\beta$ plaque formation and cytoskeletal disruption. In contrast, antioxidants, such as vitamin E, superoxide dismutase (SOD), catalase, glutathione, glutathione peroxidase, lactoferrin and transferrin, can prevent oxidative-mediated damage by scavenging and detoxifying existing free radicals or by sequestering transition metals involved in their formation. For example, SOD facilitates the formation of H_2O_2 and molecular oxygen from superoxide radicals, while catalases and glutathione peroxidases catalyze the conversion of H_2O_2 to water.

During injury, infection or aging, such processes may be disrupted. This, in turn, may lead to the excessive accumulation of free radicals or the decreased ability to defend against these toxic factors. The inability to prevent or repair such damage can result in cell death, via apoptosis or necrosis, depending on the severity of the initial insult. Therefore, maintaining a balance between the rate of reactive species formation and the rate at which such factors can be neutralized or cleared by antioxidants is important for cellular homeostasis and survival.

It has been proposed that $A\beta$ can induce oxidative stress either directly by spontaneously forming free radical oligopeptides, or indirectly by inducing reactive oxygen intermediate (ROI) production in neurons and activated MPs or astroctyes (Hensley *et al.*, 1994). Such effects may be mediated by neuronal receptors, such as RAGE or LDL-R. These receptors may act to tether potential oxidizing agents, such as $A\beta$ or AGEs, to the neuronal cell membrane where they can elicit deleterious effects. Alternatively, upon binding to RAGE or class A SRs expressed on MPs, $A\beta$ may trigger intracellular events that lead to the enhanced production and release of inducible nitric oxide synthase (iNOS), NO, superoxide, H_2O_2, hydroxyl radicals and other factors, that can contribute to tissue damage and perpetuate inflammation (Colton and Gilbert, 1987; Goodwin *et al.*, 1995; El Khoury *et al.*, 1996; Van Muiswinkel *et al.*, 1996, 1999; Yan *et al.*, 1996; McDonald *et al.*, 1997; Bianca *et al.*, 1999).

In addition to directly producing reactive species, MPs can also produce inflammatory cytokines that stimulate the production of free radicals (Dawson *et al.*, 1991). For example, both IFN-γ and TNF-α can increase the expression of NADPH oxidase, an enzyme involved in the formation of NO (Cassatella *et al.*, 1991; Chanock *et al.*, 1994; Bianca *et al.*, 1999). An important signaling molecule involved in a variety of cellular functions, including LTP and immune protection, NO is produced by activated MPs, astrocytes and endothelial cells in response to immune challenge and activation (Chao *et al.*, 1995c, 1996). Under certain conditions, NO can react with superoxide anions to form peroxynitrite (Beckman *et al.*, 1990), a powerful oxidant capable of damaging a variety of cellular molecules.

Providing additional support for the notion of oxidative-related injury in AD, transition metals that interact with free radicals to form damaging oxidants have been shown to occur at high concentrations in the AD brain (Good *et al.*, 1992). For example, aluminum, which can stimulate iron-induced lipid peroxidation, has been found to co-localize with NFT-containing neurons (Oteiza, 1994). Likewise, iron, which catalyzes the formation of hydroxyl radicals from H_2O_2 as well as the formation of AGEs, has been shown to accumulate in both NFTs and Aβ deposits. In the presence of such transition metals, AGEs and Aβ can undergo redox cycling (Baynes, 1991; Yan *et al.*, 1994, 1995) or interact with specific receptors, such as RAGE or the SR-A, to increase intracellular ROI production (Yan *et al.*, 1996). Moreover, interactions between free radicals and transition metals, such as those associated with cellular enzymes, cytoskeletal proteins and transcription factors, can interfere with normal protein phosphorylation events and disrupt cellular function. Thus, in AD, abnormal phosphorylation of the cytoskeletal protein, tau, may be a consequence of oxidative stress (Smith *et al.*, 1996). Such events can affect signal transduction pathways, including those involved in phophoinositide breakdown and DAG-mediated activation of PKC. Alterations in intracellular signaling can lead to the activation of genes responsible for apoptosis, such as p53 (Fowler, 1997). By activating poly(ADP)-ribose transferase (Buttke and Sandstrom, 1994), which aids in the polymerization of ADP-ribose to cellular proteins, reactive intermediates can also lead to the depletion of molecules required for cellular metabolism, such as NAD/NADH and ATP. Thus, whether oxidative stress causes protein and lipid modifications, directly damages cellular DNA or leads to the depletion of energy molecules, it is clear that such processes, if not counteracted, ultimately can result in severe cellular injury or loss.

6.3 Excitotoxicity

It has been proposed that excitotoxicity, which results from the chronic overactivation of excitatory amino acid (EAA) receptors (Olney, 1978; Shaw, 1994), may contribute to neuronal injury in AD and other neurodegenerative disorders. While excitotoxicity may not be the primary mechanism for Aβ-induced neuronal injury (Busciglio *et al.*, 1993), accumulating evidence suggests that the release of excitotoxins from activated MPs or injured neurons may cause secondary damage to surrounding cells (Shaw, 1994). Indeed, in culture, activated MPs have been shown to produce several factors, including glutamate, which are capable of eliciting excitotoxic damage (Lipton, 1996; Klegeris and McGeer, 1997).

Glutamate, a multifunctional EEA, is known both for its ability to act as an excitatory neurotransmitter and for its potential to cause excitotoxic injury. In order to elicit such varied effects within the CNS, glutamate interacts, with two types of receptors, ionotropic and metabotropic glutamate receptors. Ionotropic receptors, which include

NMDA, α-amino-3-hydroxy-5-methyl-4-isoxazole propionic acid (AMPA) and kainate receptors (Monaghan *et al.*, 1989), are ligand-gated ion channels involved in mediating Ca^{2+} influx from the extracellular space. In contrast, metabotropic glutamate receptors are G-protein-coupled receptors, that can stimulate the release of Ca^{2+} from intracellular stores (Bruno *et al.*, 1995). By binding to these receptors, glutamate can elicit a wide range of effects. For example, upon binding to neuronal NMDA receptors, glutamate induces an initial influx of Ca^{2+}. This, in turn, depolarizes the membrane allowing additional Ca^{2+} to enter the cell through either NMDA receptor-associated channels or VSCCs (Olney, 1990; Piani *et al.*, 1991, 1992). When properly regulated, these events aid in the propagation of electrical signals from one neuron to the next (Piani *et al.*, 1991). However, if not properly regulated, glutamate and other excitotoxins can induce a dramatic increase in intracellular Ca^{2+} levels. Such an increase in intracellular Ca^{2+} can lead to the inappropriate activation of destructive enzymes, such as the lipases, phospholipases, endonucleases and calpain, or contribute to free radical formation and mitochondrial dysfunction (Beckman *et al.*, 1990; Olney, 1990; Coyle and Puttfarcken, 1993; Lafon-Cazal *et al.*, 1993). Such events may alter neuronal gene expression (Jakoi *et al.*, 1992) or induce changes in proteins critical for normal cellular function (Shaw, 1994), causing neuronal injury (DeBoni and McLachlan, 1985; Choi *et al.*, 1987).

In addition to producing glutamate, activated MP can produce other factors, including quinolinic acid (QUIN), PAF, arachidonic acid and inflammatory cytokines, which are capable of eliciting excitotoxic injury (Lipton, 1996). Such injury may be elicited either directly through binding of these excitotoxins to EAA receptors on neurons, or indirectly through alterations in the regulatory functions of astrocytes (Olney, 1990; Coyle and Puttfarcken, 1993). For example, both QUIN and PAF have been shown to induce excessive Ca^{2+} influx, increase glutamate release and cause neuronal injury upon binding to EAA receptors (Valone and Epstein, 1988; Monaghan *et al.*, 1989; Tsuzuki *et al.*, 1989; Lindsberg *et al.*, 1991; Bito *et al.*, 1992; Clark *et al.*, 1992). In contrast, arachidonic acid and other factors may indirectly induce excitotoxic damage by altering the regulatory functions of cells involved in maintaining homeostasis within the CNS (Miller *et al.*, 1992; Bonfoco *et al.*, 1995). For example, arachidonic acid and its derivative, prostaglandin, have been shown to potentiate excitotoxic effects by impairing glutamate reuptake activity in astrocytes (Volterra *et al.*, 1994; Trottei *et al.*, 1995). Failure to clear excess glutamate, released from injured neurons or activated MPs, can cause further damage to neighboring neurons (Lipton, 1996; Sagara and Schubert, 1998). Hydroperoxyeicosatetraenoic acids (HPETEs), which are oxygenated derivatives of arachidonic acid, can also contribute indirectly to excitotoxic damage by depleting glutathione levels within neurons, making them more vulnerable to oxidative stress and apoptosis (Miller *et al.*, 1992; Nishiyama *et al.*, 1993; Buttke and Sandstrom, 1994). In addition, inflammatory cytokines, such as TNF-α, IFN-γ and IL-1 β, can potentiate the production or release of these excitotoxins (e.g. PAF and QUIN) from surrounding cells.

6.4 Apoptosis and necrosis

Depending on the intensity of the initial insult, both oxidative stress and excitotoxic injury can elicit severe neuronal injury leading to cell death via one of two pathways, necrosis or apoptosis. Necrosis, a passive, extracellularly signaled form of cell death, can be induced rapidly by either direct trauma or toxicity. This causes cellular swelling, injury to cytoplasmic organelles (mitochondria) and disruption of internal homeostatic mechanisms (Bonfoco *et al.*, 1995). In turn, such events ultimately lead to membrane lysis. Upon lysis, necrotic cells release proteases and other intracellular enzymes that injure bystander cells (Kerr and Harmon, 1991).

In contrast, apoptosis is a form of programmed cell death that can be induced by a variety of factors, including growth factor withdrawal, activation of free radical production or an increase in intracellular Ca^{2+}, which can lead to the indiscriminate activation of cellular proteases. Apoptotic cells are characterized by cell shrinkage, membrane blebbing, DNA fragmentation and nuclear condensation (Waters, 1997). Importantly, during apoptosis, membrane proteins are cross-linked in order to preserve internal and external membranes and prevent the leakage of EAAs, free radicals and proteolytic enzymes into the surrounding microenvironment. Interestingly, phosphatidylserine, expressed on the surface of apoptotic cells, triggers MP-mediated phagocytosis (Duval *et al.*, 1985). If not cleared within a certain period of time, apoptotic neurons can undergo secondary necrosis (Ankarcrona *et al.*, 1995; Bonfoco *et al.*, 1995).

Several factors, including p53, Fas receptor (CD95), B-cell leukemia-2 (Bcl-2), the Bcl-associated X protein (Bax), and transcription factors such as c-Jun, c-Fos and NF-κB are involved in regulating the cell's decision to undergo apoptosis. For example, while Bcl-2 expression acts to inhibit apoptosis and promote cell survival (Kane *et al.*, 1993; Reed, 1994; Cotman, 1998), Bax, which is expressed in both neurons and activated microglia within the AD brain, induces apoptosis (Oltvai *et al.*, 1993; MacGibbon *et al.*, 1997b). Interestingly, an up-regulation in neuronal Bax expression appears to precede tangle formation in AD (Su *et al.*, 1997). Another factor involved in regulating apoptotic signaling is NF-κB. Expressed in neurons, NF-κB is a transcriptional factor activated in response to a variety of factors, including stress, injury (Mattson *et al.*, 1997), glutamate (O'Neill and Kaltschmidt, 1997), cytokines (IL-1 β and TNF-α) (Lieb *et al.*, 1996), as well as stimulation of the Aβ receptor, RAGE (Mattson *et al.*, 1997; O'Neill and Kaltschmidt, 1997). Importantly, NF-κB can be either neuroprotective or neurotoxic depending upon the conditions surrounding its activation. For example, NF-κB can inhibit oxidative stress-induced apoptosis by stimulating production of manganese superoxide dismutase (Mn-SOD), which suppresses peroxynitrite formation and lipid peroxidation (Mattson *et al.*, 1997). In contrast, NF-κB activation may lead to toxic events that induce either neuronal or glial apoptosis (Kaltschmidt *et al.*, 1997; Akama *et al.*, 1998).

7 Laboratory and animal models for AD

There is no single animal model for AD pathogenesis that satisfactorily accounts for all the neuropathological, genetic and age-related requirements for disease (LeBlanc *et al.*, 1997; Jordan-Sciutto and Bowser, 1998). However, this section provides a brief overview of the animal and *in vitro* models currently being utilized for AD research (see Table 7.1 for an overview of a select number of murine models available for AD studies). Although there are several murine models available to study AD pathogenesis, only select models have been able to achieve high levels of APP and/or Aβ in the brain, plaque formation, glial activation and inflammatory cytokine production, hyperphosphorylation of tau, synaptic dysfunction as detected by electrophysiological techniques, and behavioral changes associated with disease (Games *et al.*, 1995; Hsiao *et al.*, 1995; Duff *et al.*, 1996;

Table 7.1 Murine models for AD studies

Genetic risk factor being modeled/phenotype	Pathology
1 Mutated *APP*	
(ii) APP23 *APP* overexpression transgenic mice C57B6 strain Swedish double mutation Murine Thy-1 promoter	APP-immunoreactive plaques (Sturchler-Pierrat *et al.* 1997); neuronal loss, synaptic abnormalities, microglial activation (Calhoun *et al.* 1998); and amyloid plaque-associated microglial activation (Stalder *et al.* 1999)
(ii) Tg2576 *APP* overexpression transgenic mice C57B6/SJL F₁ × C57B6 strain Swedish double mutation Hamster prion promoter	Increases in APP and Aβ levels, numerous Aβ plaques (Irizarry *et al.* 1997); astrocytic gliosis (Hsiao *et al.* 1995); glial expression of inflammatory cytokines (Benzing *et al.* 1999); and impaired memory (Hsiao *et al.* 1996)
(iii) PDAPP (V717F) *APP* overexpression transgenic mice C57B6 x DBA2 F₁ hybrid strain V717F mutation PDGF-β promoter	Aβ plaque formation (Games *et al.* 1995); increases in APP and Aβ levels (Johnson-Wood *et al.* 1997); long-term potentiation decay, reduced synaptic responses, loss of field potentials while exhibiting numerous amyloid plaques, neuritic dystrophy and gliosis (Larson *et al.* 1999); and behavioral disturbances (Dodart *et al.* 1999)
2 Mutated *PS1/PS2*	
(i) *PS1* overexpression transgenic mice Swiss Webster × B6D2 F₁ strain M146L and M146V mutation PDGF-β2 promoter	Early deposition of senile plaque, APP metabolism altered, Aβ deposition increased (Duff *et al.* 1996)
3 Overexpression of *ApoE4*	
(i) Plaque-producing *APP* transgenic mice with *ApoE* knockout background (Swiss Webster × C57BL/6 × DBA/2) × C57BL/6 strain V717F mutation PDGF-β promoter	Increased development of amyloid plaques (Winkler *et al.* 1999) and tau hyperphosphorylation (Cole *et al.* 1999)
4 Hyperphosphorylated tau protein	
(i) Tau overexpression transgenic mice B6D2/F₁ strain T44 isoform Murine prion promoter	Hyperphosphorylated tau and spinal cord gliosis (Ishihara *et al.* 1999)

Johnson-Wood *et al.*, 1997; Sturchler-Pierrat *et al.*, 1997; Yamada and Takashima 1997; Benzing *et al.*, 1999; Calhoun *et al.*, 1999; Cole *et al.*, 1999; Dodart *et al.*, 1999; Ishihara *et al.*, 1999; Larson *et al.*, 1999; Stalder *et al.*, 1999). With the exception of only one of these murine models, APP23, neuronal death and NFT formation have not been reproducible or been shown to correlate with cognitive decline in these models (Calhoun *et al.*, 1999). Due to these restrictions, a major obstacle is encountered when attempting to develop an animal model that can mimic all of the brain pathology and behavioral changes seen in AD.

Several hypotheses describing potential mechanisms for Aβ-induced and MP-mediated neuronal injury have been proposed. One hypothesis suggests that neuronal degeneration may initiate 'a positive feed-forward system' that leads to activation of MPs and the release of toxic factors. In turn, these factors may induce additional neuronal damage and lead to the chronic activation of brain MPs (Schmechel *et al.*, 1988; Goldgaber *et al.*, 1989). Such events can perpetuate a cycle of continued neuronal injury, amyloid deposition and inflammation. Another hypothesis proposes that an initial insult, coupled with genetic susceptibility, can induce neuronal dysfunction or injury. This, in turn, may lead to the gradual accumulation of cellular debris (e.g. insoluble Aβ fibrils) that MPs find difficult to phagocytose or digest (McGeer and McGeer, 1997). Upon reaching a threshold level, insoluble Aβ can create a huge 'phagocytolytic burden' for the MPs, leading to chronic activation and the increased production of toxic agents that induce neuronal injury (McGeer and McGeer, 1995, 1997; Chen *et al.*, 1996).

Currently, the leading hypothesis proposed to describe the progression of AD and the resultant neuropathogenicity is the 'amyloid cascade hypothesis'. This hypothesis assumes that metabolic changes in APP processing and the subsequent accumulation of APP products, such as the insoluble $Aβ_{1-42}$ fragment, are central to AD pathogenesis (Selkoe, 1996). Whether formation of the NP results from the overproduction and deposition of the amyloidogenic Aβ peptide fragments or is due to the insufficient clearance of these peptides is unknown. According to this hypothesis, the extracellular deposition of aggregated Aβ and formation of mature NPs triggers a cascade of direct and indirect neuropathological events that include tau phosphorylation, tangle formation, neuronal death, initiation of a chronic inflammatory response and activation of the classical complement pathway. Together these events lead to the pathological and clinical manifestations of disease (Eikelenboom *et al.*, 1994; Eikelenboom and Veerhuis, 1996). A variation on the 'amyloid cascade hypothesis', the 'accelerator hypothesis', postulates that activated microglia and reactive astrocytes release cytokines and amyloid-associated factors, such as apoE-ε4 and ACT, that act to accelerate Aβ aggregation and NP formation (Nilsson *et al.*, 1998). Similarly, Johnstone *et al.* (1999) propose that following Aβ deposition, astrocytes and oligodendrocytes are activated to release chemokines, that recruit microglia from the surrounding tissue and peripheral macrophages from the CNS parenchyma. Upon recruitment to areas of NP formation, Aβ may activate these cells to release cytokines and other neurotoxins, that further contribute to the inflammatory process and cause neuronal death. In contrast, Janciauskiene and Wright (1998) have proposed that Aβ may compete with apoE for LDL receptor binding, leading to the breakdown of neuronal cholesterol homeostasis and neuronal death.

Although Aβ deposition is believed to play an important role in disease pathogenicity, an alternative hypothesis suggests that destabilization of the cytoskeleton, not Aβ deposition, is the causal event in AD pathogenesis. This hypothesis states that all four of the major AD-related genes (*APP, PS1, PS2* and *ApoE*) interact in various ways with the cytoskeleton to induce pathological abnormalities. At the heart of the 'destabilization hypothesis' is hyperphosphorylated tau, which causes cytoskeletal abnormalities, such as PHFs and NFTs. Changes in the cytoskeleton can affect protein processing (especially that of APP), leading to increased Aβ deposition and ultimately synaptic loss and neuronal death (Terry, 1996). While these hypotheses postulate how individual factors may contribute to disease, both the initiating events and the final mechanisms that contribute to neuronal injury in AD remain unclear (Nilsson *et al.*, 1998).

Based on these hypotheses and other pathological and biochemical evidence, we hypothesize that Aβ priming of MP, coupled with activation by immune signals such as CD40L, could drive the neuroinflammatory events underlying AD (Figure 7.3). Mutations in the *APP, ApoE-ε4, PS1* and/or *PS2* genes may predispose an individual to abnormal APP processing, immune activation or neuronal dysfunction (Figure 7.1). Acting alone or in conjunction, these genetic conditions ultimately may contribute to NFT formation or fibrillar Aβ deposition. Interacting with receptors on MPs, perhaps RAGE or SR-A (Christie *et al.*, 1996; El Khoury *et al.*, 1996; Paresce *et al.*, 1996; Yan *et al.*, 1996; Haworth *et al.*, 1997; Murao *et al.*, 1997; El Khoury *et al.*, 1998), Aβ may then induce a series of intracellular events that alters the threshold for cellular activation. Such events can 'prime' the MPs for subsequent activation by pro-inflammatory cytokines (IL-1 β, TNF-α, IL-6 or IFN-γ), chemokines or other factors released by neighboring glial cells or trafficking lymphocytes (Kiener *et al.*, 1995) (Figure 7.2). In turn, these factors may amplify glial activation responses, producing high and sustained levels of MP secretory factors that inevitably contribute to neuronal dysfunction through distinct signaling pathways (Figure7.3).

8 Summary

AD is an age-related neurodegenerative disorder that results from a series of genetic, immune and neurochemical events that culminate in brain inflammation and neuronal death. Mutations in the major AD-related genes and interactions between their gene products can lead to the abnormal processing of APP, giving rise to the neurotoxic $Aβ_{1-42}$ peptide or, alternatively, can result in altered neuronal structure and function. Interactions between $Aβ_{1-42}$ and other AD gene products, such as ApoE-ε4, can lead to the stabilization of Aβ fibrils and the formation of dense NPs, or the disruption of neuronal lipid transport and metabolism. Such pathological abnormalities may induce an 'injury signal' that triggers a strong immune response within affected tissue. As the primary immune effector cells of the CNS, MPs play a central role in mediating this response. Upon interaction with MP receptors, such as RAGE, SR-A and LDL-Rs, Aβ can induce a cascade of intracellular signals that 'prime' the MP for subsequent activation by immune stimuli. In turn, the immunological activation of MP leads to increased cytokine production, brain inflammation and ultimately neural damage. This suggests that Aβ-primed and immune-activated MPs may play a substantial role in the disease process.

In this review, we highlighted the importance of MPs in maintaining brain homeostasis and in regulating the onset and progression of AD. We proposed that MPs affect neuroinflammatory responses associated with disease through the induction of pro-inflammatory cytokines and other neurotoxins that, in turn, affect neural function and survival. Although many of the key factors that lead to MP activation, initiation of immuno-inflammatory responses and production of neurotoxic factors are known, how these individual factors interact to induce or regulate disease remain to be elucidated. By identifying the key genetic, immune, inflammatory and neurotoxic events involved in AD and the role of MPs in such processes, we hope to unravel the mechanisms by which neuronal injury occurs. Such research may serve to identify potential therapeutic targets that can be utilized to prevent or retard the devastating neurodegeneration that is associated with AD.

Acknowledgments

We thank Drs Anuja Ghorpade and Tsuneya Ikezu for scientific discussion; Dr Jenae Limoges for excellent editorial support and suggestions; and Ms Julie Ditter and Ms Robin Taylor for outstanding administrative and secretarial support. This work was supported in part by research grants (to H.E.G.) by the National Institutes of Health USA: P01 NS31492-01, R01 NS34239-01, R01 NS34239-02, R01 NS36126-01 and P01 MH57556-01.

References

Aagaard-Tillery, K.M. and Jelinek, D.F. (1996). Phosphatidylinositol 3-kinase activation in normal human B lymphocytes. *Journal of Immunology*, **156**, 4543–54.

Abdulkadir, S.A. and Ono, S.J. (1995). How are class II MHC genes turned on and off? *FASEB Journal*, **9**, 1429–35.

Abraham, C.R., Shirahama, T. and Potter, H. (1990). Alpha 1-antichymotrypsin is associated solely with amyloid deposits containing the β-protein. Amyloid and cell localization of α1-antichymotrypsin. *Neurobiology of Aging*, **11**, 123–9.

Aisen, P.S. (1996). Inflammation and Alzheimer disease. *Molecular and Chemical Neuropathology*, **28**, 83–8.

Aisen, P.S. (1997). Inflammation and Alzheimer's disease: mechanisms and therapeutic strategies. *Gerontology*, **43**, 143–9.

Akama, K., Albanese, C., Pestell, R. and VanEldik, L. (1998). Amyloid β-peptide stimulates nitric oxide production in astrocytes through an NFκB-dependent mechanism. *Proceedings of the National Academy of Sciences USA*, **95**, 5795–800.

Akiyama, H. (1994). Inflammatory response in Alzheimer's disease. *Tohoku Journal of Experimental Medicine*, **174**, 295–303.

Akiyama, H. and McGeer, P.L. (1990). Brain microglia constitutively express β-integrins. *Journal of Neuroimmunology*, **30**, 81–93.

Akiyama, H., Ikeda, K., Kondo, H. and McGeer, P.L. (1992). Thrombin accumulation in brains of patients with Alzheimer's disease. *Neuroscience Letters*, **146**, 152–4.

Akiyama, H., Ikeda, K., Kondo, H., Kato, M. and McGeer, P.L. (1993). Microglia express the type 2 plasminogen activator inhibitor in the brain of control subjects and patients with Alzheimer's disease. *Neuroscience Letters*, **164**, 233–5.

Akiyama, H., Tooyama, I., Kondo, H., Ikeda, K., Kimura, H., McGeer, E.G. and McGeer, P.L. (1994). Early response of brain resident microglia to kainic acid-induced hippocampal lesions. *Brain Research*, **635**, 257–68.

Alderson, M.R., Armitage, R.J., Tough, T.W., Strockbine, L., Fanslow, W.C. and Spriggs, M.K. (1993). CD40 expression by human monocytes: regulation by cytokines and activation of monocytes by the ligand for CD40. *Journal of Experimental Medicine*, **178**, 669–74.

Alonso, A.C., Grundke-Iqbal, I. and Iqbal, K. (1996). Alzheimer's disease hyperphosphorylated tau sequesters normal tau into tangles of filaments and disassembles microtubules. *Nature Medicine*, **2**, 783–7.

Altstiel, L.D. and Sperber, K. (1991). Cytokines in Alzheimer's disease. *Progress in Neuropsychopharmacological and Biological Psychiatry*, **15**, 481–95.

Amaldi, I., Reith, W., Berte, C. and Mach, B. (1989). Induction of HLA class II genes by IFN-γ is transcriptional and requires a trans-acting protein. *Journal of Immunology*, **142**, 999–1004.

Andreadis, A., Wagner, B.K., Broderick, J.A. and Kosik, K.S. (1996). A tau promoter region without neuronal specificity. *Journal of Neurochemistry*, **66**, 2257–63.

Ankarcrona, M., Dypbukt, J.M., Bonfoco, E., Zhivotovsky, B., Orrenius, S., Lipton, S.A. *et al.* (1995). Glutamate-induced neuronal death: a succession of necrosis or apoptosis depending on mitochondrial function. *Neuron*, **15**, 961–73.

Araujo, D.M. and Cotman, C.W. (1992a). Basic FGF in astroglial, microglial, and neuronal cultures: characterization of binding sites and modulation of release by lymphokines and trophic factors. *Journal of Neuroscience*, **12**, 1668–78.

Araujo, D.M. and Cotman, C.W. (1992b). β-Amyloid stimulates glial cells *in vitro* to produce growth factors that accumulate in senile plaques in Alzheimer's disease. *Brain Research*, **569**, 141–5.

Arvin, B., Neville, L.F., Barone, F.C. and Feuerstein, G.Z. (1996). The role of inflammation and cytokines in brain injury. *Neuroscience and Biobehavioral Review*, **20**, 445–52.

Bales, K.R., Verina, T., Dodel, R.C., Du, Y., Altstiel, L., Bender, M. *et al.* (1997). Lack of apolipoprotein E dramatically reduces amyloid β-peptide deposition. *Nature Genetics*, **17**, 263–4.

Banati, R. B., Gehrmann, J., Schubert, P. and Kreutzberg, G.W. (1993). Cytotoxicity of microglia. *Glia*, **7**, 111–8.

Bandtlow, C.E., Meyer, M., Lindholm, D., Spranger, M., Heumann, R. and Thoenen, H. (1990). Regional and cellular co-distribution of interleukin 1 β and nerve growth factor mRNA in the adult rat brain: possible relationship to the regulation of nerve growth factor synthesis. *Journal of Cell Biology*, **111**, 1701–11.

Barnea, A., Aguila-Mansilla, N., Chute, H.T. and Welcher, A.A. (1996). Comparison of neurotrophin regulation of human and rat neuropeptide Y (NPY) neurons: induction of NPY production in aggregate cultures derived from rat but not from human fetal brains. *Brain Research*, **732**, 52–60.

Batchelor, P.E., Liberatore, G.T., Wong, J.Y., Porritt, M.J., Frerichs, F., Donnan, G.A. *et al.* (1999). Activated macrophages and microglia induce dopaminergic sprouting in the injured striatum and express brain-derived neurotrophic factor and glial cell line-derived neurotrophic factor. *Journal of Neuroscience*, **19**, 1708–16.

Baynes, J. (1991). Role of oxidative stress in development of complications in diabetes. *Diabetes*, **40**, 405–12.

Beckman, J., Beckman, T., Chen, J., Marshall, P. and Freeman, B. (1990). Apparent hydroxyl production by peroxynitrite: implications for endothelial injury form nitric oxide and superoxide. *Proceedings of the National Academy of Sciences USA*, **87**, 1620–4.

Beezhold, D.H. and Personius, C. (1992). Fibronectin fragments stimulate tumor necrosis factor secretion by human monocytes. *Journal of Leukocyte Biology*, **51**, 59–64.

Bell, M.D., Taub, D.D. and Perry, V.H. (1996). Overriding the brain's intrinsic resistance to leuko-cyte recruitment with intraparenchymal injections of recombinant chemokines. *Neuroscience*, **74**, 283–92.

Bellinger, F.P., Madamba, S. and Siggins, G.R. (1993). Interleukin 1 β inhibits synaptic strength and long-term potentiation in the rat CA1 hippocampus. *Brain Research*, **628**, 227–34.

Benjamin, R., Leake, A., McArthur, F.K., Ince, P.G., Candy, J.M., Edwardson, J.A. *et al.* (1994). Protective effect of apoE2 in Alzheimer's disease. *Lancet*, **344**, 473.

Benveniste, E.N. (1992). Inflammatory cytokines within the central nervous system: sources, func-tion, and mechanism of action. *American Journal of Physiology*, **263**, C1–16.

Benveniste, E.N. (1997a). Cytokines: influence on glial cell gene expression and function. *Chemical Immunology*, **69**, 31–75.

Benveniste, E.N. (1997b). Role of macrophages/microglia in multiple sclerosis and experimental allergic encephalomyelitis. *Journal of Molecular Medicine*, **75**, 165–73.

Benzing, W.C., Wujek, J.R., Ward, E.K., Shaffer, D., Ashe, K.H., Younkin, S.G. a*et al.* (1999). Evidence for glial-mediated inflammation in aged APP(SW) transgenic mice. *Neurobiology of Aging*, **20**, 581–9.

Berberich, I., Shu, G.L. and Clark, E.A. (1994). Cross-linking CD40 on B cells rapidly activates nuclear factor-κB. *Journal of Immunology*, **153**, 4357–66.

Bianca, V.D., Dusi, S., Bianchini, E., Dal Pra, I. and Rossi, F. (1999). β-Amyloid activates the O-2 forming NADPH oxidase in microglia, monocytes, and neutrophils. A possible inflammatory mechanism of neuronal damage in Alzheimer's disease. *Journal of Biological Chemistry*, **274**, 15493–9.

Bito, H., Nakamura, M., Honda, Z., Izumi, T., Iwatsubo, T., Seyama, Y. *et al.* (1992). Platelet-acti-vating factor (PAF) receptor in rat brain: PAF mobilizes intracellular Ca^{2+} in hippocampal neurons. *Neuron*, **9**, 285–94.

Blasko, I., Schmitt, T.L., Steiner, E., Trieb, K. and Grubeck-Loebenstein, B. (1997). Tumor necrosis factor α augments amyloid β protein (25–35) induced apoptosis in human cells. *Neuroscience Letters*, **238**, 17–20.

Blasko, I., Marx, F., Steiner, E., Hartmann, T. and Grubeck-Loebenstein, B. (1999). TNF α plus IFNγ induce the production of Alzheimer β-amyloid peptides and decrease the secretion of APPs. *FASEB Journal*, **13**, 63–8.

Blume, A.J. and Vitek, M.P. (1989). Focusing on IL-1-promotion of β-amyloid precursor protein synthesis as an early event in Alzheimer's disease. *Neurobiology of Aging*, **10**, 406–8; discussion 412–4.

Bonfoco, E., Krainc, D., Ankarcrona, M., Nicotera, P. and Lipton, S.A. (1995). Apoptosis and necrosis: two distinct events induced, respectively, by mild and intense insults with *N*-methyl-D-aspartate or nitric oxide/superoxide in cortical cell cultures. *Proceedings of the National Academy of Sciences USA*, **92**, 7162–6.

Borchelt, D.R., Thinakaran, G., Eckman, C.B., Lee, M.K., Davenport, F., Ratovitsky, T. *et al.* (1996). Familial Alzheimer's disease-linked presenilin 1 variants elevate Aβ1–42/1–40 ratio *in vitro* and *in vivo*. *Neuron*, **17**, 1005–13.

Botchkina, G.I., Meistrell, M.E., 3rd, Botchkina, I.L. and Tracey, K. J. (1997). Expression of TNF and TNF receptors (p55 and p75) in the rat brain after focal cerebral ischemia. *Molecular Medicine*, **3**, 765–81.

Boyce, J. and Shea, T. (1997). Phosphorylation events mediated by protein kinase C α and ε participate in regulation of tau steady-state levels and generation of certain 'Alzheimer-like' phospoepitopes. *International Journal of Developmental Neuroscience*, **15**, 295–307.

Brett, J., Schmidt, A.M., Yan, S.D., Zou, Y.S., Weidman, E., Pinsky, D. *et al.* (1993). Survey of the distribution of a newly characterized receptor for advanced glycation end products in tissues. *American Journal of Pathology*, **143**, 1699–712.

Bruno, V., Copani, A., Knopfel, T., Kuhn, R., Casabona, G., Dell'Albani, P. *et al.* (1995). Activation of metabotropic glutamate receptors coupled to inositol phopholipid hydrolysis amplifies NMDA-induced neuronal degeneration in cultured cortical cells. *Neuropharmacology*, **34**, 1089–98.

Burdick, D., Soreghan, B., Kwon, M., Kosmoski, J., Knauer, M., Henschen, A.Y. *et al.* (1992). Assembly and aggregation properties of synthetic Alzheimer's A4/ β amyloid peptide analogs. *Journal of Biological Chemistry*, **267**, 546–54.

Busciglio, J., Yeh, J. and Yanker, B.A. (1993). β-Amyloid neurotoxicity in human cortical culture is not mediated by excitotoxins. *Journal of Neurochemistry*, **61**, 1565–8.

Buttke, T.M. and Sandstrom, P.A. (1994). Oxidative stress as a mediator of apoptosis. *Immunology Today*, **15**, 7–10.

Buxbaum, J.D., Oishi, M., Chen, H.I., Pinkas-Kramarski, R., Jaffe, E.A., Gandy, S.E. *et al.* (1992). Cholinergic agonists and interleukin 1 regulate processing and secretion of the Alzheimer β/A4 amyloid protein precursor. *Proceedings of the National Academy of Sciences USA*, **89**, 10075–8.

Cacabelos, R., Alvarez, X.A., Fernandez-Novoa, L., Franco, A., Mangues, R., Pellicer, A. *et al.* (1994). Brain interleukin-1 β in Alzheimer's disease and vascular dementia. *Methodsand Findings in Experimental and Clinical Pharmacology*, **16**, 141–51.

Calhoun, M.E., Burgermeister, P., Phinney, A.L., Stalder, M., Tolnay, M., Wiederhold, K.H. *et al.* (1999). Neuronal overexpression of mutant amyloid precursor protein results in prominent deposition of cerebrovascular amyloid. *Proceedings of the National Academy of Sciences USA*, 96, 14088–93.

Cammer, W., Bloom, B.R., Norton, W.T. and Gordon, S. (1978). Degradation of basic protein in myelin by neutral proteases secreted by stimulated macrophages: a possible mechanism of inflammatory demyelination. *Proceedings of the National Academy of Sciences USA*, **75**, 1554–8.

Cassatella, M.A., Bazzoni, F., Amezaga, M.A. and Rossi, F. (1991). Studies on the gene expression of several NADPH oxidase components. *Biochemical Society Transactions*, **19**, 63–7

Castano, E. M., Prelli, F., Soto, C., Beavis, R., Matsubara, E., Shoji, M. *et al.* (1996). The length of amyloid-β in hereditary cerebral hemorrhage with amyloidosis, Dutch type. Implications for the role of amyloid-β 1–42 in Alzheimer's disease. *Journal of Biological Chemistry*, **271**, 32185–91.

Caux, C., Massacrier, C., Vanbervliet, B., Dubois, B., Van Kooten, C., Durand, I. *et al.* (1994). Activation of human dendritic cells through CD40 cross-linking. *Journal of Experimental Medicine*, **180**, 1263–72.

Chabot, S., Williams, G. and Yong, V.W. (1997). Microglial production of TNF-α is induced by activated T lymphocytes. Involvement of VLA-4 and inhibition by interferon-1 β. *Journal of Clinical Investigation*, **100**, 604–12.

Chanock, S.J., el Benna, J., Smith, R.M. and Babior, B.M. (1994). The respiratory burst oxidase. *Journal of Biological Chemistry*, **269**, 24519–22.

Chao, C.C., Hu, S., Molitor, T.W., Shaskan, E.G. and Peterson, P.K. (1992). Activated microglia mediate neuronal cell injury via a nitric oxide mechanism. *Journal of Immunology*, **149**, 2736–41.

Chao, C.C., Hu, S., Ehrlich, L. and Peterson, P.K. (1995a). Interleukin-1 and tumor necrosis factor-α synergistically mediate neurotoxicity: involvement of nitric oxide and of *N*-methyl-D-aspartate receptors. *Brain Behavior and Immunity*, **9**, 355–65.

Chao, C.C., Hu, S. and Peterson, P.K. (1995b). Glia, cytokines, and neurotoxicity. *Critical Reviews of Neurobiology*, **9**, 189–205.

Chao, C.C., Hu, S. and Peterson, P.K. (1995c). Modulation of human microglial cell superoxide production by cytokines. *Journal of Leukocyte Biology*, **58**, 65–70.

Chao, C.C., Hu, S., Sheng, W.S. and Peterson, P.K. (1995d). Tumor necrosis factor-α production by human fetal microglial cells: regulation by other cytokines. *Developmental Neuroscience*, **17**, 97–105.

Chao, C.C., Hu, S., Sheng, W.S., Tsang, M. and Peterson, P.K. (1995e). Tumor necrosis factor-α mediates the release of bioactive transforming growth factor-β in murine microglial cell cultures. *Clinical Immunology and Immunopathology*, **77**, 358–65.

Chao, C.C., Hu, S., Sheng, W.S., Bu, D., Bukrinsky, M.I. and Peterson, P.K. (1996). Cytokine-stimulated astrocytes damage human neurons via a nitric oxide mechanism. *Glia*, **16**, 276–84.

Chen, S., Frederickson, R.C. and Brunden, K.R. (1996). Neuroglial-mediated immunoinflammatory responses in Alzheimer's disease: complement activation and therapeutic approaches. *Neurobiology of Aging*, **17**, 781–7.

Choi, D.W., Maulucci-Gedde, M. and Kriegstein, A.R. (1987). Glutamate neurotoxicity in cortical cell culture. *Journal of Neuroscience*, **7**, 357–68.

Christie, R.H., Freeman, M. and Hyman, B.T. (1996). Expression of the macrophage scavenger receptor, a multifunctional lipoprotein receptor, in microglia associated with senile plaques in Alzheimer's disease. *American Journal of Pathology*, **148**, 399–403.

Citron, M., Diehl, T.S., Gordon, G., Biere, A.L., Seubert, P. and Selkoe, D.J. (1996). Evidence that the 42- and 40-amino acid forms of amyloid β protein are generated from the β-amyloid precursor protein by different protease activities. *Proceedings of the National Academy of Sciences USA*, **93**, 13170–5.

Clark, G., Happel, L., Zorumski, G. and Bazan, N. (1992). Enhancement of hippocampal excitatory synaptic transmission by platelet-activating factor. *Neuron*, **9**, 1211–6.

Clement, M.V. and Stamenkovic, I. (1996). Superoxide anion is a natural inhibitor of FAS-mediated cell death. *EMBO Journal*, **15**, 216–25.

Cole, G.M., Beech, W., Frautschy, S.A., Sigel, J., Glasgow, C. and Ard, M.D. (1999). Lipoprotein effects on Aβ accumulation and degradation by microglia *in vitro*. *Journal of Neuroscience Research*, **57**, 504–20.

Colton, C.A. and Gilbert, D.L. (1987). Production of superoxide anions by a CNS macrophage, the microglia. *FEBS Letters*, **223**, 284–8.

Colton, C.A., Keri, J.E., Chen, W.T. and Monsky, W.L. (1993). Protease production by cultured microglia: substrate gel analysis and immobilized matrix degradation. *Journal of Neuroscience Research*, **35**, 297–304.

Combs, C., Johnson, D., Cannady, S., Lehman, T. and Landreth, G. (1999). Identification of microglial signal transduction pathways mediating a neurotoxic response to amyloidgenic fragments of β-amyloid and prion proteins. *Journal of Neuroscience*, **19**, 928–39.

Cotman, C. (1998). Apoptosis decision cascades and neuronal degeneration in Alzheimer's disease. *Neurobiology of Aging*, **19**, S29–32.

Cotter, R., Zheng, J. and Gendelman, H.E. (1999). The role of mononuclear phagocytes in neurodegenerative disorders: lessons from multiple sclerosis, Alzheimer's disease and HIV-1 dementia. In Marwah, J. and Teitelbaum, H. (ed.), *Advances in Neurodegenerative Disorders*. Prominent Press, Scottsdale, AZ, pp. 203–41.

Cowburn, R., Fowler, C. and O'Neill, C. (1996). Neurotransmitter receptor/G-protein mediated signal transduction in Alzheimer's disease brain. *Neurodegeneration*, **5**, 483–8.

Coyle, J. and Puttfarcken, P. (1993). Oxidative stress, glutamate, and neurodegenerative disorders. *Science*, **262**, 689–95.

Das, H.K. and Lal, H. (1997). Genes implicated in the pathogenesis of Alzheimer's disease. *Frontiers in Bioscience*, **2**, 253–9.

Dash, P.K. and Moore, A.N. (1995). Enhanced processing of APP induced by IL-1 β can be reduced by indomethacin and nordihydroguaiaretic acid. *Biochemical and Biophysical Research Communications*, **208**, 542–8.

Dawson, V.L., Dawson, T.M., London, E.D., Bredt, D.S. and Snyder, S.H. (1991). Nitric oxide mediates glutamate neurotoxicity in primary cortical cultures. *Proceedings of the National Academy of Sciences USA*, 88, 6368–71.

DeBoni, U. and McLachlan, D. (1985). Controlled induction of paired helical filaments of the Alzheimer type in cultured human neurons by Glu and aspartate. *Journal of Neurological Science*, **68**, 105–18.

DeNagel, D.C. and Pierce, S.K. (1992). A case for chaperones in antigen processing. *Immunology Today*, **13**, 86–9.

De Simone, R., Giampaolo, A., Giometto, B., Gallo, P., Levi, G., Peschle, C. *et al.* (1995). The costimulatory molecule B7 is expressed on human microglia in culture and in multiple sclerosis acute lesions. *Journal of Neuropathology and Experimental Neurology*, **54**, 175–87.

De Simone, R., Levi, G. and Aloisi, F. (1998). Interferon γ gene expression in rat central nervous system glial cells. *Cytokine*, **10**, 418–22.

de Villiers, W.J., Fraser, I.P. and Gordon, S. (1994a). Cytokine and growth factor regulation of macrophage scavenger receptor expression and function. *Immunology Letters*, **43**, 73–9.

de Villiers, W.J., Fraser, I.P., Hughes, D.A., Doyle, A.G. and Gordon, S. (1994b). Macrophage-colony-stimulating factor selectively enhances macrophage scavenger receptor expression and function. *Journal of Experimental Medicine*, **180**, 705–9.

Dickson, D.W., Lee, S.C., Mattiace, L.A., Yen, S.H. and Brosnan, C. (1993). Microglia and cytokines in neurological disease, with special reference to AIDS and Alzheimer's disease. *Glia*, **7**, 75–83.

Dodart, J.C., Meziane, H., Mathis, C., Bales, K.R., Paul, S.M. and Ungerer, A. (1999). Behavioral disturbances in transgenic mice overexpressing the V717F β-amyloid precursor protein. *Behavioral Neuroscience*, **113**, 982–90.

Donnelly, R.., Friedhoff, A.J., Beer, B., Blume, A.J. and Vitek, M.P. (1990). Interleukin-1 stimulates the β-amyloid precursor protein promoter. *Cellular and Molecular Neurobiology*, **10**, 485–95.

Duff, K., Eckman, C., Zehr, C., Yu, X., Prada, C.M., Pereztur, J. *et al.* (1996). Increased amyloid-β42(43) in brains of mice expressing mutant presenilin 1. *Nature*, **383**, 710–3.

Duval, E., Wyllie, A. and Morris, R. (1985). Macrophage recognition of cells undergoing programmed cell death (apoptosis). *Immunology*, **56**, 351–8.

Eddleston, M. and Mucke, L. (1993). Molecular profile of reactive astrocytes—implications for their role in neurologic disease. *Neuroscience*, **54**, 15–36.

Eikelenboom, P. and Stam, F.C. (1982). Immunoglobulins and complement factors in senile plaques. An immunoperoxidase study. *Acta Neuropathologica*, **57**, 239–42.

Eikelenboom, P. and Veerhuis, R. (1996). The role of complement and activated microglia in the pathogenesis of Alzheimer's disease. *Neurobiology of Aging*, **17**, 673–80.

Eikelenboom, P., Zhan, S.S., van Gool, W.A. and Allsop, D. (1994). Inflammatory mechanisms in Alzheimer's disease. *Trends in Pharmacological Science*, **15**, 447–50.

El Khoury, J., Hickman, S.E., Thomas, C.A., Cao, L., Silverstein, S.C. and Loike, J.D. (1996). Scavenger receptor-mediated adhesion of microglia to β-amyloid fibrils. *Nature*, 382, 716–9.

El Khoury, J., Hickman, S.E., Thomas, C.A., Loike, J.D. and Silverstein, S.C. (1998). Microglia, scavenger receptors, and the pathogenesis of Alzheimer's disease. *Neurobiology of Aging*, **19**, S81–4.

Elkabes, S., DiCicco-Bloom, E.M. and Black, I.B. (1996). Brain microglia/macrophages express neurotrophins that selectively regulate microglial proliferation and function. *Journal of Neuroscience*, **16**, 2508–21.

Esch, F.S., Keim, P.S., Beattie, E.C., Blacher, R.W., Culwell, A.R., Oltersdorf, T. *et al.* (1990). Cleavage of amyloid β peptide during constitutive processing of its precursor. *Science*, **248**, 1122–4.

Fagan, A.M., Bu, G., Sun, Y., Daugherty, A. and Holtzman, D.M. (1996). Apolipoprotein E-containing high density lipoprotein promotes neurite outgrowth and is a ligand for the low density lipoprotein receptor-related protein. *Journal of Biological Chemistry*, **271**, 30121–5.

Faris, M., Gaskin, F., Parsons, J.T. and Fu, S.M. (1994). CD40 signaling pathway: anti-CD40 monoclonal antibody induces rapid dephosphorylation and phosphorylation of tyrosine-phosphorylated proteins including protein tyrosine kinase Lyn, Fyn, and Syk and the appearance of a 28-kD tyrosine phosphorylated protein. *Journal of Experimental Medicine*, **179**, 1923–31.

Flanders, K.C., Ren, R.F. and Lippa, C.F. (1998). Transforming growth factor-βs in neurodegenerative disease. *Progress in Neurobiology*, **54**, 71–85.

Fontana, A., Hengartner, H., de Tribolet, N. and Weber, E. (1984). Glioblastoma cells release interleukin 1 and factors inhibiting interleukin 2-mediated effects. *Journal of Immunology*, **132**, 1837–44.

Forloni, G., Demicheli, F., Giorgi, S., Bendotti, C. and Angeretti, N. (1992). Expression of amyloid precursor protein mRNAs in endothelial, neuronal and glial cells: modulation by interleukin-1. *Brain Research and Molecular Brain Research*, **16**, 128–34.

Fowler, C. (1997). The role of the phosphoinositide signalling system in the pathogenesis of sporadic Alzheimer's disease: a hypothesis. *Brain Research Review*, **25**, 373–80.

Fraser, P.E., Nguyen, J.T., McLachlan, D.R., Abraham, C.R. and Kirschner, D.A. (1993). Alpha 1-antichymotrypsin binding to Alzheimer Aβ peptides is sequence specific and induces fibril disaggregation *in vitro*. *Journal of Neurochemistry*, **61**, 298–305.

Frei, K., Siepl, C., Groscurth, P., Bodmer, S., Schwerdel, C. and Fontana, A. (1987). Antigen presentation and tumor cytotoxicity by interferon-γ-treated microglial cells. *European Journal of Immunology*, **17**, 1271–8.

Frei, K., Malipiero, U.V., Leist, T.P., Zinkernagel, R.M., Schwab, M.E. and Fontana, A. (1989). On the cellular source and function of interleukin 6 produced in the central nervous system in viral diseases. *European Journal of Immunology*, **19**, 689–94.

Fuentes, M.E., Durham, S.K., Swerdel, M.R., Lewin, A.C., Barton, D.S., Megill, J.R. *et al.* (1995). Controlled recruitment of monocytes and macrophages to specific organs through transgenic expression of monocyte chemoattractant protein-1. *Journal of Immunology*, **155**, 5769–76.

Fuller, S.J., Storey, E., Li, Q.X., Smith, A.I., Beyreuther, K. and Masters, C.L. (1995). Intracellular production of βA4 amyloid of Alzheimer's disease: modulation by phosphoramidon and lack of coupling to the secretion of the amyloid precursor protein. *Biochemistry*, **34**, 8091–8.

Fultz, M.J., Barber, S.A., Dieffenbach, C.W. and Vogel, S.N. (1993). Induction of IFN-γ in macrophages by lipopolysaccharide. *International Immunology*, **5**, 1383–92.

Furukawa, K., Barger, S.W., Blalock, E.M. and Mattson, M.P. (1996). Activation of K+ channels and suppression of neuronal activity by secreted β-amyloid-precursor protein. *Nature*, **379**, 74–8

Games, D., Adams, D., Alessandrini, R., Barbour, R., Berthelette, P., Blackwell, C. *et al.* (1995). Alzheimer-type neuropathology in transgenic mice overexpressing V717F β-amyloid precursor protein. *Nature*, **373**, 523–7.

Gehrmann, J., Matsumoto, Y. and Kreutzberg, G.W. (1995). Microglia: intrinsic immuneffector cell of the brain. *Brain Research and Brain Research Review*, **20**, 269–87.

Gelbard, H.A., Dzenko, K.A., DiLoreto, D., del Cerro, C., del Cerro, M. and Epstein, L.G. (1993). Neurotoxic effects of tumor necrosis factor α in primary human neuronal cultures are mediated by activation of the glutamate AMPA receptor subtype: implications for AIDS neuropathogenesis. *Developmental Neuroscience*, **15**, 417–22.

Gelbard, H.A., Nottet, H.S., Swindells, S., Jett, M., Dzenko, K.A., Genis, P. *et al.* (1994). Platelet-activating factor: a candidate human immunodeficiency virus type 1-induced neurotoxin. *Journal of Virology*, **68**, 4628–35.

Geng, Y.J. and Hansson, G.K. (1992). Interferon-γ inhibits scavenger receptor expression and foam cell formation in human monocyte-derived macrophages. *Journal of Clinical Investigation*, **89**, 1322–30.

Genis, P., Jett, M., Bernton, E.W., Boyle, T., Gelbard, H.A., Dzenko, K. *et al.* (1992). Cytokines and arachidonic metabolites produced during human immunodeficiency virus (HIV)-infected macrophage–astroglia interactions: implications for the neuropathogenesis of HIV disease. *Journal of Experimental Medicine*, **176**, 1703–18.

Geula, C., Wu, C.K., Saroff, D., Lorenzo, A., Yuan, M. and Yankner, B.A. (1998). Aging renders the brain vulnerable to amyloid β-protein neurotoxicity. *Nature Medicine*, **4**, 827–31.

Ghosh, A. and Greenberg, M. (1995). Calcium signaling in neurons: molecular mechanisms and cellular consequences. *Science*, **268**, 239–47.

Gillardon, F., Skutella, T., Uhlmann, E., Holsboer, F., Zimmerman, M. and Behl, C. (1996). Activation of c-Fos contributes to amyloid β-peptide-induced neurotoxicity. *Brain Research*, **706**, 169–72.

Giulian, D. (1990). Microglia, cytokines, and cytotoxins: modulators fo cellular responses after injury to the central nervous system. *Journal of Immunology and Immunopharmacology*, **10**, 15–21.

Giulian, D., Baker, T.J., Shih, L.C. and Lachman, L.B. (1986). Interleukin 1 of the central nervous system is produced by ameboid microglia. *Journal of Experimental Medicine*, **164**, 594–604.

Giulian, D., Vaca, K. and Corpuz, M. (1993). Brain glia release factors with opposing actions upon neuronal survival. *Journal of Neuroscience*, **13**, 29–37.

Goate, A., Chartier-Harlin, M.C., Mullan, M., Brown, J., Crawford, F., Fidani, L. *et al.* (1991). Segregation of a missense mutation in the amyloid precursor protein gene with familial Alzheimer's disease. *Nature*, **349**, 704–6.

Goedert, M. (1987). Neuronal localization of amyloid β protein precursor mRNA in normal human brain and in Alzheimer's disease. *EMBO Journal*, **6**, 3627–32.

Goldgaber, D., Harris, H.W., Hla, T., Maciag, T., Donnelly, R.J., Jacobsen, J.S. *et al.* (1989). Interleukin 1 regulates synthesis of amyloid β-protein precursor mRNA in human endothelial cells. *Proceedings of the National Academy of Sciences USA*, **86**, 7606–10.

Good, P., Perl, D., Bierer, L. and Schmeidler, J. (1992). Selective accumulation of aluminum and iron in the neurofibrillary tangles of Alzheimer's disease: a laser microprobe (LAMMA) study. *Annals of Neurology*, **31**, 286–292.

Goodwin, J.L., Uemura, E. and Cunnick, J.E. (1995). Microglial release of nitric oxide by the synergistic action of β-amyloid and IFN-γ. *Brain Research*, **692**, 207–14.

Gordon, S. (1995). The macrophage. *Bioessays*, **17**, 977–86.

Gottschall, P.E., Yu, X. and Bing, B. (1995). Increased production of gelatinase B (matrix metalloproteinase-9) and interleukin-6 by activated rat microglia in culture. *Journal of Neuroscience Research*, **42**, 335–42.

Gough, P.J., Greaves, D.R., Suzuki, H., Hakkinen, T., Hiltunen, M.O., Turunen, M. *et al.* (1999). Analysis of macrophage scavenger receptor (SR-A) expression in human aortic atherosclerotic lesions. *Arteriosclerosic and Thrombosic Vascular Biology*, **19**, 461–71.

Graf, D., Muller, S., Korthauer, U., van Kooten, C., Weise, C. and Kroczek, R.A. (1995). A soluble form of TRAP (CD40 ligand) is rapidly released after T cell activation. *European Journal of Immunology*, **25**, 1749–54.

Griffin, D.E. (1997). Cytokines in the brain during viral infection: clues to HIV-associated dementia. *Journal of Clinical Investigation*, **100**, 2948–51.

Griffin, W.S., Stanley, L.C., Ling, C., White, L., MacLeod, V., Perrot, L.J. *et al.* (1989). Brain interleukin 1 and S-100 immunoreactivity are elevated in Down syndrome and Alzheimer disease. *Proceedings of the National Academy of Sciences USA*, **86**, 7611–5.

Gruol, D.L. and Nelson, T.E. (1997). Physiological and pathological roles of interleukin-6 in the central nervous system. *Molecular Neurobiology*, **15**, 307–39.

Gupta, S.K., Lysko, P.G., Pillarisetti, K., Ohlstein, E. and Stadel, J.M. (1998). Chemokine receptors in human endothelial cells. *Journal of Biological Chemistry*, **273**, 4282–7.

Haass, C. and Selkoe, D J. (1993). Cellular processing of β-amyloid precursor protein and the genesis of amyloid β-peptide. *Cell*, **75**, 1039–42.

Haga, S., Akai, K. and Ishii, T. (1989). Demonstration of microglial cells in and around senile (neuritic) plaques in the Alzheimer brain. An immunohistochemical study using a novel monoclonal antibody. *Acta Neuropathologica*, **77**, 569–75.

Halliwell, B. and Gutteridge, J.M. (1985). The importance of free radicals and catalytic metal ions in human diseases. *Molecular Aspects of Medicine*, **8**, 89–193.

Hanissian, S.H. and Geha, R.S. (1997). Jak3 is associated with CD40 and is critical for CD40 induction of gene expression in B cells. *Immunity*, **6**, 379–87.

Hartmann, H., Eckert, A. and Muller, W. (1994). Disturbances of the neuronal calcium homeostasis in the aging nervous system. *Life Science*, **55**, 2011–8.

Haworth, R., Platt, N., Keshav, S., Hughes, D., Darley, E., Suzuki, H., Kurihara, Y. *et al.* (1997). The macrophage scavenger receptor type A is expressed by activated macrophages and protects the host against lethal endotoxic shock. *Journal of Experimental Medicine*, **186**, 1431–9.

Heese, K., Hock, C. and Otten, U. (1998). Inflammatory signals induce neurotrophin expression in human microglial cells. *Journal of Neurochemistry*, **70**, 699–707.

Hellendall, R.P. and Ting, J.P. (1997). Differential regulation of cytokine-induced major histocompatibility complex class II expression and nitric oxide release in rat microglia and astrocytes by effectors of tyrosine kinase, protein kinase C, and cAMP. *Journal of Neuroimmunology*, **74**, 19–29.

Henn, V., Slupsky, J.R., Grafe, M., Anagnostopoulos, I., Forster, R., Muller-Berghaus, G. *et al.* (1998). CD40 ligand on activated platelets triggers an inflammatory reaction of endothelial cells. *Nature*, **391**, 591–4.

Hensley, K., Carney, J.M., Mattson, M.P., Aksenova, M., Harris, M., Wu, J.F. *et al.* (1994). A model for β-amyloid aggregation and neurotoxicity based on free radical generation by the peptide: relevance to Alzheimer disease. *Proceedings of the National Academy of Sciences USA*, **91**, 3270–4.

Hewett, S.J., Csernansky, C.A. and Choi, D.W. (1994). Selective potentiation of NMDA-induced neuronal injury following induction of astrocytic iNOS. *Neuron*, **13**, 487–94.

Heyes, M.P., Brew, B.J., Martin, A., Price, R.W., Salazar, A.M., Sidtis, J.J. *et al.* (1991). Quinolinic acid in cerebrospinal fluid and serum in HIV-1 infection: relationship to clinical and neurological status. *Annals of Neurology*, **29**, 202–9.

Hofman, F.M., von Hanwehr, R.I., Dinarello, C.A., Mizel, S.B., Hinton, D. and Merrill, J.E. (1986). Immunoregulatory molecules and IL 2 receptors identified in multiple sclerosis brain. *Journal of Immunology*, **136**, 3239–45.

Hsiao, K.K., Borchelt, D.R., Olson, K., Johannsdottir, R., Kitt, C., Yunis, W. *et al.* (1995). Age-related CNS disorder and early death in transgenic FVB/N mice overexpressing Alzheimer amyloid precursor proteins. *Neuron*, **15**, 1203–18.

Hu, J., Ferreira, A. and Van Eldik, L.J. (1997). S100 β induces neuronal cell death through nitric oxide release from astrocytes. *Journal of Neurochemistry*, **69**, 2294–301.

Huitinga, I., van Rooijen, N., de Groot, C.J., Uitdehaag, B.M. and Dijkstra, C.D. (1990). Suppression of experimental allergic encephalomyelitis in Lewis rats after elimination of macrophages. *Journal of Experimental Medicine*, **172**, 1025–33.

Hung, A., Haas, C., Nitsch, R. *et al.* (1993). Activationof protein kinase C inhibits cellular production of the amyloid-protein. *Journal of Biological Chemistry*, **268**, 22959–62.

Huttunen, H.J., Fages, C. and Rauvala, H. (1999). Receptor for advanced glycation end products (RAGE)-mediated neurite outgrowth and activation of NF-κB require the cytoplasmic domain of the receptor but different downstream signaling pathways. *Journal of Biological Chemistry*, **274**, 19919–24.

Imamoto, K. and Leblond, C.P. (1977). Presence of labeled monocytes, macrophages and microglia in a stab wound of the brain following an injection of bone marrow cells labeled with ^{3}H-uridine into rats. *Journal of Comparative Neurology*, **174**, 255–79.

Iqbal, K. and Grundke-Iqbal, I. (1991). Ubiquitination and abnormal phosphorylation of paired helical filaments in Alzheimer's disease. *Molecular Neurobiology*, **5**, 399–410.

Ishihara, T., Hong, M., Zhang, B., Nakagawa, Y., Lee, M.K., Trojanowski, J.Q. *et al.* (1999). Age-dependent emergence and progression of a tauopathy in transgenic mice overexpressing the shortest human tau isoform. *Neuron*, **24**, 751–62.

Ishizuka, K., Kimura, T., Igata-yi, R., Katsuragi, S., Takamatsu, J. and Miyakawa, T. (1997). Identification of monocyte chemoattractant protein-1 in senile plaques and reactive microglia of Alzheimer's disease. *Psychiatry and Clinical Neuroscience*, **51**, 135–8.

Itagaki, S., McGeer, P.L., Akiyama, H., Zhu, S. and Selkoe, D. (1989). Relationship of microglia and astrocytes to amyloid deposits of Alzheimer disease. *Journal of Neuroimmunology*, **24**, 173–82.

Iwatsubo, T., Odaka, A., Suzuki, N., Mizusawa, H., Nukina, N. and Ihara, Y. (1994). Visualization of Aβ42(43) and Aβ40 in senile plaques with end-specific Aβ monoclonals: evidence that an initially deposited species is Aβ 42(43). *Neuron*, **13**, 45–53.

Jakoi, E., Sombati, S., Gerwin, C. and DeLorenzo, R. (1992). Excitatory amino acid receptor activation produces a selective and long-lasting modulation of gene expression in hippocampal neurons. *Brain Research*, **582**, 282–90.

Janciauskiene, S. and Wright, H.T. (1998). Inflammation, antichymotrypsin, and lipid metabolism: autogenic etiology of Alzheimer's disease. *Bioessays*, **20**, 1039–46

Jarrett, J.T., Berger, E.P. and Lansbury, P.T., Jr (1993). The C-terminus of the β protein is critical in amyloidogenesis. *Annals of the New York Academy of Sciences*, **695**, 144–8.

Ji, Z.S., Brecht, W.J., Miranda, R.D., Hussain, M.M., Innerarity, T.L. and Mahley, R.W. (1993). Role of heparan sulfate proteoglycans in the binding and uptake of apolipoprotein E-enriched remnant lipoproteins by cultured cells. *Journal of Biological Chemistry*, **268**, 10160–7.

Jiang, H., Burdick, D., Glabe, C.G., Cotman, C.W. and Tenner, A.J. (1994). β-Amyloid activates complement by binding to a specific region of the collagen-like domain of the C1q A chain. *Journal of Immunology*, **152**, 5050–9.

Johnson-Wood, K., Lee, M., Motter, R., Hu, K., Gordon, G., Barbour, R. *et al.* (1997). Amyloid precursor protein processing and Aβ42 deposition in a transgenic mouse model of Alzheimer disease. *Proceedings of the National Academy of Sciences USA*, 94, 1550–5.

Johnstone, M., Gearing, A.J. and Miller, K.M. (1999). A central role for astrocytes in the inflammatory response to β-amyloid; chemokines, cytokines and reactive oxygen species are produced. *Journal of Neuroimmunology*, **93**, 182–93.

Jope, R., Song, L. and Powers, R. (1997). Cholinergic activation of phosphoinositide signaling is impaired in Alzheimer's disease brain. *Neurobiology of Aging*, **18**, 111–20.

Jordan-Sciutto, K. and Bowser, R. (1998). Alzheimer's disease and brain development: common molecular pathways. *Frontiers in Bioscience*, **3**, D100–12.

Kalaria, R.N., Cohen, D.L. and Premkumar, D.R. (1996a). Cellular aspects of the inflammatory response in Alzheimer's disease. *Neurodegeneration*, **5**, 497–503

Kalaria, R.N., Harshbarger-Kelly, M., Cohen, D.L. and Premkumar, D.R. (1996b). Molecular aspects of inflammatory and immune responses in Alzheimer's disease. *Neurobiology of Aging*, **17**, 687–93.

Kaltschmidt, B., Baeuerle, P.A. and Kaltschmidt, C. (1993). Potential involvement of the transcription factor NF-κB in neurological disorders. *Molecular Aspects of Medicine*, **14**, 171–90.

Kaltschmidt, B., Uherek, M., Volk, B., Baeuerle, P.A. and Kaltschmidt, C. (1997). Transcription factor NF-κB is activated in primary neurons by amyloid β peptides and in neurons surrounding early plaques from patients with Alzheimer disease. *Proceedings of the National Academy of Sciences USA*, **94**, 2642–7.

Kane, D., Sarafian, T., Anton, R. *et al.* (1993). Bcl-2 inhibition of neural death: decreased generation of reactive oxygen species. *Science*, **262**, 1274–7.

Karras, J.G., Wang, Z., Huo, L., Howard, R.G., Frank, D.A. and Rothstein, T.L. (1997). Signal transducer and activator of transcription-3 (STAT3) is constitutively activated in normal, self-renewing B-1 cells but only inducibly expressed in conventional B lymphocytes. *Journal of Experimental Medicine*, **185**, 1035–42.

Kelly, J., Furukawa, K., Barger, S., Rengen, M., Mark, R., Blanc, E. *et al.* (1996). Amyloid β-peptide disrupts carbachol-induced muscarinic cholinergic signal transduction in cortical neurons. *Proceedings of the National Academy of Sciences USA*, **93**, 6753–8.

Kerr, J. and Harmon, B. (1991). In *Apoptosis: The Molecular Basis of Cell Death: Current Communications on Cell and Molecular Biology*. Cold Spring Harbor Laboratory Press, Cold Spring Harbor, NY, pp. 5–29.

Kerr, S.J., Armati, P.J., Guillemin, G.J. and Brew, B.J. (1998). Chronic exposure of human neurons to quinolinic acid results in neuronal changes consistent with AIDS dementia complex. *AIDS*, **12**, 355–63.

Kerschensteiner, M., Gallmeier, E., Behrens, L., Leal, V.V., Misgeld, T., Klinkert, W.E. *et al.* (1999). Activated human T cells, B cells, and monocytes produce brain-derived neurotrophic factor *in vitro* and in inflammatory brain lesions: a neuroprotective role of inflammation? *Journal of Experimental Medicine*, **189**, 865–70.

Khachaturian, Z.S. (1989). Calcium, membranes, aging, and Alzheimer's disease. Introduction and overview. A*nnals of the New York Academy of Sciences*, **568**, 1–4.

Khachaturian, Z., Phelps, C. and Buckholtz, N. (1994). The prospect of developing treatments for Alzheimer disease. In Terry, R., Katzman, R. and Bick, K. (ed.), *Alzheimer Disease*. Raven Press, New York, pp. 445–53.

Kiefer, R., Streit, W.J., Toyka, K.V., Kreutzberg, G.W. and Hartung, H.P. (1995). Transforming growth factor-β1: a lesion-associated cytokine of the nervous system. *International Journal of Developmental Neuroscience*, **13**, 331–9.

Kiener, P.A., Moran-Davis, P., Rankin, B.M., Wahl, A.F., Aruffo, A. and Hollenbaugh, D. (1995). Stimulation of CD40 with purified soluble gp39 induces proinflammatory responses in human monocytes. *Journal of Immunology*, **155**, 4917–25.

Kisilevsky, R. (1998). Amyloid β threads in the fabric of Alzheimer's disease. *Nature Medicine*, **4**, 772–3.

Klegeris, A. and McGeer, P.L. (1997). Beta-amyloid protein enhances macrophage production of oxygen free radicals and glutamate. *Journal of Neuroscience Research*, **49**, 229–35.

Klegeris, A., Walker, D.G. and McGeer, P.L. (1997). Interaction of Alzheimer β-amyloid peptide with the human monocytic cell line THP-1 results in a protein kinase C-dependent secretion of tumor necrosis factor-α. *Brain Research*, **747**, 114–21.

Koh, J.Y., Yang, L.L. and Cotman, C.W. (1990). β-Amyloid protein increases the vulnerability of cultured cortical neurons to excitotoxic damage. *Brain Research*, **533**, 315–20.

Kolson, D.L. and Pomerantz, R.J. (1996). AIDS dementia and HIV-1-induced neurotoxicity: possible pathogenic associations and mechanisms. *Journal of Biomedical Science*, **3**, 389–414.

Kooten, C.V. and Banchereau, J. (1996). CD40–CD40 ligand: a multifunctional receptor–ligand pair. *Advances in Immunology*, **61**, 1–77.

Krammer, P. *et al.* (1994). The role of APO-1-mediated apoptosis in the immune system. *Immunology Review*, **142**, 175–91.

Kreutzberg, G.W. (1996). Microglia: a sensor for pathological events in the CNS. *Trends in Neuroscience*, **19**, 312–8.

Krieger, M. and Herz, J. (1994). Structures and functions of multiligand lipoprotein receptors: macrophage scavenger receptors and LDL receptor-related protein (LRP). *Annual Review of Biochemistry*, **63**, 601–37.

Kuby, J. (1994). *Immunology*. W.H. Freeman, New York.

Kullander, K., Kylberg, A. and Ebendal, T. (1997). Specificity of neurotrophin-3 determined by loss-of-function mutagenesis. *Journal of Neuroscience Research*, **50**, 496–503.

LaDu, M.J., Falduto, M.T., Manelli, A.M., Reardon, C.A., Getz, G.S. and Frail, D.E. (1994). Isoform-specific binding of apolipoprotein E to β-amyloid. *Journal of Biological Chemistry*, **269**, 23403–6.

Lafon-Cazal, M., Pietri, S., Culcasi, M. and Bockaert, J. (1993). NMDA-dependent superoxide production and neurotoxicity. *Nature*, **364**, 535–7.

Landfield, P., Thibault, O., Mazzanti, M., Porter, N. and Kerr, D. (1992). Mechanisms of neuronal death in brain aging and Alzheimer's disease: role of endocrine-mediated calcium dyshomeostasis. *Journal of Neurobiology*, **23**, 1247–60.

Lane, P., Brocker, T., Hubele, S., Padovan, E., Lanzavecchia, A. and McConnell, F. (1993). Soluble CD40 ligand can replace the normal T cell-derived CD40 ligand signal to B cells in T cell-dependent activation. *Journal of Experimental Medicine*, **177**, 1209–13.

Larson, J., Lynch, G., Games, D. and Seubert, P. (1999). Alterations in synaptic transmission and long-term potentiation in hippocampal slices from young and aged PDAPP mice. *Brain Research*, **840**, 23–35.

Lassmann, H., Schmeid, M., Vass, K. and Hickey, W.F. (1993). Bone marrow derived elements and resident microglia in brain inflammation. *Glia*, **7**, 19–24.

Le, W.D., Xie, W.J., Kong, R. and Appel, S.H. (1997). β-Amyloid-induced neurotoxicity of a hybrid septal cell line associated with increased tau phosphorylation and expression of β-amyloid precursor protein. *Journal of Neurochemistry*, **69**, 978–85.

LeBlanc, A.C., Chen, H.Y., Autilio-Gambetti, L. and Gambetti, P. (1991). Differential APP gene expression in rat cerebral cortex, meninges, and primary astroglial, microglial and neuronal cultures. *FEBS Letters*, **292**, 1710–8.

LeBlanc, A.C., Xue, R. and Gambetti, P. (1996). Amyloid precursor protein metabolism in primary cell cultures of neurons, astrocytes, and microglia. *Journal of Neurochemistry*, **66**, 2300–10.

LeBlanc, A.C., Papadopoulos, M., Belair, C., Chu, W., Crosato, M., Powell, J. *et al.* (1997). Processing of amyloid precursor protein in human primary neuron and astrocyte cultures. *Journal of Neurochemistry*, **68**, 1183–90.

Lee, S.C., Dickson, D.W., Liu, W. and Brosnan, C.F. (1993a). Induction of nitric oxide synthase activity in human astrocytes by interleukin-1 β and interferon-γ. *Journal of Neuroimmunology*, **46**, 19–24.

Lee, S.C., Hatch, W.C., Liu, W., Kress, Y., Lyman, W.D. and Dickson, D.W. (1993b). Productive infection of human fetal microglia by HIV-1. *American Journal of Pathology*, **143**, 1032–9.

Lemere, C.A., Lopera, F., Kosik, K.S., Lendon, C.L., Ossa, J., Saido, T.C. *et al.* (1996). The E280A presenilin 1 Alzheimer mutation produces increased Aβ42 deposition and severe cerebellar pathology. *Nature Medicine*, **2**, 1146–50.

Lendon, C.L. and Goate, A.M. (1998). Genetic factors in the etiology of Alzheimer's disease. *Mediguide to Geriatric Neurology*, 1–8.

Levy-Lahad, E., Wasco, W., Poorkaj, P., Romano, D.M., Oshima, J., Pettingell, W.H. *et al.* (1995). Candidate gene for the chromosome 1 familial Alzheimer's disease locus. *Science*, **26**, 973–7.

Li, Q.X., Berndt, M.C., Bush, A.I., Rumble, B., Mackenzie, I., Friedhuber, A. *et al.* (1994). Membrane-associated forms of the βA4 amyloid protein precursor of Alzheimer's disease in human platelet and brain: surface expression on the activated human platelet. *Blood*, **84**, 133–42

Lieb, K., Fiebich, B.L., Schaller, H., Berger, M. and Bauer, J. (1996). Interleukin-1 β and tumor necrosis factor-α induce expression of α1-antichymotrypsin in human astrocytoma cells by activation of nuclear factor-κB. *Journal of Neurochemistry*, **67**, 2039–44.

Lindsberg, P., Hallenbeck, J. and Feurstein, G. (1991). Platelet-activating factor in stroke and brain injury. *Annals of Neurology*, **30**, 117–9.

Lipton, S.A., Singel, D.J. and Stamler, J.S. (1994). Neuroprotective and neurodestructive effects of nitric oxide and redox congeners. *Annals of the New York Academy of Sciences*, **738**, 382–7.

Lombardi, V.R., Garcia, M. and Cacabelos, R. (1998). Microglial activation induced by factor(s) contained in sera from Alzheimer-related ApoE genotypes. *Journal of Neuroscience Research*, **54**, 539–53.

Lopez-Ilasaca, M. (1998). Signaling from G-protein-coupled receptors to mitogen-activated protein (MAP)-kinase cascades. *Biochemical Pharmacology*, **56**, 269–77.

Lopez-Ilasaca, M., Crespo, P., Pellici, P.G., Gutkind, J.S. and Wetzker, R. (1997). Linkage of G protein-coupled receptors to the MAPK signaling pathway through PI 3-kinase γ. *Science*, **275**, 394–7.

Lorton, D., Kocsis, J.M., King, L., Madden, K. and Brunden, K.R. (1996). β-Amyloid induces increased release of interleukin-1 β from lipopolysaccharide-activated human monocytes. *Journal of Neuroimmunology*, **67**, 21–9.

Loy, R., Taglialatela, G., Angelucci, L., Heyer, D. and Perez-Polo, R. (1994). Regional CNS uptake of blood-borne nerve growth factor. *Journal of Neuroscience Research*, **39**, 339–46.

Lucas, M. and Mazzone, T. (1996). Cell surface proteoglycans modulate net synthesis and secretion of macrophage apolipoprotein E. *Journal of Biological Chemistry*, **271**, 13454–60.

Luster, A.D. (1998). Chemokines—chemotactic cytokines that mediate inflammation. *New England Journal of Medicine*, **338**, 436–45.

Ma, J., Brewer, H.B. and Potter, H. (1996). Alzheimer Aβ neurotoxicity: promotion by antichymotrypsis, apoe4; inhibition by Aβ-related peptides. *Neurobiology of Aging*, **17**, 773–80.

Ma, J., Yee, A., Brewer, H.B., Jr, Das, S. and Potter, H. (1994). Amyloid-associated proteins α1-antichymotrypsin and apolipoprotein E promote assembly of Alzheimer β-protein into filaments. *Nature*, **372**, 92–4.

MacGibbon, G., Lawlor, P., Sirimanne, E., Walton, M., Connor, B., Young, D. *et al.* (1997a). Bax expression in mammalian neurons undergoing apoptosis, and in Alzheimer's disease hippocampus. *Brain Research*, **750**, 223–34.

MacGibbon, G., Lawlor, P., Walton, M., Sirimanne, E., Faull, R., Synek, B. *et al.* (1997b). Expression of Fos, Jun, and Krox family proteins in Alzheimer's disease. *Experimental Neurology*, **147**, 316–22.

Mach, F., Schonbeck, U., Sukhova, G.K., Bourcier, T., Bonnefoy, J.Y., Pober, J.S. *et al.* (1997). Functional CD40 ligand is expressed on human vascular endothelial cells, smooth muscle cells, and macrophages: implications for CD40–CD40 ligand signaling in atherosclerosis. *Proceedings of the National Academy of Sciences USA*, **94**, 1931–6.

Mackic, J.B., Stins, M., McComb, J.G., Calero, M., Ghiso, J., Kim, K.S. *et al.* (1998). Human blood–brain barrier receptors for Alzheimer's amyloid-β1–40. Asymmetrical binding, endocytosis, and transcytosis at the apical side of brain microvascular endothelial cell monolayer. *Journal of Clinical Investigation*, **102**, 734–43.

Magnusson, A., Haug, L., Walaas, S. and Ostvold, A. (1993). Calcium-induced degradation of the IP3 receptor/calcium channel. *FEBS Letters*, **323**, 229–232.

Malik, N., Greenfield, B.W., Wahl, A.F. and Kiener, P.A. (1996). Activation of human monocytes through CD40 induces matrix metalloproteinases. *Journal of Immunology*, **156**, 3952–60.

Mallat, M. and Chamak, B. (1994). Brain macrophages: neurotoxic or neurotrophic effector cells? *Journal of Leukocyte Biology*, **56**, 416–422.

Mallat, M., Houlgatte, R., Brachet, P. and Prochiantz, A. (1989). Lipopolysaccharide-stimulated rat brain macrophages release NGF *in vitro*. *Developmental Biology*, **133**, 309–11.

Markesbery, W. and Mira, S. (1996). The neuropathology of Alzheimer's disease: diagnostic features and standardization. In Khachaturian, Z. and Radebaugh, T. (ed)., *Alzheimer's Disease: Cause(s), Diagnosis, Treatment, and Care*. CRC Press, New York, pp. 111–23.

Martin, D.P., Schmidt, R.E., DiStefano, P.S., Lowry, O.H., Carter, J.G. and Johnson, E.M., Jr (1988). Inhibitors of protein synthesis and RNA synthesis prevent neuronal death caused by nerve growth factor deprivation. *Journal of Cellular Biology*, **106**, 829–44.

Martin, J.B. (1999). Molecular basis of the neurodegenerative disorders. *New England Journal of Medicine*, **340**, 1970–80.

Marty, S., Dusart, I. and Peschanski, M. (1991). Glial changes following an excitotoxic lesion in the CNS—I. Microglia/macrophages. *Neuroscience*, **45**, 529–39.

Mattiace, L.A., Davies, P. and Dickson, D.W. (1990). Detection of HLA-DR on microglia in the human brain is a function of both clinical and technical factors. *American Journal of Pathology*, **136**, 1101–14.

Mattson, M.P., Cheng, B., Davis, D., Bryant, K., Lieberburg, I. and Rydel, R.E. (1992). β-Amyloid peptides destabilize calcium homeostasis and render human cortical neurons vulnerable to excitotoxicity. *Journal of Neuroscience*, **12**, 376–89.

Mattson, M.P., Barger, S.W., Cheng, B., Lieberburg, I., Smith-Swintosky, V.L. and Rydel, R.E. (1993a). β-Amyloid precursor protein metabolites and loss of neuronal Ca^{2+} homeostasis in Alzheimer's disease. *Trends in Neuroscience*, **16**, 409–14.

Mattson, M.P., Rydel, R.E., Lieberburg, I. and Smith-Swintosky, V.L. (1993b). Altered calcium signaling and neuronal injury: stroke and Alzheimer's disease as examples. *Annals of the New York Academy of Sciences*, **679**, 1–21.

Mattson, M.P., Goodman, Y., Luo, H., Fu, W. and Furukawa, K. (1997). Activation of NF-κB protects hippocampal neurons against oxidative stress-induced apoptosis: evidence for induction of manganese superoxide dismutase and suppression of peroxynitrite production and protein tyrosine nitration. *Journal of Neuroscience Research*, **49**, 681–97.

McDonald, D.R., Brunden, K.R. and Landreth, G.E. (1997). Amyloid fibrils activate tyrosine kinase-dependent signaling and superoxide production in microglia. *Journal of Neuroscience*, **17**, 2284–94.

McDonald, D.R., Bamberger, M.E., Combs, C.K. and Landreth, G.E. (1998). β-Amyloid fibrils activate parallel mitogen-activated protein kinase pathways in microglia and THP1 monocytes. *Journal of Neuroscience*, **18**, 4451–60.

McGeer, P.L. and McGeer, E.G. (1995). The inflammatory response system of brain: implications for therapy of Alzheimer and other neurodegenerative diseases. *Brain Research and Brain Research Review*, **21**, 195–218.

McGeer, E.G. and McGeer, P.L. (1997). The role of the immune system in neurodegenerative disorders. *Movement Disorders*, **12**, 855–8.

McGeer, P.L. and McGeer, E.G. (1998). Glial cell reactions in neurodegenerative diseases: pathophysiology and therapeutic interventions. *Alzheimer Disease and Associated Disorders*, **12**, S1–6.

McGeer, P.L., Akiyama, H., Itagaki, S. and McGeer, E.G. (1989). Immune system response in Alzheimer's disease. *Canadian Journal of Neurological Science*, **16**, 516–27.

McGeer, P.L., Rogers, J. and McGeer, E.G. (1994). Neuroimmune mechanisms in Alzheimer disease pathogenesis. *Alzheimer Disease and Associated Disorders*, **8**, 149–58.

McRae, A., Dahlström, A. and Ling, E.A. (1997). Microglia in neurodegenerative disorders: emphasis on Alzheimer's disease. *Gerontology*, **43**, 65–108.

Mecocci, P., MacGarvey, U. and Beal, M. (1994). Oxidative damage to mitochondrial DNA is increased in Alzheimer's disease. *Annals of Neurology*, **36**, 747–51.

Meda, L., Bonaiuto, C., Szendrei, G.I., Ceska, M., Rossi, F. and Cassatella, M.A. (1995a). β-Amyloid(25–35) induces the production of interleukin-8 from human monocytes. *Journal of Neuroimmunology*, **59**, 29–33.

Meda, L., Cassatella, M.A., Szendrei, G.I., Otvos, L., Jr, Baron, P., Villalba, M. *et al.* (1995b). Activation of microglial cells by β-amyloid protein and interferon-γ. *Nature*, **374**, 647–50.

Meda, L., Baron, P., Prat, E., Scarpini, E., Scarlato, G., Cassatella, M.A. *et al.* (1999). Proinflammatory profile of cytokine production by human monocytes and murine microglia stimulated with β-amyloid [25–35]. *Journal of Neuroimmunology*, **93**, 45–52.

Mennicken, F., Maki, R., de Souza, E.B. and Quirion, R. (1999). Chemokines and chemokine receptors in the CNS: a possible role in neuroinflammation and patterning. *Trends in Pharmacological Science*, **20**, 73–8.

Merrill, J.E., Koyanagi, Y. and Chen, I.S. (1989). Interleukin-1 and tumor necrosis factor α can be induced from mononuclear phagocytes by human immunodeficiency virus type 1 binding to the CD4 receptor. *Journal of Virology*, **63**, 4404–8.

Meucci, O. and Miller, R.J. (1996). gp120-induced neurotoxicity in hippocampal pyramidal neuron cultures: protective action of TGF-β1. *Journal of Neuroscience*, **16**, 4080–8.

Miller, B., Sarantis, M., Traynelis, S.F. and Attwell, D. (1992). Potentiation of NMDA receptor currents by arachidonic acid. *Nature*, **355**, 722–5.

Milward, E.A., Papadopoulos, R., Fuller, S.J., Moir, R.D., Small, D., Beyreuther, K. *et al.* (1992). The amyloid protein precursor of Alzheimer's disease is a mediator of the effects of nerve growth factor on neurite outgrowth. *Neuron*, **9**, 129–37.

Miwa, T., Furukawa, S., Nakajima, K., Furukawa, Y. and Kohsaka, S. (1997). Lipopolysaccharide enhances synthesis of brain-derived neurotrophic factor in cultured rat microglia. *Journal of Neuroscience Research*, **50**, 1023–9.

Monaghan, D., Bridges, R. and Cotman, C. (1989). The excitatory amino acid receptors. *Annual Review of Pharmacology and Toxicology*, **29**, 365–402.

Montine, T.J., Markesbery, W.R., Zackert, W., Sanchez, S.C., Roberts, L.J., 2nd and Morrow, J.D. (1999). The magnitude of brain lipid peroxidation correlates with the extent of degeneration but not with density of neuritic plaques or neurofibrillary tangles or with APOE genotype in Alzheimer's disease patients. *American Journal of Pathology*, **155**, 863–8.

Morelli, L., Giambartolomei, G.H., Prat, M.I. and Castano, E.M. (1999). Internalization and resistance to degradation of Alzheimer's Aβ1–42 at nanomolar concentrations in THP-1 human monocytic cell line. *Neuroscience Letters*, **262**, 5–8.

Mrak, R.E., Sheng, J.G. and Griffin, W.S. (1995). Glial cytokines in Alzheimer's disease: review and pathogenic implications. *Human Pathology*, **26**, 816–23.

Mucke, L., Abraham, C.R., Ruppe, M.D., Rockenstein, E.M., Toggas, S.M., Mallory, M. *et al.* (1995). Protection against HIV-1 gp120-induced brain damage by neuronal expression of human amyloid precursor protein. *Journal of Experimental Medicine*, **181**, 1551–6.

Mullan, M., Crawford, F., Axelman, K., Houlden, H., Lilius, L., Winblad, B. and Lannfelt, L. (1992). A pathogenic mutation for probable Alzheimer's disease in the APP gene at the N-terminus of β-amyloid. *Nature Genetics*, **1**, 345–7.

Mullan, M., Houlden, H., Windelspecht, M., Fidani, L., Lombardi, C., Diaz, P. *et al.* (1992). A locus for familial early-onset Alzheimer's disease on the long arm of chromosome 14, proximal to the α1-antichymotrypsin gene. *Nature Genetics*, **2**, 340–2

Murao, K., Terpstra,V., Green, S.R., Kondratenko, N., Steinberg, D., and Quehenberger, O. (1997). Characterization of CLA-1, a human homologue of rodent scavenger receptor BI, as a receptor for high density lipoprotein and apoptotic thymocytes, *Journal of Biological Chemistry*, **272**, 17551–7.

Murrell, J., Farlow, M., Ghetti, B. and Benson, M.D. (1991). A mutation in the amyloid precursor protein associated with hereditary Alzheimer's disease. *Science*, **254**, 97–9.

Nagata, S. and Golstein, P. (1995). The Fas death factor. *Science*, **267**, 1449–56.

Naito, M., Kodama, T., Matsumoto, A., Doi, T. and Takahashi, K. (1991). Tissue distribution, intracellular localization, and *in vitro* expression of bovine macrophage scavenger receptors. *American Journal of Pathology*, **139**, 1411–23.

Naito, M., Suzuki, H., Mori, T., Matsumoto, A., Kodama, T. and Takahashi, K. (1992). Coexpression of type I and type II human macrophage scavenger receptors in macrophages of various organs and foam cells in atherosclerotic lesions. *American Journal of Pathology*, **141**, 591–9.

Nathan, B.P., Bellosta, S., Sanan, D.A., Weisgraber, K.H., Mahley, R.W. and Pitas, R.E. (1994). Differential effects of apolipoproteins E3 and E4 on neuronal growth *in vitro*. *Science*, **264**, 850–2.

Neeper, M., Schmidt, A.M., Brett, J., Yan, S.D., Wang, F., Pan, Y.C. *et al.* (1992). Cloning and expression of a cell surface receptor for advanced glycosylation end products of proteins. *Journal of Biological Chemistry*, **267**, 14998–5004.

Nilsson, L., Rogers, J. and Potter, H. (1998). The essential role of inflammation and induced gene expression in the pathogenic pathway of Alzheimer's disease. *Frontiers in Bioscience*, **3**, D436–46

Nishiyama, M., Watanabe, T., Ueda, N., Tsukamoto, H. and Watanabe, K. (1993). Arachidonate 12-lipoxygenase is localized in neurons, glial cells, and endothelial cells of the canine brain. *Journal of Histochemistry and Cytochemistry*, **41**, 111–7.

O'Neill, L.A. and Kaltschmidt, C. (1997). NF-κB: a crucial transcription factor for glial and neuronal cell function. *Trends in Neuroscience*, **20**, 252–8.

Olds, J. and Alkon, D. (1991). A role for protein kinase C in associative learning. *New Biology*, **3**, 27–35.

Oleana, V.H., Salehi, A. and Swaab, D.F. (1998). Increased expression of the TIAR protein in the hippocampus of Alzheimer patients. *Neuroreport*, **9**, 1451–4.

Olney, J. (1978). Neurotoxicity of excitatory amino acids. In McGeer, E., Olney, J. and McGeer, P. (ed.), *Kainic Acid as a Tool in Neurobiology*. Raven Press, New York, pp. 95–121.

Olney, J.W. (1990). Excitotoxin-mediated neuron death in youth and old age. *Progress in Brain Research*, **86**, 37–51.

Oltvai, Z., Milliman, C. and Korsmeyer, S. (1993). Bcl-2 heterodimerizes *in vivo* with a conserved homolog, bax, that accelerates programmed cell death. *Cell*, **74**, 609–19.

Oteiza, P. (1994). A mechanism for the stimulatory effect of aluminum on iron-induced lipid peroxidation. *Archives of Biochemistry and Biophysics*, **308**, 374–379.

Pacheco, M. and Jope, R. (1996). Phosphoinositide signaling in human brain. *Progress in Neurobiology*, **50**, 255–73.

Painter, R.H. (1984). The C1q receptor site on human immunoglobulin G. *Canadian Journal of Biochemistry and Cellular Biology*, **62**, 418–25.

Panek, R.B. and Benveniste, E.N. (1995). Class II MHC gene expression in microglia. Regulation by the cytokines IFN-γ, TNF-α, and TGF-β. *Journal of Immunology*, **154**, 2846–54.

Paresce, D.M., Ghosh, R.N. and Maxfield, F.R. (1996). Microglial cells internalize aggregates of the Alzheimer's disease amyloid β-protein via a scavenger receptor. *Neuron*, **17**, 553–65.

Pazmany, T., Mechtler, L., Tomasi, T.B., Kosa, J.P., Turoczi, A. and Urbanyi, Z. (1999). Differential regulation of major histocompatibility complex class II expression and nitric oxide release by β-amyloid in rat astrocyte and microglia. *Brain Research*, **835**, 213–23.

Pericak-Vance, M.A., Bebout, J.L., Gaskell, P.C., Jr, Yamaoka, L.H., Hung, W.Y., Alberts, M.J. *et al.* (1991). Linkage studies in familial Alzheimer disease: evidence for chromosome 19 linkage. *American Journal of Human Genetics*, **48**, 1034–50.

Perlmutter, L.S., Scott, S.A., Barron, E. and Chui, H.C. (1992). MHC class II-positive microglia in human brain: association with Alzheimer lesions. *Journal of Neuroscience Research*, **33**, 549–58.

Piani, D., Frei, K., Do, K., Cuenod, M. and Fontana, A. (1991). Murine brain macrophages induce NMDA receptor mediated neurotoxicity *in vitro* by secreting glutamate. *Neuroscience Letters*, **133**, 159–62.

Piani, D., Spranger, M., Frei, K., Schaffner, A. and Fontana, A. (1992). Macrophage-induced cytotoxicity of *N*-methyl-D-aspartate receptor positive neurons involves excitatory amino acids rather than reactive oxygen intermediates and cytokines. *European Journal of Immunology*, **22**, 2429–36.

Poli, G., Bressler, P., Kinter, A., Duh, E., Timmer, W.C., Rabson, A. *et al.* (1990). Interleukin 6 induces human immunodeficiency virus expression in infected monocytic cells alone and in synergy with tumor necrosis factor α by transcriptional and post-transcriptional mechanisms. *Journal of Experimental Medicine*, **172**, 151–8.

Prehn, J.H., Backhauss, C. and Krieglstein, J. (1993). Transforming growth factor-β1 prevents glutamate neurotoxicity in rat neocortical cultures and protects mouse neocortex from ischemic injury *in vivo*. *Journal of Cerebral Blood Flow and Metabolism*, **13**, 521–5.

Prehn, J.H., Bindokas, V.P., Jordan, J., Galindo, M.F., Ghadge, G.D., Roos, R.P. *et al.* (1996). Protective effect of transforming growth factor-β1 on β-amyloid neurotoxicity in rat hippocampal neurons. *Molecular Pharmacology*, **49**, 319–28.

Pulliam, L., Herndier, B.G., Tang, N.M. and McGrath, M.S. (1991). Human immunodeficiency virus-infected macrophages produce soluble factors that cause histological and neurochemical alterations in cultured human brains. *Journal of Clinical Investigation*, **87**, 503–12.

Ranheim, E.A. and Kipps, T.J. (1993). Activated T cells induce expression of B7/BB1 on normal or leukemic B cells through a CD40-dependent signal. *Journal of Experimental Medicine*, **177**, 925–35.

Rappolee, D.A., Mark, D., Banda, M.J. and Werb, Z. (1988). Wound macrophages express TGF-α and other growth factors *in vivo*: analysis by mRNA phenotyping. *Science*, **241**, 708–12.

Reed, J. (1994). Bcl-2 and the regulation of programmed cell death. *Journal of Cellular Biology*, **124**, 1–6.

Revy, P., Hivroz, C., Andreu, G., Graber, P., Martinache, C., Fischer, A. *et al.* (1999). Activation of the Janus kinase 3-STAT5a pathway after CD40 triggering of human monocytes but not of resting B cells. *Journal of Immunology*, **163**, 787–93.

Rocamora, N., Pascual, M., Acsady, L., de Lecea, L., Freund, T.F. and Soriano, E. (1996). Expression of NGF and NT3 mRNAs in hippocampal interneurons innervated by the GABAergic septohippocampal pathway. *Journal of Neuroscience*, **16**, 3991–4004.

Roch, J.M., Shapiro, I.P., Sundsmo, M.P., Otero, D.A., Refolo, L.M., Robakis, N.K. *et al.* (1992). Bacterial expression, purification, and functional mapping of the amyloid β/A4 protein precursor. *Journal of Biological Chemistry*, **267**, 2214–21.

Rogers, J., Luber-Narod, J., Styren, S.D. and Civin, W.H. (1988). Expression of immune system-associated antigens by cells of the human central nervous system: relationship to the pathology of Alzheimer's disease. *Neurobiology of Aging*, **9**, 339–49.

Rogers, J., Schultz, J., Brachova, L., Lue, L.F., Webster, S., Bradt, B. *et al.* (1992). Complement activation and β-amyloid-mediated neurotoxicity in Alzheimer's disease. *Research in Immunology*, **143**, 624–30.

Rosenberg, G.A., Estrada, E.Y., Dencoff, J.E. and Stetler-Stevenson, W.G. (1995). Tumor necrosis factor-α-induced gelatinase B causes delayed opening of the blood–brain barrier: an expanded therapuetic window. *Brain Research*, **703**, 151–5.

Roses, A.D. (1997). Apolipoprotein E, a gene with complex biological interactions in the aging brain. *Neurobiology Disorders*, **4**, 170–85.

Roses, A.D. (1998). Apolipoprotein E and Alzheimer's disease. The tip of the susceptibility iceberg. *Annals of the New York Academy of Sciences*, **855**, 738–43.

Roses, A.D. and Saunders, A.M. (1997). ApoE, Alzheimer's disease, and recovery from brain stress. *Annals of the New York Academy of Sciences*, **826**, 200–12.

Rozemuller, J.M., Abbink, J.J., Kamp, A.M., Stam, F.C., Hack, C.E. and Eikelenboom, P. (1991). Distribution pattern and functional state of α1-antichymotrypsin in plaques and vascular amyloid in Alzheimer's disease. A immunohistochemical study with monoclonal antibodies against native and inactivated α1-antichymotrypsin. *Acta Neuropathologica*, **82**, 200–7.

Saad, B., Constam, D., Ortmann, R., Moos, M., Fontana, A. and Schachner, M. (1991). Astrocyte-derived TGF-β2 and NGF differentially regulate neural recognition molecule expression by cultured astrocytes. *Journal of Cellular Biology*, **115**, 473–84.

Sagara,Y. and Schubert, D. (1998). The activation of metabotropic glutamate receptors protects nerve cells from oxidative stress. *Journal of Neuroscience*, **18**, 6662–71.

Saito, K., Elce, J., Hamos, J. and Nixon, R. (1993). Widespread activation of calcium-activated neutral protease (calpain) in the brain in AD: a potential molecular basis of neuronal degeneration. *Proceedings of the National Academy of Sciences USA*, **90**, 2628–32.

Saitoh, T., Sundsmo, M., Roch, J.M., Kimura, N., Cole, G., Schubert, D. *et al.* (1989). Secreted form of amyloid β protein precursor is involved in the growth regulation of fibroblasts. *Cell*, **58**, 615–22.

Saitoh, T., Horsburgh, K. and Masliah, E. (1993). Hyperactivation of signal transduction systems in Alzheimer's disease. *Annals of the New York Academy of Sciences*, **695**, 34–41.

Sandbrink, R., Masters, C.L. and Beyreuther, K. (1994). APP gene family: unique age-associated changes in splicing of Alzheimer's βA4-amyloid protein precursor. *Neurobiological Disorders*, **1**, 13–24.

Santambrogio, L., Hochwald, G.M., Saxena, B., Leu, C.H., Martz, J.E., Carlino, J.A. *et al.* (1993). Studies on the mechanisms by which transforming growth factor-β (TGF-β) protects against allergic encephalomyelitis. Antagonism between TGF-β and tumor necrosis factor. *Journal of Immunology*, **151**, 1116–27.

Satoh, J., Lee, Y.B. and Kim, S.U. (1995). T-cell costimulatory molecules B7-1 (CD80) and B7-2 (CD86) are expressed in human microglia but not in astrocytes in culture. *Brain Research*, **704**, 92–6.

Saunders, A.M., Strittmatter, W.J., Schmechel, D., George-Hyslop, P.H., Pericak-Vance, M.A., Joo, S.H. *et al.* (1993). Association of apolipoprotein E allele ε4 with late-onset familial and sporadic Alzheimer's disease. *Neurology*, **43**, 1467–72.

Schellenberg, G.D. (1995). Genetic dissection of Alzheimer disease, a heterogeneous disorder. *Proceedings of the National Academy of Sciences USA*, **92**, 8552–9.

Scheuner, D., Eckman, C., Jensen, M., Song, X., Citron, M., Suzuki, N. *et al.* (1996). Secreted amyloid β-protein similar to that in the senile plaques of Alzheimer's disease is increased *in vivo* by the presenilin 1 and 2 and APP mutations linked to familial Alzheimer's disease. *Nature Medicine*, **2**, 864–70.

Schmechel, D.E., Goldgaber, D., Burkhart, D.S., Gilbert, J.R., Gajdusek, D.C. and Roses, A.D. (1988). Cellular localization of messenger RNA encoding amyloid-β-protein in normal tissue and in Alzheimer disease. *Alzheimer Disease and Associated Disorders*, **2**, 96–111.

Schmidt, A.M., Vianna, M., Gerlach, M., Brett, J., Ryan, J., Kao, J. *et al.* (1992). Isolation and characterization of two binding proteins for advanced glycosylation end products from bovine lung which are present on the endothelial cell surface. *Journal of Biological Chemistry*, **267**, 14987–97.

Schmidt, A.M., Yan, S.D., Brett, J., Mora, R., Nowygrod, R. and Stern, D. (1993). Regulation of human mononuclear phagocyte migration by cell surface-binding proteins for advanced glycation end products. *Journal of Clinical Investigation*, **91**, 2155–68.

Schubert, D., LaCorbiere, M., Saitoh, T. and Cole, G. (1989). Characterization of an amyloid β precursor protein that binds heparin and contains tyrosine sulfate. *Proceedings of the National Academy of Sciences USA*, **86**, 2066–9.

Selkoe, D.J. (1996). Amyloid β-protein and the genetics of Alzheimer's disease. *Journal of Biological Chemistry*, **271**, 18295–8.

Selkoe, D.J. (1997). Alzheimer's disease: genotypes, phenotypes, and treatments. *Science*, **275**, 630–1.

Shaw, P. (1994). Excitotoxicity and motor neurone disease: a review of the evidence. *Journal of the Neurological Sciences*, **124**, 6–13.

Sheng, J., Mrak, R. and Griffin, W. (1995). Microglial interleukin-1 α expression in brain regions in Alzheimer's disease: correlation with neuritic plaque distribution. *Neuropathology and Applied Neurobiology*, **21**, 290–301.

Sheng, J.G., Mrak, R.E. and Griffin, W.S. (1997). Neuritic plaque evolution in Alzheimer's disease is accompanied by transition of activated microglia from primed to enlarged to phagocytic forms. *Acta Neuropathologica (Berlin)*, **94**, 1–5.

Shimojo, M., Nakajima, K., Takei, N., Hamanoue, M. and Kohsaka, S. (1991). Production of basic fibroblast growth factor in cultured rat brain microglia. *Neuroscience Letters*, **123**, 229–31.

Shrikant, P., Weber, E., Jilling, T. and Benveniste, E.N. (1995). Intercellular adhesion molecule-1 gene expression by glial cells. Differential mechanisms of inhibition by IL-10 and IL-6. *Journal Immunology*, **155**, 1489–501.

Shu, U., Kiniwa, M., Wu, C.Y., Maliszewski, C., Vezzio, N., Hakimi, J. *et al.* (1995). Activated T cells induce interleukin-12 production by monocytes via CD40–CD40 ligand interaction. *European Journal of Immunology*, **25**, 1125–8.

Siman, R., Card, J.P., Nelson, R.B. and Davis, L.G. (1989). Expression of β-amyloid precursor protein in reactive astrocytes following neuronal damage. *Neuron*, **3**, 275–85.

Singh, V.K. (1996). Immune-activation model in Alzheimer disease. *Molecular and Chemical Neuropathology*, **28**, 105–11.

Sisodia, S.S., Koo, E.H., Beyreuther, K., Unterbeck, A. and Price, D.L. (1990). Evidence that β-amyloid protein in Alzheimer's disease is not derived by normal processing. *Science*, **248**, 492–5.

Smith, A.D., Johnston, C., Sim, E., Nagy, Z., Jobst, K.A., Hindley, N. *et al.* (1994). Protective effect of apo ε2 in Alzheimer's disease. Oxford Project to Investigate Memory and Ageing (OPTIMA). *Lancet*, **344**, 473–4.

Smith, M., Rudnicka-Nawrot, M., Richey, P., Praprotnik, D., Mulvihill, P., Miller, C. *et al.* (1995). Carbonyl-related posttranslational modification of neurofilament protein in the neurofibrillary pathology of Alzheimer's disease. *Journal of Neurochemistry*, **64**, 2660–6.

Smith, M., Perry, G., Richey, P., Sayre, L., Anderson, V., Beal, M. *et al.* (1996). Oxidative damage in Alzheimer's. *Nature*, **382**, 120–1.

Sozzani, S., Rieppi, M., Locati, M., Zhou, D., Bussolino, F., Proost, P. *et al.* (1994). Synergism between platelet activating factor and C-C chemokines for arachidonate release in human monocytes. *Biochemical and Biophysical Research Communications*, **199**, 761–6.

Stalder, M., Phinney, A., Probst, A., Sommer, B., Staufenbiel, M. and Jucker, M. (1999). Association of microglia with amyloid plaques in brains of APP23 transgenic mice. *American Journal of Pathology*, **154**, 1673–84.

Stout, R.D. and Suttles, J. (1996). The many roles of CD40 in cell-mediated inflammatory responses. *Immunology Today*, **17**, 487–92.

Stout, R.D., Suttles, J., Xu, J., Grewal, I.S. and Flavell, R.A. (1996). Impaired T cell-mediated macrophage activation in CD40 ligand-deficient mice. *Journal of Immunology*, **156**, 8–11.

Strauss, S., Bauer, J., Ganter, U., Jonas, U., Berger, M. and Volk, B. (1992). Detection of interleukin-6 and α2-macroglobulin immunoreactivity in cortex and hippocampus of Alzheimer's disease patients. *Laboratory Investigations*, **66**, 223–30.

Streit, W.J. and Kincaid-Colton, C.A. (1995). The brain's immune system. *Scientific American*, **273**, 54–5, 58–61.

Sturchler-Pierrat, C., Abramowski, D., Duke, M., Wiederhold, K.H., Mistl, C., Rothacher, S. *et al.* (1997). Two amyloid precursor protein transgenic mouse models with Alzheimer disease-like pathology. *Proceedings of the National Academy of Sciences USA*, **94**, 13287–92.

Su, J., Deng, G. and Cotman, C. (1997). Bax protein expression is increased in Alzheimer's brain: correlations with DNA damage, bcl-2 expression and brain pathology. *Journal of Neuropathology and Experimental Neurology*, **56**, 86–93.

Suttles, J., Milhorn, D.M., Miller, R.W., Poe, J.C., Wahl, L.M. and Stout, R.D. (1999). CD40 signaling of monocyte inflammatory cytokine synthesis through an ERK1/2-dependent pathway. A target of interleukin (Il)-4 and Il-10 anti-inflammatory action. *Journal of Biological Chemistry*, **274**, 5835–42.

Talbot, C., Lendon, C., Craddock, N., Shears, S., Morris, J.C. and Goate, A. (1994). Protection against Alzheimer's disease with apoE ε2. *Lancet*, **343**, 1432–3.

Tan, J., Town, T., Saxe, M., Paris, D., Wu, Y. and Mullan, M. (1999). Ligation of microglial CD40 results in p44/42 mitogen-activated protein kinase-dependent TNF α production that is opposed by TGF-β1 and IL-10. *Journal of Immunology*, **163**, 6614–6621.

Tancredi, V., D'Arcangelo, G., Grassi, F., Tarroni, P., Palmieri, G., Santoni, A. *et al.* (1992). Tumor necrosis factor alters synaptic transmission in rat hippocampal slices. *Neuroscience Letters*, **146**, 176–8.

Taylor, L., Marshak, D. and Landreth, G. (1993). Identification of a nerve growth factor-and epidermal growth factor-regulated protein kinase that phosphorylates the protooncogene product c-Fos. *Proceedings of the National Academy of Sciences USA*, **90**, 368–72.

Terry, R.D. (1996). The pathogenesis of Alzheimer disease: an alternative to the amyloid hypothesis. *Journal of Neuropathology and Experimental Neurology*, **55**, 1023–5.

Thery, C., Chamak, B. and Mallat, M. (1991). Cytotoxic effect of brain macrophages on developing neurons. *European Journal of Neuroscience*, **3**, 1155–64.

Thurston, V.C., Zinkowski, R.P. and Binder, L.I. (1996). Tau as a nucleolar protein in human non-neural cells *in vitro* and *in vivo*. *Chromosoma*, **105**, 20–30.

Tian, L., Noelle, R.J. and Lawrence, D.A. (1995). Activated T cells enhance nitric oxide production by murine splenic macrophages through gp39 and LFA-1. *European Journal of Immunology*, **25**, 306–9.

Tienari, P.J., Ida, N., Ikonen, E., Simons, M., Weidemann, A., Multhaup, G. *et al.* (1997). Intracellular and secreted Alzheimer β-amyloid species are generated by distinct mechanisms in cultured hippocampal neurons. *Proceedings of the National Academy of Sciences USA*, **94**, 4125–30.

Tooyama, I., Kimura, H., Akiyama, H. and McGeer, P.L. (1990). Reactive microglia express class I and class II major histocompatibility complex antigens in Alzheimer's disease. *Brain Research*, **523**, 273–80.

Tracey, K.J. and Cerami, A. (1993). Tumor necrosis factor, other cytokines and disease. *Annual Review of Cellular Biology*, **9**, 317–43.

Trottei, D., Volterra, A., Lehre, K., Rossi, D., Gjesdai, O., Racagni, G. *et al.* (1995). Arachidonic acid inhibits a purified and reconstituted glutamate transporter directly from the water phase and not via the phospholipid membrane. *Journal of Biological Chemistry*, **270**, 9890–5.

Tsuzuki, K., Iino, M. and Ozawa, S. (1989). Change in calcium permeability caused by quinolinic acid in cultured rat hippocampal neurons. *Neuroscience Letters*, **105**, 269–74.

Ueda, K., Shinohara, S., Yagami, T., Asakura, K. and Kawasaki, K. (1997). Amyloid β protein potentiates Ca^{2+} influx through L-type voltage-sensitive Ca^{2+} channels: a possible involvement of free radicals. *Journal of Neurochemistry*, **68**, 265–71.

Valone, F. and Epstein, L. (1988). Biphasic platelet-activating factor synthesis by human monocytes stimulated with IL-1 β, TNF, or IFN-γ. *Journal of Immunology*, **141**, 3945–50.

Van Muiswinkel, F.L., Raupp, S.F., de Vos, N.M., Smits, H.A., Verhoef, J., Eikelenboom, P. *et al.* (1999). The amino-terminus of the amyloid-β protein is critical for the cellular binding and consequent activation of the respiratory burst of human macrophages. *Journal of Neuroimmunology*, **96**, 121–30.

Van Muiswinkel, F.L., Veerhuis, R. and Eikelenboom, P. (1996). Amyloid β protein primes cultured rat microglial cells for an enhanced phorbol 12-myristate 13-acetate-induced respiratory burst activity. *Journal of Neurochemisty*, **66**, 2468–76.

Vitek, M.P., Snell, J., Dawson, H. and Colton, C.A. (1997). Modulation of nitric oxide production in human macrophages by apolipoprotein-E and amyloid-β peptide. *Biochemical and Biophysical Research Communications*, **240**, 391–4.

Volterra, A., Trotti, D. and Racagni, G. (1994). Glutamate uptake is inhibited by arachidonic acid and oxygen radicals via two distinct and additive mechanisms. *Molecular Pharmacology*, **46**, 986–92.

Wagner, D.H., Jr, Stout, R.D. and Suttles, J. (1994). Role of the CD40–CD40 ligand interaction in CD4+ T cell contact-dependent activation of monocyte interleukin-1 synthesis. *European Journal of Immunology*, **24**, 3148–54.

Walker, D.G., Kim, S.U. and McGeer, P.L. (1995). Complement and cytokine gene expression in cultured microglial derived from postmortem human brains. *Journal of Neuroscience Research*, **40**, 478–93.

Waters, C. (1997). Molecular mechanisms of neuronal cell death. *RBI Neurotransmisssions*, **13**, 1–7.

Webster, S. and Rogers, J. (1996). Relative efficacies of amyloid β peptide (Aβ) binding proteins in Aβ aggregation. *Journal of Neuroscience Research*, **46**, 58–66.

Weisgraber, K. and Mahley, R. (1996). Human apolipoprotein E: the Alzheimer's disease connection. *FASEB Journal*, **10**, 1485–94.

Windhagen, A., Newcombe, J., Dangond, F., Strand, C., Woodroofe, M.N., Cuzner, M.L. *et al.* (1995). Expression of costimulatory molecules B7-1 (CD80), B7-2 (CD86), and interleukin 12 cytokine in multiple sclerosis lesions. *Journal of Experimental Medicine*, **182**, 1985–96.

Winkler, K., Scharnagl, H., Tisljar, U., Hoschutzky, H., Friedrich, I., Hoffmann, M.M. *et al.* (1999). Competition of Aβ amyloid peptide and apolipoprotein E for receptor-mediated endocytosis. *Journal of Lipid Research*, **40**, 447–55.

Wisniewski, H.M., Bancher, C., Barcikowska, M., Wen, G.Y. and Currie, J. (1989). Spectrum of morphological appearance of amyloid deposits in Alzheimer's disease. *Acta Neuropathologica*, **78**, 337–47.

Wood, J.A., Wood, P.L., Ryan, R., Graff-Radford, N.R., Pilapil, C., Robitaille, Y. *et al.* (1993). Cytokine indices in Alzheimer's temporal cortex: no changes in mature IL-1β or IL-1RA but increases in the associated acute phase proteins IL-6, α2-macroglobulin and C-reactive protein. *Brain Research*, **629**, 245–52.

Xia, M.Q. and Hyman, B.T. (1999). Chemokines/chemokine receptors in the central nervous system and Alzheimer's disease. *Journal of Neurovirology*, **5**, 32–41.

Xiao, B.G., Bai, X.F., Zhang, G.X., Hojeberg, B. and Link, H. (1996). Shift from anti- to proinflammatory cytokine profiles in microglia through LPS- or IFN-γ-mediated pathways. *Neuroreports*, **7**, 1893–8.

Xiao, B.G. and Link, H. (1998). Immune regulation within the central nervous system. *Journal of Neurological Science*, **157**, 1–12.

Xu, P.T., Gilbert, J.R., Qiu, H.L., Ervin, J., Rothrock-Christian, T.R., Hulette, C. and Schmechel, D.E. (1999). Specific regional transcription of apolipoprotein E in human brain neurons. *American Journal of Pathology*, **154**, 601–11.

Yamada, T. and Takashima, A. (1997). Presenilin 1 immunostaining using well-characterized antibodies in human tissues. *Experimental Neurology*, **148**, 10–2.

Yamada, Y., Doi, T., Hamakubo, T. and Kodama, T. (1998). Scavenger receptor family proteins: roles for atherosclerosis, host defence and disorders of the central nervous system. *Cellular and Molecular Life Science*, **54**, 628–40.

Yamato, K., el-Hajjaoui, Z., Simon, K. and Koeffler, H.P. (1990). Modulation of interleukin-β RNA in monocytic cells infected with human immunodeficiency virus-1. *Jorunal of Clinical Investigation*, **86**, 1109–14.

Yan, S., Chen, X., Schmidt, A., Brett, J., Godman, G., Zou, Y. *et al.* (1994). Glycated tau protein in Alzheimer's disease: a mechanism for induction of oxidant stress. *Proceedings of the National Academy of Sciences USA*, **91**, 7787–91.

Yan, S., Yan, S., Chen, X., Fu, J., Chen, M., Kuppusamy, P. *et al*D. (1995). Non-enzymatically glycated tau in Alzheimer's disease induces neuronal oxidant stress resulting in cytokine gene expression and release of amyloid-beta peptide. *Nature Medicine*, **1**, 693–9.

Yan, S.D., Chen, X., Fu, J., Chen, M., Zhu, H., Roher, A. *et al.* (1996). RAGE and amyloid-β peptide neurotoxicity in Alzheimer's disease. *Nature*, **382**, 685–91.

Yan, S.D., Stern, D. and Schmidt, A.M. (1997). What's the RAGE? The receptor for advanced glycation end products (RAGE) and the dark side of glucose. *European Journal of Clinical Investigation*, **27**, 179–81.

Young, H. and Hardy, K. (1995). Role of interferon γ in immune cell regulation. *Journal of Leukocyte Biology*, **58**, 373–81.

Young, L., Kish, S., Li, P. and Warsh, J. (1988). Decreased brain [³H]inositol 1,4,5-trisphosphate binding in Alzheimer's disease. *Neuroscience Letters*, **94**, 198–202.

8 *Macrophages in autoimmunity and primary immunodeficiency*

J.-W. Yoon and H.-S. Jun

1 Introduction

Macrophages are a heterogeneous group of cells with common blood-borne precursors, monocytes, originating from stem cells in the bone marrow (van Furth, 1982). The monocytes migrate into various tissues where they mature and become resident macrophages. There are various subsets of macrophages, such as Kupffer cells in the liver, alveolar macrophages in the lung, microglia in the central nervous system (CNS) and synovial macrophages in the joints, with differing expressions of surface molecules and differing morphology depending upon their localization and function (Radzun *et al.*, 1988).

Macrophages play a primary role as scavenger cells. However, macrophages are also involved in immunoregulatory functions at various sites in the body. They show phagocytic activity after recognizing foreign or damaged material through cell surface receptors such as immunoglobulin, Fc receptor or complement receptor, and show cytotoxic activity through the production of toxic material such as proteinases, prostaglandins, tumor necrosis factor (TNF), interleukin (IL)-1, oxygen free radicals and nitric oxide (NO) (Nathan, 1987; Keller, 1990; Leblanc, 1990; Hartung *et al.*, 1992). In addition, macrophages can function as antigen-presenting cells to T and B lymphocytes (Unuaue, 1984; Matsumoto *et al.*, 1986; Beelen *et al.*, 1989) and generate an antigen-specific immune response. They also play a role as regulators of inflammatory responses through the production of cytokines and chemokines that attract other inflammatory cells. Macrophages also induce collagen synthesis and vessel formation by producing transforming growth factor-β (TGF-β), TNF and fibroblast growth factor (FGF) for wound healing (Leibovich *et al.*, 1987; Pierce *et al.*, 1989).

Macrophages are involved in a variety of diseases, including autoimmune diseases, immune deficiency diseases and infectious diseases through their various immune functions. In this review, we will discuss the role of macrophages in autoimmune disease and in primary immunodeficiency. Unveiling the mechanisms by which macrophages are activated and determining how they are involved in autoimmune diseases and primary immunodeficiency could be invaluable for the development of treatments for these diseases.

2 Role of macrophages in autoimmune disease

There is increasing evidence that macrophages play an important role in autoimmune diseases such as insulin-dependent diabetes mellitus (IDDM), experimental allergic encephalomyelitis (EAE) and rheumatoid arthritis (RA). Macrophages contribute to autoimmunity by processing and presenting autoantigens to T cells and by producing a variety of soluble mediators that may be involved in the induction of immune responses and have a cytotoxic effect on target cells. The cytokines produced by activated macrophages, including IL-1β, TNF-α and IL-6, contribute to the induction of the expression of adhesion molecules and the activation of T cells. In addition, these cytokines, free radicals and proteinases may exert a direct cytotoxic effect on target cells. The cytokine IL-12 is a major contributor to the creation of the Th1 immune response and, subsequently, activates autoantigen-specific cytotoxic T cells that kill target cells.

2.1 Type 1 diabetes

Type 1 diabetes, also known as insulin-dependent diabetes mellitus (IDDM), is an autoimmune disease caused by the progressive autoimmune destruction of insulin-producing pancreatic β cells (Rossini *et al.*, 1993; Bach, 1995; Yoon and Jun, 1998; Yoon *et al.*, 1998). Non-obese diabetic (NOD) mice (Makino *et al.*, 1980) and BioBreeding (BB) rats (Marliss *et al.*, 1982) are animal models that spontaneously develop autoimmune IDDM. The diabetic syndrome in these animal models is similar to IDDM in humans. Thus, NOD mice and BB rats have been widely used for studies of the pathogenic mechanisms of IDDM (Yoon *et al.*, 1995, 1999). It has been shown that the major populations of cells infiltrating the islets during the early stage of insulitis in both NOD mice and BB rats are macrophages and dendritic cells (Kolb *et al.*, 1986; Lee *et al.*, 1988a; Walker *et al.*, 1988; Voorbij *et al.*, 1989; Ziegler *et al.*, 1992; Jasen *et al.*, 1994). Electron microscope observations revealed that activated macrophages are the first infiltrates of the islets in BB rats, and that B cells, T cells and natural killer (NK) cells are not present at this initial stage (Hanenberg *et al.*, 1989). Macrophages precede invasion of the islets by T cells, NK cells and B cells (Lee *et al.*, 1988a).

The inactivation of macrophages in NOD mice and BB rats using silica or liposomal dichloromethylene diphosphonate (lip-Cl_2MDP), both toxic to macrophages, results in the prevention of insulitis (Figure 8.1) and diabetes (Oschilewski *et al.*, 1985; Lee *et al.*, 1988b,c; Jun *et al.*, 1999a). In addition, silica treatment also prevented diabetes in low-dose streptozotocin-induced diabetes (Ihm *et al.*, 1990). Further experimental results revealed that the early inactivation of macrophages by early, long-term treatment of NOD mice with silica results in the prevention of the development of β cell-specific effector T cells. However, late, short-term treatment of NOD mice with silica does not halt the destruction of β cells by pre-existing effector T cells (Ihm and Yoon, 1990). This result indicates that macrophages are needed for the generation of β cell-specific effector T cells. Further study showed that the T cells in macrophage-depleted NOD recipient mice did not destroy transplanted NOD islets, indicating that T cells in a macrophage-depleted environment lose their ability to differentiate into cytotoxic T cells that can destroy pancreatic β cells (Jun *et al.*, 1999a). However, these T cells regained their β cell-cytotoxic potential when returned to a macrophage-containing environment.

To learn why T cells in a macrophage-depleted environment lose their ability to kill β cells, the islet antigen-specific immune response and T cell activation in macrophage-depleted NOD mice were examined. There was a shift in the immune balance, a decrease in the Th1 immune response and an increase in the Th2 immune response (Figure 8.2), due to the reduced expression of the macrophage-derived cytokine IL-12. In addition, there was a deficit in T cell activation, evidenced by a significant decrease in the expression of Fas ligand and perforin (Figure 8.3). The administration of IL-12 substantially reversed the prevention of diabetes in NOD mice conferred by macrophage depletion (Jun *et al.*, 1999a). Therefore, macrophages may play an essential role in the development and activation of β cell-cytotoxic T cells that cause β cell destruction, resulting in autoimmune diabetes in NOD mice.

In addition, the role of macrophages in the development and activation of β cell cytotoxic $CD8^+$ T cells in T-cell receptor (TCR) transgenic NOD mice was examined by the adoptive transfer of splenic T cells from macrophage-depleted TCR-β transgenic NOD mice into NOD.*scid* mice (Jun *et al.*, 1999b). TCR-β transgenic NOD mice express the

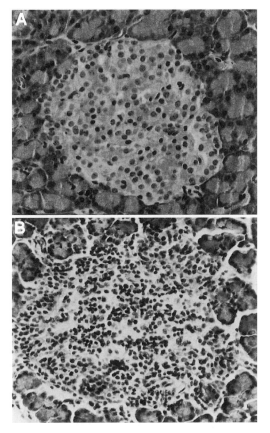

Fig. 8.1 Photomicrographs of the pancreatic islets of NOD mice. Pancreatic sections from 25-week-old female NOD mice treated with lip-C1$_2$MDP (A) or phosphate-buffered saline (PBS) (B) were stained with hematoxylin and eosin. Islets from the lip-C1$_2$MDP-treated mice are intact (A). In contrast, islets from the PBS-treated animals show severe insulitis (B). Original magnification: ×250. Reprinted with permission from The Rockefeller University Press, New York (Jun *et al.*, 1999a).

rearranged TCR-β gene derived from a diabetogenic CD8$^+$ T-cell clone, NY8.3 (Nagata and Yoon, 1992). These TCR-β transgenic NOD mice showed a 10-fold increase in the precursor frequency of β cell-specific cytotoxic T cells and a dramatically accelerated onset of IDDM (Verdaguer *et al.*, 1997). It was found that none of the NOD.*scid* recipients developed diabetes up to 10 weeks after transfer, whereas most of the NOD.*scid* recipients of splenic T cells from age-matched control TCR-β transgenic NOD mice became diabetic. When intact NOD islets were transplanted under the renal capsule of macrophage-depleted 8.3-TCR-β transgenic NOD mice, the majority of the grafted islets remained intact, whereas most of the islets grafted into age-matched, control 8.3-TCR-β transgenic NOD mice were destroyed within 3 weeks after transplantation. The depletion of macrophages in these mice resulted in a decrease in the Th1 immune response along with an increase in the Th2 immune response and a decrease in β ell-specific T-cell activation, as shown by significant decreases in the expression of FasL, CD40 ligand and perforin, as compared with control mice. As shown in NOD mice, macrophages are

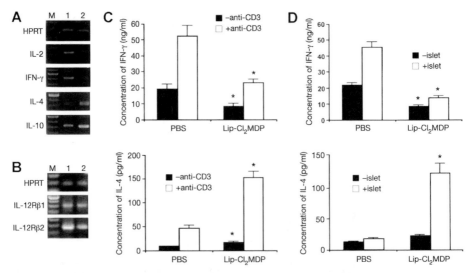

Fig. 8.2   Depletion of macrophages results in a decrease in the Th1 immune response and an increase in the Th2 immune response in NOD mice. Splenic T cells were isolated from three mice (15 weeks of age) from each group. Reverse transcriptase PCR analysis for cytokine gene expression was performed using primers specific for IL-2, IFN-γ, IL-4 and IL-10 (A) and IL-12Rβ1 and IL-12Rβ2 (B). Primers for HPRT were used as standards. M, 100-bp ladder; 1, amplified product from splenic T cells of PBS-treated NOD mice; 2, amplified product from splenic T cells of lip-C1$_2$MDP-treated NOD mice. Representative data for three independent experiments are shown. For the measurement of cytokine secretion from splenic T cell cultures, splenic T cells were isolated from lip-C1$_2$MDP- and PBS-treated NOD mice (n = 3 per group, 15 weeks of age), and activated with anti-CD3 antibody (10 µg/ml) for 2 days (C) or with irradiated NOD islets for 3 days (D). The production of cytokines was determined by ELISA. Values are shown as mean ± SD of three independent experiments. *P < 0.05 compared with the PBS-treated control group. Reprinted with permission from The Rockefeller University Press, New York (Jun *et al.*, 1999a).

absolutely required for the development and activation of β cell-cytotoxic CD8$^+$ T cells that cause β ell destruction, which leads to diabetes in 8.3-TCR-β transgenic NOD mice (Jun *et al.*, 1999b).

Although further studies to elucidate the precise mechanism of the involvement of macrophages in T-cell activation remain to be performed, our studies have shown that IL-12 secreted by macrophages may activate Th1-type CD4$^+$ T cells and, subsequently, the IL-2 and IFN-γ produced by these activated CD4$^+$ T-cells may assist in maximizing the activation of CD8$^+$ T cells (Figure 8.4). The down-regulation of islet cell-specific T-cell activation may be another major factor contributing to the impairment of the capability of T cells to kill β cells in macrophage-depleted NOD mice.

In BB rats, concanavalin A (ConA)-activated splenocytes from silica-treated diabetes-prone (DP)-BB rats do not induce insulitis or diabetes in neonate BB recipients, whereas ConA-activated splenocytes from phosphate-buffered saline (PBS)-treated BB rats do induce insulitis and diabetes in neonate BB recipients, indicating that the inactivation of macrophages by silica treatment results in loss of the ability of the splenocytes adoptively to transfer insulitis and diabetes. However, short-term silica treatment of DP-BB rats does not alter the ability of the splenocytes adoptively to transfer diabetes after ConA activation

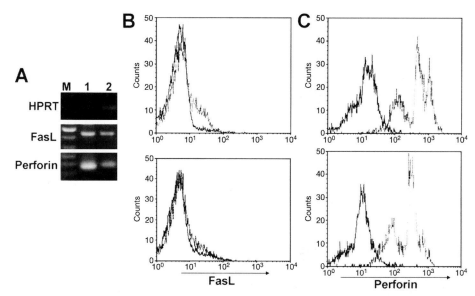

Fig. 8.3   Depletion of macrophages results in a decrease in the expression of FasL and perforin. In each group, splenic T cells were pooled from three mice (15 weeks of age) and activated with irradiated NOD islets for 72 hs. Reverse transcriptase PCR was performed using primers specific for FasL and perforin (A). Primers for HPRT were used as standards. M, 100 bp ladder; 1, amplified product from splenic T cells of PBS-treated NOD mice; 2, amplified product from splenic T cells of lip-C1$_2$MDP-treated NOD mice. Representative data from three independent experiments are shown. For FACS analysis of FasL (B) and perforin (C) expression, splenic T cells (10^6 cells) were stimulated with irradiated islets (40 islets) for 3 days and stained with biotinylated anti-FasL or anti-perforin antibodies, followed by incubation with PE–streptavidin and FITC-labeled anti-rat IgG, respectively. Solid line histograms represent cells incubated with PE–streptavidin or FITC-labeled anti-rat IgG only. Dashed line histograms represent cells stained with anti-FasL or anti-perforin antibodies. The upper panel shows the results for PBS-treated control mice and the lower panel shows the results for lip-C1$_2$MDP-treated mice. Reprinted with permission from The Rockefeller University Press, New York (Jun *et al.*, 1999a).

(Amano and Yoon, 1990). Further investigation revealed that silica treatment of DP-BB rats results in a significant decrease in the effector cell populations, including CD4$^+$ and CD8$^+$ T lymphocytes and NK cells (Amano and Yoon, 1990). The decrease in the macrophage-dependent effector T cells may result in the prevention of insulitis and diabetes in BB rats. The results of the above studies using NOD mice and BB rats indicate that macrophages are needed for the initiation of β cell-specific autoimmunity and the generation of the effector T cells that destroy pancreatic β cells (Yoon *et al.*, 1998).

Macrophages contribute directly to the destruction of β cells by the production of cytotoxic mediators such as cytokines and free radicals. When activated macrophages isolated from Wistar rats were co-cultured with islet cells, the macrophages induced the lysis of islet cells (Appels *et al.*, 1989). The islet cell lysis was mediated via the release of cytotoxic mediators, not via direct contact with macrophages (Kröncke *et al.*, 1991; Wiegand *et al.*, 1993). It has been shown that IL-1 is selectively cytotoxic to pancreatic β cells *in vitro* (Bendtzen *et al.*, 1986; Sandler *et al.*, 1991) and induces transient diabetes in normal rats (Wogensen *et al.*, 1991). It has been suggested that IL-1 receptors are

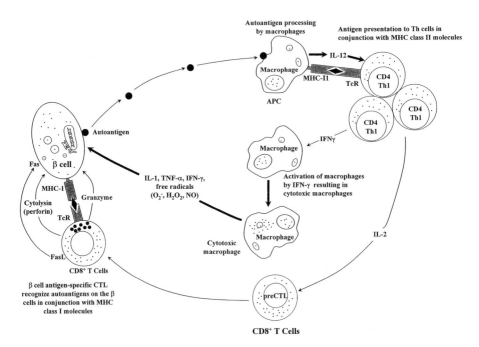

Fig. 8.4 Possible role of macrophages in the pathogenesis of autoimmune diabetes. β cell autoantigens released from the β cells during spontaneous turnover or insult by viral infection are processed by macrophages and presented to helper T cells in association with MHC class II molecules. Macrophages release IL-12, which is involved in the differentiation of Th1-type CD4⁺ T cells. While this process is taking place, β cell-specific pre-cytotoxic T cells may be recruited to the islets. These pre-cytotoxic T cells may be induced by IL-2 and other cytokines released by CD4⁺ helper T cells to differentiate into effector T cells. IFN-γ released by helper T cells may cause macrophages to become cytotoxic. Cytotoxic macrophages then release substantial amounts of β cell-toxic cytokines (including IL-1β, TNF-α and IFN-γ) and free radicals. In addition, the helper T cells secrete interleukins that activate other helper T cells, lymphocytes and cytotoxic T cells. The autoantigen-specific CD8⁺ cytotoxic T cells, as final effectors, may recognize the autoantigens expressed on many unaffected β cells in association with MHC class I molecules. These cytotoxic T cells release granzyme and perforin, which are toxic to β cells. In addition, Fas-mediated apoptosis is involved in β cell destruction. In this way, macrophages, T cells and cytokines synergistically destroy β cells, resulting in the development of autoimmune type 1 diabetes. Reprinted with permission from Academic Press, London (Yoon and Jun, 1998).

expressed on β cells (Eizirik *et al.*, 1991), and that the binding of IL-1 to IL-1 receptors induces novel mRNA transcription and protein synthesis (Hughes *et al.*, 1990).

Further studies revealed that IL-1β cytotoxicity in a certain time–dose window is preferential for β cells (Mandrup-Poulsen *et al.*, 1987a; Helqvist *et al.*, 1991). Electron microscopic observation revealed that more than 80 per cent of rat β cells showed signs of degeneration after 16 h of incubation with IL-1, while α cells did not. The destruction caused by IL-1 is potentiated by TNF (Mandrup-Poulsen *et al.*, 1987b). TNF-α inhibits insulin release and decreases the amount of insulin content in isolated mouse islets (Southern *et al.*, 1990). *In vitro* studies revealed that the cytotoxic effect of the cytokines IL-6, TNF, lymphotoxin and interferon-γ (IFN-γ) on the islets is cumulative (Rabinovitch *et al.*, 1988). These mediators, acting alone or synergistically, destroy islets *in vivo* or in cell culture (Pukel *et al.*, 1988; Appels *et al.*, 1989; Sandler *et al.*, 1990). In several studies, IL-1β and TNF-α-stimulated endogenous inducible nitric oxide synthase (iNOS) activity was revealed as a major source of β cell injury (Corbett and McDaniel, 1995). These cytokines are expressed in the insulitic lesions of NOD mice and BB rats (Jiang *et al.*, 1991; Welsh *et al.*, 1995), suggesting that the destruction of β cells may correlate with the expression of these cytokines. However, the role of TNF-α as a pro-inflammatory cytokine appears to be dependent on the time of expression. Early administration of TNF-α in NOD mice accelerated the onset of autoimmune diabetes, while late administration of this cytokine prevented the disease (Yang *et al.*, 1994). In addition, the transgenic expression of TNF-α in β cells of NOD mice early in life promoted the disease (Green *et al.*, 1998), while late transgenic expression of TNF-α reduced IDDM in NOD mice (Grewal *et al.*, 1996).

Activated macrophages generate toxic free radicals that are involved in the destruction of β cells. The toxic effect of these free radicals may be mediated by the superoxide anion and hydrogen peroxide, although the mechanisms of cell injury are not clearly understood. The β cell is very sensitive to the production of free radicals, because islet cells exhibit very low free radical scavenging activity (Malaisse *et al.*, 1982; Asayama *et al.*, 1986). It has been suggested that cytokines produced by islet-infiltrating macrophages may contribute to β cell damage by inducing the production of oxygen free radicals in the islets (Corbett and McDaniel, 1992; Faust *et al.*, 1996; McDaniel *et al.*, 1996). In macrophages, the cytokines IL-1β, TNF-α and IFN-γ induce iNOS which, in turn, generates the free radical NO from L-arginine. NO exerts a toxic effect on β cells by the induction of DNA damage. The DNA damage may activate excessive poly(ADP-ribose) polymerase (PARP), an enzyme involved in DNA repair (Satoh and Lindah, 1992), resulting in the synthesis of a large amount of poly(ADP-ribose) polymers from NAD; thereby the cellular NAD level is reduced, resulting in cell death (Uchigata *et al.*, 1982). When isolated islets were incubated with the NO donor, sodium nitroprusside, DNA strand breaks were detected within a few hours of NO exposure (Fehsel *et al.*, 1993). The expression of iNOS is not detected in the pancreatic islets without lymphocytic infiltration. Islets with advanced infiltration highly express iNOS, suggesting that the expression of iNOS may be associated with the development of diabetes in BB rats (Kleeman *et al.*, 1993). Furthermore, treatment of DP-BB rats with N^G-nitro-L-arginine-methylester significantly reduces the incidence of diabetes (Lindsay *et al.*, 1995). The treatment of NOD mice with aminoguanidine, an iNOS inhibitor, delays the onset of diabetes in adoptive transfer models (Bowman *et al.*, 1994). Recently, it was reported that the transgenic expression of iNOS in the β cells of a non-diabetic, normal strain of mice led to the development of diabetes without insulitis (Takamura *et al.*, 1998). Therefore, it appears that free radicals such as NO (generated by iNOS) may contribute to β cell destruction.

In addition to spontaneously developed autoimmune diabetes, macrophages also play an important role in virus-induced autoimmune diabetes in diabetes-resistant (DR)-BB rats. DR-BB rats do not normally develop spontaneous insulitis or diabetes. However, when DR-BB rats are infected with Kilham rat virus (KRV), one-third of the infected rats develop autoimmune diabetes similar to DP-BB rats, and an additional one-third develop insulitis without diabetes (Guberski *et al.*, 1991). KRV induces diabetes in DR-BB rats without direct infection of the β cells. Instead, KRV infects lymphoid organs such as the spleen, thymus and lymph nodes. Therefore, KRV-induced diabetes in DR-BB rats is suggested to be autoimmune-mediated, although the precise mechanisms of KRV-induced autoimmune IDDM are not well understood.

When DR-BB rats were infected with KRV, the expression of the macrophage-derived cytokines IL-12, TNF-α and IL-1β was selectively increased in the splenocytes and pancreas soon after infection. The expression of the Th1 cytokines IL-2 and IFN-γ closely correlated with an elevation in the level of IL-12. Treatment of DR-BB rats with lip-C1$_2$MDP, after infection with KRV and treatment with poly(I:C) to increase the incidence of diabetes, completely prevented the development of diabetes. In contrast, 78 per cent of KRV/poly(I:C)-injected DR-BB rats that received PBS instead of lip-C1$_2$MDP became diabetic. ConA-activated splenic lymphocytes isolated from macrophage-depleted DR-BB rats injected with KRV/poly(I:C) did not induce insulitis or diabetes in young DP-BB rats (Chung *et al.*, 1997). These results suggest that the depletion of macrophages may prevent the development of β cell-specific effector cells, resulting in the complete prevention of diabetes. Therefore, KRV infection of DR-BB rats may result in the activation of macrophages which, in turn, secrete IL-12, TNF-α and IL-1β. IL-12-activated Th1-type CD4$^+$ T cells cause the secretion of the cytokines IFN-γ and IL-2, which activate the rest of the macrophages and CD8$^+$ T cells, respectively. The toxicity of macrophage-derived cytokines and Th1-type CD4$^+$ T cell-derived cytokines to the β cells, in combination with the damage incurred from KRV antigen-specific CD8$^+$ cytotoxic T cells, may lead to the destruction of pancreatic β cells, resulting in the development of IDDM in KRV-infected DR-BB rats. It appears that the depletion of macrophages in KRV-infected DR-BB rats may reduce the selective expression of the macrophage-derived cytokines IL-12, TNF-α and IL-1β that occurs in DR-BB rats soon after KRV infection, which, in turn, down-regulates the Th1 cytokines IFN-γ and IL-2, resulting in the inhibition of CD8$^+$ cytotoxic T-cell activation. Thus, the depletion of macrophages obstructs the macrophage-mediated cascade of immune processes that lead to the destruction of β cells.

2.2 Multiple sclerosis and experimental autoimmune encephalomyelitis

Multiple sclerosis (MS) is a chronic inflammatory demyelinating disease of the CNS characterized by neurological symptoms caused by impaired nerve conduction. Experimental autoimmune encephalomyelitis (EAE) is an animal model of inflammatory disease in the CNS, and the chronic form of EAE is very similar to human MS in its clinical manifestations and pathology (Raine, 1984). In rodents and primates, EAE is induced by subcutaneous or intracutaneous injection of an encephalogenic emulsion such as whole spinal cord, purified myelin, myelin basic protein (MBP), proteolipid protein (PLP) or MBP or PLP peptides with Freund's complete adjuvant and killed *Mycobacterium tuberculosis*. After immunization, an immune response to autoantigens develops and the animals show clinical symptoms such as 'floppy tail' and paresis or paralysis of the extremities. The inflammatory lesions in the CNS contain lymphocytes and macrophages. Demyelination is associated with an inflammatory reaction that is orchestrated by activated lymphocytes, macrophages, astrocytes and microglia. Activated CD4$^+$ and CD8$^+$ T cells accumulate around small venules at the early stage of MS lesions (Hauser *et al.*, 1983). At later stages, T cells, B cells, plasma cells and activated macrophages are observed in the perivascular inflammatory site, and myelin degeneration occurs (Prineas, 1975; Prineas and Wright, 1978).

Microglia, the resident macrophages of the brain, are suggested to be derived from a bone marrow precursor of monocytic lineage (Hickey and Kimura, 1988; Perry and Gordon, 1988) and share many phenotypic markers and effector functions with blood-borne macrophages. Microglia are located close to the neurons in the gray matter and between fiber tracts in the white matter of the CNS. Microglia have multiple function in the CNS, including phagocytosis, antigen presentation and the production of cytokines, proteinases, oxygen free radicals, NO and complement components (Gordon, 1995; Gehrmann *et al.*, 1995).

Microglia/macrophages exert effector functions and are actively involved in myelin breakdown. The activated microglia express molecules such as major histocompatibility complex (MHC) class II, B7.1, B7.2 and CD40 (Hofman *et al.*, 1986; Windhagen, 1995; Gerritse *et al.*, 1996), which are involved in antigen presentation and the activation of T cells. It is considered that the activated T cells, independently of antigen specificity, can freely enter the CNS (Hickey *et al.*, 1991), and that these activated T cells and microglia are mutually activated, resulting in the recruitment of more T cells accompanied by blood-borne macrophages that are attracted by the local expression of chemokines (Karpus *et al.*, 1995; Berman *et al.*, 1996; Storch *et al.*, 1996; Pan *et al.*, 1997). The role of blood-borne macrophages in the pathogenesis of EAE has been studied by the depletion of macrophages with silica or lip-C1$_2$MDP. The depletion of macrophages using silica treatment suppressed the clinical signs of EAE and delayed the onset of the disease (Brosnan *et al.*, 1981). A later study using lip-C1$_2$MDP treatment showed the complete prevention of clinical signs of EAE (Huitinga *et al.*, 1990). It was shown that lip-C1$_2$MDP treatment did not directly affect the endogenous microglia, but eliminated peripheral blood-borne macrophages (Bauer *et al.*, 1995), and the reduction of peripheral macrophages concomitantly decreased the phagocytic microglia, suggesting that infiltrating peripheral blood-borne macrophages may be needed for the subsequent activation of microglia.

Adhesion molecules and chemokines have been considered to be involved in the trafficking of these macrophages, although the mechanisms by which macrophages cross the blood–brain barrier are not well understood. The administration of antibodies against Mac1 (CD11b) or lymphocyte function-associated antigen (LFA; CD11a), which are expressed on monocytes, significantly suppresses the clinical signs of EAE (Huitinga *et al.*, 1993; Gordon *et al.*, 1995), suggesting that the inhibition of macrophage adherence to the endothelium may prevent the disease by blocking the entry of macrophages into the CNS. The CC family of chemokines, including macrophage inflammatory protein (MIP)-1α, MIP-1β, monocyte chemoattractant peptide (MCP)-1, and regulated on activation, normal T cell expressed and secreted protein (RANTES), are known to be chemotactic for monocyte/macrophage lineage cells. In myelin oligodendrocyte glycoprotein-immunized C57BL6 mice, RANTES and MCP-1 mRNA were detected in the CNS at an early stage after immunization (Juedes *et al.* 2000). In the Lewis rat model of EAE, MCP-1 expression was correlated with disease progression. The expression of MCP-1 was increased just prior to the onset of clinical signs, peaked at the height of the disease and decreased with remission (Hulkower *et al.*, 1993). A marked increase in the expression of MCP-1 correlated with the accumulation of monocytes in CNS lesions (Berman *et al.*, 1996). In addition, MIP-1α is thought to play a role in the recruitment of macrophages in EAE. The expression of MIP-1α was induced 1–2 days prior to clinical signs of EAE and peaked at disease onset in an adoptive transfer model (Godiska *et al.*, 1995). The administration of anti-MIP-1α antibody prevented the disease and the infiltration of mononuclear cells into the CNS (Karpus *et al.*, 1995). These results suggest that the inhibition of the recruitment of mononuclear cells into the CNS by the modulation of chemokine expression prevents the disease and that macrophages play an important role in the inflammation of the CNS, leading to the development of the disease.

Microglia are activated and exert effector functions in the inflammatory site in concert with infiltrating blood-borne macrophages. The proliferation and differentiation of microglia are regulated by colony-stimulating factors produced by astrocytes. Thus, microglia show high intrinsic antigen-presenting capacities when cultured in the presence of granulocyte–macrophage colony-stimulating factor (GM-CSF) in primary glial cell cultures (Fischer *et al.*, 1993). Microglia are known to induce the expression of the IL-12 p40 subunit upon lipopolysaccharide (LPS) stimulation (Aloisi *et al.*, 1997; Stalder *et al.*, 1997), and the production of IL-12 may be regulated by IL-10 and/or other factors secreted by astrocytes (Aloisi *et al.*, 1997; Jander *et al.*, 1998). The administration of IL-12 induces relapse in EAE (Smith *et al.*, 1997), and anti-IL-12 antibodies prevent superantigen-induced and spontaneous relapses of EAE (Constantinescu *et al.*, 1998), suggesting that IL-12 derived from macrophages contributes to the exacerbation of the disease.

Microglia and macrophages produce cytokines, including IL-1β, IL-6, TNF-α, lymphotoxin (LT) and interferons that can contribute to inflammation and myelin damage within the CNS (Lee *et al.*, 1993; Walker *et al.*, 1995; Merrill and Benveniste, 1996). IL-1 is known to activate T cells and up-regulate the expression of intercellular cell adhesion molecule-1 (ICAM-1) on endothelial cells (Fabry *et al.*, 1992). IL-1β expression is detected in macrophages in the early phase of EAE, suggesting that it may induce ICAM-1 expression and, subsequently, the recruitment of macrophages to inflammatory sites in the CNS. In addition, the expression of IL-1β increases during the clinical phase of EAE and decreases during remission (Kennedy *et al.*, 1992; Bauer *et al.*, 1993). Treatment with IL-1β has been shown to increase the clinical signs of EAE, while treatment with a soluble IL-1 receptor suppresses EAE (Jacobs *et al.*, 1991), indicating that IL-1β plays a role in this disease.

TNF-α is also implicated in EAE and MS (Benveniste, 1995). It has been reported that TNF-α is highly expressed in immune cells from MS patients during the acute phases of the disease (Beck *et al.*, 1988; Rieckmann *et al.*, 1995). Similarly, TNF-α expression has been detected during the peak of clinical signs in EAE, and the source of TNF-α was found to be microglia (Renno *et al.*, 1995). The production of TNF-α by microglia may be induced by activated T cells (Chabot *et al.*, 1997). TNF-α is toxic to myelin and oligodendrocytes and destroys them *in vitro* (Selmaj and Raine, 1988). Studies using several different methods to block TNF-α demonstrated that the inhibition of TNF-α prevented EAE. The administration of anti-TNF-α antibodies prevented the adoptive transfer of EAE by MBP-reactive encephalogenic T cells (Ruddle *et al.*, 1990; Selmaj *et al.*, 1991; Korner *et al.*, 1997). TNF-α receptors (TNFRs) also have an effect on the inhibition of EAE. Treatment with bivalent human soluble TNFR1 and TNFR2 immunoglobulin (Ig) fusion protein inhibits the development of actively induced EAE. Intracranial injection of soluble TNFR–Ig has a stronger effect on inhibition of the disease than systemic administration, suggesting that TNF-α produced in local lesions in the CNS plays a major role in

EAE (Baker *et al.*, 1994; Selmaj *et al.*, 1995). The role of TNF-α in demyelinating disease was confirmed by the establishment of transgenic mice in which TNF-α is expressed constitutively in the CNS. These transgenic animals spontaneously developed a chronic inflammatory demyelinating disease at 3–8 weeks (Probert *et al.*, 1995a). Another transgenic mouse line in which TNF-α is overexpressed in the CNS showed more severe EAE, and the demyelination process proceeded chronically in the absence of T cells and was accompanied by persistent microglia/macrophage activation (Taupin *et al.*, 1997). However, studies with TNF-α knockout mice gave conflicting results. One study reported that TNF-α plays a critical role in the induction of EAE (Sean Riminton *et al.*, 1998), while another study showed that TNF-α is not required for the induction of EAE (Frei *et al.*, 1997). There is also evidence that TNF-α plays a role as an anti-inflammatory cytokine in EAE, since TNF-α knockout mice develop more severe EAE than wild-type mice (Liu *et al.*, 1998).

Free radicals produced by microglia and macrophages also damage the CNS. Myelin appears to be highly susceptible to damage induced by oxygen radicals (Konat and Wiggins, 1985). The production of free radicals in activated microglia and infiltrating macrophages in the brain increases during the clinical phase of EAE (Ruuls *et al.*, 1995). In addition, EAE is inhibited by free radical scavengers, catalase and possibly by scavenging H_2O_2. NO has been shown to be cytotoxic to myelin-forming oligodendrocytes *in vitro* (Merrill *et al.*, 1993). The expression of iNOS, an enzyme involved in NO production, is detected in the macrophages infiltrating the CNS of animals with EAE (Van Dam *et al.*, 1995), and the inhibition of iNOS by the administration of aminoguanidine ameliorates EAE (Cross *et al.*, 1994). In addition, the production of NO in the brain in EAE has been demonstrated (Lin *et al.*, 1993). These results suggest that NO may play a role in the damage of oligondendrocytes. However, recent studies using iNOS knockout mice showed the exacerbation of EAE, implicating a protective role for NO in the disease (Fenyk-Melody *et al.*, 1998; Sahrbacher *et al.*, 1998).

The matrix metalloproteinases (MMPs) are also believed to contribute to tissue destruction by degrading extracellular matrix components in MS and EAE (Gijbels *et al.*, 1992, 1993). Microglia and macrophages in MS express a variety of MMPs (Maeda and Sobel, 1996), and activated macroglia and macrophages in culture have been shown to produce MMPs (Welgus *et al.*, 1990; Colton *et al.*, 1993). Treatment with MMP inhibitor suppresses the development of EAE and reverses clinical signs of the disease (Gijbels *et al.*, 1994). In EAE, the permeability of the blood–brain barrier is enhanced; thus, the inhibition of MMP activity appears to restore normal permeability, resulting in the re-establishment of the blood–brain barrier. It has been reported that activated monocytes, by interaction with T cells, produced MMP-9 (Malik *et al.*, 1996), and that treatment with anti-CD40L abrogated MMP expression, suggesting that the activation of monocytes may occur through a CD40–CD40L interaction. Therefore, the secreted soluble mediators produced by activated microglia and macrophages, such as cytokines, free radicals and NO, along with complement and proteolytic enzymes, act synergistically to damage myelin (Figure 8.5), contributing to the development MS and EAE.

2.3 Rheumatic diseases

Macrophages have been also suggested to play an important role in autoimmune rheumatic diseases such as rheumatic arthritis (RA) and systemic lupus erythmatosus

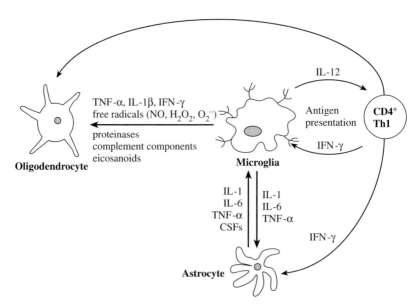

Fig. 8.5 Possible role of microglia/macrophages in the pathogenesis of EAE. Microglia/macrophages present autoantigens to CD4+ T helper T cells in association with MHC class II molecules. Microglia/macrophages release IL-12, which is involved in the differentiation of Th1-type CD4+ T cells. The activated T helper cells secrete IFN-γ. IFN-γ further activates microglia/macrophages and the activated microglia/macrophages produce IL-1β, IL-6 and TNF-α which induce astrocyte proliferation. The products of activated microglia/macrophages, such as IL-1β, IFN-γ, TNF-α, free radicals, nitric oxide, proteinases, complement components and eicosanoides, contribute to damage to oligodendrocytes through synergistic action with CD4+ T cells. Astrocytes produce colony-stimulating factors that regulate the proliferation and differentiation of microglia/macrophages as well as IL-1β, IL-6 and TNF-α.

(SLE). The role of macrophages in RA is described in detail in Chapter 9 of this volume. Here, we provide general information on the function of macrophages in the pathogenesis of autoimmune rheumatic diseases. The inflammation of the synovial tissue in RA is evidenced by the increase of cell numbers in the synovial lining. The infiltrating cells include macrophages/monocytes, T cells, B cells and plasma cells (Rooney *et al*, 1989; Bresnihan, 1992). The layer lining in normal and rheumatoid synovial tissue is composed primarily of two predominant cell populations, the macrophage-like synoviocytes (type A cells) and fibroblast-like synoviocytes (type B cells). Type A cells are macrophages, which mainly have phagocytic functions, while type B cells contain a well developed rough endoplasmic reticulum, suggesting that these cells may be involved in protein synthesis (Ziff, 1974). Type A cells are HLA class II positive and CD14 antigen positive, and type B cells are usually negative for these markers. However, in RA, a significant proportion of type B cells express HLA class II antigens (Burmester *et al.*, 1983, 1987).

In RA, bone marrow-derived peripheral blood monocytes enter into the rheumatic joint. The migration of monocytes into synovial tissue is mediated by the β2 integrins (CD11a, b, c/CD18) expressed on the monocytes and adhesion molecules expressed on the endothelia, such as endothelial–leukocyte adhesion molecule-1 (ELAM-1), vascular cell adhesion molecule-1 (VCAM-1) and ICAM-1. Consistent with this, the expression of the β2 integrins has been shown to be increased in the macrophage-like synoviocytes in RA synovial tissue. The monocytes that enter the joint are activated and differentiate into mature macrophage-like synoviocytes (Ridley *et al.*, 1990). Activated synovial macrophages are adjacent to CD4+ T cells (Janossy *et al.*, 1981). The major population of HLA-DR-positive rheumatoid synovial lining cells were found to be macrophages-like cells and were shown to present antigens to T cells, resulting in the activation of T cells (Klareskog *et al.*, 1982; Panayi *et al.*, 1992). Peripheral blood T cells are recruited through the interaction with adhesion molecules such as ELAM-1 or E-selectin expressed in RA synovial endothelium and VCAM-1 expressed on synovial macrophages (Postigo *et al.*, 1992). The macrophages in both synovial tissue and peripheral blood monocytes from RA patients show increased levels of macrophage-derived cytokines. Activated macrophages are enriched in the RA synovium, the expression of surface MHC class II is increased and the expression of macrophage-derived cytokines such as IL-1, TNF-α, IL-6, IL-8, IL-12, IL-18 and GM-CSF is increased (Saxne *et al.*, 1988; Guerne *et al.*, 1989; Xu *et al.*, 1989; Firestein *et al.*, 1990; Remick *et al.*, 1992; Gracie *et al.*, 1999). However, T cell-derived cytokines such as IL-2, IFN-γ and IL-4 are barely detectable in the RA joints, contrasting with the abundant expression of macrophage-derived cytokines (Firestein *et al.*, 1988; Symons *et al.*, 1988).

Quantitative studies of cytokine gene expression using *in situ* hybridization in the RA synovium revealed that more than 40 per cent of the macrophages express IL-1β and 15 per cent express TNF-α (Firenstein and Zvaifler, 1990). IL-1β is known to be involved in lymphocyte activation in the presence of antigen (Kumkumiam *et al.*, 1989). Blocking TNF-α by anti-TNF-α antibody therapy in RA patients significantly reduced the expression of chemokines such as IL-8 and MCP-1 and decreased inflammatory cell migration into RA joints (Taylor *et al.*, 2000). In synovial fluid from RA joints, macrophages have also shown increased expression of GM-CSF (Alvaro-Garcia *et al.*, 1990), which is known to activate MHC class II expression and augment antigen presentation function (Fischer *et al.*, 1988). In addition, it was reported that MCP-1, a chemokine that is involved in recruiting macrophages/monocytes in particular, is expressed by synovial tissue macrophages in the RA synovium (Koch *et al.*, 1992; Hachicha *et al.*, 1993). Macrophages from RA patients expressed significantly higher IL-8 than macrophages from healthy controls when the macrophages were activated with LPS (Rodenberg *et al.*, 1999). The expression of the transcription factors NK-κB and AP-1, which are involved in the transcription of most inflammatory cytokine genes, is enhanced in the macrophages of the RA synovium (Handel *et al.*, 1995). Macrophages in the RA synovium also produce proteolytic enzymes such as collagenase, gelatinase B and elastase (Jensen *et al.*, 1991; Tetlow *et al.*, 1993, 1995). Although macrophages are not the primary effector cells responsible for the degradation of matrix components, electron microscope studies showed that macrophages roughen the bony surfaces without forming resorption pits (Chang *et al.*, 1992). It was shown that the co-culture of cartilage discs with both mouse fibroblasts and macrophages resulted in a marked degradation of cartilage discs. The degradation was less effective when the discs were co-cultured with macrophages or fibroblasts alone (Janusz and Hare, 1993). In addition, macrophages are the major source of platelet-derived growth factor in the RA synovium, which contributes to the growth of fibroblast-like synoviocytes (Lafiatis *et al.*, 1989), and IL-1β and TNF-α produced from macrophages contribute to the production of proteases from fibroblast-like synoviocytes.

Therefore, the destruction of cartilage and bone in RA may be mediated by collaboratory effects of macrophage-like and fibroblast-like synoviocytes.

In different models of experimental arthritis, a large number of macrophages infiltrate the synovial membrane (Verschure *et al.*, 1989; Pelegri *et al.*, 1995). In antigen-induced arthritis in rats, freshly immigrated ED1-positive monocytes/macrophages and mature resident ED2- and ED3-positive macrophages are found (Dijkstra *et al.*, 1987; Verschure *et al.*, 1989; Damoiseax *et al.*, 1992). Similarly to human RA, synovial macrophages are activated in antigen-induced arthritis, evidenced by the expression of MHC class II molecules, the production of inflammatory cytokines and enhanced phagocytic activity (Johnson *et al.*, 1986a,b; López-Bote *et al.*, 1988; Henderson *et al.*, 1988; Smith-Oliver *et al.*, 1993). In addition, both synovial macrophages and monocytes in peripheral blood are activated in adjuvant-induced arthritis (Johnson *et al.*, 1986a,b; López-Bote *et al.*, 1988). The expression of TNF-α is significantly increased in the regional lymph nodes before the onset of arthritis in both collagen-induced and adjuvant-induced arthritis, and the increase of TNF-α expression is associated with the increase of IFN-γ (Müssener *et al.*, 1995). The transgenic expression of TNF-α results in chronic erosive arthritis (Keffer *et al.*, 1991). These results suggest that TNF-α produced from macrophages may play a crucial role in RA, and both the local and systemic production of TNF-α may play a role in RA. In contrast, IL-1β appears to play a role as an effector in local inflammation. The increase of IL-1β in the synovium is correlated with the onset of synovitis (Henderson *et al.*, 1988). The administration of IL-1β intra-arterially accelerates the development of collagen-induced arthritis (Hom *et al.*, 1988; Feige *et al.*, 1989; van de Loo *et al.*, 1995).

Strategies that neutralize macrophage-derived products or deplete macrophages have shown a preventive effect against RA. Systemic administration of antibodies against TNF-α ameliorates the disease in collagen-induced and adjuvant-induced arthritis (Piguet *et al.*, 1992; Williams *et al.*, 1992; Issekutz *et al.*, 1994). Treatment with anti-TNF-α antibodies or anti-IL-1 receptor antibodies prevents the development of arthritis in a TNF-α transgenic mouse model (Keffer *et al.*, 1991; Probert *et al.*, 1995b). Systemic administration of antibodies against IL-1α and IL-1β decreases joint inflammation and proteoglycan degradation in murine antigen- and collagen-induced arthritis (van de Loo *et al.*, 1995; Joosten *et al.*, 1996). Alternatively, the administration of cytokines such as IL-13 or IL-4 can down-regulate macrophage function by decreasing IL-1β and TNF-α, resulting in the resolution of arthritis (Allen *et al.*, 1993; Hart *et al.*, 1995). Blocking of macrophage recruitment using neutralization antibodies against MIP-1α and MIP-2 delays the onset of collagen-induced arthritis (Kasama *et al.*, 1995). The inhibition of monocyte migration by treatment with antibodies against adhesion molecules such as CD11/CD18 and very late activation antigen-4 (VLA4) reduces clinical and inflammatory signs of the disease (Issekutz and Issekutz, 1995). Reactive oxygen species such as the superoxide radical, hydrogen peroxide and hydroxyl radical, as well as reactive nitrogen species such as nitric oxide and peroxynitrite also contribute to tissue injury in RA, and thus antioxidant therapy can reduce chronic inflammation (Bauerova and Bezek, 1999). The selective depletion of macrophages using lip-C1$_2$MDP significantly reduces the clinical signs of the disease in both antigen-induced and adjuvant-induced arthritis (Camilleri *et al.*, 1995; Kinne *et al.*, 1995a). Systemic administration of lip-C1$_2$MDP does not deplete macrophages in the synovium, but does deplete macrophages in the spleen and lymph nodes (Kinne *et al.*, 1995a), and the ED3-positive macrophages, which interact with T cells, are preferentially depleted systemically. It appears that lip-C1$_2$MDP affects macrophages in the systemic circulation rather than those within inflammatory sites. Consistent with these data, local administration of lip-C1$_2$MDP is only marginally effective in arthritis (Van Lent *et al.*, 1994; Kinne *et al.*, 1995b).

Several disease-modifying antirheumatic drug therapies for the treatment of human RA are known to have antimacrophage effects. For example, gold compounds inhibit Fc and C3 receptor expression, oxygen radical generation and IL-1 production in monocytes after LPS stimulation (Scheinberg *et al.*, 1982; Harth *et al.*, 1983; Danis *et al.*, 1990) and inhibit T-cell proliferation in response to antigens or mitogens (Lipsky and Ziff, 1977). In addition, gold salt inhibits the production of IL-8 and MCP-1. Methotrexate was found to impair the chemotaxis of peripheral blood monocytes and decrease the expression of inflammatory cytokines from stimulated peripheral blood monocytes (Seitz *et al.*, 1995). The antirheumatic corticosteroids down-regulate the expression of IL-1 and IL-6 in monocytes (Amano *et al*, 1993), and dexamethasone also decreases the release of IL-8 and MCP-1 by synovial cells (Loetscher *et al.*, 1994). These drugs may regulate rheumatic disease through antimacrophage effects.

3 Role of macrophages in primary immunodeficiency disease

See also Chapter 4 for a virological perspective on HIV–macrophage interactions.

Human immunodeficiency virus (HIV) type 1 infects host cells that express both CD4 and chemokine co-receptors including CCR5 and CXR4 (Berger, 1997). These susceptible hosts are CD4$^+$ T lymphocytes, dendritic cells and mononuclear phagocytes. HIV primarily infects CD4$^+$ T cells, but rarely also infects macrophages in the blood and lymphoid tissue. The number of CD4$^+$ T cells decreases through mechanisms such as direct cytopathic effects of virus replication on CD4$^+$ T cells (Ho *et al.*, 1995) and inappropriate high levels of CD4$^+$ T cell apoptosis (Groux *et al.*, 1992). Thus, HIV infection is associated with a broad spectrum of immunological abnormalities. In general, the primary immunodeficiency in acquired immunodeficiency syndrome (AIDS) is related to the depletion of CD4$^+$ T cells, subsequently resulting in various clinical problems including opportunistic infections, degenerative neurological disease, a spectrum of malignancies and, invariably, death.

However, immunodeficiency may result not only from T cell depletion, but also from defects in the mononuclear phagocyte system, since immune function is not always correlated with CD4$^+$ T cell numbers. Mononuclear phagocytes such as tissue macrophages and blood monocytes are probably the primary cells in the body to become infected, and they live for long periods of time, whereas T cells infected with HIV die when the HIV replicates (Crowe *et al.*, 1987). Thus, macrophages provide a reservoir of ongoing viral replication and serve as vehicles for spreading HIV into many tissues, such as the brain. See also Chapter 13 for a discussion of the role of the macrophage as an HIV resevoir in the brain.

The major disease associated with infected macrophages is HIV-associated dementia complex (Price *et al.*, 1988), which is characterized by cognitive impairments including mental slowness, poor concentration, lethargy, apathy and diminished emotional responses. HIV-associated dementia is the most severe neurological complication of AIDS. The productive replication of HIV-1 in blood-derived macrophages and microglia, the brain tissue macrophages, may be the cause of the neurological impairment, since neurons, oligodendrocytes and brain microvascular endothelial cells are rarely infected. The infection of brain macrophages is associated with HIV encephalitis, which is quite different from other types of viral encephalitis. In HIV encephalitis, there is usually minimal tissue destruction and no inflammatory infiltration of the lymphocytes is observed. The neuropathological features of HIV encephalitis are multinucleated giant cell formation (giant syncytia), micronodule formation and loss of neurons (Budka *et al*, 1991; Wiley and Achim, 1994). However, the clinical symptom, HIV-associated dementia, is not tightly correlated with the presence of HIV encephalitis. Therefore, the pathological substrate of HIV-associated dementia remains to be elucidated.

Chronic HIV infection of macrophages provokes abnormal cytokine production. HIV infection of macrophages increases the production of pro-inflammatory molecules such as the eicosanoids (Nottet *et al.*, 1995), platelet-activating factor (PAF) (Gelbard *et al.*, 1994), IL-1β and TNF-α (D'Addario *et al.*, 1990, 1992; Wesselingh *et al.*, 1993; Nottet *et al.*, 1995). Human monocytes cultured in the presence of gp120 produce TNF-α, IL-1β, IL-6, macrophage colony-stimulating factor (M-CSF) and GM-CSF (Clouse *et al.*, 1991). TNF-α may damage oligodendrocytes and myelin (Selmaj and Raine, 1988) and may affect the function of neurons (Soliven and Albert, 1992). The elevated level of TNF-α in the sera of AIDS patients and the increased level of TNF-α expression in the brain of demented patients (Wesselingh *et al.*, 1993) suggest an important role for TNF-α in the pathogenesis of AIDS-associated neurological disease. TNF-α and PAF were found to be directly toxic to neuronal cells. PAF and several leukotrienes have excitatory effects on neurons (Clark *et al.*, 1992; Kato *et al.*, 1994) through an N-methyl-D-aspartate (NMDA)-mediated process and TNF-α-induced voltage-dependent Ca^{2+} currents (Soliven and Albert, 1992).

HIV infection induces high levels of transcription factor NF-κB DNA-binding activity in monocyte-derived macrophages (Nottet *et al*, 1997), which reflects the overexpression of TNF-α by HIV-infected macrophages upon activation with LPS or phorbol myristate acetate. Recently, it was reported that HIV infection of the promonocytic cell line U937 results in an increase in protein kinase activity, which in turn contributes to the enhanced activation of IκBκ and subsequent degradation of IκB α and activation of NF-κB (DeLuca *et al*, 1996; Folgueira *et al.*, 1996). In addition, HIV protease itself is known to dissociate the NF-κB–IκB complex (Riviere *et al.*, 1991), which may also contribute to NF-κB activation.

The pro-inflammatory cytokines, such as IL-1β and TNF-α, that are produced in activated HIV-infected macrophages induce the expression of adhesion molecules such as E-selectin and VCAM-1 on brain microvascular endothelial cells (Nottet *et al.*, 1996), suggesting that HIV-infected macrophages have potential for entry into the brain tissue. In fact, monocyte adhesion to brain tissue could be prevented by antibodies against E-selectin and VCAM-1. In addition, it was reported that the HIV Tat protein induced the expression of E-selectin on macrovascular endothelial cells (Hofman *et al.*, 1993). TNF-α, leukotrienes and PAF, produced by the activated HIV-infected macrophages, may increase the permeability of the blood–brain barrier (Bjork *et al.*, 1983; Black *et al.*, 1985) and help macrophages to migrate through this barrier. HIV infection of macrophages is known to up-regulate gelatinase B activity, which facilitates the digestion and invasion of basement membranes, affecting blood–brain barrier permeability (Dhawan *et al.*, 1995). In addition to adhesion molecules, chemokines may also contribute to the trafficking of macrophages to brain tissue. HIV infection of macrophages *in vitro* induces the expression of MIP-1α and less MIP-1β (Canque *et al.*, 1996). Consistent with this result, there is an increase in the expression of the β chemokines such as MIP-1α and MIP-1β in the brain tissue of AIDS patients (Schmidtmayerova *et al.*, 1996). Therefore, the enhanced expression of these chemokines in encephalitic brain tissue might contribute to further recruitment of monocytes into the brain.

HIV-infected macrophages and microglia also release soluble mediators that cause neuronal injury. HIV-infected monocytic cells such as U937 and THP-1 cells released small, heat-and cold-stable and protease-resistant molecules that were toxic to neurons from embryonic chick ciliary ganglia and embryonic rat spinal cord, when cultured with these neurons (Giulian *et al.*, 1990), and this toxic activity could be shown in human monocytes after stimulation with the HIV glycoprotein gp120 (Giulian *et al.*, 1993). This neurotoxic activity was prevented by an NMDA receptor antagonist, suggesting that the toxicity may involve the activation of NMDA receptors. In addition, a neurotoxic amine (NTox), produced from HIV-infected microglia, was found to induce neuronal injury (Giulian *et al.*, 1996). However, the culture supernatants of HIV-infected cells of either a monocytic cell line, U937, or primary monocytes were not toxic to primary rat or human neurons (Tardieu *et al.*, 1992; Bernton *et al.*, 1992). Co-cultures of HIV-infected cells and human brain cells caused neuronal damage and death (Pulliam *et al.*, 1991). These results suggest that the cytotoxic effect of HIV-infected monocytes may be mediated by direct cell contact and not by soluble mediators. Several studies have shown that HIV proteins, such as gp120 and Tat, are directly toxic to neurons (Dreyer *et al.*, 1990; Sabaiter *et al.*, 1991). The culture of rat retinal ganglion cells with gp120 markedly increased the intracellular free calcium level (Dreyer *et al.*, 1990), and this gp120-mediated calcium entry and toxicity involved the activation of neuronal NMDA receptors (Lipton, 1992; Lipton and Rosenberg, 1994).

Macrophages are also producers of arachidonic acid metabolites such as prostaglandins and thromboxane, which are involved in the induction of neurotoxic mediators such as TNF-α (Genis *et al.*, 1992). In HIV-associated dementia, the cerebrospinal fluid level of prostaglandins E_2, F_{2a} and thromboxane B_2 are elevated (Griffin *et al.*, 1994), and the *in vitro* co-culture of astrocytes and HIV-infected monocytes produced elevated arachidonic acid metabolites (Genis *et al.*, 1992).

HIV enters into the brain within blood-derived monocytes/macrophages and replicates in the macrophages and microglia in brain tissue. HIV-infected macrophages secrete proinflammatory cytokines such as IL-1β, TNF-α, IL-6 and GM-CSF, which promote the migration and activation of macrophages. In addition to these cytokines, the activated macrophages, in turn, produce eiconsanoids, proteinases and neurotoxic substances, which contribute to neuronal damage (Table 8.1). Furthermore, the interactions between HIV-infected macrophages and brain cells may lead to neuronal injury, leading to neuronal dysfunction.

Table 8.1 Secretory products from activated HIV-infected macrophages and microglia and their possible contribution to neuronal damage

Type of product	Example	Mafjor function
Cytokines	IL-1, IL-6, TNF-α, GM-CSF, M-CSF, PAF	Directly damage the neuron Induce expression of adhesion molecules on endothelial cells Increase the permeability of the blood–brain barrier
Chemokines	MCP-1, MIP-1α/β	Recruit monocytes and lymphocytes to brain tissue
Proteolytic enzymes	Gelatinase B	Affect blood–brain barrier permeability
Eicosanoids	Prostaglandins, leukotrienes, thromboxanes	Induce the neurotoxic mediator TNF-α
Neurotoxic amines	NTox	Directly damage neurons
Free radical	NO	Directly damage neurons

IL, interleukin; TNF, tumor necrosis factor-α; GM-CSF, granulocyte–macrophage colony-stimulating factor; M-CSF, macrophage colony-stimulating factor; PAF, platelet-activating factor; MCP-1, monocyte chemoattractant protein-1; MIP-1α/β, macrophage inflammatory protein-1α/β; NO, nitric oxide.

4 Summary

The importance of macrophages in the pathogenesis of autoimmune diseases such as IDDM, MS and RA and primary immunodeficiency has been investigated in *in vitro* and *in vivo* models. Animal models including the NOD mouse and BB rat for IDDM, EAE for MS, and collagen- or adjuvant-induced arthritis for RA have been used for studies on the role of macrophages in the pathogenesis of autoimmune diseases, although these animal models do not exactly mimic the human diseases. In these diseases, macrophages may contribute to the regulation of immune responses by serving as antigen-presenting cells and producers of cytokines such as IL-12, which is involved in Th1 development. In addition, macrophages may contribute directly to tissue damage in inflammatory sites by secreting toxic molecules including pro-inflammatory cytokines (IL-1β and TNF-α), proteinases, oxygen free radicals and eicosanoids. In primary immunodeficiency, the activated HIV-infected microglia, the brain macrophages, are known to play a crucial role in brain damage. Thus, there is abundant infection and activation of macrophages in HIV encephalitis. The HIV infection of blood-borne monocytes/macrophages and of microglia may result in the production of a variety of pro-inflammatory mediators, such as TNF-α, PAF and prostaglandins, and neurotoxic substances such as neurotoxic amines that damage neurons directly or indirectly. In addition, the interactions between activated macrophages and neurons also contribute to brain damage. These autoimmune diseases and immunodeficiency disease generally are ameliorated by therapeutic trials targeting macrophages or macrophage-derived soluble mediators. New information is accumulating continuously regarding the roles that macrophages play as immune effectors and producers of immunoregulatory molecules at both local and systemic levels; however, there are still many questions to be answered. Nevertheless, a clear understanding of the mechanisms of how macrophages are involved in the pathogenesis of these diseases may provide novel targets for therapeutic interventions to prevent or ameliorate these diseases.

References

Allen, J.B., Wong, H.L., Costa, G.L., Bienkowski, M.J. and Wahl, S.M. (1993). Suppression of monocyte function and differential regulation of IL-1 and IL-1ra by IL-4 contribute to resolution of experimental arthritis. *Journal of Immunology*, **151**, 4344-51.

Aloisi, F., Penna, G., Cerase, J., Menendez Iglesias, B. and Adorini, L. (1997). IL-12 production by central nervous system microglia is inhibited by astrocytes. *Journal of Immunology*, **159**, 1604–12.

Alvaro-Gracia, J.M., Zvaifler, N.J. and Firestein, G.S. (1990). Cytokines in chronic inflammatory arthritis. V. Mutual antagonism between γ-interferon and tumor necrosis factor-α on HLA-DR expression, proliferation, collagenase production and granulocyte–macrophage colony-stimulating factor production by rheumatoid arthritis synoviocytes. *Journal of Clinical Investigation*, **86**, 1790–8.

Amano, K. and Yoon, J.W. (1990). Studies on autoimmunity for initiation of β-cell destruction: V: decrease of macrophage dependent T-effector cells and natural killer cytotoxicity in silica-treated BB rats. *Diabetes*, **39**, 590–6.

Amano, Y., Lee, S.W. and Allison, A.C. (1993). Inhibition by glucocorticoids of the formation of interleukin-1α, interleukin-1β and interleukin-6: mediation by decreased mRNA stability. *Molecular Pharmacology*, **43**, 176–82.

Appels, B., Burkart, V., Kantwerk-Funke, M., Funda, J., Kolb-Bachofen, V. and Kolb, H. (1989). Spontaneous cytotoxicity of macrophages against pancreatic islet cells. *Journal of Immunology*, **142**, 3803–8.

Asayama, K., Kooy, N.W. and Burr, I.M. (1986). Effect of vitamin E deficiency and selenium deficiency on insulin secretory reserve and free radical scavenging systems in islets; decrease of islet manganosuperoxide dismutase. *Journal of Laboratory and Clinical Medicine*, **107**, 45–4564.

Bach, J.F. (1995). Insulin-dependent diabetes mellitus as a β cell-targeted disease of immunoregulation. *Journal of Autoimmunity*, **8**, 439–63.

Baker, D., Butler, D., Scallon, B.J., O'Neill, J.K., Turk, J.L. and Feldmann, M. (1994). Control of established experimental allergic encephalomyelitis by inhibition of tumor necrosis factor (TNF) activity within the central nervous system using monoclonal antibodies and TNF receptor–immunoglobulin fusion proteins. *European Journal of Immunology*, **24**, 2040–8.

Bauer, J., Berkenbosch, F., Van Dam, A.-M. and Dijkstra, C.D. (1993). Demonstration of inter-leukin-1β in Lewis rat brain during experimental allergic encephalomyelitis at the light and ultrastructural level. *Journal of Neuroimmunology*, **48**, 13–22.

Bauer, J., Huitinga, I., Zhao, W., Lassmann, H., Hickey, W.F. and Dijkstra, C.D. (1995). The role of macrophages, perivascular cells and microglial cells in the pathogenesis of experimental autoimmune encephalomyelitis. *Glia*, **15**, 437–46.

Bauerova, K. and Bezek, A. (1999). Role of reactive oxygen and nitrogen species in etiopathogenesis of rheumatoid arthritis. *General Physiology and Biophysics*, **18**, 15–20.

Beck, J., Rondot, P., Catinot, L., Falcoff, E., Kirchner, H. and Wietzerbin, J. (1988). Increased production of interferon γ and tumor necrosis factor precedes clinical manifestation in multiple sclerosis: do cytokines trigger exacerbations? *Acta Neurologia Scandinavica*, **78**, 318–23.

Beelen, R.H.J., van Rees, E.P., Bos H.J., Kamperdijk, E.W.A. and Dijkstra, D.D. (1989). Ontogeny of antigen-presenting cells. In Chaouat, G. (ed.), *The Immunology of the Fetus*. CRC Press, Florida, pp. 33–42.

Bendtzen, K., Mandrup-Poulsen, T., Nerup, J., Nielsen, J.H., Dinarello, C.A. and Svenson, M. (1986). Cytotoxicity of human *p* I7 interleukin-1 for pancreatic islets of Langerhans. *Science*, **232**, 1545–7.

Benveniste, E.N. (1995). Role of cytokines in multiple sclerosis, autoimmune encephalitis and other neurological disorders. In Aggarawal, B. and Puri, R. (ed.), *Human Cytokines: Their Role in Research and Therapy*. Blackwell, Boston, pp. 195–216.

Berger, E.A. (1997). HIV entry and tropism: the chemokine receptor connection. *AIDS*, **11** Suppl, A, S3–16.

Berman, J.W., Guida, M.P., Warren, J., Amat, J. and Brosnan, C.F. (1996). Localization of monocyte chemoattractant peptide-1 expression in the central nervous system in experimental autoimmune encephalomyelitis and trauma in the rat. *Journal of Immunology*, **156**, 3017–23.

Bernton, E.W., Bryant, H.U., Decoster, M.A., Orenstein, J.M., Ribas, J.L., Meltzer, M.S. *et al.* (1992). No direct neuronotoxicity by HIV-1 virions or culture fluids from HIV-1-infected T cells or monocytes. *AIDS Research and Human Retroviruses*, **8**, 495–503.

Bjork, J., Lindbom, L., Gerdin, B., Smedegard, G., Arfors, K.E. and Benveniste, J. (1983). Paf-acether (platelet-activating factor) increases microvascular permeability and affects endothelium–granulocyte interaction in microvascular beds. *Acta Physiologica Scandinavica*, **119**, 305–8.

Black, K.L. and Hoff, J.T. (1985). Leukotrienes increase blood–brain barrier permeability following intraparenchymal injections in rats. *Annals of Neurology*, **18**, 349–51.

Bowman, M., Simell, O., Look, Z., Luchetta, R. and Atkinson, M. (1994). Pharmokinetic and therapeutic analysis of aminoguanidine. *Diabetes*, **43** (Supplement), 235A.

Breshnihan, B. (1992). The synovial lining cells in chronic arthritis. *British Journal of Rheumatology*, **31**, 433–6.

Brosnan, C.F., Bornstein, M.B. and Bloom, B.R. (1981). The effects of macrophage depletion on the clinical and pathologic expression of experimental allergic encephalomyelitis. *Journal of Immunology*, **126**, 614–20.

Budka, H., Wiley, C.A., Kleihues, P., Artigas, J., Asbury, A.K., Cho, E.S. *et al.* (1991). HIV-associated disease of the nervous system: review of nomenclature and proposal for neuropathology-based terminology. *Brain Pathology*, **1**, 143–52.

Burmester, G.R., Dimitriu-Bona, A., Waters, S.J. and Winchester, R.J. (1983). Identification of three major synovial lining cell populations by monoclonal antibodies directed to Ia antigens and antigens associated with monocyte macrophages and fibroblasts. *Scandinavian Journal of Immunology*, **17**, 69–81.

Burmester, G.R., Jahn, B., Rohwer, R., Zacher, J., Winchester, R.J. and Kalden, J.R. (1987). Differential expression of Ia antigen by rheumatoid synovial lining cells. *Journal of Clinical Investigation*, **80**, 595–604.

Camilleri, J.P., Williams, A.S., Amos, N., Douglas-Jones, A.G. and Love, W.G. (1995). The effect of free and liposome-encapsulated clodronate on the hepatic mononuclear phagocyte system in the rat. *Clinical and Experimental Immunology*, **99**, 269–75.

Canque, B., Rosenzwajg, M., Gey, A., Tartour, E., Fridman, W.H. and Gluckman, J.C. (1996). Macrophage inflammatory protein-1α is induced by human immunodeficiency virus infection of monocyte-derived macrophages. *Blood*, **87**, 2011–9.

Chabot, S., Williams, G. and Yong, V.W. (1997). Microglial production of TNF-α is induced by activated T lymphocytes. Involvement of VLA-4 and inhibition by interferon β-1b. *Journal of Clinical Investigation*, **100**, 604–1

Chang, J.S., Quinn, J.M., Demaziere, A., Bulstrode, C.J., Francis, M.J. and Duthie, R.B. (1992). Bone resorption by cells isolated from rheumatoid synovium. *Annals of Rheumatic Disease*, **5**, 1223–9.

Chung, Y.H., Jun, H.S., Hirasawa, K., Lee, B.R., van Rooijen, N. and Yoon, J.W. (1997). Role of cytokines in the pathogenesis of Kilham rat virus-induced autoimmune diabetes in diabetes-resistant BB rats. *Journal of Immunology*, **159**, 466–71.

Clark, G.D., Happel, L.T., Zorumski, C.F. and Bazan, N.G. (1992). Enhancement of hippocampal excitatory synaptic transmission by platelet-activating factor. *Neuron*, **9**, 1211–6.

Clouse, K.A., Cosentino, L.M., Weih, K.A., Pyle, S.W., Robbins, P.B., Hochstein, H.D. *et al.* (1991). The HIV-1 gp120 envelope protein has the intrinsic capacity to stimulate monokine secretion. *Journal of Immunology*, **147**, 2892–901.

Colton, C.A., Keri, J.E., Chen, W.-T. and Monsky, W.L. (1993). Protease production by cultured microglia: substrate gel analysis and immobilized matrix degradation. *Journal of Neuroscience Research*, **35**, 297–304.

Constantinescu, C.S., Wysocka, M., Hilliard, B., Ventura, E.S., Lavi, E., Trinchieri, G. and Rostami, A. (1998). Antibodies against IL-12 prevent superantigen-induced and spontaneous relapses of experimental autoimmune encephalomyelitis. *Journal of Immunology*, **161**, 5097–104.

Corbett, J.A. and McDaniel, M.L. (1992). Does nitric oxide mediate autoimmune destruction of β-cells? Possible therapeutic interventions in IDDM. *Diabetes*, **41**, 897–903.

Corbett, J.A. and McDaniel, M.L. (1995). Intraislet release of interleukin 1 inhibits β cell function by inducing β cell expression of inducible nitric oxide synthase. *Journal of Experimental Medicine*, **181**, 559–68.

Cross, A.H., Misko, T.P., Lin, R.F., Hickey, W.F., Trotter, J.L. and Tilton, R.G. (1994). Aminoguanidine, an inhibitor of inducible nitric oxide synthase, ameliorates experimental autoimmune encephalomyelitis in SJL mice. *Journal of Clinical Investigation*, **93**, 268–90.

Crowe, S., Mills, J. and McGrath, M.S. (1987). Quantitative immunocytofluorographic analysis of CD4 surface antigen expression and HIV infection of human peripheral blood monocytes/macrophages. *AIDS Research and Human Retroviruses*, **3**, 135–45.

D'Addario, M., Roulston, A., Wainberg, M.A. and Hiscott, J. (1990). Coordinate enhancement of cytokine gene expression in human immunodeficiency virus type 1-infected promonocytic cells. *Journal of Virology*, **64**, 6080–9.

D'Addario, M., Wainberg, M.A. and Hiscott, J. (1992). Activation of cytokine genes in HIV-1-infected myelomonoblastic cells by phorbol ester and tumor necrosis factor. *Journal of Immunology*, **148**, 1222–9.

Damoiseaux, J.G.M.C., Huitinga, I., Döpp, E.A. and Dijkstra, C.D. (1992). Expression of the ED3 antigen on rat macrophages in relation to experimental autoimmune diseases. *Immunobiology*, **84**, 311–20.

Danis, V.A., Kulesz, A.J., Nelson, D.S. and Brooks, P.M. (1990). The effect of gold sodium thiomalate and auranofin on lipopolysaccharide-induced interleukin-1 production by blood monocytes *in vitro*: variation in healthy subjects and patients with arthritis. *Clinical and Experimental Immunology*, **79**, 333–40.

DeLuca, C., Roulston, A., Koromilas, A., Wainberg, M.A. and Hiscott, J. (1996). Chronic human immunodeficiency virus type 1 infection of myeloid cells disrupts the autoregulatory control of the NF-κB/Rel pathway via enhanced IκBα degradation. *Journal of Virology*, **70**, 5183–93.

Dhawan, S., Weeks, B.S., Soderland, C., Schnaper, H.W., Toro, L.A., Asthana, S.P. *et al.* (1995). HIV-1 infection alters monocyte interactions with human microvascular endothelial cells. *Journal of Immunology*, **154**, 422–32.

Dijkstra, C.D., Döpp, E.A., Vogels, I.M. C. and van Noorden, C.J.F. (1987). Macrophages and dendritic cells in antigen-induced arthritis: an immunohistochemical study using cryostat sections of the whole knee joint of rat. *Scandinavian Journal of Immunology*, **26**, 513–23.

Dreyer, E.B., Kaiser, P.K., Offermann, J.T. and Lipton, S.A. (1990). HIV-1 coat protein neurotoxicity prevented by calcium channel antagonists. *Science*, **248**, 364–7.

Eizirik, D.L., Tracey, D.E., Bendtzen, K. and Sandler, S. (1991). An interleukin-1 receptor antagonist protein protects insulin-producing β cells against suppressive effects of interleukin-1β. *Diabetologia*, **34**, 445–8.

Fabry, Z., Waldschmidt, M.M., Hendrickson, D., Love-Homan, L., Takei, F. and Hart, M.N. (1992). Adhesion molecules on murine brain macrovascular endothelial cells. Expression and regulation of ICAM-1 and Lgp55. *Journal of Neuroimmunology*, **36**, 1–11.

Faust, A., Kleemann, R., Rothe, H. and Kolb, H. (1996). Role of macrophages and cytokines in β-cell death. In Shafrir, E. (ed.), *Lessons from Animal Diabetes VI*. Birkhäuser Boston, Cambridge, pp. 47–56.

Fehsel, K., Jalowy, A., Sun, Q., Burkart, V., Hartmann, B. and Kolb, H. (1993). Islet cell DNA is a target of inflammatory attack by nitric oxide. *Diabetes*, **42**, 496–500.

Feige, U., Karbowski, A., Rordorf-Adam, C. and Pataki, A. (1989). Arthritis induced by continuous infusion of hr-interleukin-1α into the rabbit knee joint. *International Journal of Tissue Reactions*, **11**, 225–38.

Fenyk-Melody, J.E., Garrison, A.E., Brunnert, S.R., Weidner, J.R., Shen, F., Shelton, B.A. *et al.* (1998). Experimental autoimmune encephalomyelitis is exacerbated in mice lacking the NOS2 gene. *Journal of Immunology*, **160**, 2940–6.

Firenstein, G.S. and Zvaifler, N.J. (1990). How important are T cells in chronic rheumatoid arthritis? *Arthritis and Rheumatism*, **33**, 768–73.

Firestein, G.S., Townsend, K., Broide, D., Alvaro-Gracia, J., Glasebrook, A. and Zvaifler, N.J. (1988). Cytokines in chronic inflammatory arthritis. I. Failure to detect T cell lymphokines (IL-2 and IL-3) and presence of macrophage colony-stimulating factor (CSF-1) and a novel mast cell growth factor in rheumatoid synovitis. *Journal of Experimental Medicine*, **168**, 1573–86.

Firestein, G.S., Alvaro-Gracia, J.M. and Maki, R. (1990). Quantitative analysis of cytokine gene expression in rheumatoid arthritis. *Journal of Immunology*, **144**, 3347–53.

Fischer, H.G., Frosch, S., Reske, K. and Reske-Kunz, A.B. (1988). Granulocyte–macrophage colony-stimulating factor activates macrophages derived from bone marrow cultures to synthesis of MHC class II molecules and to augment antigen presentation function. *Journal of Immunology*, **141**, 3881–8.

Fischer, H.G., Bielinsky, A.K., Nitzgen, B., Daubener, W. and Hadding, U. (1993). Functional dichotomy of mouse microglia developed *in vitro*: differential effects of macrophage and granulocyte/macrophage colony-stimulating factor on cytokine secretion and antitoxoplasmic activity. *Journal of Neuroimmunology*, **45**,193–201.

Folgueira, L., Algeciras, A., MacMarran, W.S., Bren, G.D. and Paya, C.V. (1996). The Ras–Raf pathway is activated in human immunodeficiency virus-infected monocytes and participates in the activation of NF-κB. *Journal of Virology*, **70**, 2332–8.

Frei, K., Eugster, H.P., Bopst, M., Constantinescu, S.S., Lavi, E. and Fontana, A. (1997). Tumor necrosis factor α and lymphotoxin α are not required for induction of acute experimental autoimmune encephalomyelitis. *Journal of Experimental Medicine*, **185**, 2177–82.

Gehrmann, J., Matsumoto, Y. and Kreutzberg, G.W. (1995). Microglia: intrinsic immuneffector cell of the brain. *Brain Research Reviews*, **20**, 269–87.

Gelbard, H.A., Nottet, H.S.L.M., Swindells, S., Jett, M., Dzenko, K.A., Genis, P. *et al.* (1994). Platelet-activating factor: a candidate human immunodeficiency virus type 1-induced neuro-toxin. *Journal of Virology*, **68**, 4628–35.

Genis, P., Jett, M., Bernton, E.W., Boyle, T., Gelbard, H.A., Dzenko, K. *et al.* (1992). Cytokines and arachidonic metabolites produced during human immunodeficiency virus (HIV)-infected macrophage–astroglia interactions: implications for the neuropathogenesis of HIV disease. *Journal of Experimental Medicine*, **176**, 1703–18.

Gerritse, K., Laman, J.D., Noelle, R.J., Aruffo, A., Ledbetter, J.A., Boersma, W.J. *et al.* (1996). CD40–CD40 ligand interactions in experimental allergic encephalomyelitis and multiple sclero-sis. *Proceedings of the National Academy of Sciences USA*, **93**, 2499–504.

Gijbels, K., Masure, S., Carton, H. and Opdenakker, G. (1992). Gelatinase in the cerebrospinal fluid of patients with multiple sclerosis and other inflammatory neurological disorders. *Journal of Neuroimmunology*, **41**, 29–34.

Gijbels, K., Proost, P., Masure, S., Carton, H., Billiau, A. and Opdenakker, G. (1993). Gelatinase B is present in the cerebrospinal fluid during experimental autoimmune encephalomyelitis and cleaves myelin basic protein. *Journal of Neuroscience Research*, **36**, 432–40.

Gijbels, K., Galardy, R.E. and Steinman, L. (1994). Reversal of experimental autoimmune encephalomyelitis with a hydroxamate inhibitor of matrix metalloproteases. *Journal of Clinical Investigation*, **94**, 2177–82.

Giulian, D., Vaca, K. and Noonan, C.A. (1990). Secretion of neurotoxins by mononuclear phago-cytes infected with HIV-1. *Science*, **250**, 1593–6.

Giulian, D., Wendt, E., Vaca, K. and Noonan, C.A. (1993). The envelope glycoprotein of human immunodeficiency virus type 1 stimulates release of neurotoxins from monocytes. *Proceedings of the National Academy of Sciences USA*, **90**, 2769–73.

Giulian, D., Yu, J., Li, X., Tom, D., Li, J., Wendt, E. *et al.* (1996). Study of receptor-mediated neu-rotoxins released by HIV-1-infected mononuclear phagocytes found in human brain. *Journal of Neuroscience*, **15**, 3139–53.

Godiska, R., Chantry, D., Dietsch, G.N. and Gray, P.W. (1995). Chemokine expression in murine experimental allergic encephalomyelitis. *Journal of Neuroimmunology*, **58**, 167–76.

Gordon, S. (1995). The macrophage. *Bioessays*, **17**, 977–86.

Gordon, E.J., Myers, K.J., Dougherty, J.P., Rosen, H. and Ron, Y. (1995). Both anti-CD11a (LFA-1) and anti-CD11b (MAC-1) therapy delay the onset and diminish the severity of experimental autoimmune encephalomyelitis. *Journal of Neuroimmunology*, **62**, 153–60.

Gracie, J.A., Forsey, R.J., Chan, W.L., Gilmour, A., Leung, B.P., Greer, M.R. *et al.* (1999). A proinflammatory role for IL-18 in rheumatoid arthritis. *Journal of Clinical Investigation*, **104**, 1393–401.

Green, E.A., Eyon, E.E. and Flavell, R.A. (1998). Local expression of TNF α in neonatal NOD mice promotes diabetes by enhancing presentation of islet antigens. *Immunity*, **9**, 733–43.

Grewal, I.S., Grewal, K.D., Wong, F.S., Picarella, D.E., Janeway, C.A. Jr and Flavell, R.A. (1996). Local expression of transgene encoded TNFαin islets prevents autoimmune diabetes in nonobese diabetic (NOD) mice by preventing the development of auto-reactive islet-specific T cells. *Journal of Experimental Medicine*, **184**, 1963–74.

Griffin, D.E., Wesselingh, S.L. and McArthur, J.C. (1994). Elevated central nervous system prostaglandins in human immunodeficiency virus-associated dementia. *Annals of Neurology*, **35**, 592–7.

Groux, H., Torpier, G., Monte, D., Mouton, Y., Capron, A. and Ameisen, J.C. (1992). Activation-induced death by apoptosis in CD4⁺ T cells. *Journal of Experimental Medicine*, **175**, 331–40.

Guberski, D.L., Thomas, V.A., Shek, W.R., Like, A.A., Handler, E.S., Rossini, A.A. *et al.* (1991). Induction of type I diabetes by Kilham's rat virus in diabetes-resistant BB/Wor rats. *Science*, **254**, 1010–3.

Guerne, P.A., Zuraw, B.L., Vaughan, J.H., Carson, D.A. and Lotz, M. (1989). Synovium as a source of interleukin-6 *in vitro*: contribution to local and systemic manifestations of arthritis. *Journal of Clinical Investigation*, **83**, 585–92.

Hachicha, M., Rathanaswami, P., Schall, T.J. and McColl, S.R. (1993). Production of monocyte chemotactic protein-1 in human type B synoviocytes. Synergistic effect of tumor necrosis factor α and interferon-γ. *Arthritis and Rheumatism*, **36**, 26–34.

Handel, M.L., McMorrow, L.B. and Gravallese, E.M. (1995). Nuclear factor-κB in rheumatoid synovium: localization of p50 and p65. *Arthritis and Rheumatism*, **38**, 1762–70.

Hanenberg, H., Kolb-Bachofen, V., Kantwerk-Funkf, G. and Kolb, H. (1989). Macrophage infiltration precedes and is a prerequisite for lymphocytic insulitis in pancreatic islets of prediabetic BB rats. *Diabetologia*, **32**, 126–34.

Hart, P.H., Ahern, M.J., Smith, M.D. and Finlay-Jones, J.J. (1995). Regulatory effects of IL-13 on synovial fluid macrophages and blood monocytes from patients with inflammatory arthritis. *Clinical and Experimental Immunology*, **99**, 331–7.

Harth, M., Keown, P.A. and Orange, J.F. (1983). Monocyte dependent excited oxygen radical generation in rheumatoid arthritis: inhibition by gold sodium thiomalate. *Journal of Rheumatology*, **10**, 701–7.

Hartung, H.P., Jung, S., Stoll, G., Zielasek, J., Schmidt, B., Archelos, J.J. and Toyka, K.V. (1992). Inflammatory mediators in demyelinating disorders of the CNS and PNS. *Journal of Neuroimmunology*, **40**, 197–210.

Hauser, S.L., Bhan, A.K., Gilles, F.H., Hoban, C.J., Reinherz, E.L., Schlossman, S.F. *et al.* (1983). Immunohistochemical staining of human brain with monoclonal antibodies that identify lymphocytes, monocytes and the Ia antigen. *Journal of Neuroimmunology*, **5**, 197–205.

Helqvist, S., Zumsteg, U.W., Spinas, G.A., Palmer, J.P. Mandrup-Poulsen, T., Egeberg, J. *et al.* (1991). Repetitive exposure of pancreatic islets to interleukin-1β. An *in vitro* model of pre-diabetes? *Autoimmunity*, **10**, 311–8.

Henderson, B., Rowe, F.M., Bird, C.R. and Gearing, A.J.H. (1988). Production of interleukin 1 in the joint during the development of antigen-induced arthritis in the rabbit. *Clinical and Experimental Immunology*, **74**, 371–6.

Hickey, W.F. and Kimura, H. (1988). Perivascular microglial cells of the CNS are bone marrow-derived and present antigen *in vivo*. *Science*, **239**, 290–2.

Hickey, W.F., Hsu, B.L. and Kimura, H. (1991). T lymphocyte entry into the central nervous system in experimental allergic encephalomyelitis. *Journal of Neuroscience Research*, **28**, 254–60.

Ho, D.D., Neumann, A.U., Perelson, A.S., Chen, W., Leonard, J.M. and Marcowitz, M. (1995). Rapid turnover of plasma virions and CD4 lymphocytes in HIV-1 infection. *Nature*, **373**, 331–40.

Hofman, F.M., Vonhanwher, R., Dinarell, C., Mizel, S., Hinton, D. and Merrill, J.E. (1986). Immunoregulatory molecules and IL-2 receptors identified in multiple sclerosis brain. *Journal of Immunology*, **136**, 3239–45.

Hofman, F.M., Wright, A.D., Dohadwala, M.M., Wong-Staal, F. and Walker, S.M. (1993). Exogenous tat protein activates human endothelial cells. *Blood*, **82**, 2774–80.

Hom, J.T., Bendele, A.M. and Carlson, D.G. (1988). *In vivo* administration with IL-1 accelerates the development of collagen-induced arthritis in mice. *Journal of Immunology*, **141**, 834–41.

Hughes, J.H., Colca, J.R., Easom, R.A., Turk, J. and McDaniel, M.L. (1990). Interlelukin 1 inhibits insulin secretion from isolated rat pancreatic islets by a process that requires gene transcription and mRNA translation. *Journal of Clinical Investigation*, **86**, 856–63.

Huitinga, I., van Rooijen, N., de Groot, C.J.A., Uitdehaag, B.M.J. and Dijkstra, C.D. (1990). Suppression of experimental allergic encephalomyelitis in Lewis rats after elimination of macrophages. *Journal of Experimental Medicine*, **172**, 1025–33.

Huitinga, I., Damoiseauz, J.G.M.C., Döpp, E.A. and Dijkstra, C.D. (1993). Treatment with anti-CR3 antibodies ED7 and ED8 suppresses experimental allergic encephalomyelitis in Lewis rats. *European Journal of Immunology*, **23**, 709–15.

Hulkower, K., Brosnan, C.F., Aquino, D.A., Cammer, W., Kulshrestha, S., Guida, M.P. *et al.* (1993). Expression of CSF-1, c-*fms* and MCP-1 in the central nervous system of rats with experimental allergic encephalomyelitis. *Journal of Immunology*, **150**, 2525–33.

Ihm, S.H. and Yoon, J.W. (1990). Studies on autoimmunity for initiation of β-cell destruction: VI Macrophages are essential for the development of β cell-specific cytotoxic effectors and insulitis in NOD mice. *Diabetes*, **39**, 1273–8.

Ihm, S.H., Lee, K.U., Rhee, B.D. and Min, H.K. (1990). Initial role of macrophage in the development of anti-β-cell cellular autoimmunity in multiple low-dose streptozotocin-induced diabetes in mice. *Diabetes Research and Clinical Practice*, **10**, 123–6.

Issekutz, A.C. and Issekutz, T.B. (1995). Monocyte migration to arthritis in the rat utilizes both Cd11/Cd18 and very late activation antigen 4 integrin mechanisms. *Journal of Experimental Medicine*, **181**, 1197–203.

Issekutz, A.C. Maeger, A., Otterness, I. and Issekutz, T.B. (1994). The role of tumour necrosis factor-α and IL-1 in polymorphonuclear leucocyte and T-lymphocyte recruitment to joint inflammation in adjuvant arthritis. *Clinical and Experimental Immunology*, **97**, 26–32.

Jacobs, C.A., Baker, P.E., Rouz, E.R., Picha, K.S., Toivola, B., Waugh, S. *et al.* (1991). Experimental autoimmune encephalomyelitis is exacerbated by IL-1β and suppressed by soluble IL-1 receptor. *Journal of Immunology*, **146**, 2983–9.

Jander, S. and Stoll, G. (1998). Downregulation of microglial keratan sulfate proteoglycans coincident with lymphomonocytic infiltration of the rat central nervous system. *American Journal of Pathology*, **148**, 71–8.

Janossy, G., Panayi, G.S., Duke, O., Bofill, M., Poulter, L.W. and Goldstein, G. (1981). Rheumatoid arthritis: a disease of T lymphocyte/macrophage immuno-regulation. *Lancet*, **ii**, 839–42.

Janusz, M.J. and Hare, M. (1993). Cartilage degradation by cocultures of transformed macrophage and fibroblast cell lines: a model of metalloproteinase-mediated connective tissue degradation. *Journal of Immunology*, **150**, 1922–31.

Jasen, A., Homo-Delarche, R., Hooijkaas, H., Leenen, P.J., Dardenne, M. and Drexhage, H.A. (1994). Immunohistochemical characterization of monocyte–macrophages and dendritic cells involved in the initiation of insulitis and β-cell destruction in NOD mice. *Diabetes*, **43**, 667–75.

Jensen, H.S., Jensen, L.T., Saxne, T., Diamant, M. and Bendtzen, K. (1991). Human monocyte elastolytic activity, the propepides of types I and III procollagen, proteoglycans and interleukin-6 in synovial fluid from patients with arthritis. *Clinical and Experimental Rheumatology*, **9**, 391–4.

Jiang, Z. and Woda, B.A. (1991). Cytokine gene expression in the islets of the diabetic BioBreeding/Worcester rat. *Journal of Immunology*, **146**, 2990–4.

Johnson, W.J., Muirhead, K.A., Meunier, P.C., Votta, B.J., Schmitt, T.C., DiMartino, M.J. *et al.* (1986a). Macrophage activation in rat models of inflammation and arthritis: systemic activation precedes arthritis induction and progression. *Arthritis and Rheumatism*, **29**, 1122–30.

Johnson, W.J., DiMartino, M.J. and Hanna, N. (1986b). Macrophage activation in rat models of inflammation and arthritis: determination of markers of stages of activation. *Cellular Immunology*, **103**, 54–64.

Joosten, L.A.B., Helsen, M.M.A., van de Loo, F.A.J. and van den Berg, W.B. (1996). Anticytokine treatment of established type II collagen-induced arthritis in DBA/1 mice: a comparative study using anti-TNFα, anti-IL1α/β and IL-1Ra. *Arthritis and Rheumatism*, **39**, 797–809.

Juedes, A.E., Hjelmstrom, P., Bergman, C.M., Neild, A.L. and Ruddle, N.H. (2000). Kinetics and cellular origin of cytokines in the central nervous system: insight into mechanisms of myelin oligodendrocyte glycoprotein-induced experimental autoimmune encephalomyelitis. *Journal of Immunology*, **164**, 419–26.

Jun, H.S., Yoon, C.S., Zbytnuik, L., van Rooijen, N. and Yoon, J.W. (1999a). The role of macrophages in T cell-mediated autoimmune diabetes in nonobese diabetic mice. *Journal of Experimental Medicine*, **189**, 347–58.

Jun, H.S., Santamaria, P.S., Lim, H.W., Zhang, M. .L. and Yoon, J.W. (1999b). Absolute requirement of macrophages for the development and activation of β-cell cytotoxic CD8$^+$ T-cells in T-cell receptor transgenic NOD mice. *Diabetes*, **48**, 34–42.

Karpus, W.J., Lukacs, N.W., McRae, B.L., Strieter, R.M., Kunkel, S.L. and Miller, S.D. (1995). An important role for the chemokine macrophage inflammatory protein-1α in the pathogenesis of the T cell-mediated autoimmune disease, experimental autoimmune encephalomyelitis. *Journal of Immunology*, **155**, 5003–10.

Kasama, T., Strieter, R.M., Lukacs, N.W., Lincoln, P.M., Burdick, M.D. and Kunkel, S.L. (1995). Interleukin-10 expression and chemokine regulation during the evolution of murine type II collagen-induced arthritis. *Journal of Clinical Investigation*, **95**, 2868–76.

Kato, K., Clark, G.D., Bazan, N.G. and Zorumski, C.F. (1994). Platelet-activating factor as a potential retrograde messenger in CA1 hippocampal long-term potentiation. *Nature*, **367**, 175–9.

Keffer, J., Probert, L., Cazlaris, H., Georgopoulos, S., Kaslaris, E., Kioussis, D. and Kollias, G. (1991). Transgenic mice expressing human tumour necrosis factor: a predictive genetic model of arthritis. *EMBO Journal*, **10**, 4025–31.

Keller, R. (1990). Mechanisms of macrophage-mediated tumor cell killing: a comparative analysis of the role of reactive nitrogen intermediates and TNF. *International Journal of Cancer*, **46**, 682–95.

Kennedy, M.K., Torrance, D.S., Picha, K.S. and Mohler, K.M. (1992). Analysis of cytokine mRNA expression in the central nervous system of mice with experimental autoimmune encephalomyelitis reveals that IL-10 mRNA expression correlates with recovery. *Journal of Immunology*, **149**, 2495–505.

Kinne, R.W., Schmidt-Weber, C.B., Hoppe, R., Buchner, E., Palombo-Kinne, E., Nürnberg, E. *et al.* (1995a). Long-term amelioration of rat adjuvant arthritis following systemic elimination of macrophages by clodronate-containing liposomes. *Arthritis and Rheumatism*, **38**, 1777–90.

Kinne, R.W., Schmidt, C., Buchner, E., Hoppe, R., Nürnberg, E. and Emmrich, F. (1995b). Treatment of rat arthritis with clodronate-containing liposomes. *Scandinavian Journal of Rheumatology*, **23**, 83–9.

Klareskog, L. Forsum, U., Scheynius, A., Kabelitz, D. and Wigzell, H. (1982). Evidence in support of a self-perpetuating HLA-DR-dependent delayed-type reaction in rheumatoid arthritis. *Proceedings of the National Academy of Sciences USA*, **79**, 3632–66.

Kleemann, R., Rothe, H., Kolb-Bachofen, V., Xie, Q.W., Nathan, C., Martin, S. *et al*. (1993). Transcription and translation of inducible nitric oxide synthase in the pancreas of prediabetic BB rats. *FEBS Letters*, **328**, 9–12.

Koch, A.E., Kunkel, S.L., Harlow, L.A., Johnson, B., Evanoff, H.L., Haines, G.K. *et al*. (1992). Enhanced production of monocyte chemoattractant protein-1 in rheumatoid arthritis. *Journal of Clinical Investigation*, **90**, 772–9.

Kolb, H., Kantwerk, G., Treichel, U., Kurner, T., Kiesel, U., Hoppe, T. *et al*. (1986). Prospective analysis of islet lesions in BB rats. *Diabetologia*, **29** (Supplement 1), A559.

Konat, G.W. and Wiggins, R.C. (1985). Effect of reactive oxygen species on myelin membrane proteins. *Journal of Neurochemistry*, **45**, 1113–8.

Korner, H., Lemckert, F.A., Chaudhri, G., Etteldorf, S. and Sedgwick, J.D. (1997). Tumor necrosis factor blockade in actively induced experimental autoimmune encephalomyelitis prevents clinical disease despite activated T cell infiltration to the central nervous system. *European Journal of Immunology*, **27**, 1973–81.

Kröncke, K-D., Kolb-Bachofen, V., Berschick, B., Burkart, V. and Kolb, H. (1991). Activated macrophages kill pancreatic syngeneic islet cells via arginine-dependent nitric oxide generation. *Biochemistry and Biophysics Research Communications*, **175**, 752–8.

Kumkumiam, G., Lafyatis, R., Remmers, E.F., Case, J.P., Kim, S.J. and Wilder, R. (1989). Platelet-derived growth factor and interleukin-1 interactions in rheumatoid arthritis. Regulation of synoviocyte proliferation, prostaglandin production and collagenase transcription. *Journal of Immunology*, **143**, 833–7.

Lafyatis R., Remmers, E.F., Roberts, A.A.B., Yocum, D.E. and Wilder, R. (1989). Anchorage independent growth of synoviocytes from arthritic and normal joints: stimulation from exogenous platelet derived growth factor and inhibition by transforming growth factor-β and retinoids. *Journal of Clinical Investigation*, **83**, 1267–76.

Leblanc, P.A. (1990). Activated macrophages use different cytolytic mechanisms to lyse a virally infected or a tumor target. *Journal of Leukocyte Biology*, **48**, 1–12.

Lee, K.U., Kim, M.K., Amano, K., Pak, C.Y., Jaworski, M.A., Mehta, J.G. *et al*. (1988a). Preferential infiltration of macrophages during early stages of insulitis in the spontaneously diabetes-prone BB rats. *Diabetes*, **37**, 1053–8.

Lee, K.U., Pak, C.Y., Amano, K. and Yoon, J.W. (1988b). Prevention of lymphocytic thyroiditis and insulitis in diabetes-prone BB rats by the depletion of macrophages. *Diabetologia*, **31**, 400–2.

Lee, K.U., Amano, K. and Yoon, J.W. (1988c). Evidence for initial involvement of macrophage in development of insulitis in NOD mice. *Diabetes*, **37**, 989–91.

Lee, S.C., Liu, W., Dickson, D.W., Brosnan, C.F. and Berman, J.W. (1993). Cytokine production by human fetal microglia and astrocytes: differential induction by lipopolysaccharide and Il-1β. *Journal of Immunology*, **150**, 2659–67.

Leibovich, S.J., Polverini, P.J., Shephard, H.M., Wiseman, D.M., Shively, V. and Nuseir, N. (1987). Macrophage induced angiogenesis is mediated by tumor necrosis factor-α. *Nature*, **329**, 630–2.

Lin, R.F., Lin, T.S., Tilton, R.G. and Cross, A.H. (1993). Nitric oxide localized to spinal cords of mice with experimental allergic encephalomyelitis: an electron paramagnetic resonance study. *Journal of Experimental Medicine*, **178**, 643–8.

Lindsay, R.M., Smith, W., Rossiter, S.P., McIntyre, M.A., Williams, B.C. and Baird, J.D. (1995). N^W-nitro-L-arginine methyl ester reduces the incidence of IDDM in BB/E rats. *Diabetes*, **44**, 365–8.

Lipsky, P.E. and Ziff, M. (1977). Inhibition of antigen-and mitogen-induced human lymphocyte proliferation by gold compounds. *Journal of Clinical Investigation*, **59**, 455–66.

Lipton, S.A. (1992). Requirement for macrophages in neuronal injury induced by HIV envelope protein gp120. *Neuroreport*, **3**, 913–5.

Lipton, S.A. and Rosenberg, P.A. (1994). Excitatory amino acids as a final common pathway for neurologic disorders. *New England Journal of Medicine*, **330**, 613–22.

Liu, L., Marino, M.W., Wong, G., Grail, D., Dunn, A., Bettadapura, J. *et al.* (1998). TNF is a potent anti-inflammatory cytokine in autoimmune-mediated demyelination. *Nature Medicine*, **4**, 78–83.

Loetscher, P., Dewald, B., Baggiolini, M. and Seitz, M. (1994). Monocyte chemoattractant protein 1 and interleukin 8 production by rheumatoid synoviocytes: effects of anti-rheumatic drugs. *Cytokine*, **6**, 162–70.

López-Bote, J.P., Bernabeu, C., Marquet, A., Fernández, J.M. and Larraga, V. (1988). Adjuvant-induced polyarthritis: synovial cell activation prior to polyarthritis onset. *Arthritis and Rheumatism*, **31**, 769–75.

Maeda, A. and Sobel, R.A. (1996). Matrix metalloproteinases in the normal human central nervous system, microglial nodules and multiple sclerosis lesions. *Journal of Neuropathology and Experimental Neurology*, **55**, 300–9.

Makino, S., Kunimoto, K., Muraoka, Y., Mizushima, Y., Katagiri, K. and Tochino, Y. (1980). Breeding of a non-obese diabetic strain of mice. *Experimental Animals*, **29**, 1–13.

Malaisse, W.J., Malaisse-Lagae, F., Sener, A. and Pipeleers, D.G. (1982). Determinants of the selective toxicity of alloxan to the pancreatic β cell. *Proceedings of the National Academy of Sciences USA*, **79**, 927–30.

Malik, N., Greenfield, B.W., Wahl, A.F. and Kiener, P.A. (1996). Activation of human monocytes through CD40 induces matrix metalloproteinases. *Journal of Immunology*, **156**, 3952–60.

Mandrup-Poulsen, T., Egeberg, J., Nerup, J., Bendtzen, K., Nielsen, J.H. and Dinarello, C.A. (1987a). Ultrastructural studies of time-course and cellular specificity of interleukin-1 mediated islet cytotoxicity. *Acta Pathologica, Microbiologica, et Immunologica Scandinavica Section C, Immunology*, **95**, 55–63.

Mandrup-Poulsen, T., Bendtzen, K., Dinarello, C. and Nerup, J. (1987b). Human tumor-necrosis factor potentiates human interleukin 1-mediated rat pancreatic β cell-cytotoxicity. *Journal of Immunology*, **139**, 4077–82.

Marliss, E.B., Nakhooda, A.F., Poussier, P. and Sima, A.A.F. (1982). The diabetic syndrome of the BB Wistar rat: possible relevance to type 1 (insulin-dependent) diabetes in man. *Diabetologia*, **22**, 225–32.

Matsumoto, Y., Hara, N., Tanaka, R. and Fujiwara, M. (1986). Immunohistochemical analysis of the rat central nervous system during experimental allergic encephalomyelitis, with special reference to Ia-positive cells with dendritic morphology. *Journal of Immunology*, **136**, 3668–76.

McDaniel, M.L., Kwon, G., Hill, J.R., Marshall, C.A. and Corbett, J.A. (1996). Cytokines and nitric oxide in islet inflammation and diabetes. *Proceedings of the Society for Experimental Biology and Medicine*, **211**, 24–32.

Merrill, J.E. and Benveniste, E.N. (1996). Cytokines in inflammatory brain lesions: helpful and harmful. *Trends in Neuroscience*, **19**, 331–8.

Merrill, J.E., Ignarro, L.J., Sherman, M.P., Melinek, J. and Lane, T.E. (1993). Microglial cell cyto-toxicity of oligodendrocytes is mediated through nitric oxide. *Journal of Immunology*, **151**, 2132–41.

Müssener, A., Klareskog, L., Lorentzen, J.C. and Kleinau, S. (1995). TNF-α dominates cytokine mRNA expression in lymphoid tissues of rats developing collagen-and oil-induced arthritis. *Scandinavian Journal of Immunology*, **42**, 128–34.

Nagata, M. and Yoon, J.W. (1992). Studies on autoimmunity for T-cell-mediated β-cell destruction. Distinct difference in β-cell destruction between CD4⁺ and CD8⁺ T-cell clones derived from lymphocytes infiltrating the islets of NOD mice. *Diabetes*, **41**, 998—1008.

Nathan, C.F. (1987). Secretory products of macrophages. *Journal of Clinical Investigation*, **79**, 319–26.

Nottet, H.S.L.M., Jett, M., Flanagan, C.R., Zhai, Q.H., Persidsky, Y., Rizzino, A. *et al.* (1995). A regulatory role for astrocytes in HIV-1 encephalitis. An overexpression of eicosanoids, platelet-activating factor and tumor necrosis factor-α by activated HIV-1-infected monocytes is attenu-ated by primary human astrocytes. *Journal of Immunology*, **154**, 3567–81.

Nottet, H.S.L.M., Persidsky, Y., Sasseville, V.G., Nukuna, A.N., Bock, P., Zhai, Q.H. *et al.* (1996). Mechanisms for the transendothelial migration of HIV-1-infected monocytes into brain. *Journal of Immunology*, **156**, 1284–95.

Nottet, H.S.L.M., Bär, D.R., van Hassel, H., Verhoef, J. and Boven, L.A. (1997). Cellular aspects of HIV-1 infection of macrophages leading to neuronal dysfunction in *in vitro* models for HIV-1 encephalitis. *Journal of Leukocyte Biology*, **62**, 107–16.

Oschilewski, U., Kiesel, U. and Kolb, H. (1985). Administration of silica prevents diabetes in BB rats. *Diabetes*, **34**, 197–9.

Pan, Y., Lloyd, C., Zhou, H., Dolich, S., Deeds, J., Gonzalo, J.A. *et al.* (1997). Neurotactin, a mem-brane-anchored chemokine upregulated in brain inflammation. *Nature*, **387**, 611–7.

Panayi, G.S., Lanchbury, J.S. and Kingsley, G.H. (1992). The importance of the T cell in initiating and maintaining the chronic synovitis of rheumatoid arthritis. *Arthritis and Rheumatism*, **35**, 729–35.

Pelegri, C., Franch, A., Castellote, C. and Castell, M. (1995). Immunohistochemical changes in synovial tissue during the course of adjuvant arthritis. *Journal of Rheumatology*, **22**, 124–34.

Perry, V.H. and Gordon, S. (1988). Macrophages and microglia in the nervous system. *Trends in Neurosciences*, **11**, 273–7.

Pierce, G.F., Mustoe, T.A., Lingelbach, J., Masakowski, V.R., Gramates, P. and Deuel, T.F. (1989). Transforming growth factor-β reverses the glucocorticoid-induced wound-healing deficit in rats: possible regulation in macrophages by platelet-derived growth factor. *Proceedings of the National Academy of Sciences USA*, **89**, 2229–33.

Piguet, P.F., Grau, G.E., Vesin, C., Loetscher, H., Gentz, R. and Lesslauer, W. (1992). Evolution of collagen arthritis is arrested by treatment with anti-tumor necrosis factor (TNF) antibody or recombinant soluble TNF receptor. *Journal of Immunology*, **77**, 510–4.

Postigo, A.A., Garcia-Vicuna, R.G., Diaz-Gonzalez, F., Arroyo, A.G., de Landazuri, M.O., Chi-Rosso, G. *et al.* (1992). Increased binding of synovial T lymphocytes from rheumatoid arthritis to endothelial–leukocyte adhesion molecule-1 (ELAM-1) and vascular cell adhesion molecule-1 (VCAM-1). *Journal of Clinical Investigation*, **89**, 1445–52.

Price, R.W., Brew, B., Sidtis, J., Rosenblum, M., Scheck, A.C. and Cleary, P. (1988). The brain in AIDS: central nervous system HIV-1 infection and AIDS dementia complex. *Science*, **239**, 586–92.

Prineas, J.W. (1975). Pathology of the early lesion in multiple sclerosis. *Human Pathology*, **6**, 531–54.

Prineas, J.W. and Wright, R.G. (1978). Macrophages, lymphocytes and plasma cells in the perivascular compartment in chronic multiple sclerosis. *Laboratory Investigation*, **38**, 409–21.

Probert, L., Akassoglou, K., Pasparakis, M., Kontogeorgos, G. and Kollias, G. (1995a). Spontaneous inflammatory demyelinating disease in transgenic mice showing central nervous system-specific expression of tumor necrosis factor α. *Proceedings of the National Academy of Sciences USA*, **92**, 11294–8.

Probert, L., Plows, D., Kontogeorgos, G. and Kollias, G. (1995b). The type I interleukin-1 receptor acts in series with tumour necrosis factor (TNF) to induce arthritis in TNF-transgenic mice. *European Journal of Immunology*, **25**, 1794–7.

Pukel, C., Baquerizo, H. and Rabinovitch, A. (1988). Destruction of rat islet cell monolayers by cytokines. Synergistic interactions of interferon-γ, tumor necrosis factor, lymphotoxin and interleukin-1. *Diabetes*, **37**, 133–6.

Pulliam, L., Herndier, B.G., Tang, N.M. and McGrath, M.S. (1991). Human immunodeficiency virus-infected macrophages produce soluble factors that cause histological and neurochemical alterations in cultured human brains. *Journal of Clinical Investigation*, **87**, 503–12.

Rabinovitch, A., Pukel, C., Baquerizo, H. and MacKay, P. (1988). Immunological mechanisms of islet B cell destruction; cytotoxic cells and cytokines. In Shafrir, E. and Reynold, A.E. (ed.), *Frontiers in Diabetes Research. Lessons from Animal Diabetes II*. John Libbey and Co., London, pp. 52–7.

Radzun, H.J., Kreipe, H., Zavazava, N., Hansmann, M.L. and Parwaresch, M.R. (1988). Diversity of the human monocyte/macrophage system as detected by monoclonal antibodies. *Journal of Leukocyte Biology*, **43**, 41–50.

Raine, C.S. (1984). Biology of disease, analysis of autoimmune demyelination: its impact upon multiple sclerosis. *Laboratory Investigation*, **50**, 1443–8.

Remick, D.G., DeForge, L.E., Sullivan, J.F. and Showell, H.J. (1992). Profile of cytokines in synovial fluid specimens from patients with arthritis: interleukin 8 (IL-8) and IL-6 correlate with inflammatory arthritis. *Immunological Investigations*, **2**, 321–7.

Renno, T., Krakowski, M., Piccirillo, C., Lin, J.-Y. and Owens, T. (1995). TNF-α expression by resident microglia and infiltrating leukocytes in the central nervous system of mice with experimental allergic encephalomyelitis. *Journal of Immunology*, **154**, 944–53.

Ridley, M.G., Kingsley, G., Pitzalis, C. and Panayi, G.S. (1990). Monocyte activation in rheumatoid arthritis: evidence for *in situ* activation and differentiation in joints. *British Journal of Rheumatology*, **29**, 84–8.

Rieckmann, P., Albrecht, M., Kitze, B., Weber, T., Tumani, H., Broocks, A. *et al.* (1995). Tumor necrosis factor-α messenger RNA expression in patients with relapsing–remitting multiple sclerosis is associated with disease activity. *Annals of Neurology*, **37**, 82–8.

Riviere, Y., Blank, V., Kourilsky, P. and Israel, A. (1991). Processing of the precursor of NF-κB by the HIV-1 protease during acute infection. *Nature*, **350**, 625–6.

Rodenberg, R.J., van Den Hoogen, F.H., Barrera, P., van Venrooij, W.J. and van De Putte, L.B. (1999). Superinduction of interleukin 8 mRNA in activated monocyte derived macrophages from rheumatoid arthritis patients. *Annals of the Rheumatic Diseases*, **58**, 648–52.

Rooney, M., Whelan, A., Feighery, C. and Bresnihan, B. (1989). Changes in lymphocyte infiltration of the synovial membrane and the clinical course of rheumatoid arthritis. *Arthritis and Rheumatism*, **32**, 361–9.

Rossini, A.A., Greiner, D.L., Friedman, H.P. and Mordes, J.P. (1993). Immunopathogenesis of diabetes mellitus. *Diabetes Reviews*, **1**, 43–75.

Ruddle, N.H., Bergman, C.M., McGrath, K.M., Lingenheld, E.G., Grunnet, M.L., Padula, S.J. *et al.* (1990). An antibody to lymphotoxin and tumor necrosis factor prevents transfer of experimental allergic encephalomyelitis. *Journal of Experimental Medicine*, **172**, 1193–200.

Ruuls, S.R., Bauer, J., Sontrop, K., Huitinga, I., 't Hart, B.A. and Dijkstra, C.D. (1995). Reactive oxygen species are involved in the pathogenesis of experimental allergic encephalomyelitis. *Journal of Neuroimmunology*, **56**, 207–17.

Sabatier, J.M., Vives, E., Mabrouk, K., Benjouad, A., Rochat, H., Duval, A. *et al.* (1991). Evidence for neurotoxic activity of tat from human immunodeficiency virus type 1. *Journal of Virology*, **65**, 961–7

Sandler, S., Bendtzen, K., Eizirik, D.L. and Welsh, M. (1990). Interleukin-6 affects insulin secretion and glucose metabolism of rat pancreatic islets *in vitro*. *Endocrinology*, **126**, 1288–94.

Sandler, S., Eizirik, D.L., Svensson, C., Strandell, E., Welsh, M. and Welsh, N. (1991). Biochemical and molecular actions of interleukin-1 on pancreatic β-cells. *Autoimmunity*, **10**, 241–53.

Sahrbacher, U.C., Lechner, F., Eugster, H.P., Frei, K., Lassmann, H. and Fontana, A. (1998). Mice with an inactivation of the inducible nitric oxide synthase gene are susceptible to experimental autoimmune encephalomyelitis. *European Journal of Immunology*, **28**, 1332–8.

Satoh, M.S. and Lindah, T. (1992). Role of poly(ADP-ribose) formation in DNA repair. *Nature*, **356**, 356–8.

Saxne, T., Palladino, M.A., Heinega[o]rd, D., Talal, N. and Wollheim, F.A. (1988). Detection of tumor necrosis factor-α but not tumor necrosis factor-β in rheumatoid arthritis fluid and serum. *Arthritis and Rheumatism*, **31**, 1041–5.

Scheinberg, M.A., Santos, M. and Finkelstein, A.E. (1982). The effects of auranofin and sodium aurothiomalate on peripheral blood monocytes. *Journal of Rheumatology*, **9**, 366–9.

Schmidtmayerova, H., Nottet, H.S., Nuovo, G., Raabe, T., Flanagan, C.R., Dubrovsky, L. *et al.* (1996). Human immunodeficiency virus type 1 infection alters chemokine β peptide expression in human monocytes: implications for recruitment of leukocytes into brain and lymph nodes. *Proceedings of the National Academy of Sciences USA*, **23**, 700–4.

Sean Riminton D., Korner, H., Strickland, D.H., Lemckert, F.A., Pollard, J.D. and Sedgwick, J.D. (1998). Challenging cytokine redundancy: inflammatory cell movement and clinical course of experimental autoimmune encephalomyelitis are normal in lymphotoxin-deficient, but not tumor necrosis factor-deficient mice. *Journal of Experimental Medicine*, **187**, 1517–28.

Seitz, M., Loetscher, P., Dewald, B., Towbin, H., Rordorf, C., Gallati, H. *et al.* (1995). Methotrexate action in rheumatoid arthritis: stimulation of cytokine inhibitor and inhibition of chemokine production by peripheral blood mononuclear cells. *British Journal of Rheumatology*, **34**, 602–9.

Selmaj, K.W. and Raine, C.S. (1988). Tumor necrosis factor mediates myelin and oligodendrocyte damage *in vitro*. *Annals of Neurology*, **23**, 339–46.

Selmaj, K.W., Raine, C.S. and Cross, A.H. (1991). Anti-tumor necrosis factor therapy abrogates autoimmune demyelination. *Annals of Neurology*, **30**, 694–700.

Selmaj, K.W., Papierz, W., Glabinski, A. and Kohno, T. (1995). Prevention of chronic relapsing experimental autoimmune encephalomyelitis by soluble tumor necrosis factor receptor I. *Journal of Neuroimmunology*, **56**, 135–141.

Smith, T., Hewson, A.K., Kingsley, C.I., Lenoard, J.P. and Cuzner, M.L. (1997). Interleukin-12 induces relapse in experimental allergic encephalomyelitis in the Lewis rat. *American Journal of Pathology*, **150**, 1909–17.

Smith-Oliver, T., Noel, L.S., Stimpson, S., Yarnall, D.P. and Connolly, K.M. (1993). Elevated levels of TNF in the joints of adjuvant arthritic rats. *Cytokine*, **5**, 298–304.

Soliven, B. and Albert, J. (1992). Tumor necrosis factor modulates Ca^{2+} currents in cultured sympathetic neurons. *Journal of Neuroscience*, **12**, 2665–71.

Southern, D., Schulster, D. and Green, I.C. (1990). Inhibition of insulin secretion by interleukin 1-β and tumor necrosis factor-α via an L-arginine-dependent nitric oxide generation mechanism. *FEBS Letters*, **276**, 42–4.

Stalder, A.K., Pagenstecher, A., Yu, N.C., Kincaid, C., Chiang, C.S., Hobbs, M.V. *et al.* (1997). Lipopolysaccharide-induced IL-12 expression in the central nervous system and cultured astrocytes and microglia. *Journal of Immunology*, **159**, 1344–51.

Storch, M.K., Fischer-Colbrie, R., Smith, T., Rinner, W.A., Hickey, W.F., Cuzner, M.L. *et al.* (1996). Co-localization of secretoneurin immunoreactivity and macrophage infiltration in the lesions of experimental autoimmune encephalomyelitis. *Neuroscience*, **71**, 885–93.

Symons, J.A., Wood, N.C., Di Giovine, F.S. and Duff, G.W. (1988). Soluble IL-2 receptor in rheumatoid arthritis. *Journal of Immunology*, **141**, 2612–6.

Takamura, T., Kato, I., Kimura, N., Nakazawa, T., Hideto, Y., Takasawa, S. *et al.* (1998). Transgenic mice overexpressing type 2 nitric oxide synthase in pancreatic β cells develop insulin-dependent diabetes without insulitis. *Journal of Biological Chemistry*, **273**, 2493–6.

Tardieu, M., Hery, C., Peudenier, S., Boespflug, O. and Montagnier, L. (1992). Human immunodeficiency virus type 1-infected monocytic cells can destroy human neural cells after cell-to-cell adhesion. *Annals of Neurology*, **32**, 11–7.

Taupin, V., Renno, T., Bourbonniere, L., Peterson, A.C., Rodriguez, M. and Owens, T. (1997). Increased severity of experimental autoimmune encephalomyelitis, chronic macrophage/microglial reactivity and demyelination in transgenic mice producing tumor necrosis factor-α in the central nervous system. *European Journal of Immunology*, **27**, 905–13.

Taylor, P.C., Peters, A.M., Paleolog, E., Chapman, P.T., Elliott, M.J., McCloskey, R. *et al.* (2000). Reduction of chemokine levels and leukocytes traffic to joints by tumor necrosis factor α blockage in patients with rheumatoid arthritis. *Arthritis and Rheumatism*, **43**, 38–47.

Tetlow, L.C., Lees, M., Ogata, Y., Nagase, H. and Woolley, D.E. (1993). Differential expression of gelatinase B (MMP-9) and stromelysin-1 (MMP-3) by rheumatoid synovial cells *in vitro* and *in vivo*. *Rheumatology International*, **13**, 53–9.

Tetlow, L.C., Lees, M. and Woolley, D.E. (1995). Comparative studies of collagenase and stromelysin-1 expression by rheumatoid synoviocytes *in vitro*. *Virchows Archives*, **425**, 569–76.

Uchigata, Y., Yamamoto, H., Kawamura, A. and Okamoto, H. (1982). Protection by superoxide dismutase, catalase and poly(ADP-ribose) synthetase inhibitors against alloxan- and streptozoticin-induced islet DNA strand breaks and against the inhibition of proinsulin synthesis. *Journal of Biological Chemistry*, **257**, 6084–8.

Unuaue, E.R. (1984). Antigen-presenting function of the macrophage. *Annual Review of Immunology*, **2**, 395-428.

Van Dam, A.-M, Bauer, J., Man-A-Hing, W.K.H., Marquette, C., Tildres, F.J.H. *et al.* (1995). Appearance of inducible nitric oxide synthase in the rat central nervous system after rabies infection and during experimental allergic encephalomyelitis but not after administration of endotoxin. *Journal of Neuroscience Research*, **40**, 251–60.

Van de Loo, F.A.J., Joosten, L.A.B., van Lent, P.L.E.M., Arntz, O.J. and van den Berg, W.B. (1995). Role of interleukin-1, tumour necrosis factor α and interleukin-6 in cartilage proteoglycan metabolism and destruction: effect of *in situ* blocking in murine antigen- and zymosan-induced arthritis. *Arthritis and Rheumatism*, **38**, 164–72.

van Furth, R. (1982). Current view on the mononuclear phagocyte system. *Immunobiology*, **161**, 178–85.

Van Lent, P.L.E.M., van den Bersselaar, L.A.M., Holthuyzen, A.E.M., van Rooijen, N., van de Putte, L.B.A. and van den Berg, W.B. (1994). Phagocytic synovial lining cells in chronic experimental arthritis: downregulation of synovitis by Cl$_2$MDP-liposomes. *Rheumatology International*, **13**, 221–8.

Verdaguer, J., Schmidt, D., Amrani, A. anderson, B., Averill, N. and Santamaria, P. (1997). Spontaneous autoimmune diabetes in monoclonal T cell nonobese diabetic mice. *Journal of Experimental Medicine*, **186**, 1663–76.

Verschure, P.J., van Noorden, C.J.F. and Dijkstra, C.D. (1989). Macrophages and dendritic cells during the early stages of antigen-induced arthritis in rats: immunohistochemical analysis of cryostat sections of the whole knee joint. *Scandinavian Journal of Immunology*, **29**, 371–81.

Voorbij, H.A., Jeucken, P.H., Kabel, P.J., De Haan, M. and Drexhage, H.A. (1989). Dendritic cells and scavenger macrophages in pancreatic islets of prediabetic BB rats. *Diabetes*, **38**, 1623–9.

Walker, D.G., Kim, S.U. and McGeer, P.L. (1995). Complement and cytokine gene expression in cultured microglia derived from postmortem human brains. *Journal of Neuroscience Research*, **40**, 478–93.

Walker, R., Bone, A.J., Cooke, A. and Baird, J.D. (1988). Distinct macrophage subpopulations in pancreas of prediabetic BB/E rats: possible role for macrophages in pathogenesis of IDDM. *Diabetes*, **37**, 1301–4.

Welgus, H.G., Campbell, E.J., Cury, J.D., Eisen, A.Z., Senior, R.M., Wilhelm, S.M. *et al.* (1990). Neutral metalloproteinases produced by human mononuclear phagocytes: enzyme profile, regulation and expression during cellular development. *Journal of Clinical Investigation*, **86**, 1496–502.

Welsh, M., Welsh, N., Bendtzen, K., Mares, J., Standell, E., Oberg ,C. and Sandler, S. (1995). Comparison of mRNA contents of interleukin-1β and nitric oxide synthase in pancreatic islets isolated from female and male nonobese diabetic mice. *Diabetologia*, **38**, 153–60.

Wesselingh, S.L., Power, C., Glass, J.D., Tyor, W.R., McArthur, J.C., Farber, J.M. *et al.* (1993). Intracerebral cytokine messenger RNA expression in acquired immunodeficiency syndrome dementia. *Annals of Neurology*, **33**, 576–82.

Wiegand, F., Kröncke, K.-D. and Kolb-Bachofen, V. (1993). Macrophage generated nitric oxide as cytotoxic factor in destruction of alginate-encapsulated islets. Protection by arginine analogs and/or coencapsulated erythrocytes. *Transplantation*, **56**, 1206–12.

Wiley, C.A. and Achim, C. (1994). Human immunodeficiency virus encephalitis is the pathological correlate of dementia in acquired immunodeficiency syndrome. *Annals of Neurology*, **36**, 673–6.

Williams, R.O., Feldmann, M. and Maini, R.N. (1992). Anti-tumour necrosis factor ameliorates joint disease in murine collagen-induced arthritis. *Proceedings of the National Academy of Sciences USA*, **89**, 9784–8.

Windhagen, A., Newcombe, J., Dangond, F., Strand, C., Woodroofe, M.N. Cuzner, M.L. *et al.* (1995). Expression of co-stimulatory molecules B7-1 (CD80), B7-2 (CD86) and interleukin 12 cytokine in multiple sclerosis lesions. *Journal of Experimental Medicine*, **182**, 1985–96.

Wogensen, L.D., Reimers, J., Mandrup-Poulsen, T. and Nerup, J. (1991). Recombinant human interleukin-1β (IL-1) induces a transient diabetic state in normal rats (abstract). *Diabetes*, **40** (Supplement 1), 117A.

Xu, W.D., Firestein, G.S., Teatle, Y.R., Kaushansky, K. and Zvaifler, N.J. (1989). Cytokines in chronic inflammatory arthritis. 1. Granulocyte–macrophage colony-stimulating factor in rheumatoid synovial effusions. *Journal of Clinical Investigation*, **83**, 876–82.

Yang, X.D., Tisch, R., Singer, S.M., Cao, Z.A., Liblau, R.S., Schreiber, D. *et al.* (1994). Effect of tumor necrosis factor α on insulin-dependent diabetes mellitus in NOD mice. I. The early development of autoimmunity and the diabetogenic process. *Journal of Experimental Medicine*, **180**, 995–1004.

Yoon, J.W. and Jun, H.S. (1998). Insulin-dependent diabetes mellitus. In Roitt, I.M. and Delves, P.J. (ed.), *Encyclopedia of Immunology*. Academic Press, London, pp. 1390–8.

Yoon, J.W., Park, Y.H. and Santamaria, P.S. (1995). Autoimmunity of type I diabetes. In Flatt, P.R. and Ionnides, C. (ed.), *Drugs, Diet and Disease. Vol 2: Mechanistic Approaches to Diabetes*. Ellis Howard of Simon and Schuster International Group, London, pp. 57–97.

Yoon, J.W., Jun H.S. and Santamaria, P. (1998). Cellular and molecular mechanisms for the initiation and progression of β cell destruction resulting from the collaboration between macrophages and T cells. *Autoimmunity*, **27**, 109–22.

Yoon, J.W., Yoon, C.S., Lim, H.W., Huang, Q.Q., Kang, Y., Pyun, K.H. *et al.* (1999). Control of autoimmune diabetes in NOD mice by GAD expression or suppression in cells. *Science*, **284**, 1183–7.

Ziegler, A.G., Erhard, J., Lampeter, E.F., Nagelkerken, L.M. and Standl, E. (1992). Involvement of dendritic cells in early insulitis of BB rats. *Journal of Autoimmunity*, **5**, 571–9.

Ziff, M. (1974). Relation of cellular infiltration of rheumatoid synovial membrane to its immune response. *Arthritis and Rheumatism*, **17**, 313–9.

9 *Macrophages in rheumatoid arthritis*

B. Bresnihan and P. Youssef

1 Introduction

Rheumatoid arthritis (RA), with a prevalence rate of between 0.3 and 1.5 per cent, is an important cause of disability and morbidity (Wolfe, 1968). The onset of symptoms may occur at any age, with a peak between 40 and 60 years (Harris, 1997). Women are affected about three times more frequently than men. Usually, the onset is insidious and gradual over weeks to months. A more acute form, developing over days, occurs in about 15 per cent. The most prominent initial symptoms are usually stiffness, pain and swelling of several joints. The joints most frequently involved early in the course of the disease are the small joints of the feet and hands, usually in a symmetric distribution, with gradual progression to the larger joints of the upper and lower limbs and, often, the cervical spine and tempero-mandibular joints. The clinical course may be severe and progressive in some, mild and self-limiting in a small minority, or intermediate with gradual deterioration in most. Ultimately, the functional outcome will depend mainly on the degree of matrix degradation that occurs in cartilage and bone. Other characteristics of RA, usually seen in more severe disease, include subcutaneous nodules and vasculitis, and manifestations which may affect the heart, lungs and nervous system.

The cause of RA is not known. A variety of environmental factors have been considered as possible etiological agents, and there is compelling evidence to suggest that immunogenetic factors play an important role in susceptibility (Firestein, 1997). The concordance rate in monozygotic twins is between 30 and 50 per cent when one twin is affected. The association between class II major histocompatibility complex (MHC) antigens and RA has been examined in detail. Initially, HLA-DR4 was shown to be associated with RA, with a relative risk of approximately 4–5 (Stastny, 1978). As techniques and nomenclature developed, it is now known that there are several HLA-DR4 subtypes, and that the susceptibility to RA is associated with the third hypervariable region of the DR β chain, from amino acid 67 through 74 (Nepom and Nepom, 1995). The HLA-DRB1* alleles that have the strongest association with RA in many, but not all, ethnic and racial groups include DRB*0401, *0404, *0405, *0101 and *1402, each containing the shared susceptibility epitope (QKRAA).

A widely accepted paradigm for the pathogenesis of RA, based on pathophysiological and experimental evidence, is that a putative exogenous or self-antigen entering the synovium is presented to CD4$^+$ T cells (Firestein, 1997). This is followed by a cascade of events that results in a highly activated inflammatory environment in which new blood vessels proliferate and express endothelial adhesion molecules. A variety of cell populations, including macrophages, T and B cells, dendritic cells, neutrophils and mast cells, infiltrate the tissue in large numbers. Other cell populations, including fibroblasts, chondrocytes and osteoclasts, may also proliferate or become transformed. A range of pro-inflammatory and anti-inflammatory mediators, including cytokines and their inhibitors, chemokines and growth factors, are produced in abundance. The synovial membrane overgrows and begins to invade the articular cartilage as large numbers of fibroblasts and macrophages, as well as chondrocytes and osteoclasts, at the synovium–cartilage interface, secrete matrix-degrading proteolytic enzymes. These interlinking events, depending on their intensity, account for both the clinical manifestations of synovial inflammation and the degree of joint damage that follows.

2 Bone marrow and blood macrophage precursors in RA

Several bone marrow cell abnormalities have been described in RA, including markedly increased numbers of CD14⁺ macrophage precursors (Seitz *et al.*, 1992; Tomita *et al.*, 1994, 1997). Differentiation of bone marrow macrophages is stimulated by interleukin (IL)-1, tumor necrosis factor-α (TNF-α) and granulocyte–macrophage colony-stimulating factor (GM-CSF). Spontaneous generation of CD14⁺ cells from bone marrow CD14⁻ cells is accelerated in RA compared with control patients (Hirohata *et al.*, 1996). The expression of HLA-DR on bone marrow-derived CD14⁺ cells is also accelerated in RA patients compared with controls. These observations suggest that the accelerated generation of CD14⁺ cells from bone marrow progenitor cells and the accelerated maturation of such CD14⁺ cells into HLA-DR⁺ cells may play an important role in the pathogenesis of RA. Macrophage precursors were observed to be especially prominent in bone marrow adjacent to affected joints, and the number of granulocyte–macrophage colony-forming units strongly correlated with the amount of IL-1β, but not GM-CSF or IL-6, secreted by cultured synovial tissue (Kotake *et al.*, 1992). Bone marrow-derived CD14⁺ macrophage precursors from RA patients significantly increased IgM rheumatoid factor production by activated B cells, adding further support to the suggestion that these cells may have an important role in the pathogenesis of RA (Hirohata *et al.*, 1995).

Peripheral blood monocytes from patients with RA were found to be in a relatively low state of activation as determined by surface HLA-DR expression when compared with synovial fluid monocytes (Firestein and Zvaifler, 1987a). However, when peripheral blood monocytes from patients with severe RA undergoing leukapheresis were analyzed, highly enriched monocytes which constitutively released large amounts of IL-1β, TNF-α, prostaglandin E_2 (PGE_2) and neopterin were demonstrated (Hahn *et al.*, 1993). These observations indicate that cells of the monocyte/macrophage system can be highly activated in the peripheral blood of patients with active disease. Evidence of peripheral blood monocyte inhibition was observed in patients with RA receiving monoclonal anti-CD4 antibody treatment (Horneff *et al.*, 1993). Monocyte/macrophages, in addition to T-cell populations, can express CD4 on their surface. Within 1h of monoclonal antibody infusion, there was a 30 per cent decrease in the number of circulating monocytes, and a significant fall in *in vitro* production of the monocyte-derived cytokines, IL-1β and TNF-α, in those patients who demonstrated clinical benefits. In addition to very high numbers of circulating activated monocytes, large macrophage colony-forming cells, designated high proliferative potential colony-forming cells (HPP-CFC), have been demonstrated in the peripheral blood of patients with RA and other inflammatory rheumatic diseases (Horie *et al.*, 1997). HPP-CFC demonstrated characteristics of primitive hematopoietic progenitor cells. An association between circulating HPP-CFC and interstitial lung disease in RA was also noted, although the precise pathogenic significance of this association is unclear. Both peripheral blood monocytes and synovial tissue macrophages from RA patients may be transformed in the presence of either macrophage colony-stimulating factor (M-CSF) or 1,25-dihydroxyvitamin D_3 into definitive osteoclasts with the potential to cause extensive bone resorbtion (Fujikawa *et al.*, 1996).

Circulating monocytes may also have a role in tissue healing. Human cartilage glycoprotein 39 (HC gp39), initially discovered as a major secretory product of RA synovial fibroblasts, is thought to be involved in tissue remodeling events occurring in inflammatory bone and joint diseases (Nyirkos and Golds, 1990). HC gp39 production by peripheral blood monocytes and synovial tissue macrophages in RA has been demonstrated, suggesting a potential involvement in other aspects of inflammation, tissue remodeling and host defense (Kirkpatrick *et al.*, 1997).

3 Synovial tissue macrophages in RA

3.1 Synovial membrane histopathology

3.1.1 The normal synovium

The synovial membrane is the layer of tissue separating the joint cavity, containing synovial fluid, from the subsynovial fibrous joint capsule (Walsh *et al.*, 1995). The synovium is essential for normal cartilage nutrition and articular lubrication. It is normally divided into two functional compartments: (1) the lining or intimal layer and (2) the subintimal stroma containing the vasculature. The two compartments, which are unevenly distributed within the joint, are not separated by a basement membrane. The synovium is continuous with the margins of the articular cartilage and overlies the internal surface of the joint cavity. The normal synovial lining layer is two or three cells deep and is composed of two different cell populations, which are loosely organized and lack tight junctions.

Bone marrow-derived synovial tissue macrophages (type A synoviocytes) constitute approximately 10–20 per cent of the lining layer cells in normal synovium (Henderson and Edwards, 1987). The type A synoviocytes are phagocytic and can express most of the antigens characteristic of fully differentiated mature tissue macrophages. They also express cytoplasmic non-specific esterase activity (Broker *et al.*, 1990). Like other tissue macrophages, they have little capacity to proliferate. Increased numbers are recruited from the circulation during synovial inflammation. Lining layer macrophages can synthesize a wide variety of regulatory factors, including the predominant pro-inflammatory cytokines in RA, IL-1β and TNF-α.

The second cell population in the synovial lining layer is the fibroblast-like synoviocyte (FLS) (type B synoviocyte), which is particularly concentrated in the deeper parts of the lining layer (Henderson and Edwards, 1987). FLS express the collagen synthesis enzyme prolyl hydroxylase, synthesize extracellular matrix, and have the potential to proliferate. They also express uridine diphosphoglucose dehydrogenase (UDPGD) and synthesize hyaluronan, an important constituent of the synovial fluid. Furthermore, the FLS expresses CD44, the principal receptor for hyaluronan, and the vascular cell adhesion molecule-1 (VCAM-1) (Walsh *et al.*, 1995). Hyaluronan is structurally modified in rheumatoid synovial fluid and may be directly involved in the pathogenesis of RA through its angiogenic potential.

In the normal joint, a wedge-shaped tongue of synovial tissue extends from the lining layer covering the margins of articular cartilage (Allard *et al.*, 1990). The marginal tissue is immunohistochemically similar to the adjacent synovial lining layer and contains cells that possess HLA class II antigens and other antigens present on macrophages and FLS. The presence of macrophages at the normal synovium–cartilage junction highlights the capacity for recruitment of immunocompetent and inflammatory cells known to accumulate at the site of joint erosion in RA. The rich vascular network at the synovium–cartilage junction facilitates further inflammatory cell recruitment in response to pro-inflammatory signals. In the normal joint, the macrophages adjacent to cartilage are characterized by the absence of activation markers (Allard *et al.*, 1990), in contrast to the many activated synovial tissue macrophages present in the inflamed synovium (Klareskog *et al.*, 1982a; Burmester *et al.*, 1983; Allen *et al.*, 1989).

The sublining layer of the synovium separates the lining layer from the subsynovial fibrous joint capsule. The subintimal stroma is well vascularized. Cellular infiltration is sparse and the predominant cell in the sublining layer is the fibroblast (Walsh *et al.*, 1995).

3.1.2 The synovium in RA

The histopathological features of early RA were studied in patients with synovitis ranging from 3 to 30 days (Schumacher and Kitridou, 1972). Increased lining layer proliferation of up to 10 cells in depth was seen in all. Presumably, the lining layer proliferation was due mainly to macrophage accumulation, although this was not examined specifically. Perivascular lymphocyte aggregation was also prominent. Consistent with these findings was the demonstration of increased macrophage infiltration causing lining layer hyperplasia in the asymptomatic joints of patients with evolving RA (Soden *et al.*, 1989). In a further study which compared synovial tissue from symptomatic and asymptomatic joints of patients with RA, increased CD68[+] macrophage infiltration was confirmed in both the lining and sublining layers of tissue samples obtained from asymptomatic joints, but was more prominent in the tissue from symptomatic joints (Pando *et al.*, 2000). The predominance of CD68[+] macrophages in the lining layer of asymptomatic joints compared with control synovial tissue samples was also described in a study which included both patients with RA and Rhesus monkeys developing collagen-induced arthritis (Kraan *et al.*, 1998). Moreover, macrophage-derived cytokines, including IL-1β and TNF-α, were expressed abundantly in the tissues obtained from the asymptomatic joints. These immunohistochemical studies strongly suggest that macrophages begin to infiltrate the synovial tissue very early in the evolution of rheumatoid synovitis and that this occurs, perhaps in many joints, even before the emergence of clinical evidence of synovial inflammation.

The synovium in established RA is transformed into a bulky, hyperplastic, hypervascular, proliferative tissue mass (Firestein, 1997). The synovial lining layer changes from the normal depth of two or three cells to a depth of perhaps 10 or more cells and, in some, to a depth of even greater than 20 cells. This change is due partly to the accumulation of large numbers of bone marrow-derived macrophages, which migrate through the proliferating synovial blood vessels (Bresnihan, 1992; Sack *et al.*, 1994). Macrophages, which account for about 10–20 per cent of normal lining layer cells, tend to accumulate in the more superficial regions of the lining layer and can constitute 50 per cent or more of the total lining layer cells in RA (Wilkinson *et al.*, 1992). Immunohistochemical analysis of the synovial lining layer macrophages has confirmed their bone marrow origin, with features that are characteristic of mononuclear phagocytes (Athanasou and Quinn, 1991). Lining layer macrophages in RA express abundant HLA-DR and, in contrast to the normal synovium, most appear to be in an activated state (Klareskog *et al.*, 1982a; Burmester *et al.*, 1983). Synovial tissue macrophages are terminally differentiated and thought not to undergo further cell division. They can remain resident in the synovium for months, perhaps years.

The number of accumulating synovial tissue macrophages has been observed to influence the severity of disease profoundly. Thus, synovial lining layer thickness, mainly reflecting macrophage accumulation, was associated with the clinical course of RA in selected patients (Soden *et al.*, 1991), and with the degree of joint damage over 1 year (Yanni *et al.*, 1994b). The degree of joint damage over an extended period was also associated with the number of macrophages in both the lining and sublining layers, but not with other synovial tissue cell populations (Mulherin *et al.*, 1996).

Increased numbers of fibroblast-like type B synoviocytes also contribute to the hyperplastic synovial lining layer. In contrast to lining layer macrophages, these cells probably do undergo further division *in situ* in response to proliferative factors generated by the surrounding activated immunocompetent cell populations. In earlier studies, which employed techniques which involved thymidine incorporation or immunohistochemical staining of elements of nuclear proliferation, little evidence of cell division was observed. However, in studies of oncogene expression and activation in RA synovium, the evidence of fibroblast-like cell proliferation is compelling (Firestein, 1996). Synovial tissue from patients with RA demonstrated increased expression of three markers of cell proliferation, proliferating cell nuclear antigen, c-*myc* protogene and nuclear organizer regions, compared with osteoarthritis (OA) tissue samples (Qu *et al.*, 1994). This observation has been supported by several other investigators, although it does not appear to be specific to RA (Trabandt *et al.*, 1992; Ritchlin *et al.*, 1994; Roivainen *et al.*, 1995).

As RA progresses, the synovial lining layer extends across the adjacent cartilage to form the proliferating pannus, which frequently begins to invade through the cartilage surface and underlying bone. The characteristic radiographic erosion seen in RA is the result of juxta-articular cartilage and bone degradation by the invading synovial tissue at the cartilage–pannus junction (CPJ). The histopathologic appearances at the CPJ in advanced RA are varied. In some, the pannus tissue may be relatively acellular and predominantly fibrous, whereas in others the tissue at the CPJ contains different cell populations, with macrophages and fibroblasts commonly observed as the majority cell type in most pathological specimens (Bromley and Woolley, 1984). Numerous clusters of macrophages and fibroblasts frequently are observed at the leading edge where synovial tissue penetrates the degrading cartilage (Kobayashi and Ziff, 1975). These cell clusters may be separated from blood vessels, although blood vessel formation is usually prominent at the CPJ. Perivascular cellular infiltrates consisting mainly of lymphocytes, plasma cells, macrophages and fibroblasts are observed occasionally penetrating the cartilage matrix .

It is not known whether the cells that accumulate at the CPJ are predominantly activated cells migrating from the proliferative lining layer, cells newly arriving from the peripheral circulation or cells migrating through bony channels from the bone marrow. Some insights may be derived from a histopathological study of the early phases of pannus formation, in which it was observed that several layers of fibroblast-like cells initially overlaid the cartilage (Shiozawa *et al.*, 1983). Invasion of cartilage appeared to occur in the presence of macrophage-like cells accumulating in close association with the layer of fibroblasts. A pivotal role for macrophages in matrix degradation at the CPJ was supported by the demonstration of surface markers characteristic of mature activated macrophages abundantly expressed on the majority of the macrophage-like cells in the synovial lining layer and in pannus at the junction with articular cartilage (Salisbury *et al.*, 1987). Cartilage degradation is due directly to the production of tissue-degrading enzymes, including matrix metalloproteinases (MMPs) secreted mainly by fibroblasts and, to a lesser extent, by macrophages. Proteinase enzyme gene expression and secretion by fibroblasts is up-regulated by IL-1, TNF-α and other mediators which are produced locally by the accumulated macrophages. Other cells which may be seen at the CPJ and have the capacity to produce tissue-degrading enzymes include osteoclasts, chondrocytes and mast cells. However, the relative contribution of each of these cell populations to cartilage degradation remains unclear. A morphologically distinct cell type, designated the pannocyte, that shares some of the characteristics of chondrocytes and FLS has also been described (Zvaifler *et al.*, 1997). The role of this cell subpopulation also remains unclear, and it has been suggested that it may represent an earlier stage of mesenchymal cell development.

The sublining layer of the synovium is also greatly altered in RA. New blood vessel formation is a prominent feature. This facilitates the accumulation of large numbers of immunocompetent cells. Mononuclear phagocytes and lymphocytes pass through synovial venules, with T and B cells forming perivascular lymphocyte-rich infiltrates (Ishikawa and Ziff, 1976). The infiltrates contain predominantly CD4+ T cells and macrophages in close association (Klareskog *et al.*, 1981, 1982b; Forre *et al.*, 1982; Meijer *et al.*, 1982; Young *et al.*, 1984; Yanni *et al.*, 1992). B cells are relatively immobile and reside mainly in the perivascular lymphocyte-rich areas (Ishikawa and Ziff, 1976). T cells may migrate through the synovium and occupy transitional areas, often adjacent to lymphocyte-rich areas (Kurosaka and Ziff, 1983). Transitional areas contain a mixture of other cell types, including interdigitating dendritic cells, macrophages, fibroblasts, mast cells and plasma cells (Iguchi *et al.*, 1986). The abundant surface expression of the adhesion molecules CD11b and CD11c on lining and sublining layer macrophages suggested a possible role in cell-cell interactions within the inflamed synovial tissue (Allen *et al.*, 1989).

3.2 Macrophage infiltration

Macrophage recruitment into inflamed rheumatoid joints is a complex process requiring the expression of a variety of cell adhesion molecules (CAMs) on the synovial vascular endothelium, many of which are regulated by cytokines (Butcher, 1991; Springer, 1994) as well as the maintenance of a chemotactic gradient into the synovial membrane. This is best understood for neutrophils, although macrophages share similar adhesion pathways. Initially, macrophages are captured and 'roll' along the vascular endothelium, a process dependent on the selectin family of adhesion molecules (Bevilacqua and Nelson, 1993; Ley and Teddeer, 1995). Currently there are three members of the selectin family: L-selectin, E-selectin and P-selectin, so called because of their discovery on leukocytes, endothelium and platelets, respectively (Bevilacqua *et al.*, 1991).

L-selectin is constitutively functional and is expressed on circulating monocytes in RA although at lower levels than normal controls, suggesting that these cells may be activated (Bond and Hay, 1997). E-selectin expression is restricted to activated endothelial cells and is normally transient *in vitro* due to shedding and re-internalization (Bevilacqua *et al.*, 1987, 1989; Luscinskas *et al.*, 1991; Newman *et al.*, 1993). E-selectin is not expressed on normal synovium but is present on venules and capillaries in RA at higher levels than in OA (Koch *et al.*, 1991a; Munro *et al.*, 1992; Johnson *et al.*, 1993; El-Gabalawy *et al.*, 1994). Isolated synovial microvascular endothelial cells from RA demonstrate a higher surface E-selectin expression than human vascular endothelial cells when stimulated with a range of IL-1 concentrations (Abbot *et al.*, 1992).

P-selectin is stored constitutively in Weibel–Palade bodies of endothelial cells and is normally only transiently expressed on endothelium activated with histamine, thrombin or complement (Geng *et al.*, 1990), although new P-selectin synthesis can be induced by endotoxin, TNF-α and micromolar concentrations of oxidants (Patel *et al.*, 1991; Weller *et al.*, 1992). In RA, P-selectin expression is prolonged, probably due to chronic exposure to oxidative products and TNF-α (Patel *et al.*, 1991; Weller *et al.*, 1992; Johnson *et al.*, 1993). Similarly to E-selectin, P-selectin expression is limited to the vascular endothelium but unlike E-selectin it is present in normal synovium and is not up-regulated in RA when compared with OA or normal synovium (Koch *et al.*, 1991a; Johnson *et al.*, 1993). In experiments involving monocyte adhesion to frozen sections of RA synovium (Stamper–Woodruff assays), antibodies to P-selectin inhibited more than 90 per cent of the adhesion whereas antibodies to E-selectin variably blocked only 20–50 per cent of monocyte adhesion (Grober *et al.*, 1993). E-selectin expression in the RA synovial membrane is reduced by treatment with intramuscular gold, anti-TNF-α antibodies and after high dose pulse corticosteroids (Corkill *et al.*, 1991; Paleolog *et al.*, 1996). Unlike E-selectin, P-selectin expression was not altered by treatment with pulse corticosteroids.

All three selectins bind sialyl Lewis(x) (CD15s) or structures bearing this oligosaccharide (Phillips *et al.*, 1990; Walz *et al.*, 1990; Foxall *et al.*, 1992). In RA peripheral blood, CD15s is expressed in high levels on more than 99 per cent of neutrophils and more than 90 per cent of monocytes, and at low levels on 5–15 per cent of lymphocytes (Munro *et al.*, 1992). In RA synovium, only 50 per cent of neutrophils and 10 per cent of macrophages express CD15s, suggesting that this molecule is down-regulated during migration into inflamed joints (Munro *et al.*, 1992). CD15s reactivity is not seen on RA synovial vascular endothelium (Munro *et al.*, 1992).

Soluble E-selectin is found in RA serum and synovial fluid and is released from synovial vascular endothelial cells (Koch *et al.*, 1993a). In RA synovial fluid, it is present at higher levels than in OA synovial fluid and correlates directly with synovial fluid leukocyte counts (Koch *et al.*, 1993a).

The 'rolling' process slows the monocyte, allowing interaction with chemoattractant/activating factors resulting in activation and up-regulation of various β integrins and the down-regulation of L-selectin expression on the monocyte. Therefore, as expected, there is only a low level of L-selectin expression on macrophages in the rheumatoid synovial membrane (Johnson *et al.*, 1993). The β integrins mediate firm adhesion of monocytes to endothelium through protein–protein interactions with members of the immunoglobulin superfamily of CAMs. The β_1 integrins CD49d (VLA4) and 49e (VLA5) as well as the β_2 integrins CD11a, b and c are up-regulated on RA peripheral blood monocytes when compared with normal peripheral blood monocytes (Liote *et al.*, 1996). These cells also showed increased adhesiveness to a variety of surfaces and demonstrated enhanced production of IL-1 and IL-6, suggesting that they are in an activated state (Liote *et al.*, 1996). The β_2 integrins CD11b/CD18 (Mac1) and CD11c/CD18 (p150/95) are expressed at higher levels and in a greater proportion of synovial macrophages in RA than macrophages in OA or normal synovial membrane, in particular p150/95 which was only weakly detected in OA and normal synovial membrane (Allen *et al.*, 1989). The ligands for the β_2 integrins are intercellular adhesion molecule-1

(ICAM-1) and -2 (Diamond *et al.*, 1990, 1991; de Fougerolles *et al.*, 1991; Lawrence and Springer, 1991). ICAM-1 is widely expressed in the rheumatoid synovium including the vascular endothelium, synovial lining macrophages and fibroblasts as well as infiltrating leukocytes (Hale *et al.*, 1989; Gerritsen *et al.*, 1993; Johnson *et al.*, 1993; Lindsley *et al.*, 1993; Tessier *et al.*, 1993; El-Gabalawy *et al.*, 1994; Szekanecz *et al.*, 1994). ICAM-1 expression on vascular endothelium, the synovial lining and on infiltrating macrophages is significantly greater in RA and OA than in normal synovium, although there is no difference in expression between RA and OA (Johnson *et al.*, 1993; El-Gabalawy *et al*, 1994; Szekanecz *et al.*, 1994; Furuzawa-Carballeda and Alcocer-Varela, 1999). ICAM-2 is expressed on endothelial cells in RA, OA and normal synovium, as would be expected from a molecule which is constitutively expressed and not cytokine induced (El-Gabalawy *et al.*, 1994; Szekanecz *et al*, 1994). There is conflicting evidence as to whether ICAM-2 is increased in RA. Szekanecz *et al.* (1994) found no difference in the expression of ICAM-2 between RA and OA or normal synovium whereas El-Gabalawy *et al.* (1994) reported the opposite. These differences may be partially explained by the site from which synovial tissue was obtained. El-Gabalawy *et al.* obtained synovium from wrist extensor tendons, whereas Szekanecz *et al.* studied knee synovium obtained at arthroplasty, reflecting long-standing end-stage disease. The role of ICAM-2 in neutrophil trafficking in RA remains to be determined.

ICAM-1 expression can be modulated by some anti-inflammatory therapies. For example, antibodies to TNF-α as well as pulse corticosteroids reduce ICAM-1 expression in RA synovium (Paleolog *et al.*, 1996). Also, glucocorticoids reduce ICAM-1 expression on RA synovial fibroblasts *in vitro*, resulting in reduced leukocyte adhesion (Cronstein *et al.*, 1992; Tessier *et al.*, 1993, 1996).

ICAM-3 is not an endothelial ligand but is found on most leukocytes (de Fougerolles and Springer, 1992). Its role is not yet determined although it is the major ligand for α_d β_2. Szekanecz *et al.* (1994) reported that ICAM-3 (ICAM-R) was present on significantly more RA lining cells and macrophages than in OA or normals. ICAM-3, which has not been found previously on endothelial cells (de Fougerolles and Springer, 1992), was expressed on a small percentage of endothelial cells in RA and OA but not on normal endothelium. This finding was likely to be due to non-specific binding as El-Gabalawy *et al.* (1994) found no such expression. A significant role for the adhesion pathway involving α_d β_2 and ICAM-3 is suggested by the constitutive expression of α_d β_2 by synovial macrophages and macrophage-like cells and its co-expression with ICAM-3 (El-Gabalawy *et al.*, 1996).

Circulating forms of ICAM-1 have been found in normal human serum and various inflammatory states (Seth *et al.*, 1991). Soluble ICAM-1 is able to bind CD11a/CD18 and thus may have an anti-inflammatory role. Soluble ICAM-1 is present in RA peripheral blood and synovial fluid at higher levels than in OA and is increased in peripheral blood in RA vasculitis (Koch *et al*, 1993a; Mason *et al.*, 1993; Voskuyl *et al.*, 1995). In synovial fluid, levels of soluble ICAM are proportional to leukocyte counts (Koch *et al.*, 1993a).

Monocytes also express the β_1 integrins CD29/49d and CD29/49e [also very late adhesion molecules (VLAs)-4 and -5, respectively] which bind to VCAM-1. CD29/49d and 49e are expressed on macrophages in the rheumatoid synovial membrane at levels similar to those in OA and normal synovial macrophages (Johnson *et al.*, 1993). These molecules are down-regulated on RA synovial macrophages, thus favoring the retention of these cells in the synovial membrane (Johnson *et al.*, 1993). VCAM-1 is expressed on the synovial vascular endothelium and on fibroblast-like (type B) but not macrophage-like (type A) synoviocytes (van Dinther-Janssen *et al.*, 1991; Morales-Ducret *et al.*, 1992; Vonderheide and Springer, 1992; Kriegsmann *et al.*, 1995). It is expressed in RA synovial membrane at higher levels than in OA (Furuzawa-Carballeda and Alcocer-Varela, 1999).

The mechanisms of monocyte transmigration through the endothelium down a chemotactic gradient remain to be determined although homotypic binding of monocyte surface PECAM (CD31) to vascular endothelial PECAM is thought to be important (Muller *et al.*, 1993). PECAM is expressed on normal as well as RA synovial vascular endothelial cells and is not up-regulated at this site in RA compared with normal synovium (Johnson *et al.*, 1993; Szekanecz *et al.*, 1995a). However, PECAM is expressed on RA synovial macrophages and lining cells at higher levels than in non-inflamed synovium (Johnson *et al.*, 1993; Szekanecz *et al.*, 1995a). Pulse corticosteroids do not alter PECAM expression.

CD44 is present in RA synovium on vascular smooth muscle cells, synovial lining cells, macrophages and fibroblasts, and demonstrates increased expression compared with normal synovium (Demaziere and Athanasou, 1992; Johnson *et al.*, 1993). Some authors have found that expression in RA is greater than in OA (Johnson *et al.*, 1993) while others have found no difference (Haynes *et al.*, 1991). CD44 appears to be shed during migration of macrophages through activated vascular endothelium (Haynes *et al*, 1991).

3.3 Macrophage chemoattractants in RA

The β chemokines are a group of small peptides which chemoattract primarily monocytes/macrophages and lymphocytes (Baggiolini *et al.*, 1997). Several studies have identified two members of this family, monocyte chemoattractant protein-1 (MCP-1) and macrophage inflammatory protein-1α (MIP-1α), as likely β chemokines responsible for mononuclear cell accumulation into RA synovial membrane (Koch *et al.*, 1992b, 1994). The β chemokines are produced mainly by monocytes and T cells, although mast cells and other cell types such as vascular endothelium have been demonstrated to secrete these molecules (Baggiolini *et al.*, 1997). In addition to chemotaxis, β chemokines activate leukocytes to induce adhesion molecules (del Pozo *et al.*, 1996). Factors which augment the production of chemokines *in vitro* include monocyte binding to endothelium, aggregated immunoglobulin and the cytokines TNF-α, IL-1 and GM-CSF, all of which are expressed in the RA synovial membrane (Brennan *et al.*, 1991; Koch *et al*, 1992a, 1994a; Kasama *et al.*, 1993). RANTES is a chemoattractant for memory T cells as well as monocytes and is produced by RA synovial fibroblasts and macrophages. The production of RANTES by synovial tissue cells and its levels in synovial fluid in RA are similar to those in OA (Volin *et al.*, 1998).

In vivo evidence for a role for chemokines in RA comes from both animal and human studies. Mice overexpressing MCP-1 demonstrate excess tissue infiltration of monocytes/macrophages but not lymphocytes (Fuentes *et al.*, 1995). Direct injection of MCP-1 into rabbit joints results in macrophage infiltration into the synovial membrane within 6 h (Akahoshi *et al.*, 1993). Administration of neutralizing anti-MCP-1 is associated both with reduced inflammation and, significantly, with reduced joint destruction in a rabbit model of collagen-induced arthritis (Akahoshi *et al.*, 1993). Similarly, administration of anti-MIP-1α reduces inflammation in collagen-induced arthritis in mice (Kunkel *et al.*, 1996). Both molecules are found in RA serum, synovial fluid and synovial membrane at significantly higher levels than in OA and other arthritides (Koch *et al*, 1992a, 1994a; Akahoshi *et al.*, 1993). They are found in RA synovial fluid at higher levels than in serum, reflecting local production (Koch *et al.*, 1992a, 1994a). They are produced by a range of RA synovial membrane cell types in culture, including synovial macrophages and fibroblasts, although macrophages appear to be the major source (Koch *et al.*, 1992a, 1994a; Akahoshi *et al.*, 1993). In RA synovial membrane, MCP-1 and MIP-1α are present in both the lining layer and on infiltrating sublining macrophages and a subset of blood vessels (Koch *et al.*, 1992a, 1994a). The pro-inflammatory cytokines TNF-α and IL-1β stimulate their production by synovial tissue (Koch *et al.*, 1992a, 1994a; Akahoshi *et al.*, 1993). Further evidence for the role of MIP-1α in RA comes from studies which have observed that macrophages which express CCR5, the receptor for MIP-1α, accumulate in the synovial membrane and synovial fluid of patients with RA and other inflammatory arthropathies (Mack *et al.*, 1999). Also, individuals who are homozygous for the D32CCR5/D32CCR5 gene mutation which results in the expression of a truncated and non-functional CCR5, have a reduced incidence of RA (Gomez-Reino *et al.*, 1999).

There are a few reports of the effects of disease-modifying antirheumatic drugs on chemokines in RA *in vitro*. MCP-1 production by cultured synoviocytes is reduced by gold thiomalate and dexamethasone but not methotrexate or non-steroidal anti-inflammatory drugs (Loetscher *et al.*, 1994). Anti-TNF antibodies reduce CD68[+] infiltration in RA synovial membrane associated with a significant reduction in MCP-1 and a smaller reduction in MIP-1α expression (Taylor *et al.*, 2000).

3.4 Macrophage activation and regulation

Activation and differentiation of lining and sublining layer macrophages, characterized by strong HLA-DR expression, are considered to be integral events in the pathogenesis of RA (Janossy *et al.*, 1981; Klareskog *et al.*, 1982a; Allard *et al.*, 1987; Burmester *et al.*, 1987; Firestein, 1997). Following migration through synovial vessels into the perivascular areas, monocytes may encounter a variety of potential activation factors including auto- or foreign antigens, immune complexes, contact with perivascular stromal or cellular elements, cytokines and other differentiation and growth factors. Presentation of putative pathogenetic auto- or foreign antigens to T cells in the synovium is one possible mechanism whereby macrophages might contribute to the initiation or perpetuation of synovitis in RA (Burmester *et al.*, 1997). However, the exact relevance of antigen presentation in the synovium remains uncertain due to the lack of unequivocal evidence of oligoclonal T-cell proliferation and the failure to confirm the detection of any candidate auto- or foreign antigens. Moreover, it is not clear which synovial cell population is the most relevant in putative antigen presentation in RA, since synovial fibroblasts, dendritic cells, chondrocytes and B cells also have the capacity to function as antigen-presenting cells (Alsalameh *et al.*, 1991; Boots *et al.*, 1994; Thomas *et al.*, 1994). Many cytokines and other factors which are produced in abundance by RA synovium are capable of activating tissue macrophages. These include T-cell cytokines, such as interferon-γ (IFN-γ), and cytokines produced by macrophages, such as IL-1, TNF-α and GM-CSF, which may function to stimulate several macrophage functions in a paracrine or autocrine manner.

IFN-γ is present in low levels in RA synovial fluid and is minimally expressed in synovial tissue (Firestein and Zvaifler, 1987b). Therefore, its role in synovial macrophage activation is unclear. TNF-α and GM-CSF are important in stimulating several macrophage functions and in directing monocyte precursor cells to become dendritic cells (Caux *et al.*, 1992). IL-1 also stimulates several macrophage functions and induces multinucleation and bone-resorbing activity of osteoclasts which, like dendritic cells, are derived from monocyte precursor cells (Jimi *et al.*, 1999).

The perivascular areas in the synovium contain large numbers of macrophages in direct contact with activated lymphocytes (Iguchi *et al.*, 1986). It has been demonstrated *in vitro* that direct monocyte contact with activated lymphocytes results in markedly increased monocyte production of IL-1 and TNF-α, as well as MMP-1 and TIMP (Vey *et al.*, 1992; Lacraz *et al.*, 1994). These observations suggest that direct contact with cell surface antigens on activated lymphocytes may be important in macrophage activation in inflamed tissue. A number of mechanisms which may participate in synovial tissue lymphocyte–macrophage interactions in RA have been identified. The intercellular adhesion molecule receptor (ICAM-R or ICAM-3), a ligand for lymphocyte function-associated antigen 1 (LFA-1), was expressed intensely on RA synovial tissue macrophages, suggesting that it may play a role in cell contact-mediated activation. It was not expressed on normal or inflamed synovial blood vessels (El-Gabalawy *et al.*, 1994). However, a functional role for this pathway in RA has not yet been identified. In a further study, the simultaneous presence and close localization in RA synovial tissue of the co-stimulatory molecules, B7.2 (CD86, expressed on macrophages) and CD28 (on lymphocytes) suggested that their interaction may be important in sustaining synovial inflammation (Liu *et al.*, 1996). Another possible mechanism of macrophage activation by T cells is through the CD28/B7 (CD80/86) pathway (Shimoyama *et al.*, 1999). Synovial tissue T cells expressing CD28 were in close proximity to synovial cells, mostly CD14⁺, expressing B7.1 (CD80) and B7.2 (CD86). In addition, there was evidence that the synovial T cells directly induced the macrophages to produce IL-1β, IL-6 and MMP-3 *in vivo*, but this observation needs to be confirmed. Despite the demonstration of several possible T cell/macrophage co-stimulatory molecule/ligand pathways in RA synovial membrane, their relevance in pathogenetic events such as cytokine or protease production is not yet known. The accumulating evidence appears to favor a minor role for the CD40–CD40 ligand pathway (Ribbens *et al.*, 2000), and a partial role for LFA-1 and CD69 (Burger and Dayer, 1998). CD28, CTLA4, CD80 and CD86 are more likely to be associated with T-cell activation during antigen presentation by dendritic cells or B cells. Other molecules, referred to as surface-activating factors on stimulated T lymphocytes (SAFTs), which have not yet been fully characterized, are thought to be responsible for macrophage stimulation by activated T cells through cell contact (Nicod and Dayer, 1999).

Macrophages accumulating in the synovial lining layer, having migrated through perivascular areas containing large numbers of activated lymphocytes, demonstrate surface markers which indicate a greater level of maturation and activation (Mulherin *et al.*, 1996). Thus, employing a range of monoclonal antibodies which identify different stages of macrophage activation, it was observed that sublining layer macrophage expression of CD68 and CD14 was similar, and that expression of the activation/maturation markers RFD7 and BerMAC3 was notably less. However, in the lining layer, CD68 was expressed by 40 per cent of the cells, compared with only 14 per cent of cells which were

CD14⁺ (P = 0.003). It is believed that the loss of CD14 expression from tissue macrophages is a feature of increasing maturation (Broker *et al.*, 1990). CD68, RFD7 and BerMAC3 were distributed throughout all levels of the proliferative synovial lining layer, whereas CD14 was localized to the deeper lining layer. CD13, another monocyte surface activation- and maturation-related antigen present on bone marrow-derived mononuclear phagocytes (Koch *et al.*, 1991b), is up-regulated by IFN-γ and lipopolysaccharide (LPS) and is expressed abundantly by RA synovial tissue macrophages, especially those accumulating in the lining layer. Cytokine production is up-regulated in activated macrophages, and many studies have demonstrated that cytokine production by synovial tissue macrophages is maximal in the lining layer (Chu *et al.*, 1991a; Deleuran *et al.*, 1992a; Wood *et al.*, 1992a; Ulfgren *et al.*, 1995; Klimiuk *et al.*, 1997). Taken together, these observations add support to the suggestion that, following their migration through perivascular lymphocyte-rich areas, macrophages accumulating throughout the synovial lining layer represent increasingly differentiated, activated and mature cell populations. Synovial lining layer macrophages and fibroblasts, the predominant cell populations at the CPJ, are the principle effector cells in the pathophysiology of cartilage and bone degradation, though mast cells, chondrocytes and osteoclasts, having the capacity to secrete tissue-degrading enzymes, are also likely to possess important pathophysiological functions.

Steroid sex hormones may also have immunoregulatory effects. It is known that women of child-bearing age have a higher incidence of autoimmune disease than men (Sthoeger *et al.*, 1988). This discrepancy may be due partly to the immunosuppressive effects of androgens (Schuurs and Verheul, 1990). Androgen receptor-bearing cells were demonstrated in RA synovium, especially if obtained from male patients (Cutolo *et al.*, 1992). The androgen receptor-positive cells were activated macrophages, and it was suggested that androgen-induced immunosuppression in RA might be mediated through receptors on antigen-processing or antigen-presenting cells in synovial tissue.

Macrophages at the CPJ may undergo further phenotypic and functional modulation. The myeloid-related proteins (MRPs) are calcium-binding proteins expressed in high concentrations during the early differentiation of monocyte/macrophages, but are absent in mature macrophages (Odink *et al.*, 1987; Hessian *et al.*, 1993). MRP8 and MRP14 have been shown to play a role in intracellular signaling pathways during inflammation. The proteins assemble with each other to form non-covalently associated complexes in a calcium-dependent manner (Teigelkamp *et al.*, 1991). The complexes are translocated from cytosol to membrane structures and intermediate filaments, indicating a role in the interaction between cytoskeleton and membrane (Roth *et al.*, 1993). After translocation, the proteins may be secreted and observed extracellularly. This translocation correlates with inflammatory activation of monocytes, as shown by the enhanced secretion of inflammatory cytokines such as IL-1β and TN-α, and by an increase in the oxidative burst (Bhardwaj *et al.*, 1992; Lemarchand *et al.*, 1992). In RA, lining layer macrophages in tissue selected specifically from sites adjacent to the CPJ abundantly expressed MRP8, MRP14 and the heterodimer MRP8/14, in patients with active disease but not patients with inactive disease (Youssef *et al.*, 1999). These markers were not expressed on sublining layer macrophages, suggesting increased activation and differentiation of lining layer macrophages located at sites of maximal tissue degradation during active phases of RA.

3.5 Transcriptional events and gene expression by synovial tissue macrophages

Macrophages in RA synovial tissue demonstrate features of increased activation with up-regulation of numerous genes, including cytokines and chemokines (Burmester *et al.*, 1997). In inflamed tissue, a number of transcription factor families have been implicated as critical regulators of gene expression (Firestein and Manning, 1999). These include activator protein 1 (AP-1), activating transcription factor 2 (ATF2), nuclear factor-kB (NF-kB), nuclear factor of activated T cells (NF-AT), signal transducers and activators of transcription (STATs), p53 and nuclear hormone receptors. NF-kB has been implicated in enhancing the expression of genes encoding several macrophage-derived pro-inflammatory mediators, including granulocyte colony-stimulating factor (G-CSF), M-CSF and GM-CSF, TNF-A, IL-1β, IL-6, IL-8, MCP-1, and nitric oxide synthase. Specifically, it has been demonstrated that TNF-α production by RA synovial tissue macrophages is NF-kB dependent (Foxwell *et al.*, 1998). In a series of studies, NF-kB and AP-1 were found to be expressed abundantly in RA synovial tissue. Tissue from most RA patients demonstrated expression of both the p50 and p65 subunits of NF-kB in the majority of CD14$^+$ cells, in both the lining and sublining layers (Handel *et al.*, 1995). The distributions of p50 and p65 were similar. In contrast, the distributions of Jun and Fos, members of the AP-1 family, were quite different although with some overlap. The cells expressing Jun and Fos were CD14$^-$, indicating that the expression of NF-kB is much more pronounced than that of AP-1 in RA synovial tissue macrophages, and suggesting that AP-1-mediated transcription events may be associated more with synovial fibroblast activation. NF-kB expression was found to be increased in both RA and OA synovial lining layer compared with normal synovium (Han *et al.*, 1998). Jun and Fos expression in the lining layer was also significantly greater in RA than in OA. The DNA-binding activities of both NF-kB and AP-1 were significantly greater in RA than in OA. However, it is noteworthy that NF-kB expression in the synovial lining layer, when associated with acute rheumatoid synovitis, appeared to be reduced compared with chronic RA and OA (Marok *et al.*, 1996). The explanation for this observation is unclear. AP-1 also plays a pivotal role in the expression of cytokines and the MMP-1 and MMP-3 genes, which are up-regulated in synovial macrophages and fibroblasts by IL-1β and TNF-α. AP-1 DNA-binding activity in RA synovium correlated with clinical measures of disease activity (Asahara *et al.*, 1997). The precise relationships between the pathogenesis of RA and the signal transduction pathways involved in macrophage activation and cell transformation remain unclear, and a more complete understanding of these pathways may provide further opportunities for innovative therapeutic intervention.

3.6 Macrophage apoptosis in the RA synovium

Fas-mediated apoptosis is one of the characteristic forms of cell death in rheumatoid synovial tissue (Nishioka *et al.*, 1998). Apoptotic cell death is a feature of synovial tissue macrophages, fibroblasts, T cells and endothelial cells (Firestein *et al.*, 1995; Sumida *et al.*, 1997), and apoptotic cells are removed by adjacent synovial macrophages (Nakajima *et al.*, 1995). The regulation of synovial apoptosis has been studied most widely in fibroblasts and lymphocytes, and it has been suggested that defective cell death is an important mechanism in synovial proliferation (Nishioka *et al.*, 1998). Several regulatory genes which participate in the regulation of apoptosis are overexpressed due to gene mutation in RA synovial tissue. These include the p53 tumor suppressor gene, which was found to be overexpressed in lining layer fibroblasts in the early stages of disease, even in joints which do not yet appear to be clinically affected (Tak *et al.*, 1999). It remains to be determined if p53 gene mutation in RA is confined to lining layer fibroblasts or whether other synovial cell populations including macrophages, exposed to the same inflammatory environment, may also undergo p53 mutation.

3.7 Macrophage functions in the RA synovium

3.7.1 Anti-inflammatory factors

Anti-inflammatory factors which may play a significant role in the pathogenesis of RA include IL-4, -10, -11, -13 and -16, IL-1Ra and transforming growth factor-B (TGF-β). Some of these such as IL-4, IL-13 and TGF-β may have pro-inflammatory effects. The major sources of IL-10 were lining layer macrophages and T lymphocytes in the mononuclear cell aggregates (Katsikis *et al.*, 1994). *In-vitro*, IL-10 reduces the production of the pro-inflammatory cytokines IL-1 and TNF-α by rheumatoid synoviocytes and the ability of synovial macrophages to act as antigen-presenting cells (Katsikis *et al.*, 1994; Sugiyama *et al.*, 1995; Mottonen *et al.*, 1998). IL-10 reduces the production of factors produced by activated monocytes which may lead to cartilage degradation *in vitro* (van Roon *et al.*, 1996) as well as mononuclear cell migration and cartilage erosion caused by implanted RA synovial tissue on human cartilage under the skin of a SCID mouse (Jorgensen *et al.*, 1998). IL-10 also inhibits arthritis in various experimental models (Walmsley *et al.*, 1996; Lechman *et al.*, 1999). In addition, the immunoregulatory effects of dexamethasone and methotrexate are associated with an increase in IL-10 production (Constantin *et al.*, 1998; Verhoef *et al.*, 1999). Therefore, it was both surprising and disappointing that infusions of recombinant human IL-10 were no better than placebo in RA and did not alter cellular infiltration or the expression of pro-inflammatory cytokines in the synovial membrane (Smeets *et al.*, 1999).

IL-1Ra is an inhibitor of IL-1 binding to its receptors. IL-1Ra is present in RA synovial fluid at higher levels than in synovial fluid from other inflammatory arthropathies and was undetectable in synovial fluid from non-inflammatory arthropathies (Malyak *et al.*, 1993). The level of IL-1Ra was proportional to the neutrophil count, and neutrophils in synovial fluid contained IL-1Ra protein (Malyak *et al.*, 1993). Isolated human rheumatoid synovial tissue macrophages express IL-1Ra mRNA, and IL-1Ra is produced by cultured synovial tissue (Deleuran *et al.*, 1992a; Firestein *et al.*, 1992, 1994; Koch *et al.*, 1992a). Also, IL-1Ra can be demonstrated in synovial tissue and is mainly found in synovial lining cells and infiltrating macrophages and to a lesser extent in vascular endothelium (Deleuran *et al.*, 1992a; Firestein *et al.*, 1992, 1994). TNF-α and IL-1β increase IL-1Ra production by RA synoviocytes (Krzesicki *et al.*, 1993; Seitz *et al.*, 1994). Intraperitoneally administered recombinant human IL-1Ra reduces the incidence of type-II collagen-induced arthritis and streptococcal cell wall-induced but not antigen-induced arthritis in rats (Schwab *et al.*, 1991; Wooley *et al.*, 1993). Aurothiomalate increases the production of IL-1Ra in RA mononuclear cells, providing a possible mechanism of action for this disease-modifying agent (Shingu *et al.*, 1995).

It is possible that the inflammation in RA is due to an imbalance between IL-1β and IL-1Ra. Neutrophils from RA synovial fluid produce more IL-1 and less IL-1Ra than peripheral blood neutrophils (Beaulieu and McColl, 1994). The ratio of IL-1Ra to IL-1 produced by synovial cells ranges from 1.2 to 3.6, which is much less than the 10-to 100-fold increase in IL-1Ra required to inhibit IL-1 biological activity (Firestein *et al.*, 1994). Also, RA patients are defective in their ability to produce IL-1Ra after stress (Chikanza *et al.*, 1995). IL-4 and IL-10 decrease IL-1β production and IL-4 increases IL-1Ra production by cultured synovial tissue, thus increasing the IL-1Ra:IL-1 ratio (Chomarat *et al.*, 1995; Sugiyama *et al.*, 1995).

TGF-β is produced by virtually all cells of the body and consists of three isoforms, of which TGF-β₁ is the most prevalent and mediates most of its biological actions (Massague, 1990). TGF-β is produced by resting monocytes, and in increased amounts by activated monocytes and macrophages (Assoian *et al.*, 1987) as well as endothelial cells co-cultured with pericytes (Antonelli-Orlidge *et al.*, 1989). TGF-β₁, and its receptor endoglin, are found in RA and OA synovium at higher levels than in normal synovium (Brennan *et al.*, 1990; Szekanecz *et al.*, 1995b). Levels in RA synovial fluid are higher than those required to reduce vascular endothelial expression of E-selectin (Miossec *et al.*, 1990; Gamble *et al.*, 1993). TGF-β inhibits IL-1β-mediated cartilage breakdown and collagenase production in cultured rabbit articular chondrocytes and in anatomically intact articular cartilage, probably by down-regulating IL-1 receptor expression (Redini *et al.*, 1993). Intra-articular TGF-β inhibits proteoglycan degradation in a murine model of IL-1-induced arthritis but does not affect basal cartilage breakdown (van Beuningen *et al.*, 1993). It is interesting that exogenously added TGF-β does not inhibit IL-1 and TNF-α production by RA synovial mononuclear cells in culture, possibly because the TG-β inhibitory effect is maximal *in vivo* and cannot be increased *in vitro* by exogenous cytokine (Brennan *et al.*, 1990). Intra-articular administration of an anti-TGF-β antibody inhibits the acute and chronic phases of streptococcal cell wall arthritis in rats (Wahl *et al.*, 1993). Therefore, the overall effect of TGF-β on neutrophil migration is dependent on the balance between its chemotactic properties and its inhibition of endothelial activation (Sasaki *et al.*, 1992). IL-4 is either not detectable or found in small amounts in RA synovial fluid and synovial cells (Brennan *et al.*, 1990; Miossec *et al.*, 1990; Isomaki *et al.*, 1996). However IL-4 is a potent inhibitor of IL-1β and TNF-α production by cultured rheumatoid synovial tissue (Miossec *et al.*, 1992; Sugiyama *et al.*, 1995). IL-4 also increases IL-1Ra production and TNF receptor shedding by cultured rheumatoid synovial fibroblasts (Taylor, 1994; Sugiyama *et al.*, 1995). IL-4 has some pro-inflammatory effects; in particular it up-regulates and prolongs the expression of VCAM-1 on endothelial cells (Rifas and Avioli, 1999).

IL-11 is a cytokine belonging to the IL-6 family which has both pro- and anti-inflammatory potential. It is produced by synovial membrane fibroblasts and macrophages at higher levels than by OA synovial cells (Okamoto *et al.*, 1997). It is present in serum and synovial fluid of various arthritides and its circulating levels are higher in treated than active RA (Okamoto *et al.*, 1997; Hermann *et al.*, 1998; Trontzas *et al.*, 1998). IL-11 appears to act synergistically with IL-10 to inhibit TNF-α production in RA tissue. Blockade of endogenous IL-11 resulted in a twofold increase in TNF-α levels, which increased to 22-fold if endogenous IL-10 was also blocked. Addition of exogenous IL-11 inhibited spontaneous TNF-α, MMP-1 and MMP-3 production, and up-regulated TIMP-1 in RA synovial tissue (Hermann *et al.*, 1998). Recombinant human IL-11 treatment caused a significant reduction in the clinical severity of established collagen-induced arthritis, which was associated with a reduction in joint damage (Walmsley *et al.*, 1998). IL-1α and TNF-α synergistically stimulate IL-11 production by increasing PGE_2 production by synovial fibroblasts (Mino *et al.*, 1998). Indomethacin and dexamethasone decreased the level of IL-11 production by RA synovial cells by reducing PGE_2 production (Taki *et al.*, 1998).

IL-13 is produced by RA synovial fluid and synovial membrane macrophages (Isomaki *et al.*, 1996; Woods *et al.*, 1997). Recombinant IL-13 significantly reduced the production of IL-1β and TNF-α by synovial fluid macrophages and peripheral blood monocytes (Hart *et al.*, 1995; Isomaki *et al.*, 1996) and attenuated collagen-induced arthritis in mice (Bessis *et al.*, 1996). IL-13, like IL-4, also has some pro-inflammatory properties and (in synergy with TNF-α) prolongs VCAM-1 expression on RA synovial fibroblasts by increasing the half-life of VCAM-1 mRNA and increases the expression of CD16 and CD64 on RA synovial fluid macrophages (Isomaki *et al.*, 1996; Rifas and Avioli, 1999). IL-16 is produced by $CD8^+$ T cells in synovial tissue and is able to reduce IL-1 and TNF-α production by synovial tissue macrophages in synovium–SCID mouse chimeras (Klimiuk *et al.*, 1999).

3.7.2 Pro-inflammatory cytokine production

Studies of cytokine production by synovial tissue macrophages at the CPJ and at non-CPJ sites have provided interesting results. In tissue samples obtained from the CPJ of patients with late-stage RA, IL-1α-producing cells were present in abundance (Chu *et al.*, 1992). Using techniques that are highly specific for the detection of cytokine-producing cells and image analysis for quantification, CPJ tissue from a similar cohort of long-standing RA patients demonstrated IL-1α- and IL-1β-producing cells in the majority, but not in all (Ulfgren *et al.*, 2000). In contrast, in patients with early RA (disease duration <18 months), IL-1α- and IL-1β-producing macrophages were present in tissue areas adjacent to the CPJ in all, and the mean area occupied was 14.8 and 14.9 per cent, respectively. TNF-α-producing cells have also been demonstrated at the CPJ in tissues obtained from patients with long-standing RA (Chu *et al.*, 1991b). In a similar cohort of patients with long-standing RA and using highly specific and sensitive techniques, the microscopic areas occupied by TNF-α-producing macrophages were below the threshold for measurement (0.2%) or minimal in all (Ulfgren *et al.*, 2000). However, in patients with early RA (duration <18 months), all tissue samples from the CPJ demonstrated some TNF-α-producing cells. However, the mean area of tissue occupied by TNF-α-producing macrophages was only 6.8 per cent, suggesting that TNF-α-producing macrophages accumulate at the CPJ early in the course of the disease, but become less prominent in the later stages. These observations also suggest that the mean area of tissue at the CPJ occupied by IL-1β-producing macrophages in early RA is twice that of TNF-α-producing macrophages. Both IL-1 and TNF receptors are expressed abundantly on a variety of cell populations, including fibroblasts, macrophages and chondrocytes, at the site of cartilage invasion, supporting the view that a wide range of cells at the CPJ are potential targets for both IL-1β and TNF-α (Deleuran *et al.*, 1992a,b).

Tissue macrophages in RA synovium vigorously produce a large number of other cytokines and inflammatory mediators, which induce an array of biological activities ranging from induction of cell growth to cell death (Firestein, 1997). IL-6 is one of the more important (Wood *et al.*, 1992b). It can modulate both B-and T-cell functions and is a major factor in the regulation of acute phase response proteins by the liver (Gabay and Kushner, 1999). Macrophages are the major synovial source of GM-CSF, which appears to be important in inducing HLA-DR expression (Alvaro-Gracia *et al.*, 1989). A large number of chemokines produced by macrophages have been identified in RA synovial tissue. Chemokines are a family of chemoattractant peptides which are necessary for cell infiltration to inflammatory sites. They include IL-8, expressed on perivascular and scattered lining layer macrophages (Koch *et al.*, 1991c). MIP-1α, MIP-1β, MCP-1 and RANTES are other chemokines which are produced by synovial tissue macrophages (Koch *et al.*, 1992c; Hosaka *et al.*, 1994).

3.7.3 Production of other mediators

Acute phase serum amyloid A (A-SAA), the circulating precursor of amyloid A protein, is an acute phase protein which is produced by several synovial cell populations including lining layer macrophages, synoviocytes and endothelial cells (Kumon *et al.*, 1999; O'Hara *et al.*, 2000). A-SAA production increases dramatically during acute inflammation and may reach levels 1000-fold greater than normal (Gabay and Kushner 1999; Cunnane *et al.*, 2000). In addition to its role in the pathogenesis of secondary amyloidosis, A-SAA induces a number of other pathophysiological effects which may have relevance in RA synovial inflammation and joint damage. A-SAA induces migration, adhesion and tissue infiltration of circulating monocytes and polymorphonuclear leukocytes (Migita *et al.*, 1998). In addition, human A-SAA can induce IL-1β, IL-1Ra and soluble type II TNF receptor production by monocytes (Patel *et al.*, 1998). Moreover, A-SAA can induce the production of tissue-degrading enzymes by synoviocytes (Mitchell *et al.*, 1991). Synovial cell production of A-SAA is up-regulated by IL-1β and TNF-α (Kumon *et al.*, 1999; O'Hara *et al.*, 2000). The known association between a sustained acute phase response and progressive joint damage (van Leeuwen *et al.*, 1994; Cunnane *et al.*, 1999) may be the direct result of synovial A-SAA-induced effects on cartilage degradation.

Nitric oxide (NO) and inducible NO synthase (iNOS) expression has been demonstrated in RA synovial tissue, where it has been localized to lining layer macrophages and fibroblasts and to endothelial cells (Sakurai *et al.*, 1995; McInnes *et al.*, 1996; Grabowski *et al.*, 1997). NO can modulate immune and inflammatory mechanisms and, depending on its concentration, can have either pro-or anti-inflammatory effects (Stichtenoth and Frohlich, 1998). The high levels of NO produced by inflamed synovial tissue may mediate joint damage through various mechanisms including enhanced bone resorbtion (Ralston *et al.*, 1995), diminished bone proliferation (Ralston *et al.*, 1994), decreased proteoglycan synthesis (Hauselmann *et al.*, 1994), metalloproteinase release (Murell *et al.*, 1995) and the induction of chondrocyte apoptosis (Blanco *et al.*, 1995).

3.7.4 Macrophages and angiogenesis in the RA synovium

Angiogenesis, the growth and proliferation of new blood vessels, is a critical component of the pathogenesis of RA (Koch, 1998). Pathological angiogenesis in RA may persist over long periods and is dependent on many angiogenic factors, including several derived from macrophages, produced in abundance by rheumatoid synovial tissue. The regulation of angiogenesis in RA is likely to depend on the balance between angiogenic mediators and angiogenic inhibitors. One of the pivotal pro-inflammatory cytokines, TNF-α, has been demonstrated to have a dual role in experimental angiogenesis: low doses induced angiogenesis and high doses resulted in inhibition (Fajardo *et al.*, 1992). Basic fibroblast growth factor (bFGF) and angiogenin appeared to be produced by synovial tissue macrophages but were not up-regulated in RA compared with normal synovial tissue or synovium from patients with OA (Hosaka *et al.*, 1995). This observation suggested that some macrophage-derived angiogenic factors may play a role in the physiology of normal synovium and that not all are necessarily involved in pathological angiogenesis. However, others have observed bFGF expression to be increased in RA synovial fibroblasts compared with non-inflamed synovium (Nakashima *et al.*, 1994). In a further study of RA, it was observed that the majority of synovial tissue macrophages were devoid of bFGF mRNA, which was expressed predominantly by mast cells and endothelial cells, particularly those at the pannus–cartilage interface (Qu *et al.*, 1995). Therefore, the precise role of bFGF in the proliferation of synovial pannus tissue in RA remains unclear. Hepatocyte growth factor (HGF) has a variety of functions, including the induction of endothelial cell migration in culture. HGF is produced by RA, but not OA, synovial tissue macrophages and fibroblasts, is up-regulated by pro-inflammatory cytokines such as IL-1, and was proposed as an important mediator of synovial angiogenesis (Koch *et al.*, 1996). Synovial lining cells and sublining macrophages in RA and OA also produce increased amounts of vascular endothelial growth factor (VEGF), an important endothelial cell mitogen and angiogenic factor, compared with normal synovial cell populations (Koch *et al.*, 1994b; Nakashima *et al.*, 1995). VEGF in RA synovial fluid and tissue supernatants produced prominent vascular migration and proliferation, suggesting a critical role in pathological new blood vessel formation in the inflamed synovium. TGF-α and, especially, TGF-β are additional angiogenic cytokines which are also produced by synovial tissue macrophages and other synovial cell populations (Szekanecz *et al.*, 1995b). TGF-β_1 appears to be a particularly important member of the TGF family in the pathophysiology of angiogenesis in RA. It was expressed abundantly in the invading synovium at the CPJ (Chu *et al.*, 1991b). TGF-β does not appear to act directly on endothelial cells; it appears to act by recruiting other macrophages, which in turn produce angiogenic factors which can modulate endothelial cell activity (Koch, 1998). The significance of macrophage recruitment in promoting angiogenesis may relate to the macrophage-derived cytokine IL-8, a potent angiogenic factor and member of the CXC chemokine supergene family, which is produced in large quantities by RA synovial tissue (Koch *et al.*, 1992c). Angiogenic activity present in the conditioned media of inflamed human rheumatoid synovial tissue macrophages was blocked by antibodies to IL-8. Moreover, an IL-8 antisense oligonucleotide specifically blocked the production of monocyte-induced angiogenic activity. Inhibitors of angiogenesis are also produced by synovial tissue cell populations in RA and OA. Some, such as IL-10, are produced by lining layer macrophages (Katsikis *et al.*, 1994). The addition of exogenous recombinant IL-10 to RA synovial membrane cultures resulted in reduced production of IL-1β, TNF-α and IL-8, which could result in considerable downstream inhibition of angiogenesis. Thrombospondin, another angiogenesis inhibitor, is also produced by macrophages in RA synovial tissue (Koch *et al.*, 1993b).

4 The effects of treatment on synovial tissue macrophages

4.1 Conventional therapy

Treatment of RA with conventional non-targeted disease-modifying antirheumatic drug (DMARD) therapy produces quantifiable alterations in synovial tissue morphology, which include a reduction in mononuclear cell infiltration and cytokine expression (Walters *et al.*, 1987; Rooney *et al.*, 1989; Yanni *et al.*, 1994b). The numbers of sublining layer and perivascular macrophages were reduced 12 weeks after commencing treatment with gold salts. These alterations were not present at 2 weeks. In addition, neither the number of macrophages nor the percentage expressing IL-1β and TNF-α in the lining layer were altered by treatment. These observations suggest that conventional treatment of RA with gold salts has a gradual effect on perivascular macrophages and fails to modulate the activated macrophage subpopulations accumulating in the synovial lining layer and, probably, at the CPJ. They are also consistent with the limited effects of gold salt therapy on progressive joint degradation in RA. The effects of other DMARDs on macrophage functions have not been evaluated systematically.

4.2 Glucocorticoid therapy

Glucocorticoids produce their effects by a number of basic mechanisms which may act singly or in combination at multiple levels in the immune system. Glucocorticoids act by binding to a specific cytoplasmic receptor and displacing a constitutively bound heat shock protein, thereby inducing activation of the receptor through a conformational change (Beato, 1989). Intranuclear translocation of the steroid receptor complex then occurs, resulting in binding to glucocorticoid response elements in target genes. Glucocorticoid receptors have been demonstrated in normal human monocytes, neutrophils and lymphocytes (Cupps and Fauci, 1982) but are decreased in RA compared with normal subjects (Schlaghecke *et al.*, 1992).

Glucocorticoids enhance the transcription of proteins such as the lipocortins. One of the primary actions of lipocortins is to inhibit phospholipase A_2, thus inhibiting the production of eicosanoids in both human and animal tissues (Flower and Blackwell, 1979; Bomalaski and Clark, 1993) and inhibits NO production by synovial tissue (Yang *et al.*, 1998). Glucocorticoids also inhibit the transcription of cytokine genes (Beutler *et al.*, 1986; Mukaida *et al.*, 1992, 1994) as well as gene expression induced by cytokines, by interference with transcriptional factors such as CREB, AP-1 and NF-kB (Yamamato, 1985; Beato, 1989; Degitz *et al.*, 1991; Voraberger *et al.*, 1991; Funder, 1993; Read *et al.*, 1994). These transcriptional effects occur at very low doses of glucocorticoids.

Glucocorticoids also mediate transcriptional effects through protein–protein interactions on the target gene, which usually occur at higher doses of glucocorticoids. For example, the hormone–receptor complex may compete with the cAMP-mediator protein for binding to overlapping DNA regulatory sequences, resulting in an increase in expression (Akerblom *et al.*, 1988). Glucocorticoids may also act post-transcriptionally, by inducing proteins that bind to AUUUA sequences in the 3'-untranslated region of mRNA (such as ICAM-1, IL-1, IL-6, IL-8 and GMCSF mRNA), resulting in increased mRNA degradation (Shaw and Kamen, 1986; Malter, 1989; Atwater *et al.*, 1990).

Glucocorticoids directly interfere with the transcription of CAMs in response to some pro-inflammatory mediators. *In vitro*, glucocorticoids have been reported to inhibit LPS-induced synthesis of E-selectin mRNA and E-selectin and ICAM-1 protein expression (Cronstein *et al.*, 1992) as well as TNF-α-induced ICAM-1 mRNA synthesis and protein expression in synovial fibroblasts (Tessier *et al.*, 1993, 1996). Glucocorticoids interfere with gene transcription by interacting with nuclear transcription factors such as NF-kB and AP-1 (Jonat *et al.*, 1990; Mukaida *et al.*, 1994). NF-kB is an important mediator of TNF-α-induced increases in endothelial expression of E-selectin (Read *et al.*, 1994) and the ICAM-1 gene contains putative AP-1 sites as well as glucocorticoid receptor-binding sites (Degitz *et al.*, 1991; Voraberger *et al.*, 1991) which may be important response elements for pro-inflammatory cytokines and sites of glucocorticoid regulation. Also, ICAM-1 has several AUUUA-rich sequences in the 3'-untranslated region of its mRNA (Staunton *et al.*, 1988) which are possible sites at which glucocorticoids may induce mRNA instability (Shaw and Kamen, 1986; Malter, 1989). Also, Pober *et al.* (1993) have reported that increased cAMP inhibits TNF-α-induced E-selectin expression and that E-selectin has cAMP response elements in its promoter regions. Glucocorticoids have been reported to inhibit IL-1β and TNF-α production by LPS-stimulated human rheumatoid synovial explants (Bendrups *et al.*, 1993) and to inhibit IL-8 production by RA synoviocytes *in vitro* (Loetscher *et al.*, 1994) as well as peripheral blood and synovial fluid monocyte production of IL-8 and MCP-1 (Seitz *et al.*, 1991). Similarly, glucocorticoids have also been reported to inhibit the lipid mediators platelet-activating factor (PAF) and leukotriene LTB$_4$ which are important macrophage-activating factors (Tsurufuji *et al.*, 1984; Parente and Flower, 1985; Parente *et al.*, 1985). Glucocorticoids have complex effects on the production of macrophage migration inhibition factor (MIF), a pro-inflammatory mediator which increases TNF-α production by synoviocytes (Leech *et al.*, 1999). Low doses of glucocorticoids increase MIF production whereas higher doses inhibit this (Leech *et al.*, 1999, 2000). High dose intravenous pulse methylprednisolone was associated with a dramatic decrease in synovial fluid neutrophil numbers within 24 h of treatment in the presence of a peripheral blood neutrophilia (Smith *et al.*, 1988; Youssef *et al.*, 1995a, 1996). The remaining neutrophils in the synovial cavity demonstrate phenotypic changes of decreased expression of functional and structural epitopes of CD11b and increased L-selectin expression consistent with decreased activation of these cells (Youssef *et al.*, 1995). This is mediated by a reduction in cell adhesion molecules and chemotactic and activating factors in the synovial membrane and the synovial cavity. Methylprednisolone caused a rapid and substantial decrease in the expression of TNF-α and IL-8 in the lining and sublining regions of the synovial membrane as well as a decrease in levels of TNF-α and IL-8 in serum and synovial fluid, but no effect on IL-1β or IL-1Ra expression in the synovial lining (Youssef *et al.*, 1997). MP also reduced E-selectin and ICAM-1 but not P-selectin or PECAM expression on synovial endothelial cells (Youssef *et al.*, 1996b) .

4.3 Biological therapies

4.3.1 TNF-α inhibition

Anti-TNF-α therapy, administered as monoclonal anti-TNF-α antibody or as recombinant TNF receptor fusion protein, produces significant therapeutic benefits in most, though not all, patients (Elliott *et al.*, 1994; Moreland *et al.*, 1997; Maini *et al.*, 1998; Weinblatt *et al.*, 1999). The effects of anti-TNF-α treatment on synovial tissue macrophages were investigated in an open-labeled study (Taylor *et al.*, 2000). Synovial biopsies were obtained before and 2 weeks after a single 10 mg/kg infusion. There appeared to be significant reductions in the number of infiltrating CD68$^+$ macrophages in both the synovial lining and sublining layers, although this was an uncontrolled study. There were also significant reductions in synovial expression of IL-8 and the chemokine, MCP-1, in both the lining and sublining layers. There was a significant correlation between lining layer MCP-1 expression and the intensity of CD68$^+$ macrophage infiltration. If confirmed and extended, these observations may have important implications regarding the role of lining layer macrophages in the pathophysiology of synovial inflammation and joint damage. Similar studies may provide a clear rationale for targeting activated synovial tissue macrophages and their products in the development of novel therapeutic strategies.

4.3.2 IL-1β inhibition

In a randomized clinical trial, recombinant human IL-1Ra resulted in significant clinical benefits and a reduction in the rate of progressive joint damage over 24 weeks (Bresnihan *et al.*, 1998). The clinical effects were maintained and the effects on joint erosion appeared to improve in the treated patients over a further 24 weeks (Nuki *et al.*, 1997; Jiang *et al.*, 2000). In a small substudy, synovial tissue was analyzed before and after treatment (Cunnane *et al.*, 2001). Consistent reductions in the numbers of both lining and sublining layer macrophages were observed in the treated patients compared with those receiving placebo. The reduction in the number of lining layer macrophages was associated with an apparent arrest of progressive joint damage. This effect may have resulted directly from reduced macrophage accumulation in the lining layer, inhibition of IL-1β-mediated macrophage activation or down-regulation of cytokine-induced proteolytic enzyme release.

5 Macrophages in non-articular tissues in RA

5.1 Rheumatoid nodules

Histologically, rheumatoid nodules are characterized by the presence of layers of palisading cells around a central necrotic area and an outer collagenous capsule with a vascular zone and perivascular collections of inflammatory cells. Macrophages are the predominant infiltrating cell in rheumatoid nodules, making up approximately 50 per cent of the outer vascular zone and 87 per cent of the central accumulation of palisading cells (Hedfors *et al.*, 1983; Duke *et al.*, 1984; Palmer *et al.*, 1987; Athanasou *et al.*, 1988; Highton *et al.*, 1990). Macrophage accumulation is at least partly mediated by the expression of the cell adhesion molecules VCAM-1, ICAM-1, PECAM, P-selectin and E-selectin on the blood vessels in the palisading layer (Elewaut *et al.*, 1998; Wikaningrum *et al.*, 1998). E-selectin is overexpressed in nodules when compared with paired synovium from the same patients (Elewaut *et al.*, 1998; Wikaningrum *et al.*, 1998). The palisading macrophages share similar properties with synovial lining macrophage-like cells. For example, they express the CD68 antigen, prolyl hydroxylase and non-specific esterase (Edwards *et al.*, 1993) and produce the pro-inflammatory cytokines TNF-α and IL-1β as well as the inhibitory cytokine IL-1Ra (Wikaningrum *et al*, 1998). There was differential expression of these cytokines in the nodule, with IL-1β expression in perivascular macrophages in the outer layers and TNF-α expression predominating in macrophages around the central necrotic area, suggesting a role for this cytokine in the necrotic process (Wikaningrum *et al.*, 1998). Macrophages in the nodules express an activated phenotype which may be secondary to the interaction with pro-inflammatory mediators. For example, there is increased expression of β_2 integrins on a subset of palisading cell macrophages, and a subset of macrophages in proximity to the central necrotic area express the myeloid-related protein MRP8/14, which may be a marker of macrophage differentiation. With better characterization of dendritic cells within the rheumatoid nodule, it has been observed that some dendritic cells express the macrophage marker CD14 (Highton *et al.*, 2000).

5.2 Other extra-articular disease

Mononuclear cell infiltration is a histopathological feature of extra-articular manifestations of RA and may manifest as rheumatoid nodules, vasculitis and mononuclear cell tissue infiltration into tissues. Rheumatoid nodules are most commonly found subcutaneously but may be found in other organs including the lungs (Walker and Wright, 1968; Hull and mathews, 1982; Nusslein *et al.*, 1987), peripheral and central nervous systems (Markenson *et al.*, 1979; Jackson *et al.*, 1984; Bathon *et al.*, 1989), heart (Lebowitz, 1963; Ojeda *et al.*, 1986) and eyes (Barr *et al.*, 1981). Rheumatoid vasculitis is classically a pan-arteritis with infiltration of the vessel wall with mononuclear cells, and may manifest itself as peripheral neuritis, serositis (in particular pericarditis and pleuritis), visceral arteritis (especially cardiac and lung involvement), distal and large vessel arteritis and cutaneous ulceration in RA (Lebowitz, 1963; Wells, 1969; Gordon *et al.*, 1973; Moreland *et al.*, 1988; Vollertsen and Conn, 1990). Mononuclear cell infiltration may be seen in myocarditis, around the portal tracts, in the central nervous system and very rarely in glomeruli (Lebowitz, 1963; Walker and Wright, 1968; Wells, 1969; Gordon *et al.*, 1973; Markenson *et al.*, 1979; Boers *et al.*, 1987; Bathon *et al.*, 1989).

6 Summary

RA is a complex disease, the causes of which are still being elucidated. However, there is clear evidence that macrophages, and cytokines released by them, have a role to play in disease progression. A greater understanding of this role may lead to the development of novel therapeutic strategies to ameliorate the symptoms and progression of this relatively common debilitating condition.

References

Abbot, S.E., Kaul, A., Stevens, C.R. and Blake, D.R. (1992). Isolation and culture of synovial microvascular endothelial cells. Characterization and assessment of adhesion molecule expression. *Arthritis and Rheumatism*, **35**, 401–6.

Akahoshi, T., Wada, C., Endo, H., Hirota, K., Hosaka, S., Takagishi, K. *et al.* (1993). Expression of monocyte chemotactic and activating factor in rheumatoid arthritis: regulation of its production in synovial cells by interleukin-1 and tumor necrosis factor. *Arthritis and Rheumatism*, **36**, 762–71.

Akerblom, I.E., Slater, E.P., Beato, M., Baxter, J.D. and Mellon, P.L. (1988). Negative regulation by glucocorticoids through interference with a cAMP responsive enhancer. *Science*, **241**, 350–3.

Allard, S.A., Muirden, K.D., Hogg, N. and Maini, R.N. (1987). Differential expression of HLA class II antigens and macrophage subpopulations in rheumatoid pannus. *British Journal of Rheumatology*, **27**, 124–9.

Allard, S.A., Bayliss, M.T. and Maini, R.N. (1990). The synovium–cartilage junction of the normal knee: implications for joint destruction and repair. *Arthritis and Rheumatism*, **33**, 1170–9.

Allen, C.A., Highton, J. and Palmer, D.G. (1989). Increased expression of p150,95 and CR3 leukocyte adhesion molecules by mononuclear phagocytes in rheumatoid synovial membranes. Comparison with osteoarthritic and normal synovial membranes. *Arthritis and Rheumatism*, **32**, 947–54.

Alsalameh, S., Jahn, B., Krause, A., Kalden, J.R. and Burmester, G.R. (1991). Antigenicity and accessory cell function of human articular chondrocytes. *Journal of Rheumatology*, **18**, 414–20.

Alvaro-Gracia, J.M., Zvaifler, N.J. and Firestein, G.S. (1989). Cytokines in chronic inflammatory arthritis. IV. Granulocyte/macrophage colony-stimulating factor-mediated induction of class II MHC antigen on human monocytes: a possible role in rheumatoid arthritis. *Journal of Experimental Medicine*, **170**, 865–75.

Antonelli-Orlidge, A., Saunders, K.B., Smith, S.R. and D'Amore, P.A. (1989). An activated form of transforming growth factor β is produced by cocultures of endothelial cells and pericytes. *Proceedings of the National Academy of Sciences USA*, **86**, 4544.

Asahara, H., Fujisawa, K., Kobata, T., Hasunuma, T., Maeda, T., Asanuma, N. *et al.* (1997). Direct evidence of high DNA binding activity of transcription factor AP-1 in rheumatoid arthritis synovium. *Arthritis and Rheumatism*, **40**, 912–18.

Assoian, R.K., Fleurdelys, B.E., Stevenson, H.C., Miller, P.J., Madtes, D.K., Raines, E.W. *et al.* (1987). Expression and secretion of type β transforming growth factor by activated human macrophages. *Proceedings of the National Academy of Sciences USA*, **83**, 4167–71.

Athanasou, N.A. and Quinn, J. (1991). Immunocytochemical analysis of human synovial lining cells: phenotypic relation to other marrow derived cells. *Annals of the Rheumatic Diseases*, **50**, 311–5.

Athanasou, N.A., Quinn, J., Woods, C.G. and Mcgee, J.O. (1988). Immunohistology of rheumatoid nodules and rheumatoid synovium. *Annals of the Rheumatic Diseases*, **47**, 398–403.

Atwater, J.A., Wisdom, R. and Verma, I.M. (1990). Regulated mRNA stability. *Annual Review of Genetics*, **24**, 519–41.

Baggiolini, M., Dewald, B. and Moser, B. (1997). Human chemokines: an update. *Annual Review of Immunology*, **15**, 675–705.

Barr, C.C., Davis, H. and Culbertson, W.W. (1981). Rheumatoid scleritis. *Ophthalmology*, **88**, 1269–73.

Bathon, J.M., Moreland, L.W. and DiBartolomeo, A.G. (1989). Inflammatory central nervous system involvement in rheumatoid arthritis. *Seminars in Arthritis and Rheumatism*, **18**, 258–66.

Beato, M. (1989). Gene regulation by steroid hormone. *Cell*, **56**, 335–44.

Beaulieu, A.D. and McColl, S.R. (1994). Differential expression of two major cytokines produced by neutrophils, interleukin-8 and the interleukin-1 receptor antagonist, in neutrophils isolated from the synovial fluid and peripheral blood of patients with rheumatoid arthritis. *Arthritis and Rheumatism*, **37**, 855–9.

Bendrups, A., Hilton, A., Meager, A. and Hamilton, J.A. (1993). Reduction of tumor necrosis factor α and interleukin-1β levels in human synovial tissue by interleukin-4 and glucocorticoid. *Rheumatology International*, **12**, 217–20.

Bessis, N., Boissier, M.C., Ferrara, P., Blankenstein, T., Fradelizi, D. and Fournier, C. (1996). Attenuation of collagen-induced arthritis in mice by treatment with vector cells engineered to secrete interleukin-13. *European Journal of Immunology*, **26**, 2399–403.

Beutler, B., Krochin, N., Milsark, I.W., Luedke, C. and Cerami, A. (1986). Control of cachectin (tumor necrosis factor) synthesis: mechanisms of endotoxin resistance. *Science*, **232**, 977–80.

Bevilacqua, M.P. and Nelson, R.M. (1993). Selectins. *Journal of Clinical Investigation*, **91**, 379–87.

Bevilacqua, M.P., Pober, J.S., Mendrick, D.L., Cotran, R.S. and Gimbrone, M.A. (1987). Identification of an inducible endothelial–leukocyte adhesion molecule. *Proceedings of the National Academy of Sciences USA*, **84**, 9238–42.

Bevilacqua, M.P., Strengelin, S., Gimbrone, M.A. and Seed, B. (1989). Endothelial leukocyte adhesion molecule 1: an inducible receptor for neutrophils related to complement regulatory proteins and lectins. *Science*, **243**, 160–165.

Bevilacqua, M., Butcher, E., Furie, B., Furie, B., Gallatin, M., Gimbrone, M. *et al.* (1991). Selectins: a family of adhesion receptors. *Cell*, **67**, 233.

Bhardwaj, R.S., Zotz, C., Zwadlo-Klarwasser, G., Royh, J., Goebeler, M., Mahnke, K. *et al.* (1992). The calcium-binding proteins MRP8 and MRP14 form a membrane-associated heterodimer in a subset of monocyte/macrophages present in acute but absent in chronic inflammatory lesions. *European Journal of Immunology*, **22**, 1891–7.

Blanco, F.J., Ochs, R.L., Schwartz, H. and Lotz, M. (1995). Chondrocyte apoptosis induced by nitric oxide. *American Journal of Pathology*, **146**, 75–85.

Boers, M., Croonen, A.M., Dijkmans, B.A., Breedveld, F.C., Eulderink, F., Cats, A. *et al.* (1987). Renal findings in rheumatoid arthritis: clinical aspects of 132 necropsies. *Annals of the Rheumatic Diseases*, **46**, 658–63.

Bomalaski, J.S. and Clark, M.A. (1993). Phospholipase A2 and arthritis. *Arthritis and Rheumatism*, **36**, 190–8.

Bond, A. and Hay, F.C. (1997). L-selectin expression on the surface of peripheral blood leucocytes from rheumatoid arthritis patients is linked to disease activity. *Scandinavian Journal of Immunology*, **46**, 312–6.

Boots, A.M.H., Wimmers-Bertens, A.J.M.M. and Rijnders, A.W.M. (1994). Antigen-presenting capacity of rheumatoid synovial fibroblasts. *Immunology*, **82**, 268–74.

Brennan, F.M., Chantry, D., Turner, M., Foxwell, B., Maini, R. and Feldman, M. (1990). Detection of transforming growth factor-β in rheumatoid arthritis synovial tissue: lack of effect on spontaneous cytokine production in joint cell cultures. *Clinical and Experimental Immunology*, **81**, 278–85.

Brennan, F.M., Field, M., Chu, C.Q., Feldmann. M. and Maini, R.N. (1991). Cytokine expression in rheumatoid arthritis. *British Journal of Rheumatology*, **30**, 76–80.

Bresnihan, B. (1992). The synovial lining cells in chronic arthritis. *British Journal of Rheumatology*, **31**, 433–6.

Bresnihan, B., Alvaro-Gracia, J.M., Cobby, M., Doherty, M., Domljan, Z., Emery, P. *et al.* (1998). Treatment of rheumatoid arthritis with recombinant human interleukin-1 receptor antagonist. *Arthritis and Rheumatism*, **41**, 2196–204.

Broker, B.M., Edwards, J.C.W., Fanger, M.W. and Lydyard, P.M. (1990). The prevalence and distribution of macrophages bearing FcγRI, FcγRII, and FcγRIII in the synovium. *Scandinavian Journal of Rheumatology*, **19**, 123–35.

Bromley, M. and Woolley, D.E. (1984). Histopathology of the rheumatoid lesion. Identification of cell types at the sites of cartilage erosion. *Arthritis and Rheumatism*, **27**, 857–63.

Burger, D. and Dayer, J.-M. (1998). Interactions between T cell plasma membranes and mono-cytes. In Miossec, P., van den Burg, W.B. and Firestein, G.S. (ed.), *T cells in Arthritis*. Birkhauser Verlag, Basel, pp. 111–28.

Burmester, G.R., Dimitriu-Bona, A., Waters, S.J. and Winchester, R.J. (1983). Identification of three major synovial lining cell populations by monoclonal antibodies directed to Ia antigens and antigens associated with monocytes/macrophages and fibroblasts. *Scandinavian Journal of Immunology*, **17**, 69–81.

Burmester, G.R., Jahn, B., Rohwer, P., Zacher, J., Winchester, R.J. and Kalden, J.R. (1987). Differential expression of Ia antigens by rheumatoid synovial lining cells. *Journal of Clinical Investigation*, **80**, 595–604.

Burmester, G.R., Stuhmuller, B., Keyszer, G. and Kinne, R.W. (1997). Mononuclear phagocytes and rheumatoid synovitis: mastermind or workhorse in arthritis. *Arthritis and Rheumatism*, **40**, 5–18.

Butcher, E.C. (1991). Leukocyte–endothelial cell recognition: three (or more) steps to specificity and diversity. *Cell*, **67**, 1033–6.

Caux, C., Dezutter-Dambuyant, C., Schmitt, D. and Bancherau, J. (1992). GM-CSF and TNF-α cooperate in the generation of dendritic Langerhans cells. *Nature*, **360**, 258–61.

Chikanza, I.C., Roux-Lombard, P., Dayer, J.-M. and Panayi, G.S. (1995). Dysregulation of the *in vivo* production of interleukin-1 receptor antagonist in patients with rheumatoid arthritis: patho-genetic implications. *Arthritis and Rheumatism*, **38**, 642–8.

Chomarat, P., Vannier, E., Dechanet, J., Rissoan, M.C., Bancherau, J., Dinarello, C.A. *et al.* (1995). Balance of IL-1 receptor antagonist/IL-1β in rheumatoid synovium and its regulation by IL-4 and IL-10. *Journal of Immunology*, **154**, 1432–9.

Chu, C.Q., Field, M., Feldmann, M. and Maini, R.N. (1991a). Localization of tumor necrosis factor a in synovial tissues and at the cartilage–pannus junction in patients with rheumatoid arthritis. *Arthritis and Rheumatism*, **34**, 1125–32.

Chu, C.Q., Field, M., Abney, E., Zheng, R.Q.H., Allard, S., Feldmann M. *et al.* (1991b). Transforming growth factor-β1 in rheumaotid synovial membrane and cartilage/pannus junc-tion. *Clinical and Experimental Immunology*, **86**, 380–6.

Chu, C.Q., Field, M., Allard, S., Abney, E., Feldmann, M. and Maini, R.N. (1992). Detection of cytokines at the cartilage/pannus junction in patients with rheumatoid arthritis: implications for the role of cytokines in joint destruction and repair. *British Journal of Rheumatology*, **31**, 653–61.

Constantin, A., Loubet-Lescoulie, P., Lambert, N., Yassine-Diab, B., Abbal, M., Mazieres, B. *et al.* (1998). Antiinflammatory and immunoregulatory action of methotrexate in the treatment of rheumatoid arthritis: evidence of increased interleukin-4 and interleukin-10 gene expression demonstrated *in vitro* by competitive reverse transcriptase–polymerase chain reaction. *Arthritis and Rheumatism*, **41**, 48–57.

Corkill, M.M., Kirkham, B.W., Haskard, D.O., Barbatis, C., Gibson, T. and Panayi, G.S. (1991). Gold treatment of rheumatoid arthritis decreases synovial expression of the endothelial leuko-cyte adhesion receptor ELAM-1. *Journal of Rheumatology*, **18**, 1453–60.

Cronstein, B.N., Kimmel, S.C., Levin, R.I., Martiniuk, F. and Weissmann, G. (1992). A mechanism for the antiinflammatory effects of corticosteroids: the glucocorticoid receptor regulates leuko-cyte adhesion to endothelial cells and expression of endothelial–leukocyte adhesion molecule 1 and intercellular adhesion molecule 1. *Proceedings of the National Academy of Sciences USA*, **89**, 9991–5.

Cunnane, G., Grehan, S., Geoghegan, S., McCormack, C., Whitehead, A.S., Bresnihan, B. *et al.* (1999). Serum amyloid A and the development of joint damage in patients with early inflammatory arthritis. *Arthritis and Rheumatism*, **42**, S346.

Cunnane, G., Grehan, S., Geoghegan, S., McCormack, C., Shields, D., Whitehead, A.S. *et al.* (2000). Serum amyloid A in the assessment of early inflammatory arthritis. *Journal of Rheumatology*, **27**, 58–63.

Cunnane, G., Madigan, A., Murphy, E., FitzGerald, O. and Bresnihan, B. (2001). The effects of treatment with interleukin-1 receptor antagonist on the inflamed synovial membrane in rheumatoid arthritis. *Rheumatology*, **40**, 62–9.

Cupps, T.R. and Fauci, A.S. (1982). Corticosteroid-mediated immunoregulation in man. *Immunological Reviews*, **65**, 133–55.

Cutolo, M., Accardo, S., Villagio, B., Clerico, P., Indiveri, F., Carruba, G. *et al.* (1992). Evidence for the presence of androgen receptors in the synovial tissue of rheumatoid arthritis patients and healthy controls. *Arthritis and Rheumatism*, **35**, 1007–15.

de Fougerolles, A.R. and Springer, T.A. (1992). Intercellular adhesion molecule 3, a third adhesion counter-receptor for lymphocyte function-associated molecule 1 on resting lymphocytes. *Journal of Experimental Medicine*, **175**, 185–90.

de Fougerolles, A.R., Stacker, S.A., Schwarting, R. and Springer, T.A. (1991). Characterization of ICAM-2 and evidence for a third counter-receptor for LFA-1. *Journal of Experimental Medicine*, **174**, 253.

Degitz, K., Llian-Jie, L. and Caughman, S.W. (1991). Cloning and characterization of the 5′-transcriptional regulatory region of the human intercellular adhesion molecule 1 gene. *Journal of Biological Chemistry*, **266**, 14024–30.

Deleuran, B.W., Chu, C.Q., Field, M., Brennan, F.M., Mitchell, T., Feldmann, M. *et al.* (1992a). Localisation of interleukin-1α and interleukin-1 receptor antagonist in the synovial membrane and cartilage/pannus junction in rheumatoid arthritis. *British Journal of Rheumatolgy*, **31**, 801–9.

Deleuran, B.W., Chu, C.Q., Field, M., Brennan, F.M., Mitchell, T., Feldmann, M. *et al.* (1992b). Localization of tumor necrosis factor a receptors in the synovial tissue and cartilage–pannus junction in patients with rheumatoid arthritis. *Arthritis and Rheumatism*, **35**, 1170–8.

del Pozo, M.A., Sanchez-Mateos, P. and Sanchez-Madrid, F. (1996). Cellular polarisation induced by chemokines: a mechanism of leukocyte recruitment? *Immunology Today*, **17**, 127–31.

Demaziere, A. and Athanasou, N.A. (1992). Adhesion receptors of intimal and subintimal cells of the normal synovial membrane. *Journal of Pathology*, **168**, 209–15.

Diamond, M.S., Staunton, D.E., de Fougerolles, A.R., Stacker, S.A., Garcia-Aguilar, J., Hibbs, M.L. *et al.* (1990). ICAM-1 (CD54): a counter-receptor for Mac-1 (CD11b/CD18). *Journal of Cell Biology*, **111**, 3129–39.

Diamond, M.S., Staunton, D.E., Marlin, S.D. and Springer, T.A. (1991). Binding of the integrin Mac-1 (CD11b/CD18) to the third immunoglobulin-like domain of ICAM-1 (CD54) and its regulation by glycosylation. *Cell*, **65**, 961–71.

Duke, O.L., Hobbs, S., Panayi, G.S., Poulter, L.W., Rasker, J.J. and Janossy, G. (1984). A combined immunohistological and histochemical analysis of lymphocyte and macrophage subpopulations in the rheumatoid nodule. *Clinical and Experimental Immunology*, **56**, 239–46.

Edwards, J.C., Wilkinson, L.S. and Pitsillides, A.A. (1993). Palisading cells of rheumatoid nodules: comparison with synovial intimal cells. *Annals of the Rheumatic Diseases*, **52**, 801–5.

Elewaut, D., De Keyser, F., Van Damme, N., Verbruggen, G., Cuvelier, C. *et al.* (1998). A comparative phenotypical analysis of rheumatoid nodules and rheumatoid synovium with special reference to adhesion molecules and activation markers. *Annals of the Rheumatic Diseases*, **57**, 480–6.

El-Gabalawy, H., Gallatin, M., Vazeux, R., Peterman, G. and Wilkins, J. (1994). Expression of ICAM-R (ICAM-3), a novel counter-receptor for LFA-1, in rheumatoid and non-rheumatoid synovium. *Arthritis and Rheumatism*, **37**, 846–54.

El-Gabalawy, H., Canvin, J., Ma, G.M., Van der Vieren, M., Hoffman, P., Gallatin, M. *et al.* (1996). Synovial distribution of αd/CD18, a novel leukointegrin. Comparison with other integrins and their ligands. *Arthritis and Rheumatism*, **39**, 1913–21.

Elliott, M.J., Maini, R.N., Feldmann, M., Kalden, J.R., Antoni, C., Smolen, J.S. *et al.* (1994). Randomised double-blind comparison of chimeric monoclonal antibody to tumour necrosis factor α (cA2) versus placebo in rheumatoid arthritis. *Lancet*, **344**, 1105–10.

Fajardo, L.F., Kwan, H.H., Kowalski, J., Prionas, S.D. and Allison, A.C. (1992). Dual role of tumor necrosis factor-α in angiogenesis. *American Journal of Pathology*, **140**, 539–44.

Firestein, G.S. (1996). Invasive fibroblast-like synoviocytes in rheumatoid arthritis: passive responders or transformed aggressors? *Arthritis and Rheumatism* **39**, 1781–90.

Firestein, G.S. (1997). Etiology and pathogenesis of rheumatoid arthritis. In Kelley, W.N., Harris, E.D., Ruddy, S. and Sledge, C. (ed.), *Textbook of Rheumatology*. W.B. Saunders Co., Philadelphia, pp. 851–97.

Firestein, G.S. and Manning, A.M. (1999). Signal transduction and transcription factors in rheumatic disease. *Arthritis and Rheumatism*, **42**, 609–21.

Firestein, G.S. and Zvaifler, N.J. (1987a). Peripheral blood and synovial fluid monocyte activation in inflammatory arthritis. 1. A cytofluorographic study of monocyte differentiation antigens and class II antigens and their regulation by γ-interferon. *Arthritis and Rheumatism*, **30**, 857–63.

Firestein, G.S. and Zvaifler, N.J. (1987b). Peripheral blood and synovial fluid monocyte activation in inflammatory arthritis. II. Low levels of synovial fluid and synovial tissue interferon suggest that γ-interferon is not the primary macrophage activating factor. *Arthritis and Rheumatism*, **30**, 864–871.

Firestein, G.S., Beregr, A.E., Tracey, D.E., Chosay, J.G., Chapman, D.L., Paine, M.M. *et al.* (1992). IL-1 receptor antagonist protein production and gene expression in rheumatoid arthritis and osteoarthritis synovium. *Journal of Immunology*, **149**, 1054–62.

Firestein, G.S., Boyle, D.L., Yu, C., Paine, M.M., Whisenand, D.D., Zvaifler, N.J. *et al.* (1994). Synovial interleukin-1 receptor antagonist and interleukin-1 balance in rheumatoid arthritis. *Arthritis and Rheumatism*, **37**, 644–52.

Firestein, G.S., Yeo, M. and Zvaifler, N.J. (1995). Apoptosis in rheumatoid arthritis synovium. *Journal of Clinical Investigation*, **96**, 1631–8.

Flower, R.J. and Blackwell, G.J. (1979). Anti-inflammatory steroids induce biosynthesis of a phospholipase A2 inhibitor which prevents prostaglandin release. *Nature*, **278**, 456–9.

Foxall, C., Watson, S.R., Dowbenko, D., Fennie, C., Lasky, L.A., Kiso, M. *et al.* (1992). The three members of the selectin receptor family recognize a common carbohydrate epitope, the sialyl Lewis(x) oligosaccharide. *Journal of Cell Biology*, **117**, 895–902.

Foxwell B, Browne K, Bondeson J, Clarke C, de Martin R, Brennan F *et al.* (1998). Efficient adenoviral infection with IκBα reveals that macrophage tumor necrosis factor α production in rheumatoid arthritis is NF-κB dependent. *Proceedings of the National Academy of Sciences USA*, **95**, 8211–5.

Forre, O., Dobloug, J.H. and Natvig, J.B. (1982). Augmented numbers of HLA-DR-positive T lymphocytes in the synovial fluid and synovial tissue of patients with rheumatoid arthritis and juvenile rheumatoid arthritis. *In-vivo*-activated T lymphocytes are potent stimulators in the mixed lymphocyte reaction. *Scandinavian Journal of Immunology*, **15**, 227–31.

Fuentes, M.E., Durham, S.K., Swerdel, M.R., Lewin, A.C., Barton, D.S., Megill, J.R. *et al.* (1995). Controlled recruitment of monocytes and macrophages to specific organs through transgenic expression of monocyte chemoattractant protein-1. *Journal of Immunology*, **155**, 5769–76.

Fujikawa, Y., Sabokbar, A., Neale, S. and Athanasou, N.A. (1996). Human osteoclast formation and bone resorbtion by monocytes and synovial macrophages in rheumatoid arthritis. *Annals of the Rheumatic Diseases*, **55**, 816–22.

Funder, J.W. (1993). Mineralocorticoids, glucocorticoids, receptors and response elements. *Science*, **259**, 1132–3.

Furuzawa-Carballeda, J. and Alcocer-Varela, J. (1999). Interleukin-8, interleukin-10, intercellular adhesion molecule-1 and vascular cell adhesion molecule-1 expression levels are higher in synovial tissue from patients with rheumatoid arthritis than in osteoarthritis. *Scandinavian Journal of Immunology*, **50**, 215–22.

Gabay, C. and Kushner, I. (1999). Acute-phase proteins and other systemic responses to inflammation. *New England Journal of Medicine*, **40**, 448–54.

Gamble, J.R., Khew Goodall, Y. and Vadas, M.A. (1993). Transforming growth factor-β inhibits E-selectin expression on human endothelial cells. *Journal of Immunology*, **150**, 4494–503.

Geng, J.G., Bevilacqua, M.P., Moore, K.L., McIntyre, T.M., Prescott, S.M., Kim J.M. *et al.* (1990). Rapid neutrophil adhesion to activated endothelium mediated by GMP-140. *Nature*, **343**, 757–60.

Gerritsen, M.E., Kelley, K.A., Ligon, G., Perry, C.A., Shen, C.-P., Szczepanski, A. *et al.* (1993). Regulation of the expression of intercellular adhesion molecule 1 in cultured human endothelial cells derived from rheumatoid synovium. *Arthritis and Rheumatism*, **36**, 593–602.

Gomez-Reino, J.J., Pablos, J.L., Carreira, P.E., Santiago, B., Serrano, L., Vicario, J.L. *et al.* (1999). Association of rheumatoid arthritis with a functional chemokine receptor, CCR5. *Arthritis and Rheumatism*, **42**, 989–92.

Gordon, D.A., Stein, J.L. and Broder, I. (1973). The extra-articular features of rheumatoid arthritis. A systematic analysis of 127 cases. *American Journal of Medicine*, **54**, 445–52.

Grabowski, P.S., Wright, P.K., van t'Hof, R.J., Helfrich, M.H., Ohshima, H. and Ralston, S.L. (1997). Immunolocalisation of inducible nitric oxide synthase in synovium and cartilage in rheumatoid arthritis and osteoarthritis. *British Journal of Rheumatology*, **36**, 651–5.

Grober, J.S., Bowen, B.L., Ebling, H., Athey, B., Thompson, C.B., Fox, D.A. *et al.* (1993). Monocyte–endothelial adhesion in chronic rheumatoid arthritis. *Journal of Clinical Investigation*, **91**, 2609–19.

Hahn, G., Stuhlmuller, B., Hain, N., Kalden, J.R., Pfizenmaier, K. and Burmester, G.R. (1993). Modulation of monocyte activation in patients with rheumatoid arthritis by leukapheresis therapy. *Journal of Clinical Investigation*, **91**, 862–70.

Hale, L.P., Martin, M.E., McCollum, D.E., Nunley, J.A., Springer, T.A., Singer, K.H. *et al.* (1989). Immunohistologic analysis of the distribution of cell adhesion molecules within the inflammatory synovial microenvironment. *Arthritis and Rheumatism*, **32**, 22–30.

Han, Z., Boyle, D.L., Manning, A.M. and Firestein, G.S. (1998). AP-1 and NF-κB regulation in rheumatoid arthritis and murine collagen-induced arthritis. *Autoimmunity*, **28**, 197–208.

Handel, M.L., McMorrow, L.B. and Gravallese, E.M. (1995). Nuclear factor-κB in rheumatoid synovium. Localization of p50 and p65. *Arthritis and Rheumatism*, **38**, 1762–70.

Harris, E.D. (1997). Clinical features of rheumatoid arthritis. In Kelley, W.N., Harris, E.D., Ruddy, S. and Sledge, C. (ed.), *Textbook of Rheumatology*. W.B. Saunders Co., Philadelphia, pp. 898–931.

Hart, P.H., Ahern, M.J., Smith, M.D. and Finlay-Jones, J.J. (1995). Regulatory effects of IL-13 on synovial fluid macrophages and blood monocytes from patients with inflammatory arthritis. *Clinical and Experimental Immunology*, **99**, 331–7.

Hauselmann, H.J., Oppliger, L., Michel, B.A., Stefanovich-Racic, M. and Evans, C.H. (1994). Nitric oxide and proteoglycan biosynthesis by human articular chondrocytes in alginate culture. *FEBS Letters*, **352**, 361–4.

Haynes, B.F., Hale, L.P., Patton, K.L., Martin, M.E. and McCallum, R.M. (1991). Measurement of an adhesive molecule as an indicator of inflammatory disease activity. Upregulation of the receptor for hyaluronidate (CD44) in rheumatoid arthritis. *Arthritis and Rheumatism*, **34**, 1434–43.

Hedfors, E., Klareskog, L., Lindblad, S., Forsum, U. and Lindahl, G. (1983). Phenotypic characterisation of cells within subcutaneous rheumatoid nodules. *Arthritis and Rheumatism*, **30**, 729–736.

Henderson, B. and Edwards, J.C.W. (1987). *The Synovial Lining in Health and Disease*. Chapman & Hall, .London.

Hermann, J.A., Hall, M.A., Maini, R.N., Feldmann, M. and Brennan, F.M. (1998). Important immunoregulatory role of interleukin-11 in the inflammatory process in rheumatoid arthritis. *Arthritis and Rheumatism*, **41**, 1388–97.

Hessian, P.A., Edgeworth, J. and Hogg, N. (1993). MRP-8 and MRP-14, two abundant Ca(2+)-binding proteins of neutrophils and monocytes. *Journal of Leukocyte Biology*, **53**, 197–204.

Highton, J., Palmer, D.G., Smith, M. and Hessian, P.A. (1990). Phenotypic markers of lymphocyte and mononuclear phagocyte activation within rheumatoid nodules. *Journal of Rheumatology*, **17**, 1130–1136.

Highton, J., Kean, A., Hessian, P.A., Thomson, J., Rietveld, J. and Hart, D.N. (2000). Cells expressing dendritic cell markers are present in the rheumatoid nodule. *Journal of Rheumatology*, **27**, 339–46

Hirohata, S., Yanagida, T., Koda, M., Koiwa, M., Yoshino, S. and Ochi, T. (1995). Selective induction of IgM rheumatoid factors by CD14+ monocyte-lineage cells generated from bone marrow of patients with rheumatoid arthritis. *Arthritis and Rheumatism*, **38**, 384–8.

Hirohata, S., Yanagida, T., Itoh, K., Nakamura, H., Yoshino, S., Tomita, T. *et al.* (1996). Accelerated generation of CD14+ monocyte-lineage cells from the bone marrow of rheumatoid arthritis patients. *Arthritis and Rheumatism*, **39**, 836–43.

Horie, S., Nakada, K., Masuyama, J.-I., Yoshio, T., Minota, S., Wakabayashi, Y. *et al.* (1997). Detection of large colony forming cells in the peripheral blood of patients with rheumatoid arthritis. *Journal of Rheumatology*, **24**, 1517–21.

Horneff, G., Sack, U., Kalden, J.R., Emmrich, F. and Burmester, G.R. (1993). Reduction of monocyte–macrophage activation markers upon anti-CD4 treatment. Decreased levels of IL-1, IL-6, neopterin and soluble CD14 in patients with rheumatoid arthritis. *Clinical and Experimental Immunology*, **91**, 207–31.

Hosaka, S., Akahoshi, T., Wada, C. and Kondo, H. (1994). Expression of the chemokine superfamily in rheumatoid arthritis. *Clinical and Experimental Immunology*, **97**, 451–7.

Hosaka, S., Shah, M.R., Barquin, N., Haines, G.K. and Koch, A.E.. (1995). Expression of basic fibroblast growth factor and angiogenin in arthritis. *Pathobiology*, **63**, 249–56.

Hull, S. and Mathews, J.A. (1982). Pulmonary necrobiotic nodules as a presenting feature of rheumatoid arthritis. *Annals of the Rheumatic Diseases*, **41**, 21–4.

Iguchi, T., Kurosaka, M. and Ziff, M. (1986). Electron microscopic study of HLA-DR and monocyte/macrophage staining cells in the rheumatoid synovial membrane. *Arthritis and Rheumatism*, **29**, 600–13.

Ishikawa, H. and Ziff, M. (1976). Electron microscopic observations of the immunoreactive cells in the rheumatoid synovial membrane. *Arthritis and Rheumatism*, **19**, 1–14.

Isomaki, P., Luukkainen, R., Toivanen, P. and Punnonen, J. (1996). The presence of interleukin-13 in rheumatoid synovium and its antiinflammatory effects on synovial fluid macrophages from patients with rheumatoid arthritis. *Arthritis and Rheumatism*, **39**, 1693–702.

Jackson, C.G., Chess, R.L. and Ward, J.R. (1984). A case of rheumatoid nodule formation within the central nervous system and review of the literature. *Journal of Rheumatology*, **11**, 237–40.

Janossy, G., Panayi, G., Duke, O., Bofill, M., Poulter, L.W. and Goldstein, G. (1981). Rheumatoid arthritis: a disease of T-lymphocyte/macrophage immunoregulation. *Lancet*, **2**, 839–42.

Jiang, Y., Genant, H.K., Watt, I., Cobby, M., Bresnihan, B., Aitchison, R. *et al.* (2000). A multicenter, double-blind, dose-ranging, randomized and placebo-controlled study of recombinant human interleukin-1 receptor antagonist in patients with rheumatoid arthritis: radiologic progression and correlation of Genant and Larsen scoring methods. *Arthritis and Rheumatism*, **43**, 1001–9.

Jimi, E., Nakamura, I., Duong, L.T., Ikebe, T., Takahashi, N., Rodan, G.A. *et al.* (1999). Interleukin 1 induces multinucleation and bone-resorbing activity of osteoclasts in the absence of osteoblasts/stromal cells. *Experimental Cell Research*, **247**, 84–93.

Johnson, B.A., Haines, G.K., Harlow, L.A. and Koch, A.E. (1993). Adhesion molecule expression in human synovial tissue. *Arthritis and Rheumatism*, **36**, 137–46.

Jonat, C., Rahmsdorf, H.J., Park, K.-K., Cato, A.C.B., Gebel, S., Ponta, H. *et al.* (1990). Antitumour promotion and inflammation: downmodulation of AP-1 (Fos-Jun) activity by glucocorticoid hormone. *Cell*, **62**, 1189–204.

Jorgensen, C., Apparailly, F., Couret, I., Canovas, F., Jacquet, C. and Sany, J. (1998). Interleukin-4 and interleukin-10 are chondroprotective and decrease mononuclear cell recruitment in human rheumatoid synovium *in vivo*. *Immunology*, **93**, 518–23.

Kasama, T., Strieter, R.M., Standiford, T.J., Burdick, M.D. and Kunkel, S.L. (1993). Expression and regulation of human neutrophil-derived macrophage inflammatory protein 1 α. *Journal of Experimental Medicine*, **178**, 63–72.

Katsikis, P.D., Chu, C.-Q,, Brennan, F.M., Maini, R.N. and Feldmann, M. (1994). Immunoregulatory role of interleukin 10 in rheumatoid arthritis. *Journal of Experimental Medicine*, **179**, 1517–27.

Kirkpatrick, R.B., Emery, J.G., Connor, J.R., Dodds, R., Lysko, P.G. and Rosenberg, M. (1997). Induction and expression of human cartilage glycoprotein 39 in rheumatoid inflammatory and peripheral blood monocyte-derived macrophages. *Experimental Cell Research*, **237**, 46–54.

Klareskog, L., Forsum, U., Malmnas Tjernlund, U., Kabelitz, D. and Wigren, A. (1981). Appearance of anti-HLA-DR-reactive cells in normal and rheumatoid synovial tissue. *Scandinavian Journal of Immunology*, **14**, 183–92.

Klareskog, L., Forsum, U., Kabelitz, D., Ploen, L., Sundstrom, C., Nilsson, K. *et al.* (1982a). Immune functions of human synovial cells. Phenotypic and T cell regulatory properties of macrophage-like cells that express HLA-DR. *Arthritis and Rheumatism*, **25**, 488–501.

Klareskog, L., Forsum, U., Wigren, A. and Wigzell, H. (1982b). Relationships between HLA-DR-expressing cells and T lymphocytes of different subsets in rheumatoid synovial tissue. *Scandinavian Journal of Immunology*, **15**, 501–7.

Klimiuk, P.A., Goronzy, J.J., Bjornsson, J., Beckenbaugh, R.D. and Weyend, C.M. (1997). Tissue cytokine patterns distinguish variants of rheumatoid synovitis. *American Journal of Pathology*, **151**, 1311–9.

Klimiuk, P.A., Goronzy, J.J. and Weyand, C.M. (1999). IL-16 as an anti-inflammatory cytokine in rheumatoid synovitis. *Journal of Immunology*, **162**, 4293–9.

Kobayashi, I. and Ziff, M. (1975). Electron microscopic studies of the cartilage–pannus junction in rheumatoid arthritis. *Arthritis and Rheumatism*, **18**, 475–83.

Koch, A.E.. (1998). Angiogenesis: implications for rheumatoid arthritis. *Arthritis and Rheumatism*, **41**, 951–62.

Koch, A.E., Burrows, J.C., Haines, G.K., Carlos, T.M., Harlan, J.M. and Leibovich, S.J. (1991a). Immunolocalization of endothelial and leukocyte adhesion molecules in human rheumatoid and osteoarthritic synovial tissues. *Laboratory Investigation*, **64**, 13–320.

Koch, A.E., Burrows, J.C., Skoutelis, A., Marder, R., Domer, P.H., Anderson, B. *et al.* (1991b). Monoclonal antibodies detect monocyte/macrophage activation and differentiation antigens and identify functionally distinct subpopulations of human rheumatoid synovial tissue macrophages. *American Journal of Pathology*, **138**, 165–73.

Koch, A.E., Kunkel, S.L., Burrows, J.C., Evanoff, H.L., Haines, G.K., Pope, R.M. *et al.* (1991c). Synovial tissue macrophage as a source of the chemotactic cytokine IL-8. *Journal of Immunology*, **147**, 2187–2195.

Koch, A.E., Kunkel, S.L., Chensue, S.M., Haines, G.K. and Strieter, R.M. (1992a). Expression of interleukin-1 and interleukin-1 receptor antagonist by human rheumatoid synovial tissue macrophages. *Clinical Immunology and Immunopathology*, **65**, 23–9.

Koch, A.E., Kunkel, S.L., Harlow, L.A., Johnson, B., Evanoff, H.L., Haines, G.K. *et al.* (1992b). Enhanced production of monocyte chemoattractant protein-1 in rheumatoid arthritis. *Journal of Clinical Investigation*, **90**, 772–9.

Koch, A.E., Polverini, P.J., Kunkel, S.L., Harlow, L.A., DiPietro, L.A., Elner, V.M. *et al.* (1992c). Interleukin-8 as a macrophage-derived mediator of angiogenesis. *Science*, **258**, 1798–801.

Koch, A.E., Turkiewicz, W., Harlow, L.A. and Pope, R.M. (1993a). Soluble E-selectin in arthritis. *Clinical Immunology and Immunopathology*, **69**, 29–35.

Koch, A.E., Friedman, J., Burrows, J.C., Haines, G.K. and Bouck, N.P. (1993b). Localization of angiogenesis inhibitor thrombospondin in human synovial tissues. *Pathobiology*, **61**, 1–6.

Koch, A.E., Kunkel, S.L., Harlow, L.A., Mazarakis, D.D., Johnson, B., Haines, G.K. *et al.* (1994a). Macrophage inflammatory protein-1α: a novel chemotactic cytokine for macrophages in rheumatoid arthritis. *Journal of Clinical Investigation*, **93**, 921–8.

Koch, A.E., Harlow, L.A., Haines, G.K., Amento, E.P., Unemori, E.N., Wong, W.L. *et al.* (1994b). Vascular endothelial growth factor. A cytokine modulating endothelial function in rheumatoid arthritis. *Journal of Immunology*, **152**, 4149–56.

Koch, A.E., Halloran, M.M., Hosaka, S., Shah, M.R., Haskell, C.J., Baker, S.K. *et al.* (1996). Hepatocyte growth factor. A cytokine mediating endothelial migration in inflammatory arthritis. *Arthritis and Rheumatism*, **39**, 1566–77.

Kotake, S., Higaki, M., Sato, K., Himeno, S., Morita, H., Kim, J.K. *et al.* (1992). Detection of myeloid precursors (granulocyte macrophage colony forming units) in the bone marrow adjacent to rheumatoid arthritis. *Journal of Rheumatology*, **19**, 1511–6.

Kraan, M.C., Versendaal, H., Jonker, M., Bresnihan, B., Post, W.J., t'Hartm, B.A. *et al.* (1998). Asymptomatic synovitis precedes clinically manifest arthritis. *Arthritis and Rheumatism*, **41**, 1481–8.

Kriegsmann, J., Keyszer, G.M., Geiler, T., Brauer, R., Gay, R.E. and Gay, S. (1995). Expression of vascular cell adhesion molecule-1 mRNA and protein in rheumatoid synovium demonstrated by *in situ* hybridization and immunohistochemistry. *Laboratory Investigation*, **72**, 209–14.

Krzesicki, R.F., Hatfield, C.A., Bienkowski, M.J., McGuire, J.C., Winterrowd, G.E., Chapman, D.L. *et al.* (1993). Regulation of expression of IL-1 receptor antagonist protein in human synovial and dermal fibroblasts. *Journal of Immunology*, **150**, 4008–18.

Kumon, Y., Suehiro, T., Hashimoto, K., Nakatani, K. and Sipe, J.D. (1999). Local expression of serum amyloid A mRNA in rheumatoid arthritis synovial tissue and cells. *Journal of Rheumatology*, **26**, 785–90.

Kunkel, S.L., Lukacs, N., Kasama, T. and Strieter, R.M. (1996). The role of chemokines in inflammatory joint disease. *Journal of Leukocyte Biology*, **59**, 6–12.

Kurosaka, M. and Ziff, M. (1983). Immunoelectron microscopic study of the distribution of T cell subsets in rheumatoid synovium. *Journal of Experimental Medicine*, **158**, 1191–210.

Lacraz, S., Isler, P., Vey, E., Welgus, H.G. and Dayer, J.-M. (1994). Direct contact between T lymphocytes and monocytes is a major pathway for induction of metalloproteinase expression. *Journal of Biological Chemistry*, **269**, 22027–33.

Lawrence, M.B. and Springer, T.A (1991). Leukocytes roll on a selectin at physiologic flow rates: distinction from and prerequisite for adhesion through integrins. *Cell*, **65**, 859–73.

Lebowitz, W.B. (1963). The heart in rheumatoid arthritis. A clinical and pathological study of 62 cases. *Annals of Internal Medicine*, **58**, 102.

Lechman, E.R., Jaffurs, D., Ghivizzani, S.C., Gambotto, A., Kovesdi, I., Mi, Z. *et al.* (1999). Direct adenoviral gene transfer of viral IL-10 to rabbit knees with experimental arthritis ameliorates disease in both injected and contralateral control knees. *Journal of Immunology*, **163**, 2202–8.

Leech, M., Metz, C., Hall, P., Hutchinson, P., Gianis, K., Smith, M. *et al.* (1999). Macrophage migration inhibitory factor in rheumatoid arthritis: evidence of proinflammatory function and regulation by glucocorticoids. *Arthritis and Rheumatism*, **42**, 1601–8.

Leech, M., Metz, C., Bucala, R. and Morand, E.F. (2000). Regulation of macrophage migration inhibitory factor by endogenous glucocorticoids in rat adjuvant-induced arthritis . *Arthritis and Rheumatism*, **43**, 827–33.

Lemarchand, P., Vaglio, M., Mauel, J. and Markert, M. (1992). Translocation of a small cytosolic calcium-binding protein (MRP8) to plasma membrane correlates with human neutrophil activation. *Journal of Biological Chemistry*, **267**, 19379–82.

Ley, K. and Tedder, T.F. (1995). Leukocyte interaction with vascular endothelium: new insights into selectin-mediated attachment and rolling. *Journal of Immunology*, **155**, 525–8.

Lindsley, H.B., Smith, D.D., Cohick, C.B., Koch, A.E. and Davis, L.S. (1993). Proinflammatory cytokines enhance human synoviocyte expression of functional intercellular adhesion molecule-1 (ICAM-1). *Clinical Immunology and Immunopathology*, **68**, 311–20.

Liote, F., Boval-Boizard, B., Weill, D., Kuntz, D. and Wautier, J.L. (1996). Blood monocyte activation in rheumatoid arthritis: increased monocyte adhesiveness, integrin expression, and cytokine release. *Clinical and Experimental Immunology*, **106**, 13–9.

Liu, M.F., Kohsaka, H., Sakurai, H., Azuma, M., Okumura, K., Saito, I. *et al.* (1996). The presence of costimulatory molecules CD86 and CD28 in rheumatoid arthritis synovium. *Arthritis and Rheumatism*, **39**, 110–4.

Loetscher, P., Dewald, B., Baggiolini, M. and Seitz, M. (1994). Monocyte chemoattractant protein 1 and interleukin 8 production by rheumatoid synoviocytes. Effects of anti-rheumatic drugs. *Cytokine*, **6**, 162–70.

Luscinskas, F.W., Cybulsky, M.I., Kiely, J.M., Peckins, C.S., Davis, V.M. and Gimbrone, M.A., Jr (1991). Cytokine-activated human endothelial monolayers support enhanced neutrophil transmigration via a mechanism involving both endothelial–leukocyte adhesion molecule-1 and intercellular adhesion molecule-1. *Journal of Immunology*, **146**, 1617–25.

Mack, M., Bruhl, H., Jaeger, C., Cihak, J., Eiter, V., Plachy, J. *et al.* (1999). Predominance of mononuclear cells expressing the chemokine receptor CCR5 in synovial effusions. *Arthritis and Rheumatism*, **42**, 981–987.

Maini, R.N., Breedveld, F.C., Kalden, J.R., Smolen, J.S., Davis, D., Macfarlane, J.D. *et al.* (1998). Therapeutic efficacy of multiple intravenous infusions of anti-tumor necrosis factor a monoclonal antibody combined with low-dose weekly methotrexate in rheumatoid arthritis. *Arthritis and Rheumatism*, **41**, 1552–63.

Malter, J.S. (1989). Identification of AUUUA-specific messenger RNA binding protein. *Science*, **246**, 664–6.

Malyak, M., Swaney, R.E. and Arend, W.P. (1993). Levels of synovial fluid interleukin-1 antagonistin rheumatoid arthritis and other arthropathies: potential contribution from synovial fluid neutrophils. *Arthritis and Rheumatism*, **36**, 781–789.

Markenson, J.A., McDougal, J.S., Tsairis, P., Lockshin, M.D. and Christian, C.L. (1979). Rheumatoid meningitis: a localized immune process. *Annals of Internal Medicine*, **90**, 786–9.

Marok, R., Winyard, P.G., Coumbe, A., Kus, M.L., Gaffney, K., Blades, S. *et al.* (1996). Activation of the transcription factor nuclear factor-κB in human inflamed synovial tissue. *Arthritis and Rheumatism*, **39**, 583–91.

Mason, J.C., Kapahi, P. and Haskard, D.O. (1993). Detection of increased levels of intercellular adhesion molecule 1 in some patients with rheumatoid arthritis but not in patients with systemic lupus erythematosus. *Arthritis and Rheumatism*, **68**, 70–8.

Massague, J. (1990). The transforming growth factor β family. *Annual Review of Cell Biology*, **6**, 597–641.

McInnes, I.B., Leung, B.P., Field, M., Wei, X.Q., Huang, F.-P., Sturrock, R.D. *et al.* (1996). Production of nitric oxide in the synovial membrane of rheumatoid and osteoarthritis patients. *Journal of Expreimental Medicine*, **184**, 1519–24.

Meijer, C.J.L.M., de Graaff-Reitsma, C.B., Lafeber, G.J.M. and Cats, A. (1982). *In situ* localization of lymphocyte subsets in synovial membranes of patients with rheumatoid arthritis with monoclonal antibodies. *Journal of Rheumatology*, **9**, 359–65.

Migita, K., Kawabe, Y., Tominaga, M., Origuchi, T., Aoyagi, T. and Eguchi, K. (1998). Serum amyloid A protein induces production of matrix metalloproteinases by human synovial fibroblasts. *Laboratory Investigation*, **78**, 535–9.

Mino, T., Sugiyama, E., Taki, H., Kuroda, A., Yamashita, N., Maruyama, M. *et al.* (1998). Interleukin-1α and tumor necrosis factor α synergistically stimulate prostaglandin E2-dependent production of interleukin-11 in rheumatoid synovial fibroblasts. *Arthritis and Rheumatism*, **41**, 2004–13.

Miossec, P., Naviliat, M., D'Angeac, A.D., Sany, J. and Banchereau, J. (1990). Low levels of interleukin-4 and high levels of transforming growth factor β in rheumatoid synovitis. *Arthritis and Rheumatism*, **33**, 1180–7.

Miossec, P., Briolay, J., Dechanet, J., Wijdenes, J., Martinez-Valdez, H. and Banchereau, J. (1992). Inhibition of the production of proinflammatory cytokines and immunoglobulins by interleukin-4 in an *ex vivo* model of rheumatoid synovitis. *Arthritis and Rheumatism*, **35**, 874–83.

Mitchell, T.I., Coon, C.I. and Brinckerhoff, C.E. (1991). Serum amyloid A (SAA) produced by rabbit synovial fibroblasts treated with phorbol ester or interleukin-1 induces synthesis of collagenase and is neutralized by specific antiserum. *Journal of Clinical Investigation*, **87**, 1177–85.

Morales-Ducret, J., Wayner, E., Elices, M.J., Alvaro-Gracia, J.M., Zvaifler,N.J. and Firestein, G.S. (1992). Alpha 4/beta 1 integrin (VLA-4) ligands in arthritis. Vascular cell adhesion molecule-1 expression in synovium and on fibroblast-like synoviocytes. *Journal of Immunology*, **149**, 1424–31.

Moreland, L., DiBartolomeo, A. and Brick, J. (1988). Rheumatoid vasculitis with intrarenal aneurysm formation. *Journal of Rheumatology*, **15**, 845–9.

Moreland, L.W., Baumgartner, S.W., Schiff, M.H., Tindall, E.A., Fleischmann, R.M., Weaver, A.L. *et al.* (1997). Treatment of rheumatoid arthritis with a recombinant tumor necrosis factor receptor (p75)–Fc fusion protein. *New England Journal of Medicine*, **337**, 141–7.

Mottonen, M., Isomaki, P., Saario, R., Toivanen, P., Punnonen, J. and Lassila, O. (1998). Interleukin-10 inhibits the capacity of synovial macrophages to function as antigen-presenting cells. *British Journal of Rheumatology*, **37**, 1207–14.

Mukaida, N., Gussella, G.L., Kasahara, T., Ko, Y., Zacachariae, C.O.C. and Matsushima, K. (1992). Molecular analysis of the inhibition of interleukin-8 production by dexamethasone in a human fibrosarcoma cell line. *Immunology*, **75**, 674–9.

Mukaida, N., Morita, M., Ishikawa, Y., Rice, N., Okamoto, S., Kasahara, T. *et al.* (1994). Novel mechanism of glucocorticoid-mediated gene repression. Nuclear factor-κB is target for glucocorticoid-mediated interleukin 8 gene repression. *Journal of Biological Chemistry*, **269**, 13289–95.

Mulherin, D., FitzGerald, O. and Bresnihan, B. (1996). Synovial tissue macrophages and articular damage in rheumatoid arthritis. *Arthritis and Rheumatism*, **39**, 115–24.

Muller, W.A., Weigl, S.A., Deng, X. and Phillips, D.M. (1993). PECAM-1 is required for transendothelial migration of leucocytes. *Journal of Experimental Medicine*, **178**, 449–60.

Munro, J.M., Lo, S.K., Corless, C., Robertson, M.J., Lee, N.C., Barnhill, R.L. *et al.* (1992). Expression of sialyl-Lewis X, an E-selectin ligand, in inflammation, immune processes, and lymphoid tissues. *American Journal of Pathology*, **141**, 1397–408.

Murell, G.A.C., Jang, D. and Williams, R.J. (1995). Nitric oxide activates metalloprotease enzymes in articular cartilage. *Biochemical and Biophysical Research Communications*, **206**, 15–21.

Nakajima, T., Aono, H., Hasunuma, T., Yamamoto, K., Shirai, T., Hirohata, K. *et al.* (1995) Apoptosis and functional Fas antigen in rheumatoid arthritis synoviocytes. *Arthritis and Rheumatism*, **38**, 485–91.

Nakashima, M., Eguchi, K., Aoyagi, T., Yamashita, I., Ida, H., Sakai, M. *et al.* (1994). Expression of basic fibroblast growth factor in synovial tissues from patients with rheumatoid arthritis:

detection by immunohistlogical staining and *in situ* hybridisation. *Annals of the Rheumatic Diseases*, **53**, 45–50.

Nakashima, M., Yoshino, S., Ishiwata, T. and Asano, G. (1995). Role of vascular endothelial growth factor in angiogenesis of rheumatoid arthritis. *Journal of Rheumatology*, **22**, 1624–30.

Nepom, B.S. and Nepom, G.T. (1995). Polyglot and polymorphism. An HLA update. *Arthritis and Rheumatism*, **38**, 1715–21.

Newman, W., Beall, L.D. and Carson, L.W. (1993). Soluble endothelial–leukocyte adhesion mole-cule-1 (ELAM) is found in supernatants of activated endothelial cells *in vitro* and in serum of normal individuals. *Journal of Immunology*, **150**, 644–54.

Nicod, L.P. and Dayer, J.-M. (1999). Cytokines in the functions of dendritic cells, monocytes, macrophages and fibroblasts. In Theze, J. (ed.), *The Cytokine Network and Immune Functions*. Oxford University Press, Oxford, pp. 210–20.

Nishioka, K., Hasunuma, T., Kato, T., Sumida, T. and Kobata, T. (1998). Apoptosis in rheumatoid arthritis. A novel pathway in the regulation of synovial tissue. *Arthritis and Rheumatism*, **41**, 1–9.

Nuki, G., Rozman, B., Pavelka, K., Emery, P., Lookabaugh, J. and Musikic, P. (1997). Interleukin-1 receptor antagonist continues to demonstrate clinical improvement in rheumatoid arthritis. *Arthritis and Rheumatism*, **40**, S224.

Nusslein, H.G., Rodl, W., Giedel, J., Missmahl, M. and Kalden, J.R. (1987). Multiple peripheral pulmonary nodules preceding rheumatoid arthritis. *Rheumatology International*, **7**, 89–91.

Nyirkos, P. and Golds, E.E. (1990). Human synovial cells secrete a 39 kDa protein similar to a bovine mammary protein expressed during the non-lactating period. *Biochemical Journal*, **269**, 265–68.

Odink, K., Cerletti, N., Bruggen, J., Clerc, R.G., Tarcsay, L., Zwadlo, G. *et al.* (1987). Two calcium-binding proteins in infiltrate macrophages of rheumatoid arthritis. *Nature*, **330**, 80–2.

O'Hara, R., Murphy, E.P., Whitehead, A.S., FitzGerald, O. and Bresnihan, B. (2000). Acute phase serum amyloid A production by rheumatoid arthritis synovial tissue. *Arthritis Research*, **2**, 142–4.

Ojeda, V.J., Stuckey, B.G., Owen, E.T., Walters, M.N. (1986). Cardiac rheumatoid nodules. *Medical Jounal of Australia*, **144**, 92–3.

Okamoto, H., Yamamura, M., Morita, Y., Harada, S., Makino, H. and Ota, Z. (1997). The synovial expression and serum levels of interleukin-6, interleukin-11, leukemia inhibitory factor, and oncostatin M in rheumatoid arthritis. *Arthritis and Rheumatism*, **40**, 1096–105.

Paleolog, E.M., Hunt, M., Elliott, M.J., Feldmann, M., Breedveld, F.C., Maini, R.N. *et al.* (1996). Deactivation of the vascular endothelium by monoclonal anti-tumor necrosis factor α antibody in rheumatoid arthritis. *Arthritis and Rheumatism*, **39**, 1082–91.

Palmer, D.G., Hogg, N., Highton, J., Hessian, P.A. and Denholm, I (1987). Macrophage migration and maturation within rheumatoid nodules. *Arthritis and Rheumatism*, **30**, 729–36.

Pando, J.A., Duray, P., Yarboro, C., Gourley, M.F., Klippel, J.H. and Schumacher, H.R. (2000). Synovitis occurs in some clinically normal and asymptomatic joints in patients with early rheumatoid arthritis. *Journal of Rheumatology*, **27**, 1848–54.

Parente, L., Fitzgerald, M.F., Flower, R.J. and DeNucci, G. (1985a). The effect of glucocorticoids on lyso-PAF formation *in vitro* and *in vivo*. *Agents and Actions*, **17**, 312.

Parente, L. and Flower, R.J. (1985b). Hydrocortisone and 'macrocortin' inhibit the zymosan-induced release of lyso-PAF from rat peritoneal leucocytes. *Life Sciences*, **36**, 1225.

Patel, H., Fellowes, R., Coade, S. and Woo, P. (1998). Human serum amyloid A has cytokine-like properties. *Scandinavian Journal of Immunology*, **48**, 410–18.

Patel, K.D., Zimmerman, G.A., Prescott, S.M., McEver, R.P. and McIntyre, T.M. (1991). Oxygen radicals induce human endothelial cells to express GMP-140 and bind neutrophils. *Journal of Cell Biology*, **112**, 749–59.

Phillips, M.L., Nudelman, E., Gaeta, F.C., Perez, M., Singhal, A.K., Hakomori, S. *et al.* (1990). ELAM-1 mediates cell adhesion by recognition of a carbohydrate ligand, sialyl-Le^x. *Science*, **250**, 1130–2.

Pober, J.S., Slowik M.R., Deluca L.G., and Ritchie A.J. (1993). Elevated cyclic AMP inhibits endothelial cell synthesis and expression of TNF-induced endothelial leutocyte adhesion mole-cule-1, and vascular cell adhesion molecule-1, but not intercellular adhesion molecule-1, *Journal of Immunology*, **150**, 5114–23.

Qu, Z., Hernandes Garcia, C., O'Rourke, L.M., Planck, S.R., Kohli, M. and Rosenbaum, J.T. (1994). Local proliferation of fibroblast-like synoviocytes contributes to synovial hyperplasia. Results of proliferating cell nuclear antigen/cyclin, c-*myc,* and nuclear organizer region staining. *Arthritis and Rheumatism*, **37**, 212–20.

Qu, Z., Huang, X.-N,, Ahmadi, P., Andresevic, J., Planck, S.R., Hart, C.E. *et al.* (1995). Expression of basic fibroblast growth factor in synovial tissue from patients with rheumatoid arthritis and degenerative joint disease. *Laboratory Investigation*, **73**, 339–46.

Ralston, S.H., Todd, D., Helfrich, M., Benjamin, N. and Grabowski, P.S. (1994). Human osteoblast-like cells produce nitric oxide and express inducible nitric oxide synthase. *Endocrinology*, **135**, 330–6.

Ralston, S.H., Ho, L.P., Helfrich, M., Grabowski, P.S., Johnston, P.W. and Benjamin, N. (1995). Nitric oxide: a cytokine induced regulator of bone resorbtion. *Journal of Bone and Mineral Research*, **10**, 1040–9.

Read, M.A., Whitley, M.Z. and Collins, T (1994). NF-κB and Iκ-B: an inducible regulatory system in endothelial activation. *Journal of Experimental Medicine*, **179**, 503–12.

Redini, F., Mauviel, A., Pronost, S., Loyau, G. and Pujol, J.P. (1993). Transforming growth factor β exerts opposite effects from interleukin-1β on cultured rabbit articular chondrocytes through reduction of interleukin-1 receptor expression. *Arthritis and Rheumatism*, **36**, 44–50.

Ribbens, C., Dayer, J.-M. and Chizzolini, C. (2000). CD40–CD40 ligand (CD154) engagement is required but may not be sufficient for human T helper 1 cells' induction of interleukin-2-or inter-leukin-15-driven, contact-dependent, interleukin-1β production by monocytes. *Immunology*, **99**, 1–9.

Rifas, L. and Avioli, L.V. (1999). A novel T cell cytokine stimulates interleukin-6 in human osteoblastic cells. *Journal of Bone and Mineral Research*, **14**, 1096–103.

Ritchlin, C., Dwyer, E., Bucala, R. and Winchester, R. (1994). Sustained and distinctive patterns of gene activation in synovial fibroblasts and whole synovial tissue obtained from inflammatory synovitis. *Scandinavian Journal of Immunology*, **40**, 292–8.

Roivainen, A., Isomaki, P., Nikkari, S., Saario, R., Vuori, K. and Toivanen, P. (1995). Oncogene expression in synovial fluid cells in reactive and early rheumatoid arthritis: a brief report. British *Journal of Rheumatology*, **34**, 805–8.

Rooney, M., Whelan, A., Feighery, C. and Bresnihan, B. (1989). Changes in lymphocyte infiltration of the synovial membrane and the clinical course of rheumatoid arthritis. *Arthritis and Rheumatism*, **32**, 361–9.

Roth, J., Burwinkel, F., van den Bos, C., Goebeler, M., Vollmer, E. and Sorg, C. (1993). MRP8 and MRP14, S-100-like proteins associated with myeloid differentiation, are translocated to plasma membrane and intermediate filaments in a calcium-dependent manner. *Blood*, **82**, 1875–83.

Sack, U., Stiehl, P. and Geiler, G. (1994). Distribution of macrophages in rheumatoid synovial membrane and its association with basic activity. *Rheumatology International*, **13**, 181–186.

Sakurai, H., Kohsaka, H., Liu, M.-F,, Higashiyama, H., Hirata, Y., Kanno, K. *et al.* (1995). Nitric oxide production and inducible nitric oxide synthase expression in inflammatory arthritis. *Journal of Clinical Investigation*, **96**, 2357–63.

Salisbury, A.K., Duke, O. and Poulter, L.W. (1987). Macrophage-like cells of the pannus area in rheumatoid arthritic joints. *Scandinavian Journal of Rheumatology*, **16**, 263–72.

Sasaki, H., Pollard, R.B., Schmitt, D. and Suzuji, F. (1992). Transforming growth factor-β in the regulation of the immune response. *Clinical Immunology and Immunopathology*, **65**, 1–9.

Schlaghecke, R., Kornely, E., Wollenhaupt, J. and Specker, C. (1992). Glucocorticoid receptors in rheumatoid arthritis. *Arthritis and Rheumatism*, **35**, 740–4.

Schumacher, H.R. and Kitridou, R.C. (1972). Synovitis of recent onset. A clinicopathologic study during the first month of disease. *Arthritis and Rheumatism*, **15**, 465–85.

Schuurs, A.H.W.M. and Verheul, H.A.M. (1990). Effects of gender and sex steroids on the immune response. *Journal of Steroid Biochemistry*, **35**, 157–72.

Schwab, J.H., Anderle, S.K., Brown, R.R., Dalldorf, F.G. and Thompson, R.C. (1991). Pro-and anti-inflammatory roles of interleukin-1 in recurrence of bacterial cell wall-induced arthritis in rats. *Infection and Immunity*, **59**, 4436–42.

Seitz, M., Dewald, B., Gerber, N. and Baggiolini, M. (1991). Enhanced production of neutrophil-activating peptide-1/IL-8 in rheumatoid arthritis. *Journal of Clinical Investigation*, **87**, 463.

Seitz, M., Zwicker, M., Pichler, W. and Gerber, N. (1992). Activation and differentiation of myelomonocytic cells in rheumatoid arthritis and healthy individuals—evidence for antagonistic *in vitro* regulation by interferon-γ and tumor necrosis factor α, granulocyte monocyte colony stimulating factor and interleukin 1. *Journal of Rheumatology*,**19**, 1038–44.

Seitz, M., Loetscher, P., Dewald, B., Towbin, H., Ceska, M. and Baggiolini, M. (1994). Production of interleukin-1 receptor antagonist, inflammatory chemotactic proteins, and prostaglandin E by rheumatoid and osteoarthritic synoviocytes—regulation by IFN-γ and IL-4. *Journal of Immunology*, **152**, 2060–5.

Seth, R., Raymond, F.D. and Makgoba, M.W. (1991). Circulating ICAM-1 isoforms: diagnostic prospects for inflammatory and immune disorders. *Lancet*, **388**, 83–4.

Shaw, G. and Kamen, R. (1986). A conserved AU sequence from the 3′ untranslated region of GM-CSF mRNA mediates selective mRNA degradation. *Cell*, **46**, 659–67.

Shimoyama, Y., Nagafuchi, H., Suzuki, N., Ochi, T. and Sakane, T. (1999). Synovium infiltrating T cells induce excessive synovial cell function through CD28/B7 pathway in patients with rheumatoid arthritis. *Journal of Rheumatology*, **26**, 2094–101.

Shingu, M., Fujikawa, Y., Wada, T., Nonaka, S. and Nobunaga, M. (1995). Increased IL-1 receptor antagonist (IL-1ra) production and decreased IL-1β/IL-1ra ratio in mononuclear cells from rheumatoid arthritis patients. *British Journal of Rheumatology*, **34**, 24–30.

Shiozawa, S., Shiozawa, K. and Fujita, T. (1983). Morphologic observations in the early phase of the cartilage pannus junction. Light and electron microscopic studies of active cellular pannus. *Arthritis and Rheumatism*, **26**, 472–8.

Smeets, T.J., Kraan, M.C., Versendaal, J., Breedveld, F.C. and Tak, P.P. (1999). Analysis of serial synovial biopsies in patients with rheumatoid arthritis: description of a control group without clinical improvement after treatment with interleukin 10 or placebo. *Journal of Rheumatology*, **26**, 2089–93.

Smith, M.D., Ahern, M.J., Brooks, P.M. and Roberts-Thomson, P.J. (1988). The clinical and immunological effects of pulse methylprednisolone therapy in rheumatoid arthritis. III. Effects on immune and inflammatory indices in synovial fluid. *Journal of Rheumatology*, **15**, 238–41.

Soden, M., Rooney, M., Cullen, A., Whelan, A., Feighery, C. and Bresnihan, B. (1989). Immunohistological features in the synovium obtained from clinically uninvolved knee joints of patients withn rheumatoid arthritis. British *Journal of Rheumatology*, **28**, 287–92.

Soden, M., Rooney, M., Whelan, A., Feighery, C. and Bresnihan, B. (1991). Immunohistological analysis of the synovial membrane: search for predictors of the clinical course in rheumatoid arthritis. *Annals of the Rheumatic Diseases*, **50**, 673–6.

Springer, T.A. (1994). Traffic signals for lymphocyte recirculation and leukocyte emigration: the multistep paradigm. *Cell*, **76**, 301–14.

Stastny, P. (1978). Association of the B cell alloantigen DRw4 with rheumatoid arthritis. *New England Journal of Medicine*, **298**, 869–71.

Staunton, D.E., Marlin, S.D., Stratowa, C., Dustin, M.L. and Springer, T.A. (1988). Primary structure of ICAM-1 demonstrates interaction between members of the immunoglobulin and integrin supergene families. *Cell*, **52**, 925–33.

Sthoeger, Z.M., Chiorrazi, N. and Lahita, R.G. (1988). Regulation of the immune response by sex hormones. I. *In vitro* effects of estradioland testosterone on pokeweed mitogen-induced human B cell differentiation. *Journal of Immunology*, **141**, 91–8.

Stichtenoth, D.O. and Frohlich, J.C. (1998). Nitric oxide and inflammatory joint diseases. *British Journal of Rheumatology*, **37**, 246–57.

Sugiyama, E., Kuroda, A., Taki, H., Ikemoto, M., Hori, T., Yamashita, N. *et al.* (1995). Interleukin 10 cooperates with interleukin 4 to suppress inflammatory cytokine production by freshly prepared adherent rheumatoid synovial cells. *Journal of Rheumatology*, **22**, 2020–6.

Sumida, T., Hoa, T.T.M., Asahara, H., Hasunuma, T. and Nishioka, K. (1997). T cell receptor of Fas-sensitive T cells in rheumatoid synovium. *Journal of Immunology*, **158**, 1965–70.

Szekanecz, S., Haines, G.K., Lin, T.R., Harlow, L.A., Goerdt, S., Rayan, G. *et al.* (1994). Differential distribution of intercellular adhesion molecules (ICAM-1, ICAM-2, and ICAM-3) and the MS-1 antigen in normal and diseased human synovia. Their possible pathogenetic and clinical significance in rheumatoid arthritis. *Arthritis and Rheumatism*, **37**, 221–31.

Szekanecz, S., Haines, G.K., Harlow, L.A., Shah, M.R., Fong, T.W., Fu, R. *et al.* (1995a). Increased synovial expression of the adhesion molecules CD66a, CD66b, and CD31 in rheumatoid and osteoarthritis. *Clinical Immunology and Immunopathology*, **76**, 180–6.

Szekanecz, Z., Haines, G.K., Harlow, L.A., Shah, M.R., Fong, T.W., Fu, R. *et al.* (1995b). Increased synovial expression of TGF-β receptor endoglin and TGF-β1 in rheumatoid arthritis. *Clinical Immunology and Immunopathology*, **76**, 187–94.

Tak, P.P., Smeets, T.J.M., Boyle, D.L., Kraan, M.C., Shi, Y., Zhuang, S. *et al.* (1999). p53 overexpression in synovial tissue from patients with early and longstanding rheumatoid arthritis compared with patients with reactive arthritis and osteoarthritis. *Arthritis and Rheumatism*, **42**, 948–53.

Taki, H., Sugiyama, E., Mino, T., Kuroda, A. and Kobayashi, M. (1998). Differential inhibitory effects of indomethacin, dexamethasone, and interferon-γ (IFN-γ) on IL-11 production by rheumatoid synovial cells. *Clinical and Experimental Immunology*, **112**, 133–8.

Taylor, D.J. (1994). Cytokine combinations increase p75 tumor necrosis factor receptor binding and stimulate receptor shedding in rheumatoid synovial fibroblasts. *Arthritis and Rheumatism*, **37**, 232–5.

Taylor, P.C., Peters, A.M., Paleolog, E., Chapman, P.T., Elliott, M.J., McCloskey, R.V. *et al.* (2000). Reduction of chemokine levels and leukocyte traffic to joints by tumor necrosis factor α blockade in patients with rheumatoid arthritis. *Arthritis and Rheumatism, 43,* 38–47.

Teigelkamp, S., Bhardwaj, R.S., Roth, J., Meinardus-Hager, G., Karas, M. and Sorg, C. (1991). Calcium-dependent complex assembly of the myeloid differentiation proteins in MRP-8 and MRP-14. *Journal of Biological Chemistry,* **266,** 13462–7.

Tessier, P., Audette, M., Cattaruzzi, P. and McColl, S.R. (1993). Up-reguation by tumor necrosis factor α of intercellular adhesion molecule 1 expression and function in synovial fibroblasts and its inhibition by glucocorticoids. *Arthritis and Rheumatism,* **36,** 1528–39.

Tessier, P., Cattaruzzi, P. and McColl, S.R. (1996). Inhibition of lymphocyte adhesion to cytokine activated synovial fibroblasts by glucocorticoids involves the attenuation of vascular cell adhesion molecule 1 and intercellular adhesion molecule 1 gene expression. *Arthritis and Rheumatism,* **39,** 226–34.

Thomas, R., Davis, L.S. and Lipsky, P.E. (1994). Rheumatoid synovium is enriched in mature antigen-presenting dendritic cells. *Journal of Immunology,* **152,** 2613–23.

Tomita, T., Kashiwagi, M., Shimaoka, Y., Ikawa, T., Tanabe, M., Nakagawa, S. *et al.* (1994). Phenotypic characteristics of bone marrow cells in patients with rheumatoid arthritis. *Journal of Rheumatology,* **21,** 1608–14.

Tomita, T., Shimaoka, Y., Kashiwagi, N., Hashimoto, H., Kawamura, S., Lee, S.B. *et al.* (1997). Enhanced expression of CD14 antigen on myeloid lineage cells derived from the bone marrow of patients with severe rheumatoid arthritis. *Journal of Rheumatology,* **24,** 465–9.

Trabandt, A., Gay, R.E. and Gay, S. (1992). Oncogene activation in rheumatoid synovium. *Acta Pathologica, Microbiologica et Immunologica Scandinavica,* **100,** 861–75.

Trontzas, P., Kamper, E.F., Potamianou, A., Kyriazis, N.C., Kritikos, H. and Stavridis, J. (1998). Comparative study of serum and synovial fluid interleukin-11 levels in patients with various arthritides. *Clinical Biochemistry,* **31,** 673–9.

Tsurufuji, S., Kurihara, A., Kiso, S., Suzuki, Y. and Ohuchi, K. (1984). Dexamethasone inhibits generation in inflammatroy sites of the chemotactic activity attributable to leukotriene B4. *Biochemical and Biophysical Res earch Communications,* **119,** 884–90.

Ulfgren,, A.-K,, Lindblad, S., Klareskog, L., Anderson, J. and Anderson, U. (1995). Detection of cytosine-producing cells in the synovial membrane from patients with rheumatoid arthritis. *Annals of the Rheumatic Diseases,* **54,** 654–61.

Ulfgren, A.-K., Grondal, L., Lindblad, Khademi, M.S., Johnell, O., Klareskog, L. and Andersson U. (2000). Inter-individual and intra-articular variation of proinflamatory cytokines in patients with rheumatoid arthritis: potential implications for treatment. *Annals of the Rheumatic Diseases,* **59,** 439–7.

van Beuningen, H.M., van der Kraan, P.M., Arntz, O.J. and van den Berg, W.B. (1993). Protection from interleukin 1 induced destruction of articular cartilage by transforming growth factor β: studies in anatomically intact cartilage *in vitro* and *in vivo. Annals of Rheumatic Diseases,* **52,** 185–91.

van Dinther-Janssen, A.C.H.M., Horst, E., Koopman, G., Newmann, W., Scheper, R.J., Meijer, C.J.L.M. *et al.* (1991). The VLA4/VCAM-1 pathway is involved in lymphocyte adhesion to endothelium in rheumatoid synovium. *Journal of Immunology,* **147,** 4207.

van Leeuwen, M.A., van der Heijde, D.M.F.M., van Rijswijk, M.H., Houtman, P.M., van Riel, P.M., van de Putte, L.B. *et al.* (1994). Interrelationship of outcome measures and process variables in early rheumatoid arthritis. A comparison of radiologic damage, physical disability, joint counts and acute phase reactants. *Journal of Rheumatology*, **21**, 425–9.

van Roon, J.A., van Roy, J.L., Gmelig-Meyling, F.H., Lafeber, F.P. and Bijlsma, J.W. (1996). Prevention and reversal of cartilage degradation in rheumatoid arthritis by interleukin-10 and interleukin-4. *Arthritis and Rheumatism*, **39**, 829–35.

Verhoef, C.M., van Roon, J.A., Vianen, M.E., Lafeber, F.P. and Bijlsma, J.W (1999). The immune suppressive effect of dexamethasone in rheumatoid arthritis is accompanied by upregulation of interleukin 10 and by differential changes in interferon γ and interleukin 4 production. *Annals of the Rheumatic Diseases*, **58**, 49–54.

Vey, E., Zhang, J.H. and Dayer, J.-M. (1992). IFN-γ and 1,25(OH)2D3 induce on THP-1 cells distinct patterns of cell surface antigen expression, cytokine production, and responsiveness to contact with activated T cells. *Journal of Immunology*, **149**, 2040–26.

Volin, M.V., Shah, M.R., Tokuhira, M., Haines, G.K., Woods, J.M. and Koch, A.E. (1998). RANTES expression and contribution to monocyte chemotaxis in arthritis. *Clinical Immunolology and Immunopathology*, **89**, 44–53.

Vollertsen, R.S. and Conn, D.L. (1990). Vasculitis associated with rheumatoid arthritis. *Rheumatic Disease Clinics of North America*, **16**, 445–61.

Vonderheide, R.H. and Springer, T.A. (1992). Lymphocyte adhesion through very late antigen 4: evidence for a novel binding site in the alternatively spliced domain of vascular cell adhesion molecule 1 and an additional α4 integrin counter-receptor on stimulated endothelium. *Journal of Experimental Medicine*, **175**, 1433–42.

Voraberger, G., Schafer, R. and Stratowa, C. (1991). Cloning of the human gene for intercellular adhesion molecule 1 and analysis of its 5′-regulatory region: induction by cytokines and phorbol ester. *Journal of Immunology*, **147**, 2777–86.

Voskuyl, A.E., Martin, S., Melchers, I., Zwinderman, A.H., Weichselbraun, I. and Breedveld, F.C. (1995). Levels of circulating intercellular adhesion molecule-1 and -3 but not endothelial leucocyte molecule are increased in patients with rheumatoid vasculitis. *British Journal of Rheumatology*, **34**, 311–5.

Wahl, S.M., Allen, J.B., Costa, G.L., Wong, H.L. and Dasch, J.R. (1993). Reversal of acute and chronic synovial inflammation by anti-transforming growth factor β. *Journal of Experimental Medicine*, **177**, 225–30.

Walker, W.C. and Wright, V. (1968). Pulmonary lesions and rheumatoid arthritis. *Medicine*, **47**, 501.

Walmsley, M., Butler, D.M., Marinova-Mutafchieva, L. and Feldmann, M. (1998). An anti-inflammatory role for interleukin-11 in established murine collagen-induced arthritis. *Immunology*, **95**, 31–7.

Walmsley, M., Katsikis, P.D., Abney, E., Parry, S., Williams, R.O., Maini, R.N. *et al*. (1996). Interleukin-10 inhibition of the progression of established collagen-induced arthritis. *Arthritis and Rheumatism*, **39**, 495–503.

Walsh, D.A., Sledge, C.B. and Blake, D.R. (1995). Biology of the normal joint. In Kelley, W.N., Harris, E.D., Ruddy, S. and Sledge, C. (ed.), *Textbook of Rheumatology*. W.B. Saunders Co., pp. 1–22.

Walters, M.T., Smith, J.L., Moore, K., Evans, P.R. and Cawley, M.I.D. (1987). An investigation of the action of disease modifying antirheumatic drugs on the rheumatoid synovial membrane: reduction in T lymphocyte subpopulations, and HLA-DP and DQ antigen expression after gold or penicillamine therapy. *Annals of the Rheumatic Diseases*, **46**, 7–16.

Walz, G., Aruffo, A., Kolanus, W., Bevilacqua, N. and Seed, B. (1990). Recognition by ELAM-1 of the sialyl-Lex determinant on myeloid and tumor cells. *Science*, **250**, 1132–5.

Weinblatt, M.E., Kremer, J.M., Bankhurst, A.D., Bulpitt, K.J., Fleischmann, R.M., Fox, R.I. *et al.* (1999). A trial of etanercept, a recombinant tumor necrosis factor receptor:Fc fusion protein, in patients with rheumatoid arthritis receiving methotrexate. *New England Journal of Medicine*, **340**, 253–9.

Weller, A., Isenmann, S. and Vestweber, D. (1992). Cloning of the mouse endothelial selectins. Expression of both E- and P-selectin is inducible by tumor necrosis factor α. *Journal of Biological Chemistry*, **267**, 15176–83.

Wells, A.L. (1969). Extra-articular manifestations of rheumatoid arthritis. *British Medical Journal*, **4**, 173.

Wikaningrum, R., Highton, J., Parker, A., Coleman, M., Hessian, P.A., Roberts-Thompson, P.J. *et al.* (1998). Pathogenic mechanisms in the rheumatoid nodule: comparison of proinflammatory cytokine production and cell adhesion molecule expression in rheumatoid nodules and synovial membranes from the same patient. *Arthritis and Rheumatism*, **41**, 1783–97.

Wilkinson, L.S., Pitsillides, A.A., Worrall, J.G. and Edwards, J.C.W. (1992). Light microscopic characterization of the fibroblast-like synovial intimal cell (synoviocyte). *Arthritis and Rheumatism*, **35**, 1179–184.

Wolfe, A.M. (1968). The epidemiology of rheumatoid arthritis: a review. *Bulletin of Rheumatic Diseases*, **19**, 518–23.

Wood, N.C., Dickens, E., Symons, J.A. and Duff, G.W. (1992a). *In situ* hybridization of inter-leukin-1 in CD14-positive cells in rheumatoid arthritis. *Clinical Immunology and Immunopathology*, **62**, 295–300.

Wood, N.C., Symons, J.A., Dickens, E. and Duff, G.W. (1992b). *In situ* hybridization of IL-6 in rheumatoid arthritis. *Clinical and Experimental Immunology*, **87**, 183–9.

Woods, J.M., Haines, G.K., Shah, M.R., Rayan, G. and Koch, A.E. (1997). Low-level production of interleukin-13 in synovial fluid and tissue from patients with arthritis. *Clinical Immunology and Immunopathology*, **85**, 210–20.

Wooley, P.H., Dutcher, J., Widmer, M.B. and Gillis, S. (1993). Influence of a recombinant human soluble tumor necrosis factor receptor Fc fusion protein on type II collagen-induced arthritis in mice. *Journal of Immunology*, **151**, 6602–7.

Yamamato, K.R. (1985). Steroid receptor regulated transcription of specific genes and gene net-works. *Annual Review of Genetics*, **19**, 209–52.

Yang, Y.H., Hutchinson, P., Santos, L.L. and Morand, E.F. (1998). Glucocorticoid inhibition of adjuvant arthritis synovial macrophage nitric oxide production: role of lipocortin 1. *Clinical and Experimental Immunology*, **111**, 117–22.

Yanni, G., Whelan, A., Feighery, C. and Bresnihan, B. (1992). Analysis of cell populations in rheumatoid arthritis synovial tissues. *Seminars in Arthritis and Rheumatism*, **21**, 393–9.

Yanni, G., Whelan, A., Feighery, C. and Bresnihan, B. (1994a). Synovial tissue macrophages and joint erosion in rheumatoid arthritis. *Annals of the Rheumatic Diseases*, **53**, 39–44.

Yanni, G., Farahat, N.M.M.R., Poston, R.N. and Panayi, G.S. (1994b). Intramuscular gold decreases cytokine expression and macrophage numbers in the rheumatoid synovial membrane. *Annals of the Rheumatic Diseases*, **53**, 315–22.

Young, C.L., Adamson, T.C., III, Vaughan, J.H. and Fox, R.I. (1984). Immunologic characteriza-tion of synovial membrane lymphocytes in rheumatoid arthritis. *Arthritis and Rheumatism*, **27**, 32–9.

Youssef, P.P., Roberts-Thomson, P.J., Ahern, M.J. and Smith, M.D. (1995). Pulse methylpred-nisolone in rheumatoid arthritis: effects on peripheral blood and synovial fluid neutrophil surface phenotype. *Journal of Rheumatology*, **22**, 2065–71.

Youssef, P.P., Cormack, J., Evill, C.A., Peter, D.T., Roberts-Thomson, P.J., Ahern, M.J. *et al.* (1996a). Neutrophil trafficking into inflamed joints in rheumatoid arthritis and the effect of methylprednisolone. *Arthritis and Rheumatism*, **39**, 216–225.

Youssef, P.P., Triantafillou, S., Parker, A., Coleman, M., Roberts-Thomson, P.J., Ahern, M.J. *et al.* (1996b). Effects of pulse methylprednisolone on cell adhesion molecules in the synovial mem-brane in rheumatoid arthritis: reduced E-selectin and ICAM-1 expression. *Arthritis and Rheumatism*, **39**, 1970–9.

Youssef, P.P., Haynes, D., Triantafillou, S., Parker, A., Gamble, J., Coleman, M. *et al.* (1997). Effects of pulse methylprednisolone on proinflammatory mediators in peripheral blood, syn-ovial fluid and the synovial membrane in rheumatoid arthritis. *Arthritis and Rheumatism*, **40**, 1400–8.

Youssef, P.P., Roth, J., Frosch, M., Costello, P., FitzGerald, O., Sorg, C. *et al.* (1999). Expression of myeloid related proteins (MRP) 8 and 14 and the MRP 8/14 heterodimer in rheumatoid arthritis synovial membrane. *Journal of Rheumatology*, **26**, 2523–8.

Zvaifler, N.J., Tsai, V., Alsalameh, S., von Kempis, J., Firestein, G.S. and Lotz, M. (1997). Pannocytes: distinctive cells found in rheumatoid arthritis articular cartilage erosions. *American Journal of Pathology*, **150**, 1125–38.

10 *Macrophages in wound healing*

L.A. DiPietro and R.M. Strieter

1 Introduction

Normal wound repair requires the coordinated response of numerous cell types, including fibroblasts, keratinocytes, leukocytes and endothelial cells. These cells participate in an interwoven process, which includes chemotaxis, phagocytosis, mitogenesis, neovascularization and extracellular matrix (ECM) synthesis. The repair response can be viewed as four overlapping phases of hemostasis, inflammation, proliferation and resolution (Figure 10.1). Hemostasis, beginning immediately after injury, involves vasoconstriction and the formation of the fibrin clot. The inflammatory phase, marked by the influx of leukocytes, begins within hours after injury and continues for several days. The proliferative phase is paramount to the healing process, as it includes the period of active protein synthesis, cell replication and differentiation. During resolution, dynamic remodeling of the new connective tissue occurs, in tandem with a physical regression of many of the recently formed capillaries. The four phases are interdependent, and alterations within one can dramatically affect the progression of repair.

A salient feature of normal wound repair is the initial development of an acute inflammatory reaction. The inflammatory phase in wounds is characterized by the

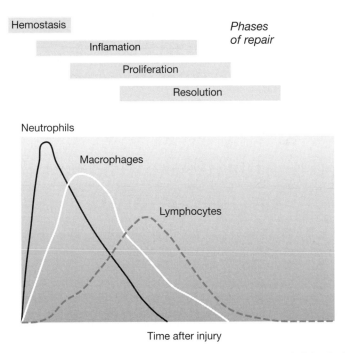

Fig. 10.1 The pattern of inflammatory cell movement into healing wounds (chart), shown in relation to the four phases of wound healing (top). Neutrophils are the first to arrive at the site of injury, and enter the wound as early as 2 h after injury. Neutrophils phagocytose debris and guard against infection by removing microbial contamination. Macrophages, derived primarily from circulating monocytes, become the predominant inflammatory cell type during the early proliferative phase of repair. Macrophages phagocytose apoptotic cells, and produce cytokines and growth factors to mediate repair. Lymphocytes, primarily T cells, enter the wound in abundance only during later phases of repair, and may contribute to the resolution of wound healing.

sequential infiltration of neutrophils, monocyte/macrophages and lymphocytes (Figure 10.1; see also Ross and Benditt, 1962). Although neutrophils are the first leukocyte in the wound, these cells are not necessary for normal wound healing (Simpson and Ross, 1972). In contrast, the tissue macrophage is believed to be particularly critical to wound healing (Leibovich and Ross, 1975).

Within the first few days after injury, circulating monocytes are recruited into the wound where they differentiate into macrophages, becoming the predominant leukocyte in the wound by day 5 (Ross and Odland, 1968). After arrival in the wound, macrophages become activated, engage in phagocytosis of debris and produce factors that regulate tissue repair (Hunt *et al.*, 1984). Macrophage-derived factors amplify the inflammatory response, and also direct the subsequent angiogenesis, fibroproliferation and deposition of ECM molecules that are requisite for appropriate repair (Clark *et al.*, 1976). The array of bioactive factors produced by wound macrophages is broad, and includes cytokines, non-protein inflammatory mediators, components of the ECM, proteinases and anti-proteinases (Rappolee *et al.*, 1988; Fukasawa *et al.*, 1989; Porras-Reyes *et al.*, 1991; Stricklin *et al.*, 1994; DiPietro *et al.*, 1996). With the appreciation that macrophages are pivotal in normal wound repair, this chapter will focus on the role of this cell in the healing of injured tissues.

2 Evidence for the importance of macrophages in wound repair

A role for leukocytes in promoting wound healing was first proposed by Dr Alexis Carrel in the early 20th century, when he demonstrated that *in vitro*, leukocytes produce factors that enhance cellular proliferation (Carrel, 1922). It was not until 1975, however, that the first direct evidence for a role for a specific leukocyte, the macrophage, was described in a wound model. In studies performed in guinea pigs, Leibovich and Ross (1975) showed that depletion of monocytes and macrophages caused significantly delayed wound repair, including a decreased clearance of fibrin and neutrophils, decreased fibroblast proliferation and immature fibrosis. This finding documented a link between inflammatory cells and tissue repair and, conceptually, was novel and exciting. Studies to demonstrate the growth-promoting properties of the macrophage then quickly followed. Activated macrophages and their conditioned media were shown to promote angiogenesis (Polverini *et al.* 1977; Koch *et al.* 1986), and wound macrophages themselves were shown to elaborate factors that stimulated both angiogenesis and collagen synthesis (Clark *et al.*, 1976; Hunt *et al.*, 1984). Today, more than 25 years after the studies of Leibovich and Ross, the role of the macrophage as an instrument of tissue repair remains an enticing area of investigation. Recent studies in new model systems provide continued support for the theory that macrophage function is critical to wound healing. For example, mice that are genetically deficient for the endothelial adhesion molecules P-selectin and E-selectin exhibit a marked decrease in wound macrophages, and demonstrate impaired wound healing (Subramanian *et al.*, 1997). New investigations further define the role of macrophages in healing, particularly for specific macrophage-derived growth factors. In some instances, certain growth factors and cytokines, such as transforming growth factor-α (TGF-α), have been shown to be dispensable for normal repair (Luettke *et al.*, 1993). As additional studies in sophisticated transgenic and knockout strains are completed, the role of the macrophage in wound healing is likely to emerge as more complex than previously imagined.

3 Monocyte recruitment into wounds

Monocyte recruitment into wounds, followed by subsequent differentiation into tissue macrophages, relies upon the sequential steps of endothelial cell activation, cell–cell interaction and migration into tissues. This movement depends upon adherence to the endothelium, as well as the establishment of a local haptotactic and chemotactic gradient for monocytes. At first glance, the rate of infiltration of each particular subpopulation of leukocyte would be expected to be proportional to the circulating leukocyte composition. Indeed, neutrophils comprise 60–70 per cent of circulating leukocytes and, as anticipated, the initial influx of cells into the wound is primarily neutrophilic. However, monocytes, which represent only about 3 per cent of circulating leukocytes, soon become the predominant inflammatory cell within wounds (Figure 10.2) (Ross and Odland, 1968). The preferential infiltration of monocytes into wounds probably results from a combination of selective endothelial adherence and a local haptotactic and chemotactic gradient that specifically favors these monocytes.

What factors within the wound attract this large number of monocytes? Certainly the array of monocyte chemoattractants within the wound is complex, as multiple types and sources of chemoattractants are present. Injury itself initiates the clotting cascade, causes

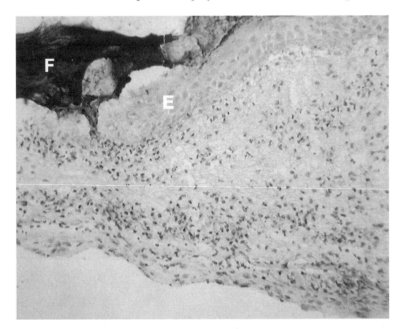

Fig. 10.2 Macrophage infiltration into a murine full-thickness excisional dermal wound at 3 days after injury. Immunohistochemical identification demonstrates abundant darkly staining macrophages within the wound bed. The number of macrophages reaches a peak at approximately 3 days after injury in this model. The locations of the advancing epithelium (E) and fibrin clot (F) are indicated.

platelet degranulation and activates complement. These initial events generate several leukocyte chemoattractants, including platelet-derived factors and complement split products. The early chemotactic factors are short lived, reaching maximum levels during hemostasis and prior to maximum monocyte infiltration. During the inflammatory phase of healing, monocyte recruitment is likely to be mediated by chemoattractants that are produced locally by both resident and newly recruited cells in the wound.

In the last decade, more than 50 leukocyte chemoattractant cytokines have been identified in human and murine systems (Keane and Strieter, 1999; Lukacs *et al.*, 1999). These cytokines are collectively termed chemokines, and are potent chemotactic factors for neutrophils, eosinophils, basophils, monocytes, mast cells, dendritic cells, natural killer (NK) cells, T and B lymphocytes. The chemokines constitute a group of related small proteins that display highly conserved cysteine amino acid residues. The chemokines are subdivided into four families on the basis of whether non-conserved amino acid residues separate the first two cysteine amino acids in the primary structure of the protein. The CXC chemokine family has the first two N-terminal cysteines separated by one non-conserved amino acid residue; the CC chemokine family has the first two N-terminal cysteines in juxtaposition; the C chemokine has one lone N-terminal cysteine amino acid; and the CX_3C chemokine has the first two N-terminal cysteines separated by three non-conserved amino acid residues. There is approximately 20–40 per cent homology between the members of the four chemokine families.

Chemokines have been found to be produced by an array of cells including monocytes, macrophages, neutrophils, platelets, eosinophils, mast cells, T and B lymphocytes, NK cells, keratinocytes, mesangial cells, epithelial cells, hepatocytes, fibroblasts, smooth muscle cells, mesothelial cells and endothelial cells. These cells can produce chemokines in response to a variety of factors, including viruses, bacterial products and cytokines. The production of chemokines by both immune and non-immune cells has been documented in numerous inflammatory conditions, and chemokines play a critical role in the recruitment of leukocytes and the pathology of several inflammatory diseases. Taken together, these findings support the contention that these cytokines may be pivotal in orchestrating inflammation in many circumstances, including the wound.

A number of studies have examined the expression and function of CC chemokines in healing wounds (Fahey *et al.*, 1990; DiPietro *et al.*, 1995, 1998; Yoak *et al.*, 1997; Gibran *et al.*, 1997). Two key CC chemokines, monocyte chemotactic protein-1 (MCP-1) and macrophage inflammatory protein-1α (MIP-1α), have been demonstrated to have distinct patterns of expression during wound repair. In a murine model of excisional wounds, MCP-1 protein levels peak at day 1, whereas MIP-1α levels are found to peak at day 3, coincident with maximum macrophage levels. Within wounds, a major cellular source for the CC chemokines is the tissue macrophage (DiPietro *et al.*, 1995, 1998). Resident and recruited macrophages appear to be instrumental in the subsequent recruitment of macrophages to the wound site (Cushing and Fogelmann, 1992; Fahey *et al.*, 1992). This concept has been substantiated recently in a murine model system. Antibody neutralization of MIP-1α resulted in a decrease in the number of wound macrophages, and also yielded a marked delay in the wound healing response. Among CC chemokines, then, MIP-1α may play a critical role in macrophage recruitment during wound repair (DiPietro *et al.*, 1998). However, the sheer redundancy of these cytokines, and their ability to recruit different subsets of leukocytes, suggest that the interplay of chemokines in wound repair may be quite complex.

4 Activation of macrophages in wounds

While recruitment of macrophages to the wound is important, the subsequent activation of macrophages is also critical to their function in mediating wound repair. Many mediators and environmental factors within the wound influence macrophage phenotype and activation status. One obvious circumstance that affects macrophages in wounds is hypoxia. As initially proposed by Hunt and colleagues, hypoxic conditions, such as those within wounds, induce changes in macrophage phenotype and protein expression (Knighton *et al.*, 1983; Lewis *et al.*, 1999). Macrophages are well adapted to survive under hypoxic conditions, and indeed have been shown to exhibit enhanced secretory activity under such circumstances. Early studies demonstrated that the exposure of macrophages to hypoxia stimulated the production of pro-angiogenic activity (Knighton *et al.*, 1983). Later studies have documented that the exposure of macrophages to hypoxic conditions leads to enhanced expression of specific growth factors and cytokines that may be important in the reparative process. Hypoxia induces the production of the angiogenic factor vascular endothelial growth factor (VEGF), as well as the angiogenic/fibrogenic factors fibroblast growth factor (FGF)-1, FGF-2 and platelet-derived growth factor (PDGF) (Kuwabara *et al.*, 1995; Xiong *et al.*, 1998). Exposure of macrophages to hypoxia also induces the production of several chemokines, including interleukin (IL)-8 and MIP-1α (Metinko *et al.*, 1992; VanOtteren *et al.*, 1995).

One macrophage function which appears to be inhibited, rather than stimulated, by hypoxia is phagocytosis (Simon *et al.*, 1991; Leeper-Woodford *et al.*, 1992). Since phagocytosis is an important function of the wound macrophage, this inhibition might be perceived as detrimental to wound repair. This dilemma magnifies the need to consider that macrophage phenotype is unlikely to be uniform throughout the wound. Within the hypoxic central area of a wound, macrophage activity may focus on the production of proliferative and chemoattractant factors. At the relatively oxygen-rich periphery, phagocytic function may dominate. Proliferative and chemoattractant factors would diffuse from the central wound to the surrounding tissue, inducing a wave of cellular migration and proliferation into the wound bed. Along the periphery, macrophages would clear the way for this proliferative response through active phagocytosis of dead cells and debris. Although this concept is appealing, documentation of such functional subpopulations of macrophages within wounds is not yet available.

The evidence that tissue hypoxia provides an important stimulus to wound macrophages is certainly strong. Yet other mediators within the wound also provide a dynamic modulation of macrophage function. Pro-inflammatory factors, such as tumor necrosis factor-α (TNF-α) and nitric oxide (NO), are present within the wound, as well as CC chemokines; these factors can stimulate monocytes. In particular, the CC chemokines may play a dual role in the wound, both recruiting and activating monocytes and macrophages. Recent studies in other systems suggest that chemokine cross-talk may be important in orchestrating the inflammatory response and its resolution (Chensue *et al.*,

1997; Tessier *et al.*, 1997). The actions of specific CC chemokines are sometimes compartmentalized into leukocyte-activating and chemoattractant activities. For example, in transgenic mice that express MCP-1 in lung alveolar epithelial cells, a second inflammatory signal by an additional CC chemokine is required to initiate activation of leukocytes (Gunn *et al.*, 1997). Theoretically then, specific chemokines may function primarily as an activating agent or a chemoattractant within the wound. Studies of the role of MIP-1α demonstrate that this CC chemokine plays an important role in the recruitment of monocytes (DiPietro *et al.*, 1998). Yet, for the most part, compartmentalization of chemokine activity has not yet been described in the context of tissue repair.

5 The wound macrophage phenotype

As indicated above, the spectrum of activating agents within wounds is complex but distinctive. The wound macrophage is therefore subjected to a unique activation pattern as a result of residence in the wound environment. Several recent studies have shown that wound macrophages are phenotypically distinct from other macrophage populations. When compared with resident peritoneal macrophages, wound-derived macrophages exhibit a decreased capacity to generate reactive oxygen intermediates (Nessel *et al.*, 1999). Wound macrophage production of NO has been shown to be modulated by the wound environment, and varies during the course of repair. Macrophages present in the early wound appear to produce high levels of inducible nitric oxide synthase (iNOS), whereas macrophages in the later phases of wound repair have been found to have reduced ability to express iNOS and produce NO (Reichner *et al.*, 1999).

Other evidence suggests that the development of phenotypic characteristics important within the wound, including the production of angiogenic, fibrogenic and inflammatory mediators, is exquisitely dependent upon the stimulus. For example, limited *in vitro* studies suggest that the manner of activation influences the pattern of production of angiogenic cytokines by macrophages. Macrophages activated by interferon-γ (IFN-γ) exhibit a pattern of expression of angiogenic factors different from macrophages activated by IL-4 and glucocorticoid (Kodelja *et al.*, 1997). This differential angiogenic activity has been defined further in functional tests. Co-cultivation of macrophages activated by IL-4 and glucocorticoid with endothelial cells was shown to induce endothelial cell proliferation at a rate approximately threefold higher than co-culture with IFN-γ activated macrophages.

The above studies suggest that the phenotype of wound macrophages is dependent upon the wound environment. Unfortunately, the specific phenotype of wound macrophages *in situ*, particularly within different locations within the wound, has not yet been investigated rigorously. This lack of *in situ* analysis is a limitation of our understanding of wound macrophage function. Many of the current concepts regarding macrophage function in wounds are derived from the study of either non-wound macrophages or macrophages that have been isolated from wounds as a total population, and subsequently subjected to tissue culture conditions. Improved *in situ* analysis will refine our knowledge of the wound macrophage phenotype.

6 The function of macrophages in wounds

6.1 Macrophage phagocytic activity in wounds

One important function of the wound macrophage is active phagocytosis. As wounds heal, new proteins are synthesized, cells replicate as necrotic tissue and apoptotic cells are removed from the site of injury. When neutrophils enter the wound, they are short lived, soon become apoptotic and subsequently are removed by phagocytosis. The efficient removal of both apoptotic cells and extracellular debris from wounds is performed primarily by macrophages (Leibovich and Ross, 1975).

Macrophage recognition and phagocytosis of senescent neutrophils is mediated by at least three characterized receptor–ligand pairs: (1) a lectin receptor with specificity for monosaccharides; (2) an integrin receptor complex with specificity for thrombospondin; and (3) a lipid receptor with specificity for phophatidylserine (Savill *et al.*, 1993). Wound macrophages, as opposed to peritoneal macrophages, appear to utilize a specific subset of these receptor–ligand pairs to recognize and phagocytose senescent neutrophils (Meszaros *et al.*, 1999). Blocking either surface lectins or the integrin receptor inhibits phagocytosis of apoptotic neutrophils by wound macrophages, while blockade of the phosphatidylserine-specific receptor has no effect on phagocytosis. In contrast, only blockade of the integrin receptor inhibits phagocytosis of apoptotic neutrophils by activated peritoneal macrophages; blockade of the other two receptors has no effect in this population. The functional importance of this change in receptor use is not yet understood. Nevertheless, the findings support the concept that the phenotype of wound macrophages is unique to this environment.

6.2 Modulation of angiogenesis by wound macrophages

During the granulation and proliferative phases of wound repair, neovascularization is exuberant and provides nutrient support for tissue regeneration. Many studies have shown that the wound macrophage is intimately involved in the stimulation of capillary growth.

Much of the current information regarding macrophage-derived pro-angiogenic factors comes from experiments performed *in vitro* with activated non-wound-derived macrophages. These studies have shown that activated macrophages produce more than 20 factors that influence endothelial cell growth, migration or morphology *in vitro*, and/or angiogenesis *in vivo* (Table 10.1) (Sunderkötter *et al.*, 1991; Keane and Strieter, 1999). Some of these mediators are known to be produced *in situ* by wound macrophages, including IL-1, TGF-α, TGF-β, PDGF, epidermal growth factor (EGF), CXC chemokines, VEGF and insulin-like growth factor-1 (IGF-1) (Rappolee *et al.*, 1988; Fahey *et al.*, 1990; Abe *et al.*, 1991; Whitby and Ferguson, 1991; Brown *et al.*, 1992). Although these studies document that wound macrophages are a source of pro-angiogenic factors, other cell types such as keratinocytes, neutrophils, eosinophils and lymphocytes have also been described to produce pro-angiogenic mediators in wounds (Brown *et al.*, 1992; Zhao *et al.*, 1993; Freeman *et al.* 1995; Hubner *et al.*, 1996). Along with multiple cellular sources, the ECM provides an additional source of growth factors. Growth factors with heparin-binding domains, such as FGF-2, are found sequestered within the ECM of normal tissue. The release of these factors after injury may contribute to the angiogenic environment (Gajdusek and Carbon, 1989). Thus, macrophages, non-

Table 10.1   Macrophage products that influence angiogenesis

1   Positive mediators
     Insulin-like growth factor-1 (IGF-1)
     Transforming growth factor-α (TGF-α)
     Basic fibroblast growth factor (FGF-2)
     Angiotropin
     Platelet-derived growth factor (PDGF)
     Platelet-derived growth factor-like compounds
     Vascular endothelial growth factor (VEGF)
     Interleukin-6 (IL-6)
     Prostaglandins
     ELR$^+$ CXC chemokines (e.g. IL-8 and ENA-78)
     Interleukin-10 (IL-10)
2   Mediators that have been observed to be both positive and negative
     Tumor necrosis factor-α (TNF-α)
     Interleukin-1(IL-1)
     Transforming growth factor-β (TGF-β)
3   Negative mediators
     Interferon-α, interferon-γ
     Thrombospondin 1 (TSP1)
     Interferon-inducible ELR$^-$ CXC chemokines (e.g. IP-10 and MIG)

macrophage cell types and growth factors sequestered in the ECM are each likely to make a substantial contribution to promoting angiogenesis in the wound.

The large number of potential pro-angiogenic factors in wounds implies that wound angiogenesis is regulated by a highly redundant and complex mechanism. Wound fluids, which are believed to be representative of the soluble milieu of wounds, contain at least eight different angiogenic factors (Cromack *et al.*, 1987; Ford *et al.*, 1989; Matsuoka and Grotendorst, 1989; Dvonch *et al.*, 1992). Surprisingly, recent studies suggest that just two factors, FGF-2 and VEGF, account for the majority of the pro-angiogenic stimulus in human wound fluids (Gupta *et al.*, 1996; Nissen *et al.*, 1996, 1998). Wound fluid obtained immediately after injury contains high levels of FGF-2; antibody neutralization of FGF-2 leads to a significant reduction in the capacity of this early fluid to stimulate endothelial cell proliferation, chemotaxis and *in vivo* angiogenesis. Because this fluid is derived at a time when macrophages are relatively rare in the wound, macrophages are unlikely to be a significant source of this initial pro-angiogenic stimulus. In late wound fluids, high levels of VEGF but low levels of FGF-2 are observed (Nissen *et al.*, 1998). In these late fluids, antibody neutralization of VEGF, but not FGF-2, nearly eliminates the pro-angiogenic capacity. Histological studies demonstrate that both macrophages and keratinocytes are prominent sources of VEGF in wounds, strongly suggesting that VEGF is a significant pro-angiogenic factor of wound macrophages. (Brown *et al.*, 1992; Nissen *et al.*, 1998).

VEGF production by macrophages within the wound may be regulated by multiple mechanisms. As mentioned above, hypoxia induces macrophage VEGF production, and thus the hypoxic environment of the wound may be important for inducing the local expression of VEGF (Shweiki *et al.*, 1992; Xiong *et al.*, 1998). VEGF synthesis and bioactivity are also regulated by lactate levels (Zabel *et al.*, 1996; Xiong *et al.*, 1998). Under conditions of hypoxia within the wound, the generation of high levels of lactate may induce the production of macrophage angiogenic activity. The wound macrophage, responding to hypoxia and lactate, generates pro-angiogenic factors until tissue oxygen and lactate levels have returned to normal.

In addition to hypoxia and lactate, NO also plays a role in regulating the activity of macrophage-derived VEGF. If the iNOS pathway is blocked, production of angiogenic activity by human monocytes is inhibited (Leibovich *et al.*, 1994). *In vivo*, suppression of iNOS production either by genetic deficiency or by treatment with iNOS inhibitors leads to severely impaired wound healing (Yamasaki, *et al.*, 1998; Stallmeyer *et al.*, 1999). However, the relevance of these *in vivo* studies specifically to macrophage function is not direct, since many other cell types within wounds, such as keratinocytes, also depend upon iNOS for proper function (Frank *et al.*, 1995; Krischel *et al.*, 1998).

Another group of angiogenic factors that are likely to influence wound capillary growth is the CXC chemokines. Although the CXC chemokines were identified originally on the basis of their chemoattractant activity, substantial evidence demonstrates that members of this family of chemokines directly modulate both physiological and pathological angiogenesis (Keane and Strieter, 1999). The CXC family of cytokines can be subdivided on the basis of the presence or absence of a Glu–Leu–Arg (ELR) motif preceding the first cysteine in the N-terminus. CXC chemokines that contain this motif (ELR⁺) exhibit significant pro-angiogenic activity. CXC chemokines that lack this motif (ELR⁻) and are interferon inducible are instead angiostatic. In healing wounds, a shift towards the production of angiogenic, ELR⁺ chemokines has been observed to coordinate with the proliferative phase of wound healing (Fivenson *et al.*, 1997). Although CXC chemokines are neutrophil chemoattractants, the angiogenic activity of the ELR⁺ CXC chemokines is distinct and dominates in the proliferative phase of wound healing. Levels of the ELR⁺ CXC chemokines peak well after maximal neutrophil infiltration and during maximal granulation tissue formation. Additional evidence for a potential role for the CXC chemokines in wound healing comes from studies of mice that constituitively express IP-10 in keratinocytes (Luster *et al.*, 1998). The overexpression of IP-10, an ELR⁻ interferon-inducible chemokine, causes significantly impaired wound healing in these mice. The wounds of IP-10-overexpressing mice displayed a more intense wound inflammation, coupled with a prolonged granulation tissue phase with impaired capillary development.

The pro-angiogenic environment of the proliferative phase eventually gives way to vascular regression. During resolution, nearly half of the newly formed capillaries regress through controlled apoptosis of existing endothelial cells (Ross and Benditt, 1962; Swift *et al.*, 1999). This suggests that perhaps an anti-angiogenic stimulus arises in the resolving wound. Macrophages may play a role in vascular regression, as this cell produces substances that are inhibitory to endothelial cell growth, including thrombospondin, ELR⁻ CXC chemokines and other less well-defined inhibitors (Jaffe *et al.*, 1985; Polverini, 1989; DiPietro and Polverini, 1993; Xiong, 1998). The role of macrophage-derived anti-angiogenic agents in wounds is highly speculative, and only minimal evidence for this concept is available currently (Polverini, 1989). However, the production of high levels of ELR⁻ CXC chemokines has been associated with a decrease in the wound proliferative response (Fivenson *et al.*, 1997). If the tissue macrophage serves as a mediator of both angiogenesis and vascular regression, a phenotypic change from a 'reparative-proliferation' profile to an 'anti-proliferative-regression' profile must occur as wound repair progresses. Additional investigations in this unexplored area would be relevant not only to normal wound repair, but also to situations in which cellular proliferation and connective tissue production are dysregulated, such as solid tumors and hypertrophic scars.

6.3 Modulation of fibrogenesis by wound macrophages

Wound macrophages influence fibrosis in a number of ways (Kovacs and DiPietro, 1994). Several macrophage-derived growth factors, such as TGF-β and PDGF, can stimulate fibroblast proliferation and collagen synthesis directly. Additionally, macrophages themselves can produce ECM components such as fibronectin, thrombospondin and other proteoglycans (Jaffe *et al.*, 1985; Nathan, 1987). Macrophages also produce numerous molecules which affect the degradation of the ECM and the wound proteinase:anti-proteinase balance, such as metalloproteinases, proteinase activators and tissue inhibitors of metalloproteinases (Fukasawa *et al.*, 1989; Welgus *et al.*, 1990; Porras-Reyes, 1991; Falcone *et al.*, 1993). These studies suggest that the wound macrophage is an active participant in the remodeling of the ECM.

Macrophage function in the wound is pleiotropic (Figure 10.3). The inter-relationships between different macrophage capabilities can be illustrated by considering the complex modulation of the wound ECM composition by macrophages. As described above, macrophages affect the eventual tissue composition of ECM both directly and indirectly. Because endothelial cell proliferation, migration and capillary formation are critically dependent upon the specific composition of the ECM, the influence of the macrophage on the ECM may directly affect angiogenesis (Ingber and Folkman, 1989). In the context of the wound, macrophages could influence angiogenesis both by production of angiogenic regulatory factors and by the modification of the ECM. Stated a different way, macrophage regulation of fibrosis influences angiogenesis, and vice versa. The inter-relationships of the many potential capacities of the wound macrophage makes it difficult to decipher precisely which functions are critical. Whether or not the macrophage is a key regulator of each of these many interwoven events is not yet known.

7 Augmentation of wound healing by alteration of macrophage function

The unique role of the macrophage in wound healing suggests that augmenting macrophage activity or the recruitment of additional macrophages would lead to markedly improved wound repair. The ability to promote macrophage function in the wound has been attempted previously by several different strategies, including the placement of additional macrophages directly into wounds, the stimulation of macrophage function with known activating agents and the direct application of purified growth factors or cytokines known to be produced by macrophages. Most of these studies have been performed at the preclinical level, but a few have reached the clinical arena.

7.1 Addition of macrophages directly to the wound

Originally, injection of macrophages into the wound of aged mice was shown to correct the age-related deficit in wound healing (Danon *et al.*, 1989). These studies have been extended to evaluate the application of autologous macrophages as a therapy for poorly healing human wounds. Monocyte-derived macrophages, obtained from peripheral blood,

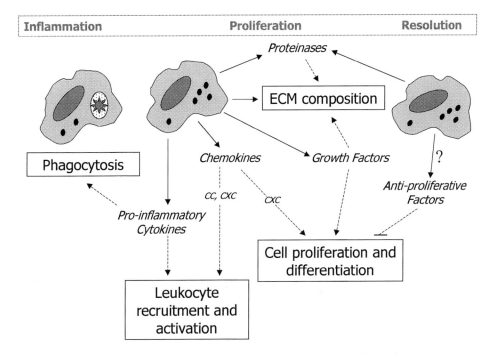

Fig. 10.3   The mutliple roles of the macrophage in the healing wound. Macrophages serve many functions within the healing wound, influencing the inflammatory, proliferative and perhaps the resolution phases of this process. Collectively, macrophages engage in all of the portrayed activities, while individual macrophages within the wound may display more limited functional attributes. Solid arrows indicate synthesis of mediators. Dashed arrows represent positive mediator effects. Dashed lines with a bar represent negative mediator effects. Speculative paths are indicated with a question mark.

have been shown to improve the healing of decubital ulcers in patients (Danon *et al.*, 1997). Similarly, the effect of adding macrophages to spinal cord injury has been examined in animal models. The implantation of autologous macrophages, pre-activated with autologous regenerative nerve, has been shown to promote the repair of transected spinal cords (Schwartz *et al.*, 1999). However, other studies have implicated the macrophage in the mediation of the acute secondary damage of spinal cord injury (Popovich *et al.*, 1999). These differences in outcome once again hint that macrophages have multiple functional capacities. The predominant effect may depend largely upon the specific manner of activation.

7.2 Addition of macrophage-stimulating agents or products directly to the wound

Due to the fact that impaired wound repair is a major clinical problem, there has been significant interest by the pharmaceutical industry in the development of agents to enhance wound healing. More than 100 published studies have described the enhancement of wound repair in a variety of animal models via the addition of either cytokines, growth factors or other substances. For some agents, the wound macrophage has been shown to mediate the pharmacological effect.

One of the first well-documented pharmacological treatments of wounds was the topical application of the macrophage-activating agent glucan (Leibovich and Danon, 1980; Browder *et al.*, 1988). Glucans are polymers of β-1,3-linked glucose, and have been demonstrated to affect numerous parameters of macrophage function, as macrophages express surface receptors for polysaccharides. Glucan treatment of wounds led to increased numbers of macrophages, and promoted fibroplasia, re-epithelialization and wound strength.

The application of specific recombinant proteins has also been examined. PDGF application has been demonstrated to have a beneficial effect on wound healing in many pre-clinical and clinical studies, and is now commercially available for clinical use to promote the repair of non-healing wounds. PDGF seems to exert its positive effect largely through the augmentation of macrophage function (Mustoe *et al.*, 1989; Pierce *et al.*, 1989). The application of PDGF augments healing of incisional wounds in rats, and this enhancement is dependent upon the recruitment of macrophages to the injury site. When rats were subjected to total body irradiation, wound macrophages were eliminated, and PDGF application had no beneficial effect. In contrast, if rats were subjected only to surface irradiation, macrophage presence in the wound was appropriate, and PDGF treatment was effective at improving repair.

More recently, the application of macrophage colony-stimulating factor was shown to accelerate wound repair via enhanced macrophage function (Wu *et al.*, 1997). The topical or systemic administration of granulocyte–macrophage colony-stimulating factor also increases the rate of wound repair, presumably by stimulation of macrophage function (Jyung *et al.*, 1994). These studies provide encouragement for the continued investigation of the use of macrophages themselves and macrophage-derived cytokines and chemokines in the treatment of recalcitrant wounds.

8 Macrophage function in special wound healing situations

Alterations in wound macrophage function are observed commonly in situations of either inadequate or hyperproliferative repair. An examination of macrophage function in aberrant repair emphasizes the importance of balanced macrophage function. If macrophage infiltration and function within the wound is extreme, a fibrotic response may ensue. Conversely, decreased macrophage infiltration or function can yield a poor reparative response.

8.1 Fetal wounds

Tissue repair in adults is often imperfect, resulting in scar formation. In contrast, wound healing in young embryos occurs rapidly, and generally without scar formation. This divergence in the repair process of the fetus and adult has attracted great attention, as a further understanding of fetal repair might be expected to provide strategies to improve wound healing in an adult. Many differences between fetal and adult repair have been documented, including changes in the manner of wound re-epithelialization, cellular composition, ECM deposition and levels of growth factors (Whitby and Ferguson, 1991; Martin *et al.*, 1993; Nodder and Martin, 1997). The inflammatory response, including macrophage infiltration, has also been shown to be significantly decreased in fetal injury.

In early embryos, platelets are absent from the wound, and both macrophage and neutrophil infiltration are greatly reduced (Adzick *et al.*, 1985; Hopkinson-Woolley *et al.*, 1994; Cowin *et al.*, 1998). Because macrophages and platelets are a prominent source of growth factors in adult wounds, the extremely efficient embryonic repair that occurs despite their relative absence remains puzzling. One explanation may be that tissue repair in the embryo is more similar to a developmental process, whereas, in adults, the inflammatory process takes center stage.

Along with the relative lack of an inflammatory response in fetal wounds, a tandem decrease in many growth factors has been observed. Remarkably, the conspicuous absence of a single growth factor, TGF-β_1, has been shown to be highly significant. Synthesis of TGF-β_1 is quite limited in the fetus, and is performed primarily by epithelial and mesenchymal cells rather than inflammatory cells (Whitby and Ferguson, 1991; Martin *et al.*, 1993). The significance of this limited expression has been demonstrated in a number of exciting studies. The addition of exogenous TGF-β_1 to fetal wounds causes a fibrotic reaction (Krummel *et al.* 1988; Lin *et al.*, 1995). Conversely, neutralization of TGF-β_1 in adult wounds yields a substantial decrease in wound scar formation (Shah *et al.*, 1992). Macrophages and several other cell types within the adult wound can produce TGF-β_1. Therefore, the specific importance of macrophage-derived TGF-β_1 to the development of scar formation in adults is not yet known. Interestingly, another member of the TGF-β family, TGF-β_3, seems to show a reverse effect, i.e. application of exogenous TGF-β_3 can reduce scarring in adult animals (Shah *et al.*, 1995).

8.2 Aging

The finding that the wounds of aged persons heal much more slowly than those of young adults is widely appreciated, having been documented in a written scientific report as early as 1916 (Du Noüy, 1916). Studies in both humans and animal model systems demonstrate age-related defects in wound re-epithelialization, angiogenesis and deposition of ECM (Holm-Pederson and Zederfeldt, 1971; Holt *et al.* 1992; Ashcroft *et al.*, 1997a; Swift *et al.*, 1999). In human cutaneous wounds, monocyte and macrophage infiltration has been described to be delayed with aging (Ashcroft *et al.*, 1998). The altered infiltration pattern seen with age is coupled with a change in the functional capacity of reparative macrophages. A large body of *in vitro* evidence suggests that, when compared with macrophages from young animals, macrophages of aged animals exhibit differences in both phagocytosis and the production of cytokines. Many of these alterations could theoretically cause a shift in the wound repair process. One connection between age-related changes in macrophages and those observed in wound repair concerns the impaired angiogenic response of aged animals (Reed *et al.*, 1998; Swift *et al.*, 1999). Aged mice exhibit delayed wound angiogenesis, in tandem with a reduction in several growth factors, including TGF-β_1, FGF-2 and VEGF. The decrease in wound VEGF is believed to derive from reduced macrophage capacity, as macrophages from aged mice produce significantly less of the pro-angiogenic mediator VEGF (Swift *et al.*, 1999). This information, in concert with studies showing that wound healing of aged animals is improved when additional macrophages are applied (Danon *et al.*, 1989), suggests that diminished macrophage function plays a role in the diminished healing response seen with age.

The influence of estrogen on macrophages may also play a role in the observed age-related changes in wound healing. Recent studies have shown that wound repair in healthy females is strongly influenced by estrogen levels, with decreased estrogen levels being associated with a delay in repair (Ashcroft *et al.*, 1997b). Hormone replacement therapy can enhance the rate of repair in post-menopausal females. This enhanced healing comes at the expense of increased scar formation, which is probably mediated by increased levels of TGF-β_1. Since macrophage function can be influenced directly by estrogen, a role for the macrophage in the estrogen-related changes in repair remains an intriguing possibility (Frazier-Jessen *et al.*, 1995).

8.3 Diabetes

Delayed wound healing is a frequent problem in patients suffering from diabetes. Many factors contribute to this delay, including hyperglycemia, decreased vascularity and tissue oxygenation, decreased growth factor levels and changes in proteinase profiles. Not surprisingly, the inflammatory response is also altered in diabetic wounds (Fahey *et al.*, 1991). An altered macrophage phenotype in diabetics has been proposed recently (Doxey *et al.*, 1998). Exposure of normal macrophages to low-density lipoprotein cholesterols and triglycerides has been shown to cause a generalized decrease in cytokine production (Chu *et al.*, 1999). These studies suggest that the serum lipid abnormalities common in diabetics can influence macrophage function and depress the healing response in diabetic individuals. Wound healing in diabetics can be greatly improved through the topical application of growth factors such as PDGF, which may assist the repair process by recruitment of inflammatory cells to the wound site (Brown *et al.*, 1994).

8.4 Fibrosis

The idea that macrophages promote fibrosis in the wound is supported by several models of pro-fibrotic diseases. For example, in a murine model of peritoneal fibrotic adhesions, fibrotic lesions develop in direct correlation to the presence of macrophages (Frazier-Jessen *et al.*, 1996). In this model, an overexpression of the CC chemokine MCP-1, and subsequent increase in macrophage infiltration, have been shown to correlate with the fibrotic response. Numerous studies of bleomycin-induced pulmonary fibrosis demonstrate the importance of the macrophage in this disease state (Smith *et al.*, 1994, 1996). These studies have defined the importance of the CC chemokines MCP-1 and MIP-1α in recruiting macrophages to the lung in this fibrotic reaction.

8.5 Trauma, hemorrhage and sepsis

Patients who experience significant traumatic events, including hemorrhage, burns or sepsis, frequently display impaired wound healing, exhibiting decreased collagen accumulation and an increase in wound healing complications (McGinn, 1973; Diegelmann *et al.*, 1986). Recent studies in animal models have documented changes in the function of peripheral macrophages, including diminished antigen presentation and decreased production of the inflammatory mediators soon after trauma/hemorrhage (McCarter *et al.*, 1998). Similarly, several studies have documented differences in peripheral monocyte/macrophage function as a result of sepsis (Ayala *et al.*, 1996). Although alterations in the function of the wound macrophage *in situ* following severe traumatic insults have not been well studied, altered cytokine production by macrophages has been implicated in the observed delay in repair (Angele *et al.*, 1999). Correction of the alteration in monocyte and macrophage function might provide an opportunity for enhancing the repair response in trauma victims.

9 Summary

The tissue macrophage has been shown to play a critical role in the wound healing process. Macrophages are essential phagocytes within the wound, and are responsible for the removal of apoptotic and dying cells. Via the production of bioactive substances, including pro-inflammatory cytokines, growth factors, proteinases and chemokines, macrophages dictate many of the inflammatory, proliferative and regenerative processes within the wound. Many circumstances of altered healing include a component of altered wound macrophage function. The application of substances to wounds that are intended to modify macrophage activity, or mimic macrophage function, will continue to demonstrate the importance of macrophages in the healing wound.

Acknowledgments

This work was supported by NIH Grants GM50875 (L.A.D.), GM 55238 (L.A.D.), CA87879 (R.M.S.), HL66027 (R.M.S.), PO1 HL67665 (R.M.S.), and P50 CA90388 (R.M.S.).

References

Abe, H., Rodgers, K.E., Ellefson, D. and DiZerega, G.S. (1991). Kinetics of interleukin-1 and tumor necrosis factor secretion by rabbit macrophages recovered from the peritoneal cavity after surgery. *Journal of Investigative Surgery*, **4**, 141–51.

Adzick, N.S., Harrison, M.R., Glick, P.L., Beckstead, J.H., Villa, R.L., Scheuenstuhl H. *et al.* (1985). Comparison of fetal, newborn, and adult wound healing by histologic, enzyme-histochemical, and hydroxyproline determinants. *Journal of Pediatric Surgery*, **20**, 315–9.

Angele, M.K. Knöferl, M.W., Ayala, A., Albina, J.E., Cioffi, W.G., Bland, K.I. *et al.* (1999). Trauma-hemorrhage delays wound healing potentially by increasing pro-inflammatory cytokines at the wound site. *Surgery*, **126**, 279–85.

Ashcroft, G.S., Horan, M.A. and Ferguson, M.W.J. (1997a). Aging is associated with reduced deposition of specific extracellular matrix components, an upregulation of angiogenesis and an altered inflammatory response in a murine incisional wound healing model. *Journal of Investigative Dermatology*, **108**, 430–7.

Ashcroft, G.S., Dodsworth, J., van Boxtel, E., Tarnuzzer, R.W., Horan, M.A., Schultz. G.S. *et al.* (1997b). Estrogen accelerates cutaneous wound healing associated with an increase in TGF-β1 levels. *Nature Medicine*, **3**, 1209–15.

Ashcroft, G.S., Horan, M.A. and Ferguson, M.W.J. (1998). Aging alters the inflammatory and endothelial cell adhesion molecule profiles during human cutaneous wound healing. *Laboratory Investigation*, **78**, 47–58.

Ayala, A., Urbanich, M.A., Herdon, C.D. and Chaudry, I.H. (1996). Is sepsis-induced apoptosis associated with macrophage dysfunction?. *Journal of Trauma-Injury Infection and Critical Care*, **40**, 568–73

Browder, W., Williams, D., Lucore, P., Pretus, H., Jones, E. and McNamee, R. (1988). Effect of enhanced macrophage function on early wound healing. *Surgery*, **104**, 224–30.

Brown, L.F., Yeo, K.T., Berse, B., Yeo, T., Senger, D.R., Dvorak, H.F. *et al.* (1992). Expression of vascular permeability factor (vascular endothelial growth factor) by epidermal keratinocytes during wound healing. *Journal of Experimental Medicine*, **176**, 1375–9.

Brown, R.L., Breeden, M.P. and Greenhalgh, D.G. (1994). PDGF and TGF-α act synergistically to improve wound healing in the genetically diabetic mouse. *Journal of Surgical Research*, **56**, 562–70.

Carrel, A. (1922). Growth-promoting function of leucocytes. *Journal of Experimental Medicine*, **36**, 385–91.

Chensue, S.W., Warmington, K., Ruth, J.H., Lukacs, N. and Kunkel, S.L. (1997). Mycobacterial and schistosomal antigen illicited granuloma formation in IFN γ and IL-4 knockout mice: analysis of local and regional cyokine and chemokine networks. *Journal of Immunology*, **159**, 3565–73.

Chu, X., Newman, J., Park, B., Nares, S., Ordonez, G. and Iacopino, A.M. (1999). *In vitro* alteration of macrophage phenotype and function by serum lipids. *Cell and Tissue Research*, **296**, 331–7.

Clark, R.A., Stone, R.D., Leung, D.Y.K., Silver, I., Hohn, D.C. and Hunt, T.K. (1976). Role of macrophages in wound healing. *Surgery Forum*, **27**, 16–8.

Cowin, C.J., Brosnan, M.P., Holmes, T.M. and Ferguson, M.W.J. (1998). Endogenous inflammatory response to dermal wound healing in the fetal and adult mouse. *Developmental Dynamics*, **212**, 385–93.

Cromack, D.T., Sporn, M.B., Roberts, A.B., Merino, M.F., Dart, L.L. and Norton, J.A. (1987). Transforming growth factor-β levels in rat wound chambers. *Journal of Surgical Research*, **42**, 622–8.

Cushing, S.D. and Fogelman, A.M. (1992). Monocytes may amplify their recruitment into inflammatory lesions by inducing monocyte chemotactic protein. *Arteriosclerosis Thrombosis*, **12**, 78–82.

Danon, D., Kowatch, M.A. and Roth, G.S. (1989). Promotion of wound repair in old mice by local injection of macrophages. *Proceeding of the National Academy of Sciences USA*, **86**, 2018–20.

Danon, D., Madjar, J., Edinov, E., Knyszynski, A., Brill, S., Diamantshtein, L. and Shinar, E. (1997). Treatment of human ulcers by application of macrophages prepared from a blood unit. *Experimental Gerontology*, **32**, 633–41.

Diegelmann, R.F., Lindblad, W.J. and Cohen, I.K. (1986). A subcutaneous implant for wound healing studies in humans. *Journal of Surgical Research* **40**, 229–37.

DiPietro, L.A. and Polverini, P.J. (1993). Angiogenic macrophages produce the angiogenic inhibitor thrombospondin 1. *American Journal of Pathology*, **143**, 678–84.

DiPietro, L.A., Polverini, P.J., Rahbe, S.M and Kovacs, E.J. (1995). Modulation of JE/MCP-1 expression in dermal wound repair. *American Journal of Pathology*, **146**, 868–75.

DiPietro, L.A., Nissen, N.N., Gamelli, R.L. Koch, A.E., Pyle, J.M. and Polverini, P.J. (1996). Thrombospondin 1 synthesis and function in wound repair. *American Journal of Pathology*, **148**, 1851–9.

DiPietro, L.A., Burdick, M., Low, Q.E., Kunkel, S.L. and Strieter, R.M. (1998). MIP-1α as a critical macrophage chemoattractant in wound repair. *Journal of Clinical Investigation*, **101**, 1693–8.

Doxey, D.L., Nares, S., Park, B., Trieu, C., Cutler, C.W. and Iacopino, A.M. (1998). Diabetes-induced impairment of macrophage cytokine release in a rat model: potential role of serum lipids. *Life Sciences*, **63**, 1127–36.

Du Noüy, P.L. (1916). Cicatrization of wounds. III. The relation between the age of the patient, the area of the wound, and the index of cicatrization. *Journal of Experimental Medicine* **24**, 461–70.

Dvonch, V.M., Murphey, R.J., Matsuoka, J. and Grotendorst. G.R. (1992). Changes in growth factor levels in human wound fluid. *Surgery*, **112**, 18–23.

Fahey, T.J., Sherry, B., Tracey, K.J., van Deventer, S., Jones, W.G., Minei, J.P. *et al.* (1990). Cytokine production in a model of wound healing: the appearance of MIP-1, MIP-2, cachectin/TNF and IL-1. *Cytokine*, **2**, 92–9.

Fahey, T.J., Sadaty, A., Jones, W.G., Barber, A., Smoller, B. and Shires, G.T. (1991). Diabetes impairs the late inflammatory response to wound healing. *Journal of Surgical Research* **50**, 308–13.

Fahey, T.J., Tracey, K.J., Tekamp-Olson, P., Cousens, L.S., Jones, W.G., Shires, G.T. *et al.* (1992). Macrophage inflammatory protein 1 modulates macrophage function. *Journal of Immunolology*, **148**, 2764–9.

Fivenson, D.P., Faria, D.T., Nickoloff, B.J., Polverini, P.J., Kunkel, S., Burdick, M. *et al.* (1997). Chemokine and inflammatory cytokine changes during chronic wound healing. *Wound Repair and Regeneration*, **5**, 310–22.

Falcone, D.J., McCaffrey, T.A., Haimovitz-Friedman, A. and Garcia, M. (1993). Transforming growth factor-β1 stimulate macrophage urokinase expression and release of matrix-bound basic fibroblast growth factor. *Journal of Cell Physiology*, **155**, 595–605.

Ford, H.R., Hoffman, R.A., Wing, E.J., Magee, M., McIntyre, L. and Simmons, R.L. (1989). Characterization of wound cytokines in the sponge matrix model. *Archives of Surgery*, **124**, 1422–8.

Frank, S., Hubner, G., Breier, G., Longaker, M.R., Greenhalgh, D.G. and Werner, S. (1995). Regulation of vascular endothelial growth factor expression in cultured keratinocytes. *Journal of Biology and Chemistry*, **270**, 12607–13.

Frazier-Jessen, M.R. and Kovacs, E.J. (1995). Estrogen modulation of JE/monocyte chemoattractant protein mRNA expression in murine macrophages. *Journal of Immunology*, **154**, 1838–45.

Frazier-Jessen, M.R., Mott, F.J., Witte, P.L. and Kovacs, E.J. (1996). Estrogen suppression of connective tissue deposition in a murine model of peritoneal adhesions formation. *Journal of Immunology*, **156**, 3036–42.

Freeman, M.R., Schneck, F.X., Gagnon, M.L., Corless, C., Soker, S., Niknejad, K. *et al.* (1995). Peripheral blood T lymphocytes and lymphocytes infiltrating human cancers express vascular endothelial growth factor: a potential role for T cells in angiogenesis. *Cancer Research*, **55**, 4140–5.

Fukasawa, M., Campeau, J.D., Yanagihara, D.L., Rodgers, K.E. and DiZerega, G.S. (1989). Mitogenic and protein synthetic activity of tissue repair cells: control by the postsurgical macrophage. *Journal of Investigative Surgery*, **2**, 169–80.

Gajdusek, C.M. and Carbon, S. (1989). Injury-induced release of basic fibroblast growth factor from bovine aortic endothelium. *Journal of Cell Physiology*, **139**, 570–9.

Gibran, N.S., Ferguson, M., Heimbach, D.M. and Isik, F.F. (1997). Monocyte chemoattractant protein-1 mRNA expression in the human burn wound. *Journal of Surgical Research*, **70**, 1–6.

Gunn, M.D., Nelken, N.A., Liao, X. and Williams, L.T. (1997). Monocyte chemoattractant protein-1 is sufficient for the chemotaxis of monocytes and lymphocytes in transgenic mice but requires an additional stimulus for inflammatory activation. *Journal of Immunology*, **158**, 376–83.

Gupta, V.K., McNeil, P.L., Riegner, C. and Howdieshell, T.R. (1996). Vascular endothelial growth factor is a key mediator of omental angiogenesis. *Surgery Forum*, **47**, 746–9.

Holm-Pederson, P. and Zederfeldt, B.. (1971). Granulation tissue formation in subcutaneously implanted cellulose sponges in young and old rats. *Scandinavian Journal of Plastic and Reconstructive Surgery*, **5**, 13–6.

Holt, D.R., Kirk, S.J., Regan, M.C., Hurson, M., Lindblad, J. and Barbul, A. (1992). Effect of age on wound healing in healthy human beings. *Surgery*, **112**, 293–8.

Hopkinson-Woolley, J., Hughes, D., Gordon, S. and Martin, P. (1994). Macrophage recruitment during limb development and wound healing in the embryonic and fetal mouse. *Journal of Cell Science*, **107**, 1159–67.

Hubner, G., Brauchle, M., Smola, H., Madlener, M., Fassler, R and Werner, S. (1996). Differential regulation of pro-inflammatory cytokines during wound healing in normal and glucocorticoid-treated mice. *Cytokine*, **8**, 548–56.

Hunt, T.K., Knighton, D.R., Thakral, K.K., Goodson, W.H. and Andrews, W.S. (1984). Studies on inflammation and wound healing: angiogenesis and collagen synthesis stimulated *in vivo* by resident and activated wound macrophages. *Surgery*, **96**, 48–54.

Ingber, D.E. and Folkman, J. (1989). Mechanochemical switching between growth and differentiation during fibroblast growth factor-stimulated angiogenesis *in vitro*: role of extracellular matrix. *Journal of Cell Biology*, **109**, 317–30.

Jaffe, E.A., Ruggiero, J.T. and Falcone, D.J. (1985). Monocytes and macrophages synthesize and secrete thrombospondin. *Blood*, **65**, 79–84.

Jyung, R.W., Wu, L., Pierce, G.F. and Mustoe, T.A. (1994). Granulocyte–macrophage colony-stimulating factor and granulocyte colony-stimulating factor: differential action on incisional wound healing. *Surgery*, **115**, 325–34.

Keane, M.P. and Strieter, R.M. (1999). The role of CXC chemokines in the regulation of angiogenesis. *Chemical Immunology*, **72**, 86–101.

Knighton, D.R., Hunt, T.K., Scheunstuhl, H. and Halliday, B.J. (1983). Oxygen tension regulates the expression of angiogenesis factor by macrophages. *Science*, **221**, 1283–5.

Koch, A.E., Polverini, P.J. and Leibovich, S.J. (1986). Stimulation of neovascularization by human rheumatoid synovial tissue macrophages. *Arthritis and Rheumatism*, **29**, 471–9.

Kodelja, V., Muller, C., Tenorio, S., Schebesch, C., Orfanos, C.E. and Goerdt, S. (1997). Differences in angiogenic potential of classically vs alternatively activated macrophages. *Immunobiology*, **197**, 478–93.

Kovacs, E.J. and DiPietro, L.A. (1994). Fibrogenic cytokines and connective tissue production. *FASEB Journal*, **8**, 854–61.

Krischel, V., Bruch-Gerharz, D., Suschek, C., Kroncke, K.D., Ruzicka, T. and Kolb-Bachofen, V. (1998). Biphasic effect of exogenous nitric oxide on proliferation and differentiation in skin derived keratinocytes but not fibroblasts. *Journal of Investigative Dermatology*, **111**, 286–91.

Krummel, T.M., Michna, B.A., Thomas, B.L., Sporn, M.B., Nelson, J.M., Salzberg, A.M. *et al.* (1988). Transforming growth factor β (TGF-β) induces fibrosis in a fetal wound model. *Journal of Pediatric Surgery*, **23**, 647–52.

Kuwabara, K., Ogawa, S., Matsumoto, M., Koga, S., Clauss, M., Pinsky, D.J. *et al.* (1995). Hypoxia-mediated induction of acidic/basic fibroblast growth factor and platelet-derived growth factor in mononuclear phagocytes stimulates growth of hypoxic endothelial cells. *Proceeding of the National Academy of Sciences USA*, **92**, 4606–10.

Leeper-Woodford, S.K. and Mills, J.W. (1992). Phagocytosis and ATP levels in alveolar macrophages during hypoxia. *American Journal of Respiratory Cell and Molecular Biology*, **6**, 326–34.

Leibovich, S.J. and Danon, D. (1980). Promotion of wound repair in mice by application of glucan. *Journal of Reticuloendothelial Society*, **27**, 1–11.

Leibovich, S.J. and Ross, R. (1975). The role of the macrophage in wound repair: a study with hydrocortisone and antimacrophage serum. *American Journal of Pathology*, **78**, 71–91.

Leibovich, S.J., Polverini, P.J., Fong, T.W., Harlow, L.A. and Koch, A.E. (1994). Production of angiogenic activity by human monocytes requires an L-arginine/nitric oxide-synthase-dependent effector mechanism. *Proceedings of the National Academy of Sciences USA*, **91**, 4190–4.

Lewis, J.S., Lee, J.A., Underwood, J.C.E., Harris, A.L. and Lewis, C.E. (1999). Macrophage responses to hypoxia: relevance to disease mechanisms. *Journal of Leukocyte Biology* **66**, 889–900.

Lin, R.Y., Sullivan, K.M., Argenta, P.A., Meuli, M., Lorenz, H.P. and Adzick, N.S. (1995). Exogenous transforming growth factor-β amplifies its own expression and induces scar formation in a model of human fetal skin repair. *Annals of Surgery*, **222**, 146–54.

Lukacs, N.W., Hogaboam, C., Campbell, E. and Kunkel, S.L. (1999). Chemokine function, regulation and alteration of inflammatory responses. *Chemical Immunology*, **72**, 102–20.

Luettke, N.C., Qiu, Th., Peiffer, R.L., Oliver, P., Smithies, O. and Lee, D.C. (1993). TGF α deficiency results in hair follicle and eye abnormalities in targeted and waved-1 mice. *Cell*, **73**, 263–78.

Luster, A.D., Cardiff, R.D., MacLean, J.A., Crowe, K. and Granstein, R.D. (1998). Delayed wound healing and disorganized neovascularization in transgenic mice expressing the IP-10 chemokine. *Proceedings of the Association of American Physicians*, **110**, 183–96.

Martin, P., Dickson, M.C., Millan, F.A. and Akhurst, R.J. (1993). Rapid induction and clearance of TGF β1 is an early response to wounding in the mouse embryo. *Developmental Genetics*, **14**, 225–38.

Matsuoka, J. and Grotendorst, G.R. (1989). Two peptides related to platelet-derived growth factor are present in human wound fluid. *Proceeding of the National Academy of Sciences USA*, **86**, 4416–20.

McCarter, M.D., Mack, V.E., Daly, J.M., Naama, H.A. and Calvano, S.E. (1998). Trauma induced alterations in macrophage function. *Surgery*, **123**, 96–101.

McGinn, F.P. (1976). Effects of haemorrhage upon surgical operations. *British Journal of Surgery*, **63**, 742–46.

Metinko, A.P., Kunkel, S.L., Standiford, J.T. and Strieter, R.M. (1992). Anoxia–hyperoxia induces monocyte-derived interleukin-8. *Journal of Clinical Investigation*, **90**, 791–8.

Meszaros, A.J., Reichner, J.S. and Albina, J.E. (1999). Macrophage phagocytosis of wound neutrophils. *Journal of Leukocyte Biology*, **65**, 35–42.

Mustoe, T.A., Purdy, J., Gramates, P., Deuel, T.F., Thomason, A. and Pierce, G.F. (1989). Reversal of impaired wound healing in irradiated rats by platelet-derived growth factor-BB. *American Journal of Surgery*, **158**, 345–50.

Nathan, C.F. (1987). Secretory products of macrophages. *Journal of Clinical Investigation*, **79**, 319–26.

Nessel, C.C., Henry, W.L. Jr, Mastrofrancesco, B., Reichner, J.S. and Albina, J.E. (1999). Vestigial respiratory burst activity in wound macrophages. *American Journal of Physiology*, **276**, R1587–94.

Nissen, N.N., Gamelli, R.L., Polverini, P.J. and DiPietro, L.A. (1996). Basic fibroblast growth factor mediates angiogenic activity in early surgical wounds. *Surgery*, **119**, 457–65.

Nissen, N.N., Polverini, P.J., Koch, A.E., Volin, M.V., Gamelli, R.L. and DiPietro, L.A. (1998). Vascular endothelial growth factor mediates angiogenic activity during the proliferative phase of wound healing. *American Journal of Pathology*, **152**, 1445–52.

Nodder, S. and Martin, P. (1997). Wound healing in embryos: a review. *Anatomy and Embryology*, **195**, 215–28.

Pierce, G.F., Mustoe, T.A., Lingelbach, J., Masakowski, V.R., Griffin, F.L., Senior, R.M. *et al.* (1989). Platelet-derived growth factor and transforming growth factor-β enhance tissue repair activities by unique mechanisms. *Journal of Cell Biology*, **109**, 429–40.

Polverini, P.J. (1989). Macrophage-induced angiogenesis; a review. In Sorg, C. (ed.), *Cytokines*. S. Karger, Basel, 1, pp. 54–73.

Polverini, P.J., Cotran, R.S., Gimbrone, M.A. and Unanue, E.R. (1977). Activated macrophages induce vascular proliferation. *Nature*, **269**, 804–6.

Popovich, P.G., Guan, Z., Wei, P., Huitinga, I., van Rooijen, N. and Stokes, B.T. (1999). Depletion of hematogenous macrophages promotes partial hindlimb recovery and neuroanatomical repair after experimental spinal cord injury. *Experimental Neurology*, **158**, 351–65.

Porras-Reyes, B.H., Blair, H.C., Jeffrey, J.J. and Mustoe, T.A. (1991). Collagenase production at the border of granulation tissue in a healing wound: macrophage and mesenchymal collagenase production *in vivo*. *Connective Tissue Research*, **27**, 63–71.

Rappolee, D.A., Mark, D., Banda, M.J. and Werb, Z. (1988). Wound macrophages express TGF-α and other growth factors *in vivo*: analysis by mRNA phenotyping. *Science*, **241**, 708–12.

Reed, M.J., Corsa, A., Pendergrass, W., Penn, P., Sage, E.H. and Abrass, I.H. (1998). Neovascularization in aged mice. Delayed angiogenesis is coincident with decreased levels of transforming growth factor β-1 and type I collagen. *American Journal of Pathology*, **152**, 113–22.

Reichner, J.S., Meszaros, A.J., Louis, C.A., Henry, W.L., Jr, Mastrofrancesco, B., Martin, B.A.. *et al.* (1999). Molecular and metabolic evidence for the restricted expression of inducible nitric oxide synthase in healing wounds. *American Journal of Pathology*, **154**, 1097–104.

Ross, R. and Benditt, E.P. (1962). Wound healing and collagen formation: fine structure in experimental scurvy. *Journal of Cell Biology*, **12**, 533–51.

Ross, R. and Odland, G. (1968). Human wound repair. II. Inflammatory cells, epithelial–mesenchymal interrelations, and fibrogenesis. *Journal of Cell Biology*, **39**, 152–68

Savill, J., Fadok, V., Henson, P. and Haslett, C. (1993). Phagocyte recognition of cells undergoing apoptosis. *Immunology Today*, **11**, 131–6.

Schwartz, M., Lazarov-Spiegler, O., Rapalino, O., Agranov, I., Velan, G. and Hadani, M (1999). Potential repair of rat spinal cord injuries using stimulated homologous macrophages. *Neurosurgery*, **44**, 1041–5.

Shah, M., Foreman, D.M. and Ferguson, M.W.J. (1992). Control of scarring in adult wounds by neutralising antibody to transforming growth factor β. *Lancet*, **339**, 213–4.

Shah, M., Foreman, D.M. and Ferguson, M.W. (1995). Neutralisation of TGF-β1 and TGF-β2 or exogenous addition of TGF-β3 to cutaneous rat wounds reduces scarring. *Journal of Cell Science*, **108**, 985–1002.

Shweiki, D., Itin, A., Soffer, D. and Keshet, E. (1992). Vascular endothelial growth factor induced by hypoxia may mediate hypoxia-initiated angiogenesis. *Nature*, **359**, 843–5.

Simon, L.M., Axline, S.G. and Pesanti, E.L. (1981). Adaptations of phagocytosis and pinocytosis in mouse lung macrophages after sustained *in vitro* hypoxia. *American Review of Respiratory Diseases*, **123**, 64–8.

Simpson, D.M. and Ross, R. (1972). The neutrophillic leukocyte in wound repair: a study with antineutrophil serum. *Journal of Clinical Investigations*, **51**, 2009–23.

Smith, R.E., Strieter, R.M., Phan, S.H., Lukacs, N.W., Huffnagle, G.B., Wilke, C.A. *et al.* (1994). Production and function of murine macrophage inflammatory protein-1α in bleomycin-induced lung injury. *Journal of Immunology*, **153**, 4704–12.

Smith, R.E., Strieter, R.M., Phan, S.H. and Kunkel, S.L. (1996). C-C chemokines: novel mediators of the profibrotic inflammatory response to bleomycin challenge. *American Journal of Respiratory Cell and Molecular Biology*, **15**, 693–702.

Stallmeyer, B., Kampfer, H., Kolb, N., Pfeilschifter, J. and Frank, S. (1999). The function of nitric oxide in wound repair: inhibition of inducible nitric oxide-synthase severly impairs wound reep-ithelialization. *Journal of Investigative Dermatology*, **113**, 1090–8.

Stricklin, G.P., Li, L. and Nanney, L.B. (1994). Localization of mRNAs representing interstitial collagenase, 72kDa gelatinase. and TIMP in healing porcine burn wounds. *Journal of Investigative Dermatology*, **103**, 352–8.

Subramaniam, M., Saffaripour, S., Van De Water, L., Frenette, P.S., Mayadas, T.N., Hynes, R.O. *et al.* (1997). Role of endothelial selectins in wound repair. *American Journal of Pathology*, **150**, 1701–9.

Sunderkötter, C., Goebeler, M., Schulze-Osthoff, K., Bhardwaj, R. and Sorg, C. (1991). Macrophage-derived angiogenesis factors. *Pharmacology and Therapeutics*, **51**, 195–216.

Swift, M.E., Kleinman, H.K. and DiPietro, L.A. (1999). Impaired wound repair and delayed angiogenesis in aged mice. *Laboratory Investigation*, **79**, 1479–87.

Tessier, P.A., Naccache, P.H., Clark-Lewis, I., Gladue, R.P., Neote, K.S. and Mecoll, S.R. (1997). Chemokine networks *in vivo*— involvement of C-X-C and C-C chemokines in neutrophil extravasation *in vivo* in response to TNF-α. *Journal of Immunology*, **159**, 3595–602.

VanOtteren, G.M., Kunkel, S.L., Standiford, J.T. and Strieter, R.M. (1995). Alterations in oxygen tension modulate the expression of tumor necrosis factor α and macrophage inflammatory protein-1α from murine alveolar macrophages. *American Journal of Respiratory Cell and Molecular Biology*, **13**, 399–409.

Welgus, H.G., Campbell, E.J., Cury, J.D., Eisen, A.Z., Senior, R.M., Wilhelm, S.M. *et al.* (1990). Neutral metalloproteinases produced by human mononuclear phagocytes. Enzyme profile, regulation. and expression during cellular development. *Journal of Clinical Investigation*, **86**, 1496–502.

Whitby, D.J. and Ferguson, M.W.J. (1991). Immunohistochemical localization of growth factors in fetal wound healing. *Developmental Biology*, **147**, 207–15.

Wu, L., Yu, Y.L., Galiano, R.D., Roth, S.I. and Mustoe, T.A. (1997). Macrophage colony-stimulating factor accelerates wound healing and upregulates TGF-β1mRNA levels through tissue macrophages. *Journal of Surgical Research*, **72**, 162–9.

Xiong, M., Elson, G., Legarda, D. and Leibovich, S.J. (1998). Production of vascular endothelial growth factor by murine macrophages: regulation by hypoxia, lactate and the inducible nitic oxide synthase pathway. *American Journal of Pathology*, **153**, 587–98.

Yamasaki, K., Edington, H.D., McClosky, C., Tzeng, E., Lizonova, A., Kovesdi, I. *et al.* (1998). Reversal of impaired wound repair in iNOS-deficient mice by topical adenoviral-mediated iNOS gene transfer. *Journal of Clinical Investigation*, **101**, 967–71.

Yoak, M.B., Haraphanahalli, S., Beaver, B.L., Dennin, D.A. and Jackman, S.H. (1997). Chemokine gene expression in a surgically wounded murine model. *Surgery Forum*, **48**, 671–3.

Zabel, D.D., Feng, J.J., Scheuenstuhl, H., Hunt, T.K. and Hussain, M.Z. (1996). Lactate stimulation macrophage-derived angiogenic activity is associated with inhibition of poly(ADP-ribose) synthesis. *Laboratory Investigation*, **74**, 644–9.

Zhao, X.M., Yeoh, T.K., Hiebert, M., Frist, W.H. and Miller, G.G. (1993). The expression of acidic fibroblast growth factor (heparin-binding growth factor-1) and cytokine genes in human cardiac allografts and T cells. *Transplantation*, **56**, 1177–82.

11 *Macrophages in tumor biology*

M. Kreutz, J. Fritsche and R. Andreesen

1 Introduction

In 1882, Elias Metchnikoff for the first time described macrophages as phagocytic cells. It is now clear that beside phagocytosis, cells of the mononuclear phagocyte system (MPS) are not only major players in natural immunity to microbial infections but also participate in host defense against malignant tumors. The MPS is found ubiquitously in all tissues and body cavities. Circulating blood monocytes are the common precursor cells of this heterogenous cell family and serve as a source for the constant renewal of tissue macrophages and dendritic cells under normal physiological conditions. The extravasation of blood monocytes markedly increases under different pathological conditions, e.g. inflammation. The tissue-adapted maturation of the infiltrating monocytes is most probably modulated by the site-specific microenvironment. Hypoxia seems to be one relevant factor for the activation and differentiation of macrophages in the microenvironment which may also, in part, be responsible for a tumor-specific phenotype of macrophages (Lewis *et al.*, 1999). However, the tumor microenvironment can differ depending on the tumor type or due to differences between the primary and metastatic site leading to different types of tumor-associated macrophages (Figure 11.1).

Most malignant tumors contain numerous macrophages as a major component of their leukocytic infiltrate (van Ravenswaay *et al.*, 1992). These so-called tumor-associated macrophages (TAMs) represent a special macrophage subpopulation and seem to be 'Janus-faced': on the one hand, TAMs can destroy neoplastic cells and present tumor-associated antigens leading to the induction of a specific immune response; on the other hand, TAMs often seem to co-exist with the malignant cells in a symbiotic manner and contribute to tumor metastasis and proliferation (Zuk and Walker, 1987; Mantovani *et al.*, 1992; Elgert *et al.*, 1998). Soluble TAM-derived cytokines may support tumor development and progression, e.g. by inducing angiogenesis. In addition, somatic hybridization of tumor cells with the inflammatory macrophage itself or aggregates of tumor cells with macrophages has been postulated to result in highly metastatic variants of the original clone and to contribute to tumor cell spread away from the site of its original transformation (Larizza *et al.*, 1984; Munzarova and Kovarik 1987; van Netten *et al.*, 1993). The extent of the macrophage infiltrate in breast carcinoma, colon carcinoma, pulmonary adenocarcinoma and lung carcinoma of cancer patients has been associated with a good or

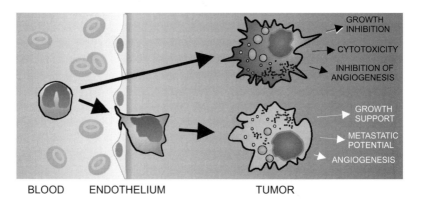

BLOOD   ENDOTHELIUM   TUMOR

Fig. 11.1   Ontogeny of tumor-associated macrophages in the tumor microenvironment.

poor prognosis, respectively (Lauder *et al.*, 1977; Luebbers *et al.*, 1985; Skinner *et al.*, 1983; Leek *et al.*, 1996; Eerola *et al.*, 1999; Takanami *et al.*, 1999). To understand this ambiguity, it may be crucial to analyze the differential ontogeny of the TAMs as circulating blood monocytes are the precursors of both the 'symbiotic' and the 'cytotoxic' macrophage. The influence of the special tumor environment on monocyte to macrophage maturation will probably modulate functional properties of TAMs and thereby determine disease progression. Thus, at least in some tumors or at certain stages of tumor progression, monocytes emigrating from the capillary bed are 'highjacked' and re-educated to serve within the machinery of the growing tumor.

2 Macrophage differentiation in a tumor spheroid—a model for TAM ontogeny

TAMs are cells that originate from monocytes infiltrating tumor tissues. To investigate the influence of a tumor environment on the activation and differentiation of monocytes, we and others developed an experimental system by co-culturing human elutriation-purified monocytes and monocyte-derived macrophages with human multicellular tumor spheroids (MCTS) as a model for non-vascularized metastases (Hauptmann *et al.*, 1993; Audran *et al.*, 1994; Konur *et al.*, 1996a; Kunz-Schughart *et al.*, 1997). In contrast to monolayer cultures of tumor cells commonly used to study monocyte–tumor interaction, this three-dimensional system provides a model which reflects more closely the complex *in vivo* situation. MCTS show growth kinetics similar to tumors *in vivo*, as well as gradients in the concentration of oxygen, pH and nutrient supply (Carlsson and Acker, 1988). Furthermore, it could be demonstrated that MCTS can produce extracellular matrix (ECM) proteins such as fibronectin, laminin, collagen and glycosaminoglycans, and show higher degrees of differentiation in comparison with the related monolayers (Sutherland *et al.*, 1986; Sutherland, 1988). Beside monocyte/macrophage co-cultures with MCTS, several *in vitro* studies used the MCTS system to analyze the interaction of tumor cells with fibroblasts (Schuster *et al.*, 1994), lymphokine-activated killer cells (Jaaskelainen *et al.*, 1989, Iwasaki *et al.*, 1990) or endothelial cells (Knuchel *et al.*, 1988).

The infiltration/migration of monocytes into MCTS seems to be regulated specifically by tumor cell factors as fibroblast MCTS were not infiltrated by monocytes/macrophages. We found that monocytes and monocyte-derived macrophages infiltrated and spread throughout the entire MCTS of the bladder carcinoma cell line J82 within 24 h (Konur *et al.*, 1996a). Similar results were obtained by Audran *et al.*, who investigated the infiltration of either stimulated or unstimulated monocyte-derived macrophages into MCTS of the lung carcinoma cell line SK-MES-1. They could demonstrate that the infiltration was inhibited by anti-ICAM (CD54) antibodies (Audran *et al.*, 1994). After 18 h co-culture, the MCTS consisted of approximately 10 per cent macrophages and 90 per cent tumor cells (Figure 11.2).

When the antigenic phenotype of monocyte-derived TAMs cultured within MCTS of the bladder carcinoma line J82 was analyzed, maturation-associated macrophage antigens (carboxypeptidase M/Max.1, CD84/Max.3 and CD51) were not expressed. In contrast, TAMs within the non-tumorigenic HCV29 spheroids expressed the normal

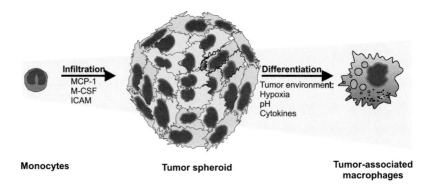

Monocytes   **Tumor spheroid**   **Tumor-associated**
                                                                        macrophages

Fig. 11.2   Infiltration and differentiation of monocytes in multicellular tumor spheroids.

maturation-associated phenotype (Konur *et al.*, 1996a). Beside the antigen expression, the cytokine response of TAMs was analyzed. TAMs in a J82 spheroid secreted spontaneously high amounts of interleukin (IL)-1β and IL-6 but low amounts of tumor necrosis factor-α (TNF-α) as compared with control macrophages differentiated without tumor contact. The secretion was enhanced further by the addition of lipopolysaccharide (LPS). The antigen profile and the cytokine pattern of TAMs within J82 spheroids are typical for monocytes, indicating a disturbed differentiation process in the J82 tumor environment (Konur *et al.*, 1996a, 1998). Since cytotoxicity of macrophages is dependent on successful differentiation, i.e. cytotoxicity is higher in mature macrophages than in monocytes (Andreesen *et al.*, 1983a), the tumor seems to suppress the differentiation process thereby protecting itself against macrophage cytotoxicity. Alterations in the differentiation pattern of monocytes/macrophages and reduced cytotoxicity of blood monocytes in cancer patients have also been reported by others (Krishnan *et al.*, 1980; Siziopikou *et al.*, 1991). A similar inhibition of differentiation could not be detected in a monolayer co-culture system with tumor cells, again supporting the notion that a MCTS/monocyte co-culture better reflects the *in vivo* situation.

   The cytotoxic capacity of different types of macrophages within MCTS was analyzed by different authors. Audran *et al.* reported cytostatic, but no cytolytic activity of infiltrating macrophages resulting in a proliferation arrest of the MCTS. Tumor cytostasis was not related to TNF-α or other soluble mediators (Audran *et al.*, 1994). Hauptmann *et al.* used MCTS of the rectum cancer cell line HRT-18 and compared the cytostatic capacity of inflammatory macrophages and resident macrophages. Both types of macrophages showed a controversial behavior in terms of cytostatic activity: inflammatory macrophages inhibited while resident macrophages stimulated tumor cell proliferation (Hauptmann *et al.*, 1993). Surprisingly, the cytostatic activity of the inflammatory macrophages was only present for 48 h. Thereafter, the phenotype of the inflammatory macrophage changed and tumor cell proliferation normalized to the control level. This indicates that the tumor environment 're-educates' the macrophage, leading to a 'symbiotic' type of TAM. The formation of reactive oxygen intermediates (ROIs) by TAMs was inhibited within MCTS of colorectal carcinomas, and this effect was transferable by tumor supernatants. However, as this inhibition was independent of the macrophage type, it does not explain the differences in tumor cytostasis (Siegert *et al.*, 1999).

3 Chemotaxis—regulation of monocyte infiltration into the tumor site

The leukocytic infiltrate of tumors consists mainly of macrophages (Elgert *et al.*, 1998) but the number of TAMs depends on the respective tumor type and stage. TAMs can play a key role in promoting tumor growth, and therefore tumor cells might benefit from attracting these cells. Tumors recruit monocytes mainly by producing the monocyte chemotactic molecules macrophage colony-stimulating factor (M-CSF) (Walter *et al.*, 1991; Savarese *et al.*, 1998) and macrophage chemotactic protein-1 (MCP-1) (Yoshimura *et al.*, 1989; Bottazzi *et al.*, 1990; Graves *et al.*, 1992).

M-CSF is a well-known hematopoetic growth factor involved in the ontogenesis of monocytes/macrophages. On the basis of alternative splicing, five different cDNAs were characterized (Fixe and Praloran, 1997). Beside its influence on the differentiation of monocytes, M-CSF is a specific chemotactic factor for monocytes/macrophages (Tang *et al.*, 1992). M-CSF transfection experiments *in vivo* revealed an induction of macrophage infiltration into the tumor site, but no tumor suppression even after macrophage stimulation with interferon-γ (IFN-γ) and/or LPS (Dorsch *et al.*, 1993). A strong expression of M-CSF has been described in tumor cells in breast carcinoma (Tang *et al.*, 1992), as well as a correlation between numbers of M-CSF-expressing cells and the amount of infiltrating monocytes (Scholl *et al.*, 1994). M-CSF is also produced by monocytes and macrophages themselves (Rambaldi *et al.*, 1987). Beside the M-CSF levels inside and at the periphery of the tumor, high M-CSF levels have been observed in the circulation of tumor patients. In patients with breast, endometrial or ovarian carcinoma, M-CSF levels in the circulation are markers for disease progression and monitoring of the response (Kacinski 1995). In addition, in these patients, high M-CSF levels correlate with a bad prognosis (Chambers *et al.*, 1995, 1997). M-CSF overexpression is also associated with p53 mutations (Asschert *et al.*, 1997).

MCP-1, along with regulated on activation, normal T cell-expressed and secreted protein (RANTES), macrophage inflammatory protein (MIP)-β and MIP-1α belongs to the CC subfamily of chemokines, a family of low molecular weight secretory proteins, which are chemotactic for monocytes, subsets of lymphocytes and natural killer (NK) cells. A positive correlation between MCP-1 and TAM levels has been demonstrated in many tumor types (Negus *et al.*, 1995; Leung *et al.*, 1997). *In vivo* studies with MCP-1-transfected adenocarcinoma cells showed an earlier and greater increase of infiltrating macrophages when compared with non-transfected cells and confirm the chemotactic influence of MCP-1 on monocytes/macrophages (Nakashima *et al.*, 1998). MCP-1 is produced not only by tumor cells, but TAMs are also a source of MCP-1 as shown for carcinoma of the lung and glioblastomas (Leung *et al.*, 1997; Wong *et al.*, 1998). In patients with ovarian carcinoma, monocytes lose their ability to respond to MCP-1 after entering the tumor site. In line with these results, a defective CC receptor 2 (CCR2) is expressed in these TAMs (Sica *et al.*, 2000a). MCP-1 also positively influences angiogenesis in invasive ductal mammary carcinomas, which is probably due to the recruitment of monocytes into the tumor site, producing angiogenic factors such as vascular endothelial growth factor (VEGF), basic fibroblast growth factor (bFGF), etc. (Goede *et al.*, 1999).

Beside M-CSF and MCP-1, TGF-β and VEGF are expressed in tumor cells and can also act as chemoattractive factors for monocytes/macrophages (Wahl *et al.*, 1987; Roberts *et al.*, 1988; Leek *et al.*, 2000).

4 The cytokine network within the tumor microenvironment—regulation of tumor growth

It is well known that several cytokines and growth factors can be detected in the sera of tumor patients. Most probably these factors are tumor-derived products and are secreted by either the tumor cells and/or the leukocytic tumor infiltrate, e.g. TAMs. TAMs are often in an activated state compared with normal tissue macrophages (Valdez *et al.*, 1990), and secretion of cytokines by TAMs is induced, for example, by tumor carbohydrate structures (Janicke and Mannel, 1990; Putz and Mannel, 1995) or soluble tumor-derived products (Evans *et al.*, 1991). The interaction of TAMs and tumor cells leads to a net result of factor production which is important for the outcome of the disease: on the one hand, paracrine and autocrine production of cytokines and growth factors can support the development of the tumor by promoting growth, angiogenesis and metastasis; on the other hand, cytokines may lead to the regression of the tumor and induce tumor cytotoxicity.

M-CSF is one of the growth factors produced by tumor cells in ovarian (Asschert *et al.*, 1997; Foti *et al.*, 1999), breast (Tang *et al.*, 1992) and lung carcinoma (Adachi *et al.*, 1994) and can also be produced by monocytes/macrophages themselves. It might act as an autocrine growth factor for some tumor cells which co-express the M-CSF receptor (Kacinski, 1995). Local M-CSF in the tumor is a chemotactic factor for infiltrating blood monocytes, and circulating M-CSF could influence monocyte recruitment from the bone marrow. In gynecological malignancies and especially in ovarian cancer, high M-CSF is a marker for disease progression and correlates with poor prognosis (Suzuki *et al.*, 1995; Chambers *et al.*, 1997). This may be due in part to its induction of urokinase-type plasminogen activator (u-PA) in macrophages, which is important for the invasion and metastasis of tumor cells (Chambers *et al.*, 1995). In addition, M-CSF can induce IL-8, known to be a potent angiogenic factor (Koch *et al.*, 1992; Hashimoto *et al.*, 1996). On the other hand, M-CSF has been reported to stimulate tumoricidal activity of monocytes *in vitro* (Suzu *et al.*, 1989) and induce TNF-α secretion (Warren and Ralph, 1986).

Similarly to M-CSF, high serum levels of IL-6 are detected in various malignancies, e.g. renal cell carcinoma (Tsukamoto *et al.*, 1992), bladder carcinoma (Seguchi *et al.*, 1992) and in malignant ascites (Moradi *et al.*, 1993; Kryczek *et al.*, 2000). Serum levels reflect the proliferative activity of tumors and the disease status in colorectal, gastric and breast carcinoma (Wu *et al.*, 1996; Kinoshita *et al.*, 1999; Zhang and Adachi 1999). For prostatic carcinoma, it has been shown that IL-6 acts as a paracrine and autocrine growth factor *in vitro* (Okamoto *et al.*, 1997). The interaction between tumor cells and macrophages could regulate the production of IL-6 in the tumor environment. Evans *et al.* measured elevated IL-6 concentrations in sera of tumor-bearing mice and demonstrated that the tumor-induced IL-1 production of macrophages in turn stimulates tumor-derived IL-6 release (Evans *et al.*, 1992). Apart from its well known capacity to induce acute phase proteins, IL-6 modulates the secretion of several macrophage products: it stimulates IL-1 receptor antagonist expression and inhibits TNF-α and IL-1 production (Aderka *et al.*, 1989; Schindler *et al.*, 1990; Tilg *et al.*, 1994).

TAMs are also a source of IL-6, but secrete low levels of IL-1β and TNF-α in ovarian carcinoma, which may be related to the high local IL-6 concentrations (Erroi *et al.*, 1989; Bernasconi *et al.*, 1995). Economou *et al.* (1988) also found decreased IL-1β production of TAM compared with healthy controls. However, in breast carcinoma, high IL-1β expression correlated with the macrophage content in the tumor (Erroi *et al.*, 1989; Jin *et al.*, 1997). Regarding the TNF-α production by TAMs and the serum level of TNF-α in cancer patients, conflicting results have been reported. Elevated levels of TNF-α were detected in the sera of some tumor patients, e.g. in liver carcinoma and ovarian carcinoma (Balkwill *et al.*, 1987; Nakazaki 1992; Moradi *et al.*, 1993), but TAMs in ovarian carcinoma release low levels of TNF-α (Bernasconi *et al.*, 1995), suggesting that tumor cells themselves may also be involved in the generation of TNF-α. The mRNA for TNF-α is expressed in ovarian carcinoma cells; however, protein expression seems to be localized primarily to a subpopulation of macrophages (Naylor *et al.*, 1993). Interestingly, tumor cells express the mRNA and protein for the p55 TNF-α receptor in ovarian and breast carcinoma, suggesting the capacity for an autocrine/paracrine interaction (Naylor *et al.*, 1993; Pusztai *et al.*, 1994). One possible mechanism could be that TAM-derived TNF-α stimulates the induction of thymidine phosphorylase expression in tumor cells, thereby regulating angiogenesis (Leek *et al.*, 1998). In contrast, other authors described recently that TNF-α leads to an autocrine self-elimination of ovarian carcinoma cells *in vitro* (Simonitsch and Krupitza, 1998) and found no correlation between serum levels of TNF-α and clinico-pathological parameters (Zhang and Adachi, 1999). In malignant melanoma, a correlation between macrophage infiltration and angiogenesis is found which may be related to the finding that TAM-derived cytokines such as TNF-α induce the production of angiogenic factors such as IL-8 and VEGF in melanoma cells (Torisu *et al.*, 2000). IL-8 production by tumor cells has also been reported in colorectal cancer, and serum levels of IL-8 were significantly higher in patients with metastases in the liver and lung (Ueda *et al.*, 1994). On the contrary, Lee *et al.* (2000) found that IL-8-transfected human ovarian cancer cells showed reduced tumorigenicity in nude mice *in vivo*.

Other factors which can be secreted by TAM include, for example, IL-10 (Yanagawa *et al.*, 1999). In addition, tumor cells produce inhibitory factors such as IL-10, TGF-β and prostaglandin E2 (PGE$_2$) (Alleva *et al.*, 1994; Elgert *et al.*, 1998). Increased amounts of IL-10 in the tumor environment in turn may down-regulate the production of cytokines such as TNF-α and IL-12 in TAMs (Sica *et al.*, 2000b). Immunosuppressive activity is not only active directly at the tumor site but can also influence peripheral mononuclear cells. Sera from patients with colorectal and ovarian but not breast carcinoma showed decreased IL-1β and TNF-β production as compared with cultures from healthy controls (Muster-Bloy *et al.*, 1996).

5 Tumor-associated macrophages and their pivotal role in angiogenesis

Angiogenesis plays a key role in tumor growth after reaching a critical size of appoximately 2 mm^3. The neovascularization guarantees the supply of the tumor and avoids hypoxia and nutrient deprivation. In addition, new blood vessels connecting the tumor with the host are one way for metastasizing tumor cells to leave the tumor and for host cells to enter the tumor. The whole process of angiogenesis can be divided into four steps: (1) digestion of components of the ECM and activation of endothelial cells; (2) migration and proliferation of endothelial cells; (3) formation of capillary tubes; and, finally, (4) differentiation. These steps are supported by factors which are derived from the tumor cells themselves, but also from infiltrating leukocytes such as TAMs. Macrophages are a major source of the angiogenic factors VEGF, bFGF, TNF-α and IL-8. The activation of TAMs and the release of these factors occur, for instance, by oxygen deprivation: hypoxia (Knighton *et al.*, 1983; Lewis *et al.*, 1999). Beside the pro-angiogenic effects of TAMs, they are also able to inhibit angiogenesis by expression of angiostatin or other anti-angiogenic factors. Therefore, in some tumors, such as adenocarcinoma of the lung, a high TAM density correlates with a high microvessel density and bad prognosis (Takanami *et al.*, 1999), yet in patients with a large cell lung carcinoma a large number of TAMs is correlated with a better survival time (Eerola *et al.*, 1999).

5.1 The support of angiogenesis by TAMs

VEGF is expressed in various cells types including TAMs (Lewis *et al.*, 1995), and its production is induced by hypoxia and TGF-β (Minchenko *et al.*, 1994; Harmey *et al.*, 1998). Up to now, four different splicing isoforms of VEGF are known to exist, resulting in different soluble or membrane/ECM-associated forms of the growth factor. For instance, two of these isoforms are bound to heparin in the ECM and are therefore inactivated (Park *et al.*, 1993; Leek *et al.*, 1994). Their activation occurs after digestion of the eECM by proteases (Plouet *et al.*, 1997). The receptors of VEGF are found mainly on endothelial cells, explaining the specific mitogenic influence of VEGF on this cell type leading to proliferation and formation of microvessels. A chemotactic effect of VEGF on macrophages was also decribed (Shen *et al.*, 1993). Furthermore, VEGF itself induces the production of various angiogenic factors, such as the serine proteases tissue-type plasminogen activator (t-PA) and u-PA (Pepper *et al.*, 1991), and collagenase (Unemori *et al.*, 1992), and acts synergistically with bFGF (Pepper *et al.*, 1992). Recently, an inverse correlation between infiltration of dendritic cells and VEGF content in gastric carcinoma tissue was found, suggesting a tumor escape mechanism mediated by VEGF (Saito *et al.*, 1998).

Another important angiogenic factor produced by TAMs and tumor cells is IL-8. This cytokine belongs to the CXC chemokine family and, like VEGF, is bound to heparin (Koch *et al.*, 1992). The spontaneous production of IL-8 in TAMs can be increased further by stimulation with granulocyte–macrophage colony-stimulating factor (GM-CSF), as shown for TAMs isolated from human ovarian cancer (Bernasconi *et al.*, 1995). *In vitro*, the release of IL-8 by matrix-digesting enzymes leads to stimulation of chemotaxis and proliferation of human umbilical vein endothelial cells. Further *in vitro* studies with conditioned media from monocytes/macrophages were performed and revealed a blockade of angiogenesis by addition of antibodies against IL-8 or TNF-α to the medium. *In vivo*, the angiogenic activity of IL-8 was verified in a rat model (Koch *et al.*, 1992). Beside its angiogenic activity, IL-8 is also discussed as an antitumor growth factor in human ovarian cancer (Lee *et al.*, 2000).

TNF-α is released by TAMs, for example in ovarian carcinoma (Naylor *et al.*, 1993; Pusztai *et al.*, 1994), and in low concentrations induces tube formation and migration (Frank 1994), but in high concentrations inhibits angiogenesis (Leek *et al.*, 1994; Sunderkotter *et al.*, 1994). TNF-α works as an angiogenic factor by stimulating the production of plasminogen activator. Plasminogen activator itself leads, via plasmin production, to the digestion of ECM and therefore to the release of angiogenic factors

(Niedbala and Stein, 1991). In addition, the levels of IL-8, VEGF, bFGF and their receptors are increased in endothelial cells after stimulation with TNF-α *in vitro*, indicating an additional indirect effect of TNF-α on angiogenesis (Yoshida *et al.*, 1997; Torisu *et al.*, 2000).

The single chain polypeptide platelet-derived endothelial cell growth factor (PD-ECGF), originally isolated from platelets, is also expressed in TAMs (Takahashi *et al.*, 1996) and acts as an pro-angiogenic mediator. Up to now, the mechanisms underlying PD-ECGF-induced angiogenesis are not clear, but evidence exists that it stimulates endothelial cell proliferation indirectly through its thymidine phosphorylase activity (Finnis *et al.*, 1993).

TGF-β produced by macrophages binds to the epidermal growth factor (EGF) receptor and is a potent inducer of angiogenesis *in vivo* (Schreiber *et al.*, 1986; Bicknell and Harris, 1991). It directly stimulates migration and proliferation of cultured endothelial cells (Sato and Rifkin, 1988) and induces the release of other angiogenic factors such as FGF and t-PA (Sato *et al.*, 1993).

bFGF is widely expressed and localized in the ECM. Apart from the expression of bFGF in stromal macrophages surrounding the tumor site, TAMs can also express this growth factor (Lewis *et al.*, 1995). It induces the proliferation and migration of endothelial cells (Connolly *et al.*, 1987), but also promotes the formation of differentiated capillary tubes *in vitro* (Montesano *et al.*, 1986).

u-PA is produced by monocyte-derived macrophages and is important for the metastasis and invasion of tumor cells (Saksela *et al.*, 1985). u-PA activates the cleavage of plasminogen to plasmin (Dvorak 1986) and plasmin in turn degrades ECM components such as fibronectin or laminin (Hildenbrand *et al.*, 1995). The ECM is involved in the control of angiogenesis through binding of angiogenic factors such as VEGF and bFGF (Nathan, 1987; (Ingber and Folkman, 1989; Hildenbrand *et al.*, 1998). Furthermore, macrophages can also secrete other matrix-degrading proteases (Polverini, 1996).

Beside the expression of pro-angiogenic factors, TAMs can also participate in the inhibition of angiogenesis by expression of anti-angiogenic factors such as thrombospondin-1 (TSP-1) and angiostatin.

5.2 The inhibition of angiogenesis by TAMs

TSP-1 is a 450 kDa disulfide-linked trimer containing three identical chains of 140 kDa, and interacts on the basis of its structure with various proteins, e.g. ECM proteins (Liu *et al.*, 1999). It is expressed by macrophages and platelets. TSP-1 represents an important anti-angiogenic factor as shown by *in vivo* studies where TSP-1 blocks neovascularization (Iruela-Arispe *et al.*, 1991). Collagenase activity, endothelial cell proliferation and migration are inhibited by TSP-1 (DiPietro and Polverini, 1993). Incubation of endothelial cells with antibodies to TSP-1 leads to an enhanced sprouting *in vitro* (Iruela-Arispe *et al.*, 1991). Investigations of human squamous carcinoma showed a correlation between decreased angiogenic activity and strongly up-regulated TSP-1 expression after stimulation with retinoic acid. This suggests a stimulus of TAMs toward an angio-inhibitory phenotype by retinoic acid treatment (Lingen *et al.*, 1996). Comparable analysis between TSP-1 and VEGF expression in endometrial carcinomas reveals a tendency toward a strong TSP-1 expression among tumors, with a weak VEGF expression indicating an inverse correlation (Salvesen and Akslen 1999).

Angiostatin, a cleavage product of plasminogen, has been shown to inhibit the proliferation of human microvascular endothelial cells and the formation of metastases (Cornelius *et al.*, 1998). TAMs influence the synthesis of angiostatin indirectly by the expression of elastase, a potent matrix metalloproteinase (MMPs) for the cleavage of plasminogen (Cornelius *et al.*, 1998). The expression of elastase in TAMs is probably induced by GM-CSF, as shown in Lewis lung carcinoma (Dong *et al.*, 1997). In addition, GM-CSF expressed by TAMs may act as an anti-angiogenic factor indirectly by stimulating the production of the anti-angiogenic protein plasminogen activator inhibitor type 2 (Joseph and Isaacs, 1998).

A further possible anti-angiogenic factor is IL-12, a heterodimeric cytokine composed of two disulfide-linked subunits of 35 and 40 kDa. IL-12 is described as a cytokine expressed in tumor-bearing host macrophages in mice (Mullins *et al.*, 1999). In a murine breast cancer model, IL-12 down-regulates VEGF expression, one of the most important factors of angiogenesis. This decrease is combined with down-regulation of MMP-9 expression and up-regulation of TIMP, an inhibitor of metalloproteinses (Dias *et al.*, 1998).

In conclusion, TAMs are a source of both pro-angiogenic and anti-angiogenic factors. Which type of activity dominates may depend on the particular tumor type and tumor microenvironment (Figure 11.3).

6   Tumor cytotoxicity of macrophages

6.1   Recognition of tumor cells by macrophages

The host defense against tumor cells can be performed by different types of immune cells: cytotoxic T cells, NK cells (Griffiths and Mueller, 1991), monocytes/macrophages (Hibbs *et al.*, 1972), dendritic cells (Fanger *et al.*, 1999) and even granulocytes (Fujimura and Torisu, 1987). Monocytes/macrophages have powerful constitutive antineoplastic properties even in the absence of specific immunity and are able to kill phenotypically diverse tumor cells. In contrast to T cells and NK cells, recognition mechanisms of monocytes and macrophages are independent of the major histocompatibility complex (MHC). They discriminate between neoplastic and normal cells and do not attack normal syngeneic cells. Precise target structures which enable macrophages to distinguish between malignant and normal cell populations are still under discussion. Common features of tumor cell membranes such as special carbohydrate structures or the abnormal presence of phospholipids such as phosphatidylserine on the outer leaflet of the membrane of tumor cells could be responsible in part for the recognition (Sharon, 1984; Fidler and Schroit, 1988). Accordingly, it has been shown that lectins can stimulate macrophage killing of tumor cells. Extracellular lectins form bridges between sugars of both cell types, thereby augmenting target cell binding of macrophages (Chattopadhyay and Bhattacharyya, 1988). Another mechanism of tumor recognition may be due to the abnormal cell growth of tumor cells. In a mouse model, only transformed fibroblasts but not untransformed fibroblasts were killed by macrophages, and cell destruction correlated with the growth potential of the target cells (Hibbs *et al.*, 1972; Piessens *et al.*, 1975). Accordingly, Horn and colleagues reported a correlation between monocyte kill and tumor cell density and proliferation. Tumor cells in a quiescent stage (G_0) of the cell

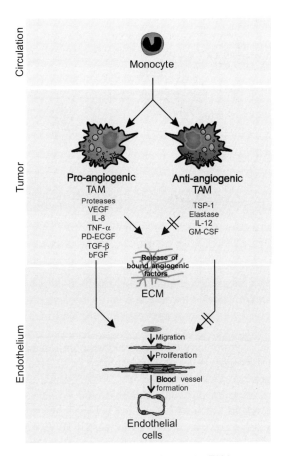

Fig. 11.3   Production of pro- and anti-angiogenic factors by TAM.

cycle were no longer susceptible to the induction of cell death by monocytes (Horn *et al.*, 1991). Membrane-bound M-CSF which is expressed on some types of tumor cells has also been suggested to be a recognition structure for macrophages (Jadus *et al.*, 1996; Zeineddine *et al.*, 1999). In addition, macrophages can bind tumor cells via Fc receptors or complement receptors if the target cells are coated by antibodies and/or complement, respectively. With respect to complement receptors, it was shown recently that β-glucans can induce killing of tumor cells. β-Glucans bind to the complement receptor type 3 (CR3, CD11b/CD18), thereby priming effector cells for the killing of tumor cells which are coated with iC3b (Yan *et al.*, 1999). Beside CD11b/CD18, other β₂ integrins also seem to be involved in tumor cell binding of monocytes (Bernasconi *et al.*, 1991). Fc receptors are very important for antibody-dependent cytotoxicity (Connor *et al.*, 1990).

6.2 Mechanisms of cytotoxicity by macrophages

Macrophages can attack neoplastic cells through contact-dependent and contact-independent mechanisms (Figure 11.4). Contact-dependent mechanisms include antibody-dependent cytotoxicity (ADCC) and antibody-independent cytotoxicity. A prerequisite for

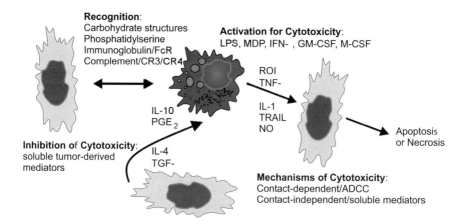

Recognition:
Carbohydrate structures
Phosphatidylserine
Immunoglobulin/FcR
Complement/CR3/CR4

Activation for Cytotoxicity:
LPS, MDP, IFN- , GM-CSF, M-CSF

ROI
TNF-

IL-10
PGE$_2$

IL-1
TRAIL
NO

Apoptosis
or Necrosis

Inhibition of Cytotoxicity:
soluble tumor-derived
mediators

IL-4
TGF-

Mechanisms of Cytotoxicity:
Contact-dependent/ADCC
Contact-independent/soluble mediators

Fig. 11.4 Different mechanisms of tumor cytotoxicity of macrophages.

ADCC is the induction of a specific immune response by B cells which generates tumor-binding antibodies. Macrophages recognize the antibody-coated tumor cell via their Fc receptors and kill them. Lysis of the target cell is attributed mainly to the secretion of hydrogen peroxide (Nathan and Cohn, 1980).

Antibody-independent cytotoxicity relies on other recognition mechanisms, e.g. carbohydrate structures on the tumor cell, but, similarly to ADCC, lysis is often based on the production of hydrogen peroxide (Nathan *et al.*, 1979). Beside cytolysis, macrophages can also induce cytostasis of tumor cells. Cytolysis and cytostasis can be mediated by soluble factors independently of a direct contact between macrophages and the tumor target. Cytotoxic/cytostatic factors such as cytokines, ROIs and nitric oxide (NO) are involved in this type of killing (Bonta and Ben-Efraim, 1993). One of the first cytokines described as an important mediator of tumor cell killing of macrophages was TNF-α (Carswell *et al.*, 1975). Even though TNF-α has the potential to act cytotoxically or cytostatically on some tumor cells *in vitro* and induce necrosis of solid tumors in some animal models *in vivo*, it can also enhance experimental metastases (Orosz *et al.*, 1993). TNF-α often acts additively or synergistically with other cytokines, namely IL-1 or IFN-γ (Feinman *et al.*, 1987; Ichinose *et al.*, 1988). IL-1 was also described to act as a cytocidal factor independently of TNF-α (Onozaki *et al.*, 1985). Despite the fact that the name of TNF-α implies an induction of tumor necrosis, TNF-α and other members of the TNF superfamily, e.g. TRAIL and fas, can induce apoptosis of the target cell (Grell *et al.*, 1994). In particular, TRAIL recently has been shown to be a cytotoxic mediator of human monocytes and dendritic cells (Fanger *et al.*, 1999; Griffith *et al.*, 1999). Other important mediators of apoptosis include NO and ROIs (Hibbs *et al.*, 1988; Aliprantis *et al.*, 1996). NO is produced by mouse macrophages, tumor cells and endothelial cells; however, it is still under discussion as to whether human macrophages are really an important source of NO (Zembala *et al.*, 1994; Weinberg *et al.*, 1995; Konur *et al.*, 1996b). Whether monocytes/macrophages kill their target cells mainly by apoptosis or necrosis is unclear. Killing mechanisms may be dependent on the respective tumor target. We found that two urothelial carcinoma cell lines, J82 and RT4, were both killed by human monocytes: J82 through the induction of apoptosis, RT4 by a cytostatic/necrotic mechanism (unpublished observations). As apoptotic tumor cells seem to inhibit macrophage cytotoxicity and even lead to a support of tumor cell growth, the choice of the death pathway may lead to an impairment of the tumor defense of macrophages (Reiter *et al.*, 1999). In addition, tumor cell death determines the capacity to induce a specific immune response by dendritic cells (Gallucci *et al.*, 1999; Sauter *et al.*, 2000). Therefore, it will be of great importance to analyze what determines the death pathway of special types of tumor cells.

6.3 Activation of macrophages for tumor cytotoxicity

Monocytes and macrophages can kill tumor cells spontaneously. During the differentiation of monocytes into macrophages, the ability to kill is increased and can be enhanced further if macrophages are stimulated with LPS, muramyl dipeptide (MDP) or IFN-γ (Doe and Henson, 1978; Sone and Fidler, 1980; Andreesen *et al.*, 1983a, 1988; Dean and Virelizier, 1983). Beside these typical macrophage activators, other substances can stimulate macrophage cytotoxicity, e.g. synthetic analogs of 2-lysophosphatidylcholine (Andreesen *et al.*, 1984), *Mycoplasma arginini* (Ribeiro-Dias *et al.*, 1999), GM-CSF (Grabstein *et al.*, 1986), M-CSF (Suzu *et al.*, 1989), glycosaminoglycans (Wrenshall *et al.*, 1999) and fibronectin (Perri *et al.*, 1982). For ADCC, an increased cytotoxicity was reported, for example after culture with M-CSF (Munn and Cheung, 1989), IL-4 (Wersall *et al.*, 1991) or stimulation with bacille Calmette–Guérin (BCG) (Koren *et al.*, 1981). To optimize the delivery of macrophage-activating stimuli such as MDP, lipsomes have been used as vehicles *in vivo* and *in vitro*. The lipid composition of the liposomes is very important to obtain a good engulfement and activation (Schroit and Fidler, 1982). Tumor cells themselves may also be involved in the activation of macrophages either by soluble factors or by membrane compounds. In the mouse system, macrophages were only primed effectively for the production of TNF-α and NO in the presence of tumor cells. Soluble tumor-derived factors seem to be responsible for this effect as no direct cell contact was necessary (Jiang *et al.*, 1992). Induction of cytokine expression through soluble tumor-derived factors was also described by Evans *et al.* (1991). Tumor cell membrane components such as carbohydrate structures are involved in the stimulation of monocytes through CD62L (Putz and Mannel, 1995).

6.4 Inhibition of tumor cytotoxicity

Even though macrophages possess, theoretically, the ability to kill tumor cells, they often seem to 'forget' about this important task. TAMs isolated from different types of tumors showed an impaired natural cytotoxic activity compared with control cells; however, they can be reactivated under certain conditions after *in vitro* culture (Mantovani *et al.*, 1980; Yanagawa *et al.*, 1985; Siziopikou *et al.*, 1991). As cytotoxicity is strongly dependent on a successful monocyte to macrophage maturation, one possible explanation for this phenomenon is that the differentiation of blood monocytes is inhibited in the tumor environment thereby generating a TAM with low cytotoxic potential (Andreesen *et al.*, 1983a, 1988; Munn and Cheung, 1989). Accordingly, TAMs generated within a tumor spheroid showed an immature phenotype (Konur *et al.*, 1996a, 1998). Other authors suggested an intrinsic maturation defect of monocytes from cancer patients (Krishnan *et al.*, 1980). The influence of the tumor on TAMs seems to depend also on the duration of the tumor contact. Suppression of macrophage tumor cytotoxicity was more pronounced in old compared with young mice and was influenced by the tumor stage (Khare *et al.*, 1999).

Soluble (tumor-derived) products have been shown to be involved in the suppression of macrophage cytotoxicity. Phosphatidylserine, which is a natural component of (tumor) membranes and widely used to enhance the uptake of liposomes with immunomodulators, inhibits macrophage tumor cytotoxicity in the murine system probably through the inhibition of NO production (Calderon *et al.*, 1994). IL-4 is another potent modulator of macrophage cytotoxicity and especially inhibits an activation-dependent tumoricidal state. This effect is mediated in part by the suppression of monokines such as IL-1 and TNF-α (Nishioka *et al.*, 1991). The same is true for IL-10, which alone or in combination with IL-4, inhibits tumor cytotoxicity of monocytes and macrophages (Nabioullin *et al.*, 1994). The suppression of hydrogen peroxide may be one mechanism of TGF-β-mediated inhibition of cytotoxicity (Tsunawaki *et al.*, 1988). The release of arachidonic acid compounds by either tumor cells or macrophages is also correlated with tumor cytotoxicity. Prostaglandins negatively regulate antitumor activity of macrophages whereas leukotrienes stimulate it (Bonta and Ben-Efraim, 1993). Accordingly, the cyclooxygenase/prostaglandin inhibitor indomethacin enhanced the cytotoxicity of macrophages and lipoxygenase/leukotriene inhibitors prevented it (Braun *et al.*, 1993; Hubbard and Erickson, 1995). However, some types of macrophage cytotoxicity seem to be resistant to prostaglandin-and IL-10-mediated blocking (Zeineddine *et al.*, 1999).

In ADCC, IL-4 increases the ADCC function of monocytes/macrophages (Wersall *et al.*, 1991), whereas IL-13 down-regulates the capacity for ADCC, most probably through the down-regulation of Fc receptors (de Waal *et al.*, 1993).

7 Regulation of a specific immune response by TAMs

It is known that T cells from cancer patients or tumor-bearing animals often are in a suppressed state, and several different mechanisms are involved in the suppression of the T cell response. One important mechanism of immunosuppression has been attributed to the down-modulation of the CD3 ζ chain in T cells which leads to defective T-cell signaling. Oxidative stress mediated by TAMs has been shown to down-modulate the CD3 z chain of the T-cell receptor complex and thereby inhibits an antigen-specific T-cell response (Otsuji *et al.*, 1996). In addition, Kono *et al.* (1996) demonstrated that hydrogen peroxide secreted by TAMs inhibits tumor-specific T-cell cytotoxicity. Even though the production of ROIs by TAMs is partially suppressed in the tumor environment (Ghezzi *et al.*, 1987; Siegert *et al.*, 1999), the oxidative stress seems to be sufficient to regulate this escape mechanism. In addition, TAM-derived cytotoxic molecules such as NO and TNF-α alter T-cell function (Alleva *et al.*, 1994; Elgert *et al.*, 1998), and Hengst *et al.* (1985), reported a correlation between the cytotoxic function and suppression of the T-cell response in human pulmonary alveolar macrophages.

Dendritic cells are important for the induction of a T-cell response, and high numbers of dendritic cells are correlated with a better prognosis in some types of malignancies (Ambe *et al.*, 1989; Zeid and Muller, 1993). Therefore, the suppression of a specific immune response may be due in part to the inhibition of dendritic cell maturation and/or infiltration into the tumor site. In gastric carcinoma, the density of dendritic cells is inversely correlated to the expression of VEGF, suggesting that VEGF may regulate dendritic cell infiltration (Saito *et al.*, 1998). Accordingly, the inhibition of VEGF improved the number and function of Langerhans cells *in vivo* (Ishida *et al.*, 1998). In breast carcinoma, immature dendritic cells reside specifically within the tumor, whereas mature cells are located peritumorally (Bell *et al.*, 1999). Two possible explanation exist for this phenomenon: first, high levels of intratumoral MIP-3α in breast carcinoma lead to an increased homing of immature cells and/or secondly, the tumor environment suppresses the maturation of dendritic cells. VEGF and other tumor-derived soluble factors such as IL-10, IL-6 or M-CSF may be responsible for the inhibition of dendritic cell differentiation in the tumor site (Ding *et al.*, 1993; Buelens *et al.*, 1995; Gabrilovich *et al.*, 1996; Menetrier-Caux *et al.*, 1998).

8 Adoptive immunotherapy—macrophage-based approaches

The systemic activation of macrophages through the use of lymphokines and synthetic analogs of MDP, as both a free and liposome-encapsulated drug, have had limited clinical effects so far, one reason being that this approach requires responsive but not 'symbiotic' macrophages at the tumor site. Thus, adoptive transfer of *ex vivo*-generated macrophages where both their differentiation and functional activation have been completed away from the 'silencing' micromilieu of the tumor may be a rationalistic and more promising way to break this type of immune tolerance (Andreesen *et al.*, 1998). More than 25 years ago, Isaac J. Fidler and colleagues in Houston pioneered the use of activated macrophages in murine models of metastatic tumor. Using the B16 melanoma model, they demonstrated that the percentage of animals cured and the suppression of pulmonary metastases depended on the *in vitro* activation as well as the number of macrophages infused (Fidler, 1974). Other groups have confirmed their findings using different tumor models, including human xenografts (Berdel *et al.*, 1980; Ortaldo *et al.*, 1986). It is important, however, to note that in these rodent studies, all types of macrophage-targeted immunotherapy were effective only in inhibiting metastasis formation, while regression of primary tumors was rarely observed (Fidler, 1985). This phenomenon might be explained by the size of the primary tumor but may also be due to the substantial differences in the functional competence of host macrophages which interact either with an established tumor or with small aggregates of metastasizing cells most often embedded in a cellular inflammatory reaction.

8.1 Adoptive immunotherapy with human macrophage cells

While murine macrophages can be obtained easily either from the peritoneal cavity or grown from bone marrow precursor cells, human studies on macrophage adoptive transfer had to wait for appropriate technology to isolate or grow human macrophages on a large scale. As blood monocytes are readily accessible and could be obtained in large quantities by leukapheresis and subsequent elutriation (Stevenson *et al.*, 1983), they were the first to be used in cancer patients (Stevenson *et al.*, 1987). In fact up to 3×10^9 monocytes can be isolated through a single apheresis processing 8–10 liters of blood. However, monocytes are still immature precursor cells which only acquire the full antineoplastic armamentarium upon further differentiation (Andreesen *et al.*, 1988, 1983b) and, secondly, when infused and having infiltrated into the tumor tissue may be 'silenced' in the same way as believed to take place in the ontogeny of TAMs. Therefore, schemes of macrophage adoptive therapy have to include terminal maturation of monocytes first, followed by functional activation with IFN-γ and re-infusion. Upon culture in the presence of autologous serum for 7 days, monocytes indeed transform to mature macrophages, as evidenced by morphology and cytochemistry (Andreesen *et al.*, 1983b), analysis of maturation-dependent antigen expression (Andreesen *et al.*, 1990a), cytokine repertoire (Scheibenbogen and Andreesen,1991) and development of both direct cell-mediated (Andreesen *et al.*, 1983a) and antibody-dependent cellular cytotoxicity (Munn and Cheung, 1989). Grown from mononuclear cells on hydrophobic Teflon foils (Andreesen *et al.*, 1983b) to which they adhere only loosely, monocyte-derived macrophages can easily be detached and recovered at day 7 and purified by elutriation from remaining lymphocytes (Brugger *et al.*, 1991) before being retransfused to the patient. Figure 11.5 depicts the scheme of macrophage adoptive immunotherapy. The recovery of macrophages from blood monocytes can be increased by the addition of GM-CSF (Eischen *et al.*, 1991). Also, serum-free conditions have been developed (Kreutz *et al.*, 1992; Vincent *et al.*, 1992.

Dose escalation studies starting with 10^5 cells were initiated in 1988 first in Freiburg (Andreesen *et al.*, 1990b) and later in Strasbourg (Faradji *et al.*, 1991). It was demonstrated in these and subsequent studies (Lopez *et al.*, 1992; Wiesel *et al.*, 1992) that *in vitro* grown MACs could be safely administered at up to 3×10^9 cells per single infusion (the maximum cell number achieved by leukapheresis) without major toxicity. Low-grade fever and flu-like symptoms were the only clinical side effects observed. Monocyte activity could be followed by an increase in serum neopterin and C-reactive protein as well as a

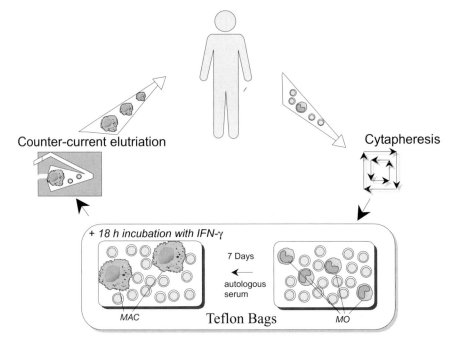

Fig. 11.5 Schematic representation of adoptive immunotherapy with human monocyte-derived macrophages.

transient cell dose-dependent rise of thrombin–antithrombin (TAT) complexes (Andreesen *et al.*, 1990b; Wiesel *et al.*, 1992), reflecting the procoagulatory activity of IFN-γ stimulated monocyte-derived macrophages. Macrophage therapies were repeated every 7–14 days, again without evidence of any cumulative toxicity. Similar dose escalation studies were performed reinfusing macrophages in the peritoneal and pleural cavities and through regional liver perfusion via selective catherization of the hepatic artery (Hennemann *et al.*, 1995). To increase the number of monocytes available for *in vitro* differentiation, GM-CSF was administered for 7 days to patients prior to leukapheresis. This allowed an increase of up to 7.3×10^9 macrophages and doubled the amount of cells to be given at a single infusion (Hennemann *et al.*, 1997). Apart from increasing the number of circulating monocytes, it could be shown by whole-blood assay that GM-CSF treatment induced functional changes in blood monocytes, e.g. an increase in TNF-α and a reduction in IL-10 secretion (Hennemann *et al.*, 1998). Furthermore, to activate the cytotoxic cytokine repertoire of macrophages, bacterial endotoxin (LPS, *Salmonella typhimurium*) was used for additional activation (Hennemann *et al.*, 1997) in one study. Here a maximal tolerated dose of 2×10^8 was established, with chills, nausea and headache being the limiting toxicities. However, no side effects were observed when patients were pre-treated with ibuprofen which allowed an increase in macrophage numbers up to 1.5×10^9 per infusion, without dose-limiting toxicity. In patients given LPS/IFN-γ-activated macrophages, a biological response could be monitored by analyzing serum levels of IL-6, IL-8 and IL-1 receptor antagonist increasing upon infusion (Hennemann *et al.*, 1997).

Labeling the autografted macrophages with [111]indium-oxine revealed that intravenously reinfused cells were retained in the lungs for 45–90 min and then pooled into liver and spleen, concentrating at or around metastatic nodules (unpublished observations). Macrophages injected intraperitoneally remained in the peritoneal cavity for more than 7 days and concentrated at sites of major tumor growth. Similarly to the slow passage through the lungs, macrophages infused via the hepatic artery were retained in the liver for about 30 min before being released into the venous circulation. Again, they seem to be localized at sites of metastasis where they could be detected for more than 7 days (Hennemann *et al.*, 1995).

The clinical evidence of an antitumor effect of macrophage adoptive therapy at present is rather limited. The reduction of malignant ascites seen in three out of seven patients treated intraperitoneally might in fact be due to non-specific inflammatory rather than antineoplastic effects, as no change in tumor activity could be detected by computed tomography or laboratory testing (Andreesen *et al.*, 1990b).

8.2 Use of monocyte-derived cells to present antigen

By changing the culture conditions, monocytes can differentiate not only into phagocytic and cytotoxic macrophages but, under the influence of IL-4, GM-CSF and TNF-α, also into highly potent antigen-presenting cells (Peters *et al.*, 1987, 1996). These monocyte-derived dendritic cells seem to be equivalent to dendritic cells derived from bone marrow progenitor cells (Meierhoff *et al.*, 1998) and have already been used succesfully as cellular vaccines in clinical trials (Nestle *et al.*, 1998); addtional data are available from several animal trials. Pulsed *in vitro* with whole tumor-derived DNA (Manickan *et al.*, 1997), tumor-associated antigenic peptides (Celluzzi *et al.*, 1996) or crude tumor lysates (Zitvogel *et al.*, 1996), or fused to generate tumor–dendritic cell hybrids (Gong *et al.*,

1997), they are injected subcutanously, intravenously or intralymphatically to initiate or boost the patient's specific immune response to the tumor (Grabbe *et al.*, 1995; Troy and Hart, 1997). Dendritic cells might even be grown from leukemic monocytes to be used as vaccines *in vivo* for generating a cytotoxic T-cell response directed against leukemia-specific fusion proteins resulting from chromosomal translocations (Smit *et al.*, 1997).

Yet, several questions remain to be answered: first of all, antigen presentation can induce both T-cell activation leading to induction of an immune response and T-cell anergy and tolerance induction (Ferrero *et al.*, 1997). Thus, it may be of crucial importance which specific type of dendritic cells is used for cellular therapy, especially as recent publications suggest an essential role for dendritic cells apparently is to decide on an immunogenic or a tolerogenic response of the recognizing T cell (Ridge *et al.*, 1996). In terms of function and phenotype, dendritic cells cultured from CD34[+] hematopoietic precursors or monocytes are quite similar (Meierhoff *et al.*, 1998), but little is known so far as to which cytokines can modulate dendritic cell biology in a way that optimizes the induction of antitumor immunity *in vivo*. A similar concern is expressed with respect to cell dose, optimal treatment schedule and the route of application.

To take the concept of antigen-presenting cells a step further, it is tempting also to explore the possible exploitation of their ability to induce cytotoxic T cells specific for tumor-associated antigens *in vitro* (Cardoso *et al.*, 1997; Nieda *et al.*, 1998) which subsequently upon expansion and activation can be used as the therapeutic cellular product. Apart from immunotherapy of tumors, other areas of medicine might benefit from dendritic cell technology: dendritic cells treated with IL-10, which down-modulates co-stimulatory molecules and suppresses mixed lymphocyte reactions, may be able to generate tolerogenic T cells (Groux *et al.*, 1996) which can be used in the setting of allogeneic bone marrow transplantation to reduce mortality from graft-versus-host disease. Also, donor-derived dendritic cells might help to reconstitute the long-lasting immunodeficiency after haplo-identical bone marrow transplantation.

9 Summary

Macrophages play an ambivalent role in cancer development and are involved in the critical balance between health and disease. Although they have the potential to mediate tumor cytotoxicity, present tumor-associated antigens to T cells and stimulate cytotoxic lymphocytes, the tumor environment seems to suppress those 'cytotoxic' macrophages, rendering the host incapable of mounting a successful antitumor response. TAMs represent a 'symbiotic' type of macrophage, promoting tumor growth and suppressing the T cell and NK cell antitumor response. The understanding of the regulatory mechanisms that control this dualism between 'symbiotic' and 'cytotoxic' macrophage may help us to tip the balance towards the 'cytotoxic' type of macrophage and thereby reactivate the antitumor functions of the immune system.

References

Adachi, N., Yamaguchi, K., Morikawa, Suzuki, T.M., Matsuda, I. and Abe, M.K. (1994). Constitutive production of multiple colony-stimulating factors in patients with lung cancer associated with neutrophilia. *British Journal of Cancer*, **69**, 125–9.

Aderka, D., Le, J.M. and Vilcek, J. (1989). IL-6 inhibits lipopolysaccharide-induced tumor necrosis factor production in cultured human monocytes, U937 cells, and in mice. *Journal of Immunology*, **143**, 3517–23.

Aliprantis, A.O., Diez-Roux, G., Mulder, L.C., Zychlinsky, A. and Lang, R.A. (1996). Do macrophages kill through apoptosis? *Immunology Today*, **17**, 573–6.

Alleva, D.G., Burger, C.J. and Elgert, K.D. (1994). Tumor-induced regulation of suppressor macrophage nitric oxide and TNF-α production. Role of tumor-derived IL-10, TGF-β, and prostaglandin E2. *Journal of Immunology*, **153**, 1674–86.

Ambe, K., Mori, M. and Enjoji, M. (1989). S-100 protein-positive dendritic cells in colorectal adenocarcinomas. Distribution and relation to the clinical prognosis. *Cancer*, **63**, 496–503.

Andreesen, R., Osterholz, J., Bross, K.J., Schulz, A., Luckenbach, G.A. and Lohr, G.W. (1983a). Cytotoxic effector cell function at different stages of human monocyte–macrophage maturation. *Cancer Research*, **43**, 5931–6.

Andreesen, R., Picht, J. and Lohr, G.W. (1983b). Primary cultures of human blood-borne macrophages grown on hydrophobic teflon membranes. *Journal of Immunological Methods*, **56**, 295–304.

Andreesen, R., Osterholz, J., Luckenbach, G.A., Costabel, U., Schulz, A. Speth, V.P. *et al.* (1984). Tumor cytotoxicity of human macrophages after incubation with synthetic analogues of 2-lysophosphatidylcholine. *Journal of the National Cancer Institute*, **72**, 53–9.

Andreesen, R., Gadd, S., Brugger, W., Lohr, G.W. and Atkins, R.C. (1988). Activation of human monocyte-derived macrophages cultured on Teflon: response to interferon-γ during terminal maturation *in vitro*. *Immunobiology*, **177**, 186–98.

Andreesen, R., Brugger, W., Scheibenbogen, C., Kreutz, M., Leser, H.G., Rehm, A. *et al.* (1990a). Surface phenotype analysis of human monocyte to macrophage maturation. *Journal of Leukocyte Biology*, **47**, 490–7.

Andreesen, R., Scheibenbogen, C., Brugger, W., Krause, S., Meerpohl, H.G., Leser, H.G. *et al.* (1990b). Adoptive transfer of tumor cytotoxic macrophages generated *in vitro* from circulating blood monocytes: a new approach to cancer immunotherapy. *Cancer Research*, **50**, 7450–6.

Andreesen, R., Hennemann, B. and Krause, S.W. (1998). Adoptive immunotherapy of cancer using monocyte-derived macrophages: rationale, current status, and perspectives. *Journal of Leukocyte Biology*, **64**, 419–26.

Asschert, J.G., Vellenga, E., Hollema, H., van-der, Z.A. and de, V.E. (1997). Expression of macrophage colony-stimulating factor (M-CSF), interleukin-6 (IL-6), interleukin-1β (IL-1β), interleukin-11 (IL-11) and tumour necrosis factor-α (TNF-α) in p53-characterised human ovarian carcinomas. *European Journal of Cancer*, **33**, 2246–51.

Audran, R., Dazord, L. and Toujas, L. (1994). Interactions between human macrophages and tumor cells in three-dimensional cultures. *Cancer Immunology and Immunotherapy*, **39**, 299–304.

Balkwill, F., Osborne, R., Burke, F., Naylor, S., Talbot, D., Durbin, H. *et al.* (1987). Evidence for tumour necrosis factor/cachectin production in cancer. *Lancet*, **2**, 1229–32.

Bell, D., Chomarat, P., Broyles, D., Netto, G., Harb, G.M., Lebecque, S. *et al.* (1999). In breast carcinoma tissue, immature dendritic cells reside within the tumor, whereas mature dendritic cells are located in peritumoral areas. *Journal of Experimental Medicine*, **190**, 1417–26.

Berdel, W.E., Bausert, W.R., Weltzien, H.U., Modolell, M.L., Widmann, K.H. and Munder, P.G. (1980). The influence of alkyl-lysophospholipids and lysophospholipid-activated macrophages on the development of metastasis of 3-Lewis lung carcinoma. *European Journal of Cancer*, **16**, 1199–204.

Bernasconi, S., Peri, G., Sironi, M. and Mantovani, A. (1991). Involvement of leukocyte (β2) integrins (CD18/CD11) in human monocyte tumoricidal activity. *International Journal of Cancer*, **49**, 267–73.

Bernasconi, S., Matteucci, C., Sironi, M., Conni, M., Colotta, F., Mosca, M. *et al.* (1995). Effects of granulocyte–monocyte colony-stimulating factor (GM-CSF) on expression of adhesion molecules and production of cytokines in blood monocytes and ovarian cancer-associated macrophages. *International Journal of Cancer*, **60**, 300–7.

Bicknell, R. and Harris, A.L. (1991). Novel growth regulatory factors and tumour angiogenesis. *European Journal of Cancer*, **27**, 781–5.

Bonta, I.L. and Ben-Efraim, S. (1993). Involvement of inflammatory mediators in macrophage antitumor activity. *Journal of Leukocyte Biology*, **54**, 613–26.

Bottazzi, B., Colotta, F., Sica, A., Nobili, N. and Mantovani, A. (1990). A chemoattractant expressed in human sarcoma cells (tumor-derived chemotactic factor, TDCF) is identical to monocyte chemoattractant protein-1/monocyte chemotactic and activating factor (MCP-1/MCAF). *International Journal of Cancer*, **45**, 795–7.

Braun, D.P., Ahn, M.C., Harris, J.E., Chu, E., Casey, L., Wilbanks, G. *et al.* (1993). Sensitivity of tumoricidal function in macrophages from different anatomical sites of cancer patients to modulation of arachidonic acid metabolism. *Cancer Research*, **53**, 3362–8.

Brugger, W., Scheibenbogen, C., Krause, S. and Andreesen, R. (1991). Large-scale production of human tumorcytotoxic macrophages grown from blood monocytes of cancer patients. *Cancer Detection and Prevention*, **15**, 407–12.

Buelens, C., Willems, F., Delvaux, A., Pierard, G., Delville, J.P., Velu, T. *et al.* (1995). Interleukin-10 differentially regulates B7-1 (CD80) and B7-2 (CD86) expression on human peripheral blood dendritic cells. *European Journal of Immunology*, **25**, 2668–72.

Calderon, C., Huang, Z.H., Gage, D.A., Sotomayor, E.M. and Lopez, D.M. (1994). Isolation of a nitric oxide inhibitor from mammary tumor cells and its characterization as phosphatidyl serine. *Journal of Experimental Medicine*, **180**, 945–58.

Cardoso, A.A., Seamon, M.J., Afonso, H.M., Ghia, P., Boussiotis, V.A., Freeman, G.J. *et al.* (1997). *Ex vivo* generation of human anti-pre-B leukemia-specific autologous cytolytic T cells. *Blood*, **90**, 549–61.

Carlsson, J. and Acker, H. (1988). Relations between pH, oxygen partial pressure and growth in cultured cell spheroids. *International Journal of Cancer*, **42**, 715–20.

Carswell, E.A., Old, L.J., Kassel, R.L., Green, S., Fiore, N. and Williamson, B. (1975). An endotoxin-induced serum factor that causes necrosis of tumors. *Proceedings of the National Academy of Sciences USA*, **72**, 3666–70.

Celluzzi, C.M., Mayordomo, J.I., Storkus, W.J., Lotze, M.T. and Falo, L.D.J. (1996). Peptide-pulsed dendritic cells induce antigen-specific CTL-mediated protective tumor immunity. *Journal of Experimental Medicine*, **183**, 283–7.

Chambers, S.K., Wang, Y., Gertz, R.E. and Kacinski, B.M. (1995). Macrophage colony-stimulating factor mediates invasion of ovarian cancer cells through urokinase. *Cancer Research*, **55**, 1578–85.

Chambers, S.K., Kacinski, B.M., Ivins, C.M. and Carcangiu, M.L. (1997). Overexpression of epithelial macrophage colony-stimulating factor (CSF-1) and CSF-1 receptor: a poor prognostic factor in epithelial ovarian cancer, contrasted with a protective effect of stromal CSF-1. *Clinics in Cancer Research*, **3**, 999–1007.

Chattopadhyay, U. and Bhattacharyya, S. (1988). Induction of tumor associated macrophage-mediated lysis of autologous tumor cells by lectins. *Neoplasma*, **35**, 321–8.

Connolly, D.T., Stoddard, B.L., Harakas, N.K. and Feder, J. (1987). Human fibroblast-derived growth factor is a mitogen and chemoattractant for endothelial cells. *Biochemical and Biophysical Research Communications*, **144**, 705–12.

Connor, R.I., Shen, L. and Fanger, M.W. (1990). Evaluation of the antibody-dependent cytotoxic capabilities of individual human monocytes. Role of FcgRI and FcgRII and the effects of cytokines at the single cell level. *Journal of Immunology*, **145**, 1483–9.

Cornelius, L.A., Nehring, L.C., Harding, E., Bolanowski, M., Welgus, H.G., Kobayashi, D.K. *et al.* (1998). Matrix metalloproteinases generate angiostatin: effects on neovascularization. *Journal of Immunology*, **161**, 6845–52.

de Waal, M., Figdor, C.G., Huijbens, R., Mohan-Peterson, S., Bennett, B., Culpepper, J. *et al.* (1993). Effects of IL-13 on phenotype, cytokine production, and cytotoxic function of human monocytes. Comparison with IL-4 and modulation by IFN-γ or IL-10. *Journal of Immunology*, **151**, 6370–81.

Dean, R.T. and Virelizier, J.L. (1983). Interferon as a macrophage activating factor. I. Enhancement of cytotoxicity by fresh and matured human monocytes in the absence of other soluble signals. *Clinical amd Experimental Immunology*, **51**, 501–10.

Dias, S., Boyd, R. and Balkwill, F. (1998). IL-12 regulates VEGF and MMPs in a murine breast cancer model. *International Journal of Cancer*, **78**, 361–5.

Ding, L., Linsley, P.S., Huang, L.Y., Germain, R.N. and Shevach, E.M. (1993). IL-10 inhibits macrophage costimulatory activity by selectively inhibiting the up-regulation of B7 expression. *Journal of Immunology*, **151**, 1224–34.

DiPietro, L.A. and Polverini, P.J. (1993). Angiogenic macrophages produce the angiogenic inhibitor thrombospondin 1. *American Journal of Pathology*, **143**, 678–84.

Doe, W.F. and Henson, P.M. (1978). Macrophage stimulation by bacterial lipopolysaccharides. I. Cytolytic effect on tumor target cells. *Journal of Experimental Medicine*, **148**, 544–56.

Dong, Z., Kumar, R., Yang, X. and Fidler, I.J. (1997). Macrophage-derived metalloelastase is responsible for the generation of angiostatin in Lewis lung carcinoma. *Cell*, **88**, 801–10.

Dorsch, M., Hock, H., Kunzendorf, U., Diamantstein, T. and Blankenstein, T. (1993). Macrophage colony-stimulating factor gene transfer into tumor cells induces macrophage infiltration but not tumor suppression. *European Journal of Immunology*, **23**, 186–90.

Dvorak, H.F. (1986). Tumors: wounds that do not heal. Similarities between tumor stroma generation and wound healing. *New England Journal of Medicine*, **315**, 1650–9.

Economou, J.S., Colquhoun, S.D., Anderson, T.M., McBride, W.W., Golub, S., Holmes, E.C. *et al.* (1988). Interleukin-1 and tumor necrosis factor production by tumor-associated mononuclear leukocytes and peripheral mononuclear leukocytes in cancer patients. *International Journal of Cancer*, **42**, 712–4.

Eerola, A.K., Soini, Y. and Paakko, P. (1999). Tumour infiltrating lymphocytes in relation to tumour angiogenesis, apoptosis and prognosis in patients with large cell lung carcinoma. *Lung Cancer*, **26**, 73–83.

Eischen, A., Vincent, F., Bergerat, J.P., Louis, B., Faradji, A., Bohbot, A. *et al.* (1991). Long term cultures of human monocytes *in vitro*. Impact of GM-CSF on survival and differentiation. *Journal of Immunological Methods*, **143**, 209–21.

Elgert, K.D., Alleva, D.G. and Mullins, D.W. (1998). Tumor-induced immune dysfunction: the macrophage connection. *Journal of Leukocyte Biology*, **64**, 275–90.

Erroi, A., Sironi, M., Chiaffarino, F., Chen, Z.G., Mengozzi, M. and Mantovani, A. (1989). IL-1 and IL-6 release by tumor-associated macrophages from human ovarian carcinoma. *International Journal of Cancer*, **44**, 795–801.

Evans, R., Kamdar, S.J. and Duffy, T.M. (1991). Tumor-derived products induce Il-1α, Il-1β, Tnfα, and Il-6 gene expression in murine macrophages: distinctions between tumor- and bacterial endotoxin-induced gene expression. *Journal of Leukocyte Biology*, **49**, 474–82.

Evans, R., Fong, M., Fuller, J., Kamdar, S., Meyerhardt, J. and Strassmann, G. (1992). Tumor cell IL-6 gene expression is regulated by IL-1α/β and TNF α: proposed feedback mechanisms induced by the interaction of tumor cells and macrophages. *Journal of Leukocyte Biology*, **52**, 463–8.

Fanger, N.A., Maliszewski, C.R., Schooley, K. and Griffith, T.S. (1999). Human dendritic cells mediate cellular apoptosis via tumor necrosis factor-related apoptosis-inducing ligand (TRAIL). *Journal of Experimental Medicine*, **190**, 1155–64.

Faradji, A., Bohbot, A., Frost, H., Schmitt-Goguel, M., Siffert, J.C., Dufour, P. *et al.* (1991). Phase I study of liposomal MTP-PE-activated autologous monocytes administered intraperitoneally to patients with peritoneal carcinomatosis. *Journal of Clinical Oncology*, **9**, 1251–60.

Feinman, R., Henriksen-DeStefano, D., Tsujimoto, M. and Vilcek, J. (1987). Tumor necrosis factor is an important mediator of tumor cell killing by human monocytes. *Journal of Immunology*, **138**, 635–40.

Ferrero, I., Anjuere, F., MacDonald, H.R. and Ardavin, C. (1997). *In vitro* negative selection of viral superantigen-reactive thymocytes by thymic dendritic cells. *Blood*, **90**, 1943–51.

Fidler, I.J. (1974). Inhibition of pulmonary metastasis by intravenous injection of specifically activated macrophages. *Cancer Research*, **34**, 1074–8.

Fidler, I.J. (1985). Macrophages and metastasis—a biological approach to cancer therapy. *Cancer Research*, **45**, 4714–26.

Fidler, I.J. and Schroit, A.J. (1988). Recognition and destruction of neoplastic cells by activated macrophages: discrimination of altered self. *Biochimica et Biophysica Acta*, **948**, 151–173.

Finnis, C., Dodsworth, N., Pollitt, C.E., Carr, G. and Sleep, D. (1993). Thymidine phosphorylase activity of platelet-derived endothelial cell growth factor is responsible for endothelial cell mitogenicity. *European Journal of Biochemistry*, **212**, 201–10.

Fixe, P. and Praloran, V. (1997). Macrophage colony-stimulating-factor (M-CSF or CSF-1) and its receptor: structure–function relationships. *European Cytokine Network*, **8**, 125–36.

Foti, E., Ferrandina, G., Martucci, R., Romanini, M.E., Benedetti,P.P., Testa, U. *et al.* (1999). IL-6, M-CSF and IAP cytokines in ovarian cancer: simultaneous assessment of serum levels. *Oncology*, **57**, 211–5.

Frank, R.N. (1994). Vascular endothelial growth factor—its role in retinal vascular proliferation. *New England Journal of Medicine*, **331**, 1519–20.

Fujimura, T. and Torisu, M. (1987). Neutrophil-mediated tumor cell destruction in cancer ascites. II. A OK-432 attracts killer neutrophils through activation of complement C5. *Clinical Immunology and Immunopathology*, **43**, 174–84.

Gabrilovich, D.I., Chen, H.L., Girgis, K.R., Cunningham, H.T., Meny, G.M., Nadaf, S. *et al.* (1996). Production of vascular endothelial growth factor by human tumors inhibits the functional maturation of dendritic cells. *Nature Medicine*, **2**, 1096–103.

Gallucci, S., Lolkema, M. and Matzinger, P. (1999). Natural adjuvants: endogenous activators of dendritic cells. *Nature Medicine*, **5**, 1249–55.

Ghezzi, P., Erroi, A., Acero, R., Salmona, M. and Mantovani, A. (1987). Defective production of reactive oxygen intermediates by tumor-associated macrophages exposed to phorbol ester. *Journal of Leukocyte Biology*, **42**, 84–90.

Goede, V., Brogelli, L., Ziche, M. and Augustin, H.G. (1999). Induction of inflammatory angiogenesis by monocyte chemoattractant protein-1. *International Journal of Cancer*, **82**, 765–70.

Gong, J., Chen, D., Kashiwaba, M. and Kufe, D. (1997). Induction of antitumor activity by immunization with fusions of dendritic and carcinoma cells. *Nature Medicine*, **3**, 558–561.

Grabbe, S., Beissert, S., Schwarz, T. and Granstein, R.D. (1995). Dendritic cells as initiators of tumor immune responses: a possible strategy for tumor immunotherapy?. *Immunology Today*, **16**, 117–21.

Grabstein, K.H., Urdal, D.L., Tushinski, R.J., Mochizuki, D.Y., Price, V.L., Cantrell, M.A. *et al.* (1986). Induction of macrophage tumoricidal activity by granulocyte–macrophage colony-stimulating factor. *Science*, **232**, 506–8.

Graves, D.T., Barnhill, R., Galanopoulos, T. and Antoniades, H.N. (1992). Expression of monocyte chemotactic protein-1 in human melanoma *in vivo*. *American Journal of Pathology*, **140**, 9–14.

Grell, M., Krammer, P.H. and Scheurich, P. (1994). Segregation of APO-1/Fas antigen- and tumor necrosis factor receptor-mediated apoptosis. *European Journal of Immunology*, **24**, 2563–6.

Griffith, T.S., Wiley, S.R., Kubin, M.Z., Sedger, L.M., Maliszewski, C.R. and Fanger, N.A. (1999). Monocyte-mediated tumoricidal activity via the tumor necrosis factor-related cytokine, TRAIL. *Journal of Experimental Medicine*, **189**, 1343–54.

Griffiths, G.M. and Mueller, C. (1991). Expression of perforin and granzymes *in vivo*: potential diagnostic markers for activated cytotoxic cells. *Immunology Today*, **12**, 415–9.

Groux, H., Bigler, M., de Vries, J.E. and Roncarolo, M.G. (1996). Interleukin-10 induces a long-term antigen-specific anergic state in human CD4+ T. *Journal of Experimental Medicine*, **184**, 19–29.

Harmey, J.H., Dimitriadis, E., Kay, E. Redmond, H.P. and Bouchier, H.D. (1998). Regulation of macrophage production of vascular endothelial growth factor (VEGF) by hypoxia and transforming growth factor β-1. *Annals of Surgical Oncology*, **5**, 271–8.

Hashimoto, S., Yoda, M., Yamada, M., Yanai, N., Kawashima, T. and Motoyoshi, K. (1996). Macrophage colony-stimulating factor induces interleukin-8 production in human monocytes. *Experimental Hematology*, **24**, 123–8.

Hauptmann, S., Zwadlo-Klarwasser, G., Jansen, M., Klosterhalfen, B. and Kirkpatrick, C.J. (1993). Macrophages and multicellular tumor spheroids in co-culture: a three-dimensional model to study tumor–host interactions. Evidence for macrophage-mediated tumor cell proliferation and migration. *American Journal of Pathology*, **143**, 1406–15.

Hengst, J.C., Kan-Mitchell, J., Kempf, R.A., Strumpf, I.J., Sharma, O.P., Kortes, V.L. *et al.* (1985). Correlation between cytotoxic and suppressor activities of human pulmonary alveolar macrophages. *Cancer Res.*, **45**, 459–463.

Hennemann, B., Scheibenbogen, C., Schumichen, C. and Andreesen, R. (1995). Intrahepatic adoptive immunotherapy with autologous tumorcytotoxic macrophages in patients with cancer. *Journal of Immunotherapy with Emphasis on Tumor Immunology*, **18**, 19–27.

Hennemann, B., Rehm, A., Kottke, A., Meidenbauer, N. and Andreesen, R. (1997). Adoptive immunotherapy with tumor-cytotoxic macrophages derived from recombinant human granulocyte–macrophage colony-stimulating factor (rhuGM-CSF) mobilized peripheral blood monocytes. *Journal of Immunotherapy*, **20**, 365–71.

Hennemann, B., Kreutz, M., Rehm, A. and Andreesen, R. (1998). Effect of granulocyte–macrophage colony-stimulating factor treatment on phenotype, cytokine release and cytotoxicity of circulating blood monocytes and monocyte-derived macrophages. *British Journal of Haematology*, **102**, 1197–203.

Hibbs, J.B.J., Lambert, L.H.J. and Remington, J.S. (1972). Control of carcinogenesis: a possible role for the activated macrophage. *Science*, **177**, 998–1000.

Hibbs, J.B.J., Taintor, R.R., Vavrin, Z. and Rachlin, E.M. (1988). Nitric oxide: a cytotoxic activated macrophage effector molecule. *Biochemical and Biophysical Research Communications*, **157**, 87–94.

Hildenbrand, R., Dilger, I., Horlin, A. and Stutte, H.J. (1995). Urokinase and macrophages in tumour angiogenesis. *British Journal of Cancer*, **72**, 818–23.

Hildenbrand, R., Jansen, C., Wolf, G., Bohme, B., Berger, S., von Minckwitz, G. *et al.* (1998). Transforming growth factor-β stimulates urokinase expression in tumor-associated macrophages of the breast. *Laboratory Investigation*, **78**, 59–71.

Horn, D., van der Bosch, J., Ruller, S. and Schlaak, M. (1991). Suppression of tumor cell susceptibility to monocyte-induced cell death by growth-inhibitory signals generated during monocyte/tumor cell interaction. *Journal of Cell Biochemistry*, **45**, 213–23.

Hubbard, N.E. and Erickson, K.L. (1995). Role of 5'-lipoxygenase metabolites in the activation of peritoneal macrophages for tumoricidal function. *Cell Immunology*, **160**, 115–22.

Ichinose, Y., Bakouche, O., Tsao, J.Y. and Fidler, I.J. (1988). Tumor necrosis factor and IL-1 associated with plasma membranes of activated human monocytes lyse monokine-sensitive but not monokine-resistant tumor cells whereas viable activated monocytes lyse both. *Journal of Immunology*, **141**, 512–8.

Ingber, D.E. and Folkman, J. (1989). How does extracellular matrix control capillary morphogenesis? *Cell*, **58**, 803–5.

Iruela-Arispe, M.L., Bornstein, P. and Sage, H. (1991). Thrombospondin exerts an antiangiogenic effect on cord formation by endothelial cells *in vitro*. *Proceedings of the National Academy of Sciences USA*, **88**, 5026–30.

Ishida, T., Oyama, T., Carbone, D.P. and Gabrilovich, D.I. (1998). Defective function of Langerhans cells in tumor-bearing animals is the result of defective maturation from hematopoietic progenitors. *Journal of Immunology*, **161**, 4842–51.

Iwasaki, K., Kikuchi, H., Miyatake, S., Aoki, T., Yamasaki, T. and Oda,Y. (1990). Infiltrative and cytolytic activities of lymphokine-activated killer cells against a human glioma spheroid model. *Cancer Research*, **50**, 2429–36.

Jaaskelainen, J., Kalliomaki, P., Paetau, A. and Timonen, T. (1989). Effect of LAK cells against three-dimensional tumor tissue. *In vitro* study using multi-cellular human glioma spheroids as targets. *Journal of Immunology*, **142**, 1036–45.

Jadus, M.R., Irwin, M.C., Irwin, M.R., Horansky, R.D., Sekhon, S., Pepper, K.A. *et al.* (1996). Macrophages can recognize and kill tumor cells bearing the membrane isoform of macrophage colony-stimulating factor. *Blood*, **87**, 5232–41.

Janicke, R. and Mannel, D.N. (1990). Distinct tumor cell membrane constituents activate human monocytes for tumor necrosis factor synthesis. *Journal of Immunology*, **144**, 1144–50.

Jiang, Y., Beller, D.I., Frendl, G. and Graves, D.T. (1992). Monocyte chemoattractant protein-1 regulates adhesion molecule expression and cytokine production in human monocytes. *Journal of Immunology*, **148**, 2423–8.

Jin, L., Yuan, R.Q., Fuchs, A., Yao, Y,. Joseph, A., Schwall, R. *et al.* (1997). Expression of interleukin-1β in human breast carcinoma. *Cancer*, **80**, 421–434.

Joseph, I.B. and Isaacs, J.T. (1998). Macrophage role in the anti-prostate cancer response to one class of antiangiogenic agents. *Journal of the National Cancer Institute*, **90**, 1648–53.

Kacinski, B.M. (1995). CSF-1 and its receptor in ovarian, endometrial and breast cancer. *Annals of Medicine*, **27**, 79–85.

Khare, V., Sodhi, A. and Singh, S.M. (1999). Age-dependent alterations in the tumoricidal functions of tumor-associated macrophages. *Tumour Biology*, **20**, 30–43.

Kinoshita, T., Ito, H. and Miki, C. (1999). Serum interleukin-6 level reflects the tumor proliferative activity in patients with colorectal carcinoma. *Cancer*, **85**, 2526–31.

Knighton, D.R., Hunt, T.K., Scheuenstuhl, H., Halliday, B.J., Werb, Z. and Banda, M.J. (1983). Oxygen tension regulates the expression of angiogenesis factor by macrophages. *Science*, **221**, 1283–5.

Knuchel, R., Feichtinger, J., Recktenwald, A., Hollweg, H.G., Franke, P., Jakse, G. *et al.* (1988). Interactions between bladder tumor cells as tumor spheroids from the cell line J82 and human endothelial cells *in vitro*. *Journal of Urology*, **139**, 640–45.

Koch, A.E., Polverini, P.J., Kunkel, S.L., Harlow, L.A., DiPietro, L.A., Elner, V.M. *et al.* (1992). Interleukin-8 as a macrophage-derived mediator of angiogenesis. *Science*, **258**, 1798–801.

Kono, K., Salazar-Onfray, F., Petersson, M., Hansson, J., Masucci, G., Wasserman, K. *et al.* (1996). Hydrogen peroxide secreted by tumor-derived macrophages down-modulates signal-transducing z molecules and inhibits tumor-specific T cell-and natural killer cell-mediated cytotoxicity. *European Journal of Immunology*, **26**, 1308–13.

Konur, A., Kreutz, M., Knuchel, R., Krause, S.W. and Andreesen, R. (1996a). Three-dimensional co-culture of human monocytes and macrophages with tumor cells: analysis of macrophage differentiation and activation. *International Journal of Cancer*, **66**, 645–652.

Konur, A., Krause, S.W., Rehli, M., Kreutz, M. and Andreesen, R. (1996b). Human monocytes induce a carcinoma cell line to secrete high amounts of nitric oxide. *Journal of Immunology*, **157**, 2109–15.

Konur, A., Kreutz, M., Knüchel, R., Krause, S.W. and Andreesen, R. (1998). Cytokine repertoire during maturation of monocytes to macrophages within spheroids of malignant and non-malignant urothelial cells. *International Journal of Cancer*, **78**, 648–53.

Koren, H.S., Meltzer, M.S. and Adams, D.O. (1981). The ADCC capacity of macrophages from C3H/HeJ and A/J mice can be augmented by BCG. *Journal of Immunology*, **126**, 1013–5.

Kreutz, M., Krause, S.W., Hennemann, B., Rehm, A. and Andreesen, R. (1992). Macrophage heterogeneity and differentiation: defined serum-free culture conditions induce different types of macrophages *in vitro*. *Research in Immunology*, **143**, 107–15.

Krishnan, E.C., Menon, C.D., Krishnan, L. and Jewell, W.R. (1980). Deficiency in maturation process of macrophages in human cancer. *Journal of the National Cancer Institute*, **65**, 273–6.

Kryczek, I., Grybos, M., Karabon, L., Klimczak, A. and Lange, A. (2000). IL-6 production in ovarian carcinoma is associated with histiotype and biological characteristics of the tumour and influences local immunity. *British Journal of Cancer*, **82**, 621–8.

Kunz-Schughart, L.A., Kreutz, M. and Knuechel, R. (1998). Multicellular speroids: a three-dimensional *in vitro* culture system to study tumor biology. *International Journal of Experimental Pathology*, **79**, 1–23.

Larizza, L., Schirrmacher, V. and Pfluger, E. (1984). Acquisition of high metastatic capacity after *in vitro* fusion of a nonmetastatic tumor line with a bone marrow-derived macrophage. *Journal of Experimental Medicine*, **160**, 1579–84.

Lauder, I., Aherne, W., Stewart, J. and Sainsbury, R. (1977). Macrophage infiltration of breast tumours: a prospective study. *Journal of Clinical Pathology*, **30**, 563–8.

Lee, L.F., Hellendall, R.P., Wang, Y. , Haskill, J.S., Mukaida, Matsushima, N.K. *et al.* (2000). IL-8 reduced tumorigenicity of human ovarian cancer *in vivo* due to neutrophil infiltration. *Journal of Immunology*, **164**, 2769–75.

Leek, R.D., Harris, A.L. and Lewis, C.E. (1994). Cytokine networks in solid human tumors: regulation of angiogenesis. *Journal of Leukocyte Biology*, **56**, 423–35.

Leek, R.D., Lewis, C.E., Whitehouse, R., Greenall, M., Clarke, J. and Harris, A.L. (1996). Association of macrophage infiltration with angiogenesis and prognosis in invasive breast carcinoma. *Cancer Research*, **56**, 4625–9.

Leek, R.D., Landers, R., Fox, S.B., Ng, F., Harris, A.L. and Lewis, C.E. (1998). Association of tumour necrosis factor α and its receptors with thymidine phosphorylase expression in invasive breast carcinoma. *British Journal of Cancer*, **77**, 2246–51.

Leek, R.D., Hunt, N.C., Landers, R.J., Lewis, C.E., Royds, J.A. and Harris, A.L. (2000). Macrophage infiltration is associated with VEGF and EGFR expression in breast cancer. *Journal of Pathology*, **190**, 430–6.

Leung, S.Y., Wong, M.P., Chung, L.P., Chan, A.S. and Yuen, S.T. (1997). Monocyte chemoattractant protein-1 expression and macrophage infiltration in gliomas. *Acta Neuropathologica*, **93**, 518–27.

Lewis, C.E., Leek, R., Harris, A. and McGee, J.O. (1995). Cytokine regulation of angiogenesis in breast cancer: the role of tumor-associated macrophages. *Journal of Leukocyte Biology*, **57**, 747–51.

Lewis, J.S., Lee, J.A., Underwood, J.C., Harris, A.L. and Lewis, C.E. (1999). Macrophage responses to hypoxia: relevance to disease mechanisms. *Journal of Leukocyte Biology*, **66**, 889–900.

Lingen, M.W., Polverini, P.J. and Bouck, N.P. (1996). Retinoic acid induces cells cultured from oral squamous cell carcinomas to become anti-angiogenic. *American Journal of Pathology*, **149**, 247–25.

Liu, Y., Thor, A., Shtivelman, E., Cao, Y., Tu, G., Heath, T.D. *et al.* (1999). Systemic gene delivery expands the repertoire of effective antiangiogenic agents. *Journal of Biological Chemistry*, **274**, 13338–44.

Lopez, M., Fechtenbaum, J., David, B., Martinache, C., Chokri, M., Canepa, S. *et al.* (1992). Adoptive immunotherapy with activated macrophages grown *in vitro* from blood monocytes in cancer patients: a pilot study. *Journal of Immunotherapy*, **11**, 209–17.

Luebbers, E.L., Pretlow, T.P., Emancipator, S.N., Boohaker, E.A., Pitts, A.M., Macfadyen, A.J. *et al.* (1985). Heterogeneity and prognostic significance of macrophages in human colonic carcinomas. *Cancer Research*, **45**, 5196–200.

Manickan, E., Kanangat, S., Rouse, R.J., Yu, Z. and Rouse, B.T. (1997). Enhancement of immune response to naked DNA vaccine by immunization with transfected dendritic cells. *Journal of Leukocyte Biology*, **61**, 125–32.

Mantovani, A., Polentarutti, N., Peri, G., Shavit, Z.B., Vecchi, A., Bolis, G. *et al.* (1980). Cytotoxicity on tumor cells of peripheral blood monocytes and tumor-associated macrophages in patients with ascites ovarian tumors. *Journal of the National Cancer Institute*, **64**, 1307–15.

Mantovani, A., Bottazzi, B., Colotta, F., Sozzani, S. and Ruco, L. (1992). The origin and function of tumor-associated macrophages. *Immunology Today*, **13**, 265–70.

Meierhoff, G., Krause, S.W. and Andreesen, R. (1998). Comparative analysis of dendritic cells derived from blood monocytes or CD34[+] hematopoietic progenitor cells. *Immunobiology*, **198**, 501–13.

Menetrier-Caux, C., Montmain, G., Dieu, M.C., Bain, C., Favrot, M.C., Caux, C. *et al.* (1998). Inhibition of the differentiation of dendritic cells from CD34(+) progenitors by tumor cells: role of interleukin-6 and macrophage colony-stimulating factor. *Blood*, **92**, 4778–91.

Minchenko, A., Bauer, T., Salceda, S. and Caro, J. (1994). Hypoxic stimulation of vascular endothelial growth factor expression *in vitro* and *in vivo*. *Laboratory Investigation*, **71**, 374–9.

Montesano, R., Vassalli, J.D., Baird, A., Guillemin, R. and Orci, L. (1986). Basic fibroblast growth factor induces angiogenesis *in vitro*. *Proceedings of the National Academy of Sciences USA*, **83**, 7297–301.

Moradi, M.M., Carson, L.F., Weinberg, B., Haney, A.F., Twiggs, L.B. and Ramakrishnan, S. (1993). Serum and ascitic fluid levels of interleukin-1, interleukin-6, and tumor necrosis factor-α in patients with ovarian epithelial cancer. *Cancer*, **72**, 2433–40.

Mullins, D.W., Burger, C.J. and Elgert, K.D. (1999). Paclitaxel enhances macrophage IL-12 production in tumor-bearing hosts through nitric oxide. *Journal of Immunology*, **162**, 6811–8.

Munn, D.H. and Cheung, N.K. (1989). Antibody-dependent antitumor cytotoxicity by human monocytes cultured with recombinant macrophage colony-stimulating factor. Induction of efficient antibody-mediated antitumor cytotoxicity not detected by isotope release assays. *Journal of Experimental Medicine*, **170**, 511–26.

Munzarova, M. and Kovarik, J. (1987). Is cancer a macrophage-mediated autoaggressive disease? *Lancet*, **1**, 952–4.

Muster-Bloy, R., Elsasser-Beile, U., Weber, W., Monting, J.S. and von Kleist, S. (1996). Immunosuppressive activity of sera from patients with colorectal and gynecological carcinomas as evaluated by impaired IFN-γ, IL-1α and TNF-α production of human peripheral mononuclear cells. *Immunobiology*, **196**, 356–62.

Nabioullin, R., Sone, S., Mizuno, K., Yano, S., Nishioka,Y., Haku, T. *et al.* (1994). Interleukin-10 is a potent inhibitor of tumor cytotoxicity by human monocytes and alveolar macrophages. *Journal of Leukocyte Biology*, **55**, 437–42.

Nakashima, E., Kubota, Y., Matsushita, R., Ozaki, E., Ichimura, F., Kawahara, S. *et al.* (1998). Synergistic antitumor interaction of human monocyte chemotactant protein-1 gene transfer and modulator for tumor-infiltrating macrophages. *Pharmacy Research*, **15**, 685–9.

Nakazaki, H. (1992). Preoperative and postoperative cytokines in patients with cancer. *Cancer*, **70**, 709–13.

Nathan, C.F. (1987). Secretory products of macrophages. *Journal of Clinical Investigation*, **79**, 319–26.

Nathan, C. and Cohn, Z. (1980). Role of oxygen-dependent mechanisms in antibody-induced lysis of tumor cells by activated macrophages. *Journal of Experimental Medicine*, **152**, 198–208.

Nathan, C.F., Silverstein, S.C., Brukner, L.H. and Cohn, Z.A. (1979). Extracellular cytolysis by activated macrophages and granulocytes. II. Hydrogen peroxide as a mediator of cytotoxicity. *Journal of Experimental Medicine*, **149**, 100–13.

Naylor, M.S., Stamp, G.W., Foulkes, W.D., Eccles, D. and Balkwill, F.R. (1993). Tumor necrosis factor and its receptors in human ovarian cancer. Potential role in disease progression. *Journal of Clinical Investigation*, **91**, 2194–206.

Negus, R.P., Stamp, G.W., Relf, M.G., Burke, F., Malik, S.T., Bernasconi, S. *et al.* (1995). The detection and localization of monocyte chemoattractant protein-1 (MCP-1) in human ovarian cancer. *Journal of Clinical Investigation*, **95**, 2391–6.

Nestle, F.O., Alijagic, S., Gilliet, M., Sun, Y., Grabbe, S., Dummer, R. *et al.* (1998). Vaccination of melanoma patients with peptide- or tumor lysate-pulsed dendritic cells. *Nature Medicine*, **4**, 328–32.

Nieda, M., Nicol, A., Kikuchi, A., Kashiwase, K., Taylor, K., Suzuki, K. *et al.* (1998). Dendritic cells stimulate the expansion of bcr-abl specific CD8[+] T cells with cytotoxic activity against leukemic cells from patients with chronic myeloid leukemia. *Blood*, **91**, 977–83.

Niedbala, M.J. and Stein, M. (1991). Tumor necrosis factor induction of urokinase-type plasminogen activator in human endothelial cells. *Biochimica et Biophysica Acta*, **50**, 427–36.

Nishioka, Y., Sone, S., Orino, E., Nii, A. and Ogura, T. (1991). Down-regulation by interleukin 4 of activation of human alveolar macrophages to the tumoricidal state. *Cancer Research*, **51**, 5526–31.

Okamoto, M., Hattori, K. and Oyasu, R. (1997). Interleukin-6 functions as an autocrine growth factor in human bladder carcinoma cell lines *in vitro*. *International Journal of Cancer*, **72**, 149–54.

Onozaki, K., Matsushima, K., Aggarwal, B.B. and Oppenheim, J.J. (1985). Human interleukin 1 is a cytocidal factor for several tumor cell lines. *Journal of Immunology*, **135**, 3962–8.

Orosz, P., Echtenacher, B., Falk, W., Ruschoff, J., Weber, D. and Mannel, D.N. (1993). Enhancement of experimental metastasis by tumor necrosis factor. *Journal of Experimental Medicine*, **177**, 1391–8.

Ortaldo, J.R., Porter, H.R., Miller, P., Stevenson, H.C., Ozols, R.F. and Hamilton, T.C. (1986). Adoptive cellular immunotherapy of human ovarian carcinoma xenografts in nude mice. *Cancer Research*, **46**, 4414–9.

Otsuji, M., Kimura, Y., Aoe, T., Okamoto, Y. and Saito, T. (1996). Oxidative stress by tumor-derived macrophages suppresses the expression of CD3 z chain of T-cell receptor complex and antigen-specific T-cell responses. *Proceedings of the National Academy of Sciences USA*, **93**, 13119–124.

Park, J.E., Keller, G.A. and Ferrara, N. (1993). The vascular endothelial growth factor (VEGF) isoforms: differential deposition into the subepithelial extracellular matrix and bioactivity of extracellular matrix-bound VEGF. *Molecualr Biology of the Cell*, **4**, 1317–26.

Pepper, M.S., Ferrara, N., Orci, L. and Montesano, R. (1991). Vascular endothelial growth factor (VEGF) induces plasminogen activators and plasminogen activator inhibitor-1 in microvascular endothelial cells. *Biochemical and Biophysical Research Communications*, **181**, 902–6.

Pepper, M.S., Ferrara, N., Orci, L. and Montesano, R. (1992). Potent synergism between vascular endothelial growth factor and basic fibroblast growth factor in the induction of angiogenesis *in vitro*. *Biochemical and Biophysical Research Communications*, **189**, 824–31.

Perri, R.T., Kay, N.E., McCarthy, J., Vessella, R.L., Jacob, H.S. and Furcht, L.T. (1982). Fibronectin enhances *in vitro* monocyte–macrophage-mediated tumoricidal activity. *Blood*, **60**, 430–5.

Peters, J.H., Ruhl, S. and Friedrichs, D. (1987). Veiled accessory cells deduced from monocytes. *Immunobiology*, **176**, 154–66.

Peters, J.H., Gieseler, R., Thiele, B. and Steinbach, F. (1996). Dendritic cells: from ontogenetic orphans to myelomonocytic descendants. *Immunology .Today*, **17**, 273–8.

Piessens, W.F., Churchill, W.H.J. and David, J. (1975). Macrophages activated *in vitro* with lymphocyte mediators kill neoplastic but not normal cells. *Journal of Immunology*, **114**, 293–9.

Plouet, J., Moro, F., Bertagnolli, S., Coldeboeuf, N., Mazarguil, H., Clamens, S. *et al.* (1997). Extracellular cleavage of the vascular endothelial growth factor 189-amino acid form by urokinase is required for its mitogenic effect. *Journal of Biological Chemistry*, **272**, 13390–13396.

Polverini, P.J. (1996). How the extracellular matrix and macrophages contribute to angiogenesis-dependent diseases. *European Journal of Cancer*, **32A**, 2430–7.

Pusztai, L., Clover, L.M., Cooper, K., Starkey, P.M., Lewis, C.E. and McGee, J.O. (1994). Expression of tumour necrosis factor α and its receptors in carcinoma of the breast. *British Journal of Cancer*, **70**, 289–292.

Putz, E.F. and Mannel, D.N. (1995). Monocyte activation by tumour cells: a role for carbohydrate structures associated with CD2. *Scandinavian Journal of Immunology*, **41**, 77–84.

Rambaldi, A., Young, D.C. and Griffin, J.D. (1987). Expression of the M-CSF (CSF-1) gene by human monocytes. *Blood*, **69**, 1409–13.

Reiter, I., Krammer, B. and Schwamberger, G. (1999). Cutting edge: differential effect of apoptotic versus necrotic tumor cells on macrophage antitumor activities. *Journal of Immunology*, **163**, 1730–2.

Ribeiro-Dias, F., Russo, M., Marzagao, B.J., Fernandes, N.F., Timenetsky, J. and Jancar, S. (1999). *Mycoplasma arginini* enhances cytotoxicity of thioglycollate-elicited murine macrophages toward YAC-1 tumor cells through production of NO. *Journal of Leukocyte Biology*, **65**, 808–14.

Ridge, J.P., Fuchs, E.J. and Matzinger, P. (1996). Neonatal tolerance revisited: turning on newborn T cells with dendritic cells. *Science*, **271**, 1723–6.

Roberts, A.B., Thompson, N.L., Heine, U., Flanders, C. and Sporn, M.B. (1988). Transforming growth factor-β: possible roles in carcinogenesis. *British Journal of Cancer*, **57**, 594–600.

Saito, H., Tsujitani, S., Ikeguchi, M., Maeta, M. and Kaibara, N. (1998). Relationship between the expression of vascular endothelial growth factor and the density of dendritic cells in gastric adenocarcinoma tissue. *British Journal of Cancer*, **78**, 1573–7.

Saksela, O., Hovi, T. and Vaheri, A. (1985). Urokinase-type plasminogen activator and its inhibitor secreted by cultured human monocyte–macrophages. *Journal of Cellular Physiology*, **122**, 125–32.

Salvesen, H.B. and Akslen, L.A. (1999). Significance of tumour-associated macrophages, vascular endothelial growth factor and thrombospondin-1 expression for tumour angiogenesis and prognosis in endometrial carcinomas. *International Journal of Cancer*, **84**, 538–43.

Sato, Y. and Rifkin, D.B. (1988). Autocrine activities of basic fibroblast growth factor: regulation of endothelial cell movement, plasminogen activator synthesis, and DNA synthesis. *Journal of Cell Biology*, **107**, 1199–205.

Sato, Y., Okamura, K., Morimoto, A., Hamanaka, R., Hamaguchi, K., Shimada, T. *et al.* (1993). Indispensable role of tissue-type plasminogen activator in growth factor-dependent tube formation of human microvascular endothelial cells *in vitro*. *Experimental Cell Researc*, **204**, 223–9.

Sauter, B., Albert, M.L., Francisco, L., Larsson, M., Somersan, S. and Bhardwaj, N. (2000). Consequences of cell death. Exposure to necrotic tumor cells, but not primary tissue cells or apoptotic cells, induces the maturation of immunostimulatory dendritic cells. *Journal of Experimental Medicine*, **191**, 423–34.

Savarese, D.M., Valinski, H., Quesenberry, P. and Savarese, T. (1998). Expression and function of colony-stimulating factors and their receptors in human prostate carcinoma cell lines. *Prostate*, **34**, 80–91.

Scheibenbogen, C. and Andreesen, R. (1991). Developmental regulation of the cytokine repertoire in human macrophages: IL-1, IL-6, TNF-α, and M-CSF. *Journal of Leukocyte Biology*, **50**, 35–42.

Schindler, R., Mancilla, J., Endres, S., Ghorbani, R., Clark, S.C. and Dinarello, C.A. (1990). Correlations and interactions in the production of interleukin-6 (IL-6), IL-1, and tumor necrosis factor (TNF) in human blood mononuclear cells: IL-6 suppresses IL-1 and TNF. *Blood*, **75**, 40–7.

Scholl, S.M., Pallud, C., Beuvon, F., Hacene, K., Stanley, E.R., Rohrschneider, L. *et al.* (1994). Anti-colony-stimulating factor-1 antibody staining in primary breast adenocarcinomas correlates with marked inflammatory cell infiltrates and prognosis. *Journal of the National Cancer Institute*, **86**, 120–6.

Schreiber, A.B., Winkler, M.E. and Derynck, R. (1986). Transforming growth factor-α: a more potent angiogenic mediator than epidermal growth factor. *Science*, **232**, 1250–3.

Schroit, A.J. and Fidler, I.J. (1982). Delivery of macrophage-augmenting factors encapsulated in liposomes for destruction of tumor metastases. *Progress in Clinical and Biological Research*, **102**, 347–55.

Schuster, U., Buttner, R., Hofstadter, F. and Knuchel, R. (1994). A heterologous *in vitro* coculture system to study interaction between human bladder cancer cells and fibroblasts. *Journal of Urology*, **151**, 1707–11.

Seguchi, T., Yokokawa, K., Sugao, H., Nakano, E., Sonoda, T. and Okuyama, A. (1992). Interleukin-6 activity in urine and serum in patients with bladder carcinoma. *Journal of Urology*, **148**, 791–4.

Sharon, N. (1984). Carbohydrates as recognition determinants in phagocytosis and in lectin-mediated killing of target cells. *Biology of the Cell*, **51**, 239–45.

Shen, H., Clauss, M., Ryan, J., Schmidt, A.M., Tijburg, P., Borden, L. *et al.* (1993). Characterization of vascular permeability factor/vascular endothelial growth factor receptors on mononuclear phagocytes. *Blood*, **81**, 2767–73.

Sica, A., Saccani, A., Bottazzi, B., Bernasconi, S., Allavena, P., Gaetano, B. *et al.* (2000a). Defective expression of the monocyte chemotactic protein-1 receptor CCR2 in macrophages associated with human ovarian carcinoma. *Journal of Immunology*, **164**, 733–8.

Sica, A., Saccani, A., Bottazzi, B., Polentarutti, N., Vecchi, A., Van Damme, J. *et al.* (2000b). Autocrine production of IL-10 mediates defective IL-12 production and NF-kB activation in tumor-associated macrophages. *Journal of Immunology*, **164**, 762–7.

Siegert, A., Denkert, C., Leclere, A. and Hauptmann, S. (1999). Suppression of the reactive oxygen intermediates production of human macrophages by colorectal adenocarcinoma cell lines. *Immunology*, **98**, 551–6.

Simonitsch, I. and Krupitza, G. (1998). Autocrine self-elimination of cultured ovarian cancer cells by tumour necrosis factor α (TNF-α). *British Journal of Cancer*, **78**, 862–70.

Siziopikou, K.P., Harris, J.E., Casey, L., Nawas, Y. and Braun, D.P. (1991). Impaired tumoricidal function of alveolar macrophages from patients with non-small cell lung cancer. *Cancer*, **68**, 1035–44.

Skinner, J.M., Jarvis, L.R. and Whitehead, R. (1983). The cellular response to human colonic neoplasms: macrophage numbers. *Journal of Pathology*, **139**, 97–103.

Smit, W.M., Rijnbeek, M., van Bergen, C.A., de Paus, R.A., Vervenne, H.A., van de Keur, M. *et al.* (1997). Generation of dendritic cells expressing bcr-abl from CD34-positive chronic myeloid leukemia precursor cells. *Human Immunology*, **53**, 216–23.

Sone, S. and Fidler, I.J. (1980). Synergistic activation by lymphokines and muramyl dipeptide of tumoricidal properties in rat alveolar macrophages. *Journal of Immunology*, **125**, 2454–60.

Stevenson, H.C., Miller, P., Akiyama, Y., Favilla, T., Beman, J.A., Herberman, R. *et al.* (1983). A system for obtaining large numbers of cryopreserved human monocytes purified by leukapheresis and counter-current centrifugation elutriation (CCE). *Journal of Immunological Methods*, **62**, 353–63.

Stevenson, H.C., Keenan, A.M., Woodhouse, C., Ottow, R.T., Miller, P., Steller, E.P. *et al.* (1987). Fate of g-interferon-activated killer blood monocytes adoptively transferred into the abdominal cavity of patients with peritoneal carcinomatosis. *Cancer Research*, **47**, 6100–3.

Sunderkotter, C., Steinbrink, K., Goebeler, M., Bhardwaj, R. and Sorg, C. (1994). Macrophages and angiogenesis. *Journal of Leukocyte Biology*, **55**, 410–22.

Sutherland, R.M. (1988). Cell and environment interactions in tumor microregions: the multicell spheroid model. *Science*, **240**, 177–84.

Sutherland, R.M., Sordat, B., Bamat, J., Gabbert, H., Bourrat, B. and Mueller-Klieser, W. (1986). Oxygenation and differentiation in multicellular spheroids of human colon carcinoma. *Cancer Research*, **46**, 5320–9.

Suzu, S., Yokota, H., Yamada, M., Yanai, N., Saito, M., Kawashima, T. *et al.* (1989). Enhancing effect of human monocytic colony-stimulating factor on monocyte tumoricidal activity. *Cancer Research*, **49**, 5913–7.

Suzuki, M., Ohwada, M., Sato, I. and Nagatomo, M. (1995). Serum level of macrophage colony-stimulating factor as a marker for gynecologic malignancies. *Oncology*, **52**, 128–33.

Takahashi, Y., Bucana, C.D., Liu, W., Yoneda, J., Kitadai, Y., Cleary, K.R. *et al.* (1996). Platelet-derived endothelial cell growth factor in human colon cancer angiogenesis: role of infiltrating cells. *Journal of the National Cancer Institute*, **88**, 1146–51.

Takanami, I., Takeuchi, K. and Kodaira, S. (1999). Tumor-associated macrophage infiltration in pulmonary adenocarcinoma: association with angiogenesis and poor prognosis. *Oncology*, **57**, 138–42.

Tang, R., Beuvon, F., Ojeda, M., Mosseri, V., Pouillart, P. and Scholl, S. (1992). M-CSF (monocyte colony stimulating factor) and M-CSF receptor expression by breast tumour cells: M-CSF mediated recruitment of tumour infiltrating monocytes? *Journal of Cell Biochemistry*, **50**, 350–6.

Tilg, H., Trehu, E., Atkins, M.B., Dinarello, C.A. and Mier, J.W. (1994). Interleukin-6 (IL-6) as an anti-inflammatory cytokine: induction of circulating IL-1 receptor antagonist and soluble tumor necrosis factor receptor p55. *Blood*, **83**, 113–8.

Torisu, H., Ono, M., Kiryu, H., Furue, M., Ohmoto, Y., Nakayama, J. *et al.* (2000). Macrophage infiltration correlates with tumor stage and angiogenesis in human malignant melanoma: possible involvement of TNFα and IL-1α. *International Journal of Cancer*, **85**, 182–8.

Troy, A.J. and Hart, D.N. (1997). Dendritic cells and cancer: progress toward a new cellular therapy. *Journal of Hematotherapy*, **6**, 523–33.

Tsukamoto, T., Kumamoto, Y., Miyao, N., Masumori, N., Takahashi, A. and Yanase, M. (1992). Interleukin-6 in renal cell carcinoma. *Journal of Urology*, **148**, 1778–81.

Tsunawaki, S., Sporn, M., Ding, A. and Nathan, C. (1988). Deactivation of macrophages by transforming growth factor-β. *Nature*, **334**, 260–2.

Ueda, T., Shimada, E. and Urakawa, T. (1994). Serum levels of cytokines in patients with colorectal cancer: possible involvement of interleukin-6 and interleukin-8 in hematogenous metastasis. *Journal of Gastroenterology*, **29**, 423–9.

Unemori, E.N., Ferrara, N., Bauer, E.A. and Amento, E.P. (1992). Vascular endothelial growth factor induces interstitial collagenase expression in human endothelial cells. *Journal of Cellular Physiology*, **153**, 557–62.

Valdez, J.C., de Alderete, N. Meson, O.E., Sirena, A. and Perdigon, G. (1990). Comparative activation states of tumor-associated and peritoneal macrophages from mice bearing an induced fibrosarcoma. *Immunobiology*, **181**, 276–87.

van Netten, J.P., Ashmead, B.J., Parker, R.L., Thornton, I.G., Fletcher, C., Cavers, D. *et al.* (1993). Macrophage–tumor cell associations: a factor in metastasis of breast cancer? *Journal of Leukocyte Biology*, **54**, 360–2.

van Ravenswaay, C., Kluin, P.M. and Fleuren, G.J. (1992). Tumor infiltrating cells in human cancer. On the possible role of CD16⁺ macrophages in antitumor cytotoxicity. *Laboratory Investigation*, **67**, 166–74.

Vincent, F., Eischen, A., Bergerat, J.P., Faradji, A., Bohbot, A. and Oberling, F. (1992). Human blood-derived macrophages: differentiation *in vitro* of a large quantity of cells in serum-free medium. *Experimental Hematology*, **20**, 17–23.

Wahl, S.M., Hunt, D.A., Wakefield, L.M., McCartney, F.N., Wahl, L.M., Roberts, A.B. *et al.* (1987). Transforming growth factor type β induces monocyte chemotaxis and growth factor production. *Proceedings of the National Academy of Sciences USA*, **84**, 5788–92.

Walter, S., Bottazzi, B., Govoni, D., Colotta, F. and Mantovan, A. (1991). Macrophage infiltration and growth of sarcoma clones expressing different amounts of monocyte chemotactic protein/JE. *International Journal of Cancer*, **49**, 431–5.

Warren, M.K. and Ralph, P. (1986). Macrophage growth factor CSF-1 stimulates human monocyte production of interferon, tumor necrosis factor, and colony stimulating activity. *Journal of Immunology*, **137**, 2281–5.

Weinberg, J.B., Misukonis, M.A., Shami, P.J., Mason, S.N., Sauls, D.L., Dittman, W.A. *et al.* (1995). Human mononuclear phagocyte inducible nitric oxide synthase (iNOS): analysis of iNOS mRNA, iNOS protein, biopterin, and nitric oxide production by blood monocytes and peritoneal macrophages. *Blood*, **86**, 1184–95.

Wersall, P., Masucci, G. and Mellstedt, H. (1991). Interleukin-4 augments the cytotoxic capacity of lymphocytes and monocytes in antibody-dependent cellular cytotoxicity. *Cancer Immunology and Immunotherapy*, **33**, 45–9.

Wiesel, M.L., Faradji, A., Grunebaum, L., Bohbot, A., Schmitt-Goguel, M., Bergerat, J.P. *et al.* (1992). Hemostatic changes in human adoptive immunotherapy with activated blood monocytes or derived macrophages. *Annals of Hematology*, **65**, 75–8.

Wong, M.P., Cheung, K.N., Yuen, S.T., Fu, K.H., Chan, A.S., Leung, S.Y. *et al.* (1998). Monocyte chemoattractant protein-1 (MCP-1) expression in primary lymphoepithelioma-like carcinomas (LELCs) of the lung. *Journal of Pathology*, **186**, 372–7.

Wrenshall, L.E., Stevens, R.B., Cerra, F.B. and Platt, J.L. (1999). Modulation of macrophage and B cell function by glycosaminoglycans. *Journal of Leukocyte Biology*, **66**, 391–400.

Wu, C.W., Wang, S.R., Chao, M.F., Wu, T.C., Lui, W.Y., P'eng, F.K. *et al.* (1996). Serum interleukin-6 levels reflect disease status of gastric cancer. *American Journal of Gastroenterology*, **91**, 1417–22.

Yan, J., Vetvicka, V., Xia, Y., Coxon, A., Carroll, M.C., Mayadas, T.N. *et al.* (1999). β-Glucan, a 'specific' biologic response modifier that uses antibodies to target tumors for cytotoxic recognition by leukocyte complement receptor type 3 (CD11b/CD18). *Journal of Immunology*, **163**, 3045–52.

Yanagawa, E., Uchida, A., Moore, M. and Micksche, M. (1985). Autologous tumor killing and natural cytotoxic activity of tumor-associated macrophages in cancer patients. *Cancer Immunology and Immunotherapy*, **19**, 163–7.

Yanagawa, H., Takeuchi, E., Suzuki, Y., Hanibuchi, M., Haku, T., Ohmoto, Y. *et al.* (1999). Production of interleukin-10 by alveolar macrophages from lung cancer patients. *Respiratory Medicine*, **93**, 666–71.

Yoshida, S., Ono, M., Shono, T., Izumi, H., Ishibashi, T., Suzuki, H. *et al.* (1997). Involvement of interleukin-8, vascular endothelial growth factor, and basic fibroblast growth factor in tumor necrosis factor α-dependent angiogenesis. *Molecular and Cellular Biology*, **17**, 4015–23.

Yoshimura, T., Yuhki, N., Moore, S.K., Appella, E., Lerman, M.I. and Leonard, E.J. (1989). Human monocyte chemoattractant protein-1 (MCP-1). Full-length cDNA cloning, expression in mitogen-stimulated blood mononuclear leukocytes, and sequence similarity to mouse competence gene JE. *FEBS Letters*, **244**, 487–93.

Zeid, N.A. and Muller, H.K. (1993). S100 positive dendritic cells in human lung tumors associated with cell differentiation and enhanced survival. *Pathology*, **25**, 338–43.

Zeineddine, N.S., Avina, M.D., Williams, C.C., Wepsic, H.T. and Jadus, M.R. (1999). Macrophages that kill glioma cells expressing the membrane form of macrophage colony stimulating factor are resistant to prostaglandin E2 and interleukin-10. *Immunology Letters*, **70**, 63–8.

Zembala, M., Siedlar, M., Marcinkiewicz, J. and Pryjma, J. (1994). Human monocytes are stimulated for nitric oxide release *in vitro* by some tumor cells but not by cytokines and lipopolysaccharide. *European Journal of Immunology*, **24**, 435–9.

Zhang, G.J. and Adachi, I. (1999). Serum interleukin-6 levels correlate to tumor progression and prognosis in metastatic breast carcinoma. *Anticancer Research*, **19**, 1427–32.

Zitvogel, L., Mayordomo, J.I., Tjandrawan, T., DeLeo, A.B., Clarke, M.R., Lotze, M.T. *et al.* (1996). Therapy of murine tumors with tumor peptide-pulsed dendritic cells: dependence on T cells, B7 costimulation, and T helper cell 1-associated cytokines. *Journal of Experimental Medicine*, **183**, 87–97.

Zuk, J.A. and Walker, R.A. (1987). Immunohistochemical analysis of HLA antigens and mononuclear infiltrates of benign and malignant breast. *Journal of Pathology*, **152**, 275–85.

12 *Macrophages in cardiovascular disease*

W. Jessup, A. Baoutina and L. Kritharides

1 Introduction

Cardiovascular disease is the term that describes diseases of the heart and blood vessels, and includes coronary heart disease (leading to heart attack and angina), cerebrovascular disease (stroke) and peripheral vascular disease (intermittent claudication and gangrene). The underlying process in all of these diseases is atherosclerosis. Atherosclerosis is a condition of major arteries, in which progressive occlusion of the vessel occurs, often starting in early adulthood and developing over many years. The occlusion results from an eccentric thickening of the internal layer (intima) of the artery wall (Figure 12.1). In advanced atherosclerotic arteries, the occlusion can be sufficiently extensive to limit blood supply to local tissues. In addition, disruption to the surface of the lesion may precipitate thrombus formation, further restricting blood supply (see Figure 12.1). In general, it is the restriction to blood supply that causes the clinical symptoms associated with atherosclerosis, such as those listed above. Atherosclerosis is a major cause of mortality and morbidity in Western societies.

2 Atherosclerosis and macrophages

2.1 The normal artery

The normal blood vessel comprises three functionally and histologically distinct layers (Figure 12.2). The outermost layer is the adventitia. This is composed mainly of connective tissue and, together with the intima, provides the mechanical strength necessary to withstand the pressures of arterial blood flow. It generally has its own blood supply (vasa

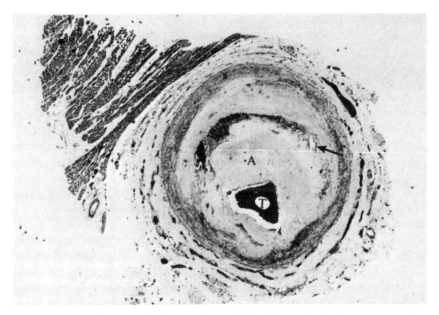

Fig. 12.1   Cross-section through a human lesion. Light micrograph of a transverse section through a human coronary artery showing almost complete occlusion of the vessel lumen with atheroma (A) and thrombus (T). Cholesterol clefts are indicated by an arrow.

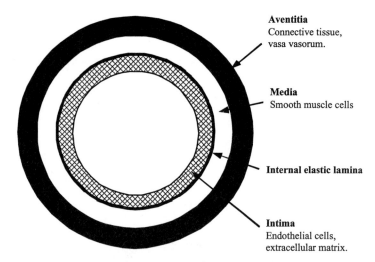

Aventitia
Connective tissue,
vasa vasorum.

Media
Smooth muscle cells

Internal elastic lamina

Intima
Endothelial cells,
extracellular matrix.

Fig. 12.2   Structure of a normal human artery. Cross-sectional diagram shows the major tissue layers (not to scale).

vasorum). The adventitia is not usually affected in atherosclerosis, although in some cases its structure may be compromised, leading to development of areas of weakness and distension (aneurysms), particularly common in major vessels such as the aorta. Within the adventitia is the media, a layer of smooth muscle cells. These also provide mechanical strength but, more importantly, control vascular tone (and thus blood pressure) by responding to contractile and relaxant stimuli. These stimuli are released by endothelial cells of the inner layer, or intima. The innermost surface of the intima is a monolayer of endothelial cells, which present a non-thrombogenic physical barrier between the blood and lower layers as well as acting as a potent source of vasoactive substances, such as endothelin and nitric oxide (NO). Between the endothelial cells and the media is a dense layer of connective tissue, the internal elastic lamina. The intima may also contain variable amounts of extracellular matrix (ECM), containing proteoglycans, elastin, collagens and the non-collagenous glycoproteins laminin and fibronectin. Proteoglycans are involved in permeability, filtration and ion exchange, collagen acts as a substratum for endothelial cell attachment, while fibronectin acts in cell–cell adhesion and cell–substrate adhesion. Laminin comprises a large proportion of the basement membrane underlying the endothelium. Macrophages and smooth muscle cells have also been identified as part of normal intima, occurring as isolated cells spread irregularly throughout the tissue.

2.2 The atherosclerotic artery

The earliest detectable event in the development of atherosclerosis is the adhesion of circulating monocytes to regions of the lumenal surface of the endothelium (Figure 12.3A). This is associated with increased expression on endothelial cells of cell adhesion molecules. Increased expression of vascular cell adhesion molecule-1 (VCAM-1) on the surface of aortic endothelial cells prior to the development of the fatty streak and increased expression of intercelluar cell adhesion molecule-1 (ICAM-1) and E-selectin on the surface of arterial endothelium, especially over sites of lipid and macrophage accu-

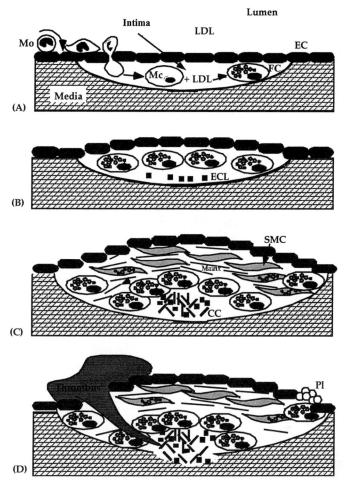

Fig. 12.3 Stages of atherosclerosis. (A) Earliest detectable changes are (i) intimal retention of low-density lipoprotein (LDL) and (ii) monocyte (Mo) adhesion to endothelium (EC), migration into the intima, differentiation to macrophages (Mc) and cholesterol accumulation to form foam cells (FC). (B) Progressive focal deposition of extracellular lipid (ECL) derived from infiltrating plasma LDL and foam cell formation leads to fatty streak formation. (C) As the lesion grows, development of a large lipid core, which includes cholesterol crystals (CC) and infiltration of smooth muscle cells (SMC) contribute to lesion volume. (D) Minor disruption to the endothelium can stimulate platelet (Pl) deposition; thrombus formation occurs when underlying tissue is exposed. (Adapted from Kritharides, 1997.)

mulation, have been reported. The atherogenic signals which mediate cell adhesion molecule expression are not known, but may include altered levels of NO and/or plasma lipoproteins and also possibly altered generation of inflammatory mediators acting on the endothelium either directly or indirectly by local production of cytokines by smooth muscle cells or macrophages. Once the initial wave of leukocytes has been recruited, these in turn may secrete other endothelial activators and chemotactic factors to enhance the response.

Certain sites within large vessels are particularly prone to the development of athero-sclerosis. These 'lesion-prone sites' are associated with sites of turbulent blood flow and accelerated penetration of plasma lipoproteins. The major plasma source of intimal lipid is low-density lipoprotein (LDL), and there is a strong correlation between plasma LDL levels and atherosclerosis in humans. The adherent macrophages migrate across the endothelium and reside in the intima. A large proportion of intimal macrophages accumu-late large intracellular deposits of lipid, which locate initially in cytoplasmic fat droplets, giving the cells a 'foamy' appearance (Figure 12.4A). The fats in such macrophage 'foam' cells comprise mainly free and esterified cholesterol.

Progressive migration of monocytes into the intima and subsequent uptake of lipid lead to the development of a foam cell-rich 'fatty streak' (Figure 12.3B) in which macrophage foam cells are organized into strata of adjacent layers rather than isolated groups of cells. At this stage, continued macrophage recruitment is evident, as the numbers of macrophages lacking lipid loading also continues to increase. Cholesteryl esters com-prise approximately three-quarters of the lipid associated with the lesion, but the lipid remains predominantly intracellular, although some extracellular lipoprotein deposits are found. At this stage, the endothelium remains intact, and such lesions are clinically silent.

As the lesion grows, the development of a large extracellular lipid core, containing cho-lesterol crystals as well as extracellular lipoproteins, becomes apparent (Figure 12.3C). This is thought to derive at least partially from necrosis of local macrophage foam cells. A fibrous cap also develops over the surface of the lipid core, in which ECM and smooth muscle cells are the main structural components. The accumulated cellular debris and extracellular lipid in the core, often accompanied by calcium deposits, can disrupt the sta-bility of the lesion structure, making it susceptible to rupture. Macrophage foam cells also constitute a large proportion of lesion volume (Figure 12.4B) surrounding the lipid core and also present at the advancing 'shoulder' edge of the lesion.

In such advanced lesions, minor disruption of the endothelium can occur, stimulating platelet deposition and formation of microthrombi (Figure 12.3D). Potent growth factors released by platelets may stimulate proliferation of cells further within the growing lesion. Rupture of the lesion may also occur at the macrophage-rich shoulder region, the fissure revealing strongly thrombogenic underlying surfaces and stimulating formation of large thrombi which may completely occlude the vessel (Figure 12.3D; see also Figure 12.1). It has been suggested that plaque rupture is also aggravated by the release of prote-olytic enzymes by macrophages that densely populate this region.

2.3 The role of macrophages in atherosclerosis

It is clear from the natural history of atherosclerosis that the macrophage is an early and persistent feature of the lesion (Gerrity, 1981) and is therefore likely to be pivotal in the disease development. Indeed, the importance of the macrophage in atherosclerosis was revealed in the osteopetrotic (op) mouse [lacking macrophage colony-stimulating factor (M-CSF) and thus severely deficient in monocytes], where profound inhibition of athero-sclerosis development was observed (Smith *et al.*, 1995; Qiao *et al.*, 1997).

The role of the macrophage in atherogenesis is likely to be multifactorial. The athero-sclerotic lesion features many characteristics of a chronic inflammatory lesion, including expression of endothelial cell adhesion molecules, monocyte margination and migration, the persistent presence of macrophages and T cells in lesions and expression of inflamma-

(A)

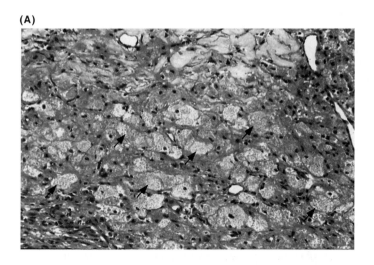

(B)

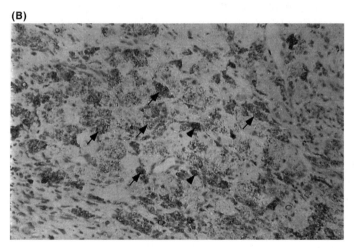

Fig. 12.4 Foam cell macrophages in human carotid atherosclerotic lesions. (A) Section of a human carotid atherosclerotic lesion stained with hematoxylin/eosin. Note the many large lipid-containing foam cells (as indicated by arrows) (magnification ×90). (B) Section of a human carotid atherosclerotic lesion stained using a mouse anti-human macrophage antibody (Ham56, Dako). Macrophages show dark staining. Note that foam cell macrophages stain diffusely (arrows), while some more densely staining non-foam cell macrophages are also present (arrowheads) (magnification ×64).

tory cytokines and growth factors (Hansson, 1994). Both macrophages and T cells express HLA-DR antigens in lesions. Epitopes expressed on modified lipoproteins (see below) have been associated with atherosclerosis, and a possible role for several microorganisms, such as herpes and *Chlamydia*, has also been suggested. However, the nature and importance of antigenic stimuli in atherosclerotic lesions remain controversial.

Macrophages in lesions may also modify the structure of extracellular macromolecules, including components of the ECM and LDL. Modulation of the ECM by macrophage-secreted proteinases and glycosidases may affect the stability of the lesion and also its interaction with local smooth muscle cells and lipoproteins. Alterations to the composition of intimal LDL, through both enzymic and non-enzymic mechanisms (Section 4.1), may regulate lipoprotein deposition in the lesion and its uptake by macrophages, thereby stimulating foam cell formation..

There is evidence that lipid loading of macrophages, a characteristic and near-unique feature of atherosclerotic lesions, profoundly affects their physiology, generally in a manner likely to promote lesion development. In this chapter, we will consider the nature of lipid deposition in foam cell macrophages, its likely origins, effects and reversal, and their impact on atherosclerosis.

3 Characteristics of macrophage foam cells in atherosclerotic plaque

3.1 Morphology of macrophage foam cells in plaque

Lipid-rich foam cell macrophages are characteristic of atherosclerosis from early fatty streak lesions, to advanced plaque (Gown *et al.*, 1986; Stary *et al.*, 1995). Macrophages without lipid droplets can also be found near the arterial lumen, whereas foam cell macrophages are observed more typically in lateral margins of the necrotic core and at the lateral edges of plaque (Stary *et al.*, 1995). Foam cells of macrophage origin may have lipid droplets stored in both cytosolic and lysosomal compartments. Differentiation of their respective sources and mechanisms of accumulation may have important implications for understanding atherogenesis.

Foam cells (predominantly macrophages) from rabbit atheroma have been separated according to their flotation density, which is determined by their lipid content (Shio *et al.*, 1978). Low-density cells (1.02 < d < 1.07) contain four times more free cholesterol, 17-fold more esterified cholesterol and 10-fold greater concentrations of lysosomal enzymes, β-glucosaminidase and β-galactosidase, than high-density cells. It is probable that other lysosomal enzymes such as proteinases are also likely to be elevated. Low-density foam cells contain two morphologically distinct types of lipid inclusions, which comprise half of the total cytoplasmic volume: (1) clear droplets without surrounding membranes; and (2) polymorphic structures, limited by a membrane containing intravacuolar debris, and containing myelin-like whorls, reticulations and crystalline inclusions (Shio *et al.*, 1978). The former represents cytosolic droplets of endogenously synthesized cholesteryl esters and the latter secondary lysosomes and residual bodies of undegraded lipid and other components. The likely origins of these deposits will be discussed below.

Within weeks of initiation of a high fat diet, lesions in experimental animals contain foam cells with prominent cytosolic lipid droplets which are surrounded by a single membrane, or no membrane, but not a true membrane bilayer. Later, macrophage foam cells contain numerous dense granules typical of lysosomes (Shio *et al.*, 1978; Schaffner *et al.*, 1980), which implies that an alteration in the distribution of cell lipids occurs with progressive cell lipid accumulation. The relative abundance of cytosolic and lysosomal lipid droplets also appears to vary within different regions in atherosclerotic plaques (Lewis *et al.*, 1988). Foam cells from early lesions, and the foam cells located on the edge of advanced lesions, principally contain cytoplasmic lipid (72 per cent of cell lipid).

Foam cell macrophages located in the center of lesions contain most lipid in secondary lysosome-like structures. The number of cytoplasmic droplets does not vary, suggesting that maximal accumulation of cytoplasmic lipid is followed by later accumulation of lipid occurring within lysosomes. Cytosolic cholesteryl esters are cell-synthesized, from either plasma membrane-derived cholesterol, endogenously synthesized cholesterol or lysosomal cholesterol (see Section 4.2). This differs from accumulation of lipid in the lysosomal compartment, which may indicate the progressive accumulation of lipoprotein-derived or other material that is resistant to lysosomal hydrolysis. The increased abundance of lysosomal lipids in advanced lesions relative to that in fatty streaks may indicate important differences in lysosomal lipid metabolism in fatty streaks and advanced plaques, such as differential accumulation of oxidized lipids (see Section 5.5).

As the shoulder region is typically the site of inflammation, erosion and rupture in lipid-rich plaques, recently infiltrated monocyte-derived foam cells may be particularly important for the evolution of acute cardiac complications such as myocardial infarction. In the core region of plaque, macrophage foam cells may show signs of cell injury, cell death and degrees of disintegration, and contribute to the high level of expression of tissue factor in this region (Stary *et al.*, 1995). This may be important, as the necrotic core contributes greatly to the thrombotic burden of plaque (Fernandez-Ortiz *et al.*, 1994). If recently infiltrated monocyte macrophages at the lesion edge and older necrotic macrophages in the core differentially contribute to the inflammatory and thrombotic complications of atherosclerosis, the respective predominance of cytosolic and lysosomal lipids in foam cells in these sites may be responsbile for these differential effects.

Cholesterol crystals and necrotic macrophages are both typical of the necrotic core. A common etiology of both core formation and cell toxicity is implied by *in vitro* studies which suggest that cellular accumulation of cytotoxic oxidized lipids, including oxysterols, could contribute to cytotoxicity within the necrotic core (Guyton *et al.*, 1990; Brown and Jessup, 1999). As atherosclerosis progresses, transition from predominantly cytosolic to predominantly lysosomal lipid accumulation coincides with the appearance of cholesterol crystals within the lysosomal compartment (Lupu *et al.*, 1987). Cell toxicity can follow the intracellular accumulation of free cholesterol in both lysosomal and cytosolic compartments (Kellner-Weibel *et al.*, 1999). Crystal formation requires the local accumulation of free cholesterol in concentrations exceeding its aqueous solubility and the absence of the opportunity for esterification. The accumulation of free cholesterol stimulates cell phospholipid (PL) synthesis and this may protect against cholesterol-induced cytotoxicity by maintaining optimal free cholesterol to PL ratios in cell membranes (Tabas, 1997). This may be associated with the formation of intracellular membrane-like whorls observed within lesion foam cells.

3.2 Protein expression by atherosclerotic lesion macrophages

Several cytokines have been identified immunohistochemically in macrophages in human atherosclerotic plaques, including platelet-derived growth factor (PDGF)-B, transforming growth factor (TGF)-β, tumor necrosis factor (TNF)-α, interleukin (IL)-1, IL-6, IL-8 and M-CSF. Elevated expression of several of these cytokines is also detected in macrophages isolated from human atheroma (for a review, see van Reyk and Jessup, 1999). Macrophages are a source of a number of enzymes implicated in ECM degradation including the matrix metalloproteinases (MMPs), components of the plasmin activation system, lysosomal proteases such as cathepsin S, heparanases and sulfatases. Several studies have demonstrated elevated expression and production of several MMPs (e.g. Galis *et al.*, 1995; Halpert *et al.*, 1996), plasmin (Raghunath *et al.*, 1995) and cathepsin S (Sukhova *et al.*, 1998) in lesion macrophages.

Alterations to the composition of the ECM may affect lipoprotein binding and retention in the intima. Macrophages also secrete other several enzymes capable of modifying LDL and stimulating its retention, including sphingomyelinase (Schissel *et al.*, 1996) and lipoprotein lipase (Mattsson *et al.*, 1993).

Macrophages are also sources of a number of proteins involved in cellular cholesterol metabolism. Apolipoprotein E (apoE) can mediate steps in reverse cholesterol transport (RCT), the process by which excess cellular cholesterol is transported from peripheral cells to the liver for degradation. ApoE protein and mRNA are present within human atherosclerotic lesions, especially in regions rich in monocyte-derived macrophage foam cells (O'Brien *et al.*, 1994). *In vitro*, macrophage apoE mRNA, apoE protein synthesis and apoE secretion all increase in response to cholesterol accumulation (Basu *et al.* 1982; Larkin *et al.*, 2000). ApoE secretion is also enhanced by apoA-I, the major protein component of high-density lipoproteins (HDLs) (Rees *et al.*, 1999). Importantly, in apoE-deficient mice, local apoE expression by bone marrow transplanted apoE +/+ macrophages diminishes atherosclerosis. The anti-atherogenic effect of apoE secretion may be due to stimulation of cell cholesterol export, enhanced binding of apoE-containing lipoproteins to hepatic receptors for cholesterol clearance, or due to local anti-inflammatory and anti-proliferative activity. In view of the diverse protective effects of local expression of apoE, factors which increase apoE secretion may restrict atherosclerosis.

3.3 Lipid composition of foam cell macrophages and cell-rich plaques

Surprisingly few studies have systematically investigated the lipid composition of human *ex vivo* foam cell macrophages; consequently, much of our current understanding is based upon animal studies and whole tissue analyses.

Cholesteryl ester is the predominant lipid fraction in all atherosclerotic lesions, representing up to 52 per cent of plaque lipid. PLs represent 14 per cent of plaque lipid, and triglycerides 9 per cent. The number of macrophages in human atherosclerotic plaques is positively correlated with the cholesteryl ester content of plaques (Felton *et al.*, 1997). Additionally, the shoulder region of plaques is associated with a greater ratio of esterified to free cholesterol which parallels the increased cellular macrophage number in this site (Felton *et al.*, 1997). PLs and cholesteryl esters, but not triglycerides, are greater at the edges of disrupted plaques than the center, consistent with a foam cell macrophage contribution to deposition of PLs and cholesteryl esters.

Studies of foam cell macrophages isolated from rabbit atheroma using monoclonal antibodies to cell surface antigens and magnetic microspheres identified that the respective major lipid classes cholesteryl esters, free cholesterol, triglycerides, phospholipids and free fatty acids, respectively, comprise 42–63, 13–17, 2–3, 19–35 and 2–3 per cent of cell lipid. Cholesteryl esters varied from two- to fivefold the amount of free cholesterol (mass) in foam cell macrophages (Mattsson *et al.*, 1991). Of cells isolated from human atherosclerotic intima, 40 per cent of mononuclear cells were CD14+. CD14+ cells were predominantly foam cells on the basis of oil-red O (neutral lipid) staining, and contained 408 ± 349 μg of cholesteryl esters/mg cell protein, 133 ± 103 μg of triglycerides/mg cell protein and 333 ± 200 µg of free cholesterol/mg cell protein (Mattsson *et al.*, 1993). Although sampling variation between and within plaque samples is significant, these data indicate that the free to esterified cholesterol ratio in human foam cells is much closer to 1:1 than suggested by data from rabbit atheroma, and also suggest that triglycerides represent a much larger proportion of total human foam cell lipid than anticipated from rabbit foam cell data or total human plaque data.

Numerous studies have identified oxidized lipids and lipoproteins in plaque. Lipid oxidation products isolated from lesions and/or lipoproteins isolated from them range from relatively early products, such as cholesteryl linoleate hydroperoxide, hydroxide and ketones, to advanced core aldehydes and isoprostanes (Hoppe *et al.*, 1997; Karten *et al.*, 1998; Niu *et al.*, 1999). Oxidized cholesterol (oxysterols) of both enzymic (mainly 27-hydroxycholesterol) and non-enzymic [mainly 7-ketocholesterol (7KC) and 7-hydroxycholesterols] origin are also elevated in plaque tissues, even when expressed relative to parent cholesterol (Brown and Jessup, 1999). Interest in the presence of oxidized lipoproteins in lesions was stimulated initially by *in vitro* evidence that they stimulate macrophage foam cell formation (see below). In addition, oxidized lipids have other biological effects on macrophages which may be of relevance to atherogenesis. These will be discussed in Section 6.

While such recent studies have measured lipid oxidation products in atherosclerotic lesions, there is actually little direct evidence of their accumulation in macrophage-derived foam cells. This is due mainly to the difficulty of isolating sufficient cells for analysis. So far, only oxysterols have been measured directly (Brown and Jessup, 1999). These are concentrated within foam cells at levels several-fold higher than in plaque as a whole, suggesting that they are either generated intracellularly and/or are selectively retained within the cell (Table 12.1). Epitopes of oxidized LDL are co-localized with macrophages and also appear to occur intracellularly, thus differing from the extracellular location of LDL epitopes in lesions (Sugiyama *et al.*, 1992). This may indicate selective intracellular accumulation of extracellularly oxidized lipoproteins, or intracellular, perhaps lysosomal, oxidation of lipoproteins after endocytosis. Ceroid and lipofuscin, insoluble lipid–protein complexes, have been identified within the lysosomes of foam cell macrophages (Hoff and Hoppe, 1995). Similar complexes are found following uptake of *in vitro* oxidized LDL. Ceroid may accumulate *in vivo* either by uptake of oxidized LDL, or by intralysosomal oxidation of LDL subsequent to its endocytosis, or a combination of both (Hoff and Hoppe, 1995).

Table 12.1   Oxysterol content of macrophage foam cells isolated from human carotid atherosclerotic plaque

Oxysterol	Concentration (as percentage of cell cholesterol)
7α-hydroxycholesterol	0.6 ± 0.3
7β-hydroxycholesterol	0.5 ± 0.1
27-hydroxycholesterol	0.7 ± 0.4
7-ketocholesterol	1.0 ± 0.7

CD14+ macrophages were isolated, subjected to cold alkaline saponification and sterols analyzed as their trimethyl silyl ether derivatives by gas chromatography–mass spectrometry with selective ion monitoring. Data are taken from Brown and Jessup (1999). Values are means ± SEM ($n = 7$). The molar ratios of oxysterol to cholesterol are expressed as a percentage. Total sterol was 2000 ± 1400 nmol/mg cell protein.

4 Mechanisms for macrophage foam cell formation

4.1 Sources of cholesterol

In all cells, cholesterol homeostasis is a delicate balance between uptake and endogenous synthesis on the one hand and metabolism and export on the other. Although cholesterol is necessary for many cellular functions, excess accumulation of free sterol must be prevented to avoid potentially toxic perturbation of membrane function and the formation of insoluble crystals. Figure 12.5 illustrates the major pathways that contribute to cholesterol accumulation in the macrophage. As in all peripheral cells, cholesterol is normally acquired either by uptake of plasma lipoproteins, principally LDL, or by endogenous synthesis (Brown *et al.*, 1980). Receptor-mediated uptake of LDL involves binding of the lipoprotein to specific cell surface LDL receptors (LDL-Rs), endocytosis, fusion with lysosomes and complete degradation of both the protein and lipid components. Lysosomal acid lipase (LAL) plays an important role in lysosomal hydrolysis of cholesteryl esters and triglycerides from endocytosed lipoproteins and generates free cholesterol, mono- and diglycerides and free fatty acids, which are transported out of the lysosomes for β-oxidation or further metabolism. Normally this enzymic activity is present in excess, and its substrates are degraded efficiently. LAL is expressed in human monocytes and macrophages and its activity is increased approximately10-fold during differentiation (Ries *et al.*, 1998). Enzymic activity is partially inhibited following endocytosis of lighly oxidized lipoproteins (i.e. containing peroxides) by macrophages (Kritharides *et al.*, 1998b), which may be of relevance in atherosclerotic intima, in which similar oxidation products are present and lysosomal lipid deposits do accumulate.

The cell has a sensitive mechanism for monitoring and maintaining cholesterol status. Membrane-bound transcription factors, called sterol regulatory element-binding proteins (SREBPs), activate the genes controlling cholesterol and fatty acid synthesis and LDL-R expression. Activation of SREBPs is cholesterol-dependent (Brown and Goldstein, 1999). In most cells, these cholesterol-sensitive mechanisms closely control the uptake and synthesis of cholesterol, through down-regulation of LDL-R expression and of the rate-limiting enzyme of cholesterol synthesis, hydroxymethylglutaryl-coenzyme A reductase (HMR), respectively. Additionally, most cells are also able to export excess cholesterol to extracellular acceptors, or to metabolize it to more readily excreted products (Section 7). In macrophages, these export pathways may be particularly important, since these scavenging phagocytic cells frequently endocytose large amounts of cholesterol-containing materials such as dead or damaged cells. Nevertheless, macrophage cholesterol balance normally is well controlled. The development of the atherosclerotic foam cell phenotype is one outstanding exception to this general observation. In this case, cholesterol accumulation clearly exceeds export, although whether the primary dysfunction lies in uptake, export or both is not known.

It is generally considered that foam cell formation involves unregulated uptake of lipoproteins using routes that bypass the cholesterol-sensitive LDL-R. Several alternative routes involving different receptors, phagocytosis or a combination of both have been identified. Central to all of these uptake routes is the chemical or physical modification of a proportion of intimal LDL, to become a ligand for one or more of the alternative pathways. The first such macrophage 'scavenger' receptor identified (now called SR-A) was shown to bind and internalize large amounts of chemically modified (acetylated) LDL,

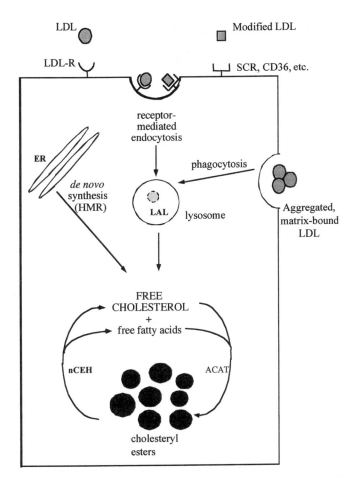

Fig. 12.5 Pathways for cholesterol accumulation in macrophage foam cells. Macrophages may accquire cholesterol either by receptor-mediated endocytosis of LDL using the LDL receptor (LDL-R) or by endogenous synthesis, in which hydroxymethylglutaryl-coenzyme A reductase (HMR) is the rate-limiting enzyme. Both routes are subject to feedback regulation by cellular cholesterol accumulation. Uptake of modified LDL by other receptors or by phagocytosis is not subject to cholesterol regulation and so can mediate foam cell formation. LDL cholesteryl esters taken up by either route are hydrolyzed in lysosomes by lysosomal acid lipase (LAL). Liberated free cholesterol partitions into cell membranes and excess cholesterol esterified by the cytosolic enzyme, acyl coenzyme A-cholesterol acyl transferase (ACAT). The products accumulate as lipid droplets in the cytoplasm. They are subject to hydrolysis by neutral cholesterol ester hydrolase (nCEH) but, in the absence of extracellular acceptors, cholesterol is re-esterified by ACAT.

converting macrophages into cholesteryl ester droplet-filled cells with a morphology similar to that of atherosclerotic foam cells (Goldstein *et al.*, 1979). This receptor also mediates uptake of oxidized LDL. Oxidized LDL is of interest as a vehicle for cholesterol loading of macrophages, because of the presence of oxidized lipoproteins in atherosclerotic lesions. Subsequently, a number of other macrophage receptors for oxidized LDL have been identified (Table 12.2; Figure 12.6). In addition, foam cell formation can be

Table 12.2 **Routes for uptake of normal and modified LDL by macrophages**

LDL modification	Receptor or other route for uptake
None	LDL-R
Chemical modification induced by:	
Oxidation	SR-A, CD-36, macrosialin/ CD68, LOX-1
Acetylation	SR-A
Aggregation induced by:	
Lipoprotein lipase	Phagocytosis
Phospholipases	
Sphingomyelinase	
Immune complex formation	
Mechanical means	
Proteoglycan association	
Mast cell granules	
Platelets	

For further details, see recent reviews (Tabas, 1999; Pentikainen *et al.*, 2000).
LDL-R, LDL receptor; SR-A, scavenger receptor type A.

induced by *in vitro* incubation of macrophages with various forms of LDL which have been physically or enzymically altered to induce either self-aggregation or association with elements of the ECM (Table 12.2). Aggregated and matrix-bound LDLs can lead to massive lipoprotein uptake, mainly by phagocytosis. These are particularly attractive candidates for stimulation of foam cell formation *in vivo*, as both aggregated and matrix-bound LDL have been directly identified in the intima.

Modifications inducing physical aggregation or retention on the ECM may involve sphingomyelinase and/or lipoprotein lipase (LPL); both enzymes are present in lesions (Tabas, 1999).

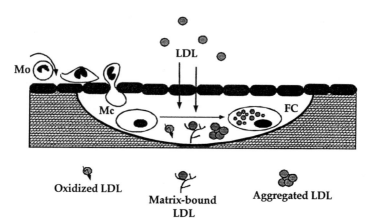

Fig. 12.6 Possible forms of modified LDL in foam cell cholesterol accumulation. Modifications to LDL which promote its uptake by macrophages are likely to occur locally in the intima. These include oxidation, binding to matrix proteoglycans and aggregation. See Section 4.1 for further details. Abbreviations are as in Figure 12.3.

4.2 Control of cellular cholesterol levels

Cholesterol is an essential component of all cell membranes, regulating both their physical state and the activity of many membrane-associated proteins, but its levels must be tightly regulated as it can be cytotoxic (Kellner-Weibel *et al.*, 1999). Cells must therefore avoid excessive accumulation of free cholesterol. In macrophages, the esterificaiton of excess cholesterol by the enzyme acyl coenzyme A:cholesteryl:acyl transferase (ACAT) provides a mechanism for sequestration of unwanted cholesterol in a relatively inert form (Figure 12.5). ACAT is active at the cytoplasmic face of the endoplasmic reticulum (ER) and its products (cholesteryl esters) accumulate in the cytoplasm as lipid droplets. Human ACAT cDNA was first identified through expression cloning and termed ACAT-1. Macrophages from ACAT-1–/– mice have a markedly reduced ability to synthesize cholesteryl esters. Subsequently, a second form of ACAT, which has 44 per cent homology with ACAT-1, has been cloned, termed ACAT-2. This is expressed mainly in liver and intestine, but does not appear of importance in macrophage cholesteryl ester synthesis. ACAT-1 is strongly expressed within macrophages of human aortic atherosclerotic lesions (Miyazaki *et al.*, 1998) as well as macrophages of several non-atherosclerotic tissues (Sakashita *et al.*, 2000). ACAT-1 protein is an integral membrane protein, located mainly in the ER. Its expression increases up to 10-fold during differentiation of human monocyte/macrophages, occurring relatively early during differentiation (within the first 2 days) (Miyazaki *et al.*, 1998). While the activity of the enzyme is affected by cholesterol levels in the cell, ACAT-1 protein levels do not change with cholesterol loading (Sakashita *et al.*, 2000). It seems that cholesterol levels affect ACAT-1 activity rather than expression.

5 Lipoprotein oxidation, macrophages and atherosclerosis

5.1 The likely importance of LDL oxidation in atherosclerosis

Oxidized lipoproteins are present in atherosclerotic lesions *in vivo*, and exert potentially pro-atherogenic effects on cells *in vitro*. However, lipoproteins isolated from lesions tend to be lightly oxidized (Niu *et al.*, 1999) and poor scavenger receptor ligands (Steinbrecher and Lougheed, 1992). It is possible that heavily oxidized LDL is generated and cleared rapidly by local macrophages but, in the absence of any supportive measurements, it appears that LDL oxidation alone cannot account for unregulated lipoprotein uptake in lesions. Therefore, other routes for the endocytosis of LDL (lightly oxidized or otherwise) are necessary. Several studies indicate that lesion lipoproteins tend to be aggregated and/or associated with ECM and may enter by phagocytosis. Binding of LDL to other molecules that stimulate aggregation and matrix association can promote both intimal retention and macrophage uptake of lipoproteins. Two recent reviews summarize several non-oxidative modifications that induce intimal lipoprotein aggregation and may induce uptake of native and lightly oxidized lipoproteins (Tabas, 1999; Pentikainen *et al.*, 2000), such as those induced by sphingomyelinase and lipoprotein lipase.

While intimal lipoprotein oxidation may not be essential for cholesterol loading, oxidation products are certainly present in lesions and have potent biological activities. Such oxidation is believed to occur locally within the intima, and to be influenced or even mediated by the cells which are in close proximity to the lipoprotein particles. The cell types present are predominantly endothelial cells and monocyte/macrophages, and also smooth muscle cells and lymphocytes as the lesion develops. The mechanisms by which such cells may influence lipoprotein oxidation have been the subject of intense interest as potential therapeutic targets. Using cultured cell systems, it has been shown that all of the above cells, including macrophages, can stimulate LDL oxidation under some circumstances; in other cases, they are able to limit the oxidative events.

5.2 Macrophage-mediated oxidation of LDL

By stimulating LDL oxidation, macrophages can exhibit pro-oxidant, potentially pro-atherogenic, activity. Despite many studies demonstrating that macrophages can promote LDL oxidation *in vitro* (Garner and Jessup, 1996), the cellular mechanism responsible has not been resolved conclusively. Several pathways have been suggested to contribute to macrophage-mediated acceleration of LDL oxidation (Figure 12.7; reviewed in Garner and Jessup, 1996). Among them are cell-mediated maintenance of transition metal ions in a reduced (and therefore highly reactive) state, involvement of cellular lipoxygenase(s) and the direct action of cell-derived oxidants (e.g. superoxide radical, hypochlorite and reactive nitrogen species).

Macrophages, through the activities of myeloperoxidase (MPO) and the respiratory burst oxidase, are potent sources of oxygen-centered free radicals (Figure 12.7). In addi-

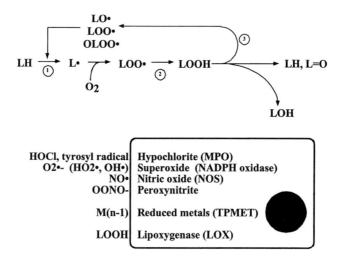

Fig. 12.7 Cell-mediated oxidation of lipoproteins; potential mechanisms. Oxidation of lipids (LH) involves abstraction of a bis-allylic hydrogen to produce a carbon-centered lipid radical (L·; reaction 1), and addition of molecular oxygen to form a peroxyl radical (LOO·). This can abstract hydrogen from a further lipid (thus propagating a chain reaction) to form relatively stable lipid hydroperoxides (LOOH; reaction 2). In the presence of reduced metals, these hydroperoxides decompose to oxygen-centered radicals (reaction 3) which can initiate further rounds of oxidation. Lipid hydroperoxides are also converted to lipid hydroxides (LOH) and ketones (L=O).
Macrophages produce several oxidants. Those capable of initiating lipid peroxidation (reaction 1) include tyrosyl radical, hydroperoxyl radical (HO2·) and peroxynitrite (OONO–). Generation of reduced metals can accelerate oxidation (reaction 3). Lipid hydroperoxides may also be generated by macrophage-derived lipoxyganses (LOX), although there is no evidence that these are secreted. See Section 5.2 for details and other abbreviations.

tion, expression of the inducible form of nitric oxide synthase (iNOS) leads to generation of large amounts of NO. This is only very weakly oxidant, but can react with superoxide radical to produce the strong oxidant, peroxynitrite. However, while *in vitro* studies have shown that most of these oxidants are capable of causing LDL oxidation in cell-free systems, macrophage-mediated LDL oxidation appears to be independent of such species (Garner and Jessup, 1996). Convincing experimental evidence suggests that the superoxide radical does not directly mediate oxidation of LDL by macrophages (reviewed in Garner and Jessup, 1996). While stimulation of the respiratory burst oxidase by zymosan accelerated monocyte- or macrophage-mediated LDL oxidation (Chisolm *et al.*, 1999, and references therein), this was also dependent on metals released from the particles and/or cells (Xing *et al.*, 1998). Interestingly, impaired superoxide production due to a deficiency in phagocyte NADPH oxidase failed to inhibit atherosclerosis in mice (Kirk *et al.*, 2000) and overexpression of superoxide dismutase did not reduce lesion development in transgenic mice. MPO-deficient monocytes oxidize LDL normally (Hiramatsu *et al.*, 1987). More recent studies suggest that MPO can stimulate LDL oxidation by generating reactive nitrogen species, such as NO·, especially under conditions related to inflammation (Hazen *et al.*, 1999). The action of these oxidants, which appears to be metal ion-independent, results in oxidative modifications to apoB and lipids. The importance of the reactive nitrogen species in macrophage-mediated lipoprotein oxidation is not clear, as enhanced generation of NO· by these cells in the presence of metals inhibits LDL oxidation (Jessup, 1996). The pro- and antioxidant action of nitric oxide and its products, however, depends on multiple factors, and the role of reactive nitrogen species in macrophage-mediated oxidation *in vivo* requires further studies.

No studies published to date have shown conclusively a role for lipoxygenase(s) (LO) in pro-oxidant activity of macrophages towards LDL, although an indirect contribution of the enzyme to macrophage-accelerated LDL oxidation has been proposed (reviewed in Kuhn and Chan, 1997). Although 15-LO mRNA and the enzyme and specific lipid oxidation products have been found in atherosclerotic lesions, overexpression of the enzyme in macrophages actually protected transgenic rabbits against atherosclerosis.

In vitro, macrophage-mediated oxidation of LDL is dependent on the presence of low, catalytic concentrations of redox-active metals such as iron or copper. This suggests that the process by which macrophages stimulate LDL oxidation *in vivo* also involves such metals (Garner and Jessup, 1996). Macrophages can directly reduce extracellular transition metal ions using a surface trans-plasma membrane electron transport (TPMET) system (Garner *et al.*, 1997) (Figure 12.8). Such reduced metals can stimulate lipoprotein oxidation by catalyzing the decomposition of peroxides (LOOH) to reactive alkoxy radicals (LO·), which initiate further rounds of lipid peroxidation either directly or via formation of peroxyl radicals (Figure 12.7; Garner and Jessup, 1996). Recent evidence suggests that TPMET contributes significantly to macrophage-mediated LDL oxidation *in vitro* (Baoutina *et al.*, 2001). Therefore, the possibility exists that metal ion-catalyzed LDL oxidation by macrophages could contribute to generation of oxidized LDL during atherosclerosis. However, this would require the availability of metals at the site of LDL oxidation in the atherosclerotic plaque. Free or loosely bound transition metal ions (iron and copper) are unlikely to be present in normal body fluids or arterial tissue, but could become available under pathological conditions, such as developing atherosclerotic lesions (Yuan, 1999). The presence of redox-active transition metal ions in plaque (Swain

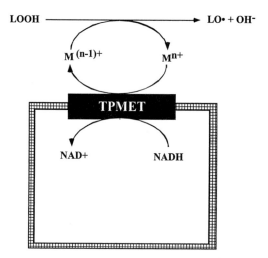

Fig. 12.8 Trans-plasma membrane electron transport (TPMET) system. A TPMET system uses intracellular reductant to reduce extracellular metals, such as copper (Cu^{2+}) and iron (Fe^{3+}). Reduced metals can stimulate lipid peroxidation by catalyzing decomposition of lipid hydroperoxides to reactive oxygen-centered radicals.

and Gutteridge, 1995) and their co-localization with ceroid and macrophages (Yuan, 1999) has been reported. Moreover, oxidative products characteristic of metal-catalyzed oxidation of LDL, both lipid and protein derived, have been identified in lesions (Fu *et al.* 1998; Niu *et al.*, 1999). Physiologically relevant forms of iron and copper (e.g. heme, ferritin and ceruloplasmin) can enhance oxidation of LDL *in vitro,* particularly under conditions related to inflammation.

Although it is generally accepted that macrophage-mediated lipoprotein oxidation *in vitro* occurs extracellularly, and does not require interaction with cellular receptors for native or modified LDL (Tangirala *et al.*, 1996), the possibility for intracellular, perhaps lysosomal, oxidation of LDL by these cells cannot be excluded. Indirect support for such oxidation *in vivo* comes from demonstration of the occurrence of epitopes of oxidized LDL (oxidized lipid–protein adducts) within lipid-laden macrophages, but not in the extracellular space in animal models of atherosclerosis (reviewed in Hoff and Hoppe, 1995). The mechanisms for such oxidation have not been elucidated, but the role of intracellular transition metal ions liberated from metal-containing proteins has been proposed (Hoff and Hoppe 1995).

5.3 Inhibitory actions of macrophages in LDL oxidation

In addition to pro-oxidant action of macrophages towards LDL, under certain conditions these cells also have activities likely to limit lipoprotein oxidation (Figure 12.9). For example, when presented with mildly oxidized LDL, macrophages remove cholesteryl ester hydroperoxides in the lipoprotein (Baoutina *et al.*, 2000). Macrophages have also been demonstrated selectively to clear cholesterol 7-hydroperoxides from oxidized LDL (Brown *et al.*, 1997) and to remove peroxides rapidly from oxidized amino acids, peptides and proteins (Fu *et al.*, 1995). Detoxification of such hydroperoxides by macrophages is protective as it converts labile hydroperoxide groups to much less reac-

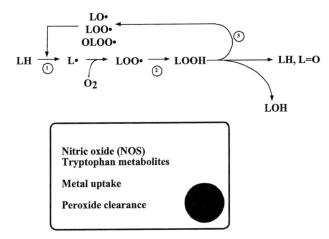

Fig. 12.9 Possible roles of macrophages in prevention of lipoprotein oxidation. Macrophages may inhibit lipid peroxidation (reactions 1 and 2; for details, see Figure 12.7) by release of antioxidants which intercept oxygen-centered radicals, converting them to more stable products incapable of initiating further oxidation, by preventing peroxide decomposition (reaction 3) by sequestration of metals or by conversion of peroxides to more stable products such as hydroxides (LOH).

tive hydroxides as the major product. Removal of cholesteryl ester hydroperoxides in LDL and of peroxidized groups on peptides and proteins is believed to occur extracellularly, while oxidized cholesterol and amino acids may penetrate the cells to be reduced intracellularly. Although the precise mechanism(s) of this activity of macrophages have not yet been fully defined, the ability of the cells to remove highly reactive and toxic peroxide molecules, capable of causing further lipid peroxidation and also possible cell toxicity, is likely to be an important protective mechanism against peroxidation. As oxidation of LDL has been implicated in atherogenesis and cholesteryl ester hydro(pero)xides, cholesterol 7-oxides and protein oxidation products have been identified in advanced atherosclerotic plaque (Fu *et al.*, 1995; Brown *et al.*, 1997; Niu *et al.*, 1999), this ability of macrophages could be considered as potentially anti-atherogenic *in vivo*.

Another example of the antioxidant activity of macrophages is their ability to inhibit *in vitro* metal-catalyzed LDL lipid peroxidation in certain media (Kritharides *et al.*m 1995a; van Reyk *et al.*, 1999). Metal sequestration and other modifications of the extracellular environment by macrophages have been suggested to contribute to such activity. In addition, it has been demonstrated that macrophages depress cell-mediated LDL lipid peroxidation and generation of a high-uptake (i.e. avidly endocytosed) form of LDL when their synthesis of NO· is elevated (Jessup, 1996), or when generation of tryptophan metabolites [e.g. 3-hydroxyanthranilic acid (3-HAA)] is increased through induction of indoleamine dioxygenase (Christen *et al.*, 1994).

5.4 Likely role of macrophages in LDL oxidation *in vivo*

In summary, macrophages can exhibit both pro- and antioxidant activities *in vitro*, the mechanisms of which are still not fully defined. These activities could be influenced by many cellular and extracellular factors (e.g. composition of extracellular fluid, number and concentration of available transition metal ions, state of activation of cells and oxidative state of LDL). Moreover, *in vitro* systems, used for modeling macrophage-mediated LDL oxidation, are quite different in many respects from the conditions in which oxidation of LDL may occur *in vivo* (e.g. with respect to pH and oxygen tension). The presence in atherosclerotic plaque and co-localization with macrophages of oxidized LDL, transition metal ions (Yuan, 1999; Swain and Gutteridge, 1995), LO and its products, MPO, iNOS, chlorinated proteins and chloro- and nitro-tyrosine, and subunits of the superoxide-generating NADH/NADPH oxidase system indicate that the contribution of any discussed mechanism of pro- and antioxidant activities of macrophages could be plausible *in vivo*. The likelihood of macrophage-mediated oxidative modification of LDL *in vivo* would depend upon the balance between these opposing activities of these cells in the complex environment of developing atherosclerotic plaque.

5.5 Metabolism of oxidized lipoproteins

Chemical support for the concept of intracellular accumulation of oxidized lipids comes from the demonstration of oxidized LDL epitopes, ceroid and oxysterols in lipid-laden macrophages in animal atherosclerosis and in patients with lysosomal dysfunction (Wolman's disease) (Hoff and Hoppe, 1995). Core aldehydes and apoB of oxidized LDL have both been shown to be resistant to lysosomal hydrolysis and to accumulate in macrophage lysosomes. Chemically characterized products of oxidation of cholesteryl linoleate, such as cholesteryl ester aldehydes, are resistant to lysosomal hydrolysis in macrophages, complex with proteins and are present in atherosclerotic lesions of humans (Hoppe *et al.*, 1997).

A number of secondary consequences may arise from accumulation of oxidized LDL in lysosomes. Human THP-1 cells exposed to oxidized LDL accumulated lipid in large swollen lysosomes and developed secondary hypertrophy of the Golgi apparatus and the *trans*-Golgi network. Additionally, uptake of mildly oxidized LDL inhibits lysosomal hydrolysis of unoxidized cholesteryl esterase, and this may relate to direct inhibitory effects of lipid hydroperoxides on cholesteryl esterases (Kritharides *et al.*, 1998b). Uptake of oxidized LDL, and intralysosomal oxidation may also perturb lysosomal integrity, with lysosomal enzyme release to the cytosol (Li *et al.*, 1998). Endocytic and secretory activities of macrophages have been altered by loading cells with oxidized LDL (Bolton *et al.*, 1997) and a number of lysosomal enzymes may be secreted in response to frustrated phagocytosis. In summary, these data suggest that mild chemical modification of LDL may secondarily perturb lysosomal function, and that more advanced oxidation products may themselves be resistant to lysosomal hydrolysis.

6 Effects of macrophage lipid accumulation on cell function

6.1 Macrophage-derived inflammatory mediators

The foam cell macrophage is an early and persistent feature of atherosclerosis and is therefore likely to play a key role in the development and progression of the disease. This may include production of inflammatory mediators and effectors such as cytokines and ECM-degrading enzymes, which are considered active agents in atherosclerosis. To determine the importance of lipid loading in lesion macrophage expression of inflammatory mediators, the effects of *in vitro* cholesterol loading of cultured macrophages has been studied. Cholesterol loading stimulates release of some, but not all cytokines and matrix-degrading enzymes (reviewed in van Reyk and Jessup, 1999). Both stimulatory and inhibitory effects of oxidized LDL (and oxidized lipid components of it) on macrophage cytokine expression have been reported (for reviews, see, for example, Brown and Jessup, 1999; van Reyk and Jessup, 1999). It should be noted that in most such studies, little attention has been given to the amounts of oxidation products that are introduced into the cells and their relevance to amounts present in lesion foam cells *in vivo*. This is an important consideration, since these compounds are generally present in foam cells in small amounts, while at high concentrations they are often toxic.

6.2 Lipoproteins and macrophage proliferation

The macrophages that accumulate in atherosclerotic lesions are derived from blood-borne monocytes that have been recruited into the intima. Local proliferation of macrophages within the vessel wall could also augment the numbers of these cells in atherosclerotic lesions. Both *in situ* tritiated thymidine incorporation and expression of proliferating cell nuclear antigen (PCNA) have shown that the rates of cell division are higher in atherosclerotic than in normal vessels, with macrophages the predominant proliferating cell type. Proliferation was greatest in lipid-rich lesions (Orekhov *et al.*, 1998) and in focal collections of lipid-laden cells of monocytic appearance (Villaschi and Spagnoli, 1983).

Lipids are established stimuli of macrophages, including cholesterol, cholesteryl esters, cardiolipin and triglycerides (Yui and Yamazaki, 1986). These stimuli are strongly enhanced when such lipids are subjected to peroxidation before exposure to the cells (Yui and Yamazaki, 1990). Perhaps not surprisingly, oxidized LDL is also mitogenic for human and murine macrophages (Yui *et al.*, 1993; Hamilton *et al.*, 1999), although the active agent is not yet established.

6.3 PPAR-α and PPAR-γ

Peroxisome proliferator-activated receptors (PPARs) are ligand-activated transcription factors belonging to the nuclear receptor superfamily. Three forms (α, δ/β and γ) have been identified, each with separate gene products and with distinct tissue distributions and patterns of expression. PPARs have roles in lipid, glucose and energy homeostasis and in regulation of differentiation. PPAR-γ is expressed in cells of the monocyte/macrophage lineage, where the level of expression is increased during differentiation and on exposure to oxidized LDL (Ricote *et al.*, 1998; Tontonoz *et al.*, 1998). In monocyte/macrophages, activation of PPAR-γ inhibits expression of several proteins including pro-inflammatory cytokines such as TNF-α, IL-6 and IL-1β. In combination with agonists of the retinoid X receptor (RXR), activation of PPAR-γ in HL60 monocytic leukemia cells causes induction of differentiation markers CD11b and CD18 (Tontonoz *et al.*, 1998). Natural ligands for PPAR-γ include lipids such as prostaglandin J2 and some polyunsaturated fatty acids such as linoleic acid. PPAR-γ is also activated by oxidized LDL, of which oxidized forms of linoleic and arachidonic acids, 9-HODE, 13-HODE and 15-HETE were efficient stimuli of PPAR-γ-mediated reporter gene transcription, while the major oxysterols were inactive (Nagy *et al.*, 1998).

PPAR-α is also expressed in macrophages (Ricote *et al.*, 1998; Tontonoz *et al.*, 1998) and reported to be present in atherosclerotic lesions but not normal vessels at levels generally more abundant than PPAR-γ (Torra *et al.*, 1999). Like PPAR-γ, its ligands include fatty acids and derivatives, including leukotriene B_4 and 8-HETE. PPAR-α activation increases hepatic uptake and esterification of free fatty acids, skeletal and cardiac fatty acid uptake and oxidation, stimulation of lipoprotein lipase, overexpression of apoA-I and apoA-II and inhibition of apoCII expression (Torra *et al.*, 1999). Its effects in macrophages are less well understood than those of PPAR-γ. It is not known if PPAR-α activation affects macrophage uptake and metabolism of fatty acids.

6.4 Reverse cholesterol transport

Macrophages loaded with copper-oxidized LDL, in which oxysterols are a significant proportion of total sterol content, exported cholesterol less readily in the presence of the extracellular acceptor apoA-I (see Section 7 for details of cholesterol efflux) than cells in which cholesterol was the only sterol accumulated (Kritharides *et al.*, 1995b). Specific enrichment of cholesterol-rich macrophage foam cells with 7KC led to a similar inhibition of cholesterol efflux (Gelissen *et al.*, 1996). Importantly, the levels of 7KC found to be inhibitory in human cells *in vitro* were in the range of those found in authentic lesion-derived foam cells. Thus, oxysterols which are present in foam cells may contribute to generation and maintenance of the foam cell phenotype by interfering with their capacity to dispose of excess cholesterol.

7 Export of cholesterol from macrophage foam cells

7.1 Routes for cholesterol disposal in foam cells

Macrophages have a limited number of mechanisms for removal of excess unesterified cholesterol (Figure 12.10). Like most peripheral cells, cholesterol export to specific extracellular acceptors, such as high-density lipoprotein (HDL), is probably the most important route, quantitatively. This is discussed further below. Such initial cholesterol removal, or cellular cholesterol efflux, is considered the first step in the RCT pathway, which ultimately delivers peripheral cholesterol to the liver for disposal through bile acid synthesis. Perturbation of the RCT pathway could contribute to the failed clearance of cell cholesterol from lesions *in vivo*. Low plasma HDL concentrations confer an increased risk of atherosclerotic coronary events, and elevation of HDL by pharmacological means decreases this risk. This is at least partly due to direct protective effects of HDL.

One other route for elimination of cholesterol from macrophages, independent of extracellular acceptors such as HDL, is the metabolism of cholesterol to 27-hydroxycholesterol (27OH) by sterol 27-hydroxylase, a mitochondrial cytochrome P450 enzyme expressed at high activity in human macrophages (Babiker *et al.*, 1997) and co-localized with macrophages in human carotid lesions (Crisby *et al.*, 1997) (Figure 12.10). 27OH is one of the most abundant oxysterols in human atherosclerotic lesions and macrophage-derived foam cells. The enzyme can hydroxylate the same methyl group three times in sequence eventually to form 3β-hydroxy-5-cholestenoic acid, and both 27OH and 3β-hydroxy-5-cholestenoic acid are synthesized by cultured macrophages in response to cholesterol loading (Lund *et al.*, 1996). The polarity of 3β-hydroxy-5-cholestenoic acid

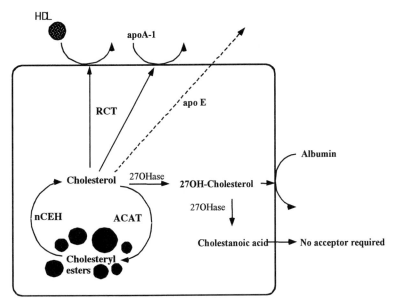

Fig. 12.10 Route for cholesterol export from macrophages. Cholesterol may be released from the plasma membrane to specific extracellular acceptors such as high-density lipoprotein (HDL) or apolipoprotein A-I (apoA-1) by the process of reverse cholesterol transport (RCT). In foam cells, cholesterol derived by hydrolysis of cholesteryl esters replaces membrane cholesterol; thus, in the presence of sufficient amounts of acceptors, foam cell formation can be reversed. In the absence of acceptors, an alternative pathway may predominate, catalyzed by sterol 27 hydroxylase (27OHase). This leads to the generation of progressively more polar sterols that can be released either to more abundant albumin, or directly without an acceptor. Secretion of endogenously synthesized apolipoprotein E (apoE) may also stimulate cholesterol export.

relative to cholesterol allows its export from macrophages even in the absence of an extracellular acceptor, and may thus be important in tissues where HDL concentrations are relatively low. Patients with cerebrotendinous xanthomatosis (who lack sterol 27-hydroxylase) die prematurely from atherosclerotic disorders, despite having normal circulating levels of cholesterol, supporting a biological role for this process.

7.2 Properties of cholesterol acceptors for macrophages

Many different molecules and particles can act as cholesterol acceptors from macrophages. These include whole HDL and its constituent apolipoproteins (A-I, A-II, E, J and A-IV) (Hara and Yokoyama, 1991). The major protein component of HDL is apoA-I and its importance in RCT is shown by the effect of depletion of apoA-I-containing particles from plasma, which greatly reduces its capacity to remove cholesterol from cells. The HDL fraction of plasma is a heterogeneous population that includes particles rich in PL and exchangeable apolipoproteins (e.g. apoA-I, apoA-II, apoE and apoJ). These also exist in equilibrium with smaller amounts of lipid-poor or lipid-free apolipoproteins such as apoA-I. The relative importance of these various plasma particles as major acceptors of cellular cholesterol in tissues such as the vessel wall remains to be determined, and is likely to vary depending on the types of acceptors available locally. *In vivo*, the most important of these for initial efflux appears to be a lipid-poor apoA-I fraction (preβ-HDL) (Castro and Fielding, 1988). In plasma, this comprises about 5 per cent of the total apoA-I pool. Similar lipid-poor apoA-I fractions are in peripheral lymph and human aorta. The majority of apoA-I in human intima is in a very high-density (lipid-poor) fraction (Smithm 1990). Apolipoproteins secreted locally are also likely to contribute to cholesterol efflux in the vascular wall. These include apoE, secreted by macrophages and smooth muscle cells, and apoJ, secreted by smooth muscle cells. Factors regulating the efflux of cholesterol have been elucidated in some detail and there have been significant recent developments in this field (Rothblat *et al.*, 1999; Rigotti and Krieger, 1999; Young and Fielding, 1999).

7.3 Mechanisms for cholesterol export from macrophages

The mechanism by which acceptors mediate cellular cholesterol export depends on their state of lipidation (Figure 12.11). PL-containing acceptors such as HDL particles may remove cholesterol by several mechanisms including aqueous diffusion and possible receptor-mediated processes involving surface proteins. In the aqueous diffusion model, free cholesterol desorbs from the cell–water interface and diffuses through the aqueous layer until it meets and is absorbed by the HDL particle. The flux of cholesterol between cells and HDL is bidirectional, the direction of net transfer of cholesterol mass being determined by the gradient in cholesterol concentration. Kinetic data indicate movement of cholesterol from the donor membrane and into the unstirred water layer before being received by the acceptor vesicle. This aqueous diffusion model is supported by various data (Phillips *et al.*, 1987) and implies that direct acceptor–cell contact is not mechanisti-

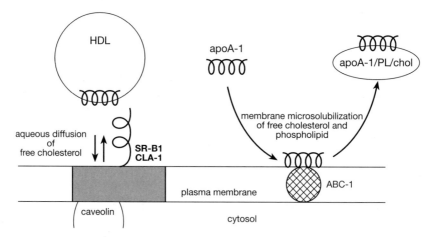

Fig. 12.11 Different mechanisms for cholesterol efflux from macrophages. Release of cholesterol to phospholipid-containing acceptors such as HDL occurs by a concentration-dependent diffusion of free cholesterol and does not require direct interaction between particle and membrane. SR-B1 promotes such efflux, apparently by facilitating cholesterol movement in the plasma membrane. SR-B1 is concentrated in specific domains of the plasma membrane called caveolae. The human homolog of SR-B1 may be CLA-1. Lipid-free apolipoprotein A-I (apoA-1) binds directly to the plasma membrane to abstract phospholipid and cholesterol (membrane microsolubilization), generating a nascent HDL particle. This process is dependent on expression of the membrane protein ABC-1, although it is not clear if direct contact between apoA-I and ABC-1 is required.

cally important. HDL-mediated efflux of cholesterol may also involve a surface receptor, SR-B1 (see below).

When cells are incubated with lipid-free (or poor) apolipoproteins, direct interaction between the apolipoprotein and the cell membrane appears to be important in cholesterol efflux (Figure 12.11). Interaction of apoA-I with cells involves transient binding of the apolipoprotein to the cell surface, followed by abstraction of plasma membrane cholesterol and PL. This results in the formation of an extracellular apoA-I–cholesterol–PL particle. Major properties of apolipoproteins which enhance cholesterol efflux are related to their surface activity such as their content of hydrophobic segments, their overall flexibility and their content of amphipathic helices. Apolipoproteins function at least to some extent by microsolubilizing plasma membrane PL (Gillotte *et al.*, 1999). Apolipoprotein-mediated efflux, as distinct from PL vesicle-mediated efflux, is an energy-requiring active cellular process. The capacity of apolipoproteins to remove cellular lipids correlates with their ability to penetrate a PL layer. Therefore, factors which affect the packing of PL also affect the ability of apoA-I to bind to the cell surface and to stimulate cholesterol and PL efflux. Cellular cholesterol enrichment enhances both cholesterol and PL efflux from macrophages to lipid-free apoA-I, and increases apolipoprotein binding to lipid bilayers. This may be related to altered ordering of lipids in the plasma membrane, since addition of cholesterol to PL monolayers increases their affinity for and capacity to bind apoA-I. Cholesterol loading also stimulates an increase in total cell PL, and this may also affect the composition of the plasma membrane with related effects on ease of cholesterol efflux. Inhibition of cholesterol efflux to apoA-I by 7KC (Section 6.4) appears to be due largely to inhibition of PL desorption from the plasma membrane to apoA-I, since 7KC also impairs PL export from cholesterol-loaded macrophages and cholesterol efflux rates are restored if HDLs (which do not require cellular PL export) are provided as acceptors (Gelissen *et al.*, 1999).

Cholesterol flux is bidirectional and is determined by the initial concentration of free cholesterol in donor and acceptor particles and the ratio of rate constants for efflux and influx. Thus, net efflux from macrophages is most marked after cholesterol enrichment and after foam cell formation (Hara and Yokoyama, 1991; Kritharides *et al.*, 1995b). The chemical cholesterol gradient between cell and acceptor remains a major determinant of net efflux achieved by diverse initiating mechanisms—including receptors such as SR-B1, apolipoprotein-mediated efflux or PL vesicles. There is significant variation between cells in their efficiency of cholesterol efflux (Rothblat *et al.*, 1999). For example, FU5Ah hepatoma cells are very fast ($t_{1/2}$ 2 h), and smooth muscle cells are relatively slow ($t_{1/2}$ 24 h). Macrophages tend to demonstrate efflux rates intermediate between these two extremes, although human macrophages appear to be especially slow (Kritharides *et al.*, 1998a), and many factors may contribute to this. Any cell cholesterol (free or esterified) accumulated in lysosomal, cytosolic or other intracellular pools will also limit cholesterol efflux, and slow intracellular processing of exogenous cholesterol appears to be particularly relevant in human macrophages (Kritharides *et al.*, 1998a).

Mobilization of cytoplasmic cholesteryl esters requires hydrolysis to free cholesterol by neutral cholesteryl ester hydrolase (nCEH) (Figure 12.10), an essential step in the process of cholesterol efflux from foam cell to extracellular acceptors, in which cholesterol export is principally at the expense of cholesteryl ester stores. Generally, it is considered that ester hydrolysis can be rate limiting, and that significant species differences in rates of cholesterol export from macrophage foam cells are related to their levels of nCEH activity (Graham *et al.*, 1996). It has been suggested that in macrophages, at least part of this activity is contributed by hormone-sensitive lipase (HSL). HSL is an enzyme of relatively broad specificity, having the ability to hydrolyze tri-, di- and monoacyl-glycerols as well as cholesteryl esters and small water-soluble substrates, being highly expressed in adipose tissue, where it is responsible for lipolysis of triglycerides. The enzyme is expressed in murine and human macrophages, although the level of expression in human macrophages is 40-fold less than in adipose cells (Reue *et al.*, 1997). Further, HSL expression seen in the THP-1 macrophage-like cell line or peripheral blood monocytes disappeared on differentiation of these cells. On the other hand, immunodepletion of HSL from macrophage homogenates removed most nCEH activity (Small *et al.*, 1989), while overexpression increased cholesteryl ester hydrolysis (Escary *et al.*, 1998). However, overexpression of HSL in mice paradoxically increased athero-sclerosis (Escary *et al.*, 1999). Thus other nCEH enzymes, such as a cholesterol-dependent form recently identified in macrophages (Ghosh, 2000), may be more important in cholesterol ester mobilization.

7.4 Plasma membrane determinants of cholesterol export

The role of discrete plasma membrane lipid domains and their associated proteins in cho-lesterol efflux is still controversial. Cell plasma membranes contain detergent-insoluble glycosphingolipid- and cholesterol-rich domains (detergent-insoluble glycolipid-enriched domains; DIGs or 'rafts'). These lateral lipid assemblies are believed to form sponta-neously due to strong hydrophobic interactions between sphingolipids (e.g. sphin-gomyelin) and cholesterol that form raft-like microdomains within a more fluid glycerophospholipid (e.g. phosphatidylcholine) environment. These assemblies are sites of association of a range of lipid-linked proteins in the plasma membrane. Some are in the form of caveolae, which are cell surface invaginations containing caveolin (a 22 kDa integral membrane protein which is important for the structural integrity of caveolae; Parton, 1996). Caveolae are abundant in adipocytes, smooth muscle cells, endothelial cells and fibroblasts, and until recently were considered deficient in lymphocytes and macrophages; however, recent studies indicate that caveolae are present in the THP-1 human macrophage-like cell line (Matveev *et al.*, 1999). Caveolae have been implicated as the source of cholesterol for primary acceptors of cell cholesterol such as preβ-HDL (Fielding and Fielding, 1997). Caveolin expression, and caveolae, are cholesterol-depen-dent, being up-regulated after accumulation of free cholesterol and down-regulated by removal of cell cholesterol or suppression of cell cholesterol synthesis. The incorporation of caveolin into lipid membranes is also cholesterol dependent. Caveolae are associated with proteins such as CD36, cytoplasmic signaling molecules, multiple glycosylphos-phatidylinositol (GPI)-linked proteins and cytoskeletal elements, so modulation of cave-olin expression by cholesterol flux could have major implications for cell function and cell signaling (Lisanti *et al.*, 1994). The secondary effects of cholesterol depletion may be equally relevant in cells which do not express caveolin but contain DIGs. DIGs are present in cells that do not express caveolin, and even in caveolin-expressing cells the bulk of DIGs exist outside of caveolae. However, at the present time, the relative impor-tance in macrophages of DIGs generally, and of caveolae in particular, remains to be determined.

Receptor-mediated processes have long been implicated in cholesterol efflux from cells but, until recently, characterization of functionally important receptors has been problematic. Two important proteins have been identified as having important roles in different aspects of the RCT pathway (Figure 12.11). The best characterized on peripheral cells is the class B type 1 scavenger receptor (SR-B1). The human homolog of rodent SR-B1 is suggested to be CLA-1. SR-B1 is important in HDL metabolism (Rothblat *et al*., 1999), mediating cholesterol delivery from HDL to the liver and adrenal gland. It is probably most important for liver uptake of HDL cholesterol. Over- or underexpression of SR-B1 and its effect on atherosclerosis in mice indicates a protective role for this protein (Trigatti *et al*., 1999).

SR-B1 expression generates a hydrophobic channel in the plasma membrane, facilitating selective uptake of cholesteryl esters from HDL, and bidirectional flux of free cholesterol. Thus it can accelerate cholesterol efflux down a concentration gradient (Rothblat *et al*., 1999). SR-B1 binds a wide range of apolipoproteins and lipoprotein particles and strongly enhances efflux to PL-containing acceptors, but does not mediate lipid-free apolipoprotein-mediated efflux. The level of SR-B1 expression has been correlated with rates of cholesterol efflux to HDL (but not to apoA-I) from several cell types (Jian *et al*., 1998), suggesting that this receptor may have a role in RCT. However, SR-B1 is poorly expressed in primary macrophages (Ji *et al*., 1997) although these cells are competent cholesterol exporters (Kritharides *et al*., 1995b). Therefore, SR-B1 is unlikely to be essential and/or rate limiting for constitutive cholesterol efflux, although its up-regulation may enhance efflux.

SR-B1 is found in caveolae (Matveev *et al*., 1999). Thus, factors that affect the expression and distribution of caveolin may indirectly determine SR-B1 expression and function. One such factor may be the density of DIGs on the cell surface. Indeed the association between SR-B1 expression and cholesterol efflux may be a reflection of a more important causal relationship between DIG concentration and cholesterol efflux rather than a primary property of SR-B1 itself.

Tangier disease (TD) is a rare condition associated with the absence of HDL, tonsillar enlargement, peripheral neuropathy and, at least in some cases, premature atherosclerosis. In TD, HDL undergoes rapid catabolism, and cells from patients with TD show normal cholesterol efflux to PL-containing acceptors (e.g. HDL) but severely impaired efflux of cholesterol and PL to lipid-free apoA-I (Oram and Yokoyama, 1996). Recently, a mutation in the ATP-binding cassette transporter 1 (ABC-1) protein has been identified in TD. ABC-1 expression is normally induced during monocyte differentiation and is up-regulated by cholesterol enrichment (Langmann *et al*., 1999), while its activity is enhanced by cAMP. As apoA-I-mediated cholesterol efflux is highly dependent upon the cholesterol enrichment of cells, and is enhanced by cAMP, this supports the importance of ABC-1 expression in apoA-I-mediated cholesterol efflux. ABC-1 and related membrane proteins have many complex biological activities including roles in multidrug resistance, transmembrane translocation of phosphatidylcholine and presentation of endogenous antigens by HLA class I molecules. Consequently, the *in vivo* effects of deficiency and overexpression in animal models may be complex, and these studies are awaited with interest.

In summary, the combination of SR-B1 and ABC-1 appears to mediate two poles of the RCT pathway. Both are involved in initial cholesterol efflux from macrophages, SR-B1 for PL-containing acceptors, and ABC-1 for apolipoprotein acceptors. SR-B1 is also important in terminal uptake of HDL lipids by the liver. These receptors may provide future therapeutics for established atherosclerosis, including reversal of macrophage foam cell formation.

8 Summary

While many cell types are involved in atherogenesis, the macrophage appears to play a central role in many aspects of lesion development. They are the major driving force in cellular cholesterol accumulation, leading eventually to the massive intra- and extracellular lipid deposition characteristic of atherosclerosis and which leads to lesion instability and clinical events. As a source of cytokines, they contribute to the infiltration and proliferation of smooth muscle cells and deposition of ECM. They are a potent potential source of oxidants that may be important in intimal lipoprotein oxidation. Macrophages are active in secretion of a range of hydrolytic enzymes that may contribute to lipoprotein modification and ECM degradation. Which of these activities are most significant in atherogenesis remain to be determined, but all present potential therapeutic targets in the prevention and reversal of atherosclerosis.

Acknowledgments

The authors acknowledge Roger T. Dean for critical comments and J. McCarroll for histology and photography. W.J., A.B. and L.K. are supported by the National Health and Medical Research Council of Australia.

References

Babiker, A. *et al.* (1997). Elimination of cholesterol in macrophages and endothelial cells by the sterol 27-hydroxylase mechanism. Comparison with high density lipoprotein-mediated reverse cholesterol transport. *Journal of Biological Chemistry*, **272**, 26253–61.

Baoutina, A., Dean, R.T. and Jessup, W. (2000). Transplasma membrane redox activity of monocytes/macrophages. *Redox Reports*, **5**, 85–6.

Baoutina, A., Dean, R.T. and Jessup, W. (2001). Transplasma membrane electron transport induces macrophage-mediated low-density lipoprotein oxidation. *FASEBJ.*, **15**, 1580–2.

Basu, S.K. *et al.* (1982). Biochemical and genetic studies of the apoprotein E secreted by mouse macrophages and human monocytes. *Journal of Biological Chemistry*, **257**, 9788–95.

Bolton, E.J., Jessup, W., Stanley, K.K. and Dean, R.T. (1997). Loading with oxidised low density lipoprotein alters endocytic and secretory activities of murine macrophages. *Biochimica et Biophysica Acta*, **1356**, 12–22.

Brown, A. and Jessup, W. (1999). Oxysterols and atherosclerosis. *Atherosclerosis*, **142**, 1–29.

Brown, A.J., Leong, S.L., Dean, R.T. and Jessup, W. (1997). 7-Hydroperoxycholesterol and its products in oxidized low density lipoprotein and human atherosclerotic plaque. *Journal of Lipid Research*, **38**, 1730–45.

Brown, M. and Goldstein, J.L. (1999). A proteolytic pathway that controls the cholesterol content of membranes, cells and blood. *Proceedings of the National Acadademy of Sciences USA*, **96**, 11041–8.

Brown, M.S., Ho, Y.K. and Goldstein, J.L. (1980). The cholesteryl ester cycle in macrophage foam cells. *Journal of Biological Chemistry*, **255**, 9344–52.

Castro, G.R. and Fielding, C.J. (1988). Early incorporation of cell-derived cholesterol into pre-β migrating high-density lipoprotein. *Biochemistry*, **27**, 25–9.

Chisolm, G.M., 3rd, Hazen, S.L., Fox, P.L. and Cathcart, M.K. (1999). The oxidation of lipoproteins by monocytes–macrophages. Biochemical and biological mechanisms. *Journal of Biological Chemistry*, **274**, 25959–62.

Christen, S., Thomas, S.R., Garner, B. and Stocker, R. (1994). Inhibition by interferon-γ of human mononuclear cell-mediated low density lipoprotein oxidation. Participation of tryptophan metabolism along the kynurenine pathway. *Journal of Clinical Investigation*, **93**, 2149–58.

Crisby, M., Nilsson, J., Kostulas, V., Bjorkhem, I. and Diczfalusy, U. (1997). Localization of sterol 27-hydroxylase immuno-reactivity in human atherosclerotic plaques. *Biochimica et Biophysica Acta*, **1344**, 278–85.

Escary, J.-L., Choy, H., Reue, K. and Schotz, M. (1998). Hormone sensitive lipase overespression increases cholesteryl ester hydrolysis in macrophage foam cells. *Arteriosclerosis, Thrombosis and Vascular Biology*, **18**, 991–8.

Escary, J.L. *et al.* (1999). Paradoxical effect on atherosclerosis of hormone-sensitive lipase overexpression in macrophages. *Journal of Lipid Research*, **40**, 397–404.

Felton, C.V., Crook, D., Davies, M.J. and Oliver, M.F. (1997). Relation of plaque lipid composition and morphology to the stability of human aortic plaques. *Arteriosclerosis, Thrombosis and Vascular Biology*, **17**, 1337–45.

Fernandez-Ortiz, A. *et al.* (1994). Characterization of the relative thrombogenicity of atherosclerotic plaque components: implications for consequences of plaque rupture. *Journal of the American College of Cardiology*, **23**, 1562–9.

Fielding, C.J. and Fielding, P.E. (1997). Intracellular cholesterol transport. *Journal of Lipid Research*, **38**, 1503–21.

Fu, S., Gebicki, S., Jessup, W., Gebicki, J.M. and Dean, R.T. (1995). Biological fate of amino acid, peptide and protein hydroperoxides. *Biochemical Journal*, **311**, 821–7.

Fu, S., Davies, M.J., Stocker, R. and Dean, R.T. (1998). Evidence for roles of radicals in protein oxidation in advanced human atherosclerotic plaque. *Biochemical Journal*, **333**, 519–25.

Galis, Z.S., Sukhova, G.K., Kranzhöfer, R., Clark, S. and Libby, P. (1995). Macrophage foam cells from experimental atheroma constitutively produce matrix-degrading proteinases. *Proceedings of the National Academy of Sciences USA*, **92**, 402–6.

Garner, B. and Jessup, W. (1996). Cell-mediated oxidation of low-density lipoprotein: the elusive mechanism(s). *Redox Reports*, **2**, 97–104.

Garner, B., van Reyk, D., Dean, R.T. and Jessup, W. (1997). Direct copper reduction by macrophages. Its role in low density lipoprotein oxidation. *Journal of Biological Chemistry*, **272**, 6927–35.

Gelissen, I., Rye, K.-A., Brown, A., Dean, R. and Jessup, W. (1999). Oxysterol efflux from macrophage foam cells: the essential role of acceptor phospholipid. *Journal of Lipid Research*, **40**, 1636–46.

Gelissen, I.C. *et al.* (1996). Sterol efflux is impaired from macrophage foam cells selectively enriched with 7-ketocholesterol. *Journal of Biological Chemistry*, **271**, 17852–60.

Gerrity, R.G. (1981). The role of the monocyte in atherogenesis: I. Transition of blood-borne monocytes into foam cells in fatty lesions. *American Journal of Pathology*, **103**, 181–90.

Ghosh, S. (2000). Cholesteryl ester hydrolase in human monocyte/macrophage: cloning, sequencing and expression of full-length DNA. *Physiological Genomics*, **2**, 1–8.

Gillotte, K.L. *et al.* (1999). Apolipoprotein-mediated plasma membrane microsolubilization. Role of lipid affinity and membrane penetration in the efflux of cellular cholesterol and phospholipid. *Journal of Biological Chemistry*, **274**, 2021–8.

Goldstein, J.L., Ho, Y.K., Basu, S.K. and Brown, M.S. (1979). Binding site on macrophages that mediates the uptake and degradation of acetylated low density lipoprotein, producing massive cholesterol deposition. *Proceedings of the National Academy of Sciences USA*, **76**, 333–7.

Gown, A.M., Tsukada, T. and Ross, R. (1986). Human atherosclerosis II. Immunocytochemical analysis of the cellular composition of human atherosclerotic lesions. *American Journal of Pathology*, **125**, 191–207.

Graham, A., Angell, A.D., Jepson, C.A., Yeaman, S.J. and Hassall, D.G. (1996). Impaired mobilisation of cholesterol from stored cholesteryl esters in human (THP-1) macrophages. *Atherosclerosis*, **120**, 135–45.

Guyton, J.R., Black, B.L. and Seidel, C.L. (1990). Focal toxicity of oxysterols in vascular smooth muscle cell culture. *American Journal of Pathology*, **137**, 425–34.

Halpert, I. *et al.* (1996). Matrilysin is expressed by lipid-laden macrophages at the sites of potential rupture in atherosclerotic lesions and localizes to areas of versican deposition, a proteoglycan for the enzyme. *Proceedings of the National Academy of Sciences USA*, **93**, 9748–53.

Hamilton, J.A. *et al.* (1999). Oxidised LDL can induce macrophage survival, DNA synthesis and enhanced proliferature response to CSF-1 and GM-GSF. *Arteriosclerosis, Thrombosis and Vascular Biology*, **19**, 98–105.

Hansson, G.K. (1994). Immunological control mechanisms in plaque formation. *Basic Research in Cardiology*, **1**, 41–6.

Hara, H. and Yokoyama, S. (1991). Interaction of free apolipoproteins with macrophages. *Journal of Biological Chemistry*, **266**, 3080–6.

Hazen, S.L. *et al.* (1999). Formation of nitric oxide-derived oxidants by myeloperoxidase in monocytes: pathways for monocyte-mediated protein nitration and lipid peroxidation *In vivo*. *Circulation Research*, **85**, 950–8.

Hiramatsu, K., Rosen, H., Heinecke, J.W., Wolfbauer, G. and Chait, A. (1987). Superoxide initiates oxidation of low density lipoprotein by human monocytes. *Arteriosclerosis*, **7**, 55–60.

Hoff, H.F. and Hoppe, G. (1995). Structure of cholesterol-containing particles accumulating in atherosclerotic lesions and the mechanisms of their derivation. *Current Opinion in Lipidology*, **6**, 317–25.

Hoppe, G., Ravandi, A., Herrera, D., Kuksis, A. and Hoff, H.F. (1997). Oxidation products of cholesteryl linoleate are resistant to hydrolysis in macrophages, form complexes with proteins and are present in human atherosclerotic lesions. *Journal of Lipid Research*, **38**, 1347–60.

Jessup, W. (1996). Oxidized lipoproteins and nitric oxide. *Current Opinion in Lipidology*, **7**, 274–80.

Ji, Y. *et al.* (1997). Scavenger receptor BI promotes high density lipoprotein-mediated cellular cholesterol efflux. *Journal of Biological Chemistry*, **272**, 20982–5.

Jian, B. *et al.* (1998). Scavenger receptor class B type I as a mediator of cellular cholesterol efflux to lipoproteins and phospholipid acceptors. *Journal of Biological Chemistry*, **273**, 5599–606.

Karten, B. *et al.* (1998). Femtomole analysis of 9-oxononanoyl cholesterol by high performance liquid chromatography. *Journal of Lipid Research*, **39**, 1508–19.

Kellner-Weibel, G. *et al.* (1999). Crystallization of free cholesterol in model macrophage foam cells. *Arteriosclerosis, Thrombosis and Vascular Biology*, **19**, 1891–8.

Kirk, E.A. *et al.* (2000). Impaired superoxide production due to a deficiency in phagocyte NADPH oxidase fails to inhibit atherosclerosis in mice. *Arteriosclerosis, Thrombosis and Vascular Biology*, **20**, 1529–35.

Kritharides, L. (1997). The pathophysiology of atherosclerosis. In Thompson, P., (ed.), *A Coronary Care Manual*. Churchill Livingston, London. pp. 49–59.

Kritharides, L., Jessup, W. and Dean, R.T. (1995a). Macrophages require both iron and copper to oxidize low-density lipoprotein in Hanks' balanced salt solution. *Archives of Biochemistry and Biophysics*, **323**, 127–36.

Kritharides, L., Jessup, W., Mander, E. and Dean, R.T. (1995b). Impaired efflux of lipids from macrophages loaded with oxidized low density lipoprotein. *Arteriosclerosis, Thrombosis and Vascular Biology*, **15**, 276–89.

Kritharides, L., Christian, A., Stoudt, G., Morel, D. and Rothblat, G.H. (1998a). Cholesterol metabolism and efflux in human THP-1 macrophages. *Arteriosclerosis, Thrombosis and Vascular Biology*, **18**, 1589–99.

Kritharides, L., Upston, J., Jessup, W. and Dean, R.T. (1998b). Accumulation and metabolism of cholesteryl linoleate hydroperoxide and hydroxide by macrophages. *Journal of Lipid Research*, **39**, 2394–405.

Kuhn, H. and Chan, L. (1997). The role of 15-lipoxygenase in atherogenesis: pro- and antiatherogenic actions. *Current Opinion in Lipidology*, **8**, 111–7.

Langmann, T. *et al.* (1999). Molecular cloning of the human ATP-binding cassette transporter 1 (hABC1): evidence of sterol-dependent regulation in macrophages. *Biochemical and Biophysical Research Communications*, **257**, 29–33.

Larkin, L., Khachigian, L.M. and Jessup, W. (2000). Regulation of apolipoprotein E production in macrophages. *International Journal of Molecular Medicine*, **6**, 253–58.

Lewis, J.C., Taylor, R.G. and Ohta, K. (1988). Lysosomal alterations during coronary atherosclerosis in the pigeon: correlative cytochemical and three-dimensional HVEM/IVEM observations. *Experimental Molecular Pathology*, **48**, 103–15.

Li, W., Yuan, X.M., Olsson, A.G. and Brunk, U.T. (1998). Uptake of oxidized LDL by macrophages results in partial lysosomal enzyme inactivation and relocation. *Arteriosclerosis Thrombosis and Vascular Biology*, **18**, 177–84.

Lisanti, M.P. *et al.* (1994). Characterization of caveolin-rich membrane domains isolated from an endothelial-rich source: implications for human disease. *Journal of Cell Biology*, **126**, 111–26.

Lund, E. *et al.* (1996). Importance of a novel oxidative mechanism for elimination of intracellular cholesterol in humans. *Arteriosclerosis, Thrombosis and Vascular Biology*, **16**, 208–12.

Lupu, F., Danaricu, I. and Siionescu, N. (1987). Development of intracellular lipid deposits in the lipid-laden cells of atherosclerotic lesions. *Atherosclerosis*, **67**, 127–42.

Mattsson, L., Bondjers, G. and Wiklund, O. (1991). Isolation of cell populations from arterial tissue using monoclonal antibodies and magnetic microspheres. *Atherosclerosis*, **89**, 25–34.

Mattsson, L., Johansson, H., Ottosson, M., Bondjers, G. and Wiklund, O. (1993). Expression of lipoprotein lipase mRNA and secretion in macrophages isolated from human atherosclerotic aorta. *Journal of Clinical Investigation*, **92**, 1759–65.

Matveev, S., van der Westhuyzen, D. and Smart, E. (1999). Co-expression of scavenger receptor-B1 and caveolin-1 is associated with enhanced selective cholesteryl ester uptake in THP-1 macrophages. *Journal of Lipid Research*, **40**, 1647–54.

Miyazaki, A. *et al.* (1998). Expression of ACAT-1 protein in human atherosclerotic lesions and cultured human monocytes–macrophages. *Arteriosclerosis, Thrombosis and Vascular Biology*, **18**, 1568–74.

Nagy, L., Tontonoz, P., Alvarez, J., Chen, H. and Evans, R. (1998). Oxidized LDL regulates macrophage gene expression through ligand activation of PPARg. *Cell*, **93**, 229–40.

Niu, X., Zammit, V., Dean, R.T., May, J. and Stocker, R. (1999). Co-existence of oxidized lipids and α-tocopherol in all lipoprotein fractions isolated from advanced human atherosclerotic plaques. *Arteriosclerosis, Thrombosis and Vascular Biology*, **19**, 1708–18.

O'Brien, K.D. *et al.* (1994). Apolipoprotein E localization in human coronary atherosclerotic plaques by *in situ* hybridization and immunohistochemistry and comparison with lipoprotein lipase. *American Journal of Pathology*, **144**, 538–48.

Oram, J.F. and Yokoyama, S. (1996). Apolipoprotein-mediated removal of cellular cholesterol and phospholipids. *Journal of Lipid Research*, **37**, 2473–91.

Orekhov, A., Andreeva, E., Mikhailova, I. and Gordon, D. (1998). Cell proliferation in normal and atherosclerotic human aorta: proliferative splash in lipid-rich lesions. *Atherosclerosis*, **139**, 41–8.

Parton, R.G. (1996). Caveolae and caveolins. *Current Opinion in Cell Biology*, **8**, 542–8.

Pentikainen, M.O., Oorni, K., Ala-Korpela, M. and Kovanen, P.T. (2000). Modified LDL—trigger of atherosclerosis and inflammation in the arterial intima. *Journal of Internal Medicine*, **247**, 359–70.

Phillips, M.C., Johnson, W.J. and Rothblat, G.H. (1987). Mechanisms and consequences of cholesterol exchange and transfer. *Biochimica et Biophysica Acta*, **906**, 223–76.

Qiao, J.H. *et al.* (1997). Role of macrophage colony-stimulating factor in atherosclerosis: studies of osteopetrotic mice. *American Journal of Pathology*, **150**, 1687–99.

Raghunath, P.N. *et al.* (1995). Plasminogen activator system in human coronary atherosclerosis. *Arteriosclerosis, Thrombosis and Vascular Biology*, **15**, 1432–43.

Rees, D., Sloane, T., Jessup, W., Dean, R.T. and Kritharides, L. (1999). Apolipoprotein A-I stimulates secretion of apolipoprotein E by foam cell macrophages. *Journal of Biological Chemistry*, **274**, 27925–33.

Reue, K., Cohen, R. and Schotz, M. (1997). Evidence for hormone-sensitive lipase mRNA expression in human monocyte–macrophages. *Arteriosclerosis, Thrombosis and Vascular Biology*, **17**, 3428–32.

Ricote, M. *et al.* (1998). Expression of the peroxisome proliferator-activated receptor g (PPARg) in human atherosclerosis and regulation in macrophages by colony stimulating fctors and oxidized low-density lipoprotein. *Proceedings of the National Academy of Sciences USA*, **95**, 7614–9.

Ries, S. *et al.* (1998). Transcriptional regulation of lysosomal acid lipase in differentiating monocytes is mediated by transcription factors Sp1 and AP-2. *Journal of Lipid Research*, **39**, 2125–34.

Rigotti, A. and Krieger, M. (1999). Getting a handle on 'good' cholesterol with the high density lipoprotein receptor. *New England Journal of Medicine*, **341**, 2011–3.

Rothblat, G.H. *et al.* (1999). Cell cholesterol efflux: integration of old and new observations provides new insights. *Journal of Lipid Research*, **40**, 781–96.

Sakashita, N. *et al.* (2000). Localization of human acyl-coenzyme A:cholesterol acyltransferase-1 (ACAT-1) in macrophages and in various tissues. *American Journal of Pathology*, **156**, 227–36.

Schaffner, T. *et al.* (1980). Arterial foam cells with distinctive immunomorphologic and histochemical features of macrophages. *American Journal of Pathology*, **100**, 57–80.

Schissel, S.L., Schuchman, E.H., Williams, K.J. and Tabas, I. (1996). Zn^{2+}-stimulated sphingomyelinase is secreted by many cell types and is a product of the acid sphingomyelinase gene. *Journal of Biological Chemistry*, **271**, 18431–6.

Shio, H., Haley, N.J. and Fowler, S. (1978). Characterization of lipid-laden aortic cells from cholesterol-fed rabbits II. Morphometric analysis of lipid-filled lysosomes and lipid droplets in aortic cell populations. *Laboratory Investigations*, **39**, 390–7.

Small, C.A., Goodacre, J.A. and Yeaman, S.J. (1989). Hormone-sensitive lipase is responsible for the neutral cholesterol ester hydrolase activity in macrophages. *FEBS Letters*, **247**, 205–8.

Smith, E.B. (1990). Transport, interactions and retention of plasma proteins in the intima: the barrier function of the internal elastic lamina. *European Heart Journal*, **11** (Supplement E), 72–81.

Smith, J.D. *et al.* (1995). Decreased atherosclerosis in mice deficient in both macrophage colony-stimulating factor (op) and apolipoprotein E. *Proceedings of the National Academy of Sciences USA*, **92**, 8264–8.

Stary, H.C. *et al.* (1995). A definition of advanced types of atherosclerotic lesions and a histological classification of atherosclerosis. A report from the Committee on Vascular Lesions of the Council on Arteriosclerosis, American Heart Association. *Arteriosclerosis, Thrombosis and Vascular Biology*, **15**, 1512–31.

Steinbrecher, U.P. and Lougheed, M. (1992). Scavenger receptor-independent stimulation of cholesterol esterification in macrophages by low density lipoprotein extracted from human aortic intima. *Arteriosclerosis, Thrombosis and Vascular Biology*, **12**, 608–25.

Sugiyama, N. *et al.* (1992). Immunohistochemical distribution of lipoprotein epitopes in xanthomata from patients with familial hypercholesterolemia. *American Journal of Pathology*, **141**, 99–106.

Sukhova, G.K., Shi, G.P., Simon, D.I., Chapman, H.A. and Libby, P. (1998). Expression of the elastolytic cathepsins S and K in human atheroma and regulation of their production in smooth muscle cells. *Journal of Clinical Investigation*, **102**, 576–83.

Swain, J. and Gutteridge, J.M. (1995). Prooxidant iron and copper, with ferroxidase and xanthine oxidase activities in human atherosclerotic material. *FEBS Letters*, **368**, 513–5.

Tabas, I. (1997). Phospholipid metabolism in cholesterol-loaded macrophages. *Current Opinion in Lipidology*, **8**, 263–7.

Tabas, I. (1999). Nonoxidative modifications of lipoproteins in atherogenesis. *Annual Reviews in Nutrition*, **19**, 123–39.

Tangirala, R.K., Mol, M.J. and Steinberg, D. (1996). Macrophage oxidative modification of low density lipoprotein occurs independently of its binding to the low density lipoprotein receptor. *Journal of Lipid Research*, **37**, 835–43.

Tontonoz, P., Nagy, L., Alvarez, J., Thomaczy, V. and Evans, R. (1998). PPAR-γ promotes monocyte/macrophage differentiation and uptake of oxidized LDL. *Cell*, **93**, 241–52.

Torra, I., Gervois, P. and Staels, B. (1999). Peroxisome proliferator-activated receptor α in metabolic disease, inflammation, atherosclerosis and aging. *Current Opinion in Lipidology*, **10**, 151–9.

Trigatti, B. *et al.* (1999). Influence of the high density lipoprotein receptor SR-BI on reproductive and cardiovascular pathophysiology. *Proceedings of the National Academy of Sciences USA*, **96**, 9322–7.

van Reyk, D.M. and Jessup, W. (1999). The macrophage in atherosclerosis: modulation of cell function by sterols. *Journal of Leukocyte Biology*, **66**, 557–61.

van Reyk, D.M., Jessup, W. and Dean, R.T. (1999). Prooxidant and antioxidant activities of macrophages in metal-mediated LDL oxidation: the importance of metal sequestration. *Arteriosclerosis, Thrombosis and Vascular Biology*, **19**, 1119–24.

Villaschi, S. and Spagnoli, L. (1983). Autoradiographic and ultrastructural studies on human fibro-atheromatous plaque. *Atherosclerosis*, **48**, 95–100.

Xing, X., Baffic, J. and Sparrow, C.P. (1998). LDL oxidation by activated monocytes: characterization of the oxidized LDL and requirement for transition metal ions. *Journal of Lipid Research*, **39**, 2201–8.

Young, S.G. and Fielding, C.J. (1999). The ABCs of cholesterol efflux. *Nature Genetics*, **22**, 316–8.

Yuan, X.M. (1999). Apoptotic macrophage-derived foam cells of human atheromas are rich in iron and ferritin, suggesting iron-catalyzed reactions to be involved in apoptosis. *Free Radical Research*, **30**, 221–31.

Yui, S., Sasaki, T., Miyazaki, A., Horiuchi, S. and Yamasaki, M. (1993). Induction of murine macrophage growth by modified LDLs. *Arteriosclerosis, Thrombosis and Vascular Biology*, **13**, 331–7.

Yui, S. and Yamazaki, M. (1986). Induction of macrophage growth by lipids. *Journal of Immunology*, **136**, 1334–8.

Yui, S. and Yamazaki, M. (1990). Augmentation of macrophage growth-stimulating activity of lipids by their peroxidation. *Journal of Immunology*, **144**, 1466–71.

13 *Macrophages in the central nervous system*

M.K. Matyszak and V.H. Perry

1 Introduction

A dominant theme in studies of the central nervous system (CNS) is the relationship between structure and function. The wide diversity of neuronal forms is believed to reflect differences in their functions. With the use of immunocytochemistry and antibodies directed against components of the plasma membrane of macrophages, it has become clear that tissue macrophages also have a wide diversity of forms (Figure 13.1). These morphological differences reflect not only adaptations of the monocyte to the local microenvironment, but also heterogeneity in functional capabilities, expression of membrane receptors and biosynthetic capacity (Gordon *et al.*, 1988). The adaptation of a monocyte appears to reach its greatest degree of morphological specialization in the microglia, the resident tissue macrophages of the CNS.

In this chapter, we have concentrated on recent studies on microglia and other macrophage populations associated with the CNS.

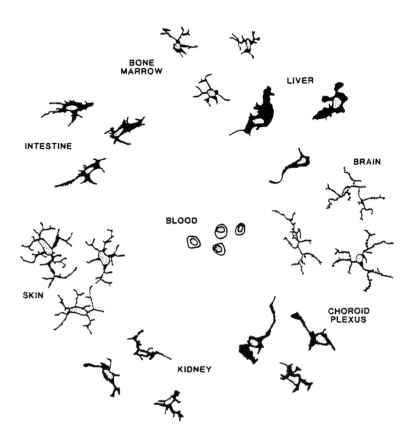

Fig. 13.1   Mononuclear phagocytes can adopt a wide range of forms, depending upon their location in a given tissue. The resident macrophages of the brain, the microglia, provide an extreme example of such specialization (see also Figure 13.4). (Reproduced from the *Journal of Cell Science*, Supplement 9, by permission of The Company of Biologists Ltd.)

2 Microglia

2.1 Origin

Microglia were first described by del Rio Hortega in 1932. He applied a silver staining method to the developing brain and described a class of cell with a morphology which changes from a simple rounded or stellate cell to that of microglia. He coined the term 'microglia' to differentiate the newly discovered cells from other glia (astrocytes and oligodendrocytes) which were known under the collective name of macroglia. There was a long-standing disagreement between researchers who believed that microglia were of monocytic origin and those who were of the opinion that microglia, like other glia cells, originated from neuroectoderm. The highly ramified and complex branching of microglia helped to fuel this controversy. The reader interested in the background to this historical debate is referred to some earlier reviews (del Rio Hortega, 1932; Ling, 1981; Jordan and Thomas, 1988).

It is now generally accepted that microglia are of bone marrow origin. Mononuclear cells enter the brain parenchyma during embryogenesis, and these macrophages are involved in the removal of cells which undergo apoptosis as a normal component of brain development. With the use of monoclonal antibody directed against the mouse macrophage antigen F4/80 (Austyn and Gordon, 1981), it has been possible to study the ontogeny of microglia in the developing retina and brain (Hume *et al.*, 1983; Perry *et al.*, 1985). In the embryonic mouse brain (at about day 16), there are F4/80[+] macrophages with a rounded or stellate form, but cells with classical microglia morphology are not found. Three to four days later, at the time of birth, larger numbers of F4/80[+] cells are present and many of these have a more ramified appearance (Figure 13.2). In the following postnatal week, the F4/80[+] cells come to resemble adult microglia (Figure 13.3). In addition to F4/80, microglia in the neonatal brain also express other plasma membrane antigens known to be present on macrophages, i.e. the Fc receptor (FcR) and the complement type 3 receptor (CR3) (Perry *et al.*, 1985). Therefore, by using antibodies directed against those macrophage markers, it has been possible to follow the differentiation of monocytes to microglia in the developing CNS.

Study of the origin of microglia has also been aided by tissue grafting experiments. Retinas from embryonic mice were transplanted into the midbrain region of newborn rats. These retinas developed relatively normal lamination; the axons grew out from the transplant to the host and made specific functional connections with visual centers of the host (Klassen and Lund, 1987). Microglia in transplanted mouse retinas were all of rat bone marrow origin as shown by labeling with antibodies specific for rat host (Perry and Lund, 1989), thus providing evidence that they were of host bone marrow origin rather than recipient origin.

More recent study of the human fetal cerebral cortex between 16 and 22 weeks of gestation has shown the correlation between the distribution of microglia and the high expression of adhesion molecules on cerebral endothelium, in particular intercellular adhesion molecule (ICAM)-1 and -2. Adhesion molecules facilitate cell entry into the brain under both normal and pathological conditions. Therefore, the high level of ICAM molecules on cerebral endothelium during development suggests that they may facilitate monocyte entry into the fetal brain and their subsequent differentiation into microglia (Rezaie *et al.*, 1997).

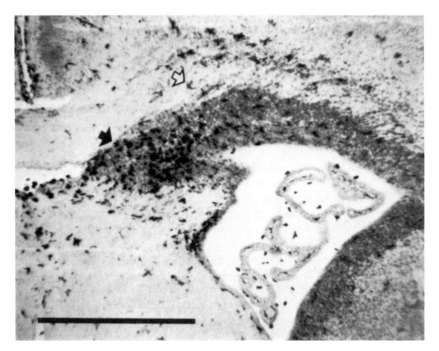

Fig. 13.2 Around the time of birth, the differentiation of macrophages recruited into the developing CNS is already underway. In the 1-day-old mouse, ramified F4/80⁺ cells (open arrow) which resemble adult microglia co-exist with macrophage-like cells (solid arrow). (Immunoperoxidase, counter-stained with cresyl violet. Scale bar, 500 μm.)

The time of the entry of monocytes into the CNS correlates with the increase in naturally occurring cell death in the retina and brain (Hume *et al.*, 1983; Perry *et al.*, 1985). Naturally occurring cell death is a major feature of CNS development. As many as 50–70 per cent of the cells generated in the embryo may degenerate during maturation, although this varies considerably from region to region (Oppenheim, 1981). It is plausible that neuronal cell death may act as a chemotactic stimulus to recruit monocytes into the developing brain, although other factors may be involved.

2.2 Morphology, phenotype and distribution

In the neonatal brain, microglia are more rounded cells, resembling the morphology of other macrophages. As mentioned in the previous section, they can be easily differentiated from other glia by surface expression of F4/80, CR3 and FcR. Also, these cells can also be labeled readily with antibodies which recognize endocytic compartments—FA/11 in mice, and ED1 in rats (Perry and Gordon, 1991). The prominence of endocytic compartments in microglia suggests that they are actively phagocytic.

During brain maturation, the macrophages in the brain parenchyma adopt the highly differentiated ramified morphology of resting microglia (Perry, 1998). Resting microglia also show a down-regulated immunophenotype sharing only a few receptors which are constitutively expressed on monocytes and other macrophages. For example, they express no major histocompatibility complex (MHC) class I and II antigens. The leukocyte

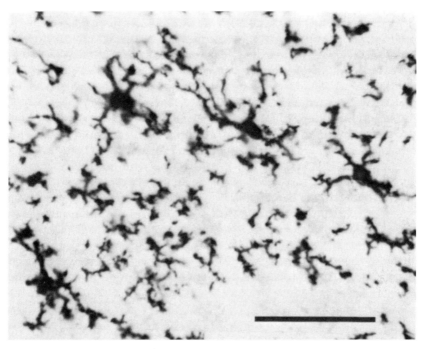

Fig. 13.3 The macrophage-specific antiserum, F4/80, reveals the elaborate morphology of resident microglia in the parietal cortex of the normal adult mouse. (Immunoperoxidase, no counter-stain. Scale bar, 50 μm.)

common antigen (CD45) in the normal rodent brain is also highly down-regulated (Perry and Gordon, 1991). A lysosomal antigen, ED1 (Sminia *et al.*, 1987), is abundant during development and later down-regulated in juvenile animals. However, microglia in the adult rodent brain retain the surface expression of F4/80 as well as CR3 and FcR. The picture changes again with the phenotype of microglia in the aged brain. The microglia there seem more activated, especially in the white matter (Perry *et al.*, 1993a). MHC molecules as well as CD45 and CD4 have been readily detected in aged rat brain. The expression of CR3 has been also found to be up-regulated and ED1 re-expressed on a large number of microglia.

When studying the distribution of microglia in the normal adult rodent brain, it becomes apparent that there are differences in microglial morphology in different parts of the brain (Lawson *et al.*, 1990a). It is possible to classify these cells into three morphological types: *radial*, *longitudinal* and *compact* microglia. The most complex cells are the *radial* microglia. These are found in the gray matter, i.e. those regions containing the cell bodies, the processes and synaptic connections of neurons. Radial microglia have from three to five primary processes which branch to give their characteristic radial appearance in two-dimensional reconstructions (Figure 13.4). Within this group, the cells vary somewhat in the length of the processes. This is partly related to the local density of microglia; smaller, more bushy cells are found in regions of higher cell density.

The second type, the *longitudinal* microglia, are found in white matter, the major fiber tracts. These cells are in many respects similar to radial cells, but their processes are

528

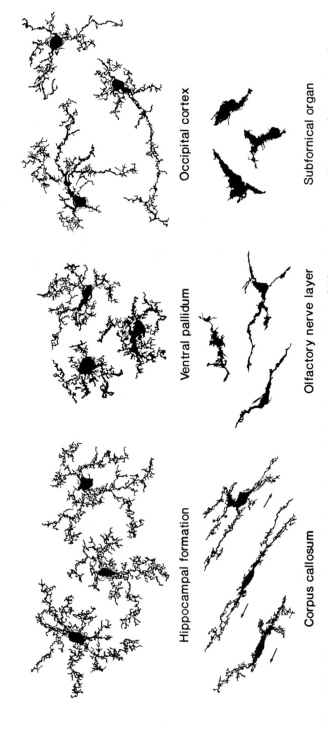

Fig. 13.4 The morphology of microglia depends upon their precise location within the CNS and can be grouped into one of three categories. *Radially branched microglia* (top row) are found in the gray matter. This is the most widespread and diverse class of microglia. *Longitudinally branched microglia* (bottom left) are characteristic of white matter. *Compact microglia* (bottom center and right) are found exlusively in areas lacking the blood–brain barrier. Cells of the olfactory nerve layer demonstrate the combined influence of adjacent nerve fibers and exposure to plasma proteins.

oriented along the long axis of the axons within a fiber tract (Figure 13.4). The third type is the *compact* microglia. They are much simpler in form than the others, having few long processes, and they are sparsely branched (Figure 13.4). These cells are found in those parts of the CNS where the blood–brain barrier is absent and the cells are exposed to plasma proteins. These areas, which include sites such as the median eminence and the subfornical organ, are known collectively as the circumventricular organs. The dramatically different forms of compact microglia may well be a direct influence of plasma proteins. Indeed, *in vitro* studies have shown that the presence of serum reduces the formation of processes by microglia (Giulian *et al.*, 1995). In addition, microglia in circumventricular organs also differ phenotypically from microglia in the white or gray matter, as shown by higher expression of a number of macrophage-associated antigens (Perry and Gordon, 1987).

The question of what makes microglia microglia still needs to be fully defined. However, there are already some important clues. For example, the differences between their morphology in the gray and white matter and that in the circumventricular organs suggests that the exclusion of plasma proteins from the brain parenchyma is important. Furthermore, the influence of other cells in the CNS is likely to be important. It has already been shown that *in vitro* co-culture of macrophages from neonatal brain with astrocytes promotes the differentiation of the macrophages into microglia (Giulian *et al.*, 1995). In another similar study, both astrocytes and astrocyte-conditioned medium have been found to promote macrophages to differentiate into cells of microglial morphology (Sievers *et al.*, 1994). The *in vitro* differentiated cells also express ion channels believed to be typical of microglia. Likewise, when ameboid microglia (the term is used for the more rounded activated microglia often seen in inflammatory conditions) and macrophages are transferred into organotypic hippocampal slice cultures, they gradually develop a ramified morphology similar to that of resting microglia (Hailer *et al.*, 1998). In the same study, when co-cultured with astrocytes, spleen macrophages down-regulated a number of surface antigens including MHC class II, leukocyte function-associated molecule 1 (LFA1) and ICAM-1. Taken together, these studies strongly suggest that the CNS microenvironment plays a pivotal role in shaping microglial cell morphology, phenotype and, ultimately, function.

Macrophages in non-CNS tissues are not usually distributed randomly. They are commonly found associated with particular tissue elements, frequently vascular endothelium or epithelium. For example, Kupffer cells of the liver line sinusoids, and macrophages of the lamina propria of the gut often surround capillaries. Some tissue macrophages may also show overt regular spacing, such as the Langerhans cells within the basal layer of the epidermis (Gordon *et al.*, 1988).

The CNS is not a homogenous organ. It has well-defined functionally distinct regions. Within these divisions, neurons differ in their morphology, connections and the type of neurotransmitter employed. We have already discussed differences in microglia morphology between white matter, gray matter and the circumventricular organs. However, it is also of interest to see whether the distribution of microglia in the adult CNS reflects, for example, the amount of natural cell death that occurred in a particular structure during development. So, for example, do regions with high levels of cell death ultimately have more microglia? These questions have been addressed in a detailed study of microglia distribution in the mouse brain (Lawson *et al.*, 1990a).

This study showed that the distribution of microglia in the normal rodent brain is heterogenous. In general, more microglia are found in the gray matter than the white matter. There is a trend for phylogenetically and ontogenetically newer structures to contain more microglia than older structures. The microglia are not scattered randomly throughout the CNS but form a quasi-regular distribution, with each cell occupying its own territory. There is a consistent pattern of distribution from animal to animal, with more than a sixfold difference in density across the CNS. In the cortical white matter, microglia represent about 5 per cent of the total glial population and, within the cortical gray matter, about 5 per cent of the total population of neurons and glia. The study found no obvious correlation between the density of microglia and the amount of developmental cell death. The distribution of microglia also did not correlate with functionally distinct subdivisions of the CNS, different neurotransmitter systems, the distribution of non-neuronal cells or the distribution and density of the vascular network. It is not known how the adult pattern emerges, whether this reflects particular sites of entry of monocytes into the CNS, selective migration pathways, regions of local proliferation or turnover or some combination of these.

The quantitative analysis performed in the same study (Lawson *et al.*, 1990a) suggested that the total number of microglia in the mouse brain is about 3.5×10^6, which on a weight-for weight basis is similar to the number of Kupffer cells in the liver. Additional measurements of the total cell surface area of microglia have shown that the cell surface area of a radial microglia is two or more times larger than that of a Kupffer cell. Thus, microglia are not only a significant population of the resident macrophage pool, but their large surface area within the CNS suggests that they might be sensitive to changes in the local milieu.

2.3 Kinetics

At present, it is not known how long monocytes live once they have entered the developing CNS and differentiated to microglial cells; whether the cells live for the lifespan of the organism; or whether senescent microglia are replaced by local division and/or incoming monocytes. In the adult CNS, neurons are post-mitotic cells and, apart from neurons of the olfactory epithelium, there is no evidence that they proliferate in the adult mammalian brain (Rakic, 1985). However, cells of the macroglial lineages continue to proliferate at low levels throughout life (Schultze and Korr, 1981; Ffrench-Constant and Raff, 1986).

A number of studies based on [³H]thymidine autoradiography have revealed that the turnover of microglia is small (McCarthy and Leblond, 1988; Lawson *et al.*, 1990b). By combining [³H]thymidine autoradiography with immunocytochemical staining, it can be determined whether the labeled cells divided or were recruited from the circulation (Lawson *et al.*, 1990b). In the latter study, the division was estimated following a single pulse of [³H]thymidine and a survival time of less than an hour. With longer survival times after a single pulse, it is possible to estimate whether there is significant monocyte entry. The work by Lawson and her colleagues has demonstrated that only a small number of microglia are labeled following a single pulse of [³H]thymidine and a one hour survival period (Figure 13.5). This shows that the turnover of microglia in the healthy brain is minimal. The [³H]thymidine-labeled, F4/80⁺ microglia were scattered, apparently at random, throughout the brain. The majority of these cells seemed in isolation, but occa-

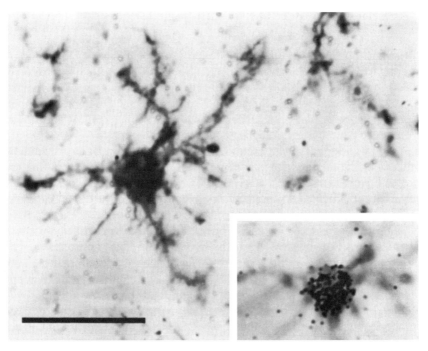

Fig. 13.5 Microglial turnover occurs in the normal adult mouse brain, albeit slowly. One hour after [³H]thymidine administration, a F4/80⁺ cell with normal resident morphology is labeled. (Immunoperoxidase. Scale bar, 25 μm.) Inset: the same cell with the plane of focus altered to display the silver grains over the nucleus.

sionally several labeled cells were found together. Quantitative analysis performed in this study revealed that the turnover of microglia is smaller that that of macrophages in other tissues such as the skin (Mackenzie, 1975) and the liver (Crofton *et al.*, 1978).

After survival times of 24 and 48 h, the numbers of [³H]thymidine-labeled F4/80⁺ cells have been somewhat greater than could have been accounted for on the basis of proliferation of the resident cells alone (Lawson *et al.*, 1990b), which strongly suggests that there is a low but continuous level of monocyte entry into the adult CNS. This is in accordance with the data described for other organs (Crofton *et al.*, 1978; Van Oud Alblas and van Furth, 1979).

The extent of monocyte traffic into the normal adult CNS is of interest in view of the possibility that these cells may act as 'Trojan horses' (Williams and Blakemore, 1990) and carry infectious agents into the CNS. Indeed, this is of particular importance in the case of human immunodeficiency virus (HIV). Microglia are the main HIV reservoir in the brain, and very probably play a major role in the development of HIV dementia (HIVD). CD4 is the major receptor for HIV entry, but in mononuclear phagocytes there are a number of co-receptors that participate in HIV entry and spread. The most important co-receptors are the chemokine receptors, CCR5, CCR3 and CXCR4. It has been shown that individuals with defective CCR5 alleles exhibit resistance to HIV-1 infection, suggesting that CCR5 has an important role *in vivo* in HIV-1 replication (He *et al.*, 1997). Likewise, antibodies to CCR5 (3A9) prevent infection of monocytes with HIV (Ghorpade *et al.*, 1998). Human microglia, as well as microglia in some rodents such as rats, express CD4. Microglia also express all three chemokine receptors (CCR3, CCR5 and CXCR4), although the level of CCR5 is higher than the level of either CCR3 or CXCR4. Using antibodies to these chemokine receptors, it has been shown that an anti-CCR5 antibody dramatically inhibited microglial infection, thus pointing to an important role for CCR5 as the co-receptor for infectivity of microglia with HIV (Albright *et al.*, 1999). Therefore, HIV uses the same receptors to infect microglia as those used to infect monocytes and macrophages.

2.4 Functions

Monocytes invade the developing CNS and play a role in removing dying neurons and their processes (Innocenti *et al.*, 1983; Perry *et al.*, 1985). Naturally occurring cell death is recognized as a major event in the development of the CNS, and as much as 50 per cent of the original neuron population generated in the embryo may degenerate before maturity (Oppenheim, 1981; Williams and Herrup, 1988). Immunohistochemically identified macrophages/microglia have been observed phagocytosing pyknotic cells at both the light and electron microscopic level. There is also evidence that during this period, infiltrating macrophages and/or immature microglia secrete interleukin-1 (IL-1) which may influence both gliogenesis and angiogenesis (Giulian *et al.*, 1988a,b). In addition, fetal microglia are likely to be important in promoting astrocyte proliferation, since they secrete growth factors for astrocytes (Giulian and Young, 1986).

There is much less known about the function of microglia in the healthy adult brain. A striking feature of adult microglia is their apparently inactive appearance. Electron microscopy studies have shown that these cells have a poorly developed biosynthetic apparatus and the perinuclear cytoplasm lacks the rich complement of organelles normally associated with macrophages (Peters *et al.*, 1976). As mentioned above, the microglial phenotype is also strongly down-regulated. The exclusion of plasma proteins from the brain parenchyma certainly explains, at least in part, the down-regulated phenotype.

However, there is some evidence that suggests that microglia continue to play a role in CNS tissue modeling (Pow *et al.*, 1989). This comes mainly from the study of magnocellular neurons. Magnocellular neurons, with their cell bodies in the hypothalamus, terminate in the posterior pituitary where they release the hormones oxytocin and vasopressin into the blood supply. At least one type of neuron in the CNS, the magnocellular neuron, is known to retain the capacity to regenerate and may be constantly growing. In the rat, approximately 20 per cent of the cells in the posterior pituitary (excluding the endothelium) are microglia. Fine processes of microglia surround endings of the magnocellular axons, particularly those parts of the neuron which have penetrated the basement membrane and lie in the perivascular space. A sequence of images has been documented showing that the microglia endocytose parts of the neurosecretory axons and digest them in lysosomal bodies (Pow *et al.*, 1989). Therefore, one of the functions of the microglia could be to 'trim' those parts of the neuron that have penetrated the basement membrane.

However, possibly the most important role that microglia play is in the defense of the CNS from injury and infection and in orchestrating inflammatory responses. Microglia responses under pathological conditions are discussed in Section 4.

3 Other macrophages in the central nervous system

In addition to the microglia within the parenchyma of the CNS, there are several other important macrophage populations at interfaces between the CNS and the blood. These include macrophages associated with the choroid plexus, leptomeninges and the microcirculation.

3.1 Choroid plexus

The choroid plexus lies within the ventricles and is responsible for the production of the cerebrospinal fluid (CSF) (Davson *et al.*, 1987). Unlike the brain parenchyma, the endothelium within the choroid plexus is fenestrated but the choroidal epithelial cells have tight junctions, preventing the free passage of large molecules from the plasma. The CSF is not simply a filtrate of plasma but is actively secreted by the choroidal cells.

There are two types of macrophage associated with the choroid plexus; the stromal macrophages which occupy the spaces between the blood vessels and the epithelial cells (Matyszak *et al.*, 1992), and epiplexus cells, also known as Kolmer cells, which reside at the apical surface of the choroid (Figure 13.6). In whole-mount preparations of mouse choroid, the stromal macrophages are regularly spaced, akin to the Langerhans cells (LCs) in the skin. Their morphology also largely resembles that of LCs. Experiments using horseradish peroxidase (HRP) tracer showed that stromal macrophages are phago-

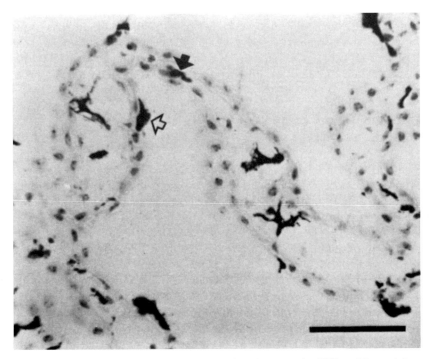

Fig. 13.6 The choroid plexus is an important interface between the CNS and the periphery and has its own distinct macrophage population. F4/80+ cells lie within the stroma (▶) as well as on the apical surface of the choroidal epithelium (⇨). Unlike microglia, these cells express MHC class II antigen. (Immunoperoxidase, counter-stained with cresyl violet. Scale bar, 50 μm.)

cytic (Matyszak *et al.*, 1992). Likewise, epiplexus cells have been shown to be phagocytic (Carpenter *et al.*, 1970; Blier and Albrecht, 1980). Both stromal macrophages and epiplexus cells express a wide range of macrophage antigens and, in contrast to microglia, have high levels of MHC antigens, CD4 and CD45 (Matyszak *et al.*, 1992).

Within the stroma of the choroid plexus, there is also a subpopulation of mononuclear cells which are F4/80 negative, but are strongly positive for MHC class II (Matyszak *et al.*, 1992). Using rat choroid plexus, it was possible to identify these cells as being OX62[+] (Matyszak and Perry, 1992a). OX62 is an antigen which is expressed on dendritic cells (DCs) (Brenan and Puklavec, 1992). Likewise, a similar population of NLDC145[+] DCs are present in the mouse choroid plexus (Agger *et al.*, 1997). DCs are the most efficient antigen-presenting cells (APCs) capable of priming naive T cells. Both stromal macrophages and resident DCs are likely to play an important role in immune responses in the ventricles as well as in the transport of the antigens from the ventricles into the local lymph nodes.

The brain lacks conventional lymphatic drainage. However, it has been shown that proteins such as ovalbumin drain from the ventricles into lymph nodes (Harling-Berg *et al.*, 1989; Cserr and Knopf, 1992). Together with CSF, they gain access to subarachnoid spaces, the cribriform plate and finally the nasal lymphatics. The proteins can be traced in the deep cervical lymph nodes. Further experiments have revealed antibodies to these proteins in the sera of experimental animals. Unlike pathogens sequestered in the brain parenchyma which can persist for months unrecognized by the immune system (Matyszak and Perry 1996b; Stevenson *et al.*, 1997), pathogens sequestered in the ventricles can drain into local lymph nodes and are readily recognized by the immune system. For example, direct intraventricular injection of bacille Calmette–Guerin (BCG) results in efficient immune priming and subsequent T cell-mediated response within the choroid plexus, at the sites of BCG deposits (Matyszak and Perry, 1996b). Likewise, immune responses are rapidly activated when influenza virus is injected into the CSF. This elicits the production of antiviral antibodies as well as priming and expansion of virus-specific CD8[+] T cells (Stevenson *et al.*, 1997).

3.2 Leptomeninges

The surface of the brain is covered by the meninges, made up of several different membranous layers. Immediately beneath the skull there is a tough connective tissue layer, the dura, and immediately beneath the dura lies the arachnoid. Between the arachnoid and the pia there is the subarachnoid space, and macrophages are found both free within the subarachnoid space and lying on the surface of the pia. These macrophages, again in contrast to microglia, express a wide range of macrophage antigens and ultrastructurally resemble typical phagocytic macrophages. They have been shown to endocytose HRP (Shabo and Maxwell, 1971). These cells are well placed to play a role in restricting the movement of antigens from the blood to the CNS compartment, and vice versa.

3.3 Perivascular macrophages

Associated with the vasculature of the CNS parenchyma there is a population of macrophages enclosed within the basement membrane and lying adjacent to the endothelium—the perivascular macrophages. Perivascular macrophages are derived from bone marrow cells, as has been demonstrated using bone marrow chimeras. In these experiments, MHC-mismatched donor cells were shown to be present in the perivascular location within 2 months after reconstitution (Hickey and Kimura, 1988). Phenotypically and morphologically, perivascular macrophages are distinct from microglia and more closely resemble macrophages in other tissues. They express many tissue macrophage-specific antigens including MHC molecules, CD45 (Graeber *et al.*, 1989) and scavenger receptor (SR; Hickey and Kimura, 1971). Perivascular macrophages can be readily identified in rats with ED2 antibody (Streit *et al.*, 1989). ED2 recognizes a membrane antigen of unknown function which is present in tissue macrophages but not in monocytes or inflammatory cells. Their phenotype and location, ideal for contact with activated T cells entering the brain, make them a prime candidate for APCs important in initiating immune responses in the CNS (Hickey and Kimura, 1971; Hickey *et al.*, 1992).

Because the number of perivascular macrophages is very low, it is difficult to purify them for *in vitro* functional studies. However, radiation bone marrow chimeras combined with experimental allergic encephalomyelitis (EAE) have been used to elicit their function *in vivo* (Lassmann *et al.*, 1993). EAE is a classical autoimmune disease which can be induced in susceptible strains of animals either by immunization with CNS antigens in complete Freund's adjuvant (Paterson, 1976), or by adoptive transfer of activated, myelin antigen-specific CD4+ T cells (Ben Nun *et al.*, 1981). Lethal irradiation of the recipient animals destroys perivascular macrophages. However, most microglia cells in the brain parenchyma survive. In their experiments, Lassman and his colleagues irradiated DA rats and subsequently reconstituted them with bone marrow from Lewis rats. Perivascular macrophages in the chimeric rats were all of Lewis rat origin. Lewis rats were used in these experiments because they are a strain known for being very susceptible to EAE. In Lewis rats, myelin basic protein (MBP) is the major autoantigen. (DA × Lewis) F_1 animals were injected intravenously with MBP-specific activated T cells of Lewis rat origin. In this experiment, the only cells in the brain which were of Lewis strain origin and which could therefore present antigen to T cells entering the brain were perivascular macrophages. F_1 animals developed EAE with a time course similar to that in normal non-chimeric Lewis rats. Therefore, this experiment provided direct evidence that perivascular macrophages are important in presenting antigen to already primed T cells, leading to the eventual induction of EAE.

4 Response of microglia to injury

One of the first responses to injury or infection in any tissue is mounted by resident macrophages. In the brain, microglia respond very rapidly to inflammatory stimuli. Indeed, there is hardly any CNS pathology in which they are not involved (Vass *et al.*, 1986; Hayes *et al.*, 1987; Shaw *et al.*, 1990; McGeer *et al.*, 1993; Perry *et al.*, 1993b; Betmouni *et al.*, 1996). Following tissue injury or infection in the brain, microglia activation generally precedes any other response.

Following a traumatic wound to the CNS, in which blood vessels and hence the blood–brain barrier are damaged, both polymorphonuclear cells and monocytes are recruited (Imamoto and Leblond, 1974). Microglia within the lesion adopt the morphology of so-called 'activated' microglia. These cells are distinct from resting microglia, resembling more standard macrophages in appearance (compare Figures 13.3 and 13.7) and phenotype. Indeed, a number of macrophage-associated antigens are up-regulated on

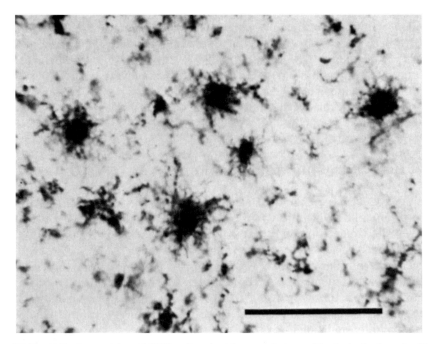

Fig. 13.7   Following an injury, F4/8O⁺ cells adopt the morphology of 'activated' microglia. These cells, in the parietal cortex of a mouse injected with kainic acid 5 days previously, are completely unlike normal resident microglia (compare with Figure 13.3). (Immunoperoxidase, no counter-stain. Scale bar, 50 μm.)

activated microglia (Perry and Gordon, 1991). Apart from their obvious role in the removal of debris, activated microglia and the inflammatory cells may play a role in re-establishing local homeostasis; in particular restoration of the blood–brain barrier. Secretion of IL-1 by recruited cells (and possibly the activated resident microglia) may promote restoration of the blood–brain barrier because IL-1 injected into the CNS has been shown to promote both angiogenesis and gliogenesis in the CNS (Giulian *et al.*, 1988b).

One of the major problems with studying activation and function of microglia following a traumatic wound to the CNS is the distinction between these and inflammatory macrophages recruited to the inflammatory sites. As discussed above, activated microglia alter their morphology dramatically, adopting a morphology which strongly resembles that of recruited macrophages. An additional difficulty comes from the fact that other inflammatory cells such as neutrophils are also recruited and will share the division of labour in the phagocytic processes.

An important feature of a local lesion in the nervous system is that damage to a fiber tract will result in degeneration at sites distant to the lesion. The segment of a nerve fiber isolated from the cell body will degenerate (Wallerian degeneration) and the parent cell body of a damaged fiber will undergo retrograde degeneration. Both Wallerian and retrograde degeneration are accompanied by microglial activation but, unlike a traumatic wound where the blood–brain barrier is bridged, at the site of retrograde degeneration the blood–brain barrier remains intact and polymorphonuclear cells are not recruited (Kernan, 1985; Kuono *et al.*, 1989). A number of models have been used to study the level of microglia activation at the site of retrograde degeneration. One of these is based on a facial nerve axotomy (Kreutzberg, 1996). After transection of the facial nerve, microglia in the nucleus proliferate and express several new surface markers including MHC class I and II. Changes in the phenotype are accompanied by a rapid change in microglial morphology, with the cells adapting a classical rod cell-shaped appearance. Similar results have been obtained in ischemic models when studying areas distant from the infarct core. The phenotypic changes on microglia in these areas were also characterized by an increased expression of CR3 and MHC class II (Schroeter *et al.*, 1999). Microglia activated at the sites of retrograde degeneration were not or were only weakly phagocytic (Kreutzberg, 1996; Schroeter *et al.*, 1999).

Another important molecule which is up-regulated on microglia following neuronal injury is the SR (Bell *et al.*, 1994). SRs are thought to promote adhesion and accumulation of macrophages at sites of deposition of modified plasma and/or extracellular matrix proteins (Fraser *et al.*, 1993). The expression of SRs on microglia has also been seen recently in the senile plaques in Alzheimer's disease and is thought to contribute to pathogenesis of this disease (Chavis *et al.*, 1996). See also Chapter 7 for further details on the role of macrophages in Alzheimer's disease.

The senile plaque, containing amyloid β (Aβ) fibrils, is a pathological hallmark of Alzheimer's disease (AD). The Alzheimer's plaques have long been associated with the presence of activated microglial cells (McGeer *et al.*, 1993). Recent studies using APP23 transgenic mice, which express human mutated Aβ precursor protein (APP), have allowed more precise assessment of microglia activation and their association with different stages of the development of plaques (Stalder *et al.*, 1999). In young APP23 mice, early amyloid deposits are already of dense core nature and are associated with a strong microglial response. Most amyloid plaques are associated with clusters of intensely Mac-1$^+$ microglia with characteristic phosphotyrosine-positive processes. No association of such activated microglia has been observed with diffuse plaques.

Although there is now good evidence that microglial activation is an important component of the pathogenesis of AD, the role of these cells in cerebral amyloidosis remains ill defined. Microglia can synthesize Aβ, but current evidence is most consistent with their phagocytic role (Kalaria, 1999). Indeed, ultrastructural studies have revealed microglia with the typical characteristics of phagocytosis being associated with dystrophic neurites rather than with amyloid fibrils (Stalder *et al.*, 1999).

A number of surface receptors involved in phagocytosis, such as complement receptor and SR, have been also reported on microglia associated with amyloid plaques, and there is now evidence that SR mediates adhesion of microglia to Aβ fibrils (Chavis *et al.*, 1996). The up-regulation of complement and scavenger receptors on microglia in amyloid plaques suggests that microglia try to remove cerebral amyloid, and are possibly involved in the transformation of Aβ into fibrils. However, the phagocytic function of microglia, although beneficial in removing amyloid deposits, also carries a risk of tissue injury. The interaction of activated microglia with amyloid deposits through SRs leads to the secretion of reactive oxygen species and cytokines by microglia and their immobilization (Chavis *et al.*, 1996). This interaction triggers the release of oxygen species such as NO (Chavis *et al.*, 1996), the pro-inflammatory cytokine IL-1β (Meda *et al.*, 1999) and various proteolytic enzymes—events that may exacerbate neuronal damage rather than incite outgrowth or repair mechanisms (Kalaria, 1999).

One of the important areas of CNS pathology, which has attracted a lot of attention, is immune-mediated responses and the function of microglia as APCs.

In immune-mediated diseases, the control of tissue-specific inflammation is largely dependent on local APCs. Therefore, understanding the interaction between local APCs and T cells is crucial for a better understanding of immune-mediated inflammatory processes including autoimmune diseases. Microglial cells are the largest population of macrophages, and therefore of potential APCs, in the brain.

In the previous section, we mentioned that microglia readily up-regulate surface expression of MHC molecules even in conditions such as neurodegeneration, where any other inflammatory stimuli are absent. The up-regulation of MHC molecules can also be seen in acute inflammation following, for example, invasion of a pathogen, as in the case of BCG (Matyszak and Perry, 1996b). The up-regulation of MHC probably results from the antigen uptake and processing which leads to *de novo* synthesis of MHC and its expression on the cell surface. It is probably of minimal consequence in the absence of T-cell responses. However, in the context of an immune response, the *de novo* synthesis of MHC by microglia will be of importance. In addition, though MHC molecules can be readily up-regulated following acute inflammation, B7 molecules are not (Windhagen *et al.*, 1995). Again, this may be different in immune-mediated responses where the presence of inflammatory cells, in particular T cells, will produce a cytokine milieu which promotes up-regulation of co-stimulatory molecules.

The engagement of T-cell receptors (TCRs), although necessary, is insufficient by itself to induce IL-2 production and T-cell proliferation. Generally, the first signal resulting from TCR engagement must be followed by co-stimulatory signals generated by the interaction between CD28 on T cells and B7 molecules on the APC (Lenschow *et al.*, 1996). There are two members of the B7 family which bind to CD28: B7.1 and B7.2. Although both B7.1 and B7.2 provide a co-stimulatory signal that allows efficient activation of CD4+ cells, a number of reports indicate the importance of B7.1 in immune responses in the CNS (Kuchroo *et al.*, 1995; Racke *et al.*, 1995). In addition to B7/CD28 co-stimulation, the interaction between CD40 and CD40L is important for T-cell priming. Blocking this interaction significantly reduces autoimmune responses in the CNS, suggesting that this interaction is also important.

As has been mentioned before, resting microglia express a minimal amount of MHC molecules. Microglia purified from human biopsies and from the brains of many strains of rodent have been also shown to express no B7.1 molecules (Ford *et al.*, 1996; Dangond *et al.*, 1997; Matyszak *et al.*, 1999). However, they express low but detectable levels of B7.2 and CD40 (Dangond *et al.*, 1997; Carson *et al.*, 1998; Matyszak *et al.*, 1999).

Some earlier *in vitro* studies have shown that microglia activated with interferon-γ (IFN-γ) can present antigens to T-cell clones (Matsumoto *et al.*, 1992; Cash *et al.*, 1993) or activated T cells (Aloisi *et al.*, 1998). However, recent evidence suggests that microglia are poor APCs. Despite the expression of MHC class II and some co-stimulation, they are unable to stimulate mixed leukocyte responses (Carson *et al.*, 1998). Microglia, both resting and those which have been partially activated with IFN-γ, are unable to stimulate an efficient antigen-specific response (Ford *et al.*, 1996; Klyushnenkova and Vanguri, 1997; Carson *et al.*, 1998; Matyszak *et al.*, 1999), and in some cases there is clear evidence that microglia inhibit T-cell proliferation (Hall *et al.*, 1999; Matyszak *et al.*, 1999).

More importantly, in tests with self-antigens such as MBP, microglia failed to present the protein to an MBP-specific T-cell line (Ford *et al.*, 1996) or *in vivo* primed T cells (Matyszak *et al.*, 1999). Furthermore, unlike DCs, in the presence of low affinity immunodominant MBP peptide (Ac1–11), microglia induced CD4$^+$ TCR Ac1–11 transgenic T-cell anergy. The anergy was preceded by a phase in which T cells were activated, as characterized by up-regulation of CD69 and IL-2 receptor (Matyszak *et al.*, 1999). Better understanding of immune responses to myelin antigens is important, because they are a prominent feature in multiple sclerosis (MS). MS is a chronic inflammatory disease and the demyelinating plaques are the hallmark of this disease. The majority of MS patients have been shown to have autoimmune responses to MBP and other myelin-associated antigens. See also Chapter 8 for further information on macrophages and MS.

One of the reasons why IFN-γ activation is insufficient to turn microglia into professional APCs became clear from studies of the changes in microglia phenotype following activation with this cytokine. Microglia activated with IFN-γ up-regulate MHC class II and also CD40, but not B7 molecules (Matyszak *et al.*, 1999). The lack of B7.1 expression and a low level of B7.2 would result in an inefficient secondary signal for T-cell activation. However, in immune-mediated responses, for example in MS or EAE lesions (EAE is a commonly used animal model for MS), microglia, in addition to MHC class II (Matsumoto and Fujiwara, 1986; Vass *et al.*, 1986; Traugott, 1987), express both B7.1 and B7.2 molecules (Williams *et al.*, 1994; De Simone *et al.*, 1995; Walker *et al.*, 1995; Windhagen *et al.*, 1995). CD40$^+$ microglia have also been seen co-localized with CD40L$^+$ T cells in MS plaques (Gerritse *et al.*, 1996). So what are the additional signals needed to induce full microglia activation?

Recent studies have shown that the co-culture of microglia with granulocyte–macrophage colony-stimulating factor (GM-CSF) induced surface expression of B7.1 (Matyszak *et al.*, 1999). This *per se* was still not sufficient to enable microglia to present MBP. What was needed to activate microglia fully was a multistep activation process involving both stimulation through cytokines (GM-CSF and IFN-γ) and cognate signaling (B7–CD28 and CD40–CD40L interactions). Fully activated microglial cells became professional APCs and were able to present native MBP to both unprimed and primed antigen-specific T cells. Co-culture of microglia with GM-CSF up-regulated the expression of co-stimulatory molecules, in particular B7.1, and MHC class II molecules. Additional activation of microglial cells with IFN-γ induced further MHC class II up-regulation and also CD40 up-regulation. Cognate CD40–CD40L interaction significantly enhanced microglial ability to prime TCR transgenic T cells, as was shown by the enhancement of T-cell proliferation, and this was essential for presentation of native MBP to *in vivo* primed CD4$^+$ T cells.

Interestingly, microglia activated with a combination of IFN-γ and lipoplysaccharide (LPS) also up-regulated B7.1, but this activation step did not restore T-cell proliferation (Matyszak *et al.*, unpublished observation). This may be explained by the recent discovery that treatment of microglia with LPS plus IFN-γ induces production of prostaglandin E$_2$ (PGE$_2$) by microglia, which results in the reduction of T-cell proliferation (Carson *et al.*, 1999).

Activated microglia also produce a number of anti-inflammatory cytokines including transforming growth factor-β (TGF-β) and IL-10. Furthermore, IL-10 production, in a synergistic fashion, is enhanced further by PGE$_2$ (Aloisi *et al.*, 1999). TGF-β is a member of a large family of growth factors which are important in cell growth and differentiation. TGF-β is also a potent inhibitor of immune responses. For example, in the CNS, it inhibits MHC class II and surface ICAM-1 expression on microglia (Shrikant *et al.*, 1996). TGF-β has also been reported to inhibit IFN-γ-induced expression of CD40, as well as CD40 mRNA production (Nguyen *et al.*, 1998). IL-10 is another well known anti-inflammatory cytokine (De Vries, 1995; Herfarth *et al.*, 1998). In EAE animals, treatment with human recombinant IL-10 or viral constructs expressing IL-10 significantly suppresses the disease (Rott *et al.*, 1994; Willenborg *et al.*, 1995). Along the same lines, IL-10 knockout animals are more susceptible to EAE (Segal *et al.*, 1998) and an increase in IL-10 production in EAE has been shown to correlate with recovery (Kennedy *et al.*, 1992). Therefore, the production of prostaglandins and anti-inflammatory cytokines may constitute an intrinsic regulatory mechanism, necessary for down-regulation of inflammation and protection against excessive tissue damage.

However, at the same time as producing anti-inflammatory cytokines and factors, activated microglia also synthesize pro-inflammatory cytokines and toxins. For example, following contact with Th1 T cells, microglia produce IL-12, a strong Th1 cytokine (Aloisi *et al.*, 1997). IFN-γ produced by Th1 T cells will induce tumor necrosis factor-α (TNF-α) transcription in microglia, which in turn suppresses IL-10 mRNA levels and IL-10 secretion (Kennedy *et al.*, 1992). As mentioned above, fully activated microglia can also present self-antigens which may inadvertently add to the chronicity of the disease. In summary, it may be that the best way to control inflammatory responses in the CNS, especially the autoimmune responses, would be to eliminate activated microglia, without inducing excessive damage to the non-activated cells.

There is increasing evidence that activated microglia may be eliminated from the pool of inflammatory cells during immune-mediated inflammatory responses in the CNS. Morphological studies have shown that both macrophages and microglia undergo apoptosis in the CNS in acute EAE lesions (White *et al.*, 1998). However, the number of microglia undergoing apoptosis is much greater than the number of inflammatory macrophages. A number of mechanisms can induce microglial death, including the involvement of TNF-α and Fas–FasL interaction. *In vitro* studies have shown that unstimulated microglia are resistant to killing through Fas–FasL interaction since they express a minimal amount of Fas. However, upon stimulation with IFN-γ and TNF-α, microglia up-regulate both mRNA and surface expression of Fas, which makes them susceptible to death by apoptosis. Both Bcl-2 and Bcl-xL (Bcl-2 and Bcl-xL act as repressors of cell death) are also down-regulated in activated cells. Interestingly, this study has shown that mRNA for FLIP was increased in activated microglia. Both viral proteins (vFLIP) and their cellular counterparts (cFLIP) block signal transduction through death receptors, including Fas (Irmler *et al.*, 1997; Thome *et al.*, 1997), therefore potentially protecting the cell from apoptosis. However, the increase in mRNA for FLIP did not protect microglia from apoptotic cell death (Spanaus *et al.*, 1998).

Fas–FasL is an important mechanism used by activated CD4+ T cells for killing target cells. CD4+ T cells up-regulate FasL during their activation. The interaction between B7.1 and CD28 results in enhanced levels of functional FasL on T cells. This suggests that T cells need to interact with APCs to enhance FasL expression, and the interaction needs to be via co-stimulatory molecules. Indeed, T-cell interaction with APCs through MHC/TCRs without additional co-stimulation results in minimal killing by T cells but is greatly enhanced in the presence of B7.1 on APCs (Thilenius *et al.*, 1999). This may be an important mechanism by which microglia function is controlled. Activated microglia up-regulate their antigen-presenting capacity by up-regulating co-stimulatory molecules and become efficient APCs. At the same time, they also up-regulate the expression of Fas which makes them a target for killing via the Fas–FasL route.

Another important advantage in the elimination of activated microglia is to minimize CNS tissue damage. As well as up-regulating Fas, activated microglia also up-regulate surface expression of FasL (Becher *et al.*, 1998), which may render these cells capable of bystander killing. For example, it has been suggested that activated microglia can kill oligodendrocytes and thus contribute to demyelination in MS lesions.

5 Summary

The resident macrophages of the CNS parenchyma are known as microglia. Monocytes enter the developing CNS and phagocytose degenerating cells and their processes, and then they differentiate to microglia. Microglia are distributed ubiquitously but heterogenously throughout the CNS and have distinct morphologies within different regions. In the normal CNS, they appear to be quiescent cells as judged by their ultrastructure and antigenic phenotype. However, microglia are exquisitely sensitive to a wide variety of pathological insults and rapidly alter their morphology and phenotype. The activation of microglia often precedes any other pathological changes, and this activation has been observed across the spectrum of inflammatory conditions from neurodegenerative diseases such as Alzheimer's disease (Chapter 7) or prion diseases, to immune-mediated diseases such as multiple sclerosis (Chapter 8). Contrary to earlier studies, recent evidence suggests that, at least in immune-mediated responses, microglia may have a regulatory function. That is, they prevent excessive inflammatory responses by controlling T-cell responses through the inhibition of T-cell proliferation, and in some cases by inducing T-cell anergy.

Acknowledgments

The work from our own laboratories reported in this review was supported by the MRC, The Wellcome Trust, British Multiple Sclerosis Society, Italian Multiple Sclerosis Society and the European Community TMR grant.

References

Agger, R., Crowley, M.T. and Witmer-Pack, M.D. (1997). The surface of dendritic cells in the mouse as studied with monoclonal antibodies. *International Review of Immunology*, **6**, 89–101.

Albright, A., Shieh, J., Itoh, T., Lee, B., Pleasure, D., O'Connor, M. *et al.* (1999). Microglia express CCR5, CXCR4, and CCR3, but of these, CCR5 is the principal coreceptor for human immunodeficiency virus type 1 dementia isolates. *Journal of Virology*, **73**, 205–13.

Aloisi, F., Penna, G., Cerase, J., Menendez, I. B. and Adorini, L. (1997). IL-12 production by central nervous system microglia is inhibited by astrocytes. *Journal of Immunology*, **159**, 1604–12.

Aloisi, F., Ria, F., Penna, G. and Adorini, L. (1998). Microglia are more efficient than astrocytes in antigen processing and in Th1 but not Th2 cells activation. *Journal of Immunology*, **160**, 4671–80.

Aloisi, F., De Simone, R., Columba-Cabezas, S. and Levi, G. (1999). Opposite effects of interferon-γ and prostaglandin E₂ on tumor necrosis factor and interleukin-10 production in microglia: a regulatory loop controlling microglia pro- and anti-inflammatory activities. *Journal of Neuroscience Research*, **56**, 571–80.

Austyn, J.M. and Gordon, S. (1981). F4/80: a monoclonal antibody directed specifically against the mouse macrophage. *European Journal of Immunology*, **11**, 805–11.

Becher, B., Barker, P.A., Owens, T. and Antel, J.P. (1998). CD95–CD95L: can the brain learn from the immune system. *Trends in Neuroscience*, **21**, 114–7.

Bell, M.D., Lopez, G.-R., Lawson, L., Hughes, D., Fraser, I., Gordon, S. *et al.* (1994). Upregulation of the macrophage scavenger receptor in response to different forms of injury in the CNS. *Journal of Neurocytology*, **23**, 605–13.

Ben Nun, A., Wekerle, H. and Cohen, I.R. (1981). The rapid isolation of clonable antigen specific T lymphocyte lines capable of mediating autoimmune encephalomyelitis. *European Journal of Immunology*, **11**, 195–9.

Betmouni, S., Perry, V.H. and Gordon, J.L. (1996). Evidence for an early inflammatory response in the central nervous system of mice with scrapie. *Neuroscience*, **74**, 1–5.

Blier, R. and Albrecht, R. (1980). Supraependymal macrophages of the third ventricle of hamster: morphological, functional and histochemical characterization *in situ* and in culture. *Journal of Comparative Neurology*, **192**, 489–504.

Brenan, M. and Puklavec, M. (1992). The MRC OX-62 antigen: a useful marker in the purification of rat veiled cells with the biochemical properties of an integrin. *Journal of Experimental Medicine*, **175**, 1457–65.

Carpenter. S.J., McCarthy, L.E. and Borison, H.I. (1970). Electron microscopic study of the epiplexus (Kolmer) cells of the cat choroid plexus. *Zeitschrift für Zellforschung Mikrosk. Anat.*, **110**, 471–86.

Carson, M.J., Reilly, C.R., Sutcliffe, J.G. and Lo, D. (1998). Mature microglia resemble immature antigen-presenting cells. *Glia*, **22**, 72–85.

Carson, M., Sutcliffe, J. and Campbel, L.I. (1999). Microglia stimulate naive T-cell differentiation without stimulating T-cell proliferation. *Journal of Neuroscience Research*, **55**, 127–34.

Cash, E., Zhang, Y. and Rott, O. (1993). Microglia present myelin antigens to T cells after phagocytosis of oligodendrocytes. *Cellular Immunology*, **147**, 129–38.

Chavis, P., Fagni, L., Lansman, J.B. and Bockaert, J. (1996). Functional coupling between ryanodine receptors and L-type calcium channels in neurons .*Nature*, **382**, 716–9.

Crofton, R.W., Diesselhoff-den-dulk, M.M.C. and van Furth, R. (1978). The origin, kinetics and characteristics of the Kupffer cells in the normal steady state. *Journal of Experimental Medicine*, **148**, 1–17.

Cserr, H. F. and Knopf, P.M. (1992). Cervical lymphatics, the blood–brain barrier and the immunoreactivity of the brain: a new view. *Immunology Today*, **13**, 507–12.

Dangond, F., Windhagen, A., Groves, C.J. and Hafler, D.A. (1997). Constitutive expression of costimulatory molecules by human microglia and its relevance to CNS autoimmunity. *Journal of Neuroimmunology*, **76**, 132–8.

Davson. H., Welch, K.. and Segal, M.B. (1987). *The Physiology and Pathophysiology of the Cerebrospinal Fluid.* Churchill Livingstone, Edinburgh.

De Simone, R., Giampaolo, A., Giometto, B., Gallo, P., Levi, G., Peschle, C. *et al.* (1995). The costimulatory molecule B7 is expressed on human microglia in culture and in multiple sclerosis acute lesions. *Journal of Neuropathology and Experimental Neurology*, **54**, 175–87.

de Vries, J.E. (1995). Immunosuppressive and anti-inflammatory properties of interleukin 10. *Annals of Medicine*, **27**, 537–41.

del Rio Hortega, P. (1932). Microglia. In Penfield, W. (ed.), *Cytology and Cellular Pathology of the Nervous System*. Paul B. Hoeber, New York, pp. 482–534.

Ffrench-Constant, C. and Raff, M.C. (1986). Proliferating bipotential glial cell progenitor cells in adult rat optic nerve. *Nature*, **319**, 499–502.

Ford, A.L., Foulcher, E., Lemckert, F.A. and Sedgwick, J.D. (1996). Microglia induce CD4 T lymphocyte final effector function and death. *Journal of Experimental Medicine*, **184**, 1737–45.

Fraser, I., Hughes, D. and Gordon, S. (1993). Divalent cation-independent macrophage adhesion inhibited by monoclonal antibody to murine scavenger receptor. *Nature*, **364**, 343–46.

Gerritse, K., Laman, J.D., Noelle, R.J., Aruffo, A., Ledbetter, J.A., Boersma, W.J.A. *et al.* (1996). CD40–CD40 ligand interactions in experimental allergic encephalomyelitis and multiple sclerosis. *Proceedings of the National Academy of Sciences USA*, **93**, 2499–504.

Ghorpade, A., Xia, M., Hyman, B., Persidsky, Y., Nukuna, A., Bock, P. *et al.* (1998). Role of the β-chemokine receptors CCR3 and CCR5 in human immunodeficiency virus type 1 infection of monocytes and microglia. *Journal of Virology*, **72**, 3351–61.

Giulian, D. and Young, D.G. (1986). Brain peptides and glial growth. II. Identification of cells that secrete glial promoting factors. *Journal of Cell Biology.*, **102**. 812–17.

Giulian, D., Young, D.G., Woodward, J., Brown, D.C. and Lachman, L.B. (1988a). Interleukin-1 is an astroglial growth factor in the developing brain. *Journal of Neuroscience*, **8**. 709–14.

Giulian, D., Woodward, J., Krebs, J.F., and Lachman, L.B. (1988b). Interleukin-1 injected into mammalian brain stimulates astrogliosis and neovascularization. *Journal of Neuroscience*, **8**, 2485–90.

Giulian, D., Li, J., Bartel, S., Broker, J., Li, X. and Kirkpatrick, J.B. (1995). Cell surface morphology identifies microglia as a distinct class of mononuclear phagocytes. *Journal of Neuroscience*, **15**, 7712–26.

Gordon. S., Perry, V.H., Rabinowitz, S., Chung. L-P., and Rosen, H. (1988). Plasma membrane receptors of the mononuclear phagocyte system. *Journal of Cell Science*, Supplement, **9**, 1–26.

Graeber, M.B., Streit, W.J., and Kreutzberg, G.W. (1989). Identity of ED2-positive perivascular cells in rat brain. *Journal of Neuroscience Research*, **22**, 103–6.

Hailer, N., Heppner, F., Haas, D. and Nitsch, R. (1998). Astrocytic factors deactivate antigen presenting cells that invade the central nervous system. *Brain Pathology*, **8**, 459–74.

Hall, G., Girdlestone, J., Compston, D. and Wing, M. (1999). Recall antigen presentation by γ-interferon-activated microglia results in T cell activation and propagation of the immune response. *Journal of Neuroimmunology*, **98**, 105–11.

Harling-Berg, C., Knopf, P.M., Merriam, J. and Cserr, H.F. (1989). Role of cervical lymph nodes in the systemic humoral immune response to human serum albumin microinfused into rat cerebrospinal fluid. *Journal of Neuroimmunology*, **25**, 185–93.

Hayes, G.M., Woodroofe, M.N. and Cuzner, M.L. (1987). Microglia are the major cell type expressing MHC class II in human white matter. *Journal of the Neurological Sciences*, **80**, 25–37.

He, J., Chen, Y., Farzan, M., Choe, H., Ohagen, A., Gartner, S. *et al.* (1997). CCR3 and CCR5 are co-receptors for HIV-1 infection of microglia. *Nature*, **385**, 645–9.

Herfarth, H.H., Bocker, U., Janardhanam, R. and Sartor, R.B.(1998). Subtherapeutic corticosteroids potentiate the ability of interleukin 10 to prevent chronic inflammation in rats. *Gastroenterology*, **115**, 856–65.

Hickey, W.F. and Kimura, H. (1988). Perivascular microglial cells of the CNS are bone marrow-derived and present antigen *in vivo*. *Science*, **239**, 290–2.

Hickey, W.F., Vass, K. and Lassmann, H. (1992). Bone marrow-derived elements in the central nervous system: an immunohistochemical and ultrastructural survey of rat chimeras. *Journal of Neuropathology and Experimental Neurology*, **51**, 246–56.

Hume, D.A., Perry, V.H. and Gordon, S. (1983). Immunohistochemical localization of a macrophage specific antigen in developing mouse retina: phagocytosis of dying neurons and differentiation of microglial cells to form a regular array in the plexiform layers. *Journal of Cell Biology*, **97**, 253–7.

Imamoto, K. and Leblond, C.P. (1974). Presence of labelled monocytes, macrophages and microglia in a stab wound of the brain following an injection of bone marrow cells labelled with ³H-uridine into rats. *Journal of Comparative Neurology*, **174**, 255–80.

Innocenti, G.M., Clarke, S. and Koppel, H. (1983). Transitory macrophages in the white matter of the developing visual cortex. II. Development and relations with axonal pathways. *Developments in Brain Research*, **11**, 55–66.

Irmler, M., Thome, M., Hahne, M., Schneider, P., Hofmann, K., Steiner, V. *et al.* (1997). Inhibition of death receptor signals by cellular FLIP. *Nature*, **388**, 190–5.

Jordan, F.L. and Thomas, W.E. (1988). Brain macrophages: questions of origin and interrelationship. *Brain Research Reviews*, **13**, 165–78.

Kalaria, R. (1999). Microglia and Alzheimer's disease. *Current Opinion in Hematology*, **6**, 15–24.

Kennedy, M.K., Torrance, D.S., Picha, K.S. and Mohler, K.M. (1992). Analysis of cytokine mRNA expression in the central nervous system of mice with experimental autoimmune encephalomyelitis reveals that IL-10 mRNA expression correlates with recovery. *Journal of Immunology*, **149**, 2496–505.

Kiernan, J.A. (1985). Axonal and vascular changes following injury to the rat's optic nerve. *Journal of Anatomy*, **141**, 139–54.

Klassen, H.J. and Lund, R.D. (1987). Retinal transplants can drive a pupillary reflex in host rat brains. *Proceedings of the National Academy of Sciences USA*, **84**, 6958–60.

Klyushnenkova, E.N. and Vanguri, P. (1997). Ia expression and antigen presentation by glia: strain and cell type-specific differences among rat astrocytes and microglia. *Journal of Neuroimmunology*, **79**, 190–201.

Kreutzberg, G.W. (1996). Microglia: a sensor for pathological events in the CNS. *Trends in Neurosciences*, **19**, 312–8.

Kuchroo, V.K., Das, M.P., Brown, J.A., Ranger, A.M., Zamvil, S.S., Sobel, R.A. *et al.* (1995). B7-1 and B7-2 costimulatory molecules activate differentially the Th1/Th2 developmental pathways: application to autoimmune disease therapy. *Cell*, **80**, 707–18.

Kuono, H., Yamamoto, T., Iwasaki, Y., Suzuki, H., Saito, T. and Terenuma, H. (1989). Wallerian degeneration induces Ia-antigen-expression in rat brain. *Journal of Neuroimmunology*, **25**, 151–9.

Lassmann, H., Schmied, M., Vass, K. and Hickey, W. F. (1993). Bone marrow derived elements and resident microglia in brain inflammation. *Glia*, **7**, 19–24.

Lawson, L.J., Perry, V.H., Dri, P. and Gordon, S. (1990a). Heterogeneity in the distribution and morphology of microglia in the normal adult mouse brain. *Neuroscience*, **39**, 151–70.

Lawson, L.J., Perry, V.H., Dri, P. and Gordon, S. (1990b). Distribution, morphology and turnover of the resident macrophages of the normal adult mouse brain. *Neuroscience Letters*, **38** (Supplement), S85.

Lenschow, D.J., Walunas, T.L. and Bluestone, J.A. (1996). CD28/B7 system of T cell costimulation. *Annual Review of Immunology*, **14**, 233–58.

Ling. E.A. (1981). The origin and nature of microglia. In Hertz, I. and Federoff, S. (ed.), *Advances in Cellular Neurobiology*, Vol. 2. Academic Press, New York, pp. 33–82.

Mackenzie, I.C. (1975). Labelling of murine epidermal Langerhans cells with H3-thymidine. *Amercan Journal of Anatomy*, **144**, 127–36.

Mato, M., Cokawara, S., Sakamoto, A., Aikawa, E., Ogawa, T., Mitsuhashi, U. *et al.* (1996). Involvement of specific macrophage-lineage cells surrounding arterioles in barrier and scavenger function in brain cortex. *Proceedings of the National Academy of Sciences USA*, **93**, 3269–74.

Matsumoto, Y. and Fujiwara, M. (1986). *In situ* detection of class I and II major histocompatibility complex antigens in the rat central nervous system during experimental allergic encephalitis. *Journal of Neuroimmunology*, **12**, 265–77.

Matsumoto, Y., Ohmori, K. and Fujiwara, M. (1992). Immune regulation by brain cells in the central nervous system: microglia but not astrocytes present myelin basic protein to encephalitogenic T cells under *in vivo*-mimicking conditions. *Immunology*, **76**, 209–16.

Matyszak, M.K. and Perry, V.H. (1996a). The potential role of dendritic cells in immune mediated inflammatory responses in the central nervous system. *Neuroscience*, **74**, 599–608.

Matyszak, M.K. and Perry, V.H. (1996b). A comparison of leucocyte responses to heat-killed bacillus Calmette–Guérin in different CNS compartments. *Neuropathology and Applied Neurobiology*, **22**, 44–53.

Matyszak, M.K., Lawson, L.J., Perry, V.H. and Gordon, S. (1992). Stromal macrophages of the choroid plexus situated at an interface between the brain and peripheral immune system constitutively express major histocompatibility class II antigens. *Journal of Neuroimmunology*, **40**, 173–81.

Matyszak, M.K., Denis-Donini, S., Citterio, S., Longhi, R., Granucci, F. and Ricciardi-Castagnoli, P. (1999). Microglia induce myelin basic protein-specific T cell anergy or T cell activation, according to their state of activation. *European Journal of Immunology*, **29**, 3063–76.

McCarthy, G.E. and Leblond, C.P. (1988). Radioautographic evidence for slow astrocyte turnover and modest oligodendrocyte production in the corpus callosum of adult mice infused with ^{3}H-thymidine. *Journal of Comparative Neurology*, **271**, 589–603.

McGeer, P.L., Kawamata, T., Walker, D.G., Akiyama, H., Tooyama, I. and McGeer, E.G. (1993). Microglia in degenerative neurological disease. *Glia*, **7**, 84–92.

Meda, L., Baron, P., Prat, E., Scarpini, E., Scarlato, G., Cassatella, M. *et al.* (1999). Proinflammatory profile of cytokine production by human monocytes and murine microglia stimulated with β-amyloid[25–35]. *Journal of Neuroimmunology*, **93**, 45–52.

Nguyen, V.T., Walker, W.S. and Benveniste, E.N. (1998). Post-transcriptional inhibition of CD40 gene expression in microglia by transforming growth factor-β. *European Journal of Immunology*, **28**, 253748.

Oppenheim, R.W. (1981). Neuronal cell death and related regressive phenomenon during neurogenesis: a selective historical review and progress report. In Cowan, W.M. (ed.), *Studies in Developmental Neurobiology: Essays in Honour of Victor Hamburger*. Oxford University Press, pp. 74–133.

Paterson, P.Y., Mescher, P.A. and Mueller-Eberhard, H.S. (eds.) (1976). *Textbook of Immunopathology.* Grune and Stratton, New York, pp. 179–213.

Perry, V.H. (1998). A revised view of the central nervous system microenvironment and major histocompatibility complex class II antigen presentation. *Journal of Neuroimmunology,* **90**, 113–21.

Perry, V.H. and Gordon, S. (1987). Modulation of the CD4 antigen on macrophages and microglia in rat brain. *Journal of Experimental Medicine,* **166**, 1138–43.

Perry, V.H. and Gordon, S. (1991). Macrophages and the nervous system. *International Review of Cytology,* **125**, 203–44.

Perry, V.H. and Lund, R.D. (1989). Microglia in retinae transplanted to the central nervous system. *Neuroscience,* **31**, 453–62.

Perry, V.H., Hume, D.A. and Gordon, S. (1985). Immunohistochemical localization of macrophages and microglia in the adult and developing mouse brain. *Neuroscience,* **15**, 313–26.

Perry, V.H., Matyszak, M.K. and Fearn, S. (1993a). Altered antigen expression of microglia in the aged rodent CNS. *Glia,* **7**, 60–7.

Perry, V.H., Andersson, P.B. and Gordon, S. (1993b). Macrophages and inflammation in the central nervous system. *Trends in Neuroscience,* **16**, 268–73.

Peters, A., Palay, S.L. and Webster, H.D. (eds.) (1991). *The fine structure of the nervous system. Neurons and their supporting cells.* Saunders, Philadelphia, pp. 304–11.

Pow, D.V., Perry, V.H., Morris, J.F. and Gordon, S. (1989). Microglia in the neurohypophysis associate with and endocytose terminal portions of neurosecretory neurons. *Neuroscience,* **33**, 567–78.

Racke, M.K., Scott, D.E., Quigley, L., Gray, G.S., Nabavi, N., Herold, D.C. *et al.* (1995). Distinct roles for B7.1(CD-80) and B7.2 (CD-86) in the initiation of experimental allergic encephalomyelitis. *Journal of Clinical Investigation,* **96**, 21952203.

Rakic, P. (1985). Limits of neurogenesis in primates. *Science,* **227**, 1054–6.

Rezaie, P., Cairns, N. and Male, D. (1997). Expression of adhesion molecules on human fetal cerebral vessels: relationship to microglial colonisation during development. *Brain Research and Developmenal Brain Research,* **104**, 175–89.

Rott, O., Fleischer, B. and Cash, E. (1994). Interleukin-10 prevents experimental allergic encephalomyelitis in rats. *European Journal of Immunology,* **24**, 1434–40.

Schroeter, M., Jander, S., Witte, O. and Stoll, G. (1999). Heterogeneity of the microglial response in photochemically induced focal ischemia of the rat cerebral cortex. *Neuroscience,* **89**, 1367–77.

Schultze, B. and Korr, H. (1981). Cell kinetic studies of different cell types in the developing and adult brain of the rat and the mouse: a review. *Cell and Tissue Kinetics,* **14**, 309—25.

Segal, B.M., Dwyer, B.K. and Shevach, E.M. (1998). An interleukin (IL)-10/IL-12 immunoregulatory circuit controls susceptibility to autoimmune disease. *Journal of Experimental Medicine,* **187**, 537–46.

Shabo, A.I. and Maxwell, D.S. (1971). The subarachnoid space following the introduction of a foreign protein: an electron microscopic study with peroxidase. *Journal of Neuropathology and Experimental Neurology,* **30**, 506–24.

Shaw, J.A., Perry, V.H. and Mellanby, J. (1990). Tetanus toxin-induced seizures cause microglial activation in rat hippocampus. *Neuroscience Letters,* **120**, 66–9.

Shrikant, P., Lee, S.J., Kalvakalanu, J., Ransohoff, R.M. and Benveniste, E.N. (1996). Stimulus-specific inhibition of ICAM-1 gene expression by TGF-β. *Journal of Immunology,* **157**, 892–900.

Sievers, J., Parwaresch, R. and Wottge, H.-U. (1994). Blood monocytes and spleen macrophages differentiate into microglia-like cells on monolayers of astrocytes: morphology. *Glia*, **12**, 245–58.

Sminia, T., De Groot, C.J.A., Dijkstra, C.D., Koetsier, J.C. and Polman, C.H. (1987). Macrophages in the central nervous system of the rat. *Immunobiology*, **174**, 43–50.

Spanaus, K.S., Schlapbach, R. and Fontana, A. (1998). TNF-α and IFN-γ render microglia sensitive to Fas ligand-induced apoptosis by induction of Fas expression and down-regulation of Bcl-2 and Bcl-xL. *European Journal of Immunology*, **28**, 4398–408.

Stalder, M., Phinney, A., Probst, A., Sommer, B., Staufenbiel, M. and Jucker, M. (1999). Association of microglia with amyloid plaques in brains of APP23 transgenic mice .*American Journal of Pathology*, **154**, 1673–84.

Stevenson, P.G., Hawke, S., Sloan, D.J. and Bangham, C.R. (1997). The immunogenicity of intracerebral virus-infection depends on anatomical site. *Journal of Virology*, **71**, 145–51.

Streit, W.J., Graeber, M.B., and Kreutzberg, G.W. (1989). Expression of Ia antigen on perivascular and microglial cells after sublethal and lethal motor neuron injury. *Experimental Neurology*, **105**, 115–26.

Thilenius, A.R.B., Sabelko-Downes, K.A. and Russell, J.H. (1999). The role of the antigen presenting cell in Fas-mediated direct and bystander killing: potential *in vivo* function of Fas in experimental allergic encephalomyelitis. *Journal of Immunology*, **162**, 643–50.

Thome, M., Schneider, P., Hofmann, K., Fickenscher, H., Meinl, E., Scaffidi, C. *et al.* (1997). Viral FLICE-inhibitory proteins (FLIPs) prevent apoptosis induced by death receptors. *Nature*, **386**, 517–21.

Traugott, U. (1987). Multiple sclerosis: relevance of class I and class II MHC-expressing cells to lesion development. *Journal of Neuroimmunology*, **16**, 283–302

Van Oud Alblas, A.B. and van Furth, R. (1979). Origin, kinetics and characteristics of pulmonary macrophages in the normal steady state. *Journal of Experimental Medicine*, **149**, 1504–18.

Vass, K., Lassmann, H., Wekerle, H. and Wisniewski, H.M. (1986). The distribution of Ia antigen in the lesions of rat acute experimental allergic encephalomyelitis. *Acta Neuropathologica*, **70**, 149–60.

Walker, W.S., Gatewood, J., Olivas, E., Askew, D. and Havenith, C.E. (1995). Mouse microglia cell lines differing in constitutive and interferon-γ-inducible antigen presenting activities for naive and memory CD4+ and CD8+ T cells. *Journal of Neuroimmunology*, **63**, 163–74.

White, C., McCombe, P. and Pender, M. (1998). Microglia are more susceptible than macrophages to apoptosis in the central nervous system in experimental autoimmune encephalomyelitis through a mechanism not involving Fas (CD95). *International Immunology*, **10**, 935–41.

Willenborg, D.O., Fordham, S.A., Cowden, W.B. and Ramshaw, I.A. (1995). Cytokines and murine autoimmune encephalomyelitis: inhibition or enhancement of disease with antibodies to select cytokines, or by delivery of exogenous cytokines using a recombinant vaccinia virus system. *Scandinavian Journal of Immunology*, **41**, 31–41.

Williams, A.E. and Blakemore, W.F. (1990). Monocyte-mediated entry of pathogens into the central nervous system. *Neuropathology and Applied Neurobiology*, **16**, 377–92.

Williams, K., Ulvestad, E. and Antel, J.P. (1994). B7/BB-1 antigen expression on adult human microglia studied *in vitro* and *in situ*. *European Journal of Immunology*, **24**, 3031–7.

Williams, R. and Herrup, K. (1988). The control of neuron number. *Annual Review of Neuroscience*, **11**, 423–53.

Windhagen, A., Newcombe, J., Dangond, F. *et al.* (1995). Expression of Il-12 and B7 costimulatory molecules in multiple sclerosis lesions. *Journal of Experimental Medicine*, **182**, 1985–96.

14 *Macrophages in reproductive biology*

H. Okamura, H. Katabuchi and H. Kanzaki

1 Introduction

Macrophages are present in every organ of the female genital tract. During the last two decades, considerable attention has been paid to macrophages and their various functions in reproductive biology. Apart from defense against specific microorganisms or antigens in collaboration with other immune cells, they are involved in a variety of homeostatic and physiological conditions through their products such as enzymes, cytokines, reactive oxygen intermediates and other biological substances. The foundation for these research achievements was laid by many functional morphological approaches. In female genital organs, they exhibit certain morphological differences, presumably attributable to the cyclical and pregnancy-induced alterations in the levels of sex steroid hormones and the immune mechanisms of embryonic–maternal interactions. In their structural diversity, the functional properties and heterogeneity of macrophages are seen in the ovaries, peritoneal cavity, fallopian tubes, endometrium and placenta.

2 Macrophages in ovaries

In the 1960s, macrophages in ovaries were first identified in atretic ovarian follicles and the regressing corpora lutea of rats using histochemical markers and electron microscopy (Lobel *et al.*, 1961, Bulmer, 1964). In 1989, it was demonstrated that they are also present within the developing follicles and the copora lutea of humans (Katabuchi *et al.*, 1989a). Macrophages appear around and within the ovarian follicles with their development, although leukocytes including macrophages are not seen around the primary follicles. They are often observed near the perifollicular capillaries of the stroma. Ultrastructurally, these macrophages are small and have no vacuoles or granules in the cytoplasm. Direct cell contact of the macrophages connects adjacent granulosa cells within the follicles. Macrophages are observed both inside and outside the corpus luteum together with other leukocytes. They are ameboid in shape with long pseudopodia. Their cytoplasm exhibits numerous electron-dense granules of variable configurations and structures. The intracellular organelles are well developed. After investigations of the distribution and fine structure of human ovarian macrophages, many studies of macrophages in normal ovaries concentrated mainly on non-human species including rats, mice, guinea pigs, hamsters and dogs because the ability to evaluate staged human specimens precisely is limited.

2.1 Macrophages in folliculogenesis and steroidogenesis

In addition to endocrine hormone passage through the bloodstream to distant sites, other forms of cellular communication such as the paracrine and autocrine systems have been proposed as local control mechanisms of follicular development since it was demonstrated that macrophages enhanced progesterone production in cultured granulosa cells in mice (Kirsch *et al.*, 1981) and in humans (Halme *et al.*, 1985). Thereafter, it has been shown that many kinds of cytokine are secreted from ovarian macrophages and their network is formed during ovarian folliculogenesis and steroidogenesis. In particular, the systems of insulin-like growth factor (IGF) (Adashi, 1993), tumor necrosis factor-α (TNF-α) (Terranova and Rice, 1997), epidermal growth factor (EGF) (Fukumatsu *et al.*, 1995, Katabuchi *et al.*, 1996) or interleukin (IL)-1 (Adashi, 1996) are documented as putative intraovarian regulators.

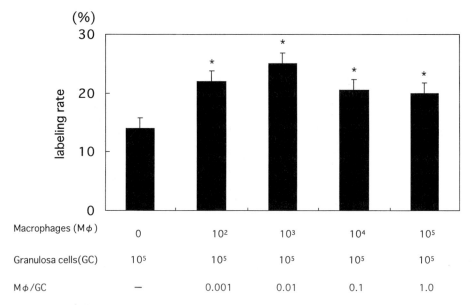

Fig. 14.1 [^{3}H]Thymidine labeling rate of rat granulosa cells in co-culture with peritoneal macrophages. *$P < 0.01$ compared with controls in granulosa cells cultured without peritoneal macrophages. (From Fukumatsu *et al.*, 1992b, with permission of *Journal of Reproduction and Fertility*.)

Using gonadotropin-primed immature female rats, macrophages can be identified in the follicles at various stages of development (Fukumatsu *et al.*, 1992b). In the proliferative capacity test of granulosa cells examined by incubation in medium containing [methyl-^{3}H]thymidine, the labeling index of granulosa cells cultured with peritoneal macrophages is highest when the ratio of macrophages to granulosa cells is 0.01 (Figure 14.1). This *in vitro* ratio is closely similar to that of macrophages to granulosa cells within the preantral and antral follicles *in vivo* (Table 14.1). Subsequently, a decrease in [methyl-^{3}H]thymidine labeling of granulosa cells of *op/op* mice was observed during follicular development (Figure 14.2) (Araki *et al.*, 1996). *Op/op* mice are characterized by reduction of monocyte/macrophage lineage cells in nearly all organs and tissues because they are deficient in the production of functional macrophage-colony stimulating factor (M-CSF) protein due to a mutation in the M-CSF gene (Yoshida *et al.*, 1990). In this natural 'knockout' species, numbers of granulosa cells and macrophages in

Table 14.1 Quantitative analysis of granulosa cells and macrophages in rat follicles

	Preantral ($n = 20$)	Antral ($n = 20$)	Mature ($n = 20$)
Diameter of largest follicle section (mm)	<0.15	0.15–0.3	>0.3
No. of follicles containing macrophages	6	17	16
No. of granulosa cells (GC)	72.8 ± 50.2	531.1 ± 379.0	1547.7 ± 402.8
No. of macrophages (M)	0.6 ± 1.1	3.7 ± 4.9	2.3 ± 2.0
M/GC	0.008	0.007	0.002

From Fukumatsu *et al.* (1992b), with permission of *Journal of Reproduction and Fertility.*

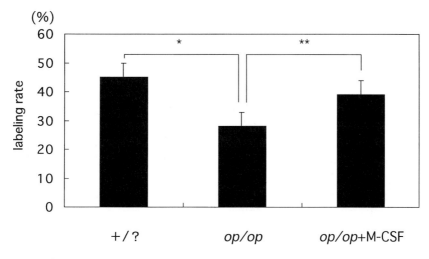

Fig. 14.2 [³H]Thymidine labeling rate of granulosa cells in antral follicles of normal littermates, *op/op* mice and M-CSF-treated *op/op* mice. *$P < 0.01$, **$P < 0.05$. (From Araki *et al.*, 1996, with permission of *Biology of Reproduction*.)

Table 14.2   Number of granulosa cells and macrophages in the antral follicles of normal littemates, *op/op* mice and M-CSF-treated *op/op* mice

	+/?	op/op	op/op+M-CSF
No. of antral follicles examined	20	20	20
No. of follicles containing macrophages	14	1	8
No. of granulosa cells per section of one follicle	525.1 ± 10.2	465.6 ± 19.7	516.3 ± 9.5
No. of macrophages per section of one follicle	1.8 ± 0.4	0.1 ± 0.1	0.6 ± 0.2

The greatest section of antral follicles with the greatest diameter in ovaries was analyzed at 19.00 h on the night of proestrus.
*P <0.01, **P <0.05.
From Araki *et al.* (1996), with permission of *Biology of Reproduction*.

antral follicles are fewer than those in the littermate controls (Table 14.2). After daily M-CSF addition, the proliferative capacity is elevated (Figure 14.2) and granulosa cells and macrophages in the antral follicles are increased in number (Table 14.2). The numbers of both antral and mature follicles in the proestrous ovary are also markedly lower compared with normal littermates and retrieved by the administration of M-CSF (Table 14.3). In addition, the number of ovulated ova in fallopian tubes is significantly smaller in *op/op* mice than in normal littermates (Figure 14.3). Such ova are markedly increased in number after daily M-CSF administration (Figure 14.3). In normal rats, M-CSF significantly increases the numbers of developing follicles and ovulated ova (Nishimura *et al.*, 1995). mRNA encoding both M-CSF and M-CSF receptors (c-*fmc* proto-oncogene product) was demonstrated in mouse granulosa cells (Arceci *et al.*, 1992). Taken together, M-CSF itself may enhance folliculogenesis and the subsequent ovulation, and/or participate in these processes by increasing macrophage numbers within follicles.

Bone marrow-derived blood monocytes are generally thought to be the precursor of these ovarian macrophages. However, the spleen has been shown recently to be one of the

Table 14.3   Number of mature and antral follicles in of normal littemates, *op/op* mice and M-CSF-treated *op/op* mice

Phenotype	No. of follicles/ovary	
	Mature	Antral
+/? (*n* = 6)	16.3 ± 1.4	77.8 ± 4.0
op/op (*n* = 6)	9.1 ± 1.5]**	39.2 ± 3.1
op/op+M-CSF (*n* = 6)	10.0 ± 1.7	55.0 ± 6.4

Growing follicles were counted in all serial sections of each ovary and analyzed at 19.00 h on the night of proestrus.
n = number of animals examined.
*P <0.01, **P <0.05.
From Araki *et al.* (1996), with permission of *Biology of Reproduction.*

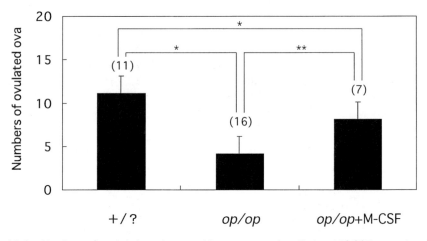

Fig. 14.3   Numbers of ovulated ova in normal littermates, *op/op* mice and M-CSF-treated *op/op* mice. Ovulated ova were counted in both Fallopian tubes at 11.00 h on the morning of metestrus. *P <0.01, **P <0.05. (From Araki *et al.*, 1996, with permission of *Biology of Reproduction.*)

sources of these macrophages. It was demonstrated that splenectomy at specific stages during the estrous cycle delays ovulation (Matsuyama *et al.*, 1987). Splenectomy was also reported to increase the levels of biologically inactive progestin in pseudopregnant rats (Saito *et al.*, 1988). These changes after splenectomy are restored by the injection of rat splenic macrophages. Moreover, it has been reported that splenic macrophages also stimulate progestin secretion from granulosa cells under the influence of an elevated level of peripheral prolactin (Yamanouchi *et al.*, 1992).

2.2 Macrophages in follicular atresia and regression of the corpus luteum

In humans, macrophages are observed in the follicular cavity when the development of the ovarian follicles is interrupted. Although light microscopic studies have shown the presence of macrophages in the cavity of atretic follicles, their ultrastrucutural characteristics have not been demonstrated, probably because of the difficulty in preparing specimens for electron microscopy. These macrophages are ultrastructurally characterized by the presence of cytoplasmic vacuoles and granules, which are delimited by a single unit membrane and lysosomal in nature (Figure 14.4a) (Katabuchi *et al.*, 1997). Both the vacuoles and the granules imply resorption of follicular fluid and phagocytosis of debris of granulosa cells.

Macrophages are increased in number during the later phase of the life span of the corpus luteum (Bulmer, 1964; Bagavandoss *et al.*, 1988; Katabuchi *et al.*, 1997). Elongated crystalline structures, presumably of cholesterol origin, and numerous lipid droplets were observed ultrastructurally in the cytoplasm of macrophages (Figure 14.4b) (Katabuchi *et al.*, 1997). These fine structures are associated with the phagocytosis of degenerating or dead lutein cells. High expression levels of mRNA for apolipoprotein E in macrophages were reported during the regression of rat luteal tissue (Nicosia *et al.*, 1992). Therefore, macrophages may be involved in steroid metabolism as well as acting as scavengers. On the other hand, ovarian macrophages may release peroxidase in the copora lutea and be involved in luteolytic action because it has been reported that reactive oxygen species may fill the role of mediators of luteolysis (Olson *et al.*, 1996). As previously stated, macrophages during the early stage of luteal development may mediate the luteotropic effect by producing and secreting several cytokines. Among them, TNF-α and IL-1 may also participate in luteal regression. These two cytokines can stimulate release of luteal prostaglandins (PGs), especially of PGF$_{2a}$ (Benyo and Pate, 1992; Townson and Pate, 1994), which inhibit adenyl cyclase activity in luteal cells (Niswender

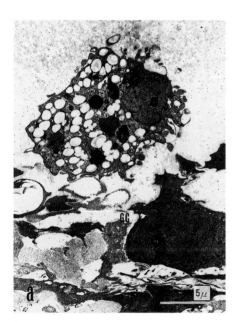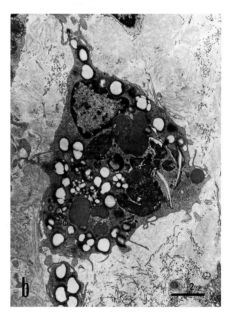

Fig. 14.4 Electron micrographs of macrophages in a human ovary. (a) Macrophages observed in an atretic follicle, at day 5 of the menstruation cycle, are large, with vacuoles and granules throughout the cytoplasm. (b) In a regressing corpora lutea, at day 5 of the menstruation cycle, macrophages contain numerous lipid droplets in the cytoplasm. Elongated crystalloid structures, presumably of cholesterol origin, are also seen. GC: granulosa cell. Lead citrate and uranyl acetate stain. Original magnification: ×1950 (a); ×2600 (b).
*$P < 0.01$, **$P < 0.05$. (From Katabuchi *et al.*, 1997, with permission of *Endocrine Journal*.)

and Nett, 1988). TNF-α and IL-1 themselves can reduce the response of luteal cells to luteotropins by inhibition of adenyl cyclase (Adashi *et al.*, 1990; Wang *et al.*, 1992; Pitzel *et al.*, 1993). Both of the macrophage-related cytokines may have distinct and yet synergistic roles depending on the phase of luteal development and regression.

3 Peritoneal macrophages

Lavage of the human peritoneal cavity, without additional stimulation, provides cellular elements such as macrophages, red blood cells, mesothelial cells and endometrial cells. The predominant cell type is macrophages, comprising approximately 50 per cent of the peritoneal fluid cell population (Burns and Shenken, 1999). The total number of peritoneal macrophages is approximately $6–7 \times 10^6$ in women without any pathological conditions (Syrop and Halme, 1987).

3.1 Cytology and classification

Peritoneal macrophages are approximately 10–15 μm in diameter. They possess appreciable cytoplasm and have an oval or slightly indented large nucleus with one or two distinct nucleoli. They are ultrastructurally characterized by projections of long filopodia and/or short microvilli from their cell surface and by the presence of several cytoplasmic vacuoles and abundant pinocytotic vesicles. The cytoplasmic vacuoles contain small amounts of homogeneous or flocculent, electron-lucid materials, and are delimited by a single unit membrane. Their cytoplasm is well developed by a Golgi apparatus, rough endoplasmic reticula, polyribosomes and many lysosomes. These fine structures are similar to those of mature macrophages observed in other organs (Fukumatsu *et al.*, 1991).

As shown in several animal species such as guinea pigs, rats, mice and rabbits, the cytochemical detection of endogenous peroxidase activity in peritoneal macrophages provides four different types of cells (Miyamura *et al.*, 1987). Their study used the glucose oxidase method to define the ultracytochemical localization of endogenous peroxidase activity and consequently showed that human peritoneal macrophages can also be classified into four subpopulations, i.e. resident, exudate, exudate-resident and peroxidase-negative (Miyamura *et al.*, 1987). Resident macrophages have peroxidase activity on the nuclear envelope and the rough endoplasmic reticulum (Figure 14.5a). Exudate macrophages exhibit peroxidase activity only in the lysosomal granules (Figure 14.5b). In exudate-resident macrophages, peroxidase activity is observed on the nuclear envelope, rough endoplasmic reticulum and lysosomal granules (Figure 14.5c). In peroxidase-negative macrophages, no endogenous peroxidase activity is detected in any organelle (Figure 14.5d). As markers of macrophage activation, increased phagocytotic ability, production of lysosomal enzymes, generation of reactive oxygen species or enhanced expression of some membrane molecules have been suggested (Burns and Schenken, 1999). Among them, several animal studies showed that exudate macrophages are an activated form because the instillation of polysaccharides (Robertson *et al.*, 1977), glucan (Burgaleta *et al.*, 1978) or thioglycollate (Fukumatsu *et al.*, 1992a) into the peritoneal cavity increases the total number of peritoneal macrophages, especially the exudate type, and that the ability to phagocytose latex spheres is highest in exudate macrophages (Fukumatsu *et al.*, 1992a).

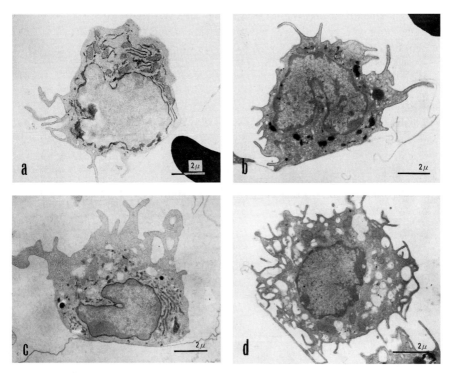

Fig. 14.5 Electron micrographs of human peritoneal macrophages. (a) Resident macrophage; peroxidase activity is evident on the nuclear envelope and rough endoplasmic reticulum. (b) Exudate macrophage; peroxidase activity is localized only in the lysosomal granules. (c) Exudate-resident macrophage; peroxidase activity is shown on the nuclear envelope, rough endoplasmic reticulum and lysosomal granules. (d) Peroxidase-negative macrophage; there appears to be no endogenous peroxidase activity. Lead citrate stain. Original magnification: ×2500 (a and b); ×3500 (c and d). (From Miyamura *et al.*, 1987, with permission of *Journal of Clinical Electron Microscopy*.)

Peritoneal macrophages defend against foreign substances and microorganisms in as much as the peritoneal cavity is open to the uterus and vagina via the oviducts. In patients with uterine leiomyoma and patent Fallopian tubes, the total number of peritoneal macrophages is 6.8×10^6 on average (Figure 14.6a) and the percentage of exudate macrophages is 3.5 per cent (Figure 14.6b). The average total number of peritoneal macrophages in patients with bilateral tubal obstruction is 9.6×10^6, which is not significantly different from that in patients with uterine leiomyoma. Therefore, retrograde menstrual blood through the tubes into the peritoneal cavity, which is often observed at laparotomy or laparoscopy, is not a stimulus in the peritoneal cavity. In contrast, patients with carcinomatous peritonitis have 47.7×10^6 peritoneal macrophages and the percentage of exudate type is 50.2 per cent; consequently, this condition is interpreted as under stimulation.

3.2 Endometriosis and peritoneal macrophages

Endometriosis, defined as the presence of ectopic endometrial glands and stroma, is a common benign gynecological condition, but its pathogenesis remains controversial, with

(a)

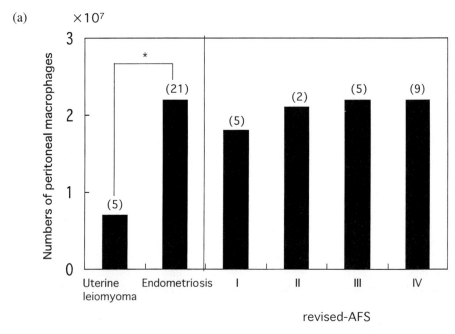

(b)

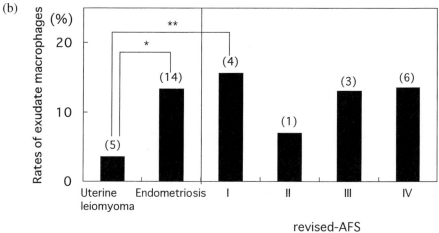

Fig. 14.6 (a) Total numbers of peritoneal macrophages in patients with pelvic endometriosis. *$P<0.025$. (b) Ratio of exudate macrophages to total peritoneal macrophages in patients with pelvic endometriosis. *$P<0.025$, **$P<0.005$. (From Fukumatsu *et al.*, 1992a, with permission of *Acta Obstetrica et Gynaecologica Japonica*.)

several theories having been put forward: the implantation theory; the metaplastic theory; and the combination theory. In all theories, peritoneal macrophages are considered to play a key role in the pathogenesis of this disease because the number of macrophages is increased in the peritoneal fluid of patients with pelvic endometriosis (Figure 14.6a) (Fukumatsu *et al.*, 1992a). In addition, the ratio of activated peritoneal macrophages is higher in patients with pelvic endometriosis than in those without (Fukumatsu *et al.*,

1992a). From studies of the ultrastructural localization of endogenous peroxidase in 14 patients with pelvic endometriosis (stage I, $n = 4$; stage II, $n = 1$; stage III, $n = 3$; stage IV, $n = 6$), the proportion of exudate macrophages was significantly larger than that in patients with uterine leiomyoma (Figure 14.6b; 13.3 per cent versus 3.5 per cent, $P < 0.025$) (Fukumatsu *et al.*, 1992a). The increase in exudate macrophages was observed even during the minimal stage of endometriosis (Figure 14.6b; 15.6 per cent versus 3.5 per cent, $P < 0.005$). Some likely functions of these activated peritoneal macrophages are the removal of sperm and the interference of ovum capture. It was reported that greater phagocytosis *in vitro* was seen in peritoneal macrophages isolated from women with endometriosis than those from fertile women or infertile women without endometriosis (Muscato *et al.*, 1982).

As a specific microenvironment, peritoneal fluid contains a large amount of cytokines/growth factors. Certain cytokines/growth factors, such as RANTES (Khorram *et al.*, 1993), transforming growth factor-β (TGF-β) (Oosterlynck *et al.*, 1994), TNF-α (Eisermann *et al.*, 1988) and monocyte chemoattractant protein-1 (MCP-1) (Akoum *et al.*, 1996; Arici *et al.*, 1997) have been suggested to induce infiltration of blood monocytes or macrophages into the pelvic cavity. However, the mechanisms that trigger their presence in the peritoneal cavity remain unresolved. A recent study demonstrated that MCP-1 protein is localized immunohistochemically in the glandular epithelium and stromal macrophages of peritoneal endometriotic lesions and that MCP-1 mRNA is also expressed in peritoneal endometriotic lesions, but not in normal pelvic peritoneum (Yih *et al.*, 2001). This suggests that endometriotic glandular epithelium and stromal macrophages are important sources of MCP-1 during the early stage of endometriotic development. Once these macrophages are recruited, they are stimulated further to secrete cytokines/growth factors, nitric oxide (NO) and other products that may influence the maintenance and progression of endometriosis. In infertile women with endometriosis, various studies reported that many different forms of cytokines/growth factors are increased in quantity (Burns and Schenken, 1999), most of which are derived from macrophages. Each cytokine/growth factor might be necessary to maintain the peritoneal cavity homeostasis if secreted in predetermined amounts. These soluble factors, however, may lead to infertility as well as endometriosis development. Some studies reported that the *in vitro* development of two-cell mouse embryos was significantly inhibited by the addition of endometriosis peritoneal fluid into the culture media, implying endometriosis-associated infertility derived from embryotoxic factors in peritoneal fluid (Morcos *et al.*, 1985; Prough *et al.*, 1990; Taketani *et al.*, 1992; Martinez-Roman *et al.*, 1997). Although endometriosis is definitely accompanied by a macrophage-mediated cytotoxicity, a wide variety of cytokines/growth factors and other substances make the pathogenesis of this disease difficult to clarify.

4 Macrophages in Fallopian tubes

Few studies of macrophages in the Fallopian tubes have been reported. However, macrophages are widely identifiable in the oviductal lumen and in the stroma and smooth muscle layer beneath the tubal epithelium during the reproductive period. During the post-menopausal period, very small numbers of macrophages were detected excluding chronic and granulomatous salpingitis or secondary peritoneal spread from carcinomas of the ovary or endometrium, where macrophages as well as lymphocytes and plasma cells are observed.

4.1 Macrophages in the oviductal lumen

Macrophages presumably migrate into the oviducts from the peritoneal cavity via the fimbrial ostia to reach the lumen. This is supported by the evidence that women with oviductal obstruction have far fewer macrophages in the oviductal lumen compared with normal women and that endometriosis patients have the highest numbers of these cells (Haney *et al.*, 1983). Macrophages make up more than 90 per cent of the cells in the oviductal lumen, with the remainder being lymphocytes (Haney *et al.*, 1983) (Figure 14.7a and b). These macrophages are indistinguishable from peritoneal macrophages by parameters such as activity of peroxidase and α-naphthyl butryrate esterase, adherence to plastic substrates, phagocytosis of latex spheres and Fc receptor-mediated phagocytois of IgG-coated sheep erythrocytes.

The cells surrounding oocytes and fertilized eggs recovered from human oviducts after ovulation are composed of macrophages, polynuclear leukocytes and red blood cells (Motta *et al.*, 1995). Similarly to the roles of ovarian macrophages in developing follicle and corpus luteum, macrophages seen among the cumulus cells may play a local role by modulating the steroid secretion of the neighboring granulosa cells (Motta *et al.*, 1995). The tubes are also the site of the fertilization of the ovum, the transport of gametes and the first cell division of the embryo. Since the development of mouse embryos is enhanced by co-culture with peritoneal macrophages (Honda *et al.*, 1994), macrophages in the oviductal lumen may exert their beneficial effects directly on embryonic develop-

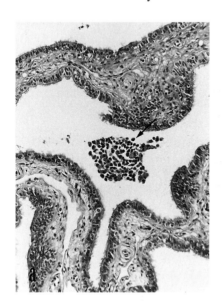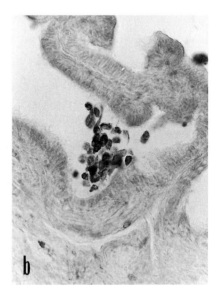

Fig. 14.7 Light micrograph and immunohistochemistry of macrophages within the lumen of the human Fallopian tube. During the secretory phase, mononuclear cells aggregate within the lumen of the Fallopian tube (a, arrow). Most of these cells are immunohistochemically positive for PM-1K, a monoclonal antibody against human monocyte/macrophage lineage cells (b). Hematoxylin and eosin stain (a); methyl green stain (b). Original magnification: ×30 (a); ×60 (b).

ment by cell–cell contact or indirectly by secretion of some embryotrophic substances. Conversely, macrophages could interfere with fertilization by engulfing and destroying normal sperm and gametes in the reproductive tract (Muscato *et al.*, 1982) or by lysing the antibody-coated sperm (London *et al.*, 1985).

4.2 Macrophages in the endosalpingeal stroma and smooth muscle layer

In 1998, the distribution and cytological characteristics of macrophages were first demonstrated within human oviductal tissue (Suenaga *et al.*, 1998). For immunohistochemical analysis, they used two monoclonal antibodies that were specific for human macrophages, namely PM-1K and PM-2K (Takeya *et al.*, 1991). PM-1K reacts with most members of monocyte/macrophage populations, corresponding to the commonly used macrophage antigen CD68. PM-2K identifies members of tissue macrophage populations and does not recognize peripheral blood monocytes. PM-1K-positive macrophages are always present in the tubal tissues and their number increases significantly during menstrual and early to mid-secretory phases (Figure 14.8). During the secretory phase, many cells of monocyte/macrophage lineage are present in the vascular lumen of the endosalpingeal stroma (Figure 14.9a), but the number of PM-2K-positive macrophages is small throughout the menstrual cycle (Figure 14.9b). During the secretory phase, macrophages ultrastructurally exhibit well-developed intracellular organelles, with only a few cytoplasmic vacuoles and granules, whereas during the menstrual phase they are characterized by cytoplasmic vacuoles and granules of various sizes and configurations.

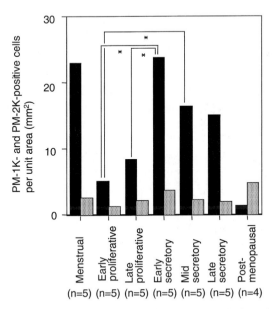

Fig. 14.8 Number of macrophages per unit area of the human Fallopian tube during the menstrual cycle. In 10 blocks along the long axis of the Fallopian tubes, the average numbers of the positive cells against PM-1K and PM-2K were calculated during various phases of the menstrual cycle. *$P <0.01$. Left: PM-1K-positive cells, right: PM-2K-positive cells. (From Suenaga *et al.*, 1998, with permission of *Acta Anatomica*.)

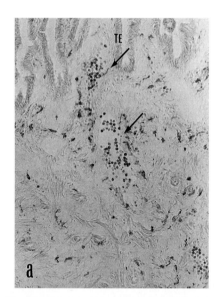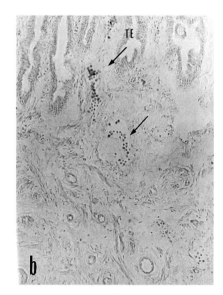

Fig. 14.9 Immunohistochemistry of macrophages located in the stroma of a human Fallopian tube. During the secretory phase, PM-1K-positive macrophages are distributed in the stroma and are also located within the vascular lumen (a, arrow). PM-2K-positive macrophages are a small population (b). TE: tubal epithelium. Methyl green stain. Original magnification: ×30 (a and b).

The role of these macrophages is not fully understood. The fine structures of tubal macrophages at the secretory phase suggest that they do not act as scavengers. During this period, the Fallopian tubes move by contraction of the smooth muscle to transport the ovum and fertilized egg through into the endometrial cavity. PGs might be produced by macrophages within the tubes and influence the smooth muscle contraction (Wilhelmsson *et al.*, 1979). However, macrophages during the menstrual phase may be involved in tissue remodeling of the tubal musculature. On the postpartum involution of the uterus, macrophages were shown to be involved in heterophagocytosis of the smooth muscle cells after their autophagocytosis (Henell *et al.*, 1983). Similarly, during this period, smooth muscle cells of the Fallopian tubes, just prior to menstruation, contain few cytoplasmic myofilaments and are characterized by electron-lucent and/or electron-dense, membrane-bound lysosomal-like granules in their cytoplasm (Fujii *et al.*, 1990); subsequently, lysosomal vacuoles and granules may be abundant in the cytoplasm of tubal macrophages during the menstrual period.

5 Endometrial/decidual macrophages

A significant number of macrophages are present in the uterine endometrium/decidua, and it is suggested that they play important role(s) in the pathophysiology of uterine function (Bulmer and Johnson, 1984). The level of macrophages is found to be relatively constant throughout the menstrual cycle in the human non-pregnant endometrium (Starkey *et al.*, 1991). Furthermore, macrophages appear as an influx of monocytes from the bone marrow into the decidua around the time of implantation. After the establishment of pregnancy, the most prominent population of basal endometrial stroma (decidua basalis) are macrophages, and they represent the largest fraction of intradecidual lymphoreticular cells (Diet *et al.*, 1992; Haller *et al.*, 1993). Macrophages during early and full-term pregnancy decidua are HLA-DR positive, and a substantial proportion also expresses DP and DQ antigens (Bulmer *et al.*, 1988a), suggesting that macrophages in decidua possess a function of antigen presentation similar to monocytes/macrophages in the peripheral blood.

5.1 Decidual macrophages and immunoregulation

During peri-implantation periods, trophoblast expression of major histocompatibility complex (MHC) and non-MHC antigens is shut off and both immunocompetent maternal cells, i.e. macrophages, dendritic cells, granulocytes, intra-epithelial lymphocytes and immunocytes, and lymphatics become sparse at the implantation site, and macrophages are abundant in decidua basalis and decidua parietalis throughout pregnancy and are closely associated with extravillous trophoblasts (Lea and Clark, 1991). After implantation, a novel population of lymphocytes, endometrial granulocytes or large granular lymphocytes (LGLs), increases very rapidly in the maternal decidual tissue. The exact role(s) of LGLs in the pregnant uterus have not been fully elucidated. However, it is suggested that interactions between decidual LGLs and macrophages, possibly mediated by soluble factors, could play a role in regulating interferon-γ (IFN-γ) secretion at the feto-maternal interface and thus contribute to the control of invasion by the fetal trophoblasts (Marzusch *et al.*, 1997). Decidual macrophages may also be attributed with an immunosuppressive function due to the secretion of PGE$_2$ (Bulmer *et al.*, 1988b). *In vitro* studies have shown that macrophages separated from early pregnancy decidua have a capacity for allo-antigen presentation and a lower capacity to produce IL-1 than their peripheral counterparts (Mizuno *et al.*, 1994). In addition, decidual macrophages produce suppressive factor(s) and exhibit a higher suppressive activity on mixed lymphocyte reactions than peripheral monocytes (Mizuno *et al.*, 1994). These findings suggest that macrophages in decidua are sufficiently activated and have roles in local immune regulation as well as controlling fetal trophoblast development and invasion into the uterus. On the other hand, these cells may be important as phagocytes and as producers of extracellular enzymes for tissue remodeling (Padykula, 1981) because ultrastructurally they have many lysosomal granules and their long cytoplasmic processes penetrate into the decidual cells with complicated interdigitations between the macrophages and decidual cells (Figure 14.10).

Macrophages in decidua also produce important substances for pregnancy maintenance or parturition. Renin, a key molecule for the generation of angiotensin II, which regulates blood pressure and fluid/electrolyte homeostasis, is known to be secreted in the endometrium. Elevated plasma renin levels during pregnancy are caused by decidua (Shaw *et al.*, 1989), and it has been revealed that macrophages in decidua express renin mRNA (Jikihara *et al.*, 1995). Platelet-activating factor (PAF) plays an important role in implantation and parturition, and a potent PAF inactivator, PAF-acetylhydrolase, is produced by macrophages in decidua (Narahara *et al.*, 1993). These findings suggest that uterine function during pregnancy might be regulated, at least partly, by macrophages distributed in decidua.

In mice, macrophages are distributed in the endometrium during the estrous cycle and early pregnancy, but there is no change in number before pregnancy, and after pregnancy

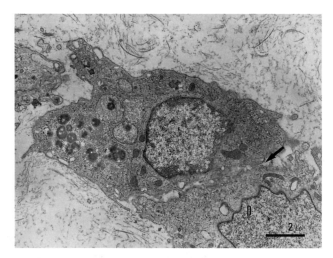

Fig. 14.10 Electron micrograph of a human decidual macrophage. The cytoplasm contains numerous lysosomes, a Golgi apparatus and rough endoplasmic reticulum. Close cell contact is noted between the macrophage and decidual cell (arrow). Eight weeks of gestation. D: decidual cell. Lead citrate and uranyl acetate stain. Original magnification: ×3500.

a significant increase in macrophage density is noted during the first stage of pregnancy (Hunt *et al.*, 1985; De *et al.*, 1991). During early pregnancy, large numbers of macrophages are observed near epithelial glands, indicating that an inflammatory-like cellular response occurs in the uterus at peri-implantation periods (De *et al.*, 1991). Macrophages are virtually absent from anti-mesometrial decidual tissue until degenerating tissue is invaded by macrophages from about day 15 of pregnancy. The metrial gland contains many macrophages until degeneration sets in, but few are seen by day 15 (Brandon, 1995). In parallel with decidualization, the density of macrophages appears to decline in the decidua with advancing gestation, and this change is due to a dilution of the macrophage population rather than a loss of individual cells, implying that macrophages do not play a major regulatory role in the success of murine pregnancy (Stewart and Mitchell, 1991). However, the significance of macrophages in the pathological situation of early embryo loss has been suggested by the study of mouse abortion models. In the resorption-prone mating of CBA/J female and DBA/2 male mice, significantly elevated numbers of macrophages are seen at the feto-maternal interface, and poly(I:C) treatment, which induces more embryo resorption in this model, shows a further increase in macrophages (Duclos *et al.*, 1994). In an endotoxin lipopolysaccharide (LPS)-induced abortion model, a moderate increase in macrophage numbers occurs in the uterus, although there is no change in their tissue distribution (Wang *et al.*, 1998). The presence of activated macrophages at implantation sites before overt embryo damage is known, and overall expression of class II MHC gene products increases in maternal and fetal tissues (Wang *et al.*, 1998). In addition, increased release of TNF-α in decidua associated with abortion was noted, which suggested that abortion may arise from infiltration/activation of scavenger cells from decidua that are likely to be macrophages (Lea *et al.*, 1998). Recently, the role of NO in early embryo loss has been suggested, and cells in decidua positive for inducible NO synthase (iNOS) in implantation sites were shown to be macrophages (Haddad *et al.*, 1995). It was also reported that IFN-γ is required for the LPS-induced abortion model in mice and that decidual macrophages from IFN-γ-deficient mice are more resistant to LPS-induced embryo loss than the wild-ype (Haddad *et al.*, 1997a). IFN-γ mRNA in macrophages is expressed simultaneously in the same embryos that also express mRNA for TNF-α and iNOS, and spontaneously increased decidual IFN-γ expression is detrimental to embryo survival (Haddad *et al.*, 1997b).

5.2 Macrophages in spiral arteries of the placental bed

As described previously, macrophages are greatly increased in number at the implantation site where they are in close contact with invasive trophoblast cells and are thought to control the invasion of trophoblasts in the decidual and myometrial segments of spiral arteries (Brosens *et al.*, 1967). Endovascular replacement by trophoblasts is essential for the maintenance of an adequate choriodecidual blood flow during normal pregnancy. In the placental bed of pre-eclamptic pregnancies, endovascular trophoblasts are restricted to the media of spiral arteries in the inner third of the myometrium, and the normal physiological changes are absent (Brosens *et al.*, 1972). Instead, the infiltration of large sized foamy macrophages is accompanied by the fibrinoid necrosis of spiral arteries (Figure 14.11a). Ultrastructurally, the smooth muscle cells and connective tissues underneath the endothelium are replaced with an electron-dense amorphous matrix. The cytoplasm of infiltrating macrophages is characterized by various sized myelinsomes, cholesterol crystals and lipid droplets (Figure 14.11b). Neutral fat and phospholipids were shown histochemically in their cytoplasm, suggesting that these macrophages may phagocytose and digest the degenerating smooth muscle tissues in arterionecrosis.

6 Villous macrophages (Hofbauer cells)

Peculiar vacuolated cells in the mesenchymal stroma of human chorionic villi were described for the first time at the end of the 19th century (Kastschenko, 1885) and have

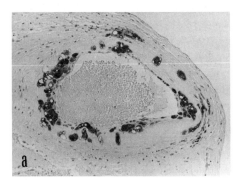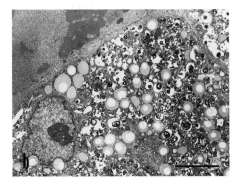

Fig. 14.11 Immunohistochemistry and electron micrograph of macrophages in the spiral artery of a patient with pre-eclampsia. (a) Large macrophages, CD68+, are infiltrated into the fibrinoid necrosis area of the spiral artery. (b) Ultrastructurally, they are 35–45 μm in size and characterized by numerous various sized granules and small lipid droplets in the cytoplasm. Thirty-eight weeks of gestation. Methyl green stain (a); lead citrate and uranyl acetate stain (b). Original magnification: ×10 (a); ×1750 (b).

been recognized as Hofbauer cells since 1903 (Hofbauer, 1903). In the second half of the 20th century, many investigators reported that these cells share ultrastructural, histochemical or immunohistochemical similarities with tissue macrophages (Boyd and Hamilton, 1970; Enders and King 1970; Katabuchi *et al.*, 1989b).

6.1 Cytological characteristics

Human villous macrophages are classified ultrastructurally into three types (Katabuchi *et al.*, 1989b). The first type of cells has few or no cytoplasmic vacuoles or granules. They are divided further into two subtypes: immature and mature. The immature cells are smaller than the other cell types. They contain poorly developed organelles in addition to polyribosomes and micropinocytotic vesicles, and their cytoplasmic processes are inconspicuous. The mature cells have copious cytoplasm and their intracytoplasmic organelles, including lysosomes, are well developed. They extend thin pseudopodia. The second type of cells are characterized by many cytoplasmic vacuoles of various sizes, thus agreeing with the cytological features of so-called Hofbauer cells. A single-unit membrane delimits the vacuoles, which appear to be empty or electron-lucent. The third type of cells are filled with numerous membrane-bound granules in the cytoplasm. These granules vary in size and in the degree of homogenous osmiophilia, and are histochemically ceroid. The vacuoles and granules are lysosomal in nature because they are proven positive by the demonstration of acid phosphatase. The immature cells increase in number during the early stage of gestation, the vacuolated cells predominate by the middle stage, and the mature cells exist persistently during the later stage. The granule-bearing cells appear through all stages, but only as a minor population.

Villous macrophages of all three types show adherence to plastic dishes, phagocytosis of latex particles and immune phagocytosis. α-Naphthyl butyrate esterase activity is demonstrated on their cell membrane, but not in the cytoplasmic vacuoles or granules. They have little or no endogenous peroxidase or lysozyme activities.

6.2 Origin

As for the origin of the fetal macrophages in the chorionic villi, some studies have suggested that they are derived from blood monocytes (Moskalewski *et al.*, 1975; King, 1987). However, no members of the monocytic or myeloid series have been recognized during the early stage of gestation when intravascular hematopoiesis occurs in the human placenta. Although macrophages are derived from monocytes originating in bone marrow hematopoiesis during postnatal life, macrophages during fetal life are known to emerge first in blood islands of the yolk sac and are differentiated from immature primitive macrophages (Takahashi and Naito, 1993).

In mouse placenta, no promonocytes or monocytes are detected in blood vessels. Primitive macrophages first appear in the mouse placenta at 10 days of gestation, then differentiate and mature into fetal macrophages (Takahashi *et al.*, 1991). This development of the primitive/fetal macrophage clusters and colonies in the mouse placenta was confirmed by culture experiments of mouse placental cell suspensions with the bone marrow stromal cell line, ST2, which is useful for investigating hematopoiesis and ontogeny *in vitro* (Ogawa *et al.*, 1988). In the soft agar culture of cell suspensions from the mouse placenta with LP3-conditioned medium, colony-forming cells were confirmed from 10 to 16 days of gestation (Takahashi *et al.*, 1991). Compared with that in the yolk sac, granulocyte/macrophage colony formation is poor in the placenta and reaches its peak 3 days after the maximal stage of yolk sac hematopoiesis at 10 days of gestation. Rather than originating from monocytes in the bone marrow, at least during the early gestational stage, human villous macrophages also travel via the circulation from immature macrophages that originate in the yolk sac (Takahashi *et al.*, 1991). During the late gestational stage, however, the monocyte/macrophage population may appear in the vessel cavities of the chorionic villi and form a different phenotype of villous macrophages.

6.3 Function

The biological roles of these macrophages are still a matter of controversy. Macrophages may be important local regulators of water, electrolytes and proteins within the core of chorionic villi (Enders and King, 1970), because vacuolated macrophages are observed mainly during the early to middle stages of gestation. Since placenta is an immunologically privileged organ and plays a major role in protecting the fetus against maternal infections and antifetal immune reactions, it has been proposed that they serve as a trap for the removal of harmful elements such as bacteria, viruses or antigen–antibody complexes (Wood and King, 1982). Since the early 1980s, cytokines have been clearly recognized to provide a major soluble intercellular signaling network in every organ of the human body. In the placenta, much attention has also been directed towards an extensive network of cytokines that are released from macrophages and other cells. In addition, their biological relationship has been clarified recently on the basis of the anatomically close location of trophoblasts and villous macrophages.

6.3.1 Villous macrophages and trophoblast growth and differentiation

Mononuclear cytotrophoblast cells form terminally differentiated syncytiotrophoblast cells. *In vitro*, cytotrophoblast cells in serum-free conditions fail to aggregate or fuse, whereas they fuse spontaneously to form multinucleated cells and concomitantly produce human chorionic gonadotropin (hCG) when cultured in medium supplemented with fetal bovine serum (Kliman *et al.*, 1986). Furthermore, cytotrophoblast cells cultured in medium containing serum from pregnant women progress to an advanced stage of trophoblast differentiation (Douglas and King, 1990). Recent investigations have shown that recombinant cytokines and growth factors, including M-CSF (Daiter *et al.*, 1992), EGF (Morrish *et al.*, 1987), vascular endothelial growth factor (VEGF) (Sharkey *et al.*, 1993) and leukemia inhibitory factor (Nachtigall *et al.*, 1996), are expressed in human placenta and/or stimulate the differentiation of trophoblasts *in vitro*. In contrast, TNF-α (Ohashi *et al.*, 1992) and TGF-β (Morrish *et al.*, 1991) are known to inhibit the differentiation of trophoblasts and their hCG secretion. The large panel of cytokines within the placental cytokine network is still in a phase of discovery and research.

More recently, a greater proliferation of cytotrophoblast cells was observed at 24 h of culture when they were cultured in villous macrophage-conditioned media than in fetal calf serum-containing media, and the numbers of aggregates were greater in villous macrophage-conditioned media than fetal calf serum-containing media at 24, 48 and 72 h of culture (Khan *et al.*, 2000a). Concentrations of both hCG and human placental lactogen (hPL) in the culture supernatants were increased at each 24 h interval over 4 days, with the concentrations at 96 h being approximately six-(hCG) and 1.5-fold (hPL) higher in villous macrophage-conditioned media than in the peritoneal macrophage-conditioned media (Figure 14.12) (Khan *et al.*, 2000a). Moreover, M-CSF and VEGF concentrations were significantly higher in villous macrophage-conditioned media than in peritoneal macrophage-conditioned media, whereas the MCP-1 concentration was higher in peritoneal macrophage-conditioned media (Figure 14.13a) (Khan *et al.*, 2000a). In accordance with the secretory pattern of the three cytokines, mRNAs of M-CSF and VEGF were

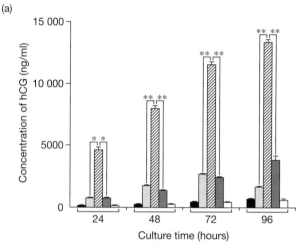

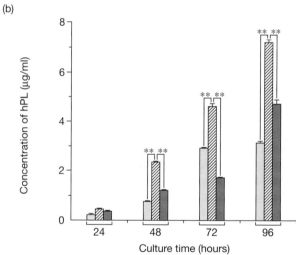

Fig. 14.12　hCG (a) and hPL (b) production from human trophoblast cells in five different culture media. *P<0.05, **P<0.001. (a) From left to right, bars represent serum-free media, 10 per cent fetal calf serum-containing media, villous macrophage culture supernatant-supplemented media, peritoneal macrophage culture supernatant-supplemented media and villous fibroblast culture supernatant-supplemented media, respectively. (b) From left to right, bars represent 10 per cent fetal calf serum-containing media, villous macrophage culture supernatant-supplemented media and peritoneal macrophage culture supernatant-supplemented media, respectively. (From Khan *et al.*, 2000a, with permission of *Biology of Reproduction*.)

strongly expressed in villous macrophages compared with those in peritoneal macrophages; in contrast, the expression of MCP-1 was stronger in peritoneal macrophages than in villous macrophages (Figure 14.13b). Taken together, it appears that villous macrophages may play a leading role in the production and secretion of some specific cytokines for the proliferation and differentiation of trophoblasts.

6.3.2 Villous macrophages and hCG degradation

Based on the use of a histochemical technique, it was reported that hCG possibly was synthesized by macrophages in human chorionic villi (Prosdocimi, 1953). However, more

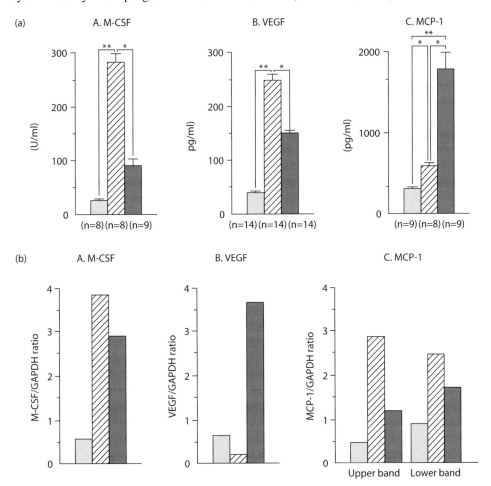

Fig. 14.13   (a) M-CSF, VEGF and MCP-1 concentrations in human villous and peritoneal macrophages. Concentrations of the three cytokines were measured after cells were cultured in serum-free media for 48 h. *P <0.05, **P <0.001. From left to right, bars represent villous fibroblast, villous macrophage and peritoneal macrophage. (b) mRNA expression of M-CSF, VEGF and MCP-1 in human villous and peritoneal macrophages. After reverse transcriptase–polymerase chain reaction (RT–PCR), ratios of each cytokine mRNA to GAPDH (glyceraldehyde-3-phosphate dehydrogenase) mRNA were calculated by computer analysis. From left to right side, bars represent whole chorinionic villi, villous macrophages and peritoneal macrophages. (From Khan *et al.*, 2000a, with permission of *Biology of Reproduction*.)

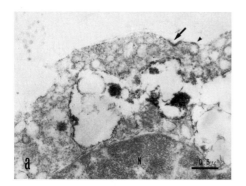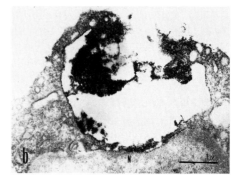

Fig. 14.14 Electron micrograph of immunoreaction products of hCG-β in a human villous macrophage. (a) HCG-β-immunoreactive products are localized in a coated pit (arrow), a coated vesicle (arrowhead) and fused multivesicular bodies of a villous macrophage. (b) Immunoreactivity is also evident within the cytoplasmic vacuole. Eight weeks of gestation. Uranyl acetate stain. N: nucleus. Original magnification: ×6000 (a and b). (From Katabuchi *et al.*, 1994, with permission of *Endocrine Journal.*)

recently, it was clearly demonstrated that they are immunohistochemically positive for the hCG-β subunit (hCG-β), but not for hCG-β C-terminal peptide (Katabuchi *et al.*, 1989b, 1994). Immunoreaction products of hCG-β were localized in coated pits, coated vesicles and multivesicular bodies (Figure 14.14a), and also within cytoplasmic vacuoles and granules (Figure 14.14b) (Katabuchi *et al.*, 1994). As reported previously (Katabuchi *et al.*, 1994), the hCG-positive vacuoles or granules show acid phosphatase activity, suggesting that villous macrophages may take up and degrade hCG locally before it enters the circulation after being secreted from trophoblasts. When isolated peritoneal macrophages are cultured in intact hCG-containing medium, the concentration of intact hCG in the supernatant decreases with time, while the concentrations of free hCG-β and hCG-β core fragment (β-CF) increase (Figure 14.15) (Khan *et al.*, 2000b). In the macrophage cytosol, the concentrations of intact hCG, free hCG-β and β-CF increase time dependently (Figure 14.15) (Khan *et al.*, 2000b). In addition, a β-CF-like substance is found in the vesicle fluid from patients with complete hydatidiform moles (Khan *et al.*, 2000b). The molar fluid β-CF was distinguishable from the β-CF in patients' urine by immunoreactivity and by elution profile on gel chromatography (Khan *et al.*, 2000b). Immunohistochemistry with anti-β-CF antibody shows a strong immunoreaction in the cytoplasm of macrophages in normal chorionic villi as well as in the molar villous stroma. The hCG/LH receptor could not be defined in villous macrophage suspension by hCG radioreceptor binding assay (Katabuchi *et al.*, 1994). However, our preliminary study has identified the presence of lectin domain-lacking hCG/LH receptor (data not shown), which was found previously in rat ovaries, but its role was not clarified (Aatsinki *et al.*, 1992). Although further studies should be performed to elucidate the exact mechanism of hCG ingestion by villous macrophages, the hCG/LH receptor isoforms on macrophages could be involved in the regulatory action of glycoprotein hormones because macrophage membrane receptors play a crucial role in biological functions such as endocytosis, altered gene expression or synthesis and release of tropic and cytotoxic products.

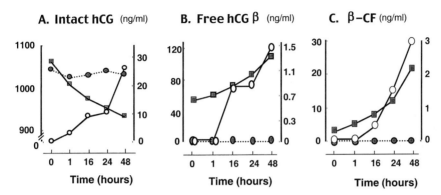

Fig. 14.15 Levels of hCG molecules in culture supernatant and cell cytosol from human peritoneal macrophages cultured with intact hCG. Peritoneal macrophages were plated at 1×10^6 per well in a culture dish and incubated in serum-free medium containing 10 µg/ml of intact hCG. (From Khan *et al.*, 2000b, with permission of *Placenta*.)

7 Summary

Macrophages are widely distributed in organs and tissues of the female genital tract and constitute an extremely versatile population of cells. Macrophages are present throughout the ovarian cycle and participate in the development and atresia of follicles and the progression and regression of luteal tissues. In particular, they may be indirectly involved in folliculogenesis and luteinization via a paracrine pathway and/or directly by cell contact with granulosa cells. Without any pathological conditions, macrophages are a predominant population of the peritoneal cavity and are classified into four types according to their ultracytochemical localization of endogenous peroxidase activity. Once the pelvic microenvironment is changed into a stimulated condition such as endometriosis, the exudate macrophages, one of the four types, is increased in number as an activated form and their cytokines/growth factors may cause cytotoxicity to sperm and ova. Macrophages located within the lumen of Fallopian tubes can play a role in the fertilization of ova, the transport of gametes and the development of the embryo; moreover, macrophages distributed in the endosalpingeal stroma and smooth muscle layer have dual functions of embryonal benefit and tubal tissue remodeling within a specific period of the menstrual cycle. Decidual macrophages also have many important roles during pregnancy and, in mice and probably in humans, products from activated macrophages in decidua may act in concert to destroy actively proliferating fetal tissues under some pathological circumstances. Macrophages in the chorionic villi are a major source of cytokines/growth factors and as yet undefined substances for the proliferation and differentiation of trophoblast cells. They also act as a local regulator of gonadotropic hormones by degrading hCG.

Macrophages are usually involved in sequential reproductive events: folliculogenesis, fertilization, implantation and gestation, and perform a vast array of physiological functions. Their distribution, structure and functional properties may be influenced by organ specificity and the local microenvironment including hormonal stimuli and immunological tolerance. Further studies are required to develop clinical therapies via a macrophage–cytokine system for treatment of pathophysiological conditions associated with female fertility and infertility, and the maintenance and termination of pregnancy.

References

Aatsinki, J.T., Pietilä, E.M., Lakkakorpi, J.T. and Rajaniemi, H.J. (1992). Expression of the LH/CG receptor gene in rat ovarian tissue is regulated by an extensive alternative splicing of the primary transcript. *Molecular and Cellular Endocrinology*, **84**, 127–35.

Adashi, E.Y. (1993). The intraovarian insulin-like growth factor system. In Adashi, E.Y. and Leung, P.C.K. (ed.), *The Ovary*. Raven Press, New York, pp. 319–35.

Adashi, E.Y. (1996). Immune modulators in the context of the ovulatory process: a role for interleukin-1. *American Journal of Reproductive Immunology*, **35**, 190–4.

Adashi, E.Y., Resnick, C.E., Packman, J.N., Hurwitz, A. and Payne, D.W. (1990). Cytokine-mediated regulation of ovarian function: tumor necrosis factor-α inhibits gonadotropin-supported progesterone accumulation by differentiating and luteinized murine granulosa cells. *American Journal of Obstetrics and Gynecology*, **162**, 889–96.

Akoum, A., Lemay, A., McColl, S., Turcot-Lemay, L. and Maheux, R. (1996). Elevated concentration and biologic activity of monocyte chemotactic protein-1 in the peritoneal fluid of patients with endometriosis. *Fertility and Sterility*, **66**, 17–23.

Araki, M., Fukumatsu, Y., Katabuchi, H., Shultz, L.D., Takahashi, K. and Okamura, H. (1996). Follicular development and ovulation in macrophage colony-stimulating factor-deficient mice homozygous for the osteopetrosis (*op*) mutation. *Biology of Reproduction*, **54**, 478–84.

Arceci, R.J., Pampfer, S. and Pollard, J.W. (1992). Expression of CSF-1/c-*fms* and SF/c-*kit* mRNA during preimplantation mouse development. *Developmental Biology*, **151**, 1–8.

Arici, A., Oral, E., Attar, E., Tazuke, S.I. and Olive, D.L. (1997). Monocyte chemotactic protein-1 concentration in peritoneal fluid of women with endometriosis and its modulation of expression in mesothelial cells. *Fertility and Sterility*, **67**, 1065–72.

Bagavandoss, P., Kunkel, S.L., Wiggins, R.C. and Keyes, P.L. (1988). Tumor necrosis factor-α (TNF-α) production and localization of macrophages and T lymphocytes in the rabbit corpus luteum. *Endocrinology*, **122**, 1185–7.

Benyo, D.F. and Pate, J.L. (1992). Tumor necrosis factor-α alters bovine luteal cell synthetic capacity and viability. *Endocrinology*, **130**, 854–60.

Boyd, J.D. and Hamilton, W.J. (1970). *The Human Placenta*. Heffer, Cambridge, pp. 228–39.

Brandon, J.M. (1995). Macrophage distribution in decidual tissue from early implantation to the periparturient period in mice as defined by the macrophage differentiation antigens F4/80, macrosialin and the type 3 complement receptor. *Journal of Reproduction and Fertility*, **103**, 9–16.

Brosens, I., Robertson, W.B. and Dixon, H.G. (1967). The physiological response of the vessels of the placental bed to normal pregnancy. *Journal of Pathology and Bacteriology*, **93**, 569–79.

Brosens, I., Robertson, W.B. and Dixon, H.G. (1972). The role of the spiral arteries in the pathogenesis of pre-eclampsia. *Obstetrics and Gynecology Annual*, **1**, 177–91.

Bulmer, D. (1964). The histochemistry of ovarian macrophages in the rat. *Journal of Anatomy (London)*, **98**, 313–9.

Bulmer, J.N. and Johnson, P.M. (1984). Macrophage populations in the human placenta and amnio-chorion. *Clinical and Experimental Immunology*, **57**, 393–403.

Bulmer, J.N., Morrison, L. and Smith, J.C. (1988a). Expression of class II MHC gene products by macrophages in human uteroplacental tissue. *Immunology*, **63**, 707–14.

Bulmer, J.N., Pace, D. and Ritson, A. (1988b). Immunoregulatory cells in human decidua: morphology, immunohistochemistry and function. *Reproduction, Nutrition, Development*, **28**, 1599–613.

Burgaleta, C., Territo, M.C., Quan, S.G. and Golde, D.W. (1978). Glucan-activated macrophages: functional characteristics and surface morphology. *Journal of the Reticuloendothelial Society*, **23**, 195–204.

Burns, W.N. and Schenken, R.S. (1999). Pathophysiology of endometriosis-associated infertility. *Clinical Obstetrics and Gynecology*, **42**, 586–610.

Daiter, E. Pampfer, S., Yeung, Y.G., Barad, D., Stanley, E.R. and Pollard, J.W. (1992). Expression of colony-stimulating factor-1 in the human uterus and placenta. *Journal of Clinical Endocrinology and Metabolism*, **74**, 850–8.

De, M., Choudhuri, R. and Wood, G.W. (1991). Determination of the number and distribution of macrophages, lymphocytes, and granulocytes in the mouse uterus from mating through implantation. *Journal of Leukocyte Biology*, **50**, 252–62.

Dietl, J., Ruck, P., Horny, H.P., Handgrentinger, R., Marzusch, K., Ruck, M. *et al.* (1992). The decidua of early human pregnancy: immunohistochemistry and function of immunocompetent cells. *Gynecologic and Obstetric Investigation*, **33**, 197–204.

Douglas, G.C. and King, B.F. (1990). Differentiation of human trophoblast cells *in vitro* as revealed by immunocytochemical staining of desmoplakin and nuclei. *Journal of Cell Science*, **96**, 131–41.

Duclos, A.J., Pomerantz, D.K. and Baines, M.G. (1994). Relationship between decidual leukocyte infiltration and spontaneous abortion in a murine model of early fetal resorption. *Cellular Immunology*, **159**, 184–93.

Eisermann, J, Gast, M.J., Pineda, J., Odem, R.R. and Collins, J.L. (1988). Tumor necrosis factor in peritoneal fluid of women undergoing laparoscopic surgery. *Fertility and Sterility*, **50**, 573–9.

Enders, A.C. and King, B.F. (1970). The cytology of Hofbauer cells. *Anatomical Record*, **167**, 231–52.

Fujii, S., Konishi, I., Katabuchi, H. and Okamura H. (1990). Ultrastructure of smooth muscle tissue in the female genital tract: uterus and oviduct. In Motta, P.M. (ed.), *Ultrastructure of Smooth Muscle*. Kluwer Academic Publishers, Dordrecht, pp. 197–220.

Fukumatsu, Y. Katabuchi, H., Miyamura, S., Matsuura, K. and Okamura, H. (1991). Peritoneal macrophages in endometriosis. In Hafez, E.S.E. (ed.), *Assisted Human Reproductive Technology*. Hemisphere Publishing Corporation, New York, pp.112–9.

Fukumatsu, Y., Katabuchi, S., Miyamura, S., Matsuura, K., Okamura, H., Naito, M. *et al.* (1992a). Activated macrophages in the peritoneal fluid of women with endometriosis: examination of the intracytoplasmic localization of endogenous peroxidase and interleukin-1. *Acta Obstetrica et Gynaecologica Japonica*, **44**, 529–36.

Fukumatsu, Y., Katabuchi, H., Naito, M., Takeya, M., Takahashi, K. and Okamura, H. (1992b). Effect of macrophages on proliferation of granulosa cells in the ovary in rats. *Journal of Reproduction and Fertility*, **96**, 241–9.

Fukumatsu, Y., Katabuchi, H. and Okamura, H. (1995). Immunohistochemical localization of epidermal growth factor and its effect on granulosa cell proliferation in rat ovary. *Endocrine Journal*, **42**, 467–73.

Haddad, E.K., Duclos, A.J., Antecka, E., Lapp, W.S. and Baines, M.G. (1997a). Role of interferon-γ in the priming of decidual macrophages for nitric oxide production and early pregnancy loss. *Cell Immunology*, **181**, 68–75.

Haddad, E.K., Duclos, A.J., Lapp, W.S. and Baines, M.G. (1997b). Early embryo loss is associated with the prior expression of macrophage activation markers in the decidua. *Journal of Immunology*, **158**, 4886–92.

Haddad, E.K., Duclos, A.J. and Baines, M.G. (1995). Early embryo loss is associated with local production of nitric oxide by decidual mononuclear cells. *Journal of Experimental Medicine*, **182**, 1143–51.

Haller, H., Radillo, O., Rukavina, D., Tedesco, F., Candussi, G., Petrovic, O. *et al.* (1993). An immunohistochemical study of leucocytes in human endometrium, first and third trimester basal decidua. *Journal of Reproductive Immunology*, **23**, 41–9.

Halme, J., Hammond, M.G., Syrop, C.H., and Talbert, L.M. (1985). Peritoneal macrophages modulate human granulosa-luteal cell progesterone production. *Journal of Clinical Endocrinology and Metabolism*, **61**, 912–6.

Haney, A.F., Misukonis, M.A. and Weinberg, J.B. (1983). Macrophages and infertility: oviductal macrophages as potential mediators of infertility. *Fertility and Sterility*, **39**, 310–5.

Henell, F., Ericsson, J.L. and Glaumann, H. (1983). An electron microscopic study of the post-partum involution of the rat uterus. With a note on apparent crinophagy of collagen. *Virchows Archiv B*, **42**, 271–87.

Hofbauer, J. (1903). Ueber das konstante Vorkommen bisher unbekannter zelliger Formelemente in der Chorionzotte der menschlichen Plazenta und über Embryotrophe. *Wiener Klinishe Wochenschrift*, **16**, 871–3.

Honda, R., Matsuura, K., Fukumatsu, Y., Kawano, T. and Okamura H. (1994). *In-vitro* enhancement of mouse embryonic development by co-culture with peritoneal macrophages. *Human Reproduction*, **9**, 692–6.

Hunt, J.S., Manning, L.S., Mitchell, D., Slanders, J.R. and Wood, G.W. (1985). Localization and characterization of macrophages in murine uterus. *Journal of Leukocyte Biology*, **38**, 255–65.

Jikihara, H., Poisner, A.M., Hirsch, R. and Handwerger, S. (1995). Human uterine decidual macrophages express renin. *Journal of Clinical Endocrinology and Metabolism*, **80**, 1273–7.

Kastschenko, N. (1885). Das menschliche Chorionepithel und dessen Rolle bei der Histogenese der Plazenta. *Archiv Anatomical Physiology (Leipzig)*, 451–80.

Katabuchi, H., Fukumatsu, Y. and Okamura, H. (1989a). Immunohistochemical and morphological observations of macrophages in the human ovary. In Hirshfield, A.N. (ed.), *Growth Factors and the Ovary*. Plenum Publishing Corporation, New York, pp. 409–13.

Katabuchi, H., Naito, M., Miyamura, S., Takahashi, K. and Okamura, H. (1989b). Macrophages in human chorionic villi. *Progress in Clinical and Biological Research*, **296**, 453–8.

Katabuchi, H., Fukumatsu, Y., Araki, M., Mizutani, H., Ohba, T. and Okamura, H. (1994). Localization of chorionic gonadotropin in macrophages of the human chorionic villi. *Endocrine Journal*, **41**, 141–53.

Katabuchi, H., Fukumatsu, Y., Araki, M., Suenaga, Y., Ohtake, H. and Okamura, H. (1996). Role of macrophages in ovarian follicular development. *Hormone Research*, **46** Supplement 1, 45–51.

Katabuchi, H., Suenaga, Y., Fukumatsu, Y. and Okamura, H. (1997). Distribution and fine structure of macrophages in the human ovary during the menstrual cycle, pregnancy and menopause. *Endocrine Journal*, **44**, 785–95.

Khan, S., Katabuchi, H., Araki, M., Nishimura, R. and Okamura, H. (2000a). Human villous macrophage-conditioned media enhance human trophoblast growth and differentiation *in vitro*. *Biology of Reproduction*, **62**, 1075–83.

Khan, S., Katabuchi, H., Araki, M., Ohba, T., Koizumi, T., Okamura, H. *et al.*, (2000b). The molar vesicle fluid contains the b-core fragment of human chorionic gonadotropin. *Placenta*, **21**, 79–87.

Khorram, O., Taylor, R.N., Ryan, I.P., Schall, T.J. and Landers, D.V. (1993). Peritoneal fluid concentrations of the cytokine RANTES correlate with the severity of endometriosis. *American Journal of Obstetrics and Gynecology*, **169**, 1545–9.

King, B.F. (1987). Ultrastructural differentiation of stromal and vascular components in early macaque placental villi. *American Journal of Anatomy*, **178**, 30–44.

Kirsch, T.M., Friedman, A.C., Vogel, R.L. and Flickinger, G.L. (1981). Macrophages in corpora lutea of mice: characterization and effects on steroid secretion. *Biology of Reproduction*, **25**,629–38.

Kliman, H.J., Nestler, J.E., Sermasi, E., Sanger, J.M. and Strauss. J.F., III (1986). Purification, characterization and *in vitro* differentiation of cytotrophoblasts from human term placentae. *Endocrinology*, **118**, 1567–82.

Lea, R.G. and Clark, D.A. (1991). Macrophages and migratory cells in endometrium relevant to implantation. *Baillieres Clinical Obstetrics and Gynecology*, **5**, 25–59.

Lea, R.G., McIntyre, S., Baird, J.D. and Clark, D.A. (1998). Tumor necrosis factor-α mRNA-positive cells in spontaneous resorption in rodents. *American Journal of Reproductive Immunology*, **39**, 50–7.

Lobel, B.L., Rosenbaum, R.M. and Deane, H.W. (1961). Enzymic correlates of physiological regression of follicles and corpora lutea in ovaries of normal rats. *Endocrinology*, **68**, 232–47.

London, S.N., Haney, A.F. and Weinberg, J.B. (1985). Macrophages and infertility: enhancement of human macrophage-mediated sperm killing by antisperm antibodies. *Fertility and Sterility*, **43**, 274–8.

Martinez-Roman, S., Balasch, J., Creus, M., Fabregues, F., Carmona, F., Vilella, R. *et al.* (1997). Immunological factors in endometriosis-associated reproductive failure: studies in fertile and infertile women with and without endometriosis. *Human Reproduction*, **12**, 1794–9.

Marzusch, K., Buchholz, F., Ruck, P., Handgretinger, R., Geiselhart, A., Engelmann, L. *et al.* (1997). Interleukin-12- and interleukin-2-stimulated release of interferon-γ by uterine CD56++ large granular lymphocytes is amplified by decidual macrophages. *Human Reproduction*, **12**, 921–4.

Matsuyama, S., Ohta, M. and Takahashi, M. (1987). The critical period in which splenectomy causes functional disorder of the ovary in adult rats. *Endocrinologica Japonica*, **34**, 849–55.

Miyamura, S., Okamura, H., Naito, M. and Takahashi, K. (1987). Ultracytochemical localization of peroxidase activity in human peritoneal macrophages. *Journal of Clinical Electron Microscopy*, **20**, 449–450.

Mizuno, M., Aoki, K. and Kinbara, T. (1994). Functions of macrophages in human decidual tissue in early pregnancy. *American Journal of Reproductive Immunology*, **31**, 180–8.

Morcos, R.N., Gibbons, W.E. and Findley, W.E. (1985). Effect of peritoneal fluid on *in vitro* cleavage of 2-cell mouse embryos: possible role in infertility associated with endometriosis. *Fertility and Sterility*, **44**, 678–83.

Morrish, D.W., Bhardwaj, D., Dabbagh, L.K., Marusyk, H. and Siy, O. (1987). Epidermal growth factor induces differentiation and secretion of human chorionic gonadotropin and placental lactogen in normal human placenta. *Journal of Clinical Endocrinology and Metabolism*, **65**, 1282–90.

Morrish, D.W., Bhardwaj, D. and Paras, M.T. (1991). Transforming growth factor β1 inhibits placental differentiation and human chorionic gonadotropin and human placental lactogen secretion. *Endocrinology*, **129**, 22–6.

Moskalewski, S., Ptak, W. and Czarnik, Z. (1975). Demonstration of cells with IgG receptor in human placenta. *Biology of the Neonate*, **26**, 268–73.

Motta, P.M., Nottola, S.A., Pereda, J., Croxatto, H.B. and Familiari, G. (1995). Ultrastructure of human cumulus oophorus: a transmission electron microscopic study on oviductal oocytes and fertilized eggs. *Human Reproduction*, **10**, 2361–7.

Muscato, J.J., Haney, A.F. and Weinberg J.B. (1982). Sperm phagocytosis by human peritoneal macrophages: a possible cause of infertility in endometriosis. *American Journal of Obstetrics and Gynecology*, **144**, 503–10.

Nachtigall, M.J., Kliman, H.J., Feinberg, R.F., Olive, D.L. Engin, O. and Arici, A. (1996). The effect of leukemia inhibitory factor (LIF) on trophoblast differentiation: a potential role in human implantation. *Journal of Clinical Endocrinology and Metabolism*, **81**, 801–6.

Narahara, H., Nishioka, Y. and Johnston, J.M. (1993). Secretion of platelet-activating factor acetyl-hydrolase by human decidual macrophages. *Journal of Clinical Endocrinology and Metabolism*, **77**, 1258–62.

Nicosia, M., Moger, W.H., Dyer, C.A., Prack, M.M. and Williams, D.L. (1992). Apolipoprotein-E messenger RNA in rat ovary is expressed in theca and interstitial cells and presumptive macrophages, but not in granulosa cells. *Molecular Endocrinology*, **6**, 978–88.

Nishimura, K., Tanaka, N., Ohshige, A., Fukumatsu, Y., Matsuura, K. and Okamura, H. (1995). Effect of macrophage colony-stimulating factor on folliculogenesis in the gonadotrophin-primed immature rats. *Journal of Reproduction and Fertility*, **104**, 325–30.

Niswender, G.D. and Nett, T.M. (1988). The corpus luteum and its control. In Knobil, E. and Neill, J.D. (ed.), *The Physiology of Reproduction*. Raven Press, New York, pp. 489–525.

Ogawa, M., Nishikawa, S., Ikuta, K., Yamamura, F., Naito, M., Takahashi, K. *et al.* (1988). B cell ontogeny in murine embryo studied by a culture system with the monolayer of a stromal cell clone, ST2: B cell progenitor develops first in the embryonal body rather than in the yolk sac. *EMBO Journal*, **7**, 1337–43.

Ohasi, K., Saji, F., Kato, M., Wakimoto, A. and Tanizawa, O. (1992). Tumor necrosis factor-α inhibits human chorionic gonadotropin secretion. *Journal of Clinical Endocrinology and Metabolism*, **74**, 130–4.

Olson, L.M., Jones-Burton, C.M. and Jablonka-Shariff, A. (1996). Nitric oxide decreases estradiol synthesis of rat luteinized ovarian cells: possible role for nitric oxide in functional luteal regression. *Endocrinology*, **137**, 3531–9.

Oosterlynck, D.J., Meuleman, C., Waer, M. and Koninckx, P.R. (1994). Transforming growth factor-β activity is increased in peritoneal fluid from women with endometriosis. *Obstetrics and Gynecology*, **83**, 287–92.

Padykula, H.A. (1981). Shifts in uterine stromal cell populations during pregnancy and regression. In Glasser, S.R. and Bullock, D.W. (ed.), *Cellular and Molecular Aspects of Implantation*. Plenum Publishing Corporation, New York, pp. 197–216.

Pitzel, L, Jarry, H. and Wuttke, W. (1993). Effects and interactions of prostaglandin F2α, oxytocin, and cytokines on steroidogenesis of porcine luteal cells. *Endocrinology*, **132**, 751–6.

Prosdocimi, O. (1953). Ricerche istochimiche per la localizzazione delle sostanze gonadotrope nel tessuto coriale normale, nella mola vescicolare e corioepitelioma. *Rivista D'ostetrica e Ginecologia Pratica (Milano)*, **35**, 133–8.

Prough, S.G., Aksel, S., Gilmore, S.M. and Yeoman, R.R. (1990). Peritoneal fluid fractions from patients with endometriosis do not promote two-cell mouse embryo growth. *Fertility and Sterility*, **54**, 927–30.

Robertson, T.A., Papadimitrou, J.M., Walters, M.N. and Wolman M. (1977). Effects of exposure of murine peritoneal exudate and resident macrophages to high molecular levan: a morphological study. *Journal of Pathology*, **123**, 157–64.

Saito, S., Matsuyama, S., Shiota, K. and Takahashi, M. (1988). Involvement of splenocytes in the control of corpus luteum function in the rat. *Endocrinologica Japonica*, **35**, 891–8.

Sharkey, A.M., Charnock-Jones, D.S., Boocock, C.A., Brown, K.D. and Smith, S.K. (1993). Expression of mRNA for vascular endothelial growth factor in human placenta. *Journal of Reproduction and Fertility*, **99**, 609–15.

Shaw, K.J., Do, Y.S., Kjos, S., Anderson, P.W., Shinagawa, T., Dubeau, L. *et al.* (1989). Human decidua is a major source of renin. *Journal of Clinical Investigation*, **83**, 2085–92.

Starkey, P.M, Clover, L.M. and Rees, M.C. (1991). Variation during the menstrual cycle of immune cell populations in human endometrium. *European Journal of Obstetrics, Gynecology and Reproductive Biology*, **39**, 203–7.

Stewart, I.J. and Mitchell, B.S. (1991). The distribution of uterine macrophages in virgin and early pregnant mice. *Journal of Anatomy*, **179**, 183–96.

Suenaga, Y., Katabuchi, H., Fukumatsu, Y. and Okamura, H. (1998). Distribution and cytological properties of macrophages in human fallopian tubes. *Acta Anatomica*, **163**, 10–9.

Syrop, C.H. and Halme, J. (1987). Peritoneal fluid environment and infertility. *Fertility and Sterility*, **48**, 1–9.

Takahashi, K. and Naito, M. (1993). Development, differentiation and proliferation of macrophages in the rat yolk sac. *Tissue and Cell*, **25**, 351–62.

Takahashi, K., Naito, M., Katabuchi, H. and Higashi K. (1991). Development, differentiation, and maturation of macrophages in the chorionic villi of mouse placenta with special reference to the origin of Hofbauer cells. *Journal of Leukocyte Biology*, **50**: 57–68.

Taketani, Y., Kuo, T.M. and Mizuno, M. (1992). Comparison of cytokine levels and embryo toxicity in peritoneal fluid in infertile women with untreated or treated endometriosis. *American Journal of Obstetrics and Gynecology*, **167**, 265–70.

Takeya, M., Tsuchiya, T., Shimokawa, K. and Takahashi, K. (1991). A new monoclonal antibody, PM-2K, specifically recognizes tissue macrophages but not blood monocytes. *Journal of Pathology*, **163**, 315–21.

Terranova, P.F. and Rice V.M. (1997). Review: cytokine involvement in ovarian processes. *American Journal of Reproductive Immunology*, **37**, 50–63.

Townson, D.H. and Pate, J.L. (1994). Regulation of prostaglandin synthesis by interleukin-1β in cultured bovine luteal cells. *Biology of Reproduction*, **51**, 480–5.

Wang, H.Z., Lu, S.H., Han, X.J., Zhou, W., Sheng, W.X., Sun, Z.D. *et al.* (1992). Inhibitory effect of interferon and tumor necrosis factor on human luteal function *in vitro*. *Fertility and Sterility*, **58**, 941–5.

Wang, Y.Y., Tawfik, O. and Wood, G.W. (1998). Endotoxin-induced abortion in mice is mediated by activated fetal macrophages. *Journal of Leukocyte Biology*, **63**, 40–50.

Wilhelmsson, L., Lindblom, B. and Wiqvist, N. (1979). The human utero-tubal junction: contractile patterns of different smooth muscle layers and the influence of prostaglandin E_2, prostaglandin $F_{2\alpha}$, and prostaglandin I_2 *in vitro*. *Fertility and Sterility*, **32**, 303–7.

Wood, G.W. and King, G.R., Jr (1982). Trapping antigen–antibody complexes within the human placenta. *Cellular Immunology*, **69**, 347–62.

Yamanouchi, K., Matsuyama, S., Nishihara, M., Shiota, K., Tachi, C. and Takahashi, M. (1992). Splenic macrophages enhance prolactin-induced progestin secretion from mature rat granulosa cells *in vitro*. *Biology of Reproduction*, **46**, 1109–13.

Yih, S., Katabuchi, H., Araki, M., Matsuura, K., Takeya, M., *et al.* (2001) Expression of monocyte chemoattractant protein-1 in peritoneal endometriotic cells *Virchow Archiv*, **438**, 70–7.

Yoshida, H., Hayashi, S., Kunisada, T., Ogawa, M., Nishikawa, S., Okamura, H. *et al.*, (1990). The murine mutation osteopetrosis is a mutation in the coding region of the macrophage colony stimulating factor gene. *Nature*, **345**, 442–4.

15 *Macrophages in gene therapy: cellular targets and gene delivery vehicles*

B. Burke, S. Sumner, P.C. Mahon and C.E. Lewis

1 Introduction

As described in various other chapters in this volume, macrophages play a central role in the immune system mainly by participating in the ingestion and killing of invading microorganisms and the presentation of antigen to T cells. In addition, they secrete over 120 different substances (Gordon, 1995) involved in host defence and inflammation. These include complement components, a wide range of cytokines and enzymes with narrow- or broad-range specificity. During infection, macrophages have the capacity to become 'activated' by cytokines and different bacterial products. These activated macrophages exhibit increased tumoricidal and microbicidal activity, and release increased levels of immune mediators.

However, macrophages (whether through 'normal' pro-inflammatory or pro-angiogenic activities, or through defects in activity, or by acting as hosts and reservoirs for pathogens) have been implicated in the onset and/or progression of various pathogenic conditions. These include the growth and spread of malignant tumors, the pronounced inflammation present in rheumatoid arthritic joints, human immunodeficiency virus (HIV) infection, chronic granulomatous disease, atherosclerosis, lysosomal storage diseases, diabetes, lupus erythematosus and Wiskott–Aldrich syndrome (reviewed by Speer and Gahr, 1989).

Many of the events regulating the activities of macrophages in such disease states have been identified. This has prompted attempts to transfer therapeutic gene constructs into macrophages to alter these activities, and thus ameliorate disease. Most studies have used gene transfer methods to manipulate gene expression in macrophages *in vitro*; however, as is often the case, attempting to replicate these studies in the more complex *in vivo* environment has proved problematic, particularly with regard to obtaining macrophage-specific transfection. Work has also begun to attempt to exploit the propensity of macrophages to infiltrate diseased tissues by using them as cellular delivery vehicles to target gene therapy to these sites.

In this chapter, we review the wide variety of methods used to transfer genes into macrophages and their precursors. Examples of how these methods have been used to attempt to alter macrophage activities *in vitro* and *in vivo* are then described. Lastly, the ways in which macrophages are being developed as cellular delivery vehicles for gene therapy are discussed.

2 Methods used for gene transfer to macrophages

Macrophages are generally known as a difficult cell type to transfect, possibly because of their many enzymic activities, many of which are related to their role, as phagocytes, in degrading ingested material. The non- (or very low) proliferative nature of these cells is also likely to be a factor, particularly when using viral vectors, several of which require cell division for chromosomal integration. There is now a growing interest in the development of efficient and reproducible methods for the transfection of primary macrophages and macrophage cell lines, partly as a means of investigating their myriad functions, but also with a view to the expression of transgenes in these cells for various therapeutic applications.

As will be seen below, several viral (adenoviruses, retro/lentiviruses, pox viruses, adeno-associated viruses and herpes viruses) and a wide array of non-viral methods have been used to transfect macrophages and their precursors. The main advantage of non-viral methods is that the time-consuming process of constructing recombinant viruses is avoided, and a large number of constructs can be tested for functionality relatively rapidly. However, viral methods generally give better transfection efficiencies (a higher percentage of cells expressing the transgene) and longer term expression (with retro/lentiviruses and adeno-associated viruses especially), particularly with primary cells.

This could be due partly to the fact that in many non-viral transfection methods, the exogenous DNA enters the macrophage by endocytosis, and is digested subsequently by nucleases in the lysosomes (following endosome–lysosome fusion). Indeed, primary macrophages are known to contain high levels of such nucleases (Nagata *et al.*, 1983), which may explain the difficulties experienced by many groups in transfecting them with non-viral methods.

2.1 Viral methods

2.1.1 Adenoviruses

Adenoviruses have become one of the most frequently used methods of gene transfer to primary macrophages due to the fact that they are capable of infecting non-dividing cells (such as macrophages) with high efficiency and of delivering reasonable longevity (up to several weeks) of transgene expression. Various studies have reported transfection efficiencies of 10–80 per cent for human macrophages, depending on cell culture conditions and the multiplicity of infection (number of infectious virus particles per cell; m.o.i.) used (Haddada *et al.*, 1993; Schneider *et al.*, 1997; De *et al.*, 1998; Heider *et al.*, 2000). It is noteworthy that adenoviruses appear to be relatively ineffective in gene transfer to monocytes, presumably due to the paucity of appropriate integrins (the receptors for adenoviruses) on monocytes (Schneider *et al.*, 1997). A recent study has solved this problem by incubating primary human monocytes in macrophage colony-stimulating factor (M-CSF) at 100 ng/ml for 72 h, resulting in increased expression of the integrins $\alpha_V\beta_3$ and $\alpha_V\beta_5$. With this method, using m.o.i.s of 100 or 50, infection rates of greater than 90 per cent were achieved (Foxwell *et al.*, 1998).

2.1.2 Retroviruses

Retroviruses (other than the lentivirus subclass) are generally considered to be ineffective in the transfection of non-proliferating or poorly proliferating cells such as primary macrophages. One explanation for this may be that such viruses are incapable of entering the nuclei of non-proliferating cells, and thus are unable to integrate their genome into the chromosomes of the infected cell, which is essential for significant levels of retroviral gene expression. Parveen and co-workers (2000) have addressed this problem by introducing a nuclear localization signal (NLS) sequence into the matrix protein of the C-type retrovirus spleen necrosis virus (SNV). This increased the ability of the SNV vector to penetrate the nucleus of macrophages, allowing more efficient infection.

There is some evidence that gene expression from integrated retroviruses often lasts only a few weeks, especially *in vivo,* which may be due to 'transcriptional silencing' caused by methylation near the promoter and integration into condensed chromatin regions in which the transgene would be inaccessible to the transcription machinery. The recent discovery of two types of DNA element, termed locus control regions (LCRs) and ubiquitously acting chromatin opening elements (UCOEs), which alter the conformation of the surrounding chromatin, offer a potential solution to the problem of insertion into transcriptionally inactive regions of chromatin (reviewed by Mountain, 2000).

CD34$^+$ bone marrow stem cell precursors of macrophages (and other leukocytes) are capable of cell division which renders them susceptible to retroviral infection. Murine leukemia viruses have been used most often, but other retroviral vectors have also been developed recently, for example based on human foamy virus, which can give a transfection efficiency of up to 80 per cent (Vassilopoulos *et al.*, 2001).

Other studies have shown that retrovirally transduced CD34$^+$ cells continue to express transgenes stably after being induced to differentiate into macrophages. In one study, long-term expression of a reporter gene in macrophages was achieved by retrovirally transducing granulocyte colony-stimulating factor (G-CSF)-mobilized peripheral blood CD34$^+$ cells in the presence of interleukin (IL)-3, IL-6, granulocyte–macrophage colony-stimulating factor (GM-CSF) and stem cell factor (SCF), prior to inducing them to differentiate into dendritic cells and macrophages with GM-CSF and tumor necrosis factor-α (TNF-α) (Chischportich *et al.*, 1999). The ability to transfect these precursor cells stably opens up the possibility of re-infusing such genetically modified stem cells into a patient, which could provide a long-term source of therapeutically modified macrophages (and other leucokytes developing from these precursors *in vivo*).

2.1.3 Lentiviruses

Other retroviruses called lentiviruses, including HIV, are able to infect and integrate into the chromosomes of non-proliferating cells, including monocyte/macrophages (Miyake *et al.*, 1998; Schroers *et al.*, 2000), and may have potential to effect stable gene transfer to such cells. In the case of HIV, sequences in the viral proteins Matrix, Vpr, Integrase and Pol have been implicated in facilitating nuclear import of the viral genome in non-dividing cells (Follenzi *et al.*, 2000). However, it should be noted that *productive* HIV infection (i.e. producing progeny virus particles) of monocytes is reported to require cell proliferation (Schuitemaker *et al.*, 1992; Schuitemaker and Miedema, 1994). There is also some evidence that lentiviral vectors are less prone to transcriptional silencing than retroviral vectors, which would be an advantage (reviewed by Mountain, 2000). Although HIV seems to offer the most effective current method for the stable transfection of DNA into macrophages, there are safety concerns over their use, even when using replication deficient variants, due to the danger of generating replication-competent viruses by recombination. However, considerable effort is going into the development of novel packaging systems, which could significantly reduce this risk (Wu *et al.*, 2000).

2.1.4 Other viruses used to transduce macrophages

A number of other viruses have been used successfully to transduce monocytes, macrophages and dendritic cells. Adeno-associated viruses (AAVs) have great potential for gene therapy, having a number of attractive features: the ability to integrate into the genome of host cells and to mediate long-term expression of transgenes (up to 2 years in mice); the ability to target both proliferating and non-proliferating cells; and stable virus particles (reviewed by Mountain, 2000). AAVs have been used recently to transduce monocytes and dendritic cells efficiently (Liu *et al.*, 2000; Ponnazhagan *et al.*, 2001). Poxviruses have also been used: a highly attenuated poxvirus, modified vaccinia Ankara (MVA), has been used to transfer genes expressing tumor-specific antibodies into

GM-CSF-activated macrophages *in vitro* in recent studies (Paul *et al.*, 2000a,b). A herpes simplex virus-1-derived vector has also been used recently to express transgenes in macrophage cell lines (Paludan, 2001).

2.1.5 Limitations of current viral vectors

A potentially important limitation on the use of retroviral/lentiviral vectors is that they impose a relatively low size limit (around 8 kb) on the amount of foreign DNA that can be incorporated. Current first-generation adenovirus vectors have a size limit similar to that for retroviruses, but there may be some scope for this to be increased in future. AAVs also suffer from this drawback, having capacity for only 4.5 kb of heterogenous DNA. In contrast, the use of pox viruses such as vaccinia is not hampered by this problem because these viruses have far larger genomes. It should be noted that the clinical use of certain viral vectors, notably adenoviruses and AAVs, may prove to be limited due to the immunogenicity of the virus-infected cells, although it is possible that less immunogenic variants, which express fewer viral proteins, could be developed.

A problem which limits the usefulness of viral vectors to transduce macrophages *in vivo* is their lack of specificity for macrophages: most of these viruses infect a broad range of cell types. However, promising recent studies have shown progress in altering the cell tropism of adenoviruses to enhance their ability to transduce target cells in disease sites. One of these studies produced a bispecific single chain antibody or 'diabody' which binds a viral protein at one end and a cell type-specific surface protein at the other (Nettelbeck *et al.*, 2001). This antibody, effectively an artificial viral cell-binding receptor, acts as an adaptor between the virus and the target cell type. Other workers, such as Krasnych *et al.* (2000, 2001), have taken the more direct route of 'genetic targeting' of adenoviruses, by genetically manipulating the adenoviral fiber proteins, protruding knob-like proteins on the exterior surface which are responsible for adenovirus–cell interactions. Such work potentially could lead to the development of adenoviruses targeted to specific cell types such as macrophages.

2.2 Non-viral methods

A number of non-viral methods have been tested for the transfer of exogenous nucleic acids (plasmid DNA, oligonucleotides and ribozymes) into macrophages, including electroporation and such non-immunogenic, synthetic DNA carriers as liposomes, lipoplexes and DEAE–dextran. However, as will be seen, these usually have both a low transfection efficiency and a short duration of transgene expression *in vitro*. They also have only limited utility for systemic application. Cationic liposome–plasmid DNA or oligonucleotide complexes, for example, are cleared rapidly from the circulation, with the highest levels of activity usually observed in organs such as the lungs, spleen and liver which have roles in the removal of heterologous matter from the bloodstream.

2.2.1 Interactions between macrophages and naked DNA

Macrophages have been shown to take up exogenous DNA, possibly via a specific transport mechanism. Most of this DNA is believed to be degraded in endosomes (Bennet *et al.*, 1985). However, exogenous DNA can, under certain conditions, be transported to the nucleus and expressed by macrophages (Stacey *et al.*, 1996; Meuli *et al.*, 2001), although in these studies the concentrations of DNA used were high, the level of expression achieved low and cell type specificity very broad.

However, there are scenarios in which constraints such as the lack of target cell specificity, and even low levels of transgene expression, may not be important, for example in genetic immunization. Condon *et al.* (1996) showed that cutaneous immunization with naked DNA, attached to microscopic particles and projected forcefully into the skin by a burst of gas from a 'gene gun', results in transfection of dendritic cells in the skin, giving potent, antigen-specific, cytotoxic T lymphocyte-mediated protective tumor immunity.

Another finding which has significance for transfection of macrophages is that these cells have specific mechanisms which sense bacterial DNA, because of the presence within it of unmethylated CpG dinucleotides (i.e. a cytosine followed by a guanine), which are rare in eukaryotic DNA (reviewed by Stacey *et al.*, 2000). Macrophages respond to such DNA by undergoing activation similar to that caused by lipopolysaccharide (LPS) (see Chapter 2). This could be a complicating factor in gene therapy protocols using plasmid DNA, or even oligonucleotides containing CpG dinucleotides, since unmethylated CpG DNA is possibly the most potent adjuvant known (Krieg, 1999). The problem possibly could be avoided by treating the DNA to be transfected with a methylase before transfection, which has been shown to be effective in the case of plasmid DNA (Stacey *et al.*, 1996).

2.2.2 Electroporation

Electroporation is a method in which a brief pulse of electricity is applied to a suspension of cells to which exogenous DNA has been added. The electric pulse causes the formation of pores in the cell membrane, allowing the cells to take up exogenous DNA which is believed to move directly into the nucleus, bypassing the endosomal degradation pathway. Various authors have noted that the conditions applied, such as the voltage and capacitance, ionic strength and temperature of the medium, and quantity of DNA added, have to be optimized for each cell type used (Weir and Meltzer, 1993). It has also been noted that the proportion of cells in S phase is important in transfection of granulocyte–macrophage progenitors (Takahashi *et al.*, 1992).

Electroporation has achieved moderate levels of transfection efficiency for both the human monocytic cell line, MonoMac 6 (40–50 per cent; B. Burke *et al.*, unpublished), and monocyte-derived macrophages (>30 per cent; Weir and Meltzer, 1993) *in vitro*, but appears less effective with pro-monocytic/leukemic cell lines (<3 per cent; Liao *et al.*, 1997; Kusumawati *et al.*, 1999). The main disadvantage of electroporation is the high level of cell death. This ranges from 5 to 60 per cent with cell lines by 72 h after electroporation (depending on the electropulsing method used; Liao *et al.*, 1997; Kusumawati *et al.*, 1999), and 30–75 per cent within 24 h with primary cells (Weir and Meltzer, 1993).

Li *et al.* (2001) used electroporation to transfect CD34$^+$ precursor cells *in vitro*, and reduced osmotic swelling and cell death using a post-pulse pelleting method and caspase inhibitors, to achieve a transfection efficiency of around 20 per cent. It remains to be seen whether this method will prove effective with macrophages. An advantage of electroporation is that a high proportion of the cells which survive may be transfected.

2.2.3 Liposomes, lipoplexes and cationic compounds

These reagents have a number of positive features—they have low toxicity, deliver DNA of essentially unlimited size and do not usually evoke an immunogenic or inflammatory response when used *in vivo*. However, attempts at using them to transfect primary macrophages or myeloid cell lines have generally yielded poor transfection efficiencies, with transgene expression lasting no more than 24 h (<5 per cent; Kusumawati *et al.*, 1999). However, when Mack *et al.* (1998) optimized their DEAE–dextran DNA transfection method for adherent primary human macrophages, they found that transgene expression could be maintained for up to 56 h.

In one study which compared the efficiency of various liposomal and non-liposomal agents for transfecting the macrophage cell line RAW 264.7, LipofectAMINE (in combination with the DNA-condensing agent protamine sulfate) was found to be the most effective, followed by Lipofectin (fourfold less), DOTAP (10-fold less) and DEAE–dextran (20-fold less) (Dokka *et al.*, 2000). Transfection efficiencies (percentage cells transfected) were not quoted, rather total luciferase activity from all transfected cells was measured. This is a common approach, but makes it impossible to assess the proportion of cells transfected, since 'high' levels of reporter gene activity could arise from a relatively small proportion of the target cells. In contrast, use of a reporter gene such as green fluorescent protein (GFP) would allow transfection efficiency to be calculated.

Cationic liposome–DNA complexes have also been shown to be capable of transfecting monocytes/macrophages *in vivo*, in the blood, liver and spleen. However, the transfection was very non-specific, with endothelial cells throughout the body being the main recipient of the transgene, with other leukocytes also transfected (Liu *et al.*, 1997; McLean *et al.*, 1997).

The use of liposomes is not restricted to the transfer of plasmid DNA. They have also been used to transfect primary macrophages with antisense oligonucleotides and ribozymes (Duzgunes *et al.*, 1999) *in vitro*. Cationic lipids have been used to deliver ribozymes to murine peritoneal macrophages *in vitro* and *in vivo* with the aim of blocking TNF-α production, achieving a 70 per cent decrease in release of this cytokine from macrophages in treated versus untreated mice (Kisich *et al.*, 1999). However, contrary to the aim of reducing TNF-α production in inflammatory disorders, administration of the lipid–RNA complexes markedly increased the numbers of peritoneal exudate cells. Also, the duration of the inhibitory effect on TNF-α was not examined, and only 6 per cent of the ribozyme was taken up by macrophages; the rest was taken up by organs such as spleen, lung, liver, pancreas and intestines.

One recent study has used a novel DNA-condensing cationic peptide, CL22, to transfect monocyte-derived dendritic cells efficiently *in vitro* with genes encoding tumor-associated antigens, and showed that these cells then protected mice from a normally lethal challenge with melanoma cells (Irvine *et al.*, 2000).

2.2.4 Receptor-mediated gene transfer

Following the detailed characterization over the last two decades of receptor expression by macrophages, some transfection methods have been adapted to target specific endocytotic pathways in these cells. Ligands such as mannose and transferrin have been incorporated into gene transfer vehicles and shown to increase the efficacy of transfection for primary macrophages (Erbacher *et al.*, 1996; Ferkol *et al.*, 1996; Simoes *et al.*, 1999). Moreover, Erbacher *et al.* produced higher reporter gene expression with human macrophages *in vitro* using mannosylated polylysine–DNA complexes than was achieved with DEAE-dextran or Lipofectin.

The main advantage afforded by the use of receptor-targeted DNA complexes is that they can be designed to target specific cell types based on the presence of cell type-specific receptors on the cell surface. This clearly has important implications for the clinic as this method potentially could allow direct injection of these complexes into the bloodstream and negate the need for *ex vivo* gene transfer. Ferkol *et al.* (1996) showed that *in vivo* gene transfer to macrophages in the liver and spleen was possible with mannosylated polylysine-conjugated plasmids, and Kawakami and co-workers (2000) showed that this was also achievable with mannosylated cationic liposomes.

2.2.5 Microorganisms as vehicles for transfection of macrophages

A number of bacterial and protozoan microorganisms have evolved the ability to infect macrophages, evade their antipathogen defence mechanisms and establish chronic infections (see Chapters 5 and 6). Clearly these organisms represent a potentially powerful method of delivering therapeutic DNA constructs to macrophages *in vivo*. A number of these intracellular microorganisms have been exploited for this purpose. Two examples are given below.

One of the main targets of *Salmonella* bacteria upon infection in humans is macrophages at the Peyer's patches in the intestines, and *Salmonella* can be manipulated easily *in vitro* to carry plasmid DNA. Paglia *et al.* (2000) have taken advantage of this to develop an attenuated (non-pathogenic) derivative of *S.typhimurium* which carries a plasmid encoding murine interferon-γ (IFN-γ) under the control of the cytomegalovirus (CMV) immediate-early promoter. In this report, the authors prove that such bacteria allowed the delivery and expression of an IFN-γ-expressing construct in macrophages *in vitro* and *in vivo*, and that treatment of IFN-γ knockout mice with this strain corrected their genetic defect.

A similar approach may be possible with *Leishmania*, a protozoan parasite which targets the lysosomes of macrophages. Although the wild-type strains of this microorganism can be highly pathogenic, attenuated mutants have been developed that can safely be used as live vaccines (Titus *et al.*, 1995). Vaccaro (2000) suggests that an attenuated *Leishmania* strain, engineered to express a therapeutic gene, could be used to infect the macrophages of individuals suffering from genetic disorders primarily affecting macrophages. Such 'symbiosis therapy' could possibly provide a tool for long-term treatment of lysosomal storage diseases (see below for further details of these disorders).

3 Macrophages as targets for gene therapy

Below, we have summarized the attempts made to use the methods for macrophage transfection described above to correct macrophage function *in vitro* and, occasionally, *in vivo*.

3.1 Malignant tumors

As outlined by Kreutz and her co-authors in Chapter 11 and reviewed recently by us (Bingle *et al.*, 2001), macrophages exert direct and indirect tumoricidal functions following stimulation with IFN-γ and LPS. They are also capable of phagocytosis of apoptotic tumor cells and presenting tumor-associated antigens to T cells.

Antigen-specific recognition and subsequent destruction of tumor cells is the goal of vaccine-based immunotherapy of cancer. Often, however, tumor antigen-specific cytotoxic T lymphocytes (CTLs) are either not available or are present in an inactive state. In addition, major histocompatibiliy (MHC) class I expression on tumor cells is often down-regulated. Either or both of these situations would allow tumors to evade CTL control. Tumor antigen-specific monoclonal antibodies, or fragments of them, have been cloned into attenuated pox viruses, and GM-CSF-activated human macrophages and cytotoxic T cells infected with such viruses acquire the ability to specifically kill tumor cells expressing those antigens *in vitro* (Paul *et al.*, 2000a,b). Whether these novel methods will be applicable *in vivo* awaits further study, but if so this method potentially could have a role in anticancer gene therapy, although the high mutation rate of cancer cells makes it likely that variants lacking the epitope being targeted might arise rapidly.

Although IFN-γ is one of the most powerful stimulants for macrophage tumoricidal activity, when this cytokine was evaluated in clinical trials using *ex vivo* adoptive cellular immunotherapy protocols, a major problem encountered was the short duration of *ex vivo* activation of macrophages: repeated injections of *ex vivo*-activated cells were required to obtain a clinical response. Various studies have tried to circumvent this problem by transfecting macrophages to overexpress activating cytokines. Nishihara *et al.* (1995) used retroviral vectors to engineer a macrophage cell line to express IFN-γ, IL-4, IL-6 or TNF-α, and showed increased *in vitro* and *in vivo* tumoricidal activity by these cells. Ringenbach *et al.* (1998) have used polyethylenimine-mediated transfection of the IFN-γ gene to enhance the tumoricidal activity of human monocytes *in vitro*. However, no attempt was made to compare the longevity *in vitro* or *in vivo* of the gene expression/activation status of these transfected cells with the activation status of cells stimulated *ex vivo* with IFN-γ.

Evidence for an indirect approach to altering macrophage function in tumors has been provided by Richter *et al.* (1993). Chinese hamster ovary (CHO) cells were stably transfected with the gene for the immunosuppressive cytokine, IL-10. When grown in mice, these cells showed reduced angiogenesis and tumorigenicity compared with untransfected cells, in both nude and SCID mice. The authors suggested that this phenomenon was linked to the marked reduction in the numbers of macrophages seen in these tumors. Although unproven, this is a plausible hypothesis as macrophages in tumors have been shown to secrete a variety of pro-angiogenic and pro-metastatic cytokines and enzymes (see Chapter 11, and Bingle *et al.*, 2001), so their elimination from tumors could suppress tumor growth.

3.2 Arthritic joints

The abundance and activation of macrophages in the inflamed synovial membrane/pannus correlates closely with the severity of rheumatoid arthritis (see Chapter 9, and Kinne *et al.*, 2000). These cells possess widespread pro-inflammatory, destructive and remodeling capabilities and contribute to the progression of acute and chronic disease. Furthermore, activation of the monocytic lineage is not locally restricted, but extends to systemic parts of the mononuclear phagocyte system. Thus, selective counter-action of macrophage activation is a possible approach to diminishing local and systemic inflammation, as well as to prevent irreversible joint damage.

Macrophage production of the potent pro-inflammatory molecule TNF-α has been implicated in the pathogenesis of inflammation in arthritic joints (reviewed by Kinne *et al.*, 2000). For this reason, Kisich *et al.* (1999) used cationic lipid-mediated delivery of ribozymes to selectively inhibit TNF-α production by murine peritoneal macrophages *in vitro* (by 80 per cent). They then went on to show that, following intraperitoneal injection of cationic lipid–ribozyme complexes, elicited peritoneal macrophages accumulated the ribozyme and their TNF release in response to LPS was reduced. Fellowes *et al.* (2000) showed that an IL-10 expression plasmid–liposome complex injected intraperitoneally in mice was taken up and expressed by macrophages in a collagen-induced model of arthritis. This led to marked and prolonged (30 days post-injection) amelioration of inflammation in the arthritic joints.

3.3 Skin wounds

Macrophages are an important source of mitogenic growth factors, pro-angiogenic cytokines, and enzymes in healing wounds (reviewed in Crowther *et al.*, 2001). A recent study has shown that it may be possible to accelerate wound healing (or correct defective wound healing) by gene transfer to macrophages in wounds. Meuli *et al.* (2001) were able to transfect fibroblasts, macrophages and adipocytes with the *LacZ* reporter gene in surgically wounded mouse skin following local injection of DNA alone or, at a much lower level, by intravenous injection of cationic liposome–DNA complexes.

3.4 Silicotic fibrosis

The finding that TNF-α release by alveolar macrophages plays a central role in the development of inflammation in silicotic fibrosis prompted Rojanasakul *et al.* (1997) to attempt to inhibit silica-induced TNF-α release by these cells using an antisense oligonucleotide for TNF-α complexed to mannosylated polylysine (which exploits the endocytotic pathway regulated by the mannose receptor on macrophages). This inhibited TNF-α production by alveolar macrophages *in vitro* in the presence of silica. Further studies are now needed to see whether systemic or local application of such complexes would be effective *in vivo*.

3.5 Atherosclerosis

This is an inflammatory disease, with the major cell types involved being macrophages, smooth muscle cells and T cells (see Chapter 12). Macrophages express low-density lipoprotein (LDL) which is atherogenic when it undergoes cell-mediated oxidation within the artery wall (Hegyi *et al.*, 2001). Oxidized LDL promotes vascular dysfunction by exerting direct cytotoxicity toward endothelial cells, increasing chemotactic properties for monocytes, transforming macrophages to foam cells via scavenger receptors (postulated to enhance their survival) and by enhancing the proliferation of various local cells (e.g. macrophages and smooth muscle cells). These events are recognized as important contributing factors in the development of atherosclerosis.

Laukkanen *et al.* (2000) used adenoviral gene transfer to make murine macrophages express a secreted form of human scavenger receptor. This inhibited their ability to degrade acetylated or oxidized LDL by up to 90 per cent, and inhibited their ability to form foam cells *in vitro*. Rekhter *et al.* (1998) used an adenovirus to introduce a reporter gene into intimal macrophages in atherosclerotic vessels in organ culture, thereby identifying them as targets for gene transfer *in vivo*.

3.6 Lysosomal storage diseases

Lysosomal storage diseases (LSDs) are a group of about 50 monogenic metabolic disorders caused by a deficiency in the intralysosomal enzymes involved in macromolecule catabolism. In afflicted patients, these defects are displayed most prominently in macrophages. Chronic granulomatous disease (CGD) is a rare inherited immunodeficiency syndrome, caused by the inability of macrophages to produce sufficient reactive oxygen metabolites. This dysfunction is due to a defect in NADPH oxidase, the enzyme responsible for the production of superoxide. It is composed of several subunits, two of which, gp91phox and p22phox, form the membrane-bound cytochrome b558, while its three cytosolic components, p47phox, p67phox and p40phox, have to translocate to the membrane upon activation (reviewed by Meischl and Roos, 1998).

Gp91phox is encoded on the X-chromosome and p22phox, p47phox and p67phox on different autosomal chromosomes, and a defect in any one of these components leads to CGD. Schneider *et al*, (1997) used adenovirus-mediated gene transfer to insert a CMV-driven form of the gp91phox gene in gp91phox-deficient macrophages. This caused more than 70 per cent of transfected cells to show respiratory burst activity both *in vitro* and *in vivo*. Thus, autologous macrophages transfected *ex vivo* or *in vivo* to express the gp91phox gene may have utility in overcoming the life-threatening infections seen in X-CGD patients.

As most of the genes encoding the normal lysosomal enzymes have now been cloned, and the size of the corresponding cDNAs found to be generally compatible with their transfer by recombinant vectors, macrophages in various forms of LSD may prove to be a viable and clinically useful target in gene therapy protocols (Poenaru, 2001).

3.7 Human immunodeficiency virus (HIV)

Monocytes and macrophages are readily infected by, and support the replication of HIV, so attempts have been made to transfect macrophages to render them resistant to this virus. Macrophages derived from the *ex vivo* differentiation of CD34$^+$ cells have been retrovirally transduced with the IFN-β gene. This enhanced their resistance to HIV infection and inhibited the replication of the virus in these cells (as well as increasing their release of IL-12 and IFN-γ which in turn would stimulate other cellular immune responses to HIV) (Cremer *et al.*, 2000).

In another study, Duzgunes *et al.* (1999) transfected macrophages *in vitro* using liposomes containing either antisense oligonucleotide to the Rev response element or a ribozyme complementary to the HIV-1 5′ long terminal repeat. Both resulted in the inhibition of HIV replication, by up to 90 per cent, in macrophages *in vitro*.

3.8 Liver disease

Kupffer cells play a significant role in the pathogenesis of many inflammatory liver diseases including early alcohol-induced liver injury. Therefore, a potential therapeutic strategy would be to modulate the activities of macrophages in the liver via a gene delivery system. Wheeler *et al.* (2001) describe how adenoviral gene transfer can be used to infect Kupffer cells in the liver *in vitro* and *in vivo*. However, many other cell types would be infected using such an approach, so some form of specific targeting, at the level of either transduction or transgene expression, would have to be devised to make this therapeutically viable.

3.9 Lung diseases

Ferkol *et al.* (1998) attempted transfer of the α1-antitrypsin gene, an inherited defect in which is a cause of the chronic lung disease emphysema, to mouse alveolar macrophages *in vivo* using mannosylated polylysine-conjugated DNA. Significant increases in the level of α1-antitrypsin were achieved in the lungs of treated mice. Inoue *et al.* (2001) administered (by direct, intratracheal inoculation) an adenovirus encoding heme oxygenase 1 (HO-1) to stimulate IL-10 secretion by alveolar macrophages in a murine model of acute lung injury induced by inhaled pathogen. HO-1 expression was found expressed not only by surface cells in the respiratory epithelium but also by alveolar macrophages.

4 Macrophages as gene delivery vehicles

It has been suggested by various authors that macrophages could be used to deliver targeted gene therapy to diseased tissues, by exploiting their natural tendency to migrate into such sites. The need for this arises from the fact that few current forms of gene delivery vehicle (viral or non-viral) have been shown to penetrate from the vasculature into diseased tissues, in which the vasculature is often disrupted.

4.1 Malignant tumors

Macrophages are frequently found in large numbers in tumors, and adoptive transfer of these cells to patients for the purposes of therapeutic gene transfer or antigen presentation has long been proposed (see reviews by Bartholeyns and Lopez, 1994; Bartholeyns *et al.*, 1996). Some of the factors which are involved in stimulating macrophage migration into tumors, and their accumulation in particular regions of tumors, are now understood, and include a range of cytokines released by tumor cells in response to such physiological stresses as hypoxia (reviewed in Chapter 11, and Bingle *et al.*, 2001).

Hypoxia (low oxygen tension) is widespread in malignant human tumors (reviewed by Vaupel *et al.*, 1989) due to their poorly organized vasculature and the faster growth of tumor cells than blood vessels. It has been shown that macrophages migrate into avascular, hypoxic sites in such tissues (Leek *et al.*, 1996). Recent reports have suggested that autologous monocytes could be differentiated into macrophages *ex vivo*, transfected with therapeutic transgenes and then re-infused into tumor-bearing patients. In practice, trafficking studies have shown that only a small proportion of such macrophages would locate to the tumor (see Section 4.5, below). Thus a method of restricting transgene expression to the tumor is required. The prime candidate to date involves the use of hypoxia response elements (HREs), short DNA sequences which bind to transcription factors called hypoxia-inducible factors (HIFs), to activate transcription.

Recently, Griffiths *et al.* (2000) used an adenoviral vector to transduce primary human macrophages with a gene encoding the pro-drug-activating enzyme cytochrome P4502B6 under the control of an HRE. Infiltration of virus-transduced macrophages into tumor spheroids (which contain hypoxia in their centres) *in vitro* resulted in a sevenfold decrease in viable tumor cells in the presence of the pro-drug cyclophosphamide compared with infiltrated spheroids not treated with the drug. However, the question of whether the basal level of cytochrome produced by the transduced macrophages in normoxic tissues would be low enough to avoid killing cells in those sites was not examined.

Carta *et al.* (2001) have engineered a construct containing the IFN-γ gene under the control of three copies of the HRE from the inducible nitric oxide synthase (iNOS) gene promoter. They transfected the ANA-1 murine macrophage cell line with this and found that although these cells secreted basal levels of IFN-γ in normoxia, secretion increased more than fivefold when cells were exposed to hypoxia *in vitro*.

It is not yet known whether HREs would be sufficiently selective for hypoxia in macrophages *in vivo*, where they would be exposed to many other stimuli and physiological stresses, to be clinically viable.

4.2 Glomerulonephritis

In a rat model of experimentally-induced glomerulonephritis, Kluth *et al.* (2001) found that rat macrophages transfected with the IL-4 gene migrated to inflamed glomeruli following injection into the renal artery. They then produced high levels of IL-4 for 4 days which caused a marked reduction in the severity of injury (i.e. inflammation, as seen by the reduced degree of albuminuria). These findings suggest that transfected macrophages could be used to treat inflammation and possibly other diseases of the kidneys.

4.3 Lysosomal storage diseases

Eto *et al.* (2000) infected macrophages using a recombinant adenoviral vector containing the human β-glucuronidase gene (HBG; a therapeutic gene for one of the LSDs) and showed that their glycosaminoglycan accumulation was markedly reduced *in vitro*. They also took macrophages from normal mice, which expressed HBG, and injected them intravenously into Sly mice (a mouse model for glucuronidase deficiency) and showed that these cells populated the liver and spleen and, in doing so, raised HBG enzyme levels in these tissues. However, they have yet to inject adenovirally infected macrophages into HBG-negative mice to see whether these cells were able to correct HBG deficiency.

4.4 Use of macrophages to synthesize/deliver therapeutic viruses

In an interesting recent development, Pastorino and co-workers (2001) produced a variant of the murine macrophage cell line, WGL5, by transducing it with a replication-defective retrovirus (bearing the reporter gene eGFP) and a helper virus. They achieved stable integration, retrovirus production and reporter gene expression. A high expressing clone was then selected. When the transduced macrophage cell line was administered subcutaneously to allogeneic mice, the macrophage-like cells formed solid tumors at these sites, as might be expected of an immortalized cell line. CD4$^+$ and CD8$^+$ T cells within the tumor were shown to be positive for the reporter gene, indicating that recombinant virus had been released from the transduced cells and was capable of infecting other cells. Transduced WGL5 cells were also administered intravenously, and found to accumulate initially in organs such as the lungs, spleen and liver, as seen in previous studies (see Section 4.5); however, after 24 h, some reporter gene expression was also observed in the brain. Whether this represents transduced WGL5 cells or free virus trafficking to the brain is not clear.

The advantage of this novel approach of using macrophages as 'virus factories' is that relatively few macrophages would need to reach the target organ to have a therapeutic effect, because of the amplification effect of each cell producing large numbers of viruses. However, there are still major obstacles to be surmounted before this approach could be viable clinically: for example, to transfer the system to primary macrophages rather than a cell line may be difficult because productive retroviral infections are thought to require cell division (Schuitemaker *et al.*, 1992; Schuitemaker and Miedema, 1994). Secondly, the DNA sequences regulating virus production would need to be modified to incorporate a second level of targeting specific to the disease or tissue being treated, to ensure that transduced macrophages which locate to non-target tissues do not produce virus and damage normal tissues. For example, using HREs as an 'on/off' switch could enable virus production to be limited to severely hypoxic tumor sites.

4.5 Homing of macrophages to diseased sites after *ex vivo* manipulation

Adoptive immunotherapy with macrophages has been attempted in a variety of studies with varying degrees of success. In a number of animal studies, infusion of *ex vivo*-activated macrophages was shown to induce tumor regression. Macrophage adoptive transfer is a relatively risk-free procedure: cancer patients have been re-infused with up to 3×10^9 *ex vivo*-activated macrophages with only mild side effects, but unfortunately these studies have shown only minimal therapeutic efficacy (reviewed by Andreesen *et al.*, 1998).

Attention began to focus on ways of enhancing the ability of adoptively transferred macrophages to kill tumor cells or ameliorate other disease states, by making use of their ability to migrate into diseased tissues to carry in therapeutic DNA constructs. Various studies have looked at macrophage trafficking after injection into a host organism, often after *ex vivo* manipulation, either genetically (e.g. using genes coding for activating cytokines such as IFN-γ) or by treatment with activating agents such as cytokines or LPS. The aim of these studies was to assess their ability to 'home' to diseased sites after local or systemic re-implantation into mice, rats or humans (Wiltrout *et al.*, 1983; Abreo *et al.*, 1985; Faradji *et al.*, 1991a,b). Homing is a fundamental requirement for their use as vehicles to target locally acting gene therapy specifically to such sites. It is clearly less important for therapeutic strategies involving *ex vivo* loading of macrophages with, for example, tumor antigens, which utilize the antigen-presenting capabilities of macrophages but do not require them to migrate to specific disease sites to perform this function.

Routes of re-implantation have included intravenous, intra-arterial, intraperitoneal and intrapleural (reviewed by Andreesen *et al.*, 1998). Macrophage homing studies (usually carried out in animal models) involve radioactive labeling of macrophages *in vitro*, with isotopes such as indium 111 or iodine 125, or by expression of a reporter gene. Typical findings are that in the short term (up to 2 h), after re-implantation, macrophages accumulate primarily in the lungs, and to a lesser extent in the liver and spleen, rather than in the target diseased tissue. Subsequently, a proportion of the labeled macrophages in the lungs return to the circulation and are carried to the liver and spleen. A small proportion of manipulated macrophages (which varies greatly between studies, ranging from 0.2 (Audran *et al.*, 1995) to 28.8 per cent (Chokri *et al.*, 1990)) following systemic administration, home to the diseased site of interest, whether it be a tumor or a wound. The presence of labeled macrophages in these sites was found to persist for at least 6–7 days in both these mouse studies. Greater success has been achieved using local administration of macrophages; for example, Chokri *et al.* (1990) reported that more than 70 per cent of locally injected macrophages homed to the tumor in mice carrying a subcutaneous melanoma.

In an intermediate means of administration between local and systemic, which could be described as 'directed systemic', cells of the rat alveolar macrophage cell line NR8383 which had been engineered to overexpress IL-4 were infused into the renal arteries of rats suffering from experimentally-induced glomerulonephritis. Infused macrophages localized to inflamed glomeruli, and the infusion resulted in a 75 per cent reduction in albuminuria, a sensitive indicator of glomerular damage (Kluth *et al.*, 2000, 2001). This means of infusion is unlikely to be possible routinely in humans, but demonstrates the potential usefulness of macrophages as a gene delivery vehicle when the problem of efficient homing to target sites can be resolved.

Parrish *et al.* (1996) showed that *ex vivo*-manipulated macrophages were capable of homing to experimentally damaged muscle, and that bone cells from a mouse transgenic for the *LacZ* reporter gene were capable of engrafting irradiated mice and providing a long-term supply of genetically-modified macrophages capable of migrating into damaged muscle sites. One of the great potential advantages of macrophage adoptive transfer would be the ability to circulate around the body after intravenous injection and seek out and target multiple diseased sites, for example tumor metastases.

Unfortunately, as described above, several studies have shown that the majority of systemically administered macrophages are trapped in organs such as the lungs, liver and spleen. However, one of the early studies, using murine peritoneal macrophages, found that the organs to which the macrophages homed was heavily influenced by the method originally used to elicit them in the peritoneal cavity. Resident macrophages and those elicited by proteose peptone or thioglycollate broth localized initially to the lungs, and then disseminated rapidly to the liver and spleen. In contrast, macrophages elicited by Brewer's thioglycollate medium localized to the lungs and remained there for at least 72 h with little or no migration to the spleen (Wiltrout *et al.*, 1983). These differences possibly are due to differences in macrophage cell surface proteins induced by the different treatments. This implies that it may be possible to target macrophages to specific organs by specific pre-treatments, or even by transfecting them with particular cell surface-expressed proteins. An example of this would be to transfect macrophages with a construct overexpressing a receptor which would cause migration into a particular type of tissue; overexpression of the receptor for macrophage chemotactic protein-1 (MCP-1), a cytokine released in large amounts by many tumors, has been proposed as a means of maximizing migration into tumors.

Another means which has been put forward to enhance macrophage targeting of diseased sites is the use of bispecific antibodies (Chokri *et al.*, 1992). These workers showed that a bispecific antibody, which bound both to Fc receptors on the surface of macrophages and also to an adenocarcinoma antigen, increased the tumor cytotoxicity of the macrophages. They proposed that this approach might also be of value in directing the migration of macrophages to particular diseased sites.

It may be that since monocytes, not macrophages, are taken up across the endothelium into both normal and pathological tissues, monocytes will prove more effective in 'homing' to such tissues. However, work in a murine model has indicated that even relatively mature *ex vivo*-manipulated murine monocytes are capable of migrating into tissues, where they undergo further maturation and cell division (Kennedy and Abkowitz, 1998).

4.6 Transcriptional targeting to overcome the lack of specificity of macrophage homing

The finding that only a small proportion of re-implanted macrophages are likely to home to the target diseased site is perhaps not surprising given the ubiquitous distribution of macrophages around the body. However, it emphasizes the need for a second level of targeting, at the transcriptional level, to ensure that genetically manipulated macrophages which locate to non-target tissues do not activate therapeutic expression. This could be achieved by using transcriptional control elements responsive to physiological states, or to secreted proteins (e.g. cytokines) associated with the diseased tissue to be targeted, where possible. An example would be the use of HREs for solid tumors, which are known often to contain regions of severe hypoxia (Vaupel *et al.*, 1989). HREs have been used to mediate hypoxia-inducible gene expression in macrophages *in vitro* (Griffiths *et al.*, 2000; Carta *et al.*, 2001); see Section 4.1. A second method, applicable to the use of macrophages as 'virus factories' (Pastorino *et al.*, 2001), would be to engineer the virus genome to contain transcriptional control elements specific for the cell type to be targeted, which would limit expression of the therapeutic gene to the selected cell or tissue type.

5 Summary

Considerable energy has been focused on modifying the activities of macrophages in a variety of diseases, and on developing their potential therapeutic utility as a delivery vehicle to carry therapeutic DNA constructs or viruses into sites of disease. It is clear that transfection methods for these cells, particularly viral methods, have made advances in recent years, and this is sure to encourage such research. However, there are still major problems to be overcome, notably the application of transfection techniques to macrophages *in vivo*, while maintaining specificity for macrophages. One way of achieving this in the future may be to combine transfection with the use of macrophage-specific promoters which would limit the impact of 'bystander' transfection of non-target cells.

One of the most exciting advances has been the development of methods to transfect the pluripotent CD34$^+$ macrophage precursor cells stably *ex vivo*, which may enable the bone marrow precursor cells of patients with inherited genetic disorders, and possibly even cancer patients, to be permanently fortified, or even replaced, with genetically modified cells. The CD34$^+$ route may turn out to be more viable clinically than transfection of monocytes or macrophages, given that it could provide the patient with a long-term, even lifelong, supply of modified macrophages without further intervention.

Regarding macrophages as delivery vehicles, there is still only limited evidence for the ability of *ex vivo*-transfected or activated macrophages to 'home' specifically to diseased tissues *in vivo* in large numbers, and this certainly requires further work. However, as things stand, a second level of targeting, at the transcriptional level, will be required for therapeutic gene expression by transfected macrophages to be limited to specific tissues or disease sites.

Acknowledgments

The authors gratefully acknowledge the support (past and/or present) of Yorkshire Cancer Research (B.B. and C.E.L.), Oxford BioMedica PLC (S.S. and P.C.M.) and the MRC, BBSRC, EPSRC and Breast Cancer Campaign (C.E.L.).

References

Abreo, K., Lieberman, L.M. and Moorthy, A.V. (1985). Distribution studies of 111 IN-oxine-labelled peritoneal mononuclear cells in tumor-bearing rats. *International Journal of Nuclear Medicine and Biology*, **12**, 53–5.

Andreesen, R., Hennemann, B. and Krause, S.W. (1998). Adoptive immunotherapy of cancer using monocyte-derived macrophages: rationale, current status, and perspectives. *Journal of Leukocyte Biology*, **64**, 419–26.

Audran, R., Collet, B., Moisan, A. and Toujas, L. (1995). Fate of mouse macrophages radiolabelled with PKH-95 and injected intravenously. *Nuclear Medicine and Biology*, **22**, 817–21.

Bartholeyns, J. and Lopez, M. (1994). Immune control of neoplasia by adoptive transfer of macrophages: potentiality for antigen presentation and gene transfer. *Anticancer Research*, **14**, 2673–6.

Bartholeyns, J., Romet-Lemonne, J.L., Chokri, M. and Lopez, M. (1996). Immune therapy with macrophages: present status and critical requirements for implementation. *Immunobiology*, **195**, 550–62.

Bennet, R.M., Gabor, G.T. and Merrit, M. (1985). DNA binding to human leucocytes: evidence for a receptor-mediated association, internalization and degradation of DNA. *Journal of Clinical Investigation*, **76**, 2182–90.

Bingle, L., Brown, N.J. and Lewis, C.E. (2002). The role of tumour-associated macrophages in the growth and metastasis of malignant human tumours. *Journal of Pathology,* **196**, 254–65.

Carta, L., Pastorino, S., Melillo, G., Bosco, M.C., Massazza, S. and Varesio, L. (2001). Engineering of macrophages to produce IFN-γ in response to hypoxia. *Journal of Immunology*, **166**, 5374–80.

Chischportich, C., Bagnis, C., Galindo, R. and Mannoni, P. (1999). Expression of the nlsLacz gene in dendritic cells derived from retrovirally transduced peripheral blood CD34+ cells. *Haematologica*, **84**, 195–203.

Chokri, M., Lallot, C., Ebert, M., Poindron, P. and Batholeyns, J. (1990). Biodistribution of indium-labelled macrophages in mice bearing solid tumours. *International Journal of Immunology*, **1**, 79–84.

Chokri, M., Girard, A., Borrelly, M.C., Oleron, C., Romet-Lemonne, J.L. and Bartholeyns, J. (1992). Adoptive immunotherapy with bispecific antibodies: targeting through macrophages. *Research in Immunology*, **143**, 95–9.

Condon, C., Watkins, S.C., Celluzzi, C.M., Thompson, K. and Falo, L.D., Jr (1996). DNA-based immunization by *in vivo* transfection of dendritic cells. *Nature Medicine*, **2**, 1122–8.

Cremer, I., Vieillard, V. and De Maeyer, E. (2000). Retrovirally mediated IFN-β transduction of macrophages induces resistance to HIV, correlated with up-regulation of RANTES production and down-regulation of C-C chemokine receptor-5 expression. *Journal of Immunology*, **164**, 1582–7.

Crowther, M., Brown, N.J., Bishop, E.T. and Lewis, C.E. (2001). Macrophage regulation of angiogenesis in wound healing and malignant tumors: role of common microenvironmental stress factors? *Journal of Leukocyte Biology*, **70**, 478–90.

De, S.K., Venkateshan, C.N., Seth, P., Gajdusek, D.C. and Gibbs, C.J. (1998). Adenovirus-mediated human immunodeficiency virus-1 Nef expression in human monocytes/macrophages and effect of Nef on downmodulation of Fcγ receptors and expression of monokines. *Blood*, **91**, 2108–17.

Dokka, S., Toledo, D., Shi, X., Ye, J. and Rojanasakul, Y. (2000). High-efficiency gene transfection of macrophages by lipoplexes. *International Journal of Pharmaceutics*, **206**, 97–104.

Duzgunes, N., Pretzer, E., Simoes, S., Slepushkin, V., Konopka, K., Flasher, D. *et al.* (1999). Liposome-mediated delivery of antiviral agents to human immunodeficiency virus-infected cells. *Molecular Membrane Biology*, **16**, 111–8.

Erbacher, P., Bousser, M.T., Raimond, J., Monsigny, M., Midoux, P. and Roche, A.C. (1996). Gene transfer by DNA/glycosylated polylysine complexes into human blood monocyte-derived macrophages. *Human Gene Therapy*, **7**, 721–9.

Eto, Y. and Ohashi, T. (2000). Gene therapy/cell therapy for lysosomal storage disease. *Journal of Inherited Metabolic Disease*, **23**, 293–8.

Faradji, A., Bohbot, A., Frost, H., Schmitt-Goguel, M., Siffert, J.C., Dufour, P. *et al.* (1991a). Phase I study of liposomal MTP-PE-activated autologous monocytes administered intraperitoneally to patients with peritoneal carcinomatosis. *Journal of Clinical Oncology*, **9**, 1251–60.

Faradji, A., Bohbot, A., Schmitt-Goguel, M., Roeslin, N., Dumont, S., Wiesel, M.L. *et al.* (1991b). Phase I trial of intravenous infusion of *ex-vivo*-activated autologous blood-derived macrophages in patients with non-small-cell lung cancer: toxicity and immunomodulatory effects. *Cancer Immunology and Immunotherapy*, **33**, 319–26.

Fellowes, R., Etheridge, C.J., Coade, S., Cooper, R.G., Stewart, L., Miller, A.D. *et al.* (2000). Amelioration of established collagen induced arthritis by systemic IL-10 gene delivery. *Gene Therapy*, **7**, 967–77.

Ferkol, T., Perales, J.C., Mularo, F. and Hanson, R.W. (1996). Receptor-mediated gene transfer into macrophages. *Proceedings of the National Academy of Sciences USA*, **93**, 101–5.

Ferkol, T., Mularo, F., Hilliard, J., Lodish, S., Perales, J.C., Ziady, A. *et al.* (1998). Transfer of the human α1-antitrypsin gene into pulmonary macrophages *in vivo*. *American Journal of Respiratory Cell and Molecular Biology*, **18**, 591–601.

Follenzi, A., Ailles, L.E., Bakovic, S., Geuna, M. and Naldini, L. (2000). Gene transfer by lentiviral vectors is limited by nuclear translocation and rescued by HIV-1 pol sequences. *Nature Genetics*, **25**, 217–22.

Foxwell, B., Browne, K., Bondeson, J., Clarke, C., de Martin, R., Brennan, F. *et al.* (1998). Efficient adenoviral infection with IκBα reveals that macrophage tumor necrosis factor α production in rheumatoid arthritis is NF-κB dependent. *Proceedings of the National Academy of Sciences USA*, **95**, 8211–5.

Gordon, S. (1995). The macrophage. *Bioessays*, **17**, 977–86.

Griffiths, L., Binley, K., Iqball, S., Kan, O., Maxwell, P., Ratcliffe, P. *et al.* (2000). The macrophage—a novel system to deliver gene therapy to pathological hypoxia. *Gene Therapy*, **7**, 255–62.

Haddada, H., Lopez, M., Martinache, C., Ragot, T., Abina, M.A. and Perricaudet, M. (1993). Efficient adenovirus-mediated gene transfer into human blood monocyte-derived macrophages. *Biochemical and Biophysical Research Communications*, **195**, 1174–83.

Hegyi, L., Hardwick, S.J., Siow, R.C. and Skepper, J.N. (2001). Macrophage death and the role of apoptosis in human atherosclerosis. *Journal of Hematotherapy and Stem Cell Research*, **10**, 27–42.

Heider, H., Verca, S.B., Rusconi, S. and Asmis, R. (2000). Comparison of lipid-mediated and adenoviral gene transfer in human monocyte-derived macrophages and COS-7 cells. *Biotechniques*, **28**, 260–5, 268–70.

Inoue, S., Suzuki, M., Nagashima, Y., Suzuki, S., Hashiba, T., Tsuburai, T. *et al.* (2001). Transfer of heme oxygenase 1 cDNA by a replication-deficient adenovirus enhances interleukin 10 production from alveolar macrophages that attenuates lipopolysaccharide-induced acute lung injury in mice. *Human Gene Therapy*, **12**, 967–79.

Irvine, A.S., Trinder, P.K., Laughton, D.L., Ketteringham, H., McDermott, R.H., Reid, S.C. *et al.* (2000). Efficient nonviral transfection of dendritic cells and their use for *in vivo* immunization. *Nature Biotechnology*, **18**, 1273–8.

Kawakami, S., Sato, A., Nishikawa, M., Yamashita, F. and Hashida, M. (2000). Mannose receptor-mediated gene transfer into macrophages using novel mannosylated cationic liposomes. *Gene Therapy*, **7**, 292–9.

Kennedy, D.W. and Abkowitz, J.L. (1998). Mature monocytic cells enter tissues and engraft. *Proceedings of the National Academy of Sciences USA*, **95**, 14944–9.

Kinne, R.W., Brauer, R., Stuhlmuller, B., Palombo-Kinne, E. and Burmester, G.R. (2000). Macrophages in rheumatoid arthritis. *Arthritis Research*, **2**, 189–202.

Kisich, K.O., Malone, R.W., Feldstein, P.A. and Erickson, K.L. (1999). Specific inhibition of macrophage TNF-α expression by *in vivo* ribozyme treatment. *Journal of Immunology*, **163**, 2008–16.

Kluth, D.C., Erwig, L.P., Pearce, W.P. and Rees, A.J. (2000). Gene transfer into inflamed glomeruli using macrophages transfected with adenovirus. *Gene Therapy*, **7**, 263–70.

Kluth, D.C., Ainslie, C.V., Pearce, W.P., Finlay, S., Clarke, D., Anegon, I. *et al.* (2001). Macrophages transfected with adenovirus to express IL-4 reduce inflammation in experimental glomerulonephritis. *Journal of Immunology*, **166**, 4728–36.

Krasnykh, V.N., Douglas, J.T. and van Beusechem. V.W. (2000). Genetic targeting of adenoviral vectors. *Molecular Therapy*, **1**, 391–405.

Krasnykh, V., Belousova, N., Korokhov, N., Mikheeva, G. and Curiel, D.T. (2001). Genetic targeting of an adenovirus vector via replacement of the fiber protein with the phage T4 fibritin. *Journal of Virology*, **75**, 4176–83.

Krieg, A.M.J. (1999). Direct immunologic activities of CpG DNA and implications for gene therapy. *Journal of Gene Medicine*, **1**, 56–63.

Kusumawati, A., Commes, T., Liautard, J.P. and Widada, J.S. (1999). Transfection of myelomonocytic cell lines: cellular response to a lipid-based reagent and electroporation. *Analytical Biochemistry*, **269**, 219–21.

Laukkanen, J., Lehtolainen, P., Gough, P.J., Greaves, D.R., Gordon, S. and Yla-Herttuala, S. (2000). Adenovirus-mediated gene transfer of a secreted form of human macrophage scavenger receptor inhibits modified low-density lipoprotein degradation and foam-cell formation in macrophages. *Circulation*, **101**, 1091–6.

Leek, R.D., Lewis, C.E., Whitehouse, R., Greenall, M., Clarke, J. and Harris, A.L. (1996). Association of macrophage infiltration with angiogenesis and prognosis in invasive breast carcinoma. *Cancer Research*, **15**, 4625–9.

Li, L.H., McCarthy, P. and Hui, S.W. (2001). High-efficiency electrotransfection of human primary hematopoietic stem cells. *FASEB Journal*, **15**, 586–8.

Liao, H.S., Kodama, T., Doi, T., Emi, M., Asaoka, H., Itakura, H. *et al.* (1997). Novel elements located at –504 to –399 bp of the promoter region regulated the expression of the human macrophage scavenger receptor gene in murine macrophages. *Journal of Lipid Research*, **38**, 1433–44.

Liu, Y., Mounkes, L.C., Liggitt, H.D., Brown, C.S., Solodin, I., Heath, T.D. *et al.* (1997). Factors influencing the efficiency of cationic liposome-mediated intravenous gene delivery. *Nature Biotechnology*, **15**, 167–73.

Liu, Y., Santin, A.D., Mane, M., Chiriva-Internati, M., Parham, G.P., Ravaggi, A. and Hermonat, P.L. (2000). Transduction and utility of the granulocyte–macrophage colony-stimulating factor gene into monocytes and dendritic cells by adeno-associated virus. *Journal of Interferon and Cytokine Research*, **20**, 21–30.

Mack, K.D., Wei, R., Elbagarri, A., Abbey, N. and McGrath, M.S. (1998). A novel method for DEAE-dextran mediated transfection of adherent primary cultured human macrophages. *Journal of Immunological Methods*, **211**, 79–86.

McLean, J.W., Fox, E.A., Baluk, P., Bolton, P.B., Haskell, A., Pearlman, R. *et al.* (1997). Organ-specific endothelial cell uptake of cationic liposome–DNA complexes in mice. *American Journal of Physiology*, **273**, H387–404.

Meischl, C. and Roos, D. (1998). The molecular basis of chronic granulomatous disease. *Springer Seminars in Immunopathology*, **19**, 417–34.

Meuli, M., Liu, Y., Liggitt, D., Kashani-Sabet, M., Knauer, S., Meuli-Simmen, C. *et al.* (2001). Efficient gene expression in skin wound sites following local plasmid injection. *Journal of Investigative Dermatology*. **116**, 131–5.

Miyake, K., Suzuki, N., Matsuoka, H., Tohyama, T. and Shimada, T. (1998). Stable integration of human immunodeficiency virus-based retroviral vectors into the chromosomes of nondividing cells. *Human Gene Therapy*, **9**, 467–75.

Mountain, A. (2000). Gene therapy: the first decade. *Trends in Biotechnology*, **18**, 119–28.

Nagata, Y., Diamond, B. and Bloom, B.R. (1983). The generation of human monocyte/macrophage cell lines. *Nature*, **306**, 597–9.

Nettelbeck, D.M., Miller, D.W., Jerome, V., Zuzarte, M., Watkins, S.J., Hawkins, R.E. *et al.* (2001). Targeting of adenovirus to endothelial cells by a bispecific single-chain diabody directed against the adenovirus fiber knob domain and human endoglin (CD105). *Molecular Therapy*, 3, 882–91.

Nishihara, K., Barth, R.F., Wilkie, N., Lang, J.C., Oda, Y., Kikuchi, H. *et al.* (1995). Increased *in vitro* and *in vivo* tumoricidal activity of a macrophage cell line genetically engineered to express IFN-γ, IL-4, IL-6, or TNF-α. *Cancer Gene Therapy*, **2**, 113–24.

Paglia, P., Terrazzini, N., Schulze, K. and Guzman, C.A. (2000). Colombo MP. *In vivo* correction of genetic defects of monocyte/macrophages using attenuated *Salmonella* as oral vectors for targeted gene delivery. *Gene Therapy*, **7**, 1725–30.

Paludan, S.R. (2001). Requirements for the induction of interleukin-6 by herpes simplex virus-infected leukocytes. *Journal of Virology*, **75**, 8008–15.

Parrish, E.P., Cifuentes-Diaz, C., Li, Z.L., Vicart, P., Paulin, D., Dreyfus, P.A. *et al.* (1996). Targeting widespread sites of damage in dystrophic muscle: engrafted macrophages as potential shuttles. *Gene Therapy*, **3**, 13–20.

Parveen, Z., Krupetsky, A., Engelstadter, M., Cichutek, K., Pomerantz, R.J. and Dornburg, R. (2000). Spleen necrosis virus-derived C-type retroviral vectors for gene transfer to quiescent cells. *Nature Biotechnology*, **18**, 623–9.

Pastorino, S., Massazza, S., Cilli, M., Varesio, L. and Bosco, M.C. (2001). Generation of high-titer retroviral vector-producing macrophages as vehicles for *in vivo* gene transfer. *Gene Therapy*, **8**, 431–41.

Paul, S., Bizouarne, N., Dott, K., Ruet, L., Dufour, P., Acres, R.B. *et al.* (2000a). Redirected cellular cytotoxicity by infection of effector cells with a recombinant vaccinia virus encoding a tumor-specific monoclonal antibody. *Cancer Gene Therapy*, **7**, 615–23.

Paul, S., Snary, D., Hoebeke, J., Allen, D., Balloul, J.M., Bizouarne, N. *et al.* (2000b). Targeted macrophage cytotoxicity using a nonreplicative live vector expressing a tumor-specific single-chain variable region fragment. *Human Gene Therapy*, **11**, 1417–28.

Poenaru, L. (2001). From gene transfer to gene therapy in lysosomal storage diseases affecting the central nervous system. *Annals of Medicine*, **33**, 28–36.

Ponnazhagan, S., Mahendra, G., Curiel, D.T. and Shaw, D.R. (2001). Adeno-associated virus type 2-mediated transduction of human monocyte-derived dendritic cells: implications for *ex vivo* immunotherapy. *Journal of Virology*, **75**, 9493–501.

Rekhter, M.D., Simari, R.D., Work, C.W., Nabel, G.J., Nabel, E.G. and Gordon, D. (1998). Gene transfer into normal and atherosclerotic human blood vessels. *Circulation Research*, **82**, 1243–52.

Richter, G., Kruger-Krasagakes, S., Hein, G., Huls, C., Schmitt, E., Diamantstein, T. *et al.* (1993). Interleukin 10 transfected into Chinese hamster ovary cells prevents tumor growth and macrophage infiltration. *Cancer Research*, **53**, 4134–7.

Ringenbach, L., Bohbot, A., Tiberghien, P., Oberling, F. and Feugeas, O. (1998). Polyethylenimine-mediated transfection of human monocytes with the IFN-γ gene: an approach for cancer adoptive immunotherapy. *Gene Therapy*, **5**, 1508–16.

Rojanasakul, Y., Weissman, D.N., Shi, X., Castranova, V., Ma, J.K. and Liang, W. (1997). Antisense inhibition of silica-induced tumor necrosis factor in alveolar macrophages. *Journal of Biological Chemistry*, **272**, 3910–4.

Schneider, S.D., Rusconi, S., Seger, R.A. and Hossle, J.P. (1997). Adenovirus-mediated gene transfer into monocyte-derived macrophages of patients with X-linked chronic granulomatous disease: *ex vivo* correction of deficient respiratory burst. *Gene Therapy*, **4**, 524–32.

Schroers, R., Sinha, I., Segall, H., Schmidt-Wolf, I.G., Rooney, C.M., Brenner, M.K. *et al.* (2000). Transduction of human PBMC-derived dendritic cells and macrophages by an HIV-1-based lentiviral vector system. *Molecular Therapy*, **1**, 171–9.

Schuitemaker, H. and Miedema, F. (1996). Viral and cellular determinants of HIV-1 replication in macrophages. *AIDS*, **10** Supplement A, S25–32.

Schuitemaker, H., Kootstra, N.A., Fouchier, R.A., Hooibrink, B. and Miedema, F. (1994). Productive HIV-1 infection of macrophages restricted to the cell fraction with proliferative capacity. *EMBO Journal*, **13**, 5929–36.

Simoes, S., Slepushkin, V., Pretzer, E., Dazin, P., Gaspar, R., Pedroso de Lima, M.C. *et al.* (1999). Transfection of human macrophages by lipoplexes via the combined use of transferrin and pH-sensitive peptides. *Journal of Leukocyte Biology*, **65**, 270–9.

Speer, C.P. and Gahr, M. (1989). The monocyte–macrophage system in the human. *Monatsschrift Kinderheilkunde*, **137**, 390–5.

Stacey, K.J., Sweet, M.J. and Hume, D.A. (1996). Macrophages ingest and are activated by bacterial DNA. *Journal of Immunology*, **157**, 2116–22.

Stacey, K.J., Sester, D.P., Sweet, M.J. and Hume, D.A. (2000). Macrophage activation by immunostimulatory DNA. *Current Topics in Microbiology and Immunology*, **247**, 41–58.

Takahashi, M., Furukawa, T., Tanaka, I., Nikkuni, K., Aoki, A., Kishi, K. *et al.* (1992). Gene introduction into granulocyte–macrophage progenitor cells by electroporation: the relationship between introduction efficiency and the proportion of cells in S-phase. *Leukocyte Research*, **16**, 761–7.

Titus, R.G., Gueiros-Filho, F.J., de Freitas, L.A.R. and Beverley, S.M. (1995). Development of a safe live *Leishmania* vaccine line by gene replacement. *Proceedings of the National Academy of Sciences USA*, **92**, 10267–71

Vaccaro, D.E. (2000). Symbiosis therapy: the potential of using human protozoa for molecular therapy. *Molecular Therapy*, **2**, 535–8.

Vassilopoulos, G., Trobridge, G., Josephson, N.C. and Russell, D.W. (2001). Gene transfer into murine hematopoietic stem cells with helper-free foamy virus vectors. *Blood*, **98**, 604–9.

Vaupel, P., Kallinowski, F. and Okunieff, P. (1989). Blood flow, oxygen and nutrient supply, and metabolic microenvironment of human tumours: a review. *Cancer Research*, **49**, 6449–65.

Weir, J.P. and Meltzer, M.S. (1993). Transfection of human immunodeficiency virus type 1 proviral DNA into primary human monocytes. *Cellular Immunology*, **148**, 157–65.

Wheeler, M.D., Yamashina, S., Froh, M., Rusyn, I. and Thurman, R.G. (2001). Adenoviral gene delivery can inactivate Kupffer cells: role of oxidants in NF-κB activation and cytokine production. *Journal of Leukocyte Biology*, **69**, 622–30.

Wiltrout, R.H., Brunda, M.J., Gorelik, E., Peterson, E.S., Dunn, J.J., Leonhardt, J. *et al.* (1983). Distribution of peritoneal macrophage populations after intravenous injection in mice: differential effects of eliciting and activating agents. *Reticuloendothelial Society*, **34**, 253–69.

Wu, X., Wakefield, J.K., Liu, H., Xiao, H., Kralovics, R., Prchal, J.T. *et al.* (2000). Development of a novel trans-lentiviral vector that affords predictable safety. *Molecular Therapy*, **2**, 47–55.

16 *Use of mathematical models to simulate and predict macrophage activity in diseased tissues*

H.M. Byrne and M.R. Owen

1 Introduction

The key role played by macrophages in developmental biology, normal physiology and the progression of many diseases is now well accepted, and is underlined by the range of subjects already discussed in this book. Whilst the involvement of macrophages in, for example, angiogenesis (Bennet and Schulz, 1993; Polverini *et al.*, 1977), bacterial and parasitic infections (see Chapters 5 and 6) and human immunodeficiency virus (HIV) infection (see Chapter 4, and Wodarz *et al.*, 1999) is undisputed, their precise function is not always well understood. For example, on the basis of current, experimental evidence, it is not clear whether the presence of macrophages within solid tumors is a good prognostic indicator: in breast carcinoma, extensive macrophage infiltration is significantly associated with poor prognosis (Leek *et al.*, 1996), whereas in other cancers the association between infiltration and prognosis has not been established. The difficulty in making general predictions about macrophage behavior is undoubtedly linked to their multifaceted nature: an individual macrophage is capable of performing a large repertoire of functions, with a combination of its location, activation status and the stimuli to which it is being subjected controlling the action that is undertaken. Faced with such a complex cell, the prospect of using mathematical techniques to provide additional insight into the role that macrophages play in human biology may appear alternately naive and infeasible. However, closer inspection of the phenomena in which macrophages are implicated reveals several common features that can, and should, be exploited when developing mathematical models. For example, the preferential (or chemotactic) migration of macrophages to hypoxic sites at which they are activated to express angiogenic factors such as vascular endothelial growth factor (VEGF) is characteristic of not only wound healing but also tumor angiogenesis and rheumatoid arthritis. Equally, the ability of macrophages to engulf and destroy foreign bodies is integral to the immune system's ability to combat bacterial and parasitic infections and is often compromised by HIV infection.

The main aim of this chapter is to discuss the ways in which mathematical modeling and analysis can aid progress in understanding macrophage function in diseased tissues. This will be achieved by explaining the different levels of insight that mathematical techniques provide. For example, statistical tests are widely used to identify correlations between observed phenomena. At a more involved level, a mathematical model may be developed to describe the fundamental mechanisms underlying a given set of *in vivo* or *in vitro* experimental data. Parameters are introduced into the model to denote the rates at which the different physical processes occur, for example the rates of macrophage influx, proliferation and decay in diseased tissue. Parameter estimates are obtained by varying the model parameters until the best fit to the experimental data is attained—this is usually equivalent to minimizing the discrepancies or errors between the experimental data and the values predicted by the corresponding model. A common feature of statistical analysis and parameter estimation is that the biology drives the mathematics. In each case, a hypothesis is stated and the mathematics is used to test that hypothesis. For example, the statistical analysis determines whether a postulated correlation exists between observed phenomena and the parameter fitting indicates whether a pre-defined model provides a realistic description of the experimental data. The next level of complexity that mathematical modeling can provide, and the aspect on which attention will focus in this chapter, is independent insight. By independent insight, we mean that the mathematical model generates theoretical predictions that could not have been anticipated in advance of developing the mathematical model and whose validation requires further experimental work.

Given that relatively few diseases in which macrophages are involved have, as yet, benefitted from mathematical analyses, a related objective of this chapter is to indicate, where possible, directions for future mathematical research. In practice, this may be achieved more readily by exploiting features of macrophage function that are common to several diseases. For example, the model of macrophage infiltration into hypoxic regions of avascular spheroids presented in Section 3.2 may be *adapted* to describe macrophage infiltration into wound spaces or *extended* to test the feasibility of using genetically engineered macrophages to target the notoriously therapy-resistant hypoxic tumor sites with anti-angiogenic and cytotoxic chemicals (see Chapter 15 for details).

In order to reflect the areas on which most mathematical modeling has focused, the diseases on which attention is concentrated in the remainder of this chapter are cancer and HIV infection. Before reviewing the mathematical work in these fields, we will start with a general discussion of the complementary insight that mathematical modeling may provide in Medicine.

2 The role of mathematical modeling in Medicine

The mathematical technique with which experimentalists are most familiar is probably statistical analysis, for example Chi-square or Mann–Whitney non-parametric tests. Such tests may be used to establish whether a particular intervention produces a statistically significant effect, for example whether the administration of a drug leads to the cure of a disease. In this way, Negus *et al.* (1998) were able to show that monocyte migration in response to monocyte chemoattractant protein 1 (MCP-1) is significantly inhibited under hypoxia. Statistics may also be used to identify correlations between observable phenomena. For example, Leek *et al.* (1999) found that the degree of necrosis in invasive carcinoma of the breast was positively correlated with both macrophage infiltration and angiogenesis.

Having established, with statistical significance, the existence of correlations between observable phenomena, it is natural to ask why such correlations arise. Through the development of a mathematical model that reproduces the observed behavior, it is possible to predict the physical mechanisms underlying such correlations and, thereby, stimulate further biological experiments that test these hypotheses and validate the model. In this way, mathematical modeling has the potential to provide valuable insight into a wide range of complex biological systems, including those in which macrophages play a role.

The first step in the design of a mathematical model is to identify the biological features of interest and, hence, to determine those features on which to focus. Decisions regarding which mechanisms to retain and which to neglect should be made jointly by the mathematician and biologist and should reflect the degree of biological detail under consideration. As an example, consider a subconfluent population of proliferating cells. Suppose we wish to estimate how long it will take for the population to reach confluence. At one level, we could write down an exceedingly complex model which takes account of the details of mitosis, including the phases of the cell cycle, the machinery of DNA synthesis, cytokinesis, and so on. Alternatively, we could model the population as having an intrinsic cell division rate, which may, for example, be modulated by contact inhibition.

Clearly the simple approach would be more appropriate in the first instance. From this example, we note that the first modeling steps invariably involve making a number of assumptions that should be clearly stated.

Once the mechanisms of interest have been identified, the relevant physical variables should be apparent. For the example of cells growing to confluence, the only variable needed when developing the simple model is the cell number. However, in order to pursue the complex case, we would also need to consider the concentrations of the large number of intracellular chemicals regulating mitosis, with separate equations describing each of the desired variables formulated from descriptions of the underlying biological mechanisms.

When embarking upon a program of mathematical modeling, it is useful to have an overview of the modeling cycle depicted in Figure 16.1. The key point here is that modeling is a continuous process that does not end with the first set of model predictions. Rather, it is an iterative process whose success relies heavily on ongoing interactions between the biologist and modeler. By working together, they can interpret the model predictions in a biological context, identify the limitations of the model predictions and suggest ways in which the limitations can be eliminated in new models. In addition, independent biological experiments carried out to test the mathematical hypotheses may suggest other model refinements, and so the cycle continues.

Another noteworthy issue is that different mathematical models may provide alternative explanations of a given data set. For example, logistic and Gompertzian growth laws may yield equally good descriptions of an avascular tumor's growth kinetics. Decisions regarding which model is more appropriate require close collaboration between the biologist and mathematician.

3 Macrophage dynamics in tumors

It is well known that most solid tumors are highly heterogenous, containing a variety of populations of normal and abnormal cell types. Whilst malignant cells drive the tumor's

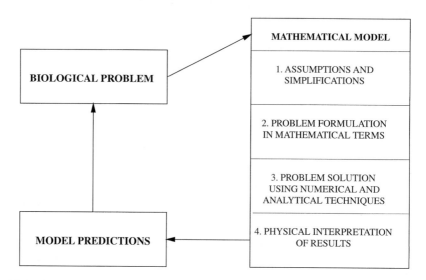

Fig. 16.1 Schematic diagram illustrating the stages involved in the modeling cycle.

growth, normal tissue cells may continue to proliferate, and the additional recruitment of other cells, including lymphocytes, macrophages and endothelial cells, is well documented (see Chapter 11). In the context of this tumor infiltrate, macrophages are referred to as tumor-associated macrophages (TAMs). TAMs frequently form a significant proportion of the total mass of a tumor, over 50 per cent in many cases of breast carcinoma (O'Sullivan and Lewis, 1994). They can influence tumor angiogenesis, growth rates, connective tissue formation and dissolution, and the killing of malignant cells. Like tumor cells, TAMs release a range of factors which alter their own and other cells' activity. The details of this regulation are important for predicting tumor survival, and for assessing the feasibility of treatments designed to manipulate the balance between pro- and antitumor effects. (For detailed reviews of the different interactions and their mechanisms, see Hamilton and Adams, 1987; Mantovani, 1989, 1990; Esgro *et al.*, 1990; Mantovani *et al.*, 1992.) It is important to stress that macrophages form only one part of the complex interaction between tumors and the immune system. Depending on the function of the many components of the immune system, the net effect may be to stimulate or inhibit tumor growth (Prehn, 1994). It is this complex network of interactions which mathematical modeling can help to unravel. Specific components of the system can be studied in isolation, or within subsets of the network. For example, we know that the net effect of macrophages on solid tumors is a balance between competing pro- and antitumor influences. Before studying these effects together, it is instructive to focus on the antitumor role played by macrophages, in order to establish whether they are capable of eradicating a tumor. As we show in the next section, this is relatively easy to accomplish in a mathematical model.

It is worth noting that many different mathematical approaches have been used to model different aspects of tumor biology, such as mitotic and apoptotic regulation (Wheldon, 1975; Michelson and Leith, 1991; Sherratt and Norwak, 1992; Markovitch, 1993; Tomlinson and Bodner, 1995), and the growth of avascular multicell spheroids (Greenspan, 1972; Chaplain and Sleeman, 1993; Byrne and Chaplain, 1995). A variety of detailed models of tumor immunology have also been proposed; for a review, see Adam and Bellomo (1997); for additional references, see Owen and Sherratt (1997).

3.1 Antitumor effects and imunotherapy

In this section, we present a mathematical model that describes the proliferation of cells within a tumor, the aggregation of macrophages and one of the main antitumor effects of macrophages, tumor cell cytolysis. Key stages of this process that are included in the model are the activation of macrophages and their subsequent binding to, and lysis of, tumor cells. Analysis of the model indicates that, whilst such an immune response is incapable of tumor eradication, the addition of exogenous macrophage-activating factors may lead to successful treatment if the tumor burden at the start of treatment is small enough.

As variables for our model, we use population densities of macrophages, l; tumor cells, m; normal cells, n; and macrophage–tumor cell complexes, c. In order to minimize complexity, we assume that all macrophages are identical, a simplification that could be relaxed in future models. For example, we might distinguish between activated and quiescent macrophages; preliminary work along these lines indicates that such extensions do not alter the fundamental conclusions (Owen, 1997). The final variable that we consider is the concentration of a chemical regulator, f, which is responsible for macrophage activation, proliferative control and stimulating their influx from the bloodstream. Whilst in practice different chemicals control each of these processes, we choose to treat them as a single generic variable called 'macrophage-activating factor' (MAF). This is a reasonable simplification, since the relevant regulators all derive primarily from tumor cells.

In simple terms, when activated by appropriate chemicals, macrophages will lyse tumor cells in preference to normal cells (Hamilton and Adams, 1987; Mantovani, 1990). They form a complex with the tumor cells, and kill them by secreting cytolytic factors (Mantovani, 1990). In our model, we assume that complex formation is the rate-limiting step in tumor cell lysis, and that its rate is directly proportional to the concentration of the MAF, f, and the macrophage and tumor cell densities. We also assume that, after tumor cell lysis, the complexes release viable macrophages to the tumor environment (Esgro *et al.*, 1990). Schematically, these processes can be represented in the following form:

$$f + l + m \xrightarrow{k_1} c + f \quad \text{and} \quad c \xrightarrow{k_2} l + \text{debris},$$

where the positive constants k_1 and k_2 denote, respectively, the rates at which complexes form and cell lysis occurs. We remark that there are, as yet, no definitive experimental data detailing this tumor cell destruction process: we have considered several alternative formulations (e.g. distinguishing between activation and complex formation, and allowing degradation of the MAF). Our results suggest that these changes do not alter the qualitative features of the model kinetics (Owen, 1997). As with our discussion above regarding whether to consider a single homogenous macrophage population, this highlights a key strength of mathematical modeling: the ability easily to test alternative and/or more complex mechanisms. Such flexibility also facilitates the distillation of complex dynamics into a minimal set of processes that adequately represent the system in question. We note also that details of ligand–receptor binding and signal transduction could be included in our mathematical model. However, in this case, they would probably offer little new insight.

To illustrate the modeling process, we now explain how the mechanistic description of tumor cell lysis presented above can be formulated in mathematical language, and incorporated into a model that describes interactions between populations of normal and tumor cells, the latter possessing a proliferative advantage over their normal counterparts. The mathematical framework used here is that of *ordinary differential equations*, with the governing equations developed by applying a mass balance law. This law states that the rate of change of each variable is determined by the rates at which it is produced and eliminated from the system. We start by stating the equation governing the tumor cell density m and then interpret each of the terms.

$$\begin{pmatrix} \text{rate of change of} \\ \text{tumor cell} \\ \text{density} \end{pmatrix} = \begin{pmatrix} \text{rate of} \\ \text{cell division} \end{pmatrix} - \begin{pmatrix} \text{rate of} \\ \text{binding to} \\ \text{macrophages} \end{pmatrix} - \begin{pmatrix} \text{rate of} \\ \text{cell death} \end{pmatrix},$$

$$\frac{dm}{dt} = \boxed{\frac{\xi\delta(N + N_e)m}{N + l + m + n}} - k_1 flm - \delta m .$$

The first, boxed term represents the rate at which the tumor cells proliferate. It includes four *parameters*, ξ, δ, N and N_e, which have the following interpretation: ξ represents the proliferative advantage of tumor cells compared with normal cells; δ denotes the proliferation rate per cell of normal cells at normal densities (so that $\xi > 1$ means tumor cells proliferate at a higher rate than normal cells); N_e denotes the normal cellular density in the tissue; and N measures the decrease in proliferation rate as the cellular density increases, which is due to nutrient depletion and contact inhibition—thus the term $(N + 1 + m + n)^{-1}$ means that the proliferation rate per cell decreases as the total population increases. The factor m reflects the fact that the rate of change of the whole population is the proliferation rate per cell, multiplied by the number of cells.

$$
\begin{pmatrix} \text{rate of change of} \\ \text{tumor cell} \\ \text{density} \end{pmatrix} = \begin{pmatrix} \text{rate of} \\ \text{cell division} \end{pmatrix} - \begin{pmatrix} \text{rate of} \\ \text{binding to} \\ \text{macrophages} \end{pmatrix} - \begin{pmatrix} \text{rate of} \\ \text{cell death} \end{pmatrix},
$$

$$
\frac{dm}{dt} = \frac{\xi\delta(N + N_e)m}{N + l + m + n} - \boxed{k_1 flm} - \delta m .
$$

The boxed term now represents the binding and lysis scheme outlined above. The rate at which tumor cells bind to macrophages is assumed to be proportional to the concentration of MAF (f), the density of macrophages (l) and the density of tumor cells (m), with constant of proportionality k_1. This is an example of the *law of mass action*, which says that *the rate of a reaction is proportional to the product of the concentrations of the reactants*, and is widely used in many areas of biochemistry. For example, there are a variety of models for ligand–receptor binding in which each biochemical reaction occurs at a rate which depends on the concentrations of certain reactants (Waters *et al.*, 1990; Murray, 1991). This law is also used in the HIV model in Section 4, to determine the rate at which infected cells meet and infect susceptible cells.

The final term in the tumor cell density equation reflects the assumption that tumor cells have a natural life span and, hence, die at a constant rate, δ, say. This is a simplification, since, in practice, cell death is a highly regulated process.

In the rest of this section, no further mathematical equations are presented (details can be found in Owen and Sherratt, 1999). Instead, we write 'word equations' which encapsulate the relevant biological processes.

Perhaps the most important factor influencing TAMs is their recruitment to the tumor site by diffusible chemoattractants produced within the tumor: the chemoattractants cause circulating monocytes to adhere to capillary walls and enter the tissue, where they mature into macrophages. Experimental investigations have identified a number of tumor-derived macrophage chemoattractants, including MCP-1, -2 and -3 (Bottazzi *et al.*, 1983; Van Damme *et al.*, 1992) and macrophage colony-stimulating factor (M-CSF) (Wang *et al.*, 1987, 1988). An important correlation has been identified between the extent of chemotactic activity and the proportion of TAMs within tumors (Bottazzi *et al.*, 1983, 1985, 1992; Walter *et al.*, 1991). We would expect an appropriate mathematical model not only to exhibit this feature but also to suggest why it arises.

Being mindful of the chemotactic influx of TAMs, when modeling the macrophage density we make the following assumptions: (1) macrophages proliferate only in the presence of the MAF f (Bottazzi *et al.*, 1990), at a rate which is directly proportional to f; (2) nutrient depletion by all cell types limits macrophage proliferation; (3) the normal background level of tissue macrophages is maintained by a constant influx from the bloodstream; (4) there is an additional influx of macrophages which increases linearly with the MAF concentration; and (5) macrophages die at a constant rate, i.e. they have a natural life span. Combining these terms gives the following word equation for the macrophage density:

$$\begin{pmatrix} \text{rate of change of} \\ \text{macrophage} \\ \text{density} \end{pmatrix} = \begin{pmatrix} \text{rate of} \\ \text{cell division} \end{pmatrix} + \begin{pmatrix} \text{rate of} \\ \text{influx} \end{pmatrix}$$

$$+ \begin{pmatrix} \text{rate of} \\ \text{release from lysed} \\ \text{tumor cells} \end{pmatrix} - \begin{pmatrix} \text{rate of} \\ \text{binding to} \\ \text{tumor cells} \end{pmatrix} - \begin{pmatrix} \text{rate of} \\ \text{cell death} \end{pmatrix}.$$

The dynamics of normal cells are assumed to be similar to those of the tumor cells, except that normal cells do not undergo lysis. Thus the normal cells satisfy the following word equation:

$$\begin{pmatrix} \text{rate of change of} \\ \text{normal cell} \\ \text{density} \end{pmatrix} = \begin{pmatrix} \text{rate of} \\ \text{cell division} \end{pmatrix} - \begin{pmatrix} \text{rate of} \\ \text{cell death} \end{pmatrix}.$$

The sole source of MAF is taken to be tumor cells, and we assume a constant secretion rate per tumor cell. Of course, in practice, macrophages may also produce MAF; for simplicity, we assume here that the tumor cells are the dominant source of MAF production. Natural decay is assumed to be the only mechanism by which MAF is eliminated from the system. Combining these effects leads to the following word equation:

$$\begin{pmatrix} \text{rate of change of} \\ \text{MAF} \end{pmatrix} = \begin{pmatrix} \text{rate of} \\ \text{production by} \\ \text{tumor cells} \end{pmatrix} - \begin{pmatrix} \text{rate of} \\ \text{natural} \\ \text{decay} \end{pmatrix}.$$

When modeling the rate of change of complex density, we equate the rate of complex formation to the rate at which tumor cells bind to macrophages (i.e. $k_1 flm$). We assume that complexes are eliminated when lysis is complete. In addition, complexes may disappear if the cells that constitute the complex die before lysis is completed. Combining these terms gives the following word equation for the complexes:

$$\begin{pmatrix} \text{rate of change} \\ \text{of complex density} \end{pmatrix} + \begin{pmatrix} \text{rate at which} \\ \text{tumor cells bind} \\ \text{to macrophages} \end{pmatrix} - \begin{pmatrix} \text{rate of} \\ \text{lysis} \end{pmatrix} - \begin{pmatrix} \text{rate of} \\ \text{cell death} \end{pmatrix}.$$

Before solving the above equations, we must establish estimates for the parameters associated with each of the processes included in the model (e.g. the proliferation rate of normal cells can be estimated from their doubling time). A discussion of parameter estimates is included in Owen and Sherratt (1998), and summarized in the Appendix.

Figure 16.2 illustrates the growth dynamics generated by the above model when a small population of tumor cells is introduced into a region of normal tissue. Due to their proliferative advantage over the normal cells, the tumor cells increase in density and the normal cells are gradually eliminated. Concomitant with this, there is an increase in the concentration of MAF, which leads to an increase in the formation of macrophage–tumor cell complexes and the recruitment of additional macrophages. As more MAF is produced, the newly recruited macrophages also form complexes and the free macrophage population falls. Meanwhile, the increasing number of tumor cells deprives the normal cells of space and nutrients, and so the normal cell density falls. This process eventually levels off when the maximum sustainable tumor cell population is reached.

Whilst the model simulation presented in Figure 16.2 shows that, for a particular set of parameter values, macrophages are incapable of halting the tumor's growth, it would be more useful to make general statements about the system, which are valid for wide ranges of parameter values. In fact, it is possible to prove mathematically (Owen and Sherratt,

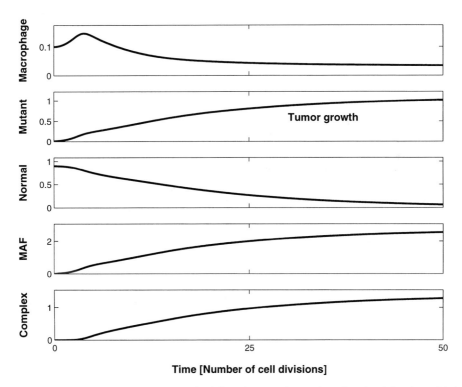

Fig. 16.2   Typical results showing that the influx of macrophages from the circulation is unable to check the tumor's growth. The parameters are $\alpha = 0.01$, $\beta = 5.0$, $\delta_c = 0.5$, $\delta_f = 2.0$, $\delta_l = 0.1$, $N = 1$, $l = 0.01$, $k_1 = 10.0$, $k_2 = 0.2$, $\sigma = 25$, $\xi = 2.0$, and the initial conditions are $(l, m, n, f, c) = (0.1, 0.01, 0.9, 0, 0)$.

1998) that, given the mechanisms included in the model, this is the only possible outcome. However, the same analysis indicates that the composition of a tumor may change dramatically as the parameter values are varied. For example, if the macrophages are highly active, they may become the dominant cell type within the tumor and, hence, reduce the tumor burden.

The mathematical analysis presented in Owen and Sherratt (1998) also leads to the following intuitive explanation of why the macrophage response is not effective at eliminating the tumor. Recall that the basic processes leading to tumor cell lysis are: production of MAF by tumor cells; activation of macrophages by MAF; and binding of activated macrophages to tumor cells. Now suppose that the density of tumor cells is very small. Then the MAF concentration will also be small and, in consequence, only a small number of macrophages are likely to become activated *and* bind to tumor cells. If the tumor were even smaller, this number would decrease even further. In other words, a small tumor does not generate enough macrophage activity to eradicate it. Such reasoning indicates how the problem may be overcome—the addition of exogenous activating factors would eliminate this double dependency. In the next section, we show how the mathematical model may be modified to include this approach and then investigate its clinical relevance.

3.1.1 Immunotherapy

The only equation that needs to be altered to account for the addition of exogenous MAF is the word equation for the MAF, which now becomes:

$$
\begin{pmatrix} \text{rate of change of} \\ \text{MAF concentration} \end{pmatrix} = \begin{pmatrix} \text{rate of} \\ \text{production by} \\ \text{tumor cells} \end{pmatrix} - \begin{pmatrix} \text{rate of} \\ \text{natural} \\ \text{decay} \end{pmatrix} + \boxed{\begin{pmatrix} \text{rate of} \\ \text{addition of} \\ \text{exogeneous MAF} \end{pmatrix}}
$$

We remark that modifications of this type are much easier to accomplish mathematically than experimentally.

Analysis of the extended model indicates that the addition of sufficient levels of exogenous MAF (e.g. lipopolysacharride or interferon-γ; Allavena *et al.*, 1990; Colombo *et al.*, 1992; Fidler and Kleinerman, 1993) can eradicate a tumor successfully. Figure 16.3 shows how the rate at which exogenous MAF is added to the tumor affects its growth, with the control case (no exogenous MAF) included for comparison. When MAF is added at moderate levels (4×10^{-9} M/cell division time), the tumor persists with only a slight reduction in tumor cell density. When a slightly higher rate (5×10^{-9} M/cell division time) is employed, the effect is more pronounced and the tumor regresses rapidly. The significant transition from one type of behavior to another (namely persistence to regression) that results from a small change in the addition rate is termed a bifurcation. When designing treatment protocols, it is important to be aware of and, where possible, to identify such transition points in order to maximize the efficacy of the treatment. In practice, the identification of such bifurcation points requires realistic mathematical modeling and accurate parameter estimates.

Another important factor in the response to therapy is the tumor burden at the start of treatment. The simulations presented in Figure 16.4 reinforce this point. They show that if treatment is administered whilst the tumor is sufficiently small, then the tumor regresses; otherwise it persists.

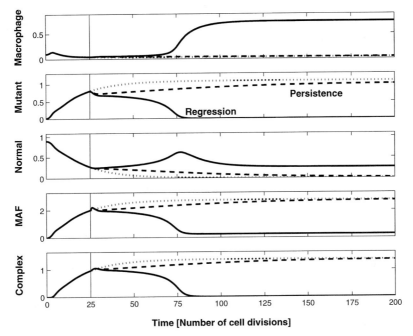

Fig. 16.3 Model simulations showing the effect that exogenous addition of MAF has on tumor growth. Solutions are shown for the control case (no exogenous MAF, dotted line) and for two different rates of exogenous addition (4×10^{-9} M/cell division time, dashed lines; and 5×10^{-9} M/cell division time, solid lines), with treatment starting at $t = 25$. When the treatment level is sufficiently high (solid lines), the tumor regresses; otherwise it persists (dashed lines). The parameter values and initial conditions are the same as those used in Figure 16.2.

Taken together, the model simulations presented in Figures 16.3 and 16.4 suggest two alternative strategies for improving a tumor's response to therapy: either increase the amount of exogenous MAF being administered or use surgery to reduce the inital size. The results also suggest that surgery to excise a tumor should be followed by a course of immunotherapy: the addition of sufficiently high levels of exogenous MAF will eradicate any tumor fragments or secondary tumors within the patient.

3.2 Macrophage infiltration into solid tumors

The mathematical model discussed in the previous section treated the tumor as a spatially uniform entity, through which macrophages were evenly distributed. In practice, even very small tumors are spatially heterogenous. Consider, for example, a well-developed avascular spheroid: proliferating cells are localized in the outer rim, necrotic cells are concentrated at the center, and hypoxic cells occupy the intermediate region. Given that hypoxic cells are believed to be a dominant source of macrophage chemoattractants such as MCP-1, when developing realistic models of macrophage migration, details of a tumor's spatial structure should be taken into account. In this section, we present a mathematical model that describes the spatial distribution of macrophages that migrate into tumor spheroids via a combination of random motion and chemotaxis. Random motion describes the tendency of cells to move away from regions of high density to areas of lower density. As such, it tends to smooth out spatial variations in cell density.

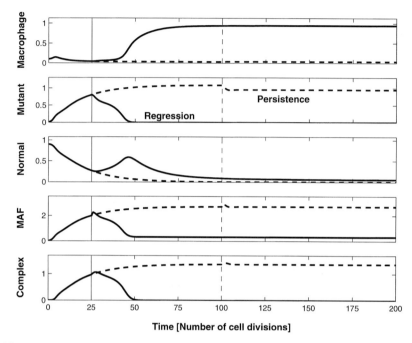

Fig. 16.4 Model simulations showing the effect that the tumor burden at the start of treatment has on its response to treatment. If treatment commences when the tumor is sufficiently small ($t = 25$, solid lines), then the tumor regresses, whereas if treatment is delayed until the tumor is larger ($t = 100$, dashed lines), then the tumor persists. The parameter values and initial conditions are identical to those employed in Figure 16.2.

Chemotaxis is the process by which cells move in response to gradients in chemical stimuli. For example, macrophages are known to move up gradients of MCP-1, -2 and -3, and this response has been quantified experimentally (see below).

The model developed below is used to determine whether observed differences in infiltration patterns into spheroids from two tumor cell lines may be due to differences in their rates of expression of chemoattractant, with one cell line (HEPA-1 spheroids) expressing chemoattractant and the second (C4 spheroids) not (Leek *et al.*, 1997).

Details of the macrophage infiltration experiments on which the model is based are contained in Leek *et al.* (1997). Typical results, which show the penetration depth of macrophages after 2, 4, 6 and 12 h co-culture with 10 day spheroids, are presented in Figure 16.5. They show that the macrophages migrate into the HEPA-1 spheroids more rapidly than into the C4 spheroids, and are consistent with the hypothesis that, unlike the HEPA-1 spheroids, the C4 spheroids do not express macrophage chemoattractants.

Before continuing, the following points should be noted when interpreting the experimental data presented in Figure 16.5. First, the sizes of the C4 and HEPA-1 spheroids are different, the HEPA-1 spheroids being larger and possessing larger necrotic cores. Secondly, the spheroids continue to grow during the experiments. Thirdly, the number of macrophages within the spheroids increases during the experiments, but not in a predictable manner. Finally, the data are subject to experimental errors, so that some of the

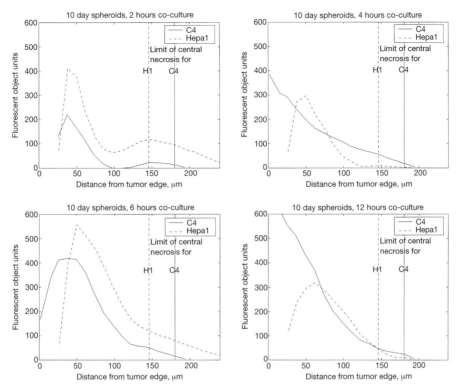

Fig. 16.5 Series of figures showing the pattern of infiltration of macrophages into 10-day spheroids cultured from C4 and HEPA-1 tumor cells lines. Macrophages migrate into the HEPA-1 spheroids more rapidly than into C4 spheroids, their motion being facilitated by chemotaxis. Data reproduced from Leek *et al.* (1997).

measurements are less reliable than others (see, for example, the distribution of macrophages within the C4 spheroids after 12 h co-culture). Each of these factors makes it difficult to state, with confidence, the mechanisms responsible for the different infiltration patterns seen in Figure 16.5. One advantage of using a mathematical model is that these discrepancies may be eliminated.

3.2.1 The mathematical model

When developing a mathematical model to describe macrophage infiltration, we assume that the macrophage chemoattractant is produced by hypoxic tumor cells and that, during the experiments, the tumor does not grow, i.e. its spatial structure is fixed. In view of these assumptions, the minimal set of variables needed to develop the model is the oxygen concentration, the chemoattractant concentration and the macrophage density (the oxygen concentration is needed to locate the hypoxic regions of the tumor which act as sources of macrophage chemoattractant). The model consists of equations that describe how the spatial distribution of the three variables changes over time. These equations are derived by applying the Principle of Conservation of Mass. This principle relates the rate of change of a particular species (e.g. the oxygen concentration) within a region to the net flux of the species into the region (i.e. the rate at which it enters the region) and the net rate of production there, that is:

$$\begin{pmatrix} \text{rate of change} \\ \text{of species, } X \end{pmatrix} = \begin{pmatrix} \text{net flux of } X \\ \text{into the region} \end{pmatrix} + \begin{pmatrix} \text{net rate of} \\ \text{production of } X \\ \text{within region} \end{pmatrix}.$$

When applying mass conservation to the oxygen concentration, which is externally supplied to the spheroid, we assume that diffusion drives its motion, or flux, into the tumor and that it is consumed by live tumor cells as it diffuses towards the spheroid's center. Oxygen levels may be diminished further by natural decay. Combining these effects yields the following word equation:

$$\begin{pmatrix} \text{rate of change} \\ \text{of oxygen} \\ \text{concentration} \end{pmatrix} = \begin{pmatrix} \text{flux due to} \\ \text{diffusion} \end{pmatrix} - \begin{pmatrix} \text{rate of} \\ \text{consumption by} \\ \text{live tumor cells} \end{pmatrix} - \begin{pmatrix} \text{rate of} \\ \text{natural} \\ \text{decay} \end{pmatrix}.$$

The following equation for the chemoattractant concentration is derived in a similar manner:

$$\begin{pmatrix} \text{rate of change} \\ \text{chemoattractant} \\ \text{concentration} \end{pmatrix} = \begin{pmatrix} \text{flux due to} \\ \text{diffusion} \end{pmatrix} + \begin{pmatrix} \text{rate of} \\ \text{production by} \\ \text{hypoxic tumor cells} \end{pmatrix} - \begin{pmatrix} \text{rate of} \\ \text{natural} \\ \text{decay} \end{pmatrix}.$$

Finally, neglecting macrophage proliferation and death (they occur over a longer time scale than the experiments; Leek *et al.*, 1997), and assuming that random motion and chemotaxis are the dominant mechanisms of macrophage movement within the spheroid, mass conservation applied to the macrophages leads to the following equation:

$$\begin{pmatrix} \text{rate of change of} \\ \text{macrophage} \\ \text{density} \end{pmatrix} = \begin{pmatrix} \text{flux due to} \\ \text{random} \\ \text{motion} \end{pmatrix} + \begin{pmatrix} \text{flux due to} \\ \text{chemotaxis} \end{pmatrix}.$$

Here, we assume that macrophage motility is regulated by the oxygen concentration, and is therefore minimal in the necrotic core.

Our mathematical model of macrophage infiltration consists of the three word equations stated above. In order to generate numerical solutions that reproduce the experimental results, the word equations must be rewritten in mathematical form, in much the same way as the word equation for the tumor cell density presented in Section 3.1 was rewritten as a differential equation. This process entails relating the various mechanisms to specific functions that may be determined from independent experiments. For example, denoting the oxygen concentration by c and its half-life by λ_c, we write

$$\begin{pmatrix} \text{rate of natural decay} \\ \text{of oxygen concentration} \end{pmatrix} = \lambda_c c.$$

The expression describing the rate at which tumor cells consume oxygen is more involved and may be derived in the following way. Recall that only live tumor cells consume oxygen. We assume that a cell's viability is determined by the local oxygen concentration, with live cells occupying regions where the oxygen level exceeds the (experimentally determined) value C_{live} and necrotic cell death prevailing elsewhere. Live cells are categorized further according to whether they proliferate: where the oxygen level exceeds a second threshold value, C_{hyp} cells proliferate whereas in the intermediate region, where $C_{live} < C < C_{hyp}$ the cells do not proliferate—they produce chemoattractant. We assume that all live cells consume oxygen at a basic, constant rate α but that proliferating cells consume additional amounts of oxygen at a rate βc. Combining these assumptions, we deduce that an appropriate mathematical formulation for the rate at which live cells consume oxygen is

$$\left(\begin{array}{c} \text{rate of oxygen consumption} \\ \text{by live tumor cells} \end{array} \right) = \begin{cases} \alpha + \beta c & \text{if } c > C_{hyp} \\ \alpha & \text{if } C_{live} < c < C_{hyp} \\ 0 & \text{if } C_{live} < c < C_{hyp} \end{cases}.$$

It is not always possible to obtain accurate estimates of all parameters appearing in a mathematical model. Where gaps appear, it may be possible to make inferences about some of the parameter values. For example, since oxygen molecules are much smaller than proteins (e.g. the chemoattractant MCP-1) that are smaller than individual cells (e.g. macrophages), we anticipate that oxygen molecules will diffuse much more rapidly than MCP-1 molecules that will diffuse more quickly than macrophages. We combine this physical insight with experimental measurements, which indicate that the diffusion coefficient for oxygen is approximately 10^{-10} cm²/s to estimate that the diffusion coefficient for the chemoattractant will be about 10^{-12} cm²/ and that of the macrophages approximately 10^{-14} cm²/s. These estimates were used to obtain the numerical simulations presented below. In addition, guided by Negus *et al.*'s experimental results which showed that monocyte migration is dramatically inhibited under hypoxia (Negus *et al.*, 1998), we assume that the macrophage random motility and chemotaxis coefficients diminish as the oxygen level decreases, becoming negligible when necrosis is initiated.

3.2.2 Numerical results and model predictions

The simulations presented in Figure 16.6 were obtained by solving the model equations numerically and are typical of the infiltration patterns that the model generates. The simulations show that macrophage infiltration is enhanced by the presence of a spatially varying chemoattractant and are in good qualitative agreement with the experimental results presented in Figure 16.5. In more detail, when only random motion governs macrophage migration, the macrophage density decreases steadily from the tumor's outer edge towards the necrotic core (since macrophages cannot survive within the fluid-filled necrotic core, only a small number of macrophages ever penetrate into that core). During the early stages of infiltration, the distribution profiles of macrophages migrating via random motion and chemotaxis are similar to those of macrophages migrating by random motion alone. However, under chemotaxis, the macrophages eventually accumulate at the necrotic margin, where the source of chemoattractant is strongest.

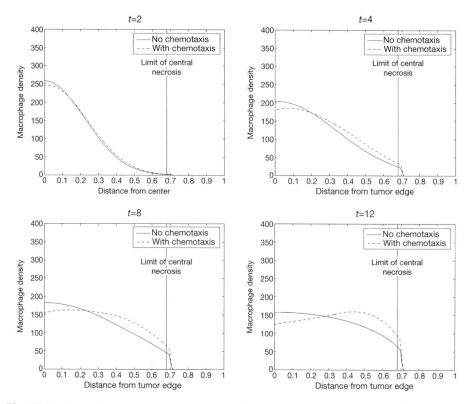

Fig. 16.6 Numerical results showing how the pattern of macrophage infiltration into tumor spheroids is affected by chemotaxis.

As stated above, the numerical simulations are in good qualitative agreement with the experimental results of Leek *et al.* (1997). By comparing Figures 16.5 and 16.6, we conclude that the different patterns of macrophage infiltration into C4 and HEPA-1 tumor spheroids may be due to differences in their rates of production of macrophage chemoattractant. In more detail, infiltration into the C4 spheroids, which produce minimal levels of chemoattractant, is dominated by random motion, whereas migration into the HEPA-1 spheroids, which produce significant amounts of chemoattractant, is controlled by a combination of random motion and chemotaxis.

In the infiltration experiments of Leek *et al.* (1997), the fluid surrounding the spheroids acted as a source of vital nutrients (e.g. oxygen and glucose) and macrophages. In practice, this fluid is either allowed to settle or agitated continuously. The simulations presented in Figure 16.6 pertain to experiments in which the medium was unstirred. In such cases, macrophages present in the fluid that do not adhere to the spheroid surface rapidly settle at the bottom of the chamber in which the experiment is being performed. Since macrophage proliferation and death are negligible during the time scale of the experiments, we deduce that, in such cases, the number of macrophages present within a spheroid will remain constant throughout the experiment. In contrast, if the surrounding fluid is agitated, then the macrophages do not settle at the bottom of the chamber, but may continue to adhere to the spheroid surface, so there will be a progressive increase in the number of macrophages within a spheroid during an experiment. These key differences between the agitated and static experiments may be incorporated into the mathematical model by suitable specification of the boundary conditions—boundary conditions are equations which state what happens to the model variables at the endpoints of the region of interest. For example, a boundary condition that states that the oxygen concentration is continuous across the tumor boundary corresponds to assuming that oxygen levels in the fluid adjacent to the tumor are the same as those just inside it.

The boundary conditions used to generate the numerical simulations presented in Figure 16.6 were altered to describe agitated experiments, with continuous delivery of macrophages into the spheroids, and the results are presented in Figure 16.7. As before, the speed of macrophage infiltration is enhanced in the presence of a chemoattractant. The effect of having a continuous source of macrophages entering through the outer tumor leads to a more pronounced and rapid reduction in the macrophage distribution within the tumor. Otherwise, the pattern of infiltration is similar to that observed when there is no ongoing source of macrophages. In the absence of chemoattractants, the macrophage density decreases steadily from the outer tumor boundary towards the necrotic core. As in Figure 16.6, the initial profiles of macrophages migrating by random

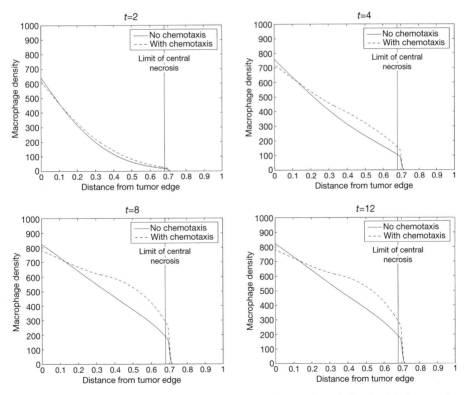

Fig. 16.7 Numerical results showing how the pattern of macrophage infiltration into tumor spheroids changes when there is continuous delivery of macrophages onto the surface of the spheroids. This corresponds to experiments in which the fluid medium is agitated continuously, so that macrophages cannot simply settle at the bottom of the container.

motion and chemotaxis are similar to those migrating by random motion alone. Eventually, under chemotaxis, the macrophages accumulate at the necrotic margin, the dominant source of chemoattractant.

There are many ways in which our model of macrophage infiltration could be adapted and improved. For example, by extending the model to include multiple populations of macrophages (e.g. normal and genetically engineered macrophages), it should be possible to test the efficacy of therapies involving macrophages which have been genetically engineered to release anti-angiogenic or cytotoxic chemicals under hypoxia (see Chapter 15).

3.2.3 Estimating macrophage motility parameters

The qualitative agreement between the experimental results and model simulations presented in the previous section suggests that the mathematical model provides a good description of the physical mechanisms that control macrophage infiltration into spheroids. Further agreement can only be achieved by using physically realistic parameter values in the model simulations. In practice, these may be obtained from experiments involving, for example, the Boyden chamber assay which is widely used to estimate parameters associated with cell migration. Owen and Sherrat (1997) used experimental data from Boyden chamber assays carried out by Sozzani *et al.* (1991) to estimate the random motility and chemotaxis coefficients μ and χ, respectively, for monocytes moving in response to MCP-1.

Estimates for the monocyte motility parameters were made by varying μ and χ within a mathematical model, which represents the specific experimental scenario and is identical to the infiltration model of the previous section, apart from the simplifying assumption that the oxygen level throughout the chamber is constant. With $\chi = 0$ held fixed, the value of μ used in the model was varied until the numerical simulations predicted the same number of cells migrating through the filter as recorded in the experiments. The corresponding value of μ was taken to be the correct random motility coefficient for a given level of MCP-1. Using these values of μ, the chemotaxis coefficient χ was then estimated in the same way, from experiments in which the MCP-1 levels in the upper and lower wells were different (the resulting chemical gradient established in the chamber stimulated chemotactic motion). A brief summary of the experimental data and parameter estimates is presented in Table 16.1.

Table 16.1   Calculated motility parameters for monocytes responding to MCP-1

MCP-1 ($\times 10^{-10}$ M) Lower well	Upper well	Filter	Cells counted	μ (m^2/s)	χ (m^2/s/M)	$\chi \times$ filter conc^n(m^2/s)
0	0	0	20 ± 3	4.61×10^{-15}	0	0
1	1	1	57 ± 8	1.04×10^{-14}	0	0
5	5	5	36 ± 6	6.82×10^{-15}	0	0
10	10	10	12 ± 1	3.54×10^{-15}	0	0
1	0	0.5	48 ± 3	7.51×10^{-15}	6.22×10^{-3}	3.11×10^{-13}
5	0	2.5	62 ± 7	9.06×10^{-15}	1.98×10^{-3}	4.95×10^{-13}
10	0	5	75 ± 4	6.82×10^{-15}	2.59×10^{-3}	12.95×10^{-13}

Taken from Owen and Sherrat (1997).
The experimental data are taken from the Boyden chamber experiments of Sozzani *et al.* (1991), showing the number of migrated monocytes counted in five oil fields, for different concentrations of recombinant MCP-1 in the upper and lower wells.

Estimates of μ varied from 4.61×10^{-15} to 1.04×10^{-14} m²/s and estimates of χ varied from 1.98×10^{-3} to 6.22×10^{-3} m²/s/M. In separate experiments, Kuratsu *et al.* (1993) obtained *in vivo* measurements of MCP-1 levels in patients with and without tumors which varied in the range 0.2–6.3 ng/ml. This range is in good agreement with the range of MCP-1 levels used by Sozzani *et al.* (1991), i.e. 0.5–10 ng/ml. Hence we deduce that the motility parameters calculated from the Boyden chamber data are appropriate for describing monocyte migration into spheroids *in vitro* and also migration into tumors *in vivo*.

More generally, we would advocate caution when using parameter estimates obtained from *in vitro* experiments to infer *in vivo* values: there may be significant differences between the two situations. Nevertheless, if we assume that macrophage motility is dictated by the relative contributions of random and directed movement, and that the relative importance of these two effects is conserved in a variety of different environments, then the *in vitro* experiments may still be used to estimate their relative importance in macrophage migration *in vivo*.

3.2.4 Combining antitumor effects and infiltration to generate spatial heterogeneity

In the previous sections, we described a spatially uniform model for macrophage–tumor interactions, and a spatially structured model for infiltration. Here we combine both approaches in order to develop a mathematical description of the antitumor activities of macrophages, which includes a detailed accounting for the location and movement of cells of each type within the tumor. For example, if a certain type of tumor produces macrophage-activating factors, then in regions of high tumor cell density we would expect there to be more of those factors, and hence an increased rate of macrophage activation. In contrast, macrophages in regions of low tumor cell density would remain unactivated. Similarly, cell densities and chemical concentrations at a given location will vary as cells proliferate, die, bind, produce protein, etc., and as cells migrate to that location from nearby.

The word equation for the macrophage population which incorporates local phenomena (e.g. binding to tumor cells and cell death) and spatial motion is obtained by combining the macrophage equations used in Sections 3.1 and 3.2. It is written in the following way:

$$\begin{pmatrix} local \text{ rate of change of} \\ \text{macrophage density} \end{pmatrix} = \begin{pmatrix} \text{rate of} \\ \text{cell division} \end{pmatrix} + \begin{pmatrix} \text{rate of} \\ \text{influx} \end{pmatrix}$$

$$+ \begin{pmatrix} \text{rate of} \\ \text{release from lysed} \\ \text{tumor cells} \end{pmatrix} - \begin{pmatrix} \text{rate of} \\ \text{binding to} \\ \text{tumor cells} \end{pmatrix} - \begin{pmatrix} \text{rate of} \\ \text{cell death} \end{pmatrix}$$

$$+ \boxed{\begin{pmatrix} \text{flux due to} \\ \text{random} \\ \text{motion} \end{pmatrix} + \begin{pmatrix} \text{flux due to} \\ \text{chemotaxis} \end{pmatrix}}$$

In a similar way, we include random motion of all the other cell species in the model presented in Section 3.1, and diffusion of the chemical regulator. Note that whilst this extended model for macrophage antitumor effects has these spatial interactions in common with the model for infiltration of Section 3.2, we have not included oxygen concentration.

Recall that a fundamental aim of mathematical modeling is to make new predictions that were not obvious otherwise. So far, we have seen that the model including cytolysis of tumor cells reproduces experimental observations of increased macrophage infiltration in response to increased chemoattractant production. More importantly, the model gives an explanation of why this cytolysis should be ineffective at eradicating a tumor, and suggests ways of optimizing therapies that aim to boost the natural immune response. Here, we describe a completely novel prediction that arises from the inclusion of the spatial interactions described above, namely the generation of heterogeneity within a tumor. Analysis and numerical simulation of the extended model show that random cellular movement and the diffusion of chemical regulators can lead to the development of patterns, which have the form of regions of macrophage aggregation with very few cancer cells, and corresponding regions with very low macrophage content, but many cancer cells. Figure 16.8 shows how, mathematically, the patterns are very regular, but we expect that in real tumors the structure would be much less ordered due to other interactions.

Having predicted such behavior mathematically, the next challenge is to explain it intuitively—if we can explain it in terms of the biology then we can be confident that it is not simply a mathematical artifact. In this case, we feel that we have come up with a biologically motivated explanation of how a dense region of tumor cells can become isolated. Suppose we start with a homogenous tumor, in which the different cell types are uniformly intermixed, except for a small region containing cancer cells. This region will produce a larger concentration of MAF than elsewhere. The MAF will rapidly diffuse away from the aggregate, causing enhanced macrophage activation and recruitment in

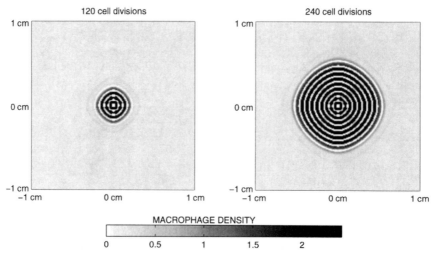

Fig. 16.8 Numerical simulation showing that the model for macrophage antitumor activity may generate spatial pattern when all physical variables undergo random motion. The parameters are the same as in Figure 16.2, except for $\sigma = 30$ and the new parameters which govern the spatial movement: $D_l = D_m = D_n = 5$, $D_f = 500$, $D_c = 2.5$.

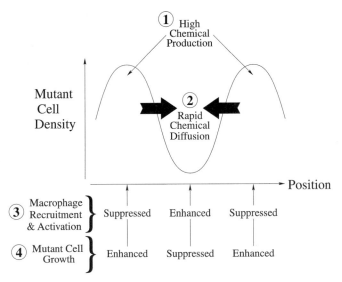

Fig. 16.9 An intuitive explanation for the development of spatial inhomogeneities within a tumor, due to interactions with macrophages. A locally elevated tumor cell density is reinforced by the consequently elevated chemical regulator production (1): if the chemical diffuses sufficiently quickly (2), then local macrophage recruitment and activation will be suppressed (3), and, hence, tumor cell growth enhanced (4). Correspondingly, non-local recruitment and activation of macrophages will be enhanced, and tumor cell growth suppressed.

the neighboring regions, which will in turn suppress the net rate of tumor expansion there. In the meantime, tumor cell lysis and the concomitant reduction in MAF production mean that macrophage activation and recruitment in the aggregate are severely curtailed, allowing those cancer cells to escape from cytolysis and proliferate further. In this way, a dense region of tumor cells may form, with a high macrophage density surrounding it. This intuitive explanation, which derives directly from the mathematical model studied here, is summarized in Figure 16.9.

Now that we have predicted regular patterns mathematically, and understand the intuition behind this prediction, we naturally move on to consider the next layer of complexity, namely the effect of macrophage chemotaxis. Again the modeling presents a novel prediction—that macrophage chemotaxis can lead to complex structural changes as time progresses, as illustrated in Figure 16.10. Macrophages move to a region in response to chemoattractants, lyse tumor cells and then move away again as a result of their own effect at that location, namely the reduction in tumor cell number, and therefore reduced chemoattractant production there.

Whilst there may be some contention regarding the importance of tumor cell lysis which is at the heart of the model discussed above, the same type of dynamics are thought to be present in the case of interactions between macrophages and the vasculature—macrophages move to hypoxic regions, induce vascularization and therefore move away again once oxygenation is sufficient. Thus the basic mechanism is that a macrophage moves in response to a stimulus which it down-regulates indirectly as a result of the functions it performs when it reaches the stimulus.

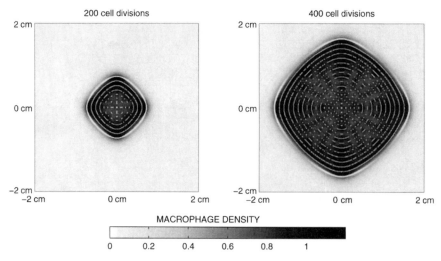

Fig. 16.10 Numerical simulation of the model for macrophage antitumor activity, with random motion of all variables and macrophage chemotaxis, using motility parameters estimated from the Boyden chamber data of Sozzani *et al.* (1991). The solution in space is shown after 200 and 400 cell divisions. Macrophage chemotaxis causes the tumor to become irregular in both space and time. The parameters are the same as in Figure 14.8, except for $\xi = 2.8$, $\sigma = 58$, $D_I = 40$, $D_f = 10\,000$.

4 Macrophages as a primary site for HIV infection

Apart from cancer, another disease involving macrophages that has been the subject of mathematical investigation is HIV infection (Nelson and Perelson, 1992; Nowak and Bangham, 1996; deBoer and Perelson, 1998). Here the ability of the virus to infect macrophages and T cells during the early stages of the disease is believed to play a central role in its progression. Recent mathematical modeling, which focused on the different ways in which the virus infects macrophages and T cells, led Wodarz *et al.* (1999) to predict that initial HIV infection predominantly involves macrophages since they are less resistant to the virus than T cells. The infected macrophages act as a reservoir from which aggressive viral strains, with the ability to infect T cells, may emerge. In the following sections, we retrace the sequence of mathematical steps that led Wodarz *et al.* (1999) to generate their hypotheses. In essence, they developed two, similar mathematical models that describe HIV interactions with macrophages and T cells. After investigating the behavior of the simple models, they were combined in order to study macrophage–HIV–T cell interactions.

4.1 Macrophage–HIV interactions

The first model developed by Wodarz *et al.* (1999) focuses on macrophage–HIV interactions and distinguishes uninfected and infected macrophages. We note that no distinction is made between macrophages that are circulating in the bloodstream and those that have extravasated: this assumption is made to minimize the complexity of the model and to focus on the interaction dynamics between the different cell types. Word equations describing how the number of uninfected and infected macrophages changes over time may be derived using the principles introduced in the previous sections. Following this approach, the word equation that we write to describe the rate of change of uninfected macrophages is given by:

$$
\left(\begin{array}{c} \text{rate of change of} \\ \text{uninfected} \\ \text{macrophages} \end{array} \right) = \left(\begin{array}{c} \text{rate of} \\ \text{production of} \\ \text{uninfected} \\ \text{macrophages} \end{array} \right) - \left(\begin{array}{c} \text{rate of} \\ \text{viral} \\ \text{infection} \end{array} \right) - \left(\begin{array}{c} \text{rate of} \\ \text{cell} \\ \text{death} \end{array} \right).
$$

The corresponding equation for the infected macrophages is written as

$$
\left(\begin{array}{c} \text{rate of change of} \\ \text{uninfected} \\ \text{macrophages} \end{array} \right) = \left(\begin{array}{c} \text{rate of} \\ \text{viral} \\ \text{infection} \end{array} \right) - \left(\begin{array}{c} \text{rate of} \\ \text{cell} \\ \text{death} \end{array} \right).
$$

As in Section 3, we rewrite the word equations in the mathematical language of differential equations, denoting by $x(t)$ and $y(t)$ the numbers of uninfected and infected macrophages at time t. In formulating the differential equations, assumptions are made about the way in which the various physical processes occur. For example, since neither activation nor mitosis is necessary for macrophage infection (Stevenson and Gendelman, 1994; Stevenson, 1996), it is assumed that the virus is transmitted by contact between infected and uninfected macrophages at a constant rate, β say. In addition, we assume that uninfected macrophages are produced at a constant rate λ and die at a rate d whilst infected macrophages (or antigens) die at a rate α. Combining these ideas, we obtain the following systems of differential equations:

$$
\left. \begin{array}{l} \dfrac{dx}{dt} = \lambda - dx - \beta xy \\[2mm] \dfrac{dy}{dt} = \beta xy - ay \end{array} \right\}.
\qquad 16.1
$$

By studying Equation 16.1, it is possible to show that the final outcome of this model depends only on the value of the virus reproduction ratio $R_0 = \lambda\beta/ad$: if $R_0 < 1$, then the virus is completely eliminated whereas, if $R_0 > 1$, then a viral infection is established. This simple result may be used to predict the effect that changes in the model parameters have on the success of the HIV virus to establish an infection within an individual's macrophages. For example, an increase in the rate of production of uninfected macrophages (λ) or the rate of cell–cell contact (β) will increase R_0 and, thereby, improve the virus' ability to establish an infection. Conversely, an increase in the death rate of either the uninfected or infected macrophages (d or a) will diminish R_0, making it harder for the virus to persist.

Obviously the above model of macrophage–HIV interactions is overly simplistic. For example, in real situations, antigens encounter other immune response cells, such as cytotoxic T lymphocytes (CTLs), which may bind to, and lyse, the infected macrophages. Additionally, such contact may stimulate the CTLs to increase their division rate. By introducing a third equation to describe how the number of CTLs changes over time, the model presented above may be extended and used to investigate the effect that interactions between CTLs and infected macrophages have on the disease's progression. As for the original model, it is possible to show that if the reproductive ratio satisfies $R_0 < 1$ then the virus is eliminated and if $R_0 > 1$ then it persists. However, the type of infection that is established when $R_0 > 1$ now depends crucially on the rate at which antigens stimulate CTL proliferation. If this rate falls below a threshold value, then the CTL response eventually disappears and the virus incubates within the infected macrophages, unchallenged by the CTLs. Conversely, if the rate at which antigens stimulate CTL proliferation exceeds a threshold value, then a permanent CTL response to the HIV virus will be mounted.

4.2 HIV–T cell interactions

Since HIV can only infect *activated* T cells (Wodarz *et al.*, 1999), when modeling HIV–T cell interactions distinctions between inactive (or resting) cells, uninfected activated cells and infected cells (or antigens) must be made. Three equations, which describe how the number of cells of each type changes over time, and are similar, in form, to Equation 16.1, may be derived by balancing the rates of production, conversion and death of each cell population (for details see Wodarz *et al.*, 1999). Analysis of the resulting mathematical model shows that, as for macrophage–HIV interactions, if the T cell reproductive ratio is large enough ($R_0 > 1$), then a viral infection is established. However if $R_0 < 1$, then, in contrast to the macrophage–HIV model, persistence of the virus may occur. The ability of the virus to establish an infection now depends on the initial composition of the T-cell population, i.e. the numbers of resting T cells, uninfected activated T cells and antigens. If the initial viral load is low, then the model predicts that the virus is unable to activate enough T cells to establish a persistent infection. Conversely, if the initial viral load is high, then sufficient numbers of T cells are activated to establish a persistent infection. As a general rule, the minimal viral load needed to establish a persistent infection *decreases* as the number of activated T cells initially present *increases* (see Figure 1 of Wodarz *et al.*, 1999 for details).

As for the model of HIV–macrophage dynamics, the model of HIV–T cell interactions may be extended to include a lytic CTL response. Analysis of the new, four-equation model reveals the following results. As in the absence of a CTL response, the initial levels of the constituent cells play a key role in the virus' ability to establish an infection. For example, a persistent infection will only be established if the initial viral load exceeds a (lower) threshold value. However, when a CTL response is triggered, if the initial viral load is too high (i.e. it exceeds an upper threshold value), then the virus is eliminated. In this case, the high initial viral load stimulates a rapid and strong CTL response that suppresses the virus and reduces the number of antigens below the level needed for persistence (Wodarz *et al.*, 1999). As the initial number of CTLs present increases, the upper viral load threshold decreases, reducing the range of initial viral loads with which a persistent infection can be established. Eventually, if the initial number of CTLs is large enough, it becomes impossible to establish an infection. Changing the initial number of uninfected activated T cells produces a similar effect on the virus' dynamics as changing the initial number of CTLs.

4.3 Macrophage–HIV–T cell interactions

In the previous two sections, we identified conditions under which an HIV virus can establish a persistent infection in either macrophages or T cells. The only condition required for macrophage infection was that the reproduction ratio $R_0 > 1$. In contrast, the conditions necessary for a persistent T-cell infection were more stringent, depending not only on the parameter values but also on the initial composition of the T-cell population and the initial viral load. In this section, the HIV–macrophage and HIV-T–cell models are combined in order to determine whether the presence of a viral strain capable of infecting macrophages facilitates persistence of a second viral strain within the T cells (Wodarz *et al.*, 1999). When the models are combined, interactions between the two viral strains are mediated by the immune response in the following way: specifically, resting T cells may be activated when they come into contact with infected macrophages. Depending on whether the effect of a CTL response is included, the resulting model consists of five or six equations that describe the evolution of uninfected and infected macrophages, resting T cells, uninfected and infected activated T cells and, possibly, CTLs. Since analysis of the resulting model is necessarily complex, we will simply focus on the key results.

When there is no CTL response, there are four possible outcomes: (1) both viruses are eliminated from the macrophages and T cells; (2) only the macrophage-infecting virus persists; (3) only the T cell-infecting virus persists; and (4) both viral strains establish persistent infections. By focusing on the solution for which only the macrophage-infecting virus survives, it is possible to show that increasing the replication rate of the T cell viral strain above a threshold value makes the macrophage-only infection unstable (i.e. unlikely to be observed in practice), and, in so doing, renders T-cell infection more likely to occur. Alternatively, varying the initial conditions appropriately may improve the likelihood of establishing a persistent infection within the T cells; since the pattern that emerges is similar to that discussed for the HIV–T cell model, it is not discussed further here.

When a CTL response is included in the model, infected macrophages and T cells are assumed to stimulate CTL proliferation at different rates. Similarly, CTLs are assumed to kill infected macrophages and T cells at different rates. As in the absence of a CTL response, the replication rate of the T cell-infecting virus plays a central role in establishing a permanent T-cell infection. However, the effectiveness of the CTL response is also important. A high rate of CTL proliferation in response to infected macrophages inhibits the T cell-infecting virus by reducing the viral load and, thereby, reducing the number of activated, susceptible T cells. In contrast, if the rate at which CTLs kill infected macrophages is high, then the number of CTLs falls and viral invasion of the T cells is promoted.

Whilst undoubtedly complex, the model of HIV infection that we have discussed is a simplification of what happens *in vivo*, and there are many ways in which it could be extended. One important feature, which could be included, is related to the ability of the macrophage-infecting virus to produce mutant viral strains that are capable of infecting the T-cell populations.

5 Topics ripe for mathematical modeling

There are a number of areas of active research in macrophage biology that are now at a stage where they would benefit from mathematical modeling. Several of these areas are discussed briefly below.

5.1 Wound healing

Macrophages perform a range of functions during the many interdependent stages of wound healing (Polverini *et al.*, 1977; Bennet and Schulz, 1993). Initially, they act as phagocytes, engulfing dead cells and any bacteria that are present in the wound space; they also play an integral role in angiogenesis (the formation of a new vasculature) by expressing a range of cytokines such as VEGF that stimulate the proliferation and direct the motion of endothelial cells into the wound space. There are a number of mathematical models that address aspects of wound healing, including angiogenesis (Pettet *et al.*, 1996a,b; Olsen *et al.*, 1997), scar formation (Dale *et al.*, 1994, 1996; Olsen *et al.*, 1995) and the infiltration of fibroblasts in dermal thickness wounds (Dallon *et al.*, 1999). As we have remarked before, there are also a number of similarities between the mechanisms by which macrophages are recruited to sites of tissue damage or hypoxia, be that in the context of tumor biology, arthritis or wound healing. There is clearly considerable scope for extending previous wound healing models to include macrophage dynamics, and equally for adapting the models for macrophage infiltration, described earlier in this chapter, to the wound healing scenario.

5.2 Macrophage activation

Whilst macrophages may be activated to perform a vast array of functions, the manner in which they interpret different, and frequently conflicting, stimuli is still unknown. For example, whilst binding of a certain protein to a receptor on the macrophage's membrane may induce a response, the precise outcome may depend on the rates of a number of different steps in the signal transduction pathway. These rates may in turn be influenced by other stimuli to which the macrophage is being subjected. With multiple, conflicting stimuli, the outcome may be even less transparent. Mathematical modeling is an ideal tool with which to unravel such complexity. For example, if a mathematical model that represents a proposed signal pathway produces the same response to a prescribed stimulus as observed experimentally, then we would anticipate that the proposed pathway may be operational. In practice, several equally plausible pathways may be identified in this way, but the flexibility of the mathematical approach can be used to guide the design of further biological experiments that distinguish between the alternatives. In this way, mathematics and biology can work together.

As a simple example, consider the situation in which both pro-inflammatory [e.g. interleukin (IL)-1, tumor necrosis factor-α (TNF-α) and anti-inflammatory (e.g. IL-10) cytokines are produced by, and act on, macrophages. The interaction between these cytokines and their receptors is governed by a variety of feedback mechanisms, and functions as a kind of switch between quiescent and inflammatory responses. Whilst some preliminary models have been discussed by Wilson *et al.* (1998), there is still much to be done before we understand how this cytokine network functions under normal and pathological conditions.

5.3 Arthritis

Arthritic joints are known to contain significant numbers of infiltrating macrophages, and the mechanisms by which macrophages appear are believed to be similar to those regulating their infiltration into solid tumors (Mapp *et al.*, 1995; Bischof *et al.*, 2000). In particular, increased cell proliferation at the surface of a joint leads to synovial thickening and the creation of hypoxic regions. Under hypoxia, fibroblasts and other cells present in the synovium secrete a range of chemicals including VEGF and MCP-1 which stimulate chemotactic infiltration of macrophages. Whilst no mathematical models specifically addressing macrophage involvement in arthritis have been developed, the similarities between this situation and macrophage infiltration into tumor spheroids could easily be exploited and existing models of macrophage infiltration into spheroids adapted to describe their infiltration into arthritic joints.

5.4 Atherosclerosis

Atherosclerosis is a life-threatening condition that causes thickening and hardening of the arteries. Macrophages play a key role in several facets of the disease. For example, they absorb low-density lipoproteins and become foam cells. When localized in an atherosclerotic plaque, they also release growth factors that stimulate proliferation of smooth muscle cells and cause the plaque to become fibrotic. The resulting reduction in blood flow leads to heart disease and stroke (Babeav *et al.*, 1999; deVilliers and Smart, 1999). These features of macrophage function represent new areas for mathematical modeling. Whilst some progress has been made in modeling the formation of atherosclerotic plaques, to our knowledge the role of macrophages in atherosclerosis has yet to be investigated using mathematical techniques.

6 Discussion

Our goal in this chapter has been to introduce the techniques of mathematical modeling as applied to macrophage biology. We have shown how separate components of biological systems can be studied in isolation, and then combined to develop more realistic descriptions in a way that enables understanding of the simpler systems to be carried forward, generating significant new insight. As well as describing specific topics in macrophage biology and the type of results that can obtained using mathematics, we have presented an overview of the modeling process, i.e. the way in which the identification of pertinent biological mechanisms can be translated into mathematical language. This process has been illustrated with a range of examples, with differing levels of complexity. Whilst the involvement of mathematics in the study of macrophage biology is still in its infancy, we hope that we have demonstrated the importance of its involvement in interdisciplinary research.

The simplest models that we have described are those for HIV infection, which stem from a long tradition of epidemiological modeling. The most basic approach is to consider two populations, in this case of cells, one of which is uninfected (often called the susceptibles), the other infected. The rate at which susceptibles become infected depends on the frequency with which they meet infected cells, and this is determined by the law of mass action. The law of mass action is based upon the classical approach to chemical reactions, and relies upon the assumption that the rate at which different populations contact each other depends on both their densities and concentrations. Intuitively, the contact rate increases as the density of each species increases—if there are large numbers of infected macrophages and susceptibles, there will be many contacts between them.

Conversely, if there are few of each, the number of contacts will be small. Each time contact is made, there is a probability that the virus is transmitted. These infection dynamics underpin the HIV models, and must be supplemented by terms representing the production of new, uninfected cells, cell death and any other salient features. Even this simple approach shows how the establishment of viral infection in macrophages depends on biologically relevant parameters such as the rate of production of uninfected macrophages.

The next level of model complexity that we have discussed is that in Section 3.1 for the antitumor activity of macrophages. This model includes proliferation dynamics for a number of cell types, as well as chemical regulation and interactions between different cells. Intuitively, it would seem that if tumor cells can stimulate macrophages to cytotoxicity then the activated macrophages should be able to eliminate a tumor. In this chapter, we have presented a mathematical model that not only indicates that this is not the case, but also helps us to understand why. To reiterate, we could consider a single tumor cell with a proliferative advantage, which produces macrophage-activating factors—what do you think the chances would be that there is a macrophage near enough to respond to this signal, find the tumor cell, bind to it and kill it? This 'double dependency' on the tumor cell population means that it becomes less and less effective at stimulating its own demise as it decreases in size. Mathematically, this double dependency appears as a 'second order non-linearity'. Success would be far more likely if there were a macrophage population already primed, or *activated* to the tumoricidal state: such activation would remove one level of dependence on the number of tumor cells, and coincides with current ideas for macrophage-mediated immunotherapy (Allavena *et al.*, 1990; Colombo *et al.*, 1992; Fidler and Kleinerman, 1993). Indeed, adaptation of our original model to include the exogenous addition of macrophage-activating factors such as interferon-γ indicated that such an approach can lead to eradication. A crucial *prediction* of the mathematical analysis is that success or failure depends on the initial tumor burden when treatment begins, so that other means of reducing this burden, for example surgery, may be necessary prior to treatment. Our analysis also indicated that a careful calculation of the system parameters may enable the model to be used to optimize such therapies.

At this point, we draw an important mathematical distinction between models that describe the way in which biological variables change over time, and those which address both spatial and temporal dynamics. The former are sometimes known as compartmental models, since they deal with the rate of change of a physical quantity within a compartment (e.g. the number of infected macrophages in a patient). Clearly there may be situations where location is significant. This is exemplified by the case of tumor growth, where many features are dependent on distance from a blood supply. The model, presented in Section 3.2, which describes the infiltration of macrophages into avascular tumor spheroids, is an example of this next level of complexity. This kind of model enables us to say not only how many macrophages are in the tumor, but also *where* they are; such detailed knowledge has important implications for optimizing cancer therapies.

In Section 3.3, we showed that the rapid diffusion of chemical regulators in comparison with cell movement, combined with the antitumor effects of macrophages, could lead to the appearance of hot spots of high tumor cell density. In practice, interactions with a variety of other factors mean that regular patterns such as those presented in Figure 16.8 do not occur. However, there is evidence for the existence of dense clusters of macrophages, whose location is thought to be related to the tumor cytotoxic role of macrophages (Kerrebijn *et al.*, 1994). This supports our view that the interaction between macrophages and tumor cells is a potential mechanism for generating spatial heterogeneity. In the 1950s and 1960s, the potential of the immune system to eliminate tumors spontaneously was widely debated (Baldwin, 1955); more recently, this 'immune surveillance hypothesis' has been widely disputed and remains controversial. Attention has switched to more complex regulatory effects of the immune system on tumor progression (Matzinger, 1994), such as the role of macrophages in tumor angiogenesis (Lewis *et al.*, 1995). Our work provides a link between these old and new philosophies. We have shown that while the tumoricidal activity of macrophages is insufficient to eliminate tumors, it can have important implications for their structure. This work is important because this is the first explicit model mechanism which leads naturally to irregularity in tumor composition.

Recent biological developments indicate that the number of macrophages in breast carcinoma is closely correlated with prognosis, and that macrophages may be linked to a complex spatio-temporal variation in blood supply and tissue oxygenation. Macrophage hot spots are situated away from regions of high vascular density, implying that macrophages actively migrate away from the blood vessels (Leek *et al.*, 1996). Macrophages themselves promote angiogenesis (Lewis *et al.*, 1995), so that they will encourage new vascular hot spots to develop. If the macrophages then move away or die, we have the ingredients for a constantly changing spatio-temporal picture. Although current models do not include interactions with the tumor vasculature, they represent the first steps towards a thorough mathematical description of this complex system.

The modeling techniques described throughout this chapter are typical of those employed when mathematics is used to investigate biological problems. As we have outlined previously, many of the existing models could be adapted or extended to study other aspects of macrophage biology, such as their role in wound healing, arthritis and atherosclerosis.

We have now seen that biology and medicine can benefit from mathematics at several, conceptually different levels. At one level, mathematics is simply an abstract tool being used to find a non-mathematical answer to a non-mathematical question, for example does cell kill increase with increasing drug dosage? At another level, mathematics is more than a tool: it plays an integral role in formulating and answering questions of interest, for example what is the relationship between drug dose and cell kill? Finally, mathematics has the potential to provide new and complementary biological insight and, thereby, stimulate further biomedical research (by suggesting, for example, the way in which a particular drug up-regulates cell death and how this rate increases with dosage). Other advantages of modeling stem from the relative ease and reproducibility with which mathematical experiments can be carried out. Indeed, mathematical simulations may be viewed as clean experiments in which parameter manipulations are transparent—this is not always the case in biological experiments, where it can be difficult to vary a single parameter in isolation. In this respect, mathematical simulations may be viewed as thought experiments, with which to test the feasibility of proposed investigations in the laboratory, and which may, at the same time, reduce the number of time-consuming, technically difficult and often expensive experiments being performed.

7 Summary

Mathematical modeling is a powerful tool which, when used in collaboration with Biology, can provide valuable mechanistic insight into a variety of biological problems, including macrophage dynamics in tumors, and HIV infection. As quantitative studies of macrophage biology become more important, mathematical modeling can be expected to play an increasingly important role in the analysis of the data generated, and in establishing the response of macrophages to multiple stimuli. Ultimately, we envisage the application of mathematical modeling techniques to every aspect of macrophage dynamics described in this book.

Acknowledgments

The authors are grateful to Professor Claire Lewis for informative discussions, and to Catherine Kelly for the production of Figures 16.5, 16.6 and 16.7.

References

Adam, J A. and Bellomo, N. (1997). *A Survey of Models for Tumor–Immune System Dynamics*. Birkhäuser.

Allavena, P., Peccatori, F., Maggioni, D., Sironi, M., Colombo, N., Lissoni, A. *et al.* (1990). Intraperitoneal recombinant γ-interferon in patients with recurrent ascitic ovarian carcinoma: modulation of cytotoxity and cytokine production in tumor-associated effectors and major histocompatibility antigen expression on tumour cells. *Cancer Research*, **50**, 7318–323.

Babaev, V.R., Fazio, S., Gleaves, L.A , Carter, K.J., Semenkovich, C.F. and Linton, M F. (1999). Macrophage lipoprotein lipase promotes foam cell formation and atherosclerosis *in vivo*. *Journal of Clinical Investigation*, **103**, 1697–705.

Baldwin, R W. (1995). Immunity to methylcholanthrene induced tumours in inbred rats following atrophy and regression of implanted tumours. *British Journal of Cancer*, **9**, 652–7.

Bennet, N.T. and Schulz, G.S. (1993). Growth factors and wound healing: part II. Role in normal and chronic wound healing. *American Journal of Surgery*, **166**, 74–81.

Bischof, R.J, Zafiropoulos, D., Hamilton, J.A. and Campbell, I.K. (2000). Exacerbation of acute inflammatory arthritis by the colony-stimulating factors CSF-1 and granulocyte macrophage (GM)-CSF: evidence of macrophage infiltration and local proliferation. *Clinical Experiments in Immunology*, **119**, 361–7.

Bottazzi, B., Polentarutti, N., Acero, R., Balsari, A., Boraschi, D., Ghezzi, P. *et al.* (1983). Regulation of the macrophage content of neoplasms by chemoattractants. *Science*, **220**, 210–2.

Bottazzi, B., Ghezzi, P., Taraboletti, G., Salmona, M., Colombo, N., Bonnazzi, C. *et al.* (1985). Tumor-derived chemotactic factor(s) from human ovarian carcinoma: evidence for a role in the regulation of macrophage content of neoplastic tissues. *International Journal of Cancer*, **36**, 167–73.

Botazzi, B., Erba, E., Nobili, N., Fazioli, F., Rambalid, A. and Mantovani, A. (1990). A paracrine circuit in the regulation of the proliferation of macrophages infiltrating murine sarcomas. *Journal of Immunology,* **144**, 2409–12.

Bottazzi, B., Walter, S., Govoni, D., Colotta, F. and Mantovani, A. (1992). Monocyte chemotactic cytokine gene transfer modulates macrophage infiltration, growth and susceptibility to IL-2 therapy of a murine melanoma. *Journal of Immunology*, **148**, 1280–5.

Byrne, H.M. and Chaplain, M.A.J. (1995). Growth of nonnecrotic tumors in the presence and absence of inhibitors. *Mathematical Biosciences*, **130**, 151–11.

Chaplain, M.A.J. and Sleeman, B.D. (1993). Modelling the growth of solid tumours and incorporating a method for their classification using nonlinear elasticity theory. *Journal of Mathematical Biology*, **31**, 431–79.

Colombo, N., Peccatori, F., Paganin, C., Bini, S., Brandely, N., Mangioni, C. *et al.* (1992). Anti-tumor and immunomodulatory activity of intraperitoneal IFN-γ in ovarian carcinoma patients with minimal residual tumor after chemotherapy. *International Journal of Cancer*, **51**, 42–6.

Dale, P.D., Maini, P.K. and Sherratt, J.A. (1994). Mathematical modelling of corneal epithelial wound healing. *Mathematical Biosciences*, **124**, 127–47.

Dale, P.D., Maini, P.K. and Sherratt, J.A. (1996). A mathematical model for collagen fiber formation during fetal and adult dermal wound-healing. *Proceedings of the Royal Society of London, Series B: Biological Sciences*, **263**, 653–60.

Dallon, J.C., Sherratt, J.A. and Maini, P.K. (1999). Mathematical modelling of extracellular matrix dynamics using discrete cells: fibre orientation and tissue regeneration. *Journal of Theoretical Biology*, **199**, 449–71.

deBoer, R.J. and Perelson, A.S. (1998). Target cell limited and immune control models of HIV infection: a comparison. *Journal of Theoretical Biology*, **190**, 201–14.

deVilliers, W.J.S. and Smart, E.J. (1999). Macrophage scavenger receptors and foam cell formation. *Journal of Leukocyte Biology*, **66**, 740–6.

Esgro, J.J., Whitworth, P. and Fidler, I.J. (1990). Macrophages as effectors of tumor immunity. *Immunology and Allergy Clinics of North America*, **10**, 705–29.

Fidler, I.J. and Kleinerman, E.S. (1993). Therapy of cancer metastasis by systemic activation of macrophages: from the bench to the clinic. *Research in Immunology*, **144**, 284–7.

Greenspan, H.P. (1972). Models for the growth of a solid tumour by diffusion. *Studies in Applied Mathematics*, **51**, 317–40.

Hamilton, T.A. and Adams, D.O. (1987). Mechanisms of macrophage-mediated tumor injury. In den Otter, W. and Ruitenberg, E.J. (ed.), *Tumor Immunology—Mechanisms, Diagnosis, Therapy*. Elsevier Science Publishers B.V., pp. 89–107.

Kerrebijn, J.D., Balm, A.J.M., Knegt, P.P., Meeuwis, C.A. and Drexhage, H.A. (1994). Macrophage and dendritic cell infiltration in head and neck squamous-cell carcinoma—an immunohisto-chemical study. *Cancer Immunology and Immunotherapy*, **38**, 31–7.

Kuratsu, J., Yoshizato, K., Yoshimura, T., Leonard, E.J., Takeshima, H. and Ushio, Y. (1993). Quantitative study of monocyte chemoattractant protein-1 (MCP-1) in cerebrospinal fluid and cyst fluid from patients with malignant glioma. *Journal of the National Cancer Institute*, **85**, 1836–9.

Leek, R.D., Lewis, C.E., Whitehouse, R., Greenall, M., Clarke, J. and Harris, A.L. (1996). Association of macrophage infiltration and angiogenesis and prognosis in invasive breast carcinoma. *Cancer Research*, **56**, 1836–9.

Leek, R.D., Lewis, C.E. and Harris, A.L. (1997). The role of macrophages in tumour angiogenesis. In Bicknell, R., Lewis, C.E. and Ferrara, N. (ed.), *Tumour Angiogenesis*. Oxford University Press, Oxford, pp. 81–99.

Leek, R.D., Landers, R.J., Harris, A.L. and Lewis, C.E. (1999). Necrosis correlates with high vascular density and focal macrophage infiltration in invasive carcinoma of the breast. *British Journal of Cancer*, **79**, 991–5.

Lewis, C.E., Leek, R., Harris, A. and McGee, J.O.D. (1995). Cytokine regulation of angiogenesis in breast cancer—the role of tumor-associated macrophages. *Journal of Leukocyte Biology*, **57**, 747–51.

Mantovani, A. (1989). Cytotoxic killing of tumour cells by monocytes. In Zembala, M. and Asherson, C.L. (ed.), *Human Monocytes*. Academic Press, London, pp. 303–311.

Mantovani, A. (1990. Tumour-associated macrophages. *Current Opinion in Immunology*, **2**, 689–92.

Mantovani, A., Bottazzi, B., Colotta, F., Sozzani, S. and Ruco, L. (1992). The origin and function of tumor-associated macrophages. *Immunology Today*, **13**, 265–70.

Mapp, P.I., Grootvold, M.C. and Blake, D.R. (1995). Hypoxia, oxidative stress and rheumatoid arthritis. *British Medical Bulletin*, **51**, 419–36.

Markovitch, S. (1993). The particular role of cell loss in timour growth. *Mathematical and Computer Modelling*, **18**, 83–9.

Matzinger, P. (1994). Tolerance, danger, and the extended family. *Annual Review of Immunology*, **12**, 991–1045.

Michelson, S. and Leith, J. (1991). Autocrine and paracrine growth factors in tumor growth: a mathematical model. *Bulletin of Mathematical Biology*, **53**, 639–56.

Murray, J.D. (1991). *Mathematical Biology*. Springer-Verlag, Berlin.

Negus, R.P., Turner, L., Burke, F. and Balkwill, F.R. (1998). Hypoxia down-regulates MCP-1 expression: implications for macrophage distribution in tumours. *Journal of Leukocyte Biology*, **63**, 758–65.

Nelson, G.W. and Perelson, A.S. (1992). A mechanism of immune escape by slow-replicating HIV strains. *Journal of Acquired Immune Deficiency Syndromes*, **5**, 82–93.

Nowak, M.A. and Bangham, C.R.M. (1996). Population dynamics of immune responses to persistent viruses. *Science*, **272**, 74–9.

Olsen, L, Sherratt, J.A. and Maini, P.K. (1995). A mechanochemical model for adult dermal wound contraction and the permanence of the contracted tissue displacement profile. *Journal of Theoretical Biology*, **177**, 113–28.

Olsen, L., Sherratt, J.A., Maini, P.K. and Arnold, F. (1997). A mathematical model for the capillary endothelial cell–extracellular matrix interactions in wound-healing and angiogenesis. *IMA Journal of Mathematics Applied to Medicine and Biology*, **14**, 261–81.

O'Sullivan, C. and Lewis, C.E. (1994). Tumor-associated leukocytes—friends or foes in breast carcinoma. *Journal of Pathology*, **172**, 229–35.

Owen, M.R. (1997). Mathematical modelling of the macrophage invasion of tumours and juxtacrine signalling in epidermal wound healing. PhD thesis, University of Warwick.

Owen, M.R. and Sherratt, J.A. (1997). Pattern formation and spatiotemporal irregularity in a model for macrophage–tumour interactions. *Journal of Theoretical Biology*, **189**, 63–80.

Owen, M.R. and Sherratt, J.A. (1998). Modelling the macrophage invasion of tumours: effects on growth and composition. *IMA Journal of Mathematics Applied to Medicine and Biology*, **15**, 165–85.

Owen, M.R. and Sherratt, J.A. (1999). Mathematical modelling of macrophage dynamics in tumours. *Mathematical Models and Methods in Applied Sciences*, **9**, 513–39.

Pettet, G.J., Byrne, H.M., McElwain, D.L.S. and Norbury, J. (1996a). A model of wound-healing and angiogenesis in soft tissue. *Mathematical Biosciences*, **136**, 35–63.

Pettet, G.J., Chaplain, M.A.J., MCElwain, D.L.S. and Byrne, H.M. (1996b). On the role of angiogenesis in wound-healing. *Proceedings of the Royal Society of London, Series B: Biological Sciences,* **263**, 1487–93.

Polverini, P.J., Cotran, R.S., Gimbrone. M A., Jr and Unanue, E.R. (1977). Activated macrophages induce vascular proliferation. *Nature*, **269**, 804–6.

Prehn, R.T. (1994). Stimulatory effects of immune reactions upon the growth of untransplanted tumours. *Cancer Research*, **54**, 908–14.

Sherratt, J.A. and Nowak, M.A. (1992). Oncogenes, anti-oncogenes and the immune response to cancer: a mathematical model. *Proceedings of the Royal Socieyt of London, Series B: Biological Sciences*, **248**, 261–71.

Sozzani, S., Luini, W., Molino, M., Jilek, P., Bottazzi, B., Cerletti, C. *et al.* (1991). The signal transduction pathway involved in the migration induced by a monocyte chemotactic cytokine. *Journal of Immunology*, **147**, 2215–21.

Stevenson, M. (1996). Portals of entry—uncovering HIV nuclear transport pathways. *Trends in Cell Biology*, **6**, 9–15.

Stevenson, M. and Gendelman, H.E. (1994). Cellular and viral determinants that regulate HIV-1 infection in macrophages. *Journal of Leukocyte Biology*, **56**, 278–88.

Tomlinson, I.P.M. and Bodmer, W.F. (1995). Failure of programmed cell death and differentiation as causes of tumors: some simple mathematical models. *Proceedings of the National Academy of Science USA*, **92**, 11130–4.

van Damme, J., Proost, P., Lenaerts, J.P. and Opdenakker, G. (1992). Structural and functional identification of two human, tumor-derived monocyte chemotactic proteins (MCP-2 and MCP-3) belonging to the chemokine family. *Journal of Experimental Medicine*, **176**, 59–65.

Walter, S., Bottazi, B., Govoni, D., Colotta, F. and Mantovani, A. (1991). Macrophage infiltration and growth of sarcoma clones expressing different amount of monocyte chemotactic protein/JE. *International Journal of Cancer*, **49**, 431–5.

Wang., J.M., Colella, S., Allavena, P. and Mantovani, A. (1987). Chemotactic activity of human recombinant granulocyte–macrophage colony-stimulating factor. *Immunology*, **60**, 439–44.

Wang, J.M., Griffin, J.D., Rambaldi, A., Chen, Z.G. and Mantovani, A. (1988). Induction of monocyte migration by recombinant macrophage colony-stimulating factor. *Journal of Immunology*, **141**, 575–9.

Waters, C.M., Oberg, K.C., Carpenter, G. and Overholser, K.A. (1990). Rate constants for binding, dissociation, and internalization of EGF: effect of receptor occupancy and ligand concentration. *Biochemistry*, **29**, 3563–9.

Wheldon, T.E. (1975). Mitotic autoregulation of normal and abnormal cells: alternative mechanisms for the derangement of growth control. *Journal of Theoretical Biology*, **53**, 421–33.

Wilson, M., Seymour, R. and Henderson, B. (1998). Bacterial perturbation of cytokine networks. *Infection and Immunity*, **66**, 2401–9.

Wodarz, D., Lloyd, A.L., Jansen, V.A.A. and Nowak, M.A. (1999). Dynamics of macrophage and T cell infection by HIV. *Journal of Theoretical Biology*, **196**, 101–13.

Appendix: some mathematical details

The model for macrophage antitumor effects, given by the word equations in the main text, is written mathematically as a set of five differential equations:

$$\frac{\partial l}{\partial t} = D_l \nabla^2 l - \chi_l \nabla \left(l \nabla f \right) + \frac{\alpha f l (N+1)}{N + l + m + n} + I(1 + \sigma f) - k_1 f lm + k_2 c - \delta_l l$$

$$\frac{\partial m}{\partial t} = D_m \nabla^2 m + \frac{\xi m (N+1)}{N + l + m + n} - m - k_1 f lm$$

$$\frac{\partial n}{\partial t} = D_n \nabla^2 n + \frac{n(N+1)}{N + l + m + n} - n$$

$$\frac{\partial f}{\partial t} = D_f \nabla^2 f + \beta m - \delta_f f$$

$$\frac{\partial c}{\partial t} = D_c \nabla^2 c + k_1 f lm - k_2 c - \delta_c c .$$

There are insufficient experimental data available to determine all the model parameters. We list here generic order of magnitude estimates, with brief justifications. All the phenomena described in this chapter occur for ranges of parameters within these estimates.

α 10^{-2}: macrophages are a mature form of blood monocyte, which reside in tissues and do not normally proliferate. With certain stimuli, including some tumor-derived chemicals, they may proliferate, but at a low level (Bottazzi *et al.*, 1990), particularly in humans (Mantovani *et al.*, 1992).

N 10^1: N is a measure of the initial growth rate, and of the subsequent response to crowding, and should be of the same order of magnitude as the normal cell turnover time.

I 10^{-2}: $I < \delta_l$ must hold for the normal tissue steady state to be non-negative. In addition, the proportion of macrophages in normal tissue is relatively small.

σ 10^0–10^2: s represents the macrophage influx in response to macrophage-activating factors, and will, therefore, depend on the tumor cell line under consideration.

k_1, k_2 10^0–10^2: activation, complex formation and lysis have time scales of hours (Hamilton and Adams, 1987).

δ_l 10^{-1}: macrophages survive in tissue for significantly longer than normal cells.

ξ 10^{-1}: represents the growth advantage of tumor cells, and thus must be greater than one; however, tumor cell growth should still be of the same order of magnitude as for normal cells.

β, δ_f 10^0–10^1: the chemical production and decay rates should be of the same order of magnitude, and the chemical regulator is expected to decay at a faster rate than normal cells die.

δ_c 10^{-1}–10^0: the complex death rate is expected to be similar in magnitude to the death rates of its constituent cells, namely macrophages (10^{-1}) and tumor cells (10^0).

The coefficients governing random motility of macrophages, tumor cells, normal cells and complexes are assumed to be constant, and independent of any of the variables. In practice, we expect that these coefficients will vary with density, and perhaps also with the local concentration of regulatory chemicals. In addition, the random motility coefficients of the different cell types are assumed to be similar in magnitude, with values in the region of 10^{-15} m^2/s. Since we measure time in terms of cell divisions and space in terms of typical cell lengths, these figures give rescaled coefficients $D_l = D_m = D_n = 5$. Being much smaller in size, chemical regulators are expected to diffuse substantially faster than cells moving by random motion. However, since increasing D_f leads to a pattern-forming bifurcation, we treat it as a free parameter. Concerning the random motion of complexes, it is not clear whether the formation of a complex renders the cells immobile, or simply reduces their ability to undergo random motion. Since the complex consists of two cells, we halve the value for the random motility coefficient of unbound cells, giving $D_c = 2.5$. Whilst this choice is purely intuitive, the qualitative nature of the solutions does not depend on the particular value, even if it is set to zero. Regarding macrophage chemotaxis, we have described in the main text how estimates of the chemotaxis parameters may be obtained from experimental data.

Index